ETHICAL ISSUES IN MODERN MEDICINE

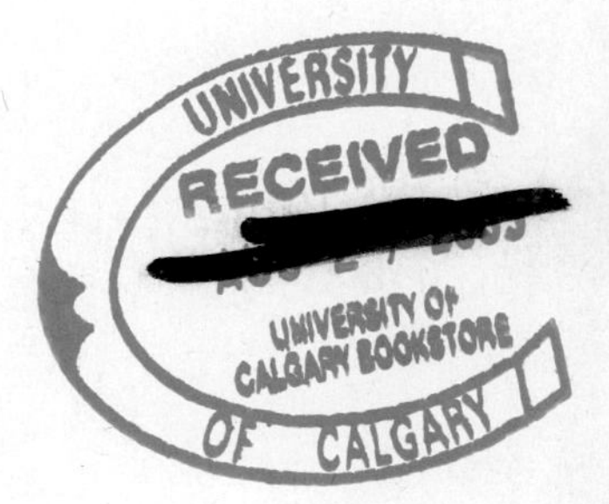

ETHICAL ISSUES IN MODERN MEDICINE

SIXTH EDITION

Bonnie Steinbock

State University of New York—Albany

John D. Arras

University of Virginia

Alex John London

Carnegie Mellon University

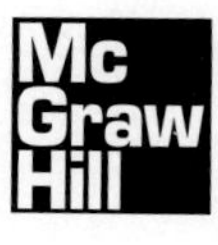

Boston Burr Ridge, IL Dubuque, IA Madison, WI New York San Francisco St. Louis
Bangkok Bogotá Caracas Kuala Lumpur Lisbon London Madrid Mexico City
Milan Montreal New Delhi Santiago Seoul Singapore Sydney Taipei Toronto

McGraw-Hill Higher Education

A Division of The ***McGraw-Hill*** *Companies*

ETHICAL ISSUES IN MODERN MEDICINE

Published by McGraw-Hill, a business unit of The McGraw-Hill Companies, Inc., 1221 Avenue of the Americas, New York, NY, 10020.

This book is printed on acid-free paper.

1 2 3 4 5 6 7 8 9 0 DOC/DOC 0 9 8 7 6 5 4 3 2

ISBN 0-7674-2016-0

Publisher: *Kenneth King*
Associate editor: *Jon-David Hague*
Marketing manager: *Greg Brueck*
Project manager: *Jean R. Starr*
Production supervisor: *Susanne Riedell*
Coordinator of freelance design: *Mary E. Kazak*
Cover design: *Sarah Studnicki*
Cover image: *© Dan Chavkin/Getty Images*
Typeface: *9/11 Palatino*
Compositor: *GAC Indianapolis*
Printer: *R.R. Donnelley and Sons Company*

Library of Congress Cataloging-in-Publication Data

Steinbock, Bonnie.
Ethical issues in modern medicine / Bonnie Steinbock, John D. Arras, Alex John London.—6th ed.
p. cm.
Includes index.
ISBN 0-7674-2016-0 (alk. paper)
1. Medical ethics. I. Arras, John. II. London, Alex John. III. Title.
R724.E788 2003
174′.2—dc21

2002067870

Manufactured in the United States of America
10 9 8 7 6 5 4 3 2 1

www.mhhe.com

For
Susan Vermazen
and
Gabriel Arnell and Luke Wright
and
John, Elaine, and Tracy London

CONTENTS

PREFACE

Welcome to the sixth edition of *Ethical Issues in Modern Medicine.* The three-year interval between this and the last edition has brought major changes both to the field of bioethics and to the editorial chain gang responsible for this book. To begin with personnel, Bonnie Steinbock and John Arras are pleased to introduce our new co-editor, Alex John London of Carnegie-Mellon University. Alex is not entirely a newcomer to this text, since he contributed significantly to the fifth edition as John's graduate research assistant before emerging from the University of Virginia with his Ph.D. in philosophy. Since then, Alex's star has begun to rise in the bioethics firmament, and we are confident that his addition to the editorial team will only enhance the tradition of depth and rigor that has become a hallmark of this collection.

The sixth edition began under the stewardship of our trusted editor, Ken King, who was also responsible for the fifth edition. With the acquisition of Mayfield Publishing Company by McGraw-Hill, Ken gave over the reins to Jon-David Hague. Though we miss Ken's unique combination of philosophical judgment and sharp business sense, we are delighted with our new editor and the production team at McGraw-Hill.

The other significant change in personnel has stemmed from John Arras's decision to assume more of an advisory role on this and subsequent editions and to leave most of the hard work to Bonnie and Alex. After toiling on five editions of this book between 1977 and 1999, John decided to devote himself to other projects while still maintaining an important voice in decisions over content. Thus, Bonnie and Alex have rewritten all the introductions, updated the bibliographies, and prepared the manuscript for publication, while John continued to play his usual role of helping to select the best available readings for this anthology. Alex took charge of editing Parts One (The Professional-Patient Relationship), Two (Allocation, Social Justice, Health Policy), and Five (Experimentation on Human Subjects); and Bonnie took primary responsibility for Part Three (Defining Death, Foregoing Life-Sustaining Treatment, and Euthanasia) and for the greatly expanded Part Four (Reprogenetics). Although we carved up primary responsibility for the various Parts in this fashion, the final choices over the table of contents have remained, as always, a delightfully collaborative enterprise.

In keeping with our tradition of viewing each new edition as an occasion for a major overhaul of the book, we have made some far-reaching changes in the text to reflect both important developments in medicine and biotechnology and new emphases within the field of bioethics. The most dramatic change in the text tracks the newly emerging confluence of human genetics and reproductive ethics in an entirely new Part Four entitled "Reprogenetics." Materials that were presented in former editions under the separate rubrics of genetics and reproduction are merged here in order to highlight the ways in which our new knowledge of the human genome is being brought to bear on reproductive decisions. Particularly noteworthy here are two entirely new sections devoted to "Carrier Screening, Prenatal Testing, and Reproductive Decisions" and "Mapping the Human Genome: Implications for Genetic Testing, Genetic Counseling, and Genetic Interventions." This Part also includes a brace of new articles on the hotly contested issues of stem cell research and human cloning.

Another important feature of this edition is our decision to move the Part on "Allocation, Social Justice, and Health Policy" from the end to (near) the beginning of the book. We have done this in order to reflect our conviction that the issues debated within this Part are absolutely central to bioethics and health policy. So rather than relegating them to the back of the book, as is so often done in such anthologies, we have moved these questions of justice up front and center. We have also incorporated a new article into this Part devoted to the importance of the social determinants of health and disease. Although we continue to stress the importance of the debate over the right to health care, we firmly believe that there's more to health than health care. We are thus convinced that bioethics must broaden its horizons to encompass not only a concern for individual health, but also a justice perspective on the conditions that enhance or undermine the public's health.

Through the years the editors of this text have taken great pride in two important pedagogical features of each succeeding edition: namely, the inclusion of rich case studies that provide grounding for the longer, more analytical articles, and a judicious balancing of conflicting moral and political points of view. This edition sustains both traditions. We include here for the first time some pivotal cases in the history of research ethics (including the infamous Tuskegee Syphilis Study), as well as new case material (much of it written expressly for this volume) devoted to such issues as genetic testing and misattributed paternity, the recent but already famous *Wendland* case involving the discontinuation of artificial nutrition and hydration, and the troubling Kennedy-Krieger lead paint study on children in poverty sponsored by Johns Hopkins University. Likewise, our tradition of moral and political inclusivity continues with robust new debates on truth-telling, the discontinuation of life-sustaining treatments (featuring specially written articles by the opposed attorneys in the *Wendland* case), the right to die vs. the duty to die, cloning and stem cell research, and the conduct of placebo-controlled clinical research trials in developing countries.

Although we try in our periodic revisions to abide by the maxim, "If it ain't broke, don't fix it!", we have a hard time resisting the allure of absolutely first-rate bioethical scholarship. As a result, we have ended up including almost forty new articles. Although the largest cluster of these exciting new papers have gone into the entirely new Part devoted to "reprogenetics," all of the other Parts have been revitalized by the addition of some really excellent new writing on such themes as disclosing error in medicine, caring for the indigent, cost-effectiveness analysis, access to enhancement technologies, brain death, abortion, and research on children. Although there is always room for improvement—a fact that will weigh more heavily on us when we start planning for the next edition—we are confident that the book before you represents the state of the art in contemporary bioethical scholarship and debate.

Each new edition of this text engenders scores of new debts to those who have helped make this book what it has become, and now is the time for the editors to express our profound gratitude to one and all. John Arras no longer presides over the actual construction of the book, so his debts are fewer this time around. Still, he wishes to thank his indefatigable and indispensable administrative assistant, Carolyn Randolph, as well as his two most recent graduate assistants, Robert Crouch and Jennifer Flynn. John delights in being able to dedicate this volume to his two new grandsons, Luke and Gabriel. (No, John isn't getting any older, but he does worry about his aging daughters.)

Bonnie wishes to thank Lori Knowles and Erik Parens, the co-principal investigators on the Reprogenetics project at the Hastings Center. They, and the group's members, provided her with an unforgettable learning experience. She also thanks Erik for his advice on the sixth edition. It was his idea to combine the various issues in reproduction and genetics into one humongous Reprogenetics chapter, reflecting the increasing convergence of these areas. Bonnie also thanks Ann Willey of the New York State Department of Health and Eric Juengst of Case Western Reserve University for their willingness to read and correct the Reprogenetics introduction. They have spared her much embarrassment. She is especially grateful to Eric Juengst who patiently answered her questions about genetics and gave so many helpful suggestions for articles, we almost had to make him a co-editor.

Alex wishes to thank John and Bonnie for the generous trust they have placed in him, for the sagacity of their advice, the warmth of their friendship, and the levity of their wit. In addition, Alex wishes to thank the numerous contributors to this collection who were so willing to share their encouragement and insight with him throughout this process. Thanks to Jennifer Crossan, who remains unsurpassed in her photocopying prowess and unflappable willingness to rummage through the stacks of near-by libraries, and to Wilfried Sieg for his enlightened leadership and support. Most of all, thanks to Tracy London for her patience and impeccable sense of proper grammatical form.

We are indebted as well to the following individuals for their thoughtful review of the last edition and their suggestions for this edition: Insoo Hyun, Western Michigan University; Leslie Francis, University of Utah; Debra Penna-Fredericks, St. Louis University; Gabriel Palmer, Youngstown State University; Mary Mahowald, University of Chicago; and Michael Henry, St. John's University.

THE CONTRIBUTORS

Felicia Ackerman, Ph.D.,
is professor of philosophy at Brown University in Providence, Rhode Island.

David B. Allen, M.D.,
is professor of pediatrics, director of pediatric endocrinology, and director of the pediatric residency program at the University of Wisconsin Children's Hospital and Medical School in Madison.

Marcia Angell, M.D., F.A.C.S.,
is a senior lecturer in social medicine at the Harvard Medical School and former editor-in-chief of The New England Journal of Medicine.

George J. Annas, J.D., M.P.H.,
is professor and chair of the Health Law Department, Boston University School of Public Health, and Professor, Boston University School of Medicine and School of Law.

Paul S. Appelbaum, M.D.,
is AF Zeleznik distinguished professor of psychiatry, chairman of psychiatry, and director of law and psychiatry program at the University of Massachusetts Medical School.

John D. Arras, Ph.D.,
is the William and Linda Porterfield professor of bioethics and professor of philosophy at the University of Virginia, Charlottesville.

Adrienne Asch, Ph.D.,
is the Henry R. Luce professor in biology, ethics, and the politics of human reproduction at Wellesley College in Massachusetts.

Margaret A. Battin, M.F.A., Ph.D.,
is distinguished professor of philosophy and adjunct professor of internal medicine in the Division of Medical Ethics at the University of Utah.

Françoise Baylis, Ph.D.,
is associate professor, Departments of Bioethics and Philosophy, Dalhousie University, Halifax, Canada.

Martin Benjamin, Ph.D.,
is professor of philosophy at Michigan State University in East Lansing.

Jeffrey R. Botkin, M.D., M.P.H.,
is a pediatrician and professor of pediatrics and medical ethics at the University of Utah.

Allan Brandt, Ph.D.,
is the Amalie Moses Kass professor of the history of medicine at the Harvard Medical School.

Dan W. Brock, Ph.D.,
is the Charles C. Tillinghast, Jr., university professor and professor of philosophy and biomedical ethics, and the director

of the Center for Biomedical Ethics at Brown University in Providence, Rhode Island.

Baruch A. Brody, Ph.D.,
is professor of philosophy at Rice University and director of the Center for Ethics at Baylor College of Medicine, Texas.

Howard Brody, M.D., Ph.D.,
is professor and director of the Center for Ethics and Humanities in the Life Sciences at Michigan State University in East Lansing, Michigan.

Allen Buchanan, Ph.D.,
is professor of philosophy at the University of Arizona, Tucson.

Keith Burton
is managing director at Golin/Harris International in Chicago. He was a freelance journalist when he made the 1985 documentary, "Dax's Case."

Norman L. Cantor, J.D.,
is professor of law and Justice Nathan Jacobs Scholar at the Rutgers University School of Law in Newark, New Jersey.

Jean-Claude Chevrolet, M.D.,
is head of the Medical Intensive Care Division, University Hospital Geneva, Switzerland.

Carl Cohen, Ph.D.,
is professor of philosophy at the University of Michigan in Ann Arbor.

Francis S. Collins, M.D., Ph.D.,
is a physician-geneticist and the director of the National Human Genome Research Institute, Washington, D.C.

Robert A. Crouch, M.A.,
is a doctoral student in philosophy at the University of Virginia, Charlottesville.

Norman Daniels, Ph.D.,
is professor of ethics and population health in the Department of Population and International Health, Harvard School of Public Health.

David M. Danks, Ph.D.,
former director at the Murdoch Institute for Research into Birth Defects Limited, Royal Children's Hospital in Melbourne, Australia, is retired.

Rebecca S. Dresser, J.D.,
is professor of law and ethics in medicine at Washington University, St. Louis, Missouri.

Ronald Dworkin, L. L. B.,
is Quain professor of jurisprudence at University College, London, and professor of law and philosophy at New York University.

David M. Eddy, M.D., Ph.D.,
is senior advisor for health policy and management at Kaiser Permanente of Southern California.

Mark Eibert, J.D.,
is a trial lawyer and patients' rights advocate in California.

Stuart Eisendrath, M.D.,
is professor of clinical psychiatry at the University of California in San Francisco.

Bernice S. Elger, M.D., M.A.,
is an internist at the Institute of Legal Medicine, University of Geneva.

H. Tristram Engelhardt, Ph.D., M.D.,
is professor of medicine and community medicine at Baylor College of Medicine in Houston, Texas.

Leonard M. Fleck, Ph.D.,
is professor of philosophy, center for ethics and Humanities in the Life Sciences, and in the Philosophy Department, Michigan State University, East Lansing.

Norman Fost, M.D.,
is professor of pediatrics and the director of the Program in Medical Ethics at the University of Wisconsin, Madison.

Benjamin Freedman, Ph.D.,
was professor at the McGill Centre for Medicine, Ethics, and Law, Montreal, Canada, and clinical ethicist at the Sir Mortimer B. Davis-Jewish General Hospital, Montreal.

Abraham Fuks, M.D., C.M.,
is dean of the Faculty of Medicine at McGill University.

Leonard H. Glantz, JD,
is professor of health law at Boston University School of Public Health.

Marthe R. Gold, MD, MPH,
is professor of community health and social medicine at the City University of New York Medical School.

Alan Goldman, Ph.D.,
is professor of philosophy at the University of Miami, Florida.

Michael A. Grodin, MD,
is professor of health law, psychiatry, socio-medical sciences and community medicine, Boston University Schools of Public Health and Medicine.

John Hardwig, Ph.D.,
is professor of philosophy and department head at the University of Tennessee in Knoxville.

Deborah S. Hellman, M.A., J.D.,
is associate professor of law at the University of Maryland, Baltimore.

Samuel Hellman, M.D.,
is the A.N. Pritzker distinguished service professor in the department of Radiology and Cellular Oncology at the Cancer Research Center of the University of Chicago School of Medicine.

Kathy Hudson, Ph.D.,
is director, Office of Policy and Public Affairs of the National Human Genome Research Institute, Washington, D.C.

Albert R. Jonsen, Ph.D.,
is professor emeritus of ethics in medicine in the Department of Medical History and Ethics, University of Washington, Seattle. He chaired the department from 1987–1998.

Eric T. Juengst, Ph.D.,
is an associate professor of biomedical ethics at the Case Western Reserve University School of Medicine in Cleveland, Ohio.

Leon R. Kass, M.D., Ph.D.,
is the Addie Clark Harding professor in the Committee on Social Thought and the College at the University of Chicago and the Roger and Susan Hertog fellow at the American Enterprise Institute.

Jay Katz, M.D.,
is Elizabeth K. Dollard professor emeritus of law, medicine, and psychiatry and Harvey L. Karp professorial lecturer in law and psychoanalysis at Yale Law School in New Haven, Connecticut.

Sara Ann Ketchum, Ph.D., J.D.,
is an attorney in the Tax Division of the Department of Justice, in Washington, D.C. The views expressed here are hers and not those of her employer.

Saul Krugman, M.D.,
was professor and chairman of pediatrics at New York University Medical Center.

Bruce Landesman, Ph.D.,
is professor of philosophy at the University of Utah.

Norman Levinsky, M.D.,
is professor of medicine and physiology, and associate provost at the Boston University Medical Center.

Margaret Olivia Little, Ph.D.,
is an associate professor in the Philosophy Department, and a senior research scholar in the Kennedy Institute of Ethics, at Georgetown University in Washington, D.C.

Alex John London, Ph.D.,
is an assistant professor in the Philosophy Department and the Center for the Advancement of Applied Ethics at Carnegie Mellon University in Pittsburgh, Pennsylvania.

Ruth Macklin, Ph.D.,
is professor of bioethics at Albert Einstein College of Medicine in the Bronx, New York.

Sarah Marchand
is a doctoral candidate in philosophy at University of Wisconsin, Madison.

Wendy K. Mariner, JD, LLM, MPH,
is professor of health law, Boston University School of Public Health.

Maurie Markman, M.D.,
is director of the Cleveland Clinic Taussig Cancer Center in Cleveland, Ohio, and chairman of the Department of Hematology/Oncology at The Cleveland Clinic Foundation, where he holds the Lee and Jerome Burkons Research Chair in Oncology.

Don Marquis, Ph.D.,
is professor of philosophy at the University of Kansas, Lawrence.

Paul Menzel, Ph.D.,
is professor of philosophy at Pacific Lutheran University.

Steven H. Miles, M.D.,
is professor of bioethics and medicine in the Department of Medicine and Center for Bioethics at the University of Minnesota, Minneapolis.

E. Haavi Morreim, Ph.D.,
is professor in the Department of Human Values and Ethics at the University of Tennessee College of Medicine, Memphis.

Alvin H. Moss, M.D.,
is professor of medicine and director of the Center for Health Ethics and Law at West Virginia University, Morgantown.

Thomas H. Murray, Ph.D.,
is president of The Hastings Center, a bioethics research institute in Garrison, New York.

Thomas Nagel, Ph.D.,
is professor of law and professor of philosophy at New York University.

Lawrence J. Nelson, Ph.D., J.D.,
is adjunct associate professor of philosophy and of women and gender studies and Faculty Scholar, Markkula Center for Applied Ethics at Santa Clara University, California.

Erik Nord, Ph.D.,
is senior researcher, National Institute of Public Health, Oslo, Norway.

Robert Nozick, Ph.D.,
was the Arthur Kingsley Porter professor of philosophy and Pellegrino University professor at Harvard University in Cambridge, Massachusetts.

Julie Gage Palmer, J.D.,
is lecturer in law at the University of Chicago Law School.

Jose-Luis Pinto-Prades, Ph.D.,
is professor of economics at Pompeu Fabra University, Barcelona, Spain.

Timothy E. Quill, M.D.,
is associate chief of medicine at the Genesee Hospital, a professor of medicine and psychiatry at the University of Rochester School of Medicine and Dentistry, and a primary care internist in Rochester, New York.

John Rawls, Ph.D.,
is professor emeritus of philosophy at Harvard University in Cambridge, Massachusetts.

Nancy K. Rhoden, J.D.,
was professor of law at the University of North Carolina at Chapel Hill, and a co-editor of the third edition of Ethical Issues in Modern Medicine.

Jeffrey Richardson, Ph.D.,
is professor of economics and director of the Health Economics Unit of the Centre for Health Program Evaluation at Monash University, Australia.

John A. Robertson, J.D.,
holds the Vinson & Elkins chair of law at the University of Texas School of Law in Austin, Texas, and is the chair of the Ethics Committee of the American Society of Reproductive Medicine.

Lainie Friedman Ross, M.D., Ph.D.,
is associate professor in the Department of Pediatrics and the College at the University of Chicago. She is also an assistant director of the MacLean Center for Clinical Medical Ethics at the University of Chicago where she is the director of the ethics case consultation service.

David J. Rothman, Ph.D.,
is Bernard Schoenberg professor of social medicine and director of the Center for the Study of Society and Medicine, Columbia College of Physicians and Surgeons, Columbia University.

Sheila M. Rothman, Ph.D.,
is professor of public health in the Sociomedical Sciences Division of the Joseph L. Mailman School of Public Health, and deputy director of the Center for the Study of Society and Medicine College of Physicians and Surgeons, Columbia University.

Maura A. Ryan, Ph.D.,
is associate provost and associate professor of Christian Ethics, University of Notre Dame in Indiana.

Thomas Scanlon, Ph.D.,
is professor of philosophy at Harvard University in Cambridge, Massachusetts.

Mark Siegler, M.D.,
is Lindy Bergman distinguished service professor of medicine and director of the MacLean Center for Clinical Medical Ethics at the University of Chicago.

Wesley J. Smith, J.D.,
is an author, attorney, and consumer advocate. His most recent book is Culture of Death: The Assault on Medical Ethics in America.

Bonnie Steinbock, Ph.D.,
is professor of philosophy at the University at Albany, State University of New York.

Judith Jarvis Thomson, Ph.D.,
is professor of philosophy at the Massachusetts Institute of Technology in Cambridge, Massachusetts.

Peter A. Ubel, M.D.,
is director of the Program for Improving Health Care Decisions at the University of Michigan and Ann Arbor Veterans Administration Medical Center.

Robert M. Veatch, Ph.D.,
is professor of medical ethics at the Kennedy Institute of Ethics at Georgetown University in Washington, D.C.

Robert Wachbroit, Ph.D.,
is a research scholar at the Institute for Philosophy and Public Policy at the School of Public Affairs, the University of Maryland.

LeRoy Walters, Ph.D.,
is professor of philosophy at Georgetown University, and the Joseph P. Kennedy, Sr. Professor of Christian Ethics at the Kennedy Institute of Ethics in Washington, D.C.

David Wasserman, J.D.,
is a research scholar at the Institute for Philosophy and Public Policy at the School of Public Affairs, the University of Maryland.

Charles Weijer, M.D., Ph.D.,
is associate professor of medicine, Department of Bioethics Dalhousie University, Halifax, Canada.

Lowell Weiss, B.A.,
a former speechwriter for President Bill Clinton, is an executive at the Morino Institute in Reston, Virginia.

Robert B. White, M.D.,
is professor emeritus of psychiatry at the University of Texas Medical Branch at Galveston.

Daniel Wikler, Ph.D.,
is professor of ethics and population health in the Department of Population and International Health, Harvard School of Public Heath.

Benjamin S. Wilfond, M.D.,
is the head of the Bioethics Research Section of the Medical Genetics Branch of the National Human Genome Research Institute and the head of the Genetics Section in the Department of Clinical Bioethics at the Warren G. Magnuson Clinical Center of the National Institutes of Health, Washington, D.C.

Sidney M. Wolfe, M.D.,
is director of the Public Citizen Research Group in Washington, D.C.

MORAL REASONING IN THE MEDICAL CONTEXT

BONNIE STEINBOCK / JOHN D. ARRAS / ALEX JOHN LONDON

BIOETHICS: NATURE AND SCOPE

Doctor Deborah Brody was not looking forward to Jim Lasken's next visit. Mr. Lasken, a 40-year-old former postman, devoted husband, and father of two teenagers, was at a critical juncture in his treatment for amyotrophic lateral sclerosis, a progressive and ultimately fatal degenerative disease of the nervous system, known to most people as Lou Gehrig's disease. Dr. Brody had been seeing Mr. Lasken for the past ten years, during which time his condition had been steadily deteriorating. Mr. Lasken was now in very bad shape. In the past three years he had lost the ability to walk, work, dress himself, and sit up without supports. He was now incontinent, and could only speak a few short words at a time, and only with agonizing difficulty. Mr. Lasken's psychological state had tracked his physical decline. Although he had kept up a brave front as many of his faculties declined over the first years of his illness, Mr. Lasken was becoming more and more despondent as his condition worsened. Dr. Brody suspected that Mr. Lasken was in a deep depression, but, given his life prospects, she could not really blame him.

Dr. Brody dreaded Mr. Lasken's next visit not simply because he was seriously ill and getting progressively worse, but because Mr. Lasken had been asking her to help him "end it." As he and his wife, Jane, had explained, his life had become unbearable. He could no longer enjoy his former hobbies, he could no longer communicate with anyone without enduring monumental frustration and fatigue, he knew he was a tremendous burden to his family, and was well aware that things were just going to get worse. It had become clear, in fact, that Mr. Lasken would soon have to be hooked up to a mechanical ventilator to do his breathing for him, or else he would drown in his own secretions.

This was apparently the last straw. Mr. Lasken was now adamant: he saw no point in either going on the respirator or dying a slow, wasting death without it. He wanted to die now, and he wanted Dr. Brody to help him. "Give me a shot," he implored, "it's all you can do for me now. My life is over."

Dr. Brody now had a serious problem. Should she help her patient commit suicide? Indeed, since Mr. Lasken could no longer actively do anything to take his own life, the doctor would have to do it herself, engaging in what is called "active euthanasia." She knew that it was against the law in her

---

Editors' note: Although this essay represents a complete reworking and expansion of the introduction from previous editions of this book, the authors gratefully acknowledge the enduring contributions of Robert Hunt, coeditor of the first edition, to these pages.

state either to assist someone in a suicide or directly to kill another person, but could such an act be ethically permitted if the patient were sufficiently desperate and helpless? Supposing that *someone* might be justified in performing euthanasia, was this the sort of thing that a *doctor* could or should do? As a physician, she empathized with her patient's pain, isolation, and desperation, and would have done just about anything to alleviate his terrible suffering. "A big part of my job is to combat suffering, not just death," she thought. "If my patient's mental and physical suffering can only be ended by death, and if his life is no longer of any use to him, why should I not help him?" On the other hand, she recalled the Hippocratic Oath, a version of which she took upon graduation from medical school, which condemned giving patients "deadly drugs." The message, transmitted from one generation of doctors to the next, was that physicians are supposed to be healers, not killers.

Dr. Brody's dilemma is also society's problem. More and more individuals are claiming that just as they have a right to control what happens to their own bodies during life, so they have a right to control the timing and manner of their deaths. Celebrated cases, like that of Dr. Kevorkian in Michigan, focus public attention on the question of whether the laws that currently constrain Dr. Brody should be changed. Given appropriate circumstances, checks, and balances, should doctors be given legal permission to prescribe deadly drugs for their suicidal patients? Should they be allowed to kill outright? What are the social implications of allowing individuals such a right to die? Should these practices become widespread, what would be the likelihood of abuse and the "slippery slope" toward killing the mentally infirm, the elderly, and the poor?

Problems of this sort lie at the heart of contemporary bioethics, the field introduced by this anthology. Like its parent disciplines, moral philosophy and religious ethics, bioethics is a study of moral conduct, of right and wrong. As such, it is inescapably *normative*. As opposed to some historical or social scientific approaches to moral conduct that emphasize description of the way the world is, or causal conjectures about why it is the way it is, bioethics inquires about the rightness or wrongness of various actions, character traits, and social policies. Thus, instead of fixing on such issues as the history of physicians' participation in their patients' suicides, or the way in which their attitudes are shaped by age, gender, specialty, and so on, "bioethicists" typically ask whether assisted suicide or euthanasia can be morally justified, whether either practice would be good social policy, and whether these practices are compatible with the character traits of a good physician. (This is not to say, however, that good normative reasoning can or should take place without careful attention to empirical details, which often prove crucial to the careful resolution of practical moral problems.)

In addition to these straightforward normative concerns, bioethicists are also increasingly interested in what philosophers call "metaethical" themes. That is, they are concerned not just with the question, say, of whether assisted suicide is morally justified, but also with broader and more abstract questions bearing on the nature of moral justification and the kind of thinking that supports it. As we shall see near the end of this essay, some bioethicists might claim, for example, that the justifiability of physician-assisted suicide must be sought in the articulation and application of various moral theories or principles, while others might claim that justification must proceed the other way around, beginning with concrete and unmistakable instances of good and bad behavior, and then gradually developing principles that capture and distill our most fundamental moral responses to cases. It is a question, in other words, of whether ethical thought should proceed from the "top down" or from the "bottom up."

SOURCES OF BIOETHICAL PROBLEMS AND CONCERNS

Since its birth in the early 1970s, the contemporary bioethics movement has grown from a mere blip on the radar of public consciousness to a major academic- and service-oriented profession with its own research centers, journals, conferences, and degree programs. Not a week goes by, it seems, without some controversial biomedical case or issue making its way into the nation's headlines and talk shows: "Gene for Homosexuality Discovered!" "Parents Insist on Treatment for Baby Without a Brain!" "Patients Subjected to Radiation Experiments Without

Their Consent!" "Dr. Kevorkian Strikes Again!" Why are we beset in this present age with so many fundamental and fascinating questions?

Technological Innovation

Obviously, much of the ferment in contemporary biomedical ethics is due to the unrelenting pace of technological advance. The story is by now familiar: Clever physicians, researchers, and technicians discover newer and better ways to do things, such as sustaining the lives of terminally ill patients, diagnosing fetal abnormalities in utero, and facilitating conception for infertile couples. Before we know it, however, these new techniques and services begin to take on lives of their own, expanding well beyond the problems and patients for whom they were originally intended.

Cardiopulmonary resuscitation, for example, originally intended for otherwise healthy victims of drowning or electrocution, has gradually and unceremoniously become a violent and final "rite of passage" for many aged, moribund patients in our nation's hospitals. The administration of artificial nutrition and hydration, originally intended as a temporary bridge to the restoration of patients' digestive functioning, now is routinely delivered to thousands of patients who have irretrievably lost all higher brain functions.

Prenatal diagnosis, originally intended for fetuses at high risk of a metabolic or genetic disorder, is now routinely offered to, and sought by, many women in their late twenties or early thirties who are at no special health risk. The availability of this technology has thus expanded choice, while simultaneously imposing new pressures on many women by altering their definition of an "acceptable risk" during pregnancy.

Finally, in vitro fertilization (IVF), originally developed to aid infertile married couples, is now offered to single women, to adult daughters volunteering to serve as surrogate mothers for their own mothers' children (i.e., to be the mothers of their own siblings), and to postmenopausal women in their late forties and fifties. In conjunction with the newly developed techniques of embryo freezing and "embryo splitting," a kind of cloning, IVF might soon make it possible for a woman grown from a split embryo to give birth to her own previously frozen identical twin.

Needless to say, problems such as these, as they spawn new possibilities for remaking ourselves, our families, and our society, call into question the adequacy of our traditional ways of thinking. In some instances, it is clear that scientific and technological developments have brought about a change in values and moral beliefs. As Emmanuel Mesthene has remarked, "By adding new options . . . technology can lead to changes in values in the same way that the appearance of new dishes on the heretofore standard menu of one's favorite restaurant can lead to changes in one's tastes and choices of food."[1] Often, what science and technology make possible soon becomes permissible and, eventually, normal and expected. For example, when the use of anesthesia during childbirth was introduced around 150 years ago, it was condemned as morally wrong. Women were "supposed" to suffer through labor: it was "unnatural" if they did not. But what *could* be done *was* done, and eventually those beliefs were revised.

In the more recent past, we have noted a change in attitude toward heart transplants; at first, many people had moral reservations about this procedure, not because it was new and risky, but because the heart was associated with the soul or personality. Today, although heart transplants continue to raise social policy problems, this particular moral reservation has completely vanished.

Most readers may feel comfortable about the attitudinal changes just mentioned, but in other areas the influence of technology on values and morals has had more controversial results. For example, developments in medical knowledge and techniques have played a major role in reshaping cultural and legal attitudes toward contraception and abortion, and more recent developments—e.g., the "abortion pill," RU 486, and long-acting contraceptives such as Norplant—promise to erode traditional moral qualms even further. Yet not everyone believes that these developments constitute an unalloyed good; some regard them as a profound insult to their

1. Emmanuel Mesthene, "The Role of Technology in Society," in *Technology and Man's Future*, edited by A. Teich (New York: St. Martin's Press, 1972), 137.

conception of the sanctity of life, while others suspect that they will be coercively targeted at vulnerable minority groups. And what about the near future? Already there is widespread concern regarding the ethical implications of techniques and procedures that are still in their developmental stages. Will developments in genetic knowledge made possible by the human genome project and advances in reproductive technologies help usher in a "brave new world"? Is there, perhaps, some knowledge that we ought not try to seek? Or are our reservations about such matters as in vitro fertilization for women old enough to be grandmothers as time-bound and unwarranted as those of the people who opposed anesthesia and heart transplants?

As Nicholas Rescher has pointed out, the phenomenon of value change is a complex one, and technological developments may lead to "value restandardization."[2] The value of good health may not have changed position in our hierarchy of values, but as a result of technology the standard of what constitutes good health may have been revised considerably upward. As technology increases the possibilities in life, as values diversify and expectations rise, abnormalities—and common conditions—that were once taken for granted come to be viewed as pathological conditions requiring treatment and/or prevention. It is, after all, a comparatively recent assumption that medical relief can and should be sought for such conditions as acne, obesity, short stature, crooked teeth, small breasts, and the failure to achieve orgasm.

In addition to curing disease, medicine is now increasingly capable of *optimizing* more or less normal conditions that nevertheless can be improved upon. Drugs like Prozac, for example, promise a future in which individuals might not merely manage clinical depression better, but also alter their personalities in significantly positive ways. Having problems with self-esteem? Having trouble mustering the courage to ask for that promotion? "Cosmetic psychopharmacology" may be able to provide just what you need.[3]

2. Nicholas Rescher, "What Is Value Change? A Framework for Research," in *Values and the Future*, edited by K. Baier and N. Rescher (New York: Free Press, 1969).

3. Peter Kramer, *Listening to Prozac* (New York: Viking, 1993).

Related to all these issues is, of course, the restandardization of what constitutes adequate health care. Today we expect not only to be cured of ills that were previously incurable, but also to be prevented from experiencing a variety of infirmities and misfortunes that were once the common lot of humankind. And we feel wronged if these expectations go unfulfilled. Driven by the pressure of consumer demand, treatments that many might regard today as "frills," such as in vitro fertilization and cosmetic personality-altering drugs, may well be regarded tomorrow as essential ingredients in the "pursuit of happiness."

The impact of technology on our value systems is also seen in the fact that the development of new knowledge and techniques may blur, rather than sharpen, the very concepts that are central to our norms and values. The advent of organ transplantation and critical-care technologies, for example, has forced physicians and society at large to rethink the very meanings of life and death. The traditional "definition" of life as the presence of respiration and heartbeat has been replaced in every U.S. state over the past twenty years by the notion of whole-brain death, yet few people, even today, can identify a noncontroversial philosophical rationale for the new law's insistence that the entire brain, both "higher" and "lower," must have ceased functioning irreversibly for a patient to be dead. As a result, the moral and legal status of patients with no higher brain functions, those in persistent vegetative states, poses an ongoing challenge to the current approach to brain death. If a patient has permanently lost the capacity for any kind of thought, feeling, and human interaction—if, to put it somewhat crudely, "no one is home"—why not consider him or her to be dead? (Issues such as this also raise methodological questions: e.g., Is the definition of death primarily a matter of discovery, death being some kind of brute fact with contours that merely need better tracing, or is it, rather, something that the citizens of a political community must *invent* for themselves?)

The definition of death is perhaps the most salient conceptual puzzle served up by the new medicine, but it is by no means the only one. Similar issues are posed by the advent of new reproductive technologies (Is a woman who donates an egg to another woman the "mother" of the child born? Is she a mother in any sense that matters?), the human genome project (Is the otherwise healthy 20-year-old carrier of a gene associated with the development of coronary artery disease in later life "diseased" in some sense?), and, of course, abortion (Is the fetus a "person" or full-fledged human being deserving of our respect and protection, is it merely a clump of cells, or is it perhaps something in-between?).

Finally, technology drives the bioethical agenda by virtue of its phenomenal success in addressing medical needs and desires. Hundreds of years ago, when medicine could offer little more than bleeding, blistering, and purging—when the leech represented the cutting edge of biotechnology—there weren't many "tragic choices" to be made. With the advent of technological success, however, has come the need to pay for increasingly expensive curative, diagnostic, and palliative procedures, access to which is increasingly perceived as a matter of right. But as costs skyrocket and as the demand for access spreads, the inevitability of limits and priority-setting gradually comes into focus. Assuming that meeting every conceivable health care need would either break the bank or devour funds earmarked for other important societal needs—such as food, shelter, education, transportation, and the arts—the question of the explicit rationing of health care acquires real seriousness and urgency. Can we afford to pay for a patient's third organ transplant, for his or her experimental bone marrow transplant for advanced cancer, or for the short but otherwise normal child's synthetic growth hormone injections? Can we afford these things when millions of people lack basic health insurance and decent preventive and primary care? Conceived in their broadest framework, these questions ask how our health care system might be reformed so as to provide universal access to a good package of "basic" services, without either bankrupting society or destroying the doctor-patient relationship.

Other Sources of Bioethical Problems

Although the urgency and frequency of bioethical controversies owe much to the magnitude and pace of technological change, there are other factors at work driving the recent explosion of bioethical issues. Some medical-moral problems of long standing, such as the limits of confidentiality, truth-telling, and euthanasia, have more to do with the ethics of human relationships—with what we owe to one another and may (or may not) do to one another—than with the advent of new technologies. More important than technology in reshaping the physician-patient relationship are such widespread social phenomena as the increasing demand, modeled on the civil rights movement, for patients' rights to information and health care; the growing distrust of professional privilege; women's critiques of male dominance within medicine; and the assimilation of medicine to our consumerist and entrepreneurial culture.

Even here, however, it remains true that advances in biology and medicine have often given a characteristically modern spin to some of these traditional problems. Truth-telling, for example, is perhaps now more important and more difficult an obligation than ever before, due in large measure to the vast proliferation of possible treatments and diagnostic interventions available to physicians and their patients. Likewise, our traditional norms governing the confidentiality of medical information are sorely tested when new genetic tests reveal serious abnormalities not only in patients coming for diagnosis and/or treatment, but also, of necessity, in some of their family members as well.

Still, many highly controversial practices require surprisingly little technological assistance in threatening our fundamental values and established customs. Artificial insemination with donated sperm, for example, allows infertile married couples to have children, but it also enables single women and lesbian partners to give birth without the presence of a male spouse; in addition, it makes possible the practice of so-called surrogate motherhood, in which, for example, a woman agrees to be inseminated with the sperm of the husband of a childless marriage. For some, these developments signal serious threats to the welfare of children and to the institution of marriage, the very bedrock of our society; for others, they merely represent the next logical step in the growth of reproductive rights for all individuals, whether they be married or single, straight or gay, fertile or infertile. Ironically, at the heart of this impassioned debate about rights, marriage, and society lies the most ordinary of technological means: the humble turkey baster.

CHALLENGES TO ETHICAL THEORY

The issues raised in the preceding section pose challenging factual, conceptual, and moral problems. People often have strong feelings about some of these issues (for example, abortion and euthanasia). On some issues, many of us do not know what to think (for example, IVF for older women, or using children born without a higher brain as sources of transplantable organs). The assumption in philosophical bioethics is that careful analysis can help us at least make progress on some of these issues, if not resolve all of them. However, some are skeptical about this assumption. They believe, for a variety of reasons, that ethical disputes are, in principle, unresolvable by rational means.

Moral Nihilism

Princeton philosopher Gilbert Harman defines "moral nihilism" as "the doctrine that there are no moral facts, no moral truths, and no moral knowledge."[4] Extreme nihilists think that nothing is right or wrong; that morality, like religion, is an illusion that should be abandoned. This implies that torturing, raping, and killing a young child is not wrong—something few people could accept. More moderate nihilists do not recommend abandoning morality, but, rather, offer a theory about the meaning of moral terms that explains why there are no moral facts, truths, or knowledge.

Ethics and Feelings

The theory of moral language that is offered by moderate moral nihilists is known as "emotivism." Emotivists believe that moral utterances do not express facts, or tell us anything about how the world is. Rather, they express our feelings. Therefore, such statements are not—indeed, cannot be—true or false, any more than "Go, Yankees!" is true or false. The sentence, "Abortion is wrong," does not say anything about abortion, but rather expresses someone's negative feelings about abortion.

4. Gilbert Harman, *The Nature of Morality: An Introduction to Ethics* (New York: Oxford University Press, 1977), 11.

How plausible is this thesis about moral language? Undoubtedly, moral claims often do express feelings, but it is debatable that that is all they do. Consider Dr. Brody's quandary. She might ask herself, "I wonder if euthanasia is wrong." In an emotivist analysis, this can only mean, "I wonder if I have negative feelings about euthanasia." Is this Dr. Brody's question? It seems rather that she wonders what she *thinks* about euthanasia. Should she be motivated by her empathy for her patient and her desire to alleviate his suffering? Or should she act according to that part of the Hippocratic oath that requires doctors to be healers, not killers? What would be the larger implications for society if doctors were to engage in terminating their patients' lives? Dr. Brody's internal debate is of a kind familiar to most of us. In other words, when we face a moral dilemma, instead of trying to resolve our puzzlement by an introspective attempt at ascertaining which of our feelings is really the strongest, we tend to look "outward" at various external or objective aspects and implications of the alternatives in order to determine which is right.

We do not deny a relationship between feelings and ethical decisions, for moral issues often, if not always, provoke deep emotional responses. But to assign feelings ultimate authority in these matters is, we think, to put the cart before the horse. Our feelings may provoke us to moral inquiry, but the inquiry does not terminate there.

Ethics and Culture

Another form of moderate moral nihilism denies the possibility of moral truth *independent of a particular culture*. This view, known as "ethical relativism," says that morality is relative to the society one lives in and the way one was brought up. The rightness or wrongness of an action or practice cannot be determined apart from the cultural or social context in which it occurs.

Support for ethical relativism comes from three sources. First, it stems from an observation that different cultures have different moral beliefs and practices. However, simply noting moral differences in various cultures does not establish ethical relativism. Ethical relativism goes beyond noting that cultures differ in their moral beliefs and practices; it maintains that when there are moral differences, no one is right (or wrong). According to relativism, right and wrong are always relative to, and determined by, culture.

A reason for thinking that morality is always relative to culture is that there does not seem to be any way to prove that an ethical belief or practice is right (or wrong). Infanticide, for example, is treated as murder in our culture, but is accepted or tolerated in others. Who's to say who's right? The inability to prove an ethical belief is contrasted with the ability to prove factual claims. If we come across people who think that the Earth is flat, we can (in principle) show them that it is round. Note that the difference between ethics and science is not that ethics has a monopoly on disagreement. There are plenty of heated disagreements among scientists. However, scientists agree (in principle) about what kinds of evidence would settle a dispute. There is no such agreement in ethics. In other words, we do not have a decision procedure for resolving ethical disputes. This is the second source of support for ethical relativism.

The above two reasons offered in support of relativism make observations about the world, and then offer a theory about the nature of reality that is consistent with these observations. We might characterize these as intellectual reasons for relativism. The third reason for relativism is quite different. It offers a moral reason for adopting relativism: namely, that relativism promotes tolerance toward people who hold moral beliefs different from one's own. This apparently was the motivation of nineteenth-century anthropologists who wished to prevent Western imperialists from imposing their culture on indigenous peoples.

Assume that we accept the plausible claim that different cultures do in fact differ in their moral beliefs. (Even this statement can be questioned, but let us accept it for the sake of argument.) What about the second support for relativism, that there is no decision procedure in ethics? This claim seems most plausible when we think of controversial issues, such as abortion or euthanasia, about which intelligent people of good will can disagree. Suppose, however, we think instead of a practice that virtually everyone thinks is wrong: for example, slavery. In the eighteenth and nineteenth centuries, slavery was often justified on the grounds that the Africans were inherently inferior to their European masters, incapable of learning or governing themselves. This is a "factual" claim, and it is clearly false. Indeed, had the slaves really been incapable of learning, laws prohibiting the teaching of reading to slaves would have been pointless—there were no laws outlawing the teaching of reading to cows, for example. These and other justifications of slavery are clearly false and self-serving.

Slavery can also be criticized as inconsistent with other fundamental values, such as the equality of all men (or as we would say today, all human beings), as proclaimed in the Declaration of Independence. It seems likely that the discrepancy between the value of equality and the practice of slavery was a motivation for the abolition of slavery, along with its recognition as cruel, exploitative, and unjust. These terms also have considerable factual content, so that it is not "just a matter of opinion" whether a practice is cruel, exploitative, or unjust.

A further point against relativism (parallel to the argument we presented against emotivism) is that it gives an inaccurate account of the meaning of certain moral claims, notably those of moral reformers. According to relativism, right and wrong are always relative to culture. What a culture (or the majority of a culture) thinks is right is right—for them. However, a moral reformer challenges the conventional beliefs of his or her own culture. For example, Martin Luther King, Jr., said that segregation was wrong. According to relativism, this can only mean that segregation is considered wrong by his culture, which was obviously false in the American South in the 1950s. Of course King was not claiming that his culture *regarded* segregation as wrong. He was making the very different claim that segregation *was* wrong. (Indeed, if his culture already believed that segregation was wrong, he would not have had to demonstrate and go to jail for his beliefs!) Relativism simply cannot make sense of the claims of moral reformers. Since we do understand the claims of moral reformers, and at least sometimes are influenced by them, it seems that relativism cannot be true.

Despite these considerations, ethical relativism holds sway with many people, perhaps because the alternative seems terribly arrogant. One often hears the following sort of argument: "How can anyone say that another person's values are wrong? Who are you to tell me that you're right and I'm wrong?

What makes you an authority? Everyone has a right to an opinion." However, we must be careful here. To say that everyone has a right to an opinion is not to say that every opinion is right. One can certainly agree that people have a right to their moral views without being a relativist. Indeed, if we think that everyone has the right to an opinion, we are *not* relativists. For "everyone has the right to an opinion" is itself a moral value. According to relativism, this moral value (like any other) is only true for societies that believe it. But not all cultures accept freedom of thought as a basic value. What if a culture believes in complete conformity of thought, and in brutal suppression of nonconformity? What if they practice conversion by the sword? Can we say that they are wrong to do this, that they ought to be tolerant? Not if we are relativists. Tolerance, then, is not a value that relativists can consistently promote, for tolerance, like all other moral values, is only right in cultures that think it right.

Finally, relativism not only prevents us from criticizing the brutal and intolerant practices of others, it also does not permit us to criticize our own past. We cannot say that slavery or child labor or the oppression of women were mistakes, since this implies an objective moral standard according to which we can evaluate our past practices. There is no moral progress, only moral change. This is another reason for rejecting ethical relativism, at least in its most extreme form.

At the same time, relativism has two things to recommend it, which we believe can be incorporated into a nonrelativist approach. First, the relativist is right to point out that morality occurs in a cultural context. Before presuming to judge another culture's practices and beliefs, we would do well to try to understand them "from the inside." We may still decide ultimately that a practice is wrong, but we are not entitled to make this judgment without understanding the practice in context. Second, relativism encourages multiple perspectives on and solutions to moral problems. Both of these insights are present in "multiculturalism." As we understand it, multiculturalism is *not* an uncritical acceptance of the values and practices of all other cultures. Rather, it is the awareness that there are a range of different ways to live, which offer different solutions to the problems faced by human beings, combined with a recognition that our own solutions—practices, institutions, values, and moral rules—may not be the best ones. Multiculturalism is a welcome corrective to an unfortunate tendency of Western civilization to assume superiority and to dismiss other ways of life as inferior and backward.

One can, however, be a multiculturalist without being a relativist. Indeed, it is only if one *rejects* relativism that one can meaningfully say such things as, "Our culture's attitude toward nature is domineering, exploitative, and wasteful. We could learn something from Native Americans." Multiculturalism requires an open mind toward the customs and beliefs of other cultures, but such open-mindedness need not, and should not, be uncritical. It is entirely consistent with a conception of morality as amenable to rational considerations, and the conviction that there can be better or worse moral justifications.[5]

MORAL THEORIES AND PERSPECTIVES

How are we to assess moral reasons and arguments? Intuitively, most of us can probably recognize good—or especially bad—moral reasoning, but in complicated situations we are often left wondering whether a consideration is pertinent. Is assisted suicide wrong because it helps someone to kill him- or herself, and killing is wrong? Or is it right because it helps someone to do what he or she reasonably wants to do, and thus promotes autonomy? To answer questions of this sort, we need "a framework within which agents can reflect on the acceptability of actions and can evaluate moral judgments and moral character."[6] Such a framework is known as an "ethical theory."

---

5. Robert K. Fullinwider, "Ethnocentrism and Education in Judgment," *Report from the Institute for Philosophy & Public Policy* 14 (1994): 6–11. See also Charles Taylor et al., *Multiculturalism and "The Politics of Recognition"* (Princeton, NJ: Princeton University Press, 1992); and Amy Gutmann, "The Challenge of Multiculturalism in Political Ethics," *Philosophy and Public Affairs* 22, no. 3 (Summer 1993): 171–206.

6. Tom Beauchamp and James F. Childress, *The Principles of Biomedical Ethics*, 4th ed. (New York: Oxford University Press, 1994), 44.

Traditionally, ethical theories tend to be reductionist; that is, they offer one idea as the key to morality, and attempt to reduce everything to that one idea. For example, classical utilitarians maintain that right actions are those that promote the greatest happiness of the greatest number, while Kantians tell us that right actions are those that can be consistently willed universally. Each theory claims to have discovered the single, overarching standard of morality or right action. In a typical introduction to ethical theory class, each theory is presented and subjected to devastating criticism. The unfortunate result is that students frequently conclude that all of the theories are wrong—or worse, are pretentious nonsense.

In recent years, a number of philosophers have come to doubt that any normative theory can plausibly claim to be *the* correct theory. It may be that moral reality is sufficiently complex that any one theory gives only partial insight. Utilitarians are certainly right that achieving human happiness is an important goal of morality, but nonconsequentialists are also right in insisting, first, that other values such as justice and autonomy are also important, and second, that these values cannot be reduced to happiness. We conclude that it is a mistake to view the various theoretical alternatives as mutually exclusive claims to moral truth. Instead, we should view them as important but partial contributions to a comprehensive, although necessarily fragmented, moral vision.

Utilitarianism

Jeremy Bentham (1748–1832) and John Stuart Mill (1806–1873) are generally credited with developing the first detailed and systematic formulation of the ethical theory known as "utilitarianism." The heart of utilitarianism is "the greatest happiness principle," which, as Mill puts it, "holds that actions are right in proportion as they tend to promote happiness; wrong as they tend to produce the reverse of happiness."[7] The greatest happiness principle is also known as the principle of utility. The utility of an action is determined by its tendency to produce or promote happiness. Actions that result in happiness have positive utility; those that create misery have negative utility. Clearly, many actions can create both conditions. An act that is pleasurable now (not going to the dentist) can cause considerable suffering later on; and often the happiness of some persons (car thieves) is purchased at the expense of unhappiness for others. The right action is the one that, on balance, promotes the most happiness, or the greatest amount of pleasure over pain.

The first thing to note about utilitarianism is that it is a "consequentialist" theory. That is, it judges the rightness and wrongness of an action by its consequences, or what will happen if the action is or is not performed. Second, utilitarianism's theory of value says that good consequences are those that produce or promote happiness or pleasure, bad consequences those that produce or promote the reverse. As we will see, both consequentialism and utilitarianism's theory of value have lately come under attack.

There are several advantages to utilitarianism. It provides us with a decision procedure for deciding what to do: namely, whichever action produces, on balance, the greatest net amount of happiness. Moreover, happiness is alleged to be something empirical, something both measurable and comparable. In principle, therefore, utilitarianism provides definite answers to the question of how we ought to act.

Features of Utilitarianism As we indicated earlier, utilitarianism is a form of consequentialism, and thus it holds that the results of actions are the *only* relevant feature in assessing actions. Considerations of an agent's intentions, feelings, or convictions are seen as irrelevant to the question, "What is the right thing to do?" Similarly, utilitarianism regards the question of whether a given course of action conforms to established social norms or ethical codes as relevant only to the extent that such conformity has a bearing on the production of happiness or unhappiness. Departing from established social codes typically has adverse consequences for the rule-breaker, and these consequences must be considered in deciding whether departing from the norm is the right thing to do.

Another important feature of utilitarianism is its impartiality. The utilitarian does not say, "The

7. John Stuart Mill, *Utilitarianism* (New York: Liberal Arts Press, 1957), 10.

goodness of an action is determined by the amount of happiness it produces *for me*." Rather, the good is determined by the overall net happiness achieved. The utilitarian considers his or her own happiness, but no more and no less than the happiness of others. In weighing the effects of an action, utilitarianism maintains that we must take into consideration all of the parties concerned and that all parties shall be given equal consideration. Thus, utilitarianism is committed to the value of equality.

How far does this equality extend? In the nineteenth century, women were not considered the equals of men. Women were largely under the control of their fathers before marriage, and their husbands after. They could not vote, and their ability to own property was greatly restricted. Mill rejected such inequality. He supported equal rights for women and opposed slavery. Indeed, Mill thought that any creature capable of being happy or miserable—"all sentient creation so far as possible"—was deserving of moral concern. Contemporary utilitarians, like Peter Singer, have argued that nonhuman animals should count equally with humans, and that therefore painful experimentation on animals is wrong.

Utilitarianism has been influential not only in expanding our notion of "who counts" morally, but also in focusing attention on long-term, as well as short-term, results. Many decisions and actions performed today have an impact on the future. Remoteness in time is not, in principle, a reason to ignore a consequence, any more than is remoteness in space (although, of course, our knowledge about the future is less certain than our knowledge of the present). This is particularly important when we think of issues such as genetic engineering and gene therapy, which may have a profound impact on the genetic makeup of people in future generations. Utilitarianism espouses a prudent moral doctrine that requires us to think carefully about what we should do, and to consider not only the immediate effects of our actions, but also their long-term consequences.

To summarize the advantages of utilitarianism, first, it reduces vagueness by providing a single criterion of right action: namely, the promotion of human happiness. Moreover, happiness, whether understood as pleasure or as preference satisfaction, is something that can be empirically measured. Utilitarianism thus provides an objective standard for judging whether an action is right or wrong, and a method for resolving moral disputes. Finally, and more importantly, the principle of utility is derived from the very point of morality, which is to improve the lot of human beings living together. Morality does not relate to the satisfaction of some abstract or arbitrary code; rather, it relates to the improvement of the human condition, which means alleviating suffering and increasing happiness.

That the point of morality is to promote human welfare may seem boringly obvious, but it was regarded as quite radical in the nineteenth century, and not only because of its egalitarian implications. In addition, the focus on human happiness seemed to conflict with Christian teachings; for example, those teachings espousing the value of suffering. As we noted earlier, anesthesia during childbirth was condemned in the nineteenth century as unnatural and contrary to biblical teachings ("In sorrow shalt thou bring forth children"). Even today the suffering of terminally ill patients is valued by some Catholic theologians, who regard the opportunity to identify with and participate in Christ's suffering on the cross as a positive good. Utilitarians are likely to have little patience with such views. Utilitarianism regards suffering and sacrifice as having moral value only if they promote overall happiness. Suffering and sacrifice have no intrinsic moral worth.

Objections to Utilitarianism Utilitarianism has been subjected to numerous objections, four of which we will consider here. One objection is to utilitarianism's theory of value: namely, the claim that happiness is the greatest good, the ultimate end. Critics have maintained that this theory leaves out many other "goods," such as health, friendship, creativity, intellectual attainment, and so forth. Mill agreed that these things are all valuable, but argued that they are valuable because they contribute to a happy life, one as rich as possible in enjoyment and as free as possible from pain. However, it remains questionable whether all values are commensurable; that is, whether all values can be reduced to happiness, however happiness is interpreted. And even if it were possible to reduce the plurality of values to a single value, happiness, is it possible to compare and weigh the happiness of one person against that of another? What if an action will make one person intensely happy but leave several people somewhat depressed? Exactly how are we to arrive at the right utilitarian solution? Moreover, some people feel things more intensely than others. Should we pay attention to the strength of desires? On the one hand, it seems that we should, since the intensity of an individual's happiness or unhappiness affects the total amount, and utilitarianism tells us to maximize happiness. On the other hand, this gives an advantage to the passionate over the phlegmatic that seems to violate Bentham's dictum that everyone counts for one, nobody for more than one.

A second objection to utilitarianism is that it requires us to calculate the probable consequences of every action, and this task is impossible. The sheer calculations alone would prevent anyone from doing anything. In response, it should be noted that both Bentham and Mill thought of utilitarianism primarily as a guide to legislative policy, rather than as a guide to individual behavior. No one thinks it unreasonable to ask for impact studies on the likely consequences of legislation. These are sometimes called "cost-benefit" analyses, and they are the direct descendants of classical utilitarianism.

Being utilitarians in our private lives does not mean that we must calculate all the consequences of every act, which would be impossible. Instead, we can rely on what Mill calls secondary principles, like "Don't lie," and "Don't harm others." We know from centuries of experience that adherence to these secondary principles promotes the greatest happiness for all, while departure from them causes insecurity and misery.

A more recent criticism of utilitarianism (or consequentialism generally) concerns the theory of responsibility it implies. For nonconsequentialists, it can be very significant whether an outcome occurs because of something *I did*, whereas for consequentialists all that matters ultimately is *what happens*. This has led some consequentialists to reject a time-honored distinction in medicine, the distinction between killing and "letting die." Many doctors believe that it is permissible for them to stop treatment when death is desirable; for example, in the case of a terminally ill patient in a great deal of pain who wants to die. However, they think it would be wrong (as well as illegal) actively to kill a patient in that same situation. Utilitarians, by contrast, are likely to regard killing and letting die as morally equivalent, since the outcome—a desirable death—is achieved in both cases (see Part 3, Section 5).

A final major criticism of utilitarianism is that it is inadequate as a moral theory because it conflicts with some of our most basic moral intuitions.

> Suppose we could greatly increase human happiness and diminish misery by occasionally, and perhaps secretly, abducting derelicts from city streets for use in fatal but urgent medical experiments. If utilitarian considerations were decisive, this practice might well be justifiable, even desirable. Yet it is surely wrong. Such a case suggests that we cannot always explain good and bad simply in terms of increasing or decreasing overall happiness.[8]

A utilitarian might respond by denying the premise that we could in fact promote the greatest happiness by abducting derelicts for medical experiments. He or she might argue that this fails to take into consideration all the negative side effects of such a policy: the impossibility of keeping it secret, the terror of the derelicts not yet abducted, the risk of mistake and abuse, the psychological effect on the doctors performing the experiments, etc. It is precisely because of such long-range negative consequences that policies like informed consent are rational from a utilitarian viewpoint. Still, it seems possible that, in special circumstances, the good effects could outweigh the bad. Some utilitarians will acknowledge that in such circumstances it would be right to use derelicts in fatal medical experiments (while reminding us that such circumstances are extremely unlikely to obtain, and it is even less likely that we can be sure that they do). However, they maintain that the fact that this practice would conflict with many people's deeply held moral convictions is not a worthwhile criticism of utilitarianism. Many utilitarians are quite skeptical of "deeply held moral convictions," which they regard as often no more than irrational superstitions.

8. Christina and Fred Sommers, eds., *Vice and Virtue in Everyday Life: Introductory Readings in Ethics,* 2nd ed. (San Diego, CA: Harcourt Brace Jovanovich, 1989), 80.

Others, attracted by the virtues of utilitarianism, are nevertheless disturbed by the possibility of conflicts with justice and other basic moral practices, such as telling the truth and keeping promises. Rule-utilitarianism may be seen as one attempt to counter this objection.

Rule-Utilitarianism versus Act-Utilitarianism

Mill left unresolved the question whether the greatest happiness principle is to be applied to specific acts or to general kinds of acts. It has been suggested that if we apply the principle to kinds of acts, we can avoid some of the criticisms of utilitarianism. The version of utilitarianism that is primarily concerned with the consequences of specific acts has become known as "act-utilitarianism," while the version primarily concerned with the consequences of general policies is called "rule-utilitarianism."

Act-utilitarianism tells us to apply the principle of utility directly to the particular act in question. Suppose a doctor is faced with the question whether it would be morally right to help a terminally ill patient to die. An act-utilitarian would seek to determine which alternative in this particular case would maximize happiness and/or minimize suffering. Relevant considerations would include the possibility of recovery, whether the patient really wanted to die or was in a depression that might be alleviated, the impact on the patient's family, the impact on the doctor, and so forth.

By contrast, rule-utilitarianism uses the principle of utility not to decide which acts to perform or avoid, but rather to formulate and justify moral rules. The correct moral rules are those that promote the greatest happiness of the greatest number. Faced with a decision about how to act, rule-utilitarianism tells us that we are not to appeal directly to the principle of utility. Rather, we are to consider whether this action falls under a rule that is justified by the principle of utility. Rule-utilitarianism would direct Dr. Brody to ask whether a general rule permitting assisted suicide would maximize happiness. Here, an important consideration would be whether such a practice would start us down a "slippery slope" and threaten the lives of terminally ill patients who do not really want to die, but who, for various reasons, are either afraid of being a burden to their families, or have families that want to get rid of them. Thus, a rule-utilitarian might argue that while helping *this* patient to die might maximize happiness (or minimize misery), it would nevertheless be wrong, because the consequences of a general policy of assisting suicide would be disastrous.

The difference between act- and rule-utilitarianism is *not* that only the latter appeals to moral rules. Both act- and rule-utilitarians use rules to guide their behavior. Rather, the difference lies in the way each group regards moral rules. For the act-utilitarian, rules are *summaries of past experience*. They're what we might call "rules of thumb": handy guides to the future based on past experience. Since it's often difficult to know what will maximize happiness in a particular situation, and since people are likely to be prejudiced by their own self-interest in their calculations, rules help us decide what to do.

Rules are regarded differently by rule-utilitarians. Rules are not just devices to help us figure out what will maximize happiness in a particular case. The rules themselves are justified on the grounds that having these particular rules maximizes happiness. But once we decide what the best rules are (that is, which ones are most likely to maximize happiness over the long run), then those are the rules we should follow, even if following them in a particular situation doesn't maximize happiness.

Thus, the rule-utilitarian can apparently avoid the sorts of situations that make act-utilitarianism unsatisfactory to many. In brief, the rule-utilitarian agrees with the act-utilitarian that the value of just practices resides in their tendency to promote happiness; but he will not agree that it is permissible to perform an unjust act in order to maximize happiness.

Is Rule-Utilitarianism an Improvement over Act-Utilitarianism? Act-utilitarians make this criticism of rule-utilitarianism: It makes no sense for a utilitarian to insist that a rule that will have less than optimal consequences should be followed simply because the rule maximizes happiness *in general*. J. J. C. Smart gives the following example. A good rule of thumb in a chess game is that you shouldn't sacrifice your queen for a pawn. But if, in a particular game of chess, you could checkmate your opponent by sacrificing your queen for a pawn, it would be absurd to stick dogmatically to the "Never sacrifice your queen for a pawn" rule. Smart thinks rule-utilitarianism is guilty of the same absurdity. Just as checkmating your opponent is the whole point of chess, so maximizing happiness is the whole point of utilitarian morality. It would not be rational from the standpoint of utility to refuse to break a moral rule when by doing so you could maximize welfare. For this reason, Smart calls rule-utilitarianism "superstitious rule worship."[9]

A related objection to rule-utilitarianism is that it collapses into act-utilitarianism. For whenever an act-utilitarian would say it was right to *break* a moral rule, it seems that the rule-utilitarian would generally agree, but instead say that the rule should be *modified*. Suppose, for example, that the only way to save someone's life is by telling a lie. An act-utilitarian would say that it was right to lie in such circumstances. But what would a rule-utilitarian say? That it is wrong to lie, knowing that the result will be an avoidable death? Surely not. A rule-utilitarian would say that the original rule, "Don't lie," is too crude. A better rule would be, "Don't lie, except to save a life." Moreover, it is likely that there is more than one exception to the "Don't lie" rule. That is, the rule most likely to maximize happiness probably allows for several situations in which lying is morally right. But now it seems that whatever would lead the act-utilitarian to break the rule would lead the rule-utilitarian to modify the rule. Thus, the two versions give exactly the same advice; they are "extensionally equivalent," so rule-utilitarianism cannot be an improvement over act-utilitarianism. On the other hand, if the rule-utilitarian holds fast to the original rule, even when modifying it would have better results, he or she deviates from utilitarianism and is guilty of Smart's charge of "rule-worship."

In response, a rule-utilitarian might say that the criticism of extensional equivalence reflects a naive view of the operation of social rules and policies. While the considerations that lead an act-utilitarian to break a rule in a particular case can perhaps be articulated, it is much less easy to formulate a general policy that covers all the relevant exceptions. Consider the case study with which we began. A rule-utilitarian would not only consider whether it would be right for Dr. Brody to help Mr. Lasken kill himself, but also whether doctors generally ought to be able to make decisions of this kind. For it is clear that this is not a one-of-a-kind situation; there are lots of Jim Laskens and Deborah Brodys. Should doctors make such decisions on a case-by-case basis? That approach has the advantage of allowing the individual doctor to decide whether the patient's pain outweighs the general rule against killing. The disadvantage of that approach, however, is that most people, including doctors, are not perfect happiness optimizers. There are bound to be mistakes. Some patients who are not terminally ill will be killed, as will some who could have been helped with psychiatric treatment or better pain medicine. Some doctors may be unduly influenced by relatives who want the patient's life to be over when the patient does not. More disturbing, in times of cost-cutting, might there not be a tendency to regard the terminally ill as "expendable" and not worth spending money on, even if a sick individual does not want to die? The problem is not so much that we cannot say when assisted suicide would and would not be justified (though this too is difficult to specify in advance); rather, it is that the practice of this policy on a large scale may result in many unnecessary and undesirable deaths. The question, then, is whether the need for such a policy is outweighed by the risk of mistake and abuse. These rule-utilitarian considerations do not seem to be captured by an act-utilitarian approach, which looks only at the consequences of a specific act. Therefore, rule-utilitarianism does not collapse into act-utilitarianism.

Nevertheless, rule-utilitarianism acknowledges that it is, in principle, possible that a practice we ordinarily think of as completely immoral (such as slavery) might, in unusual circumstances, promote the greatest happiness and would therefore be right. Moreover, the factor that determines whether a practice maximizes happiness (for example, whether the number of people made miserable was sufficiently small) seems morally irrelevant. How can it be right to ride roughshod over the rights of a few people simply to make the majority happy? It is considerations of this kind that lead some people to

9. J. J. C. Smart, "Extreme and Restricted Utilitarianism," in *Theories of Ethics*, edited by Philippa Foot (Oxford: Oxford University Press, 1967), 177.

reject utilitarianism altogether and opt for something completely different.

Kantian Ethics

Utilitarian ethics has a strong appeal. The utilitarian says, "*Surely* consequences are terribly important. Whenever we act, we are trying to bring about certain states of affairs and avoid others. It is right to bring about happiness, and wrong to create misery. How can there be any other criterion of right and wrong? What *makes* lying and cheating wrong, if not that they cause misery?"

At the same time, it seems that there are some things we must not do, even if doing them would accomplish great good. What if we could maximize happiness by deliberately hurting innocent people or by violating their rights? Surely this would be wrong. It seems to matter not just *what* happens, but *how* it comes about.

Kantian ethics, so titled from its most illustrious exponent, Immanuel Kant (1724–1804), captures this intuitive conviction. Whereas Mill said that the right act is the one with the best consequences, Kant argued that consequences can never make an action right or wrong. An action that brings about the greatest amount of happiness might still be wrong. Good consequences can never make a wrong action right, and one must never act wrongly in order to bring about good consequences. In other words, the ends do not justify the means.

In addition to rejecting consequentialism, Kant also rejects the view that pain is intrinsically bad and pleasure intrinsically good. According to Kant, the badness of pain depends on whether it is deserved. It is morally right that the wicked should suffer and morally wrong that they should prosper. Kant rejects the utilitarian view that the pleasure experienced by a sadist is an intrinsic good, albeit one which can be outweighed by the suffering of his victim. The sadist's pleasure has absolutely no moral worth. Indeed, pain and pleasure, which play so prominent a role in utilitarian ethics, have a relatively minor role in Kantian ethics. As we saw earlier, Mill and Bentham extended moral concern to all sentient beings. By contrast, Kant considers our capacity to experience pleasure and pain as fairly insignificant morally. Of far greater importance is our rationality: our ability to think, to plan our lives, to be motivated by abstract considerations. This is allegedly what separates us from the rest of creation, giving human beings a central and special moral status. As animals, we are subject to the laws of nature, physical and psychological. However, unlike other animals, human beings are rational beings, or persons.

For Kant, rational beings have a special moral standing because of their ability to act on the basis of reason and to conform their behavior to the moral law. Kant argues that many of the common ends that people pursue, such as health, wealth, education, and the like, are only valuable because of their place in the projects of rational beings. In contrast, the value of persons does not depend on the way they fit into the projects of other rational beings. Persons have intrinsic worth and must be treated as ends in themselves and not merely as a means to some other end. Because the source of this dignity lies in rational nature, Kant also argues that morality requires that all persons must be treated equally.

To contrast the value of persons as ends in themselves with the value of the ends that depend on the projects of persons, Kant says that rational beings possess dignity, as opposed to a use-value. Consider the way that Kant differs from the consequentialist over the question of whether it would be morally right to prevent the deaths of five innocent people, each of whom needs an organ transplant, by killing another innocent person and distributing his or her vital organs. According to utilitarianism, this would be right, since it results in a net gain of four lives. Of course, this reasoning fails to take into consideration the side effects we mentioned earlier in the theoretical use of derelicts in urgent medical experiments. For a utilitarian, the moral question turns on whether the negative side effects outweigh the benefit of saving four lives. On a Kantian approach, however, to kill an innocent person for his or her organs is a paradigm case of treating a person as a mere means, and could never be justified. The fact that the killing is done from altruistic motives, or that it would result in a net saving of lives, does not change the fact that it would be murder, which is intrinsically wrong. Kant did not claim that we should *ignore* the consequences of actions; that would be absurd. Other things being equal, we should of course try to bring about good consequences, if we can do so without doing anything morally wrong. We should consider the consequences of a proposed action only after determining that the action is morally permissible.

How then are we to identify morally permissible and impermissible actions? Most people already have a pretty good idea of the kinds of actions that are wrong. We learn to distinguish right from wrong from our parents, teachers, and playmates. We know that lying, breaking promises, cheating, stealing, and hurting others are wrong—and if someone does not know these things by the time he or she is seven or eight, a course in moral philosophy is unlikely to be of help. What a moral theory can do is provide an explanation of *why* these things are wrong. What makes them wrong? As we've seen, the utilitarian explanation is that the actions we normally regard as wrong—lying, cheating, stealing, killing—promote unhappiness. The trouble with this explanation is that it seems possible, in a particular case, that no one gets hurt by an act of lying or cheating, or that the negative consequences of such an act are outweighed by the positive. Suppose I can get away with cheating without anyone finding out; would that make it morally acceptable? Kant would say of course not, it's still cheating. The important thing is not the consequences of the act, but the kind of act it is. An action could bring about the best nonmoral consequences—e.g., save the most number of lives, make the most people happy— and still be morally wrong because it is unjust or dishonest.

Another reason Kant rejects consequentialism is that what happens is often not within our control and so is not something for which we can be praised, blamed, or held at all responsible. A physician may administer a drug that kills a patient due to unknown and unforeseeable side effects. Though the outcome is disastrous, surely the physician does not act immorally. Kant holds that if you act rightly, you are not responsible for any bad effects that occur. (Utilitarians distinguish between rightness and moral blameworthiness. They say that what the physician did was wrong, though it was not his fault and he should not be *blamed*.)

According to Kant, the fact that an action is likely to promote happiness or human welfare has nothing to do with whether anyone has a moral duty to do it. Duty must be entirely independent of consequences, for if it were otherwise, moral imperatives could only be "hypothetical." That is, they would tell us only, "*If* you want to achieve *x*, then do *y*." If someone does not want to achieve *x*, or does not care if *x* occurs, then he or she has no reason to do *y*. Morality, Kant held, is clearly *not* like this. Morality tells us, "Do *y*, whatever you may happen to want or feel." In other words, morality yields "categorical," rather than mere hypothetical, imperatives.

Imperatives (commands) can be either hypothetical or categorical, depending on the implicit principle contained within them. For example, "Treat people with respect," is a hypothetical imperative if the rationale for respecting others is to gain their friendship. Interpreted as a hypothetical imperative, this maxim tells us to treat others with respect *if* we want their friendship. However, some people do not care about gaining others' friendship. If "Treat others with respect" were only a hypothetical imperative, it would not apply to those who are indifferent to others. Since morality is clearly not conditional in this way, however, Kant argued that morality cannot consist of hypothetical imperatives. Instead, morality consists of categorical imperatives: commands that are valid for rational agents as such, independent of the feelings and desires they happen to have. Moreover, because morality consists of these categorical imperatives devoid of empirical content, it can have necessity; it can tell us what we *must* do, what we are obligated to do, what it is our duty to do.

To find out whether a proposed action is consistent with duty, and morally permissible, the right question to ask, Kant says, is not, "What are the likely consequences of doing (or not doing) this action?" but rather, "*Can I, as a rational agent, consistently will that everyone in a similar situation should act this way?*" If we convert this question into an imperative, we get "Act always on that maxim (or principle) that you can consistently will as a principle of action for everyone similarly situated." Kant calls this rule the "categorical imperative," and it is the foundation of his ethical system. If the proposed action is one that would be wrong if done generally, then the particular action is wrong, too—even if it would not, in the case at hand, have harmful consequences. What matters is that the maxims of these actions cannot be consistently universalized. While it may seem entirely abstract and formal, universalization is, in part, a mechanism for ensuring equal respect for persons. It achieves this by not allowing us to make exceptions of ourselves, but requires us always to act only on principles that we could consistently will that everyone follow.

Kant thought that consistency and universality are clearly part of our concept of morality and duty. In trying to explain why we ought to do certain things (like voting) or refrain from doing others (like cheating), we are liable to ask, "What would happen if everyone acted that way?" But note that we do not regard it as a rebuttal if it is pointed out that not everyone *will* act that way. Universalization requires us to abstract from the actual circumstances and to refrain from making exceptions of ourselves. This test of right action is considered so important that many moral philosophers hold that a person "has a morality" only if that person is willing to universalize his or her moral judgments.[10]

Universalization is only one aspect of Kantian ethics. Equally important is Kant's insistence that persons must always be treated as "ends in themselves" and never merely as means. This means that in our dealings with others, we are to realize that they have their own goals, aims, and projects. We are never to treat other people as if they do not matter or count, or as if they exist simply to fulfill our purposes. This Kantian idea is reflected in the insistence that patients and research subjects must give informed consent before they can be treated or used in experiments. We also show respect for persons by telling them the truth, even when such knowledge might be painful, and by allowing them to make their own moral choices, even when we think they will choose unwisely. Thus, Kantian ethics has been a strong force against the medical paternalism that held sway until fairly recently.

If a proposed action fails either the universalization test or the respect for persons test, then it is contrary to duty and must not be done. Kantian ethics can help us determine what we must not do; but how are we to decide what we should do? For often in deciding what to do, we are faced with a range of alternatives, none of which conflict with duty and all of which are morally permissible. Kantian ethics does not provide a decision procedure for deciding which out of all morally permissible acts is the right act. It thus gives the individual a great deal more latitude than does utilitarianism, which commands us to choose the act that has the best consequences. At the same time, Kantian ethics gives proportionately less guidance. This can be viewed as a deficiency, but it can also be viewed as an advantage, in that it allows for more individual autonomy.

How would a Kantian resolve Dr. Brody's dilemma? May Dr. Brody end the life of a suffering and seriously ill patient who requests such help? To answer this question, we need to ask whether it is morally permissible for Mr. Lasken to engineer his own death. For no one can have a duty to help another person do something that is morally wrong. Thus, we first have to consider the question of the morality of suicide. Kant himself thought that suicide violated the categorical imperative. His argument is as follows: Suicides kill themselves to spare themselves the pain of living. However, the desire to avoid pain is intrinsic to self-preservation. Committing suicide is thus acting from both self-preservation and self-destruction at the same time, and so is self-contradictory. Kant's argument here seems extremely murky. It is far from clear why it is self-contradictory to prefer death to life under horrible conditions.

Does suicide violate the requirement of respect for persons? Persons are worthy of respect, according to Kant, because they are ends in themselves. This rather obscure formulation alludes to the fact that persons are not mere things which are simply subject to natural laws, but rather rational agents with their own goals and ends. Moreover, rational natures are capable of assessing their own goals and desires, of deciding whether they want to pursue a certain goal or have a particular desire. (Philosophers call these wants about wants "second-order desires.") This ability to assess our desires and goals, and to act on those assessments, makes us *autonomous*. Autonomy, for Kant, is not simply a matter of the ability to make choices (as it is often portrayed in the medical context). Autonomy is the ability to formulate and follow laws that we would

10. See, for example, William Frankena, *Ethics,* 2nd ed. (Englewood Cliffs, NJ: Prentice Hall, 1972), 113–114.

be willing to have everyone follow, that is, universal laws. It is because human beings are autonomous that they have dignity and are worthy of respect.

Would acceding to Mr. Lasken's request to be killed violate the principle of respect for humanity, and thus be contrary to duty? Certainly, pressuring Mr. Lasken to die, or taking advantage of his vulnerable situation, would be ruled out by Kantian ethics. As Onora O'Neill puts it, "We use others as *mere means* if what we do reflects some maxim *to which they could not in principle consent*."[11] Deception, coercion, and exploitation are all wrong because they treat others as mere means. We are assuming, however, that Mr. Lasken genuinely wants to die and is not being deceived, coerced, or exploited. Does helping him to die fail to respect his humanity? A possible Kantian objection might be that in choosing to die in order to avoid pain, the prospective suicide treats himself as merely a sentient being, no more than an animal. In creating a maxim that derives solely from his animal nature, he fails to respect his own humanity or rational nature. However, Jim Lasken might respond that he wants to end his life, and to get Dr. Brody's help in doing so, not simply to avoid pain, but also to avoid the certain deterioration of his mental powers, the subsequent loss of rationality, and the gradual erosion of his own sense of dignity and meaning. This reasoning should have considerable weight from a Kantian perspective. Kant's absolute opposition to rational suicide seems more a product of the conventional morality of his time than a requirement of the categorical imperative in either of its formulations.

It appears that a Kantian, even if not the historical Kant, could in principle support assisted suicide and voluntary euthanasia as promoting autonomy and self-determination. On the other hand, it is possible that a policy of voluntary euthanasia would lead to the devaluing of human life, and ultimately the nonvoluntary killing of the weak, the vulnerable, and the poor. If so, this would violate the values of autonomy and respect for persons, which would lead Kantians to oppose euthanasia. (Remember that Kantians do not ignore consequences; they simply do not regard consequences themselves as determinative of right and wrong.)

Thus, we may expect to find Kantians—as well as utilitarians—on both sides of the euthanasia issue, depending on their factual predictions and their conceptions of basic moral concepts, such as autonomy and personhood. This conclusion will be discouraging for anyone who expects ethical theories to provide handy-dandy formulas for resolving moral issues. But ethical theories are not meant to provide formulas; instead, they provide frameworks for trying to reach workable solutions to complex and difficult questions.

Social Contract Theory

Any ethical theory must answer two fundamental questions. The first is about the content of our moral obligations: What are we required to do? The second is about our motivation for acting: Why are we required to do it? The social contract approach to ethics gives related answers to these questions. Our obligations are determined by the agreements we have made, and we ought to fulfill our obligations because we have agreed to them.[12]

There are two basic forms of contemporary social contract theory. Philosopher Will Kymlicka explains their difference this way:

> One approach stresses a natural equality of physical power, which makes it mutually advantageous for people to accept conventions that recognize and protect each other's interests and possessions. The other approach stresses a natural equality of moral status, which makes each person's interests a matter of common or impartial concern. This impartial concern is expressed in agreements that recognize each person's interests and moral status.[13]

Kymlicka calls proponents of the mutual advantage theory "Hobbesian contractarians," and proponents of the impartial theory "Kantian contractarians,"

11. Onora O'Neill, "The Moral Perplexities of Famine and World Hunger," in *Matters of Life and Death: New Introductory Essays in Moral Philosophy*, 2nd ed., edited by Tom Regan (New York: Random House, 1986), 322.

12. Will Kymlicka, "The Social Contract Tradition," in *A Companion to Ethics*, edited by Peter Singer (Oxford: Basil Blackwell, 1993), 186.

13. Ibid., 188.

because Hobbes and Kant inspired and foreshadowed these two forms of contract theory.

Hobbesian Contractarianism Hobbesian contractarianism is a form of moral nihilism in its rejection of objective (or real) moral values. There is nothing inherently right or wrong about the goals one chooses to pursue, or the means one uses to pursue these goals. However, unless there are restrictions on the goals people pursue and the means by which they pursue them, the world is a threatening, dangerous place. Everyone is better off restricting his or her own liberty to injure others, so long as the others do likewise. Harming others is not inherently wrong in this view, but it is to our mutual advantage to accept conventions that define such harm as wrong.[14]

Hobbesian contractarianism replicates a good deal of ordinary morality, but not all of it. For one thing, it is clear that there is no mutual advantage in bargaining with those who are too weak to pose a threat of retaliation. Thus, Hobbesian contractarianism leaves out defenseless human beings, such as babies and the disabled.[15] This departure from everyday morality is no argument against Hobbesian contractarianism since, as Kymlicka points out, the theory denies that we have any natural duties to others; it is, as we said, a form of moral nihilism. Hobbesian contractarianism may be the best we can do in a world without natural duties or objective values.[16]

How would a Hobbesian contractarian approach the problem of doctor-assisted suicide? The question is whether it is to everyone's mutual advantage to allow doctors to kill (or help to die) their terminally ill patients who request such help. On the one hand, it would appear irrational to rule out an option that a great many people apparently wish to have at the end of life. On the other hand, when we become terminally ill, we do not want doctors killing us for cost-control, to convenience our relatives, etc. Thus, the Hobbesian contractarian analysis looks a great deal like a rule-utilitarian analysis.

14. Ibid., 189.

15. David Gauthier, *Morals by Agreement* (Oxford: Oxford University Press, 1986), 286.

16. Kymlicka, 191 (see note 12).

Kantian Contractarianism The best-known exponent of Kantian contractarianism is John Rawls. According to Rawls, people matter not because they can harm or benefit others (as in the Hobbesian view), but because they are ends in themselves (as Kant held). Everyone is entitled to equal consideration, and this basic notion of equality gives rise to a natural duty to promote a just society. A just society is one based on fair principles. However, the social contract approach creates a problem in attempting to derive fair principles. The problem is that, in a bargaining situation, the strong have a clear advantage over the weak, which is intuitively unfair. Rawls's solution to the problem of natural inequality is a hypothetical social contract whereby a society chooses its basic social principles from the standpoint of "the original position."

In the original position, all parties are under a "veil of ignorance." That is, while they know that they are human and have basic human needs, they are deprived of all knowledge of their special characteristics. No one knows if he or she is rich or poor, black or white, male or female, or politically liberal or conservative. This ignorance prevents people from tailoring social principles to their own advantage.

In the original position, each contractor is motivated by self-interest; that is, each is trying to do the best for him- or herself. But since no one knows what his or her position in society eventually will be, this self-interest amounts to acting impartially. To promote my own good, I must put myself in the shoes of every member of society and see what promotes his or her good, since I may end up being any one of these members.[17] It would be contrary to my own self-interest to choose a society that permitted slavery, since I might be a slave. Of course, it might turn out that I get to be a master, in which case I would be better-off living in a slave-owning society. However, one cannot know one's place in advance. Rawls thinks that it would be irrational to opt for a slave-owning society, since being a slave in a slave-owning society is much worse than living as a free person in a society that prohibits slavery. Similarly, individuals in the original position could not choose a caste system, since they might turn out to

17. Kymlicka, 192 (see note 12).

be untouchables; they could not choose a male-dominated society, since they might turn out to be women. The very arrangements we intuitively reject as unfair turn out to be irrational from the perspective of the original position.

Rawls goes on to argue that rational people in the original position would choose two basic principles to guide and determine the institutions of their society. The first principle is a principle of liberty. It maintains that everyone is to have as much liberty as possible, consonant with everyone else's having the same amount of liberty. This principle would be chosen from the standpoint of the original position because it would be irrational to choose a principle that gives some people more liberty than others. After all, you might end up being one of the people with less liberty.

The second principle is a principle of equality. It has two parts. The first part is a principle of distribution, often referred to as the "difference principle." It says that all goods should be equally distributed, except where an unequal distribution makes everyone, especially the worst off, better off. Why would choosers in the original position opt for equal distribution? Because if you don't know your position in society, it would be irrational to choose a distribution in which some have enormous wealth and others are impoverished. True, you might be Donald Trump, but it's better to forgo the chance for great wealth than to risk being impoverished. At the same time, it would be irrational to insist on absolute equal distribution if an unequal distribution would make everyone better off. (For example, it is in the best interests of the worst off to have an adequate supply of well-trained brain surgeons who are paid much more than the average person, if this inequality is the necessary incentive for them to set aside so many years for training.)

The second part of the principle of equality is a principle of equality of opportunity. Everyone is to have equal opportunity in achieving the various offices and roles in society; they are all to be open to everyone. Rawls's principle of fair equality of opportunity has been used by Norman Daniels as the basis for a universal right to health care.[18] The basic idea is that sickness and disability prevent us from functioning normally and deprive us of the opportunity to compete on an equal basis with others for the goods in society. While we can strive to keep ourselves healthy through various means (e.g., abstaining from smoking, following a low-fat diet, exercising regularly), for the most part, we have no control over becoming sick or disabled. The sick and the disabled are therefore at a considerable and unfair disadvantage. Those who do not get the medical attention that can restore "normal species-functioning" are thus doubly disadvantaged, first by "nature's lottery," and second by social arrangements that give some, but not others, access to health care. If equal opportunity is to be a reality, we must guarantee universal access to health care. Moreover, the concept of "normal species-functioning" is a guide for what kinds of treatment should be provided. Vaccination and eyeglasses are obvious candidates, while cosmetic surgery is not.

Rawls requires that his principle of liberty take precedence over his principle of equality. He states that the claims of liberty must be satisfied before social and economic inequalities can be contemplated, and that departures from the principle of equal liberty cannot be justified or made good by greater social and economic advantages.[19] The elements of the principle of equality are similarly ordered: Rawls sees that genuinely fair equality of opportunity (as opposed to merely formal access) must be guaranteed before we can address ourselves to social or economic inequalities.

If we compare Rawls's vision of "justice as fairness" with utilitarianism, we see some striking differences. The most dramatic difference concerns the respective theories of the "good" and the "right," and the way these important moral concepts are related. Utilitarian theories define the good independently of the right: first the good is defined as happiness, then the right is defined as that which maximizes happiness. Because justice is defined as a function of utility, it cannot limit the claims of utility. By contrast, Rawls sees the concepts of right and justice as preceding the concept of the good.[20] He

18. See Norman Daniels, *Just Health Care* (Cambridge: Cambridge University Press, 1985).

19. John Rawls, *A Theory of Justice* (Cambridge, MA: Harvard University Press, 1971), 61.

20. Ibid., 31.

states that for desires to have any value or to play any role in ethical calculations, they must accord with the principles of justice.

Rawls's theory of justice has been criticized as embodying problematic notions of rationality—in particular, a fundamental aversion to risk. Why assume that a rational person behind the veil of ignorance would opt for the equality of the difference principle? A gambler might be willing to take a relatively small risk of being impoverished for the chance of becoming very wealthy. Is this obviously irrational? A related criticism is that the contract does no real work. As we have seen, and as Rawls acknowledges, there can be different interpretations of the original position. A risk-aversive interpretation, which yields the difference principle, is not the only possible one. According to Rawls, we decide which interpretation of the original position is most suitable by determining which interpretation yields principles that match our convictions of justice. But, as Kymlicka points out, "if each theory of justice has its own account of the contracting situation, then we have to decide *beforehand* which theory of justice we accept, in order to know which description of the original position is suitable."[21] If this is so, then the contract cannot be used to establish the correct theory of justice. Nevertheless, contracting from an original position has some useful purposes. The veil of ignorance is a vivid expression of the moral requirement of our commitment to others, and of putting ourselves in their shoes. It dramatizes the claim that we would accept a certain principle, however it affected us. As Kymlicka says, "In these and other ways, the contract device illuminates the basic ideas of morality as impartiality, even if it cannot help defend those ideas."[22]

So how would a Kantian contractarian, or Rawlsian, approach Dr. Brody's dilemma? The principle of liberty requires that each individual have the maximum liberty possible, consistent with equal liberty for others. That requirement seems to argue in favor of allowing people to choose the time and manner of their death at the end of their life, in order to avoid great suffering, as well as financial loss for their families. At the same time, Rawls is concerned to protect the weak and vulnerable who cannot bargain on their own behalf. That would militate against a policy that could have a discriminatory impact on the elderly, the disabled, and the poor. Thus, a Rawlsian would be likely to approve of a policy of doctor-assisted suicide if it promoted the value of individual autonomy, but not if it violated equal respect for persons. (Rawls's own view on physician-assisted suicide is given in "The Philosophers' Brief" in Part 3, Section 5.)

RELIGIOUS ETHICS

We noted above that religious ethics is one of the parent disciplines of bioethics. We are not suggesting that "religious ethics" is an ethical theory in the same sense as utilitarianism and Kantian ethics; religious beliefs do not, in general, imply any one particular ethical orientation. Some Christians take a utilitarian approach, while others have views closer to Kantianism. Although there are certainly ethical directives inherent in religious belief (e.g., "Do unto others as you would be done by"), each of these directives can be compatible with very different ethical theories.

Some religious traditions have been more influential than others in bioethics; for example, Roman Catholic moral thought. One reason for this influence is that the Roman Catholic Church is characterized by considerable unanimity. There is, on a number of issues, an official Church doctrine—this is not generally true of Protestantism, which has a great many denominations, or Judaism, which is divided into Orthodox, Conservative, Reform, and Reconstructionist. Another reason for the more powerful influence of Roman Catholicism is that it includes a well-developed, written body of thought on medical-moral issues, which has had considerable influence on prevailing attitudes (even among many non-Catholics), as well as on legal doctrine regarding a wide range of biomedical ethical issues. Lastly, the Catholic tradition includes an alternative ethical theory—known as natural law ethics—that provides principles for interpreting the general ethical directives of the Christian faith.

Natural Law Theories

Natural law theorists offer an account of the human good and ethical duty that contrasts sharply with

21. Kymlicka, 193 (see note 12).
22. Ibid.

the views of both utilitarianism and Kantianism on these issues. Utilitarianism defines the good in terms of happiness or the satisfaction of desire, while Kant repudiated all ethical theories based in any way upon desire or inclination. In contrast to utilitarianism, natural law ethicists insist that the human good cannot be reduced to a mere function of what people happen to desire. In this view, things are not good because we desire them; rather, we desire them, or should desire them, because they are good.

But natural law ethics is also opposed to Kantian ethics in that it is based on a conception of human nature. Kant insists that the categorical imperative must be empty of all empirical content; otherwise it could not have the necessity characteristic of the moral law. But what else, if not a concern for human welfare, can ethics possibly be founded upon, and how can it have any motivational force? Why, asks the natural law theorist, should we desire to be moral in the first place and follow the dictates of morality, unless such behavior holds out some prospect of promoting human well-being and happiness?

Natural law theorists thus agree with utilitarians that ethics must be grounded in a concern for the human good. But they agree with Kantians that the good cannot be defined simply in terms of what people "happen" to want. Instead, there is a good for human beings that, based on their nature, is objectively desirable.

Catholic theologians conceive of natural law as the law inscribed by God into the nature of things—as a species of divine law. According to this conception, the Creator endows all things with certain potentialities or tendencies that serve to define their natural end; the fulfillment of a thing's natural tendencies constitutes the specific "good" of that thing. The natural potential of an acorn is to become an oak. But what is the natural potential of human beings? Like Kant, the natural law theorist focuses on what makes human beings distinctive, what separates us from the rest of the natural world—namely, the ability to reason. Through our ability to reason, we can participate actively in God's plan. However, natural law ethics is distinct from Kantian ethics in that natural law ethicists do not attempt to empty their theories of all empirical content. On the contrary, our moral obligations are derived from a conception of the good life for human beings. For example, the Catholic Church opposes both abortion and birth control because these are inconsistent with a conception of sexuality as expressed within monogamous marriage only, and primarily oriented toward its natural end or purpose, procreation.

The most general moral precept of the natural law is "do good and avoid evil." Evil must always be avoided, even if avoiding evil will bring about great harm. As St. Paul put it, "Do not evil that good may come." The commission of an evil deed, such as the murder of an innocent person, can never be condoned, even if it is intended to advance the noblest of ends.

The Doctrine of the Double Effect

The doctrine of the double effect (DDE) was formulated in response to the recognition that an act may have both a good and a bad effect. Are we to shun such an action because of its bad effect? For example, administering morphine to a dying cancer patient may be necessary to ease his or her pain, but it may also depress respiration and hasten death. Must a doctor refrain from using the most effective pain medication because it might also kill the patient? Would this count as "doing evil (causing death) that good (relieving pain) may come"?

According to Catholic doctrine, the permissibility of the action depends largely on whether the bad effect is intended, or merely foreseen and permitted to happen. In addition, it must also be the case that

1. The act itself is not intrinsically wrong.
2. The good effect is produced directly by the action and not by the bad effect.
3. The good effect is sufficiently desirable to compensate for allowing the bad effect.[23]

Applying these conditions, the use of pain-relieving drugs that may also shorten life can be justified. The physician's purpose is not to kill, but rather to ease pain, although he or she foresees that death is a possible, or even likely, result. Giving drugs for pain relief is not intrinsically wrong; indeed, it is a central function of the physician. The

23. "Double Effect," *New Catholic Encyclopedia*.

good effect—the relief of pain—is produced directly by the administering of the drug, and not by the bad effect: namely, the patient's death. And lastly, when a patient is both terminally ill and suffering, the desirability of relieving suffering compensates for the shortening of his or her life. Thus, the DDE can be a useful tool for justifying an action that has a bad effect.

Double-effect reasoning has sometimes been incorrectly and speciously used. Someone who shoots a person at point-blank range cannot use the DDE to mitigate his or her responsibility, saying, "I didn't mean to kill him, only to get him out of the way." One is guilty of killing a person even if death is not desired in itself, but only as a means to achieve an end. A Michigan jury used such specious reasoning in their acquittal of Dr. Jack Kevorkian, who was accused of violating the state's assisted-suicide law when he helped a terminally ill man to die by carbon monoxide poisoning. The law made an exception for physicians who administer pain-relieving drugs that may cause death. The jury accepted Kevorkian's argument that he did not intend to cause the man's death, but only to relieve his suffering. This reasoning, however, is a perversion of the DDE. Carbon monoxide, unlike morphine, is never offered as a means of pain relief. It has no medical use at all. It causes death, and death causes cessation of pain, but this is bringing about the good effect by means of the bad effect, which violates the second condition of the DDE. Thus, the DDE cannot be used to justify Dr. Kevorkian's act or to sustain his claim that he did not intend to cause the man's death. After the acquittal, law professor Yale Kamisar characterized the jury's decision as "confused." However, it seems likely that the decision was less the result of confusion about the appropriate application of double-effect reasoning, and more the result of their belief that Dr. Kevorkian was *right* in doing what he did and should not be punished.

Critics of the DDE argue that the principle is confusing and difficult to apply. It is not always easy to know whether a result is intended or merely foreseen, or whether it is brought about (impermissibly) by means of the bad effect or (permissibly) by the morally neutral action. The concepts of "means" and "intention" need to be made clearer before the DDE can give clear guidance.

Some theorists doubt that the DDE has moral significance even if it can be clearly and correctly applied. They note that the whole point of the doctrine is to avoid the counterintuitive implications of an absolutist ethic that insists that some acts (like directly causing the death of an innocent person) are absolutely wrong, regardless of reason or context. However, why should we assimilate garden-variety murder with causing the death of a terminally ill patient who wants to die? The solution, these critics say, is to recognize that causing death is not always wrong. If death is desirable, why should it make any difference *how* death is brought about—whether indirectly, by pain relief, or directly, by carbon monoxide?

Ordinary versus Extraordinary Treatment

Another influential distinction devised by Catholic medical ethicists is the distinction between "ordinary" and "extraordinary" treatment. Ordinary treatment is considered obligatory, while there is no obligation to provide extraordinary treatment. How are these two types of treatment to be best defined?

This question is complicated because there are various different grounds that have been used to distinguish ordinary and extraordinary treatments. For example, "ordinary" treatment may be viewed as routine or standard care, while "extraordinary" treatment is considered unusual. This distinction has the advantage of providing an empirical definition, based on current medical practice. However, it is not clear that this basis has moral significance. If a treatment is helpful to a patient, what difference does it make that it is unusual, or even unique? For this reason, some people prefer to think of the distinction between ordinary and extraordinary treatment as being a distinction between "beneficial" and "nonbeneficial" treatment.

Understood this way, the ordinary/extraordinary distinction is context dependent. Treatment such as a respirator may be ordinary in one context (e.g., to sustain a patient through a severe bout with a respiratory disease), but extraordinary in another (e.g., to sustain the life of a severely brain-damaged patient in a persistent vegetative state [PVS]). This makes the normative assumption that a PVS individual is not benefited by continued existence with no hope of recovery to consciousness. Someone who regards biological life itself as valuable will not agree that the use of a respirator to sustain the life of a PVS patient is "nonbeneficial," and so will not classify the treatment as extraordinary. However, this reasoning raises serious doubts about the usefulness of the distinction. If our moral views determine whether a treatment is to be classified as ordinary or extraordinary, the distinction itself cannot provide moral guidance.

Despite this difficulty, doctors and laypeople alike often use terms like "extraordinary" and "heroic" to characterize treatment they regard as inappropriate. Rather than regarding these classifications as morally significant in themselves, it is important to understand the moral presuppositions lying behind them. It is these presuppositions—not the shorthand labels that stand for them—that need discussion and debate (see "In the Matter of Claire C. Conroy," Part 3, Section 4).

"RIGHTS-BASED" APPROACHES

The idea that, simply by virtue of being human, people can have rights regardless of the legal system under which they live, has ancient roots. The Stoic philosophers recognized the possibility that actual human laws might be unjust. They contrasted conventional laws with an unvarying natural law to which everyone had access through individual conscience and by which actual laws could be judged.[24] Later, the spread of the Roman Empire provided a system of law that applied to all people, whatever their tribe, race, or nationality. Christianity also incorporated the idea of natural law as the paramount standard by which all social institutions and laws should be judged.

However, neither the ancient Greeks, nor the Romans, nor the medieval Christians made the transition to natural rights. The notion of natural rights had its heyday in the seventeenth century, with writers like Grotius, Pufendorf, and Locke. Rights also played a crucial role in the American and French revolutions in the late eighteenth century. However, states Brenda Almond, "In the nineteenth and early twentieth centuries, . . . appeal to rights was eclipsed by movements such as utilitarianism and Marxism, which could not, or would not, accommodate them."[25]

Appeal to natural rights revived in the aftermath of World War II, during the Nuremberg trials. Some theorists argued that since the actions of the accused were not contrary to German law (indeed, were required by it), the trials had no legal basis, but were merely a cynical attempt by the victors to punish the losers. Others maintained that the trials were a return to principles of legality and justice in the aftermath of Nazi barbarism, and that these principles have their foundation in both international and natural law.

Natural or human rights unquestionably occupy an important role in contemporary international moral and political debate. Apartheid, the death penalty, and female genital mutilation, to take just a few examples, have all been condemned as violations of human rights. Discussions of abortion, euthanasia, access to health care, the treatment of animals and the environment, and our obligations to future generations are typically framed in terms of conflicting moral rights.

Some see "rights talk" as unnecessary and vague. Bentham regarded the notion of moral—as opposed to legal—rights as "nonsense," and the notion of natural rights as "nonsense on stilts."[26] According to Bentham and other legal positivists, legal rights can be explained as claims that will be upheld by the power of the state. Legal rights can be identified because they stem from legislative acts or judicial decisions. So-called moral rights have no such legitimation, and it is partly for this reason that positivists regard them as empty rhetoric. According to utilitarianism, to say that someone has a moral right to something is only a shorthand way of saying that he or she *ought* to have it, and ought to be protected in his or her possession of it. There is, then, a role for moral rights in utilitarianism, but it

24. Brenda Almond, "Rights," in *A Companion to Ethics*, edited by Peter Singer (Basil Blackwell, 1993), 259.

25. Ibid.

26. From *Anarchical Fallacies: Being an Examination of the Declaration of Rights Issued During the French Revolution*. Cited in Ronald Dworkin, *Taking Rights Seriously* (Cambridge, MA: Harvard University Press, 1977), 184.

is completely derivative from the principle of utility. To some extent, rights can serve as barriers against the application of overall utility. For example, utilitarians might, on grounds of utility, take property rights very seriously. They will agree that individuals should not be deprived of their property, unless this is essential to the general welfare, and even then there should be compensation. In other words, while utilitarians reject the Lockean idea of a "natural right to property," they are likely to agree that there are good utilitarian reasons to create something very like our existing system of property rights.

Rights-based critics of utilitarianism maintain that its conception of rights gives insufficient protection to individuals, whose happiness may be sacrificed for the benefit of the many. In *Taking Rights Seriously*, Ronald Dworkin offers a penetrating critique of the positivist analysis of law, as well as the utilitarian morality intimately linked to it. Rather than seeing rights as a device to achieve net utility, Dworkin sees rights as "trumps," as claims that supersede other kinds of claims. Similarly, Robert Nozick conceives of rights as "side constraints," which place limits on the things we may do to achieve goals.

In *Anarchy, State, and Utopia*, Nozick presents a libertarian view that is fundamentally opposed to utilitarianism.[27] He thus joins Kant, Rawls, and Dworkin in this opposition, holding that an action that is unfair or that violates someone's rights cannot be right, even if it does achieve the greatest net happiness. Happiness might be maximized by forcing people to volunteer their time to work in hospitals, or by making them donate blood or spare kidneys, but they have no obligation to do so according to Nozick; indeed, they have a right not to do so.

Nozick is equally opposed to Rawls's contractarianism. The central question of distributive justice is, "How should the goods of society be distributed?" According to Nozick, this question misconceives the issue because it implies that the goods of society—money, property, services—are there simply to be distributed, like manna fallen from the heavens. Instead, these goods already belong to people who have invested their labor in them, been given them, or traded something for them. Taking goods away from those who are entitled to them violates their rights, and so is fundamentally unfair.

Another important feature of libertarianism is the distinction between negative and positive rights. Libertarians maintain that the only rights are negative rights: rights to be left alone, rights not to be interfered with. They reject positive rights—rights to be helped—because recognition of such rights would infringe on the freedom of individuals to spend their time and money as they choose. An example of a positive right is a right to an education. Libertarians oppose taxation generally on the grounds that it deprives individuals of their legitimate property; thus, they oppose taxation for the creation and support of public schools. However, they recognize the need for an army to defend a country from foreign enemies, for a police force to protect citizens against aggression and attack, and for a legal system to uphold contractual agreements. Taxation to support these purposes is regarded as legitimate.

Libertarians reject the idea of a right to health care, since health care is regarded as a positive right—a right to be given certain treatment. However, it is not clear why they assume this distinction to have such moral significance. If it is legitimate to tax people for a police force that will protect their lives, why isn't it equally legitimate to tax people to provide them with health care, which is also often necessary for survival?

Perhaps the biggest objection to libertarianism is that it works to the disadvantage of those who, through no fault of their own, are born into poverty. Poverty limits people's life chances. The poor typically get substandard health care, inferior schools, and inadequate housing. These disadvantages make it unlikely that they will have an equal opportunity to obtain the goods of society: jobs, money, and material goods. Rawls attempts to compensate for life's initial unfairness, but libertarianism reinforces it.

In a rights-based approach, the fundamental question in our opening case study would be whether Mr. Lasken has a right to end his life, and to ask his doctor for help in doing so. Those who

27. Robert Nozick, *Anarchy, State, and Utopia* (New York: Basic Books, 1974).

oppose voluntary euthanasia and physician-assisted suicide maintain that Lasken has no such right. They see a distinction between the established right to refuse medical treatment and an affirmative right to seek help in dying. However, this interpretation was disputed for the first time by a federal judge on May 3, 1994, when Judge Barbara F. Rothstein found Washington state's assisted-suicide law unconstitutional. Rothstein held that the law places an undue burden on the Fourteenth Amendment interests of terminally ill, mentally competent patients. Moreover, she found that the law "unconstitutionally distinguishes between two similarly situated groups," namely, those on life support and those not on life support. Washington permits terminally ill patients to hasten their deaths by allowing removal of life-support systems, yet bars physicians from giving medication that would bring about the same results. Rothstein wrote that from "a constitutional perspective, the court does not believe that a distinction can be drawn between refusing life-sustaining medical treatment, and physician-assisted suicide by an uncoerced, mentally competent, terminally ill adult."[28]

Rights play an important role in moral discourse. Without the notion of individual rights, it would be difficult—if not impossible—to express our convictions about informed consent, protections for research subjects, and other such issues. However, this should not lead us to conclude that the application of individual rights is always appropriate, or that such rights are the only relevant factors.

The area of treatment refusal presents an obviously inappropriate instance of invoking the right to self-determination. Suppose that a patient enters an emergency room screaming from the pain of severe burns. The attending physicians conclude that, although her burns are serious, she will recover if given immediate and sustained treatment. Suddenly the patient, on the verge of shock, rebuffs the efforts of the medical staff on the grounds that she has a right to "die with dignity." Clearly, in this sort of case it would be wrong for the medical staff to honor the claimed right to refuse treatment. Not only is the woman mistaken in her belief that she is about to die, regardless of treatment, but her capacity for self-determination has itself been substantially impaired or temporarily eclipsed by her recent trauma. To honor her refusal would be tantamount to treating this incompetent person as though she were competent, with morally disastrous results.

The above example demonstrates limits to the scope of the right of self-determination, namely, that it should be restricted to competent individuals. Conflicts between individual rights and the welfare of other persons—including, on occasion, the welfare of the entire community—constitute another set of problematic issues of libertarianism. For example, some libertarians argue that people should have the right to do whatever they please, so long as they do not violate anyone's rights. On a small-scale, interpersonal level, this principle is extremely problematic. Imagine a jilted lover who decides on impulse to marry another woman, not because he loves her, but merely to spite the woman who rejected him. We might all agree that this man has a right to marry whomever he chooses, but is "having a right" the same as "doing the right thing"? Obviously not, since the decision to marry out of spite will predictably inflict great suffering upon his unsuspecting bride.

On a broader social scale, libertarians often assert that individual freedom should include the right to shoot heroin, smoke crack cocaine, and take any other accurately labeled drug, so long as an individual freely chooses to do so. If our liberty is to mean anything, so the argument goes, it must encompass the right to take risks. To allow the government to decide what we may or may not put into our own bodies is to give up control over them. It is analogous to slavery.[29]

The trouble with a libertarian approach to the drug problem is that it ignores social consequences and focuses only on individual rights. Drugs have destroyed many inner-city neighborhoods. Some of the related problems—such as crime due to illegal trafficking—might be solved by legalization, but

28. *National Law Journal* (May 16, 1994): A6.

29. Walter Block, "Drug Prohibition: A Legal and Economic Analysis," in *Drugs, Morality, and the Law*, edited by Steven Luper-Foy and Curtis Brown (New York: Garland Publishing, Inc.), 199–216.

not all of them would. Drug addiction has contributed to a skyrocketing rate of child abuse and neglect, because addicts—especially crack addicts—make notoriously poor parents. In addition, drug abuse by pregnant women is connected with dramatic increases in infant mortality, congenital syphilis, and HIV-positive infants. Serious students of the drug problem realize that hard questions remain even after the right of the individual to go to the devil has been invoked. What, for example, is the causal connection, if any, between unemployment, poverty, and ghetto conditions on the one hand, and hard drug addiction on the other? Would not an important consideration be if widespread use of drugs could be shown to reinforce racism and poverty? When unthinkingly waved as a trump, the right to self-determination can mask injustice and justify inequity.

We also need to ask what the effect of legalization on access and consumption would be. Some say that it would have little effect, since it is already so easy to obtain drugs in certain areas. At the same time, it should be remembered that three times as many Americans abuse alcohol as use illegal drugs, largely because of availability. From a public health perspective, if the end result of legalization is higher addiction rates, this is a serious argument against it. Astonishingly, this consideration has no bearing at all on a libertarian view. For the libertarian, the level of addiction in society is irrelevant; the only thing that matters is whether the individual has made a free and voluntary decision to use drugs. Once again, the individual's freedom is everything, and the impact on society is ignored.[30]

Rights are important, for they protect individuals from—as Mill called it—"the tyranny of the majority." Nevertheless, an overemphasis on rights can sometimes exacerbate conflict. For example, to justify criminal punishment of women who use drugs during pregnancy, conservatives appeal to fetal rights. At the other extreme, some feminists and civil libertarians insist that a woman has a right to control her own body during pregnancy, regardless of the harm she causes to her future child. A recognition that mother and fetus are a unit, whose interests are generally promoted together, might be preferable to a rigid rights-based approach.

COMMUNITARIAN ETHICS

For all their differences, Hobbes, Mill, Kant, Rawls, Gauthier, and Nozick share the belief, bequeathed to us by the Enlightenment philosophers of the eighteenth century, that people should find moral rules in the application of reason to practical conduct. For this tradition, which we shall call "liberal individualism," ethical truth must be sought not in the vagaries of history, tradition, and religious faith, but rather in the universal tenets of rationality. Whether ethical norms are conceived in terms of enlightened self-interest, maximized utility, or the recognition of autonomy and human rights, they are viewed by this tradition as objective and universal, applicable to all times and places.

Another important theoretical strand connecting these theorists is their commitment to the individual as the unique focal point of moral concern. In utilitarianism, the collective preferences of each individual determine right and wrong. Everyone is to count as one, and nobody for more than one. However, the interest of the community as a whole may conflict with any particular individual's interest. Thus, a perennial problem for utilitarianism is the conflict between individual rights and the welfare of society as a whole. By contrast, "rights-based" Kantian and contractarian moral theory, as well as Nozick's brand of libertarianism, are committed to the notion that the rights and dignity of the individual should never (or rarely) be sacrificed to the interests of the larger society. Indeed, the whole point of social organization, of the "social contract," according to this tradition is the advancement of the *individual's* interests, rights, and happiness.

An important corollary of this view is the claim that, since different individuals will naturally have different values and conflicting visions of the good life, a truly liberal society will not—indeed cannot justifiably—adopt any particular conception of the good life to the exclusion or diminution of others.[31]

30. Bonnie Steinbock, "Drug Prohibition: A Public-Health Perspective," in *Drugs, Morality, and the Law*, 233–234.

31. Ronald Dworkin, "Liberalism," in *A Matter of Principle* (Cambridge, MA: Harvard University Press, 1985), 181–204.

Thus, a liberal society must remain "neutral" with regard to these competing conceptions of value and the good. To do otherwise—for example, by imposing a religion-based test on what kind of literature people should be allowed to read—amounts to a serious form of tyranny.

This ethical consensus on rationalism and individualism has had a profound impact on the development of contemporary biomedical ethics. Recently, however, the consensus has been challenged by a number of critics who can usefully, if somewhat uneasily, be lumped under the common banner of "communitarianism."[32] According to communitarian ethical theorists, all of our guiding ethical norms, rules, principles, theories, and virtues can be traced to distinct ethical traditions and ways of life. They argue that it is impossible for us to "bootstrap" ourselves outside of time and space in order to discover some eternal realm of ethical insight. Rather, they claim, history, tradition, and concrete moral communities are the real wellsprings of our moral thought, judgment, and action. As Aristotle put it, we are social beings; our values, our conceptual schemes, our very identities are engendered, shaped, and nurtured within the confines of community.

Within this countertradition, ethical truth is thus particular, not universal. In contrast to the liberal claim that society must remain neutral vis-à-vis competing conceptions of the good life, communitarians argue that if any progress is to be made on a host of public controversies, ranging from pornography to the treatment of dying patients, we will have to begin not with abstract statements of rights, nor with an attempt to promote the good of all by promoting the good of each, but rather with some conception of common meanings, with a vision of what we take to be a "good society." Necessarily, our conception of this good society will crucially depend upon our own history, traditions, institutions, and customs.

Communitarians reject both the rationalism of liberalism's approach to method and their claim to value neutrality. In opposition to individualistic utilitarianism, they offer the idea of a "common good." That is, where utilitarianism looks to the welfare of all individuals taken together, communitarianism looks to the *shared* values, ideals, and goals of a community. Where utilitarianism asks, "Which policies will produce the greatest happiness, on balance, of all of the individuals in society?" communitarianism asks, "Which policies will promote the kind of community in which we want to live?" The difference is subtle, but real. Against rights-based approaches, communitarians reject the penchant for elevating the individual above the social group or community. According to communitarians, the tendency of liberalism to focus so insistently on individual rights—to the exclusion of other social interests—can give rise to circumstances that a good society would not, and should not, tolerate.[33] Take, for example, the practice of some very large corporations with deep community roots—firms employing thousands of workers in relatively small cities—of simply pulling up stakes to search for cheaper labor markets in Mexico. In a society that gives pride of place to rights of ownership, such companies are given total freedom of movement; but the social costs of such rights and freedom can be enormous and often devastating to the affected communities, adding to unemployment, poverty, and the disintegration of neighborhoods and families. A good society, it is argued, would focus not only on individual rights, but also on the good of the larger community.

The dominance of liberal individualism within bioethics has recently been challenged on a number of fronts. Daniel Callahan has brought a communitarian perspective to debates over health care issues,

32. See, for example, Alasdair MacIntyre, *After Virtue* (Notre Dame, IN: University of Notre Dame Press, 1981). Reprinted in *Contemporary Moral Problems*, 4th ed., edited by James E. White (St. Paul, MN: West Publishing Company, 1994). See also Michael Sandel, *Liberalism and the Limits of Justice* (Cambridge: Cambridge University Press, 1982); Charles Taylor, "Atomism," in *Philosophical Papers*, vol. 2 (Cambridge: Cambridge University Press, 1982); Michael Walzer, *Spheres of Justice* (New York: Basic Books, 1983); Shlomo Avineri and Avner de-Shalit, eds., *Communitarianism and Individualism* (Oxford: Oxford University Press, 1992); and, for a good general overview, Stephen Mulhall and Adam Swift, *Liberals and Communitarians* (Oxford: Basil Blackwell, 1992).

33. See, e.g., Mary Ann Glendon, *Rights Talk: The Impoverishment of Political Discourse* (New York: Free Press, 1991).

such as rationing and reform (see Part 2, Section 2). According to Callahan, the combination of our desire to provide universal access to care, the burgeoning cost of high-tech medicine, and the sharp rise in the population of the elderly force some very hard choices that may decide who will live. Instead of starting, in standard liberal fashion, with individual wants, needs, interests, and rights, Callahan urges us to begin by asking what kind of society we wish to have—or as one of his book titles puts it, "What kind of life?"[34] To get at this big question, Callahan must confront some other very difficult and controversial questions, such as, What ought to be the goals and virtues of elderly persons? Should they seek individual happiness, or devote themselves to the education and welfare of future generations? And what ought to be the goals of medicine at various stages of the life cycle? Should medicine seek, at great expense, to forestall death for the very old with the latest high-tech devices, or should it merely try to provide dignified terminal *care?* Clearly, all this talk about goals and virtues necessarily implicates us in a quest for common meanings and values. Rather than ruling such questions off-limits due to the strictures of liberal neutrality, Callahan claims simply that we *must* address them as a community if we are to act responsibly. Failure to do so, thus allowing each person to chart his or her own course, could well vindicate individual freedom of the elderly at the expense of the young.

How might a communitarian interpret our case of physician-assisted suicide? This is a difficult question to answer in light of the remarkable diversity among communitarian thinkers. For communitarians such as Alasdair MacIntyre, the emphasis upon history, traditional practices, and virtues leads to the wholesale abandonment of liberal individualism and the embrace of a rather "conservative" political agenda. More moderate communitarians, on the other hand, some of whom are politically quite "progressive," stress the importance of social meanings and communal values while attempting to preserve a more modest role for the language of individual rights.

Some communitarians, then, might approach the case of Dr. Brody and Mr. Lasken by stressing the customary and time-honored prohibition of assisted suicide and euthanasia in all Western societies. They might argue that, in spite of individuals' strong claims to liberty in this area, the claims of society are stronger. The needs of many suicidal patients might well be met in ways other than by killing them, and society will be a better place if it acknowledges the sanctity and inviolability of human life. A similar argument might be mounted by physicians who could point to their own traditional professional commitments and values: "We heal; we don't kill. That's who we are as doctors; that's how we have always been."

An alternative communitarian reading of the case might reach the same conclusion, but for very different reasons. One could argue, for example, that even though individuals have a powerful claim of self-determination in this matter, the social costs of allowing a right of assisted suicide in a society distinguished by widespread poverty, lack of access to health care, and discrimination against vulnerable minority groups would be prohibitive. While the first communitarian response to our case has a distinctly conservative political flavor, the second might issue from a highly progressive, even Marxist, critique of existing social relationships.

An overall evaluation of communitarianism is an exceedingly complicated matter, due to the disparate character of the theorists and theories lumped under its banner. For the purposes of this brief introduction, however, we venture the following conclusions and recommendations. (1) We agree with the claim that all ethical principles, rules, and virtues grow out of concrete historical traditions and derive their meaning and weight from those traditions. Thus, although our moral principles might extend very far indeed in both space and time, they are not the products of disembodied "reason." (2) The emphasis upon the communal dimension of our moral lives should be viewed as a welcome corrective to the largely asocial invocation of individual rights. We should worry a lot more

34. Daniel Callahan, *What Kind of Life?* (New York: Simon and Schuster, 1990). See also his *Setting Limits* (New York: Simon and Schuster, 1987). For a recent attempt to develop a comprehensive communitarian theory of bioethics, focusing specifically on end-of-life and access to health care issues, see Ezekiel Emanuel, *The Ends of Human Life: Medical Ethics in a Liberal Polity* (Cambridge, MA: Harvard University Press, 1991).

about the "ecology of rights,"[35] the kind of society, neighborhood, and family life within which rights are developed and claimed.

On the negative side, (3) the more hardcore communitarians' wholesale rejection of liberal rights in favor of traditional practices and virtues is especially problematic. Curbing the socially destructive invocation of property rights is one thing, but limiting the freedom of individuals, in the name of communal values, to read pornography, obtain contraceptives, have abortions, or engage in homosexual relationships is, to us, a more disturbing prospect.[36] Finally, (4) it must be noted that an emphasis upon community, neighborhood, family, and traditional values will always express a preference for some *particular conception* of family, neighborhood, and community. For minority groups and women struggling to assert their own, quite varied, conceptions of individual and cultural identity, the communitarian impulse must learn to appreciate and respect such differences within our increasingly cosmopolitan societies.[37]

FEMINIST ETHICS

Just as communitarianism started as a critique of certain assumptions in liberal theory, so too the idea of a feminist ethic stems, in part, from a critique of traditional ethical theories as representing the experiences of men, not women. Feminist approaches to morality seek to correct this underlying bias.

Feminism is not a monolithic theory; thus, there is no one definition of "feminist ethics." Rather, feminism incorporates a variety of social and political beliefs, and there are even differing conceptions of feminism itself. All varieties of feminism are characterized by a concern for the welfare of all women, and a belief that women have historically been—and continue to be—oppressed by patriarchal societies. As Alison Jaggar writes, "Feminist approaches to ethics are distinguished by their explicit commitment to rethinking ethics with a view to correcting whatever forms of male bias it may contain."[38] They all seek to unmask and challenge the oppression, discrimination, and exclusion that women have faced. Feminist approaches to ethics are political, in the sense that they are keenly aware of imbalances of power between women and men, rich and poor, healthy and disabled, white people and people of color, and first world and third world peoples.

Feminist approaches to ethics are also marked by attention to the so-called private sphere, including reflection on intimate relations, such as affection and sexuality, which were ignored by modern moral theory until quite recently. Finally, feminist ethics, rather than seeing women as less fully developed versions of men, insists on taking the moral experience of all women seriously. Modern feminists also warn against the tendency to make generalizations about "women" based on the experience of the relatively small group of middle-class white women. Many feminists today emphasize that sexual oppression is only one form of oppression, and that all forms—whether based on gender, class, race, or disability—must be acknowledged and fought.

Some issues, such as abortion and reproductive technology, are traditionally conceived as "women's issues," and many feminists have written on these topics. However, feminist approaches to bioethics are not limited to this sphere; feminist thought has influenced thinking about the health professional-patient relationship, informed consent, experimental trials, disability, access to health care, and other issues.[39]

One issue that divides feminists is whether virtue is "gendered"; that is, whether there are

35. Mary Ann Glendon, 136–144 (see note 33).

36. See Amy Gutmann, "Communitarian Critics of Liberalism," *Philosophy and Public Affairs* 14 (1985): 308–322.

37. See Iris Marion Young, *Justice and the Politics of Difference* (Princeton, NJ: Princeton University Press, 1990); and Marilyn Friedman, "Feminism and Modern Friendship: Dislocating the Community," *Ethics* 99 (1989): 275–290.

38. Alison M. Jaggar, "Feminist Ethics: Some Issues for the Nineties," in *Contemporary Moral Problems*, 4th ed., edited by James E. White (St. Paul, MN: West Publishing Company, 1994), 61.

39. See Susan Wolf, ed., *Feminism and Bioethics: Beyond Reproduction* (New York: Oxford University Press, 1995); Helen B. Holmes and Laura Purdy, eds., *Feminist Perspectives in Medical Ethics* (Bloomington: Indiana University Press, 1992); and Susan Sherwin, *No Longer Patient* (Philadelphia, PA: Temple University Press, 1992).

virtues that are specifically female and male. Many feminists reject this approach, as the idea of "feminine virtues"—including selflessness, devotion to family needs, and submissiveness to men—has long been linked with the oppression of women. Nevertheless, many nineteenth-century women, including many who were concerned with women's emancipation, believed not only that there were specifically female virtues, but also that women were morally superior to men and that society could be transformed through the influence of women. Today, some feminists regard many of the evils of society—war, violence, racism, the destruction of the environment—as the result of specifically male faults, such as aggression.[40] They believe that the "feminine" virtues of kindness, generosity, helpfulness, and sympathy can serve as a corrective to these evils.

A related issue on which feminists divide is the meaning of sexual equality. Are men and women treated equally when they are treated the same? Jaggar states that "By the end of the 1960s, most feminists in the United States had come to believe that the legal system should be sex-blind, that it should not differentiate in any way between women and men."[41] However, this version of equality does not always promote women's interests. A notorious example is "no-fault" divorce settlements that divide family property equally between husband and wife. Here, equal distribution leaves many women much worse off financially, because women—who often shoulder most of the family responsibilities, such as housework and caring for children—typically have much lower job qualifications and less work experience than men. Divorce settlements that do not take social realities into account are egregiously unfair, and moreover reinforce sexual inequality. At the same time, the alternative way of seeking equality, by providing women with special legal protection, appears to promote sexual stereotypes.

Feminists continue to debate the correct interpretation of equality, even while some feminists reject the entire concept of equality as part of an "ethic of justice" that is characteristically masculine, relying on rules and abstracting from particular, concrete situations, instead of responding to immediately perceived needs.[42] Such feminists suggest an alternative "ethic of care,"[43] stressing connectedness, the importance of human relationships, empathy, and an acknowledgment of dependency. It shares with virtue ethics the conviction that undue emphasis on moral rules obscures the crucial role of moral insight, virtue, and character in determining how to deal with ethical issues.

Some feminists have claimed that the ethic of caring fails to give enough attention to moral principles. Virginia Held reminds us that "an absence of principles can be an invitation to capriciousness."[44] Moreover, issues such as economic justice "cry out for relevant principles. Although caring may be needed to motivate us to act on such principles, the principles are not dispensable."[45] Without such principles, the claims of those unrelated to us, or different from us, may go unheeded. Moreover, it is not clear that an ethic of care would ensure the rights of women to equality and fair treatment.[46]

The emphasis on the importance of emotions is seen by many (and not just feminists) as a welcome balance to the sort of moral theory that completely ignores feeling. At the same time, taking emotion as a guide can often degenerate into a "do what feels good" kind of subjective relativism.[47] The problem of relativism remains a difficult one for feminism. On the one hand, many feminists join with postmodernists and communitarians in rejecting the Enlightenment notion of a universal morality, valid for all people at all times and places. This notion ignores the particularity most feminists regard as essential and too long ignored by Western ethics. On the other

40. Mary Daly, *Gyn/Ecology: The Metaethics of Radical Feminism* (Boston, MA: Beacon Press, 1978).

41. Jaggar, 63 (see note 38).

42. Ibid., 64.

43. Carol Gilligan, *In a Different Voice: Psychological Theory and Women's Development* (Cambridge, MA: Harvard University Press, 1982); Nell Noddings, *Caring: A Feminine Approach to Ethics and Moral Education* (Berkeley: University of California Press, 1984).

44. Virginia Held, "Feminism and Moral Theory," in *Contemporary Moral Problems*, 4th ed., edited by James E. White (St. Paul, MN: West Publishing Company, 1994), 75.

45. Ibid.

46. Ibid., 76. See also Joan Tronto, *Moral Boundaries: A Political Argument for an Ethic of Care* (New York: Routledge, 1993).

47. Jaggar, 68 (see note 38).

hand, however, feminists are understandably concerned that their critique of the oppression of women not be dismissed as a single point of view.[48]

The problem of relativism for feminists is poignantly posed by the practice of clitoridectomy, or female "circumcision." This practice, common among certain groups in Africa, involves the excision of the clitoris. Sometimes the vulva is sewn up as well. The clitoris is removed to reduce sexual pleasure and remove temptation to sexual activity; the lips of the vulva are sewn up to ensure that the young woman will remain a virgin until her marriage. The circumcision is usually done when a girl reaches puberty, although it is also often performed on very young children. It is performed without anesthesia, using unsterilized razor blades, while the girl is held down by older women. It frequently causes life-threatening blood loss and infection. It can lead to painful intercourse, infertility, and difficult childbirth.

> Ironically, the frigidity or infertility caused by the mutilation leads many husbands to shun their brides .... Doctors throughout Africa recognize the harmful effects of female circumcision but feel powerless to stop a practice so entrenched in custom and tradition. Many organizations are campaigning against it, and the new African Charter on the Rights of Children includes items condemning circumcision. Governments in Sudan and elsewhere have passed laws against it, but they are seldom enforced.[49]

Despite this opposition, many Africans continue to regard female circumcision as an important cultural and religious ritual.

The practice of female circumcision poses a dilemma for feminists. On the one hand, feminism is committed to multiculturalism, that is, to the view that no culture has a monopoly on the right way to live, and that the voices of all people must be heard. On the other hand, feminists must reject a practice they regard as patently contrary to the interests of women. Not only is clitoridectomy painful and dangerous, but its justification stems from suppositions antithetical to feminist thought: that women are male property, that female virginity must be preserved, that women ought not to have sexual feelings, that adultery is a male prerogative, and so forth. Is there a way out of the dilemma, a way to remain faithful to feminist ideals without rejecting multiculturalism?

We think that there is a way out. As suggested earlier, we need to develop an interpretation of multiculturalism that does not imply relativism. Keeping an open mind about the practices of other cultures, and attempting to understand them "from within," does not commit us to unqualified acceptance of these practices, particularly when they conflict with our deepest values and principles. For feminists, a core value is the conviction that women are full human persons, entitled to equality and justice. Clitoridectomy is not compatible with the recognition of women as free and equal members of society; indeed, it contributes to women's oppression, and is thus opposed by many African women and men. Western feminists can support these Africans in this struggle, and not be guilty of arrogance, smugness, or cultural imperialism.

VIRTUE ETHICS

In light of the problems facing consequentialist and deontological moral theories, the last fifty years or so have witnessed a growing interest in what is called "virtue ethics." Virtue ethics does not represent a single distinctive moral theory. Rather, it is a label for a family of moral theories that are specially concerned with or that give special priority to the role of the virtues in the moral life. In fact, one of the main challenges facing theories of this kind is to differentiate themselves from the moral theories we have already discussed. After all, a utilitarian like Mill will value the moral virtues on the grounds that they motivate those who possess them to reliably perform actions that maximize the overall good. Contractarians like Hobbes will value them because of the way they contribute to our ability to cooperate with one another and to form a stable community.[50] In fact, virtue plays a central role in

48. Ibid., 67.

49. *Time* (Fall 1990), 39. Cited in Joel Feinberg, *Freedom and Fulfillment: Philosophical Essays* (Princeton, NJ: Princeton University Press, 1992), 199.

50. For an analysis of the role of moral virtues in Hobbes's moral philosophy and a contrast of this view with those of Plato and Aristotle, see Alex John London, "Virtue and Consequences: Hobbes on the Value of the Moral Virtues," *Social Theory and Practice* (Spring 1998).

Kant's moral philosophy. For Kant, the good will is the only thing unconditionally good, and virtue is what makes the good will good. Virtue is the strength of the will's commitment to performing actions from the motive of duty, and it is, therefore, the condition for the goodness of anything the will does. To begin with, then, it will be useful to mark a very general contrast between the role the virtues play in these moral theories and the more central place they occupy in virtue ethics.

According to an act-consequentialist moral theory, the right action is the one that produces the best consequences. In order to be practically useful, such theories must provide us with a meaningful account of the relevant consequences and how they are to be calculated or measured. Similarly, according to a deontological moral theory, the right action is the one specified by a particular rule of some sort. In order to be of any practical benefit, such theories must supply us with the appropriate set of rules or with some procedure or criteria by which we can generate the relevant rules. In contrast, the right action in a virtue-theoretic account is the one that the virtuous person would perform. In order to be practically useful, this sort of theory must tell us who the virtuous people are and it must give us an account of the nature and number of whatever virtues it recognizes.[51] Unlike consequentialist or rule-based theories, then, virtue ethics begins with an account of the moral virtues and then links the possession of these traits to the ability to reliably perform certain kinds of actions and, importantly, to an inability to perform certain others. As a result, moral theories in this family may differ in the kinds of things they count as virtues and vices, the number of virtues and vices they recognize, their reasons why the virtues are valuable, and the relationship of the virtues to right actions.

Contemporary virtue ethicists tend to see themselves as carrying on or working within a tradition of moral philosophy that begins with Aristotle. According to Aristotle, the priorities reflected in the choices we make in our lives reveal our conception of the good life, or human flourishing—what Aristotle calls "*eudaimonia.*" We may disagree about the nature of the good life, but we can all agree that it is around some conception of happiness or doing well that we structure our various activities and give a distinctive shape to our lives. As a result, a central question for Aristotle is, What is the best life for a person to lead?

For Aristotle, a candidate for this highest good must not be something that others bestow upon us. Rather, it must be proper to its possessor and not easily taken away (1095b26-27).[52] Because honor or fame fail both of these tests, the life dedicated to their pursuit is ruled out as a candidate for the good life. Similarly, any candidate for the highest good must be a final good in the sense that we choose other things for the sake of it, but we don't choose it for the sake of anything else (1097a30). As a result, the life of money making is ruled out. In addition, the candidate must be self-sufficient in the sense that the presence of it alone makes life desirable and worth living (1097b ff). In Aristotle's view, the virtues of temperance, courage, justice, wisdom, and practical reason represent the excellent states of our emotional and intellectual faculties. Because each of these traits represents the proper development of some human faculty, they are valuable for themselves (1097b2-5, 1144a1-7). But Aristotle believes that the virtues are also valuable for the activities that they produce and that happiness, or the highest human good, is a life of activity that consists in the exercise of such well-developed emotional and intellectual faculties under the guidance of our distinctly human capacity for rationality.

To cultivate the virtues, however, one must first perform actions that are noble and good. Noble and just actions have a kind of symmetry or balance about them—they are a mean between unacceptable extremes—and the only way to cultivate character states that share this symmetry is to repeatedly perform virtuous actions. To understand

51. This way of contrasting virtue ethics with consequentialist and deontological moral theories is explained at length by Rosalind Hursthouse in "Normative Virtue Ethics," in *How Should One Live One's Life?* edited by Roger Crisp (New York: Oxford University Press, 1996), 19–36.

52. These numbers refer to the page and line numbers of Bekker's edition of Aristotle's works. They are the standard method of citing particular passages in the works of Aristotle and can be found in the margins of the text of most translations.

what is right, noble, and just, however, one must have received a proper upbringing. One must have cultivated good habits, such as consideration for others, truthfulness, and self-control, because one becomes just and temperate by first doing just and temperate things. But virtue isn't simply a matter of practice or mere habit. Rather, it is only by acting in certain ways that we can come to understand what is noble and just and why this is so. Those who lack appropriate role models or guardians to instruct them will be unable to appreciate these things. Furthermore, Aristotle thinks that right, noble, and just actions are of such a diverse nature that they cannot be adequately captured by a set of rules or decision procedures. As a result, one cannot rely solely on some external theory or decision principle to determine which actions one ought to perform. To reliably perform the right action, one must cultivate the virtues for oneself and rely on one's experience and ability to appreciate and judge such things for oneself.

This does not mean that one will not be able to explain why something was the right thing to do given a particular situation. To the contrary, the virtuous person will be able to bring out the salient features of a situation and to say why some action is morally acceptable. This ability to appreciate the facts of a situation and to justify acting in one way rather than another, however, is quite different from the ability to give a general and practically useful account of the features that are morally important to situations in general and of what makes an action right and noble such that nonvirtuous people could use this account as a guide to action. For Aristotle, the only reliable way to understand what must be done, and to ensure that one is sufficiently willing to act on this understanding, is to become a just person oneself.

In this reading of Aristotle, the virtues play a central role in his ethical theory for several reasons. First, because they represent the excellent states of important human emotional and intellectual capacities, they are valuable in their own right. Second, the virtues play an important role in human flourishing, since the exercise of these well-developed states of our faculties is what Aristotle regards as happiness, or *eudaimonia*. Third, the virtues play an important epistemological role in the good life—namely, without the virtues, one will not fully understand what makes an action noble and just, or be able to appreciate the morally relevant factors of complicated situations. Fourth, the moral virtues provide the motivation for consistently performing the right actions since the person who possesses them will not only understand what makes them noble and just, but will also take pleasure in acting well and will do so for its own sake and not for the sake of some external consideration. Those who lack the proper upbringing will regard such actions as painful, to be done only to avoid punishment or to gain some advantage, such as obtaining money, power, or friends.

Some contemporary versions of virtue ethics differ from Aristotle on one or more of these points. For example, Aristotle says that the right action is the one that the virtuous person would perform because the virtuous person "judges each thing rightly" and "things appear to him as they truly are," so that what sets the virtuous person apart from others is that "he sees the truth in each thing, being himself the norm and measure of the noble and the pleasant" (1113a26-35 cf. 1176a12-19). We can use the virtuous person as a standard or measure of what is right because she understands why some action is right and just and can be counted on to reliably perform such actions. The virtuous person is thus an epistemological guide to determining which actions are right. But the rightness of those actions is not a product of the fact that they are the actions virtuous people would perform, although some contemporary virtue theorists embrace this view.

According to these theorists, the virtues are of primary importance to the moral life because they are the primary locus of moral value. As such, the virtuous are the norm and measure of what is right and good precisely because actions derive whatever moral value they possess from their relationship to the virtues. If an action is one that the virtuous person would perform, then this makes the action right and just.[53] The value of the action is therefore determined by the judgment of the virtuous person. One major problem for a view of this

53. A version of this view can be found in Rosalind Hursthouse, "Virtue Theory and Abortion," *Philosophy & Public Affairs* 20 (1991): 223–246.

sort lies in explaining the grounds on which virtuous agents make their initial judgment. On what grounds do they decide whether an action is the right one? Certainly it cannot be simply because it is the action they did in fact choose. This would make their judgment seem arbitrary and capricious. But if it is because it is the action they *should* choose, then we want to know what it is about the action that makes it worthy of choice. In either case it looks like such a theory will either turn out to be arbitrary and unhelpful or it will have to advert to some explanation of the value of an action that reaches beyond its relation to the judgment of the virtuous themselves.

Similarly, many contemporary virtue ethicists differ from Aristotle in rejecting the view that the virtues are excellent states of our cognitive and affective faculties. For example, Alasdair MacIntyre argues that the virtues should not be thought of as timeless, human excellences. Rather, they are acquired human qualities that allow us to achieve goods internal to those cultural roles and practices that can be shaped into a coherent vision of the good life within a particular community.[54] As such, cultural traditions, community membership, and role obligations play a crucial part in determining which kinds of human qualities are virtues and what kinds of activities count as virtuous activities.

In MacIntyre's view, Dr. Brody has to ask herself whether assisting in suicide is consistent with the goods that are internal to the practice of medicine in late twentieth-century America and the obligations that she has taken on in her role as physician. On the one hand, Dr. Brody is committed to ameliorating pain and suffering, but she is also aware that doctors have traditionally conceived of themselves as the agents of health, not death. She also knows that there may be considerable consequences to a choice to assist Mr. Lasken's suicide, and she has to weigh these consequences against her own well-being and self-interest. Is it fair that Mr. Lasken cannot receive help in ending his suffering until his condition degenerates to the point that his life is being sustained by machines, the support of which it might then be permissible to withdraw? Is it acceptable for her to lie or dissemble in order to help Mr. Lasken and avoid going to jail, or to comfort or assuage him if she decides not to come to his aid?

These are difficult questions, and the fact that virtue ethics does not provide us with easy answers to them is not peculiar to this ethical theory. Even so, critics are generally nonplussed by the advice to do whatever the virtuous person would do, especially in situations where compassion, fidelity, courage, prudence, and self-interest seem to be at odds with one another. What critics demand is some way of ranking the virtues and their hold on us so that people like Dr. Brody will know how to negotiate such conflicts. In the eyes of critics, without such a ranking, virtue ethics will never entirely substitute for a more principled approach.

Yet the fact that the virtue ethicist relies on the good judgment of the virtuous person to negotiate such apparent conflicts should not detract from the fact that the consequentialist and the deontologist face very similar problems. The consequentialist must provide Dr. Brody with an account of the relevant consequences and with a procedure by which to weigh or measure them without running afoul of our deepest intuitions about this case. Similarly, the deontologist must produce a set of rules or decision procedures flexible enough to accommodate the nuances of the situation. So it appears that with each of these theories as well, Dr. Brody is going to have to exercise her deliberative skills to do what is right for Mr. Lasken and for herself.

Nevertheless, the virtue-based approach to cases like this does have certain advantages. For example, it brings out a variety of prima facie concerns, each of which makes a serious claim on us and demands that we apply ourselves to finding a judicious way to address each of them as best we can. It also brings out the way in which a physician must be committed to her patients and to her craft. The goal and goods of medicine require physicians to take chances for their patients—to have the courage to attend to them even when this may conflict with their own self-interest. Willingness to expose oneself to risk, including disease and sickness, is part of what it means to be a physician. As Arnold Relman puts it, "the risk of contracting the patient's disease is one of the risks that is inherent in the profession

54. Alasdair MacIntyre, *After Virtue*, 2nd ed. (Notre Dame, IN: University of Notre Dame Press, 1984), 191.

of medicine. Physicians who are not willing to accept that risk . . . ought not to be in the practice of medicine."[55] Although there are limits to the duty to put oneself at risk, a virtue-based approach establishes a strong presumption in favor of the duty to treat over doctors' rights to decide whom to treat and what risks to take.[56] Indeed, one of the shortcomings of a narrowly contractualist approach to the doctor-patient relationship, an approach that specifies numerous duties *within* that relationship, is its silence on the question of whether doctors have moral and professional obligations to *establish* relationships with needy, dangerous, or HIV-infected patients.

NONMORAL CONSIDERATIONS

The dizzying array of moral theories and perspectives presented above make it hard enough to decide how to act in a given situation. We suggested that it is not a question of determining which moral theory is correct; all of them contribute to an extraordinarily complex moral reality. Still, in deciding what to do, one must decide when utilitarian considerations should prevail, or when one ought to adhere to absolutist principles; when to appeal to principles and when to seek guidance in virtues; when to abide by universal, impartial considerations and when to concentrate on personal relationships and feelings.

As if the moral dimension of decision making were not complicated enough, there is another dimension we have not so far discussed: the "nonmoral" dimension. How should we think about the political, personal, prudential, economic, or legal implications of our actions? According to one school of thought, moral reasons are the "best" reasons; they always "trump" other considerations. Thus, if it would be morally right to do something, then one ought to do it, even if it would have adverse nonmoral consequences. More recently, philosophers like Bernard Williams[57] and Susan Wolf[58] have argued that one is sometimes entirely justified in overriding impartial moral reasons to pursue a significant personal goal or defining relationship. Conceivably, many of the considerations left out of traditional ethics can be recovered if we take seriously the idea, advocated by feminists and others, that personal relations and feelings are as important to ethics as universal and impartial principles. Nevertheless, however broadly ethics is conceived, there will always be the possibility of conflict between moral and nonmoral considerations. In such cases, how are we to decide what to do?

Consider, once again, Dr. Brody. Suppose she decides that the morally right thing to do is to help Mr. Lasken. Helping him is breaking the law. She could be prosecuted and go to jail; even if she is not convicted, she could lose her license to practice medicine. It seems clear that these are important considerations and that it would be absurd (as opposed to noble) for Dr. Brody to completely ignore them. Whether her personal risk should override her view of the morally right action depends, in part, on the degree of the risk. If the risks of discovery, prosecution, and punishment are sufficiently low, and if she believes that it is morally right to help Mr. Lasken, Dr. Brody should perhaps be willing to risk legal and professional repercussions. In other situations, doing the morally right thing might ask too much of a person. The hard thing in life is having the wisdom to figure out when nonmoral actions are justified.

MODES OF MORAL REASONING

The above survey of moral theories suggests the richness and diversity of our repertoire of ethical language and concepts. The task for this section is to show how these disparate and sometimes conflicting elements of morality figure into the moral judgments that we make. What should we *do* with all this ethical "raw material"?

55. *Cardiovascular News* (August 1987): 7.

56. Norman Daniels argues that a virtue-based approach to the question of the duty to treat implies a contractualist theory. See "Duty to Treat or Right to Refuse?" *Hasting Center Report* 21, no. 2 (1991): 36–46.

57. Bernard Williams, *Ethics and the Limits of Philosophy* (Cambridge, MA: Harvard University Press, 1985).

58. Susan Wolf, "Moral Saints," *Journal of Philosophy* (August 1982): 419–439.

Many of the enumerated theoretical perspectives—such as utilitarianism, Kantianism, and rights-based theories—articulate basic moral values, principles, and rules at a fairly high level of abstraction. We are told, for example, to maximize happiness, respect persons, honor patients' rights to confidentiality, and so on. But we are also told—for example, by the partisans of an ethic of care—to deemphasize such abstractions in favor of a heightened caring responsiveness to individual people and situations. An important question arises, then, about precisely how these generalities are, or should be, brought to bear in specific cases. In the language of the philosophical tradition, it is a question about the relationship between the universal and the particular.

This is also a question about the nature of moral justification. In pointing out the importance of happiness, personhood, rights, virtues, caring, etc., each of the above theories contributes to our search for ethical *warrants* or reasons that tend to *justify* our actions. When called upon to justify or defend individual actions or social policies, how do—or how should—we respond? Insofar as it makes sense to pursue ethical certitude about our actions, where does such certitude lie: in our philosophical or religious theories, in our pretheoretical convictions of right and wrong generated by our history and culture, or perhaps in some combination of these two areas?

The Principles Approach

One tempting response to these questions is to hold that justification in ethics is a matter of deducing the best and most comprehensive ethical theory from the foregoing list, and deriving this theory's correct conclusions. Thus, one should throw in his or her lot with, say, utilitarianism or Kantianism and then "apply" this theoretical framework to the facts at hand. Understood in this way, bioethics has been described as a kind of "applied ethics," as though philosophers and theologians do all the ethical heavy lifting, while others simply apply their findings to this or that set of factual circumstances. Tempting as it is in its simplicity, this conception of bioethics must nevertheless be rejected.

First, although this approach identifies philosophical theory as the ultimate locus of moral certitude, it is far from clear what the "best and most comprehensive" ethical theory is. Indeed, after centuries of moral debates, we still disagree, sometimes vehemently, about justice and the nature of the good life. Second, as we have seen in the application of various theories to our case of physician-assisted suicide, theories are often stated at such a high level of generality (e.g., "Maximize happiness," "Respect persons") that they are capable of generating contradictory answers to the same moral questions. Third, this way of understanding "theory"—i.e., as an abstract construction built upon one or two overarching values—tends to obscure the extraordinary richness and diversity of the moral life. So, even if one of the enumerated "standard" theories were miraculously to attract a consensus, the result would be more impoverishing than liberating. To repeat, ethical theories as we understand them are best viewed as partial perspectives on a complex moral reality.

A powerful alternative to theory-driven approaches to bioethics emphasizes the role in moral reasoning of a small cluster of middle-level ethical principles. Instead of pursuing difficult and highly divisive foundational issues, the partisans of the "principles approach" (or "principlism") begin with our common moral experience and the manifest importance of keeping a short list of moral duties. Originally developed by Professors Tom Beauchamp and James Childress in their justly influential book, *The Principles of Biomedical Ethics*,[59] and later endorsed by prestigious governmental ethics commissions,[60] the method of principlism rapidly became the dominant mode of "doing bioethics" in the United States.

Stated in their popular tongue-twisting, Latinate formulations, these norms include the principles of autonomy, beneficence, nonmaleficence, and justice. In simpler terms, the core principles of bioethics bid us to (1) respect the capacity of individuals to

59. Beauchamp and Childress, *The Principles of Biomedical Ethics* (see note 6).

60. National Commission for the Protection of Human Subjects of Biomedical and Behavioral Research, *The Belmont Report: Ethical Principles and Guidelines for the Protection of Human Subjects of Research* (Washington, DC: U.S. Government Printing Office, 1978).

choose their own vision of the good life and act accordingly; (2) foster the interests and happiness of other persons and of society at large; (3) refrain from harming other persons; and (4) act fairly, distribute benefits and burdens in an equitable fashion, and resolve disputes by means of fair procedures.

In contrast to the partisans of applied moral theory, who tend to reduce the sources of normative guidance and criticism to a single overarching value (for example, Kantian respect for persons or the maximization of utility), the principlists settle for a small cluster of "middle level" norms, each one consistent with a number of ethical theories, no one of which enjoys automatic supremacy over the others. They reject the notion that serious moral conflict can always be resolved by appeal to a higher moral standard provided by some ultimate theory. Instead, they frankly admit the necessity of "weighing and balancing" the various principles against one another in each concrete moral situation.

While each principle articulates a serious moral duty, these duties are not absolute. They are, in the words of the late philosopher W. D. Ross, prima facie obligations.[61] This means that the ethical principles are indeed binding, but on any given occasion one principle may eclipse another with which it conflicts. So we say that a given principle is binding prima facie, or "at first blush," but that in the final analysis, all things having been considered, the pull of another principle might turn out to be even stronger. Importantly, however, even when a principle is outweighed, it usually continues to exert a strong moral pull on our behavior; it does not simply become irrelevant.

The conflict between the demands of confidentiality and the protection of public health in the context of AIDS provides a useful example of how principlism could be applied. On the one hand, physicians swear an oath to uphold the confidentiality of their patients. Since Hippocrates, this duty has been utterly central to the vocation of physicians. Without assurances that their often embarrassing secrets are safe with the doctor, patients will be reluctant to speak frankly about their symptoms or medical history, and in some cases may avoid seeking medical attention to the detriment of their condition. A doctor's violations of confidentiality thus might be seen as violating the principles of beneficence and nonmaleficence.

The principle of autonomy provides further warrant for a doctor's confidentiality. Patients have a right to determine who knows what about their medical history. When physicians or nurses share this information with others who do not have a legitimate medical need to know, they rob their patients of control over information that is rightfully theirs. Combined, then, the principles of autonomy, beneficence, and nonmaleficence make an exceedingly strong case for respecting patient confidentiality.

But now suppose that you are a physician caring for a bisexual male infected with the HIV/AIDS virus. Your patient admits to having regular unprotected sex with his fiancée, who does not suspect his HIV status, yet he insists upon absolute confidentiality out of a (well-founded) fear of losing her. On one hand, you feel the pull of your duty to respect confidentiality; but, on the other hand, your patient's behavior is placing another human being in mortal peril and you are in a unique position to protect this unsuspecting, vulnerable person.

This ethical dilemma, discussed at greater length in Part 1, Section 3, effectively illustrates the prima facie character of the principles approach. As a physician, you are clearly bound by your duty of confidentiality, but you are also bound to prevent grave harm to highly vulnerable people, especially when you are in a unique position to do so. According to principlism, you cannot simply invoke a supreme value that always wins; you must instead undertake the difficult task of weighing and balancing conflicting values. In this case, you might decide that the principle of autonomy is outweighed by the prevention of harm to others. The risk is great, the projected harm exceedingly grave, and your patient's insistence upon his autonomy might be discounted as self-contradictory and hypocritical in light of his irresponsible disregard of his fiancée's autonomy, as well as her life.

On balance, then, your prima facie duty to respect your patient's confidentiality might fall short as a duty *all things considered* in this particular situation. But this does not mean either that these rival concerns will always prevail in similar circumstances or

61. W. D. Ross, *The Right and the Good* (Oxford: Clarendon Press, 1930).

that confidentiality simply becomes irrelevant once it is outweighed. If your patient is an HIV-infected woman who (credibly) claims that her abusive, drug-taking, and possibly HIV-infected boyfriend will kill her should he discover her secret, you will most likely find another way to solve the problem than by violating your patient's confidentiality. And even when you decide that, all things considered, confidentiality must yield to another principle, such as the prevention of harm, confidentiality continues to exert moral influence by setting the terms of legitimate disclosure. Even though the bisexual's fiancée has a right to know the truth, the same cannot be said of his employer, the other patients in your waiting room, or the members of your weekly poker game.

Objections to the Principles Approach

In spite of its enormous success, the method of principlism has recently been criticized on a number of fronts. Although some of these objections lack merit, others pose important challenges to principlism. As we shall see, principlism has nevertheless proved itself remarkably adaptive in responding to many of these complaints.[62]

1. Principlism Is Mechanistic and Vacuous. Although astute commentators like Beauchamp and Childress have wielded principlism in a thoughtful, carefully nuanced, and fruitful manner, in less-skilled hands this method has tended to degenerate into a ritualistic incantation of empty abstractions. Bioethical literature abounds with superficial claims that "the principle of autonomy (or of beneficence, or of the 'best interests' of the patient) *requires* that we do such and such." The problem with this common locution is that it ignores the difficulty (or the vacuousness) of passing immediately from very abstract statements of principle to very concrete conclusions about what to do here and now. Quite apart from the vexing problem of rank ordering *competing* principles in morally complex situations, we first have to determine what these abstract formulations of principle actually mean.

What does it mean, for example, to invoke the moral principle that caregivers should always seek the "best interests" of all patients, including severely impaired newborns? How are the interests of such a child to be assessed, and according to which conception of the good? Some argue that life is sacred and that continued life is always in the child's interest; others contend that a life of constant suffering is not a life worth living; while still others advance a conception of the good based on more complex notions of human flourishing and dignity, which might sanction nontreatment decisions even given the absence of pain and suffering.[63]

Whatever the merit of these individual suggestions, the point is that unless we *interpret* "the principles of bioethics," they will merely play the role of empty "chapter headings,"[64] doing little, if any, actual work in moral analysis. Unless we furnish principles with a definite shape and content—*Which* principle of justice? *Which* conception of autonomy?—they will merely lend a patina of objectivity to bioethical debates while masking the need to pin down arguments and choices defining the substance of those principles.

2. Principlism Founders on the Problem of Moral Conflict. Other critics call attention to principlism's inability or unwillingness to provide a rationally defensible framework for settling conflicts between competing principles. Clearly, such critics have a point here. Unlike utilitarians or Rawlsians who could settle, at least to their own satisfaction, the inevitable conflicts of the moral life using some overarching principle of "lexical ordering," the principlists forthrightly admit that their moral principles do not come with pre-established theoretical weights; consequently, conflicts have to be settled through a subtle process of weighing and balancing of principles in the midst of real cases, an approach

62. The following account of the role of principles and cases in moral argument is based upon John Arras's more extensive discussion in "Principles and Particularity: The Roles of Cases in Bioethics," *Indiana Law Journal* 69, no. 4 (Symposium on Emerging Paradigms in Bioethics, Fall 1994): 983–1014.

63. See Ezekiel Emanuel, *The Ends of Human Life,* 70–87 (see note 34).

64. K. Danner Clouser and Bernard Gert, "A Critique of Principlism," *Journal of Medicine and Philosophy* 15 (1990): 227.

to conflict resolution that some philosophers regard as excessively subjective. We believe, however, that there is wisdom in the principlists' modesty. Their critics have neither established the clear superiority of any monistic theory, such as utilitarianism, nor have they produced a convincing account of why, within more pluralistic systems, certain favored values such as utility or liberty should *always* prevail over all other competing values in a myriad of convoluted real world situations.

3. Principlism Is Deductivistic. Another group of critics, the partisans of a more "case-driven" mode of analysis, object to the apparently unidirectional movement from principles to cases within principlism. While later editions of Beauchamp's and Childress's *The Principles of Bioethics* address this criticism, earlier editions gave the distinct impression that theory justifies principles, that principles justify moral rules, and that rules justify moral judgments in particular cases.[65]

This "top down" conception of moral reasoning has been faulted for ignoring the pivotal role of intuitive, case-based judgments of right and wrong. To be sure, the judgments in question are not to be confused with just any responses to cases, no matter how prejudiced, ill-considered, or subject to coercion they might be. Rather, the critics have in mind something more akin to John Rawls's notion of "considered" moral judgments;[66] i.e., those judgments about whose genesis and moral rectitude we feel most confident, such as that slavery is wrong. It is precisely these judgments, they claim, that give concrete meaning, definition, and scope to our moral principles, thus providing us with critical leverage in refining their articulation.

The ultimate point of this criticism is that the relationship between principles and cases is dialectical or reciprocal: the principles provide normative guidance and the cases provide considered judgments that, in turn, help shape the principles, which then provide more precise guidance. Another way of putting this, following Rawls's terminology, is that principles and cases exist together in creative tension or "reflective equilibrium."[67] One can thus insist on a robust role for principles in moral reasoning without being committed to a "top down" or deductivistic approach.[68]

Casuistry or "Case-Based" Reasoning

The renaissance of casuistry, or "case-based" reasoning, in practical ethics has stressed the pivotal role of the particularity of cases while de-emphasizing the role of theory and routinized appeals to "the principles of bioethics."[69] According to its leading proponents, a casuistical method must begin with a typology or grouping of cases around paradigmatic instances of a moral rule or principle. In the area of research ethics, for example, the atrocities of Nazi medicine still serve to exemplify unethical dealing with human subjects. From this signal case, one then branches out to analogous cases of greater complexity and difficulty, such as research on children or the demented elderly, proceeding by a method akin to "moral triangulation." As one goes from case to case, responding to the particularities of different settings, treatments, and categories of research subjects, principles emerge and become increasingly refined and complex.

Crucially, the casuists contend that whatever "weight" a principle might have vis-à-vis competing principles must be determined not in the abstract, but rather in response to the particularities

65. Beauchamp and Childress, *The Principles of Biomedical Ethics*, 1st edition (New York: Oxford University Press, 1979), 5.

66. Rawls, 47 (see note 19).

67. Ibid., 20ff, 48–50.

68. The principlists' response to this line of criticism has been to embrace it, over time, with increasing forthrightness and enthusiasm. Although they may have been slower than others to discern the formative and critical roles of case analysis with regard to principles and theories, Beauchamp and Childress (4th ed.) now embrace reflective equilibrium as *the* methodology of principlism, and emphatically denounce deductivism for precisely the same reasons given by their critics. See Chapters 1–2 (see note 6).

69. See, e.g., Albert Jonsen and Stephen Toulmin, *The Abuse of Casuistry* (Berkeley: University of California Press, 1988); John D. Arras, "Getting Down to Cases: The Revival of Casuistry in Bioethics," *Journal of Medicine and Philosophy* 16 (1991): 29–51; and Baruch Brody, *Life and Death Decision Making* (New York: Oxford University Press, 1988).

of individual cases.[70] Suppose, for example, that physicians and nurses at a nursing home wish to study the refusal to eat of many elderly patients with Alzheimer's disease. Further suppose that informed consent to participate in the study cannot be expected from this impaired patient population. According to the dictates of our paradigm case—e.g., the infamous and lethal experiments of the Nazi doctors—the principle of respect for persons always requires the free and informed consent of the research subject. But according to the casuists, whether the principle of autonomy should prevail over the principle of beneficence in nursing home research—a result that many consider the primary lesson of Nazi research atrocities—will be determined in the context of a nuanced investigation into the "who" (enslaved ethnic populations versus patients with Alzheimer's disease); the "what" (experiments designed to kill versus studying and filming patients' eating behaviors); the "where" (death camps versus a regulated nursing home with a competent research review board); and the "when" (after capture and before execution versus after the consent of family, the loss of decision-making capacity, and the approval and ongoing oversight of an ethics committee). Rather than assigning a timeless relative weight to a certain principle, casuistry holds that the weight lies in the details. In this hypothetical situation, a proposed protocol might be so far removed from our paradigm of unethical research, and the potential benefits to future patients might be so great, that our moral approval may be justified even without the patient's consent.

Presented in this way, the casuistical method obviously has much in common with the method of the common law. Indeed, given the pivotal and ubiquitous role of legal cases in the recent history of bioethics—a history punctuated by such names as Karen Quinlan, Claire Conroy (see Part 3, Section 4), and Nancy Cruzan, (Part 3, Section 4)—it was entirely natural for bioethicists to begin drawing parallels between case-based reasoning in ethics and in law. In both casuistry and law, we seem to reason from the "bottom up" (from specific cases to fleshed-out principles) rather than from the "top down" (as in most versions of applied ethics); the principles themselves are consequently "open textured," always subject to further revision and specification; and our final judgments usually turn on a fine-grained analysis of the particularities of the case.

To many ethicists, this account of reasoning in both ethics and law accurately describes how we actually think, both in clinical situations and in the classroom; that is, we tend to see cases, which serve as a kind of shorthand, as exemplars for moral analysis and assessment. "This is a Quinlan-type case, except instead of a ventilator the issue is a feeding tube (or antibiotics, or the sustainment of minimal conscious awareness, or a family insisting that everything be done, etc.). How does each different variable alter the case? Is it so different that it should dictate an alternative result?" Instead of ritualistically invoking the mantra of principles, casuistic ethicists thus urge us all to conform our rhetoric to our actual practice.

Just as the casuists insist that the weight of principles resides in the details, they also insist that moral certainty resides in our responses to paradigmatic cases, rather than in abstractions of theory or principle. We are much more confident in our knowledge that torturing and killing Jews to learn about hypothermia is wrong than we are in our assessment of which moral theory or constellation of moral principles best explains why. We would, in fact, be much more likely to switch our allegiance to a different moral theory or set of principles than to change our judgment on what the Nazi doctors did. Indeed, were a moral theory to approve of the Nazis' experiments, we would most likely take that specific judgment as sufficient reason to reject the theory.

Although some extreme casuists reject principles entirely, more moderate versions of casuistry make room for principles, theories, and cultural norms, while still insisting on the priority of the particular. Instead of imposing a false choice between principles and responses to cases, these ethicists envision, in the words of Martha Nussbaum, a "process of loving conversation between rules and concrete responses, general conceptions and unique cases, in which the general articulates the particular and is in

70. Albert Jonsen, "Of Balloons and Bicycles, or the Relationship between Ethical Theory and Practical Judgment," *Hastings Center Report* 21 (1991): 14–16.

turn further articulated by it."[71] Principles play a role, then, but rarely—if ever—as mere axioms from which to deduce moral conclusions. Indeed, whatever validity or usefulness general principles might have depends upon the insight, moral sensitivity, and casuistical skill that mediate their "application" to the particulars of a case.

At this point it should be clear that principlism and the emerging paradigm of casuistry are not necessarily as antithetical as their respective partisans often suggest. On the contrary, chastened principlists who have abandoned deductivism, and moderate casuists who admit a role for principles and general norms, could endorse Martha Nussbaum's dictum with equal enthusiasm; it is, after all, just another way of calling for reflective equilibrium between principles and cases.

According to this emerging consensus, then, moral justification lies not in the correspondence between our moral theories and some sort of moral bedrock, such as nature or God's will; rather, justification resides in the coherence or "fit" among the whole network of our considered judgments and the principles and rules that emanate from them. Insofar as our most confident moral judgments cohere with the system of norms built upon them, they can be considered justified. Contrary to deductivism, moral certainty does not lie in either principles or theory; and contrary to extreme casuistry, certainty does not lie only in our responses to paradigmatic cases. Instead, we believe that any moral certitude lies at the intersection between our abstract norms and our responses to cases.

Judgments that conflict with well-established moral norms, even judgments that might have once seemed unassailable, should be subjected to further scrutiny. Even though it might have once been "plain as day" that African Americans deserve second-class status or that doctors should never assist patients to commit suicide, the principles of respect for persons or individual autonomy might well prompt us to rethink—and in some cases reject—what was once thought to be our moral bedrock. By the same token, as we have seen, principles develop out of reflection on our considered judgments and acquire their precise meaning and weight within the crucible of contextualized judgments.

It should be noted, however, that even though we speak of reflective "equilibrium" and the "system" of coherent judgments and general norms, the moral life will always be more dynamic and less tidy than these terms imply. The uneasy balance between particular judgments and general norms will most likely never reach equilibrium. Our considered judgments are in a state of constant, if glacially slow, flux, and our concepts, principles, and rules are always merely provisional—always subject to further expansion in scope, specification of meaning, and fluctuation in importance vis-à-vis other general norms. The best we can hope for, then, is a constant striving for greater and greater coherence. Complete coherence—a total seamless system of morality—is most likely beyond our grasp, kept out of reach by both the limitations of our mental capacities and the inherent fragmentation among the values that constitute our complicated moral lives.

71. Martha Nussbaum, "The Discernment of Perception: An Aristotelian Conception of Private and Public Rationality," in *Love's Knowledge: Essays on Philosophy and Literature* (New York: Oxford University Press, 1990), 95.

PART ONE

FOUNDATIONS OF THE HEALTH PROFESSIONAL-PATIENT RELATIONSHIP

The success of scientific medicine, the growing impersonality of the medical setting, and the rise of consumerism—together with the recent emergence of managed care—have combined to shake the foundations of the traditional doctor-nurse-patient relationship. The burgeoning number of medical malpractice suits alone provides eloquent testimony of profound changes taking place both in our expectations of medical science and in our awareness of patients' rights. What responsibilities and rights *should* attach to the roles of nurse, doctor, and patient? And how should health professionals think about the inevitable conflicts of duty that arise from the intersection of their specific roles? Part 1 is devoted to the exploration of these questions. Although clarifying the moral foundations of the health professional-patient relationship is an interesting and important task in its own right, the resolution of these basic issues will also shed welcome light on the biomedical problems raised in subsequent parts of the text.

AUTONOMY, PATERNALISM, AND MEDICAL MODELS

The relationship between health professionals and patients is mediated in complex ways by an array of values and social norms. Sometimes these norms are explicit and overt, as when physicians take an oath to look after the welfare of their patients. In many cases, however, these values remain largely implicit and unarticulated, embedded in the culture and the institutions in which we work, learn, or live, and in the roles that persons inhabit within those institutions. Sometimes sociologists, social psychologists, anthropologists, and other social scientists seek to understand these norms, to explain their origins and the myriad ways in which they actually shape the expectations, responses, emotions, and other dispositions of the persons who are affected by them. Understanding this factual information is also of fundamental importance for bioethics, because medicine and the biosciences are not isolated fields that operate on an ideal frictionless plane. They are concrete social activities that take place within specific institutions, with their own histories and traditions.

For the ethicist, however, this information is not the end of the inquiry. Rather, it provides the background against which a more fundamental set of questions is posed: How *ought* we to think about the bond uniting health care providers and patients? How *ought* we to organize the larger concrete social institutions in which this bond is forged? What are the values that *ought* to shape the way people perceive and respond to others in these settings? Consider the different values implicit in the metaphors that have been used to describe the relationship between health care providers and patients: parent/child, teacher/student, seller/buyer, priest/penitent, oppressor/victim, friends, contractors. Understanding, for example, that a particular way of conceiving of the "patient" shapes the way we are disposed to perceive and respond to persons so labeled is but one extremely important step in a process of critical reflection in which latent norms are made explicit so that they can be discussed and evaluated publicly. The choice between these and other possible "models" of the provider-patient relationship will profoundly shape both our outlook on medical ethics generally and our views on particular controversies.

Not long ago, the patient-provider relationship was conceived almost exclusively in terms of a patient-centered consequentialism that traced its roots back to the Hippocratic tradition. Section 1 begins with the formative text of this tradition. If we turn to the Hippocratic oath, we see that the doctor pledges to "apply dietetic measures for the benefit of the sick according to [his] ability and judgment," and he promises to keep his patients from "harm and injustice." This "moral core" of the oath admirably commits the physician above all else to the health and well-being of his patients—as opposed, for example, to the advancement of medical science, profits, or cost containment. Unlike utilitarianism, a form of consequentialism that instructs agents to evaluate the consequences of their actions for some large social group, patient-centered consequentialism enjoins providers to evaluate their conduct based on its consequences for the welfare of the individual patient. Perhaps the most controversial element of traditional Hippocratic ethics, however, is the way it identifies the patient's welfare with physical health. This strikingly narrow way of thinking about a person's welfare allows the patient to be conceived of as a largely passive recipient of the physician's expert ministrations which are determined by the principles of his art and his own "ability and judgment."

On this model, physicians are thought to be better suited to make health-related decisions for their patients than are the patients themselves because the patient's welfare is defined in terms of physical health, a subject about which physicians and other health professionals have special technical knowledge. As a result, the medical tradition based on this oath has hardly considered lying or shielding the patient from the truth a form of "injustice," as the following passage from the "Decorum," another Hippocratic text, strikingly shows: "Perform [these duties] calmly and adroitly, concealing most things from the patient while you are attending to him. Give necessary orders with cheerfulness and serenity, turning his attention away from what is being done to him; sometimes remove sharply and emphatically, and sometimes comfort with solicitude and attention, revealing nothing of the patient's future or present condition."

This model, however, is highly paternalistic because it entails that health care providers can legitimately restrict or dictate the conduct of even competent adults for the sake of that person's own good. On the traditional model, the physician's duty to tell the truth to patients is subordinated to, and derived from, the more fundamental duty to "do no harm." If, in the physician's judgment, telling the truth would result in depression or otherwise adversely impact the care of a patient, then the physician would be duty bound to withhold such information.

In the 1960s and 70s, however, the prevailing paternalism of American medicine was subjected to increased public scrutiny as a broad range of reform movements encouraged the public to question the authority of many dominant social institutions and the values imbedded in the roles those institutions assigned to persons. Also during these decades, a number of prominent research scandals came to light in which physicians had performed medical experiments on vulnerable populations such as the indigent, elderly patients of the Jewish Chronic Disease Hospital who were injected with live cancer cells without their consent, the mentally retarded children of the Willowbrook State School who were purposefully infected with hepatitis, or the 600 poor, African American males whose syphilis was deliberately left untreated for 40 years so that a generation of physician researchers could study the natural history of the disease (see Part 5, Section 1). High-profile revelations like these fueled distrust of the authority wielded by the medical profession, and out of the resulting scrutiny there emerged a trenchant and multifaceted critique of medical paternalism.

The question of truth-telling became a lightning rod for criticism as an increasingly skeptical public began to question the assumptions of traditional medical practice. Some critics attempted to refute the paternalistic approach to truth-telling on its own terms, by demonstrating through opinion polls and empirical research that many patients want to be told the truth. Contrary to the assumption that physicians are well qualified to assess the risks and benefits of withholding the truth, it was argued that they rarely possess good evidence for their customary refusal to disclose the truth and that they have no special training to make such difficult value-laden decisions regarding what is really best for patients and their families. As Alan Goldman points out in "The Refutation of Medical Paternalism," this view equates welfare with physical health, ignoring the fact that how people value health is itself shaped by their broader values and life projects. Doctors and patients do not always share the same values or aim at the same treatment goals. Whereas many physicians tend to regard the extension of life as the predominant value, their patients might well value the quality of their future life more than its quantity.

On a more fundamental level, though, Goldman argues that paternalism fails to recognize the independent value of self-determination and the respect that people are entitled to as "choosing beings." Because the traditional view leaves no room for self-determination as an important aspect of a patient's welfare, it fails to treat patients as the *moral* equals of their physicians by denying them the information they need to make informed decisions about their own person. Without sufficient information upon which to base a judgment, a patient's consent to treatment will not be informed, and in the absence of informed consent a patient's self-determination is effectively thwarted. From this perspective, the physician always has a strong duty to be truthful with patients—a duty that is grounded ultimately on the patient's dignity as a choosing being. All the various tried and true forms of deceit—from outright lying, to withholding information, to using medical jargon ("no need to worry; it's just a little carcinoma")—undermine the status of the patient as an autonomous agent.

In the vast majority of cases, respecting patient autonomy by engaging the patient's own powers of deliberation, choice, and agency is not just consistent with the desire to benefit the patient, but is itself a means of doing so. As a result, the importance of respect for autonomy is widely recognized in contemporary medicine and can fairly be described as the cornerstone of contemporary bioethics. Nevertheless, this does not mean that many of the central views and values of the Hippocratic tradition have disappeared. Rather, they persist even today, only they tend now to be expressed, not in direct opposition to the value of respect for autonomy, but within the debate over what it means to respect autonomy in practice and where to draw the boundaries where the pursuit of this goal should give way to other values such as beneficence or nonmaleficence.

This is illustrated nicely in the case study, "Beneficence Today, or Autonomy (Maybe) Tomorrow?" in which a health care team disagrees over whether to wake a heavily sedated patient on a ventilator in order to inform her that she has terminal cancer and perhaps less than three months to live. For Bernice S. Elger, the fact that waking Monica may cause her physical distress and informing her of her terminal condition may cause psychological pain is of secondary importance in comparison to the need to give her a chance to make informed decisions about how she wants to face her illness and order her life in her remaining days. In contrast, Jean-Claude Chevrolet likens waking Monica and asking her to choose between several bleak options to subjecting her to a pointless medical intervention. For Chevrolet, Monica's situation is so bleak that her best interests would not be served by subjecting her to physical and mental anguish under the name of respect for her autonomy.

In this instance, Elger and Chevrolet agree that in ordinary situations, health care providers cannot legitimately restrict or dictate the conduct of competent adults for the sake of that person's own good. Their disagreement thus presupposes a common rejection of traditional medical paternalism. For Chevrolet, however, this is an extraordinary case. His suggestion that waking Monica to get her consent would be analogous to administering a pointless treatment harkens back to the well-worn idea in Hippocratic ethics that information ought to be treated like any other tool in the physician's black bag; it should be used sparingly and only to advance therapeutic goals. If Chevrolet thinks that this is a case in which it does not make sense to pursue the goal of facilitating patient autonomy, it may be because he conceives of the value of this goal in terms of its ultimate contribution to patient welfare. In most cases, respect for autonomy is an important element in achieving the more fundamental aim of ministering to the welfare of the patient, but not in this case. Similarly, if Elger thinks that it does make sense to try to facilitate Monica's ability to make important decisions about the end of her life, it may be because she thinks that the contribution of autonomy to patient welfare outweighs the physical and emotional distress that will come with it. Alternatively, however, it may be that Elger gives independent weight to the value of autonomy, quite apart from its contribution to patient welfare, and that her commitment to wake Monica is rooted not in a concern for her state of being (i.e., for her welfare), but for Monica as a person.

Placing respect for autonomy at the core of the provider-patient relationship represents the ideal of treating both providers and patients as responsible moral agents capable of making important decisions that will have a bearing on their lives. This has given rise to a model of the provider-patient relationship based on the metaphor of a contract or covenant. Contrary to the paternalistic or Hippocratic model, the patient is the party within the "contractual" relationship charged with making important value-laden decisions that will affect the overall direction of treatment. The physician is responsible for presenting the available treatment options to the patient and carrying out the details of the agreed-upon plan of care with professional expertise. Importantly, the physician retains his or her moral integrity within the contractual model and is not reduced to a mere "body mechanic" or "engineer" doing the bidding of patients. Since a contractual relationship is a two-way street, the physician may decide to terminate the relationship if, for example, the patient makes unreasonable demands or is flagrantly noncompliant with treatment (Veatch 1972). This contractual understanding of the physician-patient relationship has proven to be a powerful counterpoint to traditional physician ethics.

The idea that the value of respecting patient autonomy is richer and more complex than is captured by simple juxtapositions of "autonomy versus paternalism" is explored further by Ezekiel and Linda Emanuel in "Four Models of the Physician-Patient Relationship." The Emanuels present a typology of various models of the physician-patient relationship, including (1) the paternalistic model, (2) the informative model, (3) the interpretive model, and (4) the deliberative model. They also point out that all of the above models, excluding, of course, all frankly coercive approaches, accept some notion of autonomy, ranging from the mere acceptance of the doctor's recommendations to the more robust notion of moral learning and development in the deliberative model. Although there are few proponents of bald-faced paternalism today, there remains widespread debate about the nature and limits of autonomy, how it should be related to other aspects of a person's welfare, and how to respect it in the complex world of contemporary medicine.

Important threads of this debate are illustrated by the Emanuels. While their first model is the familiar Hippocratic approach, the second and third together constitute what others would call the "contractual approach." Their version of the informative model, however, makes a sharp distinction between facts and values, assigning the patient the role of decision maker concerning values and relegating the physician to the role of providing expert factual information to the patient. In this respect, it deviates from standard conceptions of the contractual model because it tends to reduce the physician to a mere tool of the patient's wishes.

The interpretive model, like the standard contractual approach, lodges final decision-making authority in the patient, but it emphasizes the problematic nature of discovering what the patient's values and preferences really are. Advocates of the contractual model often seem to assume, quite erroneously, that patients always know exactly how they feel and what they want in enormously complex and emotionally trying circumstances. In this interpretive model, by contrast, the doctor's role is analogous to that of a counselor who engages the patient in a mutual effort to understand what the patient's values really are and to discern which medical interventions will best advance those values.

The Emanuels' deliberative model encompasses the information-sharing and interpretive efforts of the previous models, but goes one controversial step further in recommending that the patient choose the "best" or "most admirable" course involving health-related values. Here the doctor's role is that of a teacher or moral guide who, though shunning coercive methods, recommends to the patient the medically best choice. For example, instead of simply laying out all the pros and cons of gluttony and smoking, a "deliberative" physician will directly recommend that the patient eat in moderation and stop smoking altogether. The directive aspect of their favored deliberative model, however, remains a point of controversy. Many readers might well wonder how physicians are to distinguish in-practice recommendations based upon "health-related values," which are permitted in this model, from those recommendations based on the physician's personal moral code, which are not permitted.

At one extreme, one must avoid confusing the need to respect physicians and patients as moral equals with the idea that physicians and patients are equally well situated in terms of their information, social position, familiarity with medical institutions, and other important personal and social capacities. The effective autonomy of many patients is compromised by illness, poverty, lack of education, social position, or by differences in cultural or ethnic background. For some, this means that respecting patient autonomy must involve actively facilitating a person's capacities for self-determination, rather than blithely assuming that they already exist.

At the other extreme, one must avoid holding an overintellectualized and one-dimensional view of what it means to be autonomous. In "Offering Truth," Benjamin Freedman argues that autonomous persons may decide that they want to be shielded from the truth or that they want to delegate responsibility for their care to loved ones. Rather than a zero-sum game, Freedman argues that responsible providers can offer their patients the opportunity to decide how much of the truth they want to be told and that this represents a reasonable middle ground between unjustified paternalism and a conception of respect for autonomy that bludgeons unprepared or vulnerable patients with blunt discussions of difficult news. This strategy also attempts to mediate cultural differences that may exist between groups that prize communal decision making and familial membership over individualism by offering patients an opportunity to decide which norms they are most comfortable with.

INFORMED CONSENT

The ethical cornerstone of the contractual and interpretive models is their insistence that the patient should make value-laden decisions bearing on his or her body and future life. The philosophical basis for this position is based on two distinct values: advancement of the patient's well-being and respect for the patient's autonomy. Partisans of the contractual and interpretive models contend that the patient, if adequately informed, is usually the best judge of his or her own best interests and should therefore possess the ultimate decision-making authority. Moreover, as Goldman points out, most of us value the ability to make decisions on our own behalf, quite apart from the consequences.

This ethical ideal of self-determination has received legal sanction in the doctrine of informed consent. As articulated by Justice Cardozo in a justly celebrated formulation in the case of *Schloendorff* v. *Society of New York Hospital* (1914), "Every adult human being of adult years and sound mind has a right to determine what shall be done with his own body. . . ." In order to consent freely, the patient must not be subject to any coercion or undue influence; and in order that the patient's consent be *informed*, the patient must, as we shall see in the readings, receive adequate information on which to base his or her choice. A final threshold condition for informed consent, in the words of Cardozo, is that the patient have a "sound mind" (a requirement that is addressed in Part 3, Section 2).

How much information is required in order to render the patient's consent truly informed? The law's attempt to answer this difficult question can be found in the 1972 California Supreme Court case of *Cobbs* v. *Grant*.

Mr. Cobbs, the plaintiff, had the misfortune of experiencing a number of remote "maloccurrences" incidental to his original surgery for a peptic ulcer. Since none of his physicians had warned him of any of these risks, Mr. Cobbs sued on the ground that his right to informed consent had been violated.

At the time he brought suit, however, the hapless Cobbs had little reason to think that his claim would hold up in court. In determining the scope of a physician's duty to inform patients, most American jurisdictions had adopted a "professional standard" approach that placed lay claimants at a severe disadvantage. Under this rule, a physician's conduct in disclosing information was to be judged by the standards actually observed by members of the local medical community. If it was not common practice to disclose a given risk, then the patient could not recover damages for breach of informed consent. Under this legal doctrine, good medical practice (as defined by the local medical community) made good law.

Cobbs sued nonetheless, arguing that the "professional standard" approach placed too much discretion in the hands of physicians. Happily for Cobbs, he again found himself on the cutting edge, but this time of a revolution in the law of informed consent. His case, *Cobbs* v. *Grant*, along with several others decided in the early 1970s, made the patient's right of self-determination the measure of the doctor's duty to reveal. Doctors were found to have a duty to disclose "all information relevant to a meaningful decisional process." Instead of asking, "What do physicians ordinarily disclose around here?" the *Cobbs* court asked, "What information would a competent patient need to make a reasonable decision?"

In response to those critics who debunk the informed consent requirement as a sheer impossibility, presiding Judge Mosk noted that a "minicourse" in medicine is not required, nor is a useless list of remote minor risks. Simply put, the patient must be told what a reasonable person would need to know about the procedure and its attendant risks in order to make a rational decision on the basis of his or her own values. In a passage strongly influenced by the contractual model, Mosk noted that the physician's expert *medical function* is limited to describing the nature of the procedure and its risks; the actual decision must incorporate those risks, must weigh them against a patient's values, hopes, and fears, and must therefore be left to the patient.

Against this historical background, in Section 2 we present two case studies designed both to probe the moral dimensions of informed consent law and to update the legal standard as enunciated in *Cobbs*. In the 1993 legal case *Arato* v. *Avedon*, the plaintiffs attempted to extend the law as articulated in *Cobbs* by charging that physicians had a duty to disclose not merely the risks of a certain medical procedure, but also the statistical likelihood of the patient's survival. Miklos Arato was a successful electrical contractor and real estate developer who was diagnosed at the age of 42 with pancreatic cancer. Acting on the advice of his physicians, Mr. Arato consented to an aggressive experimental course of surgery with combined chemotherapy and radiation. His doctors had informed him of the grave nature of this particular disease; the experimental nature of the treatment, including its risks and benefits; the incurable nature of the illness should it recur after surgery; and the option of doing nothing. However, they did not inform him of the very low statistical probability (approximately 1–5 percent) of patients with his diagnosis living another five years. Unfortunately, Mr. Arato died about one year after his surgery.

Mr. Arato's wife and family sued the physicians on the ground that their failure to reveal such a low statistical probability gave the patient false hopes of survival and prevented him from properly ordering his financial affairs to avoid the failure of his business enterprises. They claimed that, had he been properly informed, Mr. Arato would not have consented to such a rigorous and painful course of experimental treatment and would have had time to put his affairs in order. This lawsuit thus attempted to push the established boundaries of informed consent law in two ways. First, it attempted to expand physicians' duty of disclosure to include relevant prognostic information, preferably in the form of statistical odds of survival; second, it would have expanded the range of information deemed "material" to the patient's decision to include data concerning the relevance of his medical condition to his *nonmedical* interests, including his financial affairs. Although the California Court of Appeal sided with Mr. Arato's family, arguing that his consent was meaningless in the absence of some statistical information on the virulence of his particular cancer, the state Supreme Court reversed the decision and sided with the jury in refusing to impose these additional informational requirements on physicians. Students should ask themselves as they read this excerpt from the Supreme Court's decision whether this result is consistent with the spirit of an autonomy-inspired legal doctrine of informed consent.

In our second case study, "Antihypertensives and the Risk of Temporary Impotence," John D. Arras shows how difficult problems of information sharing arise not merely in high-profile surgical cases such as *Cobbs* and *Arato*, but also in the course of the undramatic and mundane practice of primary care medicine. This case asks whether a physician should inform a patient with high blood pressure that a cheap and effective medication also poses a very small risk of inducing temporary impotence, a risk that would be magnified by the very act of informing the patient.

The ethical and legal challenges posed by cases such as these have elicited a wide range of critical responses. Here we present two especially thoughtful but diverging critical responses from Jay Katz and Howard Brody. In his article "Informed Consent—Must It Remain a Fairy Tale?" Katz contends that the ethical ideal of self-determination at the core of informed consent has been resisted by medicine and distorted by the law. Contrary to those who view the advent of informed consent as the triumph of patient autonomy over medical paternalism, Katz shows how the framework of malpractice law has systematically betrayed the ethical ideal of self-determination out of deference to medical professionalism. Notwithstanding a brief flirtation with autonomy in cases like *Cobbs*, Katz argues that the law has fallen far short of its promise in reshaping the doctor-patient relationship. At most, he says, the law has created an expanded *duty to warn* rather than a more supportive context for patient decision making.

Although Katz would agree with critics who charge that the law's capacity for fundamental reform of the doctor-patient relationship is quite limited, and that real progress will most likely come (if at all) from a different kind of medical education, he nevertheless claims that the doctrine of informed consent has posed some very powerful and disturbing questions for the medical profession. In particular, he asks doctors to question whether their opposition to informed consent stems not merely from patients' alleged incompetence to handle harsh truths, but also perhaps from their own deep-seated reluctance to admit the widespread existence of medical uncertainty both to their patients and to themselves. For Katz, the ethical ideal of informed consent, as opposed to its legalistic trappings, is an appeal to the medical profession to discover new ways of relating to patients, new modes of communication that might foster hope on the basis of mutual respect rather than deceit.

Two points are particularly noteworthy about Katz's article. First, in stark contrast to courts and physicians, who tend to view informed consent either as a mere recitation of potential risks or, worse yet, as the signing of a form, Katz envisions true informed consent as a kind of searching conversation between patient and physician. Second, as to whether physicians ought to be required to converse with their patients about statistical probabilities, Katz sides with the lower court in *Arato* in holding that physicians should be required to inform patients of their dire prognosis and that patients have a right to make decisions not only about their bodies, but also about their lives.

In "Transparency: Informed Consent in Primary Care," physician-ethicist Howard Brody concurs with Katz that the courts' emphasis on a mere duty to warn patients of possible maloccurrences sends the wrong message to practicing physicians, prompting them only to ask, "Have I *told* the patient of everything that could possibly go wrong?" Moreover, Brody agrees with Katz that the notion of a conversation between doctor and patient nicely captures the ethical essence of the informed consent requirement. Brody worries, however, that this conversational norm is notoriously vague and slippery, thus making it difficult for physicians to determine just when they have properly discharged their legal duty to disclose. Although as an ethical matter it might be clear to a physician when any particular conversation has lasted sufficiently long and covered a sufficient number of topics for a patient to make a responsible decision, as a legal matter, Brody contends, such a subjective standard does not set for physicians a sufficiently determinate standard. So, without abandoning Katz's commitment to conversation, Brody suggests an alternative legal norm based on the notion of "transparency," which, he claims, should be especially useful in the context of primary care medicine, the field of Arras' case study. Brody contends that disclosure should be considered adequate when the physician's basic thinking about a decision and recommendation has been made clear or transparent to the patient. Thus, the doctor's duty is not merely to disclose what other reasonable practitioners would disclose, nor what a putative "reasonable patient" would want to know. Instead, the doctor must make her own reasoning clear to the patient, and then invite the patient to ask questions. The physician should facilitate the level of conversational participation desired by the patient. Although Brody's proposal has a number of virtues, including a somewhat more determinate legal standard than the one advocated by Katz, in practice it could conceivably reintroduce medical paternalism through the back door. While it would clearly obligate physicians to reveal the nature, gravity, and likelihood of any risks they considered in making up their own minds about any particular recommendations, Brody's standard could lead some physicians, such as Dr. Black in Arras' case study, to remain silent on aspects of a decision that they might dismiss as insignificant—such as the remote possibility of temporary, reversible impotence—but that any given patient might consider to be very important indeed.

CONFLICTING PROFESSIONAL ROLES AND RESPONSIBILITIES

The relationship between health professionals and patients provides the background against which the foregoing controversies are set. This might lead some readers to conclude that this context provides the sole source of the health professional's moral obligations. Such a conclusion, however, would be seriously mistaken. Although the Hippocratic tradition in medicine would have us believe that the physician's only obligation is to his or her patient, such a view ignores the complex relationships that obtain between health workers, as members of distinctive professions, and the social and cultural settings in which those professions exist. Even a cursory look at the Hippocratic oath belies this convenient image. Before the "moral core" of the oath in which the physician pledges to keep the sick from "harm and injustice," the physician binds himself to honor "him who has taught me this art as equal to my parents and to live my life in partnership with him, and if he is in need of money to give him a share of mine." Already in this ancient document there is an awareness of responsibilities that physicians incur, not in their role as healers, but insofar as they are members of a particular profession.

It is a fact of contemporary professional life that the health professional's obligations to his or her patients often conflict with duties to other parties—such as other members of the health care team, the patient's family, other patients, or persons who might be harmed in some way by the patient. In addition, physicians and other health professionals are increasingly employed by large institutions such as the armed forces, prisons, insurance companies, and corporations—whose goals have more to do with killing, retribution, and profits than with healing. When health workers act as "double agents" on behalf of both patients and agencies of social control, how should they resolve the inevitable conflicts of loyalty stemming from their conflicting roles? While we might think it appropriate for company physicians to report workers who pose a health hazard to other employees or to the public at large, what are we to think when psychiatrists are required to warn third parties about the violent tendencies of their patients, or when physicians are asked to administer capital punishment by means of lethal injections?

Section 3 explores some of the dimensions along which these conflicts may occur. In "Errors in Medicine: Nurturing Truthfulness," Françoise Baylis examines some of the considerations that prevent health care providers from openly revealing the occurrence of medical errors to their patients. The considerations are emblematic of the way that individual caregivers struggle, often in isolation, with their own fallibility and with a medical culture that tends to treat errors as moral as well as technical failures. A recent report on medical errors issued by the Institute of Medicine estimated that between 44,000 and 98,000 people die in U.S. hospitals annually as a result of medical errors. If these figures are accurate, medical mistakes surpass motor vehicle accidents, breast cancer, and AIDS as a cause of death in the United States. As a result, the Institute of Medicine report has generated a maelstrom of controversy and brought a public spotlight to the question of whether and to what extent medical professionals are obligated to disclose the occurrence of mistakes to patients or their families. It has also raised the issue of how mistakes ought to be dealt with inside the medical profession.

Disclosing medical mistakes can isolate a caregiver, making him or her subject to recrimination and scapegoating from colleagues while opening up the possibility of litigation from patients. In fact, many health professionals avoid disclosing mistakes to patients out of a fear of being sued, even though many patients report that a key factor in their decision to litigate was the perception that caregivers were being less than candid with them. Undoubtedly, the pursuit of individual excellence is a laudable and exemplary goal, but the activities of physicians, nurses, and other caregivers are often structured by larger systems, protocols, or routines which it may be possible to redesign in order to minimize the likelihood of error. The process of examining and testing these systems can only begin, however, with the recognition of deficiencies, and this will require a change in the way the medical profession, and the public it serves, think about fallibility. Sweeping mistakes under the institutional rug can foster a perception of concealment and incubate resentment that may erode public trust and rob health care teams of their best chance to learn and improve.

At the heart of the current controversy over how best to respond to medical errors is the need to facilitate open communication about human failings while safeguarding the fragile bond of trust between patients and health professionals. This trust is strained in a different way when the physician's duty to maintain confidentiality is pitted against the protection of third parties.

The obligation on the part of health professionals to maintain the confidentiality of patient information is grounded in part in the patient's right to control sensitive information about him- or herself—i.e., his right to privacy. Just as patients have a right to decide what happens to their bodies, they have a right to keep certain facts about themselves private. It is also grounded in the vital protection it provides, both to the interests of patients and to the very existence of the health professional-patient relationship. Due to the sensitive nature of the information shared in the medical context, patients are highly vulnerable to serious harm should that information fall into the hands of others. This is especially true of persons suffering from conditions that may be stigmatized by negative social stereotypes or associations. Given the still pervasive discrimination against persons who are HIV positive, for instance, medical confidentiality helps to shield patients from the loss of employment, insurance, and important human relationships.

Perhaps the most important function of confidentiality is to maintain the very possibility of a productive relationship between physicians and patients. If prospective patients distrust the willingness of physicians to keep secrets, they may not seek help in the first place. Even if they do enter into a treatment relationship, a lack of trust will often prevent patients from revealing important but potentially embarrassing information about clinical signs and symptoms. The caregiver's ability to heal and guide the patient thus depends on the maintenance of trust, but in the absence of confidentiality there can be no trust. Hence, confidentiality is a basic requirement of medical practice.

Although some might claim that this duty imposes an *absolute* requirement of fidelity to patients, it can conflict with equally compelling values and obligations, such as the duty to protect innocent third parties from harm. In the famous *Tarasoff* case, for example, psychotherapists were found to have a positive *legal duty* to violate confidentiality in order to protect a young woman, Tatiana Tarasoff, from the murderous intentions of their patient, Prosenjit Poddar. The California Supreme Court ruled that the public interest in safety and the peril to the woman's life outweighed the medical values of confidentiality and free communication between therapist and patient. Given the presence of a "determinate threat," the court ruled that therapists had a duty to exercise "reasonable care" to protect the intended victim.

In the *Tarasoff* case, the severity of the threatened harm was very grave (i.e., death), but its predictability became the point of heated debate within both the court and the psychiatric profession. Recognizing the difficulty of predicting dangerous behavior, the court merely required therapists to exercise "that reasonable degree of skill, knowledge, and care ordinarily possessed and exercised [by therapists] under similar circumstances." But critics of the court contended that psychiatrists and psychologists possessed no special "professional skill" of predicting violence and claimed that the court's ruling would prompt therapists to vastly overestimate the likelihood of violence.

The problems associated with accurately predicting possible harms to third parties arise again in "Please Don't Tell." For commentator Leonard Fleck, the likelihood that Consuela would contract HIV from caring for her brother Carlos is too remote to license breaching Carlos's confidentiality in order to inform her of his HIV-positive status. Instead, health professionals can discharge their duty to exercise reasonable care by instructing Consuela in the use of universal precautions, providing her with the necessary gloves, masks, goggles, and gowns, and insisting that she practice these measures when caring for Carlos.

Fleck is quick to note that, while members of the health care team treating Carlos have an obligation to safeguard information about his HIV-positive status and his sexual orientation, his sister would be under no such obligation, even though she would be acting as his nurse. For commentator Marcia Angell, however, the fact that Consuela is providing a service that normally would be provided by the health system entitles her to be informed of information that is material to her choice to care for her brother. In fact, Angell worries that not informing Consuela of her brother's HIV status would constitute a form of deception and would rob her of the chance to decide for herself what risks she is willing to assume in caring for her brother. Beneath Angell's assessment of this case lurks a tension between fulfilling the special duties that health professionals owe to their patients and fulfilling one's more general moral obligations to persons as such. Protecting Carlos's confidentiality respects his right to privacy. But is it achieved at the cost of deceiving or acting paternalistically toward Consuela, who is not a patient in this case, but who will be assuming the responsibilities of caring for Carlos at home?

Even if we conclude that medical professionals may set aside their oath of confidentiality in such cases, they will still have to confront a number of problems as they exercise their discretion or duty to warn. For example, when should efforts to persuade be abandoned and confidentiality finally violated? To whom does the provider owe this duty—only to named family members or named sexual partners or more broadly to friends and associates or all sexual partners the patient may have (with the added obligation to discover the identities of these persons)? As we consider the concrete implications of questions like these, the worries expressed by Justice Clark in the striking dissent to the majority in *Tarasoff* become more salient. In particular, will the imposition of a duty to warn deter those who are most in need of help from seeking it? Justice Clark's essentially rule-consequentialist argument is that a duty to violate the confidentiality of dangerous persons will most likely lead to more violence, not less, and that continued contact with health care professionals and voluntary persuasion are the best strategies for dealing with most conflicts between confidentiality and possible harms to third parties.

These cases pit the confidentiality of one patient against possible harms to nonpatient third parties. Advances in genetics and information sciences, however, may challenge the way we think about the provider-patient relationship as they expand the scope of the personal information that can be gathered in the health care setting, and the number of people regarded as "patients." In "Disclosing Misattributed Paternity" Lainie Friedman Ross discusses the ethical issues that arise when genetic tests for heritable medical conditions reveal that the male partner in a relationship is not the biological father of a child. As Ross notes, several recent studies show that genetic counselors are extremely reluctant to inform the male partner of misattributed paternity, even though his genetic material was used in the testing process and the resulting information may have important implications for his future procreative choices. Although, in such cases, each party contributes genetic material for testing, do genetic counselors have separate obligations to protect the confidentiality of each party individually? Even if they do, does the obligation to respect the woman's confidentiality justify withholding information from the male party that was gained in part through testing of his genetic material? To what extent, if any, should the decisions of counselors in these cases be based on estimates of the likely consequences that disclosing such information will have on the relationship between, or the individual well-being of, the persons involved? Similarly, how, if at all, should our deliberations about these issues take account of gender inequalities that persist in contemporary American culture?

When multiple persons with possibly diverging interests have the status of patient in a single case, as above, or when a patient poses a credible threat to the welfare of other persons, health professionals quickly find themselves struggling to honor conflicting moral obligations. While it may be possible to regard the sort of conflicts canvassed so far as relatively exceptional intrusions into the provider-patient relationship, there are other more systematic conflicts that cannot be so regarded. For many

Americans, managed care is perceived as threatening to undermine the ethical foundations of the provider-patient relationship by sacrificing the legitimate interests of patients at the altar of cost containment and, worse yet, corporate profit.

The traditional doctor-patient relationship has been well described as resting on an ethic of "personal care" (Fried 1974). According to this conception, the patient's vulnerability combines with the physician's expertise to yield a *fiduciary* relationship; that is, a relationship based not upon mere self-interest but on loyalty and concern for those in need. According to this ethic, well articulated by Norman Levinsky in "The Doctor's Master," the physician's primary loyalty is to the individual patient, not to the population at large or to other utilitarian abstractions such as "future patients" or "the future of medical science." When physicians have strayed from this ethic of personal care—as they did in Nazi Germany by forcing Jews and Gypsies to serve as subjects in lethal medical experiments (see Part 5, Section 1)—the results have tended to be scandalous and morally disastrous.

Today a serious and pervasive threat to this ethic of personal care is perceived to stem not so much from the errant motives of unethical researchers as from changes in the very organization and financing of health care. Gone are the days of unfettered "fee for service" medicine when doctors would be generously reimbursed for just about any kind of medical care they ordered for patients. While this system encouraged doctors always to do more for their patients, it was also a horribly wasteful and expensive system, full of incentives to overtreat. In its place, we have witnessed the birth and development of alternative financial arrangements, such as "managed care," in which public and private insurers exercise strict control over doctors' medical choices, and "health maintenance organizations" (HMOs), in which doctors are given incentives to contain costs by the prudent shepherding of medical resources.

Very recently, the demonizing of managed care has become something of a public, bipartisan blood sport and, while it would be unwise to overlook the ethical concerns generated by this new economic dispensation, it would be equally unwise to dismiss the very real ethical rationale behind such efforts at cost containment. As we will see in Part 2, the demand to increase access to health care, together with the high cost of new medicines and technologies, gives rise to an ethical imperative to control costs. Continued profligate spending will seriously undermine efforts to extend needed care to those who cannot presently gain access to it. How to expand access to quality health care while controlling costs in a way that is equitable, however, is a difficult and hotly debated issue. Of special concern is how to implement cost reduction strategies without systematically undermining the physician's duty of personal care to present, individual patients.

Suppose that you are the physician confronted by the dilemma sketched in "The HMO Physician's Duty to Cut Costs." You have concluded that an entirely patient-centered ethic of personal care would dictate prescribing the two drugs for your patient, one very cheap and the other very expensive. On the other hand, the HMO's physicians are under constant pressure to rein in costs by prescribing cheaper drugs whenever possible. You think your patient would be better off with the more expensive drug, but only marginally so. As a physician, you ask, "Is the small extra benefit worth the $400 cost differential per year? Would it be worth, say, an additional $16,000 spread out over the next 40 years?" Would it make a difference in your thinking if the managed care company would pass along a portion of the savings directly to you if you were able to decrease costs for this patient, and similarly for other patients in your practice?

According to Norman Levinsky, the doctor can and should serve only one "master," and that is the patient. Others might worry about cost containment and the percentage of the national budget spent on health care, but for Levinsky the doctor's entire loyalty belongs to the individual patient. E. Haavi Morreim, on the other hand, contends that the social and economic system that once supported Levinsky's ideal no longer exists, and that the doctor's traditional aloofness from the grubby realities of cost is no longer a tenable attitude. She argues that "fiscal scarcity"—i.e., the fact that there isn't enough money to pay for everything that medical science might provide for everyone—necessitates serious cost constraints, and that meaningful constraints will require some compromises with patient care at the bedside. Morreim concludes that the moral question for physicians today "is no longer whether to participate in cost containment, . . . but how to do so in morally credible ways."

The influence of managed care on the economics of medicine also raises troubling issues for the contractual model of the health professional-patient relationship. In a very important sense, the contractual model was not intended to replace the patient-centeredness of the traditional doctor-patient relationship, but to provide a corrective to a paternalism that often denied persons their dignity as free and equal moral agents in the name of ministering to their welfare. In fact, one could argue that the goal of the contractual model was to make the provider-patient relationship genuinely patient-centered by ensuring that patients themselves played a more active role in determining the course of their care. The contractual model was not intended to replace the fiduciary relationship between providers and patients with a standard, arm's length relationship that governs business contracts.

The more we see the provider-patient relationship as mediated by the terms of the actual contracts that patients and physicians each make with managed care companies or other third parties, however, the more the traditional physician-patient relationship looks like an ordinary business relationship. Perhaps one of the most disturbing consequences of this move is its implications for the most vulnerable and needy members of society. In "What Are We Teaching About Indigent Patients?" Steven H. Miles illustrates the way that current organizational and fiscal bureaucracies can conspire with the incentives to practice economically responsible medicine in order to produce a system that lavishes care on wealthy citizens while denying even the most basic services to the indigent.

For Miles, the point is not that we should expect the altruism and beneficence of medical professionals to fill the gaps of a medical system that fails to reach significant portions of the population. It is, rather, that we must not lose sight of the duties incurred by medical professionals to care for those in need, even when fulfilling this duty is attended by certain costs or dangers. One of the most serious deficiencies of the contractual model, then, is its inability to represent what Miles sees as an obligation not just to care for those with whom one contracts, but to enter into health care relationships with the vulnerable and the needy.

A fundamental question raised by this criticism of the contractual model, however, concerns the reasons we might have, if any, for treating health, or health care as morally special. Why not treat health care like other valuable commodities that are left to be distributed by the free market? It is to these issues that we turn in Part 2.

SECTION 1

AUTONOMY, PATERNALISM, AND MEDICAL MODELS

THE HIPPOCRATIC OATH

I swear by Apollo Physician and Asclepius and Hygieia and Panaceia and all the gods and goddesses, making them my witness, that I will fulfil according to my ability and judgment this oath and this covenant:

To hold him who has taught me this art as equal to my parents and to live my life in partnership with him, and if he is in need of money to give him a share of mine, and to regard his offspring as equal to my brothers in male lineage and to teach them this art—if they desire to learn it—without fee and covenant; to give a share of precepts and oral instruction and all the other learning to my sons and to the sons of him who has instructed me and to pupils who have signed the covenant and have taken an oath according to the medical law, but to no one else.

I will apply dietetic measures for the benefit of the sick according to my ability and judgment; I will keep them from harm and injustice.

I will neither give a deadly drug to anybody if asked for it, nor will I make a suggestion to this effect. Similarly I will not give to a woman an abortive remedy. In purity and holiness I will guard my life and my art.

I will not use the knife, not even on sufferers from stone, but will withdraw in favor of such men as are engaged in this work.

Whatever houses I may visit, I will come for the benefit of the sick, remaining free of all intentional injustice, of all mischief and in particular of sexual relations with both female and male persons, be they free or slaves.

What I may see or hear in the course of the treatment or even outside of the treatment in regard to the life of men, which on no account one must spread abroad, I will keep to myself holding such things shameful to be spoken about.

If I fulfil this oath and do not violate it, may it be granted to me to enjoy life and art, being honored with fame among all men for all time to come; if I transgress it and swear falsely, may the opposite of all this be my lot.

From Ludwig Edelstein, *Ancient Medicine: Selected Papers of Ludwig Edelstein*. Owsei Temkin and C. Lillian Temkin, eds., Baltimore, MD: Johns Hopkins University Press, 1967.

THE REFUTATION OF MEDICAL PATERNALISM

Alan Goldman

In the case of doctors the question is whether they have the authority to make decisions for others that they would lack as nonprofessionals. The goal of providing optimal health treatment may be seen to conflict in some circumstances with the otherwise overriding duties to tell the patient the truth about his condition or to allow him to make decisions vitally affecting his own interests. Again the assumption of the profession itself appears to be that the doctor's role is strongly differentiated in this sense. The Principles of Medical Ethics of the American Medical Association leaves the question of informing the patient of his own condition up to the professional judgment of the physician, presumably in relation to the objective of maintaining or improving the health or well-being of the patient.[1] I shall concentrate upon these issues of truth telling and informed consent to treatment in the remainder of this chapter. They exemplify our fundamental issue because the initially obvious answer to the question of who should make decisions or have access to information vital to the interests of primarily one person is that person himself.[2]

Rights are recognized, we have said, partially to permit individuals control over their own futures. Regarding decisions vital to the interests of only particular individuals, there are three main reasons why such decisions should normally be left to the individuals themselves, two want-regarding and one ideal-regarding. First is the presumption of their being the best judges of their own interests, which may depend upon personal value orderings known only to them. There is often a temptation for others to impose their own values and preferences, but this would be less likely to produce satisfaction for the individuals concerned. The second reason is the independent value of self-determination, at least in regard to important decisions (in medical contexts decisions may involve life and death alternatives, affect the completion of major life projects, or affect bodily integrity). Persons desire the right or freedom to make their own choices, and satisfaction of this desire is important in itself. In addition, maximal freedom for individuals to develop their own projects, to make the pivotal choices that define them and to act to realize them, allows for the development of unique creative personalities, who become sources of new value in the goods they create and that they and others enjoy.

Resentment as well as overall harm is therefore generally greater when caused by a wrong, even if well-meaning, decision of another than when caused to oneself. There is greater chance that the other person will fail to realize one's own values in making the decision, and, when this happens, additional resentment that one was not permitted the freedom to decide. Thus, since individuals normally have rights to make decisions affecting the course of their lives and their lives alone, doctors who claim authority to make medical decisions for them that fall into this self-regarding category are claiming special authority. The normally existing right to self-determination implies several more specific rights in the medical context. These include the right to be told the truth about one's condition, and the right to accept or refuse or withdraw from treatment on the basis of adequate information regarding alternatives, risks and uncertainties. If doctors are permitted or required by the principle of providing optimal treatment, cure or health maintenance for patients sometimes to withhold truth or decide on their own what therapeutic measures to employ, then the Hippocratic principle overrides important rights to self-determination that would otherwise obtain, and the practice of medicine is strongly role differentiated.

This is clear enough in the case of informed consent to therapy; it should be equally clear in the case of withholding truth, from terminally ill patients for

---

From *The Moral Foundations of Professional Ethics* by Alan Goldman, Rowman and Littlefield, 1980. Reprinted by permission of the publisher.

Editors' note: Sections of this essay have been omitted, and the notes have been renumbered.

example. The right violated or overridden when truth is withheld in medical contexts is not some claim to the truth per se, but this same right to self-determination, to control over decisions vital to the course of one's life. In fact, it seems on the face of it that there is a continuum of medical issues in which this right figures prominently. These range from the question of consent to being used as a subject in an experiment designed primarily to benefit others, to consent to treatment intended as benefit to the patient himself, to disclosure of information about the patient's condition. In the first case, that of medical experimentation, if the consent of subjects is required (as everyone these days admits it is), this is partly because the duty not to harm is stronger than the duty to provide benefits. Hence if there is any risk of harm at all to subjects, they cannot be used without consent, even if potential benefits to others is great. But consent is required also because the right to self-determination figures independently of calculations of harms and benefits. Thus a person normally ought not to be used without his consent to benefit others even if he is not materially harmed. This same right clearly opposes administration of treatment to patients without their consent for their own benefit. It opposes as well lying to patients about their illnesses in order to save them distress.

What is at least prima facie wrong with lying in such cases is that it shifts power to decide future courses of action away from the person to whom the lie is told.[3] A person who is misinformed about his own physical condition may not complete certain projects or perform certain actions that he would choose to perform in full knowledge. If a person is terminally ill and does not know it, for example, he may fail to arrange his affairs, prepare himself for death, or may miss opportunities to complete projects or seek certain experiences always put off before. Being lied to can reduce or prevent from coming into view options that would otherwise be live. Hence it is analogous to the use of force, perhaps more coercive than the use of force in that there is not the same chance to resist when the barrier is ignorance. The right to know the truth in this context then derives from the right to make for oneself important decisions relating primarily to one's own welfare and to the course of one's life. If the doctor's authority is to be augmented beyond that of any nonprofessional, allowing him to override these important rights in contexts in which this is necessary to prevent serious harm to the patient's health, then his position appears to meet in a dramatic way our criteria for strong role differentiation.

THE CASE FOR MEDICAL PATERNALISM

Since the primary rights in potential conflict with the presumed fundamental norm of medical ethics are rights of patients themselves, and since the norm seeks to serve the health needs of patients themselves, arguments in favor of strong role differentiation in this context are clearly paternalistic. We may define paternalism as the overriding or restricting of rights or freedoms of individuals for their own good. It can be justified even for competent adults in contexts in which they can be assumed to act otherwise against their own interests, values, or true preferences. Individuals might act in such self-defeating ways from ignorance of the consequences of their actions, from failure to weigh the probabilities of various consequences correctly, or from irrational barriers to the operation of normal short-term motivations. Paternalistic measures may be invoked when either the individual in question, or any rational person with adequate knowledge of the situation, would choose a certain course of conduct, and yet this course is not taken by the individual solely because of ignorance, carelessness, fear, depression, or other uncontroversially irrational motives.[4]

Paradigm Cases

It will be useful in evaluating arguments for strong role differentiation for doctors to look first at criteria for justified paternalism in nonmedical cases, in order to see then if they are met in the medical context. In approaching the controversial case of withholding truth from patients, we may begin with simpler paradigm cases in which paternalistic behavior is uncontroversially permissible or required. We can derive a rule from these cases for the justification of such conduct and then apply the rule to decide this fundamental question of medical ethics.

The easiest cases to justify are those in which a person is acting against even his immediate desires out of ignorance: Dick desires to take a train to New York, is about to board the train for Boston on the other side of the platform, and, without time to warn him, he can only be grabbed and shoved in the other direction. Coercing him in this way is paternalistic, since it overrides his right of free movement for his own good. "His own good" is uncontroversial in interpretation in this easiest case. It is defined by his own clearly stated immediate and long-range preferences (the two are not in conflict here). Somewhat more difficult are cases in which persons voluntarily act in ways inconsistent with their long-range preferences: Jane does not desire to be seriously injured or to increase greatly her chances of serious injury for trivial reasons; yet, out of carelessness, or just because she considers it a nuisance and fails to apply statistical probabilities to her own case, she does not wear a helmet when riding a motorcycle. Here it might be claimed that, while her action is voluntary in relation to trivial short-term desires, it is nevertheless not fully voluntary in a deeper sense. But to make this claim we must be certain of the person's long-range preferences, of the fact that her action is inconsistent with these preferences (or else uncontroversially inconsistent with the preferences of any rational person). We must predict that the person herself is likely to be grateful in the long run for the additional coercive motivation. In this example we may assume these criteria to be met. For rational people, not wearing a helmet is not an essential feature in the enjoyment of riding a motorcycle, even if people ride them primarily for the thrill rather than for the transportation. The chances are far greater that a rider will at some time fall or be knocked off the cycle and be thankful for having a helmet than that one will prefer serious head injury to the inconvenience of wearing protection that can prevent such injury. Therefore we may justifiably assume that a person not wearing a helmet is not acting in light of her own true long-range values and preferences.

As the claim that the individual's action is not truly voluntary or consistent with his preferences or values becomes more controversial, additional criteria for justified paternalism must come into play. They become necessary to outweigh the two considerations mentioned earlier: the presumption that individuals know their own preferences best (that interference will be more often mistaken than not), and that there is an important independent value to self-determination or individual freedom and control (the latter being true both because persons value freedom and because such freedom is necessary to the development of genuinely individual persons). The additional criteria necessary for justifying paternalism in more controversial cases relate to the potential harm to the person from the action in question: it must be relatively certain, severe, and irreversible (relative to the degree of coercion contemplated). These further criteria are satisfied as well in the case of motorcycle helmets, because the action coerced is only a minor nuisance in comparison to the severity of potential harm and the degree of risk.

It is important for the course of the later argument to point out that these additional criteria relating to the harm that may result from self-regarding actions need not be viewed in terms of a simple opposition between allowing freedom of action and preventing harm. It is not simply that we can override a person's autonomy when in our opinion the potential harm to him from allowing autonomous decision outweighs the value of his freedom. His right to self-determination, fundamental to individuality itself, bars such offsetting calculations. The magnitude of harm is rather to be conceived as *evidence* that the person is not acting in accord with *his own* values and preferences, that he is not acting autonomously in the deepest sense. A rights-based moral theory of the type I am assuming as the framework for this study will view the autonomy of the individual as more fundamental than the particular goods he enjoys or harms he may suffer. The autonomous individual is the source of value for those other goods he enjoys and so not to be sacrificed for the sake of them. The point here is that cases of justified paternalism, even where the agent's immediate or short-term preferences are overridden, need not be viewed as reversing that order of priority.

Criteria for justified paternalism are also clearly satisfied in certain medical contexts, to return to the immediate issue at hand. State control over physician licensing and the requirement that prescriptions be obtained for many kinds of drugs are medical cases in point. Licensing physicians prevents some quacks from harming other persons, but also limits these persons' freedom of choice for their own good. Hence it is paternalistic. We may assume that no rational person would want to be treated by a quack or to take drugs that are merely harmful, but that many people would do so in the absence of controls out of ignorance or irrational hopes or fears. While controls impose costs and bother upon people that may be considerable in the case of having to see a doctor to obtain medication, these are relatively minimal in comparison to the certainty, severity and irreversibility of the harm that would result from drugs chosen by laymen without medical assistance. Such controls are therefore justified, despite the fact that in some cases persons might benefit from seeing those who could not obtain licenses or from choosing drugs themselves. We can assume that without controls mistakes would be made more often than not, that serious harm would almost certainly result, and that people really desire to avoid such harm even given additional costs.

There is another sense too in which paternalistic measures here should not be viewed as prevention of exclusively self-regarding harm by restriction of truly autonomous actions. The harm against which laymen are to be protected in these cases, while deriving partly from their own actions in choosing physicians or drugs, can be seen also as imposed by others in the absence of controls. It results from the deception practiced by unqualified physicians and unscrupulous drug manufacturers. Hence controls, rather than interfering with autonomous choice by laymen, help to prevent deceptive acts of others that block truly free choice.[5] This is not to say that some drugs now requiring prescriptions could not be safely sold over the counter at reduced cost, or that doctors have not abused their effective control over entrance to the profession by restraining supply in relation to demand, maintaining support for exorbitant prices. Perhaps controls could be imposed in some other way than by licensing under professional supervision. This issue is beyond our scope here. The point for us is that some such restraints appear to be necessary. Whichever form they take, they will be paternalistic, justifiably so, in their relation to free patient choice.

We have now defined criteria for justified paternalism from considering certain relatively easy examples or paradigm cases. The principal criterion is that an individual be acting against *his own* predominant long-range value preferences, or that a strong likelihood exist that he will so act if not prevented. Where either clause is controversial, we judge their truth by the likelihood and seriousness of the harm to the person risked by his probable action. It must be the case that this harm would be judged clearly worse from the point of view of the person himself than not being able to do what we prevent him from doing by interfering. Only if the interference is in accord with the person's real desires in this way is it justified. Our question now is whether these criteria are met in the more controversial medical cases we are considering, those of doctors' withholding truth or deciding upon courses of treatment on their own to prevent serious harm to the health of their patients.

Application of the Criteria to Medical Practice

The argument that the criteria for justified paternalism are satisfied in these more controversial medical cases begins from the premise that the doctor is more likely to know the course of treatment optimal for improving overall health or prolonging life than is his patient. The patient will be comparatively ignorant of his present condition, alternative treatments, and risks, even when the doctor makes a reasonable attempt to educate him on these matters. More important, he is apt to be emotional and fearful, inclined to hold out false hope for less painful treatments with little real chance of cure, or to despair of the chance for cure when that might still be real. In such situations it again could be claimed, as in the examples from the previous subsection, that patient choice in any event would not be truly voluntary. A person is likely to act according to his true long-range values only when his decision is calm, unpressured, and informed or knowledgeable. A seriously ill person is unlikely to satisfy these conditions for free choice. Choice unhindered by others is nevertheless not truly free when determined by internal factors, among them fear, ignorance, or other irrational motivation, which result in choice at variance with the individual's deeper preferences. In such circumstances interference is not to be criticized as restrictive of freedom.

The second premise states that those who consult doctors really desire to be cured above all else. Health and the prolonging of life may be assumed (according to this argument) to have priority among values for any rational person, since they are necessary conditions for the realization of almost every other personal value. While such universally necessary means ought to have priority in personal value orderings, persons may again fail to act on such orderings out of despair or false hope, or simply lack of knowledge, all irrational barriers to genuinely voluntary choice. When they fail to act rationally in medical contexts, the harm may well be serious, probable and irreversible. Hence another criterion for justified paternalism appears to be met; we have another sign that the probable outcome in these circumstances of unhindered choice is not truly desired, hence the choice not truly voluntary.

While it is possible that a doctor's prognosis might be mistaken, this can be argued to support further rather than weaken the argument for paternalism. For if the doctor is mistaken, this will infect the patient's decision-making process as well, since his appreciation of the situation can only fall short of that of his source of information. Furthermore, bad prognoses may tend to be self-fulfilling when revealed, even if their initial probability of realization is slight. A positive psychological attitude on the part of the patient often enhances chances for cure even when they are slight; and a negative attitude, which might be incurred from a mistaken prognosis or from fear of an outcome with otherwise low probability, might increase that probability. In any case it can be argued that a bad prognosis is more likely to depress the patient needlessly than to serve a positive medical purpose if revealed. The doctor will most likely be able to convince the patient to accept the treatment deemed best by the doctor even after all risks are revealed. The ability to so convince might well be conceived as part of medical competence to provide optimal treatment. If the doctor knows that he can do so in any case, why needlessly worry or depress the patient with discussion of risks that are remote, or at least more remote or less serious than those connected with alternative treatments? Their revelation is unlikely to affect the final decision, but far more likely to harm the patient. It therefore would appear cruel for the doctor not to assume responsibility for the decision or for remaining silent on certain of its determining factors.

Thus all the criteria for justified paternalism might appear to be met in the more controversial cases as well. The analogies with our earlier examples appear to support overriding the patient's right to decide on the basis of the truth by the fundamental medical principle of providing optimal care and treatment. Let us apply this argument more specifically to . . . the case of withholding truth when no other medical decisions remain to be made, when the question is what to tell the terminally ill patient for example. Here recognition of an absolute right of the patient is likely to result in needless mental suffering and even in some cases hasten death. The dying patient is likely to realize at a certain point that he is dying without having to be informed. If he does realize it, blunt and open discussion of the fact may nevertheless be depressing. What appear to be pointless deceptive games played out between patients and relatives in avoiding such discussion may actually express delicate defense mechanisms whose solace may be destroyed by the doctor's intrusion. When the doctor has no reason to predict such detrimental effects, then perhaps he ought to inform. But why do so when this is certain to cause needless additional suffering or harm? To do so appears not only wrong, but cruel.

We certainly are justified in lying to a person in order to prevent serious harm to another. If I must lie to someone in order to save the life of another whom the first person might kill if told the truth (even if the killing would be nonintentional), there is no doubt at all that I should tell the lie or withhold the information. Rights to be told the truth are not absolute, but, like all rights, must be ordered in relation to others. If I may lie to one person to save another from harm, why not then when the life of the person himself might be threatened or seriously worsened by the truth, as it might be in the medical contexts we are considering? Why should the fact that only one person is involved, that only the person himself is likely to be harmed by the truth, alter the duty to deceive or withhold information in order to prevent the more serious harm? If it is replied that when only one person is involved, that person is likely to know the best course of action for himself, the answer is that in medical contexts this claim appears to be false. The doctor is likely to be better informed than the patient about his condition and the optimal treatments for it.

Thus there are two situations in which the doctor's duty not to harm his patient's health or shorten his life might appear to override otherwise obtaining rights of the patients to the full truth. One is where the truth will cause direct harm—depression or loss of continued will to live. The other is where informing may be instrumentally harmful in leading to the choice of the wrong treatment or none at all. Given that information divulged to the patient may be harmful or damaging to his health, may interfere with other aspects of optimal or successful treatment, it is natural to construe what the doctor tells the patient as an aspect of the treatment itself. As such it would be subject to the same risk-benefit analysis as other aspects. Doctors must constantly balance uncertain benefits and risks in trying to provide treatment that will maximize the probability of cure with least damaging side effects. Questions regarding optimal treatment are questions for medical expertise. Since psychological harm must figure in the doctor's calculations if he is properly sensitive, since it may contribute as well to physical deterioration, and since what he says to a patient may cause such harm, it seems that the doctor must construe what he *says* to a patient as on a par with what he *does* to him, assuming full responsibility for any harm that may result. Certainly many doctors do so conceive of questions of disclosure. A clear example of this assimilation to questions regarding treatment is the following:

> From the foregoing it should be self-evident that what is imparted to a patient about his illness should be planned with the same care and executed with the same skill that are demanded by any potentially therapeutic measure. Like the transfusion of blood, the dispensing of certain information must be distinctly indicated, the amount given consonant with the needs of the recipient, and the type chosen with the view of avoiding untoward reactions.[6]

When the patient places himself in the care of a physician, he expects the best and least harmful treatment, and the physician's fundamental duty, seemingly overriding all others in the medical context, must be to provide such treatment. Indeed the terminology itself, "under a physician's care," suggests acceptance of the paternalistic model of strong role differentiation. To care for someone is to provide first and foremost for that person's welfare.[7] The doctor ministers to his patient's needs, not to his immediate preferences. If this were not the case, doctors would be justified in prescribing whatever drugs their patients requested. That a person needs care suggests that, at least for the time being, he is not capable of being physically autonomous; and given the close connection of physical with mental state, the emotional stress that accompanies serious illness, it is natural to view the patient as relinquishing autonomy over medical decisions to the expert for his own good. Being under a physician's care entails a different relationship from that involved in merely seeking another person's advice.

THE REFUTATION OF MEDICAL PATERNALISM

In order to refute an argument, we of course need to refute only one of its premises. The argument for medical paternalism, stripped to its barest outline, was:

1. Disclosure of information to the patient will sometimes increase the likelihood of depression and physical deterioration, or result in choice of medically inoptimal treatment.
2. Disclosure of information is therefore sometimes likely to be detrimental to the patient's health, perhaps even to hasten his death.
3. Health and prolonged life can be assumed to have priority among preferences for patients who place themselves under physicians' care.
4. Worsening health or hastening death can therefore be assumed to be contrary to patients' own true value orderings.
5. Paternalism is therefore justified: doctors may sometimes override patients' prima facie rights to information about risks and treatments or about their own conditions in order to prevent harm to their health.

The Relativity of Values: Health and Life

The fundamentally faulty premise in the argument for paternalistic role differentiation for doctors is that which assumes that health or prolonged life must take absolute priority in the patient's value orderings. In order for paternalistic interference to be justified, a person must be acting irrationally or inconsistently with his own long-range preferences. The value ordering violated by the action to be prevented must either be known to be that of the person himself, as in the train example, or else be uncontroversially that of any rational person, as in the motorcycle helmet case. But can we assume that health and prolonged life have top priority in any rational ordering? *If* these values could be safely assumed to be always overriding for those who seek medical assistance, then medical expertise would become paramount in decisions regarding treatment, and decisions on disclosure would become assimilated to those within the treatment context. But in fact very few of us act according to such an assumed value ordering. In designing social policy we do not devote all funds or efforts toward minimizing loss of life, on the highways or in hospitals for example.

If our primary goal were always to minimize risk to health and life, we should spend our entire federal budget in health-related areas. Certainly such a suggestion would be ludicrous. We do not in fact grant to individuals rights to minimal risk in their activities or to absolutely optimal health care. From another perspective, if life itself, rather than life of a certain quality with autonomy and dignity, were of ultimate value, then even defensive wars could never be justified. But when the quality of life and the autonomy of an entire nation is threatened from without, defensive war in which many lives are risked and lost is a rational posture. To paraphrase Camus, anything worth living for is worth dying for. To realize or preserve those values that give meaning to life is worth the risk of life itself. Such fundamental values (and autonomy for individuals is certainly among them), necessary within a framework in which life of a certain quality becomes possible, appear to take precedence over the value of mere biological existence.

In personal life too we often engage in risky activities for far less exalted reasons, in fact just for the pleasure or convenience. We work too hard, smoke, exercise too little or too much, eat what we know is bad for us, and continue to do all these things even when informed of their possibly fatal effects. To doctors in their roles as doctors all this may appear irrational, although they no more act always to preserve their own health than do the rest of us. If certain risks to life and health are irrational, others are not. Once more the quality and significance of one's life may take precedence over maximal longevity. Many people when they are sick think of nothing above getting better; but this is not true of all. A person with a heart condition may decide that important unfinished work or projects must take priority over increased risk to his health; and his priority is not uncontroversially irrational. Since people's lives derive meaning and fulfillment from their projects and accomplishments, a person's risking a shortened life for one more fulfilled might well justify actions detrimental to his health. . . .

To doctors in their roles as professionals whose ultimate concern is the health or continued lives of patients, it is natural to elevate these values to ultimate prominence. The death of a patient, inevitable as it is in many cases, may appear as an ultimate defeat to the medical art, as something to be fought by any means, even after life has lost all value and meaning for the patient himself. The argument in the previous section for assuming this value ordering was that health, and certainly life, seem to be necessary conditions for the realization of all other goods or values. But this point, even if true, leaves open the question of whether health and life are of ultimate, or indeed any, intrinsic value, or whether they are valuable *merely* as means. It is plausible to maintain that life itself is not of intrinsic value, since surviving in an irreversible coma seems no better than death. It therefore again appears that it is the quality of life that counts, not simply being alive. Although almost any quality might be preferable to none, it is not irrational to trade off quantity for quality, as in any other good.

Even life with physical health and consciousness may not be of intrinsic value. Consciousness and health may not be sufficient in themselves to make the life worth living, since some states of consciousness are intrinsically good and others bad. Furthermore, if a person has nothing before him but pain and depression, then the instrumental worth of being alive may be reversed. And if prolonging one's life can be accomplished only at the expense of incapacitation or ignorance, perhaps preventing lifelong projects from being completed, then the instrumental value of longer life again seems overbalanced. It is certainly true that normally life itself is of utmost value as necessary for all else of value, and that living longer usually enables one to complete more projects and plans, to satisfy more desires and derive more enjoyments. But this cannot be assumed in the extreme circumstances of severe or terminal illness. Ignorance of how long one has left may block realization of such values, as may treatment with the best chance for cure, if it also risks incapacitation or immediate death.

Nor is avoidance of depression the most important consideration in such circumstances, as a shallow hedonism might assume. Hedonistic theories of value, which seek only to produce pleasure or avoid pain and depression, are easily disproven by our abhorrence at the prospect of a "brave new world," or our unwillingness, were it possible, to be plugged indefinitely into a "pleasure machine." The latter prospect is abhorrent not only from an ideal-regarding viewpoint, but, less obviously, for want-regarding reasons (for most persons) as well. Most people would in fact be unwilling to trade important freedoms and accomplishments for sensuous pleasures, or even for the illusion of greater freedoms and accomplishments. As many philosophers have pointed out, while satisfaction of wants may bring pleasurable sensations, wants are not primarily *for* pleasurable sensations, or even for happiness more broadly construed, per se. Conversely, the avoidance of negative feelings or depression is not uppermost among primary motives. Many people are willing to endure frustration, suffering, and even depression in pursuit of accomplishment, or in order to complete projects once begun. Thus information relevant to such matters, such as medical information about one's own condition or possible adverse effects of various treatments, may well be worth having at the cost of psychological pain or depression.

The Value of Self-Determination

We have so far focused on the inability of the doctor to assume a particular value ordering for his patient in which health, the prolonging of life, or the avoidance of depression is uppermost. The likelihood of error in this regard makes it probable that the doctor will not know the true interests of his patient as well as the patient himself. He is therefore less likely than the patient himself to make choices in accord with that overall interest, and paternalistic assumption of authority to do so is therefore unjustified. There is in addition another decisive consideration mentioned earlier, namely the independent value of self-determination or freedom of choice. Personal autonomy over important decisions in one's life, the ability to attempt to realize one's own value ordering, is indeed so important that normally no amount of other goods, pleasures or avoidance of personal evils can take precedence. This is why it is wrong to contract oneself into slavery, and another reason why pleasure machines do not seem attractive. Regarding the latter, even if people were willing to forgo other goods for a life of constant pleasure, the loss in variety of other values, and in the creativity that can generate new sources of value, would be morally regrettable. The value of self-determination explains also why there is such a strong burden of proof upon those who advocate paternalistic measures, why they must show that the person would otherwise act in a way inconsistent with his own value ordering, that is, irrationally. A person's desires are not simply evidence of what is in his interest—they have extra weight.

Especially when decisions are important to the course of our lives, we are unwilling to relinquish them to others, even in exchange for a higher probability of happiness or less risk of suffering. Even if it could be proven, for example, that some scientific method of matching spouses greatly increased chances of compatibility and happiness, we would insist upon retaining our rights over marriage decisions. Given the present rate of success in marriages, it is probable that we could in fact find some better method of matching partners in terms of increasing that success rate. Yet we are willing to forgo increased chances of success in order to make our own choices, choices that tend to make us miserable in the long run. The same might be true of career choices, choices of schools, and others central to the course of our lives. Our unwillingness to delegate these crucial decisions to experts or computers, who might stand a better chance of making them correctly (in terms of later satisfactions), is not to be explained simply in terms of our (sometimes mistaken) assumptions that we know best how to satisfy our own interests, or that we personally will choose correctly, even though most other people do not. If our retaining such authority for ourselves is not simply irrational, and I do not believe it is, this can only be because of the great independent value of self-determination. We value the exercise of free choice itself in personally important decisions, no matter what the effects of those decisions upon other satisfactions. The independent value of self-determination in decisions of great personal importance adds also to our reluctance to relinquish medical decisions with crucial effects on our lives to doctors, despite their medical expertise.

Autonomy or self-determination is independently valuable, as argued before, first of all because we value it in itself. But we may again add to this want-regarding or utilitarian reason a second ideal-regarding or perfectionist reason. What has value does so because it is valued by a rational and autonomous person. But autonomy itself is necessary to the development of such valuing individual persons or agents. It is therefore not to be sacrificed to other derivative values. To do so as a rule is to destroy the ground for the latter. Rights in general not only express and protect the central interests of individuals (the raison d'être usually emphasized in their exposition); they also express the dignity and inviolability of individuality itself. For this reason the most fundamental right is the right to control the course of one's life, to make decisions crucial to it, including decisions in life-or-death medical contexts. The other side of the independent value of self-determination from the point of view of the individual is the recognition of him by others, including doctors, as an individual with his own possibly unique set of values and priorities. His dignity demands a right to make personal decisions that express those values. . .

NOTES

1. American Medical Association, *Principles of Medical Ethics.*
2. I restrict discussion for the time being to competent adults. I assume for now that if they have rights to information or to make their own decisions in medical contexts, then parents or guardians, not doctors, have these same rights in relation to children or the mentally incapacitated.
3. Compare Sissela Bok, *Lying* (New York: Pantheon, 1978), pp. 18–19.
4. See Gerald Dworkin, "Paternalism," in R. Wasserstrom, ed., *Morality and the Law* (Belmont, Cal.: Wadsworth, 1971).
5. Compare Norman Cantor, "A Patient's Decision to Decline Life-Saving Medical Treatment: Bodily Integrity Versus the Preservation of Life," in T. Beauchamp and S. Perlin, eds., *Ethical Issues in Death and Dying* (Englewood Cliffs, N.J.: Prentice-Hall, 1978), pp. 208–209.
6. Bernard Meyer, "Truth and the Physician," in Beauchamp and Perlin, eds., op. cit., p. 160.
7. Compare A. R. Jonsen, "Do No Harm: Axiom of Medical Ethics," *Philosophy and Medicine* 3 (1977): 27–41, p. 30.

BENEFICENCE TODAY, OR AUTONOMY (MAYBE) TOMORROW?

Monica, a forty-nine-year-old divorced mother of two children in their early twenties, was admitted to the hospital for acute respiratory insufficiency on a Friday evening. She is a heavy smoker and had experienced dyspnea for several weeks previously, but had not sought medical advice. Chest x-ray revealed several abnormalities and a bronchoscopy was scheduled for Monday morning.

On Saturday evening Monica's difficulty breathing worsened and during a heavy cough of sudden onset she became cyanotic and nearly lost consciousness. The physician on call performed an emergency intubation and transferred her to the intensive care unit, where she was heavily sedated. On Sunday, a bronchoscopy was performed, revealing a large, tumor-like mass in her trachea. Biopsies were taken from the mass, and from a palpable lymph node. On Monday the pathologist confirmed the presence of tumor cells and a diagnosis was made of a poorly differentiated squamous cell carcinoma of the lungs metastatic to the lymph node.

The multidisciplinary treatment team agreed that the tumor is inoperable (by either surgery or laser) and chemotherapy and radiation therapy are of unproven benefit. Monica cannot be extubated because the tumor will immediately obstruct her airway, and tracheostomy would be very risky—and probably not feasible—given the size of the tumor. Implanting a stent would also be difficult with so advanced a tumor. The team believes Monica's life expectancy is no more than three months.

The team discussed the following alternatives for Monica's care: they could withdraw life-sustaining measures; continue mechanical ventilation and heavy sedation but not treat any complications, such as infection, that arise; persuade (or coerce) the surgeon to implant a stent without consulting Monica; or wake Monica so that the team could discuss the diagnosis and prognosis with her and ascertain her preferences among the treatment alternatives.

The team is concerned that Monica will not really be able to make an informed, autonomous decision if they wake her. They worry that being intubated without sedation will impose further suffering for Monica, only to allow them to impart a grim prognosis. Should they wake her, or should they make treatment decisions on her behalf?

COMMENTARY

Bernice S. Elger

When Monica lost consciousness she knew only that she was in the hospital to be treated for an acute lung problem. We do not know why she did not seek treatment earlier—did she perhaps fear lung cancer? Even if she did, she cannot be supposed to be aware of the severity of her illness and of the small amount of time left to her to live.

The principle of autonomy, so central to modern biomedical ethics, clearly dictates that Monica should have the opportunity to decide about her future. While there are limits to imposing suffering on patients in order to grant them autonomy in decisionmaking, only patients themselves can know exactly what those limits are. Would Monica prefer to be awakened from sedation at all? If so, would she want to participate in the medically, ethically, and psychologically difficult decision about her treatment options?

Reducing sedation in an intubated patient like Monica in order to allow her to be informed about her situation and to communicate her preferences will induce significant physical and psychological suffering. The coughing and vomiting reflex caused by the tube cannot be completely inhibited and makes the patient very uncomfortable. Learning in such a difficult moment that she is going to die soon of lung cancer is likely to be very painful psychologically. Monica's willingness to accept this suffering will depend on her individual threshold of pain and her ability to cope with both pain and learning that she is near death. Perhaps even more importantly, it will depend on whether there are important things in her life that she would like to accomplish before she dies. Many patients would like at least to say goodbye to their loved ones or clarify a relationship after a recent dispute. Monica might want to make a will or indicate how and by whom her affairs should be handled after her death.

Monica, it seems, has not previously expressed preferences about end of life care either in a living will or orally to a relative, friend, or physician, and there is no way to know her desire except by waking her. Discussion with her children or someone else who knows her well might be helpful, but individuals in close emotional contact with patients in situations like Monica's can too easily be influenced by an overwhelming desire to protect the patient from suffering. In the absence of written or oral directives, not waking Monica would be an unjustified form of hard paternalism.

The harm done to her by waking her should be kept to a minimum. She should know her diagnosis and prognosis, and that she can at any time delegate decisionmaking power to another person and receive sedating medication. Without the attempt, she would not be in a good position to know how it feels to be on a ventilator while conscious and whether she is able to tolerate this for the sake of a last contact with her family and friends.

At this stage it is not necessary to tell her the details about heroic or experimental treatment options. Only if Monica chooses to participate in decisions about her care must she then choose between refusing or accepting aggressive therapy at all, and if she wants treatment, how aggressive her care should be. One could imagine her, for example, wanting the surgeon to attempt to place a stent, even if chances of success are slim, to enable her to spend her last days more comfortably and gain time to think about her future.

When deciding about Monica's participation in the treatment decision, caregivers are right to be concerned about whether she will truly be competent to make decisions in this complex situation. If we accept a sliding scale of competency, however, we can make the case that she can be the ultimate decisionmaker: since there is no clearly "best" alternative among the treatment possibilities, Monica will not be in a position of asking doctors to do something "irrational" or "dangerous" and thus will not have to "prove" her competency on the highest standards. Physicians concerned about the distress of asking Monica to make a decision on her own could also recommend the treatment that a majority of the team has decided is most adequate in her situation and ask Monica whether she consents.

Monica has a right to be informed to a degree that she herself determines according to her ability and willingness to cope with suffering. The team should wake her. Unless she declares that she does not want to know, she should be told that the decision she faces is difficult and that at any time she may designate another person or group to make decisions in her place.

COMMENTARY

Jean-Claude Chevrolet

Strong arguments can be made justifying the preeminence of autonomy in any situation and they seem easily accepted by anyone, at least on theoretical grounds. Nonetheless, Monica's caregivers, even after a thorough discussion of the ethical dimensions of the situation, and after having obtained expert medical opinions, could not see concretely how to proceed. They could not immediately accept causing what they believed would be a great amount of suffering to their patient for what they estimated to be a very poor result—that is, to offer benefits primarily to others, including Monica's family and other associates—without any certainty that this suffering could lead to an autonomous decision by Monica herself.

The question for Monica's caregivers, then, is whether autonomy becomes overvalued when it conflicts with other values, and what the conditions are or should be for applying the "therapeutic privilege" of not informing Monica of her diagnosis and prognosis in her own best interest. When the possibility was discussed of waking Monica so that she could decide what to do next, her physicians and nurses were really afraid that when faced with physical suffering and a horrible prognosis, she would not in fact be in any position to make an autonomous decision on any possible issue. They worried that the conditions for autonomous choice—that is, being able to act intentionally, with understanding, and without controlling influences—simply could not be met in this situation.

Of course, not respecting Monica's autonomy must be well justified because it clearly represents a decision that could be characterized as strong paternalism. The caregivers have to be sure, of course, that their own psychological distress in the case of waking Monica for respecting her autonomy and asking her to choose between several horrible options would not influence their own medical and ethical judgment. If this could not be assumed or were not the case, the real ethical dilemma would indeed be the clash between autonomy and beneficence. But Monica faces so short a life expectancy, and the quality of that life can be presumed to be so miserable, that caregivers may ask whether waking her just for the purpose of letting her choose among her horrible options isn't similar to the use of extraordinary means—that is, therapeutic tools and resources that have no reasonable chance of succeeding and could even be considered malpractice. They might ask whether the best analogy isn't to withholding a pointless treatment, in which case Monica's best interest could not be served by clinging to the ethical principle of autonomy.

It takes courage to decide that waking Monica only to impose on her a question that is impossible to answer, in conditions that could not permit sound judgment, is not the ethically best course of action. But Monica's best interests will not be served by a charade of autonomy.

FOUR MODELS OF THE PHYSICIAN-PATIENT RELATIONSHIP

Ezekiel J. Emanuel and Linda L. Emanuel

During the last two decades or so, there has been a struggle over the patient's role in medical decision making that is often characterized as a conflict between autonomy and health, between the values of the patient and the values of the physician. Seeking to curtail physician dominance, many have advocated an ideal of greater patient control. Others question this ideal because it fails to acknowledge the potentially imbalanced nature of this interaction when one party is sick and searching for security, and when judgments entail the interpretation of technical information. Still others are trying to delineate a more mutual relationship. This struggle shapes the expectations of physicians and patients as well as the ethical and legal standards for the physician's duties, informed consent, and medical malpractice. This struggle forces us to ask, What should be the ideal physician-patient relationship?

We shall outline four models of the physician-patient interaction, emphasizing the different understandings of (1) the goals of the physician-patient interaction, (2) the physician's obligations, (3) the role of patient values, and (4) the conception of patient autonomy. To elaborate the abstract description of these four models, we shall indicate the types of response the models might suggest in a clinical situation. Third, we shall also indicate how these models inform the current debate about the ideal

---

From *Journal of the American Medical Association* 267, no. 16, April 22/29, 1992: 2221–2226.

Editors' note: Author's notes have been deleted. Students who wish to follow up on sources should consult the original article.

physician-patient relationship. Finally, we shall evaluate these models and recommend one as the preferred model.

As outlined, the models are Weberian ideal types. They may not describe any particular physician-patient interactions but they highlight, free from complicating details, different visions of the essential characteristics of the physician-patient interaction. Consequently, they do not embody minimum ethical or legal standards, but rather constitute regulative ideals that are "higher than the law" but not "above the law."

THE PATERNALISTIC MODEL

First is the *paternalistic* model, sometimes called the parental or priestly model. In this model, the physician-patient interaction ensures that patients receive the interventions that best promote their health and well-being. To this end, physicians use their skills to determine the patient's medical condition and his or her stage in the disease process and to identify the medical tests and treatments most likely to restore the patient's health or ameliorate pain. Then the physician presents the patient with selected information that will encourage the patient to consent to the intervention the physician considers best. At the extreme, the physician authoritatively informs the patient when the intervention will be initiated.

The paternalistic model assumes that there are shared objective criteria for determining what is best. Hence the physician can discern what is in the patient's best interest with limited patient participation. Ultimately, it is assumed that the patient will be thankful for decisions made by the physician even if he or she would not agree to them at the time. In the tension between the patient's autonomy and well-being, between choice and health, the paternalistic physician's main emphasis is toward the latter.

In the paternalistic model, the physician acts as the patient's guardian, articulating and implementing what is best for the patient. As such, the physician has obligations, including that of placing the patient's interest above his or her own and soliciting the views of others when lacking adequate knowledge. The conception of patient autonomy is patient assent, either at the time or later, to the physician's determinations of what is best.

THE INFORMATIVE MODEL

Second is the *informative* model, sometimes called the scientific, engineering, or consumer model. In this model, the objective of the physician-patient interaction is for the physician to provide the patient with all relevant information, for the patient to select the medical interventions he or she wants, and for the physician to execute the selected interventions. To this end, the physician informs the patient of his or her disease state, the nature of possible diagnostic and therapeutic interventions, the nature and probability of risks and benefits associated with the interventions, and any uncertainties of knowledge. At the extreme, patients could come to know all medical information relevant to their disease and available interventions and select the interventions that best realize their values.

The informative model assumes a fairly clear distinction between facts and values. The patient's values are well defined and known; what the patient lacks is facts. It is the physician's obligation to provide all the available facts, and the patient's values then determine what treatments are to be given. There is no role for the physician's values, the physician's understanding of the patient's values, or his or her judgment of the worth of the patient's values. In the informative model, the physician is a purveyor of technical expertise, providing the patient with the means to exercise control. As technical experts, physicians have important obligations to provide truthful information, to maintain competence in their area of expertise, and to consult others when their knowledge or skills are lacking. The conception of patient autonomy is patient control over medical decision making.

THE INTERPRETIVE MODEL

The third model is the *interpretive* model. The aim of the physician-patient interaction is to elucidate the patient's values and what he or she actually wants, and to help the patient select the available medical interventions that realize these values. Like the informative physician, the interpretive physician provides the patient with information on the nature of the condition and the risks and benefits of possible interventions. Beyond this, however, the interpretive physician assists the patient in elucidating and articulating his or her values and in determining what medical interventions best realize the specified values, thus helping to interpret the patient's values for the patient.

According to the interpretive model, the patient's values are not necessarily fixed and known to the patient. They are often inchoate, and the patient may only partially understand them; they may conflict when applied to specific situations. Consequently, the physician working with the patient must elucidate and make coherent these values. To do this, the physician works with the patient to reconstruct the patient's goals and aspirations, commitments and character. At the extreme, the physician must conceive of the patient's life as a narrative whole, and from this specify the patient's values and their priorities. Then the physician determines which tests and treatments best realize these values. Importantly, the physician does not dictate to the patient; it is the patient who ultimately decides which values and course of action best fit who he or she is. Neither is the physician judging the patient's values; he or she helps the patient to understand and use them in the medical situation.

In the interpretive model, the physician is a counselor, analogous to a cabinet minister's advisory role to a head of state, supplying relevant information, helping to elucidate values, and suggesting what medical interventions realize these values. Thus the physician's obligations include those enumerated in the informative model but also require engaging the patient in a joint process of understanding. Accordingly, the conception of patient autonomy is self-understanding; the patient comes to know more clearly who he or she is and how the various medical options bear on his or her identity.

THE DELIBERATIVE MODEL

Fourth is the *deliberative* model. The aim of the physician-patient interaction is to help the patient determine and choose the best health-related values that can be realized in the clinical situation. To this end, the physician must delineate information on the patient's clinical situation and then help elucidate the types of values embodied in the available options. The physician's objectives include suggesting why certain health-related values are more worthy and should be aspired to. At the extreme, the physician and patient engage in deliberation about what kind of health-related values the patient could and ultimately should pursue. The physician discusses only health-related values, that is, values that affect or are affected by the patient's disease and treatments; he or she recognizes that many elements of morality are unrelated to the patient's disease or treatment and beyond the scope of their professional relationship. Further, the physician aims at no more than moral persuasion; ultimately, coercion is avoided, and the patient must define his or her life and select the ordering of values to be espoused. By engaging in moral deliberation, the physician and patient judge the worthiness and importance of the health-related values.

In the deliberative model, the physician acts as a teacher or friend, engaging the patient in dialogue on what course of action would be best. Not only does the physician indicate what the patient could do, but, knowing the patient and wishing what is best, the physician indicates what the patient should do—what decision regarding medical therapy would be admirable. The conception of patient autonomy is moral self-development; the patient is empowered not simply to follow unexamined preferences or examined values, but to consider, through dialogue, alternative health-related values, their worthiness, and their implications for treatment.

COMPARING THE FOUR MODELS

Importantly, all models have a role for patient autonomy; a main factor that differentiates the models is their particular conceptions of patient autonomy. Therefore, no single model can be endorsed because it alone promotes patient autonomy. Instead the models must be compared and evaluated, at least in part, by evaluating the adequacy of their particular conceptions of patient autonomy.

The four models are not exhaustive. At a minimum, there might be added a fifth: the *instrumental* model. In this model, the patient's values are irrelevant; the physician aims for some goal independent of the patient, such as the good of society or the furtherance of scientific knowledge. The Tuskegee syphilis experiment and the Willowbrook hepatitis study (see Part 5, Section 1) are examples of this model. As the moral condemnation of these cases reveals, this model is not an ideal, but an aberration. Thus we have not elaborated it herein.

A CLINICAL CASE

To make tangible these abstract descriptions and to crystallize essential differences among the models, we will illustrate the responses they suggest in a clinical situation, that of a 43-year-old premenopausal woman who has recently discovered a breast mass. Surgery reveals a 3.5-cm ductal carcinoma with no lymph node involvement that is estrogen receptor positive. Chest roentgenogram, bone scan, and liver function tests reveal no evidence of metastatic disease. The patient was recently divorced and has gone back to work as a legal aide to support herself. What should the physician say to this patient?

In the paternalistic model a physician might say, "There are two alternative therapies to protect against recurrence of cancer in your breast: mastectomy or radiation. We now know that the survival with lumpectomy combined with radiation therapy is equal to that with mastectomy. Because lumpectomy and radiation offers the best survival and the best cosmetic result, it is to be preferred. I have asked the radiation therapist to come and discuss radiation treatment with you. We also need to protect you against the spread of the cancer to other parts of your body. Even though the chance of recurrence is low, you are young, and we should not leave any therapeutic possibilities untried. Recent studies involving chemotherapy suggest improvements in survival without recurrence of breast cancer. Indeed, the National Cancer Institute (NCI) recommends chemotherapy for women with your type of breast cancer. Chemotherapy has side effects. Nevertheless, a few months of hardship now are worth the potential added years of life without cancer."

In the informative model, a physician might say, "With node-negative breast cancer there are two issues before you: local control and systemic control. For local control, the options are mastectomy or lumpectomy with or without radiation. From many studies we know that mastectomy and lumpectomy with radiation result in identical overall survival, about 80 percent 10-year survival. Lumpectomy without radiation results in a 30 percent to 40 percent chance of tumor recurrence in the breast. The second issue relates to systemic control. We know that chemotherapy prolongs survival for premenopausal women who have axillary nodes involved with tumor. The role for women with node-negative breast cancer is less clear. Individual studies suggest that chemotherapy is of no benefit in terms of improving overall survival, but a comprehensive review of all studies suggests that there is a survival benefit. Several years ago, the NCI suggested that for women like yourself, chemotherapy can have a positive therapeutic impact. Finally, let me inform you that there are clinical trials, for which you are eligible, to evaluate the benefits of chemotherapy for patients with node-negative breast cancer. I can enroll you in a study if you want. I will be happy to give you any further information you feel you need."

The interpretive physician might outline much of the same information as the informative physician, then engage in discussion to elucidate the patient's wishes, and conclude, "It sounds to me as if you have conflicting wishes. Understandably, you seem uncertain how to balance the demands required for receiving additional treatment, rejuvenating your personal affairs, and maintaining your psychological equilibrium. Let me try to express a perspective that fits your position. Fighting your cancer is important, but it must leave you with a healthy self-image and quality time outside the hospital. This view seems compatible with undergoing radiation therapy but not chemotherapy. A lumpectomy with radiation maximizes your chance of surviving while preserving your breast. Radiotherapy fights your breast cancer without disfigurement. Conversely, chemotherapy would prolong the duration of therapy by many months. Further, the benefits of chemotherapy in terms of survival are smaller and more controversial. Given the recent changes in your life, you have too many new preoccupations to undergo months of chemotherapy for a questionable benefit. Do I understand you? We can talk again in a few days."

The deliberative physician might begin by outlining the same factual information, then engage in a conversation to elucidate the patient's values, but continue, "It seems clear that you should undergo radiation therapy. It offers maximal survival with minimal risk, disfigurement, and disruption of your life. The issue of chemotherapy is different, fraught with conflicting data. Balancing all the options, I think the best one for you is to enter a trial that is investigating the potential benefit of chemotherapy for women with node-negative breast cancer. First, it ensures that you receive excellent medical care. At this point, we do not know which therapy maximizes survival. In a clinical study the schedule of follow-up visits, tests, and decisions is specified by leading breast cancer experts to ensure that all the women receive care that is the best available anywhere. A second reason to participate in a trial is altruistic; it allows you to contribute something to women with breast cancer in the future who will face difficult choices. Over decades, thousands of women have participated in studies that inform our current treatment practices. Without those women, and the knowledge they made possible, we would probably still be giving you and all other women with breast cancer mastectomies. By enrolling in a trial you participate in a tradition in which women of one generation receive the highest standard of care available but also enhance the care of women in future generations because medicine has learned something about which interventions are better. I must tell you that I am not involved in the study; if you elect to enroll in this trial, you will initially see another breast cancer expert to plan your therapy. I have sought to explain our current knowledge and offer my recommendation so you can make the best possible decision."

Lacking the normal interchange with patients, these statements may seem contrived, even caricatures. Nevertheless, they highlight the essence of each model and suggest how the objectives and assumptions of each inform a physician's approach to his or her patients. Similar statements can be imagined for other clinical situations such as an obstetrician discussing prenatal testing or a cardiologist discussing cholesterol-reducing interventions.

THE CURRENT DEBATE AND THE FOUR MODELS

In recent decades there has been a call for greater patient autonomy or, as some have called it, "patient sovereignty," conceived as patient *choice* and *control* over medical decisions. This shift toward the informative model is embodied in the adoption of business terms for medicine, as when physicians are described as health care providers and patients as consumers. It can also be found in the propagation of patient rights statements, in the promotion of living-will laws, and in rules regarding human experimentation. For instance, the opening sentences of one law state: "The Rights of the Terminally Ill Act authorizes an adult person to *control* decisions regarding administration of life-sustaining treatment. . . . The Act merely provides one way by which a terminally-ill patient's *desires* regarding the use of life-sustaining procedures can be legally implemented" (emphasis added). Indeed, living-will laws do not require or encourage patients to discuss the issue of terminating care with their physicians before signing such documents. Similarly, decisions in "right-to-die" cases emphasize patient control over medical decisions. As one court put it:

> The right to refuse medical treatment is basic and fundamental. . . . Its exercise requires no one's approval. . . . *[T]he controlling decision belongs to a competent informed patient.* . . . It is not a medical decision for her physicians to make. . . . *It is a moral and philosophical decision that, being a competent adult, is [the patient's] alone.*[1] (emphasis added)

Probably the most forceful endorsement of the informative model as the ideal inheres in informed consent standards. Prior to the 1970s, the standard for informed consent was "physician based." Since 1972 and the *Canterbury* case, however, the emphasis has been on a "patient-oriented" standard of informed consent in which the physician has a "duty" to provide appropriate medical facts to empower the patient to use his or her values to determine what interventions should be implemented.

> True consent to what happens to one's self is the informed exercise of a choice, and that entails an opportunity to evaluate knowledgeably the options available and the risks attendant upon each. . . . *[I]t is the prerogative of the patient, not the physician, to determine for himself the direction in which his interests seem to lie.* To enable the patient to chart his course understandably, some familiarity with the therapeutic alternatives and their hazards becomes essential.[2] (emphasis added)

SHARED DECISION MAKING

Despite its dominance, many have found the informative model somewhat "arid." The President's Commission and others contend that the ideal relationship does not vest moral authority and medical decision-making power exclusively in the patient but must be a process of shared decision making constructed around "mutual participation and respect." The President's Commission argues that the physician's role is "to help the patient understand the medical situation and available courses of action, and the patient conveys his or her concerns and wishes." Brock and Wartman[3] stress this fact-value "division of labor"—having the physician provide information while the patient makes value decisions—by describing "shared decision making" as a collaborative process

> in which both physicians and patients make active and essential contributions. Physicians bring their medical training, knowledge, and expertise—including an understanding of the available treatment alternatives—to the diagnosis and management of patients' conditions. Patients bring knowledge of their own subjective aims and values, through which risks and benefits of various treatment options can be evaluated. With this approach, selecting the best treatment for a particular patient requires the contribution of both parties.

Similarly, in discussing ideal medical decision making, Eddy[4] argues for this fact-value division of labor between the physician and patient as the ideal:

> It is important to separate the decision process into these two steps. . . . The first step is a question of facts. The anchor is empirical evidence. . . . [T]he second step is a question not of facts but of personal values or preferences. The thought process is not analytic but personal and subjective. . . . [I]t is the patient's preferences that should determine the decision. . . . Ideally, you and I [the physicians] are not in the picture. What matters is what Mrs. Smith thinks.

This view of shared decision making seems to vest the medical decision-making authority with the patient while relegating physicians to technicians "transmitting medical information and using their technical skills as the patient directs." Thus, while the advocates of "shared decision making" may aspire toward a mutual dialogue between physician and patient, the substantive view informing their ideal reembodies the informative model under a different label.

Other commentators have articulated more mutual models of the physician-patient interaction. Prominent among these efforts is Katz's *The Silent World of the Doctor and Patient*. Relying on a Freudian view in which self-knowledge and self-determination are inherently limited because of unconscious influences, Katz views dialogue as a mechanism for greater self-understanding of one's values and objectives. According to Katz, this view places a duty on physicians and patients to reflect and communicate so that patients can gain a greater self-understanding and self-determination. Katz's insight is also available on grounds other than Freudian psychological theory and is consistent with the interpretive model.

OBJECTIONS TO THE PATERNALISTIC MODEL

It is widely recognized that the paternalistic model is justified during emergencies when the time taken to obtain informed consent might irreversibly harm the patient. Beyond such limited circumstances, however, it is no longer tenable to assume that the physician and patient espouse similar values and views of what constitutes a benefit. Consequently, even physicians rarely advocate the paternalistic model as an ideal for routine physician-patient interactions.

OBJECTIONS TO THE INFORMATIVE MODEL

The informative model seems both descriptively and prescriptively inaccurate. First, this model seems to have no place for essential qualities of the ideal physician-patient relationship. The informative physician cares for the patient in the sense of competently implementing the patient's selected interventions. However, the informative physician lacks a caring approach that requires understanding what the patient values or should value and how his or her illness impinges on these values. Patients seem to expect their physician to have a caring approach; they deem a technically proficient but detached physician as deficient, and properly condemned. Further, the informative physician is proscribed from giving a recommendation for fear of imposing his or her will on the patient and thereby competing for the decision-making control that has been given to the patient. Yet, if one of the essential qualities of the ideal physician is the ability to assimilate medical facts, prior experience of similar situations, and intimate knowledge of the patient's view into a recommendation designed for the patient's specific medical and personal condition, then the informative physician cannot be ideal.

Second, in the informative model, the ideal physician is a highly trained subspecialist who provides detailed factual information and competently implements the patient's preferred medical intervention. Hence, the informative model perpetuates and accentuates the trend toward specialization and impersonalization within the medical profession.

Most importantly, the informative model's conception of patient autonomy seems philosophically untenable. The informative model presupposes that persons possess known and fixed values, but this is inaccurate. People are often uncertain about what they actually want. Further, unlike animals, people have what philosophers call "second-order desires," that is, the capacity to reflect on their wishes and to revise their own desires and preferences. In fact, freedom of the will and autonomy inhere in having "second-order desires" and being able to change our preferences and modify our identities. Self-reflection and the capacity to change what we want often require a "process" of moral deliberation in which we assess the value of what we want. And this is a process that occurs with other people who know us well and can articulate a vision of who we ought to be that we can assent to. Even though changes in health or implementation of alternative interventions can have profound effects on what we desire and how we realize our desires, self-reflection and deliberation play no essential role in the informative physician-patient interaction. The informative model's conception of autonomy is incompatible with a vision of autonomy that incorporates second-order desires.

OBJECTIONS TO THE INTERPRETIVE MODEL

The interpretive model rectifies this deficiency by recognizing that persons have second-order desires and dynamic value structures and placing the elucidation of values in the context of the patient's medical condition at the center of the physician-patient interaction. Nevertheless, there are objections to the interpretive model.

Technical specialization militates against physicians cultivating the skills necessary to the interpretive model. With limited interpretive talents and limited time, physicians may unwittingly impose their own values under the guise of articulating the patient's values. And patients, overwhelmed by their medical condition and uncertain of their own views, may too easily accept this imposition. Such circumstances may push the interpretive model toward the paternalistic model in actual practice.

Further, autonomy viewed as self-understanding excludes evaluative judgment of the patient's values or attempts to persuade the patient to adopt other values. This constrains the guidance and recommendations the physician can offer. Yet in practice, especially in preventive medicine and risk-reduction interventions, physicians often attempt to persuade patients to adopt particular health-related values. Physicians frequently urge patients with high cholesterol levels who smoke to change their dietary habits, quit smoking, and begin exercise programs before initiating drug therapy. The justification given for these changes is that patients should value their health more than they do. Similarly, physicians are encouraged to persuade their human immunodeficiency virus (HIV)–infected patients who might be engaging in unsafe sexual practices either to abstain or, realistically, to adopt "safer sex" practices. Such appeals are not made to promote the HIV–infected patient's own health, but are grounded on an appeal for the patient to assume responsibility for the good of others. Consequently, by excluding evaluative judgments, the interpretive model seems to characterize inaccurately ideal physician-patient interactions.

OBJECTIONS TO THE DELIBERATIVE MODEL

The fundamental objections to the deliberative model focus on whether it is proper for physicians to judge patients' values and promote particular health-related values. First, physicians do not possess privileged knowledge of the priority of health-related values relative to other values. Indeed, since ours is a pluralistic society in which people espouse incommensurable values, it is likely that a physician's values and view of which values are higher will conflict with those of other physicians and those of his or her patients.

Second, the nature of the moral deliberation between physician and patient, the physician's recommended interventions, and the actual treatments used will depend on the values of the particular physician treating the patient. However, recommendations and care provided to patients should not depend on the physician's judgment of the worthiness of the patient's values or on the physician's particular values..As one bioethicist put it:

> The hand is broken; the physician can repair the hand; therefore the physician must repair the hand—as well as possible—without regard to personal values that might lead the physician to think ill of the patient or of the patient's values. . . . [A]t the level of clinical practice, medicine should be value-free in the sense that the personal values of the physician should not distort the making of medical decisions.[5]

Third, it may be argued that the deliberative model misconstrues the purpose of the physician-patient interaction. Patients see their physicians to receive health care, not to engage in moral deliberation or to revise their values. Finally, like the interpretive model, the deliberative model may easily metamorphose into unintended paternalism, the very practice that generated the public debate over proper physician-patient interaction.

THE PREFERRED MODEL AND THE PRACTICAL IMPLICATIONS

Clearly, under different clinical circumstances, different models may be appropriate. Indeed, at different times, all four models may justifiably guide physicians and patients. Nevertheless, it is important to specify one model as the shared, paradigmatic reference; exceptions to use other models would not be automatically condemned, but would require justification based on the circumstances of a particular situation. Thus, it is widely agreed that in an emergency where delays in treatment to obtain informed consent might irreversibly harm the patient, the paternalistic model correctly guides physician-patient interactions. Conversely, for patients who have clear but conflicting values, the interpretive model is probably justified. For instance, a 65-year-old woman who has been treated for acute leukemia may have clearly decided against reinduction chemotherapy if she relapses. Several months before the anticipated birth of her first grandchild, the patient relapses. The patient becomes torn about whether to endure the risks of reinduction chemotherapy in order to live to see her first grandchild or whether to refuse therapy, resigning herself to not seeing her grandchild. In such cases, the physician may justifiably adopt the interpretive approach. In other circumstances, where there is only a one-time physician-patient interaction without an ongoing relationship in which the patient's values can be elucidated and compared with ideals, such as in a walk-in center, the informative model may be justified.

Descriptively and prescriptively, we claim that the ideal physician-patient relationship is the deliberative model. We will adduce six points to justify this claim. First, the deliberative model more nearly embodies our ideal of autonomy. It is an oversimplification and distortion of the Western tradition to view respecting autonomy as simply permitting a person to select, unrestricted by coercion, ignorance, physical interference, and the like, his or her preferred course of action from a comprehensive list of available options. Freedom and control over medical decisions alone do not constitute patient autonomy. Autonomy requires that individuals critically assess their own values and preferences; determine whether they are desirable; affirm, upon reflection, these values as ones that should justify their actions; and then be free to initiate action to realize the values. The process of deliberation integral to the deliberative model is essential for realizing patient autonomy understood in this way.

Second, our society's image of an ideal physician is not limited to one who knows and communicates to the patient relevant factual information and competently implements medical interventions. The ideal physician—often embodied in literature, art, and popular culture—is a caring physician who integrates the information and relevant values to make a recommendation and, through discussion, attempts to persuade the patient to accept this recommendation as the intervention that best promotes his or her overall well-being. Thus, we expect the best physicians to engage their patients in evaluative discussions of health issues and related values. The physician's discussion does not invoke values that are unrelated or tangentially related to the patient's illness and potential therapies. Importantly, these efforts are not restricted to situations in which patients might make "irrational and harmful" choices but extend to all health care decisions.

Third, the deliberative model is not a disguised form of paternalism. Previously there may have been category mistakes in which instances of the deliberative model have been erroneously identified as physician paternalism. And no doubt, in practice, the deliberative physician may occasionally lapse into paternalism. However, like the ideal teacher, the deliberative physician attempts to *persuade* the patient of the worthiness of certain values, not to *impose* those values paternalistically; the physician's aim is not to subject the patient to his or her will, but to persuade the patient of a course of action as desirable. In the *Laws*, Plato[6] characterizes this fundamental distinction between persuasion and imposition for medical practice that distinguishes the deliberative from the paternalistic model:

> A physician to slaves never gives his patient any account of his illness. . . . [T]he physician offers some orders gleaned from experience with an air of infallible knowledge, in the brusque fashion of a dictator. . . . The free physician, who usually cares for free men, treats their disease first by thoroughly discussing with the patient and his friends his ailment. This way he learns something from the sufferer and simultaneously instructs him. Then the physician does not give his medications until he has persuaded the patient; the physician aims at complete restoration of health by persuading the patient to comply with his therapy.

Fourth, physician values are relevant to patients and do inform their choice of a physician. When a pregnant woman chooses an obstetrician who does not routinely perform a battery of prenatal tests or, alternatively, one who strongly favors them; and when patients seek an aggressive cardiologist who favors procedural interventions or one who concentrates therapy on dietary changes, stress reduction, and life-style modifications, they are, consciously or not, selecting a physician based on the values that guide their medical decisions. And, when disagreements between physicians and patients arise, there are discussions over which values are more important and should be realized in medical care. Occasionally, when such disagreements undermine the physician-patient relationship and a caring attitude, a patient's care is transferred to another physician. Indeed, in the informative model the grounds for transferring care to a new physician is either the physician's ignorance or incompetence. But patients seem to switch physicians because they do not "like" a particular physician or that physician's attitude or approach.

Fifth, we seem to believe that physicians should not only help fit therapies to the patients' elucidated values, but should also promote health-related values. As noted, we expect physicians to promote certain values, such as "safer sex" for patients with HIV or abstaining from or limiting alcohol use. Similarly, patients are willing to adjust their values and actions to be more compatible with health-promoting values. This is in the nature of seeking a caring medical recommendation.

Finally, it may well be that many physicians currently lack the training and capacity to articulate the values underlying their recommendations and persuade patients that these values are worthy. But, in part, this deficiency is a consequence of the tendencies toward specialization and the avoidance of discussions of values by physicians that are perpetuated and justified by the dominant informative model. Therefore, if the deliberative model seems most appropriate, then we need to implement changes in medical care and education to encourage a more caring approach. We must stress understanding rather than mere provisions of factual information in keeping with the legal standards of informed consent and medical malpractice; we must educate physicians not just to spend more time in physician-patient communication but to elucidate and articulate the values underlying their medical care decisions, including routine ones; we must shift the publicly assumed conception of patient autonomy that shapes both the physician's and the patient's expectations from patient control to moral development. Most important, we must recognize that developing a deliberative physician-patient relationship requires a considerable amount of time. We must develop a health care financing system that properly reimburses—rather than penalizes—physicians for taking the time to discuss values with their patients.

CONCLUSION

Over the last few decades, the discourse regarding the physician-patient relationship has focused on two extremes: autonomy and paternalism. Many have attacked physicians as paternalistic, urging the empowerment of patients to control their own care. This view, the informative model, has become dominant in bioethics and legal standards. This model embodies a defective conception of patient autonomy, and it reduces the physician's role to that of a technologist. The essence of doctoring is a fabric of knowledge, understanding, teaching, and action, in which the caring physician integrates the patient's medical condition and health-related values, makes a recommendation on the appropriate course of action, and tries to persuade the patient of the worthiness of this approach and the values it realizes. The physician with a caring attitude is the ideal embodied in the deliberative model, the ideal that should inform laws and policies that regulate the physician-patient interaction.

Finally, it may be worth noting that the four models outlined herein are not limited to the medical realm; they may inform the public conception of other professional interactions as well. We suggest that the ideal relationships between lawyer and client, religious mentor and laity, and educator and student are well described by the deliberative model, at least in some of their essential aspects.

NOTES

1. *Bouvia v. Superior Court*, 225 Cal Rptr 297 (1986).
2. *Canterbury v. Spence*, 464 F2d 772 (D.C. Cir 1972).
3. Brock DW, Wartman SA. When competent patients make irrational choices. *N Engl J Med*. 1990; 322:1595–1599.
4. Eddy DM. Anatomy of a decision. *JAMA*. 1990; 263:441–443.
5. Gorovitz S. *Doctors' Dilemmas: Moral Conflict and Medical Care*. New York, NY: Oxford University Press Inc; 1982:chap 6.
6. Plato; Hamilton E, Cairns H, eds; Emanuel EJ, trans. *Plato: The Collected Dialogues*. Princeton, NJ: Princeton University Press; 1961:720 c–e.

OFFERING TRUTH

One Ethical Approach to the Uninformed Cancer Patient

Benjamin Freedman

Medical and social attitudes toward cancer have evolved rapidly during the last 20 years, particularly in North America.[1,2] Most physicians, most of the time, in most hospitals, accept the ethical proposition that patients are entitled to know their diagnosis. However, there remains in my experience a significant minority of cases in which patients are never informed that they have cancer or, although informed of the diagnosis, are not informed when disease progresses toward a terminal phase. Although concealment of diagnosis can certainly occur in cases of other terminal or even nonterminal serious illnesses, it seems to occur more frequently and in more exacerbated form with cancer because of the traditional and cultural resonances of dread associated with cancer.

These cases challenge our understanding of and commitment to an ethical physician-patient relationship. In addition, they are observably a significant source of tension between health-care providers. When the responsible physician persists in efforts to conceal the truth from patients, consultant physicians, nurses, social workers, or others may believe that they cannot discharge their functions responsibly until the patient has been told. Alternatively, when a treating physician decides to inform the patient of his or her diagnosis, strong resistance from family members who have instigated a conspiracy of silence may be anticipated.

This article outlines one approach, employed in my own ethical consultations and at some palliative care services or specialized oncology units. This approach, offering truth to patients with cancer, affords a means of satisfying legal and ethical norms of patient autonomy, ameliorating conflicts between families and physicians, and acknowledging the cultural norms that underlie family desires.

COMMON FEATURES OF CASES

Mrs A is a woman in her 60s with colon cancer, with metastatic liver involvement and a mass in the abdomen. She is not expected to survive longer than weeks. Other than a course of antibiotics, which she was just about to complete, no active treatment is indicated or intended. She is alert. She knows that she has an infection; her family refuses to inform her that she has cancer. The precipitating cause of the ethical consultation, requested by the newly assigned treating physician (Dr H), is his ethical discomfort with treating Mrs A in this manner.

When one is confronted with a case of concealment, it is worth wondering how it came about that everyone but the patient has been told of the diagnosis, so that similar situations may be avoided in the future. Often, a diagnosis is defined in the course of surgery and disclosed to waiting relatives; this may most appropriately be handled by a prior understanding with the patient, communicated to the family, as to whether and how much they will be told before the patient awakens. But there are at least two other major ways in which a situation of concealment might develop.

A patient might be admitted in medical crisis, at a time when he or she is obtunded and incapable of being informed of his or her condition and treatment options. Law and ethics alike require that the medical team inform and otherwise deal with the person who is most qualified to speak on the patient's behalf (usually, the next of kin), until the patient has recovered enough to speak for himself or herself. Unfortunately for this plan, though, a patient will often fail to cross, at one moment, the bright line from incompetent to competent. Consequently, patterns of communicating with the relative instead of with the patient may persist beyond the intended period. Such situations have their own momentum. Later disclosure to the patient will need to deal both with the burden of providing bad news and with the fact that this information has been concealed from the patient up to that point.

A second typical way in which concealment develops is the following. A patient with close family ties is always attended by a relative (commonly, spouse or child) at medical appointments. Before a firm diagnosis is established, that relative manages to elicit a promise from the physician not to tell the patient should the tests show that the patient has cancer. Faced with a distraught and deeply caring relative, the physician goes along, at least as a temporizing tactic, only to discover, as described above, how the situation develops its own inertia. The cycle may be broken in a number of ways. Sometimes the physician simply decides to call a halt to concealment; often the patient's care is transferred to another physician who has not been a party to the conspiracy, as had happened with Mrs A.

As clinical ethicist, I met with Dr H and the relevant family members (husband, daughter, and son). Most of the discussion was held with the son; the husband, a first-generation Greek-Canadian immigrant, knows little English and was at any rate somewhat withdrawn. As expected, they are a close family, deeply solicitous of the patient, and convinced that she will suffer horribly were she to be told she has cancer. They confirmed my sense that the Greek cultural significance of cancer equals death—something that in this case is in all likelihood true.

At this time the family was willing to sign any document we wanted them to, assuming all responsibility for the decision to conceal the truth from Mrs A. "Do us this one favor" was a plea that punctuated the discussion.

Although other factors, such as the context of treatment and the patient's own idiosyncratic personality, may cause the same kind of problem in communication, my experience suggests the situation is often, as here, mediated by cultural factors. As one text on ethnic factors in family counseling puts it, "Greek Americans do not believe that the truth shall make you free, and the therapist should not attempt to impose the love of truth upon them."[3] (And compare Dalla-Vorgia et al.[4]) I often find other immigrant families of Mediterranean or Near Eastern origin reacting similarly, for example, Italian families and those of Sephardic Jews who have immigrated from Morocco. In all cases, in my experience, there is a special plea on the part of families to respect their cultural pattern and tradition. Health-care providers often feel the force of this claim and its corollary: informing the patient would be an act of ethical and cultural imperialism. Moreover, the family not uncommonly feels strongly enough that legal action is threatened unless their wishes are respected. Mrs A's family, in fact, threatened to sue at one point when they were told that Mrs A's diagnosis would be revealed.

TELLING FAMILIES WHY THE PATIENT SHOULD BE INFORMED

By the time a clinical ethical consultation is requested, the situation has often become highly charged emotionally. In addition to the unpleasantness of threats of legal action, there may have been some physical confrontation.

> Mrs S was a Sephardic woman in her 70s with widespread metastatic seedings in the pleura and pericardium from an unknown primary tumor. Her family insisted that she not be informed of her diagnosis and prognosis. Suffering from a subjective experience of apnea, she was to have a morphine drip begun to alleviate her symptoms. The family physically expelled the nurse from the room. If their mother were to learn she was getting morphine, they said, she would deduce that her situation was grave.

Such aberrant behavior cannot fairly be understood without realizing that these families may be acting out of uncommonly deep concern for the well-being of the patient, as they (perhaps misguidedly) understand it. The health-care team shares the same ultimate goal, to care for the patient in a humane, decent, caring manner. This commonality can serve as the basis for continuing discussion, as in the above case of Mrs A, the Greek patient.

> Discussion with the family was long and meandering. The usual position of the health-care team was explained in some detail: patients in our institution are generally told their diagnosis; we are accustomed to telling patients that they have cancer, and we know how to handle the varied normal patient reactions to this bad news; patients do not (generally) kill themselves immediately on being told, or die a voodoo death, in spite of the family's fears and cultural beliefs about patient reaction to this diagnosis. Patients have a right to this information and may have the need to attend to any number of tasks pending death: to say goodbye, to make arrangements, to complete unfinished business. As her illness progresses, decisions will likely need to be made about further treatment, for example, of infections or blockages that develop. Already, one of Mrs A's kidneys is blocked and her urine is backing up. If the mass should obstruct her other kidney, for example, should a catheter be placed directly into the kidney or not? These decisions of treatment management for dying patients are dreadful and should if possible be made by the patient, with awareness of her choices and prospects. In addition, Mrs A is very likely already suspicious that she is gravely ill, and we have no means of dealing with her fears without the ability to speak to her openly. Finally, the fears that the family expresses about the manner of informing her—"How can we tell our mother, 'You have cancer, it will kill you in weeks'"—are groundless: she must be told that she is very ill, but we would never advise telling her she has a period of *x* weeks to live—a statement that is never wise or medically sound—nor will we try to remove her hope.

The physician or other health-care provider may be primarily motivated by the ethical principle of respect for patient autonomy, grounding a patient's right to know of his or her situation, choices, and likely fate. Connected with this may be the correct belief that any consent to treatment that the patient provides without having an opportunity to learn the reason for that treatment is legally invalid. To be properly informed, consent must be predicated on information about the nature and consequences of treatment, which must in turn be understood in the context of the patient's illness. A patient cannot validly consent to the passing of a tube into the kidney without being informed that her urinary tract is blocked, or of the reason for that blockage.

These reasons, so determinative for the physician, often carry no weight with the family. In Mrs A's case, for example, the family pledged to sign anything we would like to free us of liability. Our response, that their willingness cannot affect either our moral or legal obligation, which vests in the patient directly, was similarly unpersuasive; nonetheless, it was a fact and had to be said.

The direct negative impact on the patient's care and comfort that results from her being left in the dark represents more in the way of common ground between family and health-care provider. It is often quite clear that failure to reveal the truth causes a variety of unfortunate psychosocial results. As in all such cases, we highlighted for Mrs A's family the strong possibility that she already suspects she is ill and dying of cancer but is unable to speak about this with them because all of us, in our concealment and evasions, had not given her "permission" to broach the topic. Mrs A is dying, but there are things worse than dying, for example, dying in silence when one needs to speak.

It is also important to emphasize to families that the patient may have "unfinished business" that he or she would like to complete. For example, after one of my earliest consultations of this nature, the patient in question chose to leave the hospital for several weeks to revisit his birthplace in Greece.

Finally, it is sometimes the case that the failure to discuss with the patient his or her diagnosis can directly result in inadequate or inappropriate medical care. Mrs S, above, was denied adequate comfort measures because the institution of morphine might tip her off to her condition. In another case, the son and daughter-in-law of a patient insisted that she not receive chemotherapy for an advanced but treatable blood cancer so that she would be spared the knowledge of her disease and the side effects of treatment. In such cases, great injury is added to the insult of withholding the truth from a patient. Often, it is this prospect that serves as the trigger to mobilize the health-care team to seek an ethical consultation.

OFFERING TRUTH TO THE UNINFORMED PATIENT WITH CANCER

A patient's knowledge of diagnosis and prognosis is not all-or-nothing. It exists along a continuum, anchored at one end by the purely theoretical "absolute ignorance" and at the other by the unattainable "total enlightenment." Actual patients are to be found along this continuum at locations that vary in response to external factors (verbal information, nonverbal clues, etc) as well as internal dynamics, such as denial.

The approach called here "offering truth" represents a brief dance between patient and health-care provider, a pas de deux, that takes place within that continuum. When offering truth to the patient with cancer, rather than simply ascertaining that the patient is for the moment lucid, and then proceeding to explain all aspects of his or her condition and treatment, both the physician(s) and I attempt repeatedly to ascertain from the patient how much he or she wants to know. In dealing with families who insist that the patient remain uninformed, I explain this approach, a kind of compromise between the polar stances. I also explain that sometimes the results are surprising, as indeed happened with Mrs A.

> In spite of all the explanations we provided to Mrs A's family of the many reasons why it might be best to speak with her of her illness, they continued to resist. Mrs A, the son insisted, would want all the decisions that arise to be made by the physicians, whom they all trusted, and the family itself.
>
> If their assessment of Mrs A is correct, I pointed out, we have no problem. Dr H agrees with me that while Mrs A has a *right* to know, she does not have a *duty* to know. We would not force this information on her—indeed, we cannot. Patients who do not want to know will sometimes deny ever having been told, however forthrightly they have been spoken to. So Mrs A will be offered this information, not have it thrust on her—and if they are right about what she wants, and her personality, she will not wish to know.
>
> Mrs A was awake and reasonably alert, although not altogether free of discomfort (nausea). She was told that she had had an infection that was now under control, but that she remains very ill, as she herself can tell from her weakness. Does she have any questions she wants to ask; does she want to talk? She did not. We repeated that she remains very ill and asked if she understands that—she did. Some patients, it was explained to her, want to know all about their disease—its name, prognosis, treatment choices, famous people who have had the disease, etc—while others do not want to know so much, and some want to leave all of the decisions in the hands of their family and physicians. What would she like? What kind of patient is she? She whispered to her daughter that she wants to leave it alone for now.
>
> That seemed to be her final word. We repeated to her that treatment choices would need to be made shortly. She was told that we would respect her desire, but that if she changed her mind we could talk at any

time; and that, in any event, she must understand that we would stay by her and see to her comfort in all possible ways. She signified that she understood and said that we should deal with her children. Both Dr H and I understood this as explicitly authorizing her children to speak for her with respect to treatment decisions.

The above approach relies on one simple tactic: a patient will be offered the opportunity to learn the truth, at whatever level of detail that patient desires. The most important step in these attempts is to ask questions of the patient and then listen closely to the patient's responses. Since the discussion at hand concerns how much information the patient would like to receive, here, unlike most physician-patient interchanges, the important decisions will need to be made by the patient.

Initiating discussion is relatively easy if the patient is only recently conscious and responsive; it is more difficult if a conspiracy of silence has already taken effect. The conversation with the patient might be initiated by telling him or her that at this time the medical team has arrived at a fairly clear understanding of the situation and treatment options. New test results may be alluded to; this is a fairly safe statement, since new tests are always being done on all patients. These conversational gambits signal that a fresh start in communication can now be attempted. (At the same time it avoids the awkwardness of a patient's asking, "Why haven't you spoken to me before?")

The patient might then be told that, before we talk about our current understanding of the medical situation, it is important to hear from the patient himself or herself, so that we can confirm what he or she knows or clear up any misunderstanding that may have arisen. The patient sometimes, with more than a little logic, responds, "Why are you asking me what is wrong? You're the doctor, you tell me what's wrong." A variety of answers are possible. A patient might be told that we have found that things work better if we start with the patient's understanding of the illness; or that time might be saved if we know what the patient understands, and go from there; or that whenever you try to teach someone, you have to start with what they know. Different approaches may suggest themselves as more fitting to the particular patient in question. The important thing is to begin to generate a dynamic within which the patient is speaking and the physician responding, rather than vice versa. Only then can the pace of conversation and level of information be controlled by the patient. The structure of the discussion, as well as the content of what the physician says, must reinforce the message: We are now establishing a new opportunity to talk and question, but you as the patient will have to tell us how much you want to know about your illness.

The chief ethical principle underlying the idea that patients should be offered the truth is, of course, respect for the patient's personal autonomy. By holding the conversation, the patient is given the opportunity to express autonomy in its most robust, direct fashion: the clear expression of preference. Legal systems that value autonomy will similarly protect a physician who chooses to offer truth and to respect the patient's response to that offer; "a medical doctor need not make disclosure of risks when the patient requests that he not be so informed."[5] A patient's right to information vests in that patient, to exercise as he or she desires; so that a patient's right to information is respected no less when the patient chooses to be relatively uninformed as when full information is demanded.[6] This stance is entirely consistent with the recent adoption of the widely noted (and even more widely misconstrued) Patient Self-Determination Act.[7] The major innovation this entails has been to involve institutions in the process of informing patients of their rights. However, the Patient Self-Determination Act has not changed state laws about informed consent to treatment in any way,[8] and as such the basic question here addressed—a physician's responsibility to inform patients of their diagnoses—remains entirely unaffected.

When offering truth, we are forced to recognize that patients' choices should be respected not because we or others agree with those choices (still less, respected *only* when we agree with those choices), but simply because those are the patient's choices. Indeed, the test of autonomy comes precisely when we personally disagree with the path the patient had chosen. If, for example, patient choice is respected only when the patient chooses the most effective treatment, when respecting those choices we would be respecting only effective therapeutics, not the person who has chosen them.

Many physicians hold to the ideal of an informed, alert, cooperative, and intelligent patient.

But the point of offering truth—rather than inflicting it—is to allow the patient to choose his or her own path. As a practical matter, of course, it could scarcely be otherwise. A physician with fanatic devotion to informing patients can lecture, explain, even harangue, but cannot force the patient to attend to what the physician is saying, or think about it, or remember it.

Families need to confront the same point. Ambivalence and conflict are often observed among family members concerning whether the patient who has not been informed "really" knows (or suspects, etc), and by offering the patient the opportunity to speak, this issue may be settled. More fundamentally, though, the concealing family—which is after all characterized by deep concern for the patient's well-being—will rarely (has never, in my experience to date) maintain that even if the patient demands to know the truth, the secret should still be kept. The family rather relies on the patient's failure to make this explicit demand as his or her tacit agreement to remain ignorant. Families can be helped to see that there may be many reasons for the patient's failure to demand the truth (including the fact that the patient may believe the lies that have been offered). If the patient wishes to remain in a state of relative ignorance, he or she will tell us that when asked; and if the patient states an explicit desire to be informed, families will find it hard to deny his or her right to have that desire respected.

Some families, naturally enough, suspect chicanery, that this approach is rigged to get the patient to ask for the truth. To them I respond that my experience proves otherwise: to my surprise and that of the physicians, some patients ask to leave this in the family's hands; to the surprise of families, some patients who seemed quietistic in fact strongly wish to be told the truth (which many of them had already suspected). We cannot know what the patient wants until we ask, I tell them, and we all want to do what the patient wants.

Having held the discussion, it is important to move on to its resolution as soon as possible.

> I met with Mrs S's children, together with a nurse, medical resident, and medical student, for about an hour and a half; the treating oncologist also made a brief appearance. The discussion featured a lengthy and eloquent exposition by the resident of why Mrs S needs to be spoken to, and a passionate and equally eloquent appeal by one son to respect the different culture from which they come. Finally, I introduced the idea that we offer her the truth, and then follow her lead. This was agreed to by the family, and I left.

The medical student thanked me some days later and told me the rest of the story. The tension that had existed between health-care team and family had largely dissipated; as the student put it, "People were able to look each other in the eye again." Mrs S was lucid but fatigued that evening; for that reason, and probably because they had already spent so much time talking at our meeting, the family delayed the agreed-on discussion. Unexpectedly, Mrs S did not survive the night.

CONCLUSION

The problem of the uninformed patient with cancer can be described in many different ways, for example, as faulty physician-patient communication; as an obstacle to good medical care; as a cause of stress among hospital staff; and as a failure to respect patient autonomy. A dimension at least as important as these, but rarely acknowledged, is the clash it may represent between diverse cultures and their basic moral commitments.

The approach presented above reflects an effort to maintain accepted standards of the physician-patient relationship while respecting the cultural background and requirements of families. This form of respect involves reasonable accommodation to these cultural expectations but should not be confused with uncritical acquiescence. The critical question is, perhaps, this: How should we react to a family that refuses to allow the patient an offering of truth, that maintains that discussion itself to be contrary to cultural norms? Under those circumstances, I believe the offering must be made notwithstanding family demands. My reasons have as much to do with my beliefs about the nature of ethnic and religious moral norms themselves as with the view that in cases of conflict, our public morality (as concretized in law) should prevail.

First, I believe that members of a cultural community are as prone to mistaking what their own norms require of them as we within the broader culture are to mistaking our own moral obligations. The norm of protecting the patient clearly requires rather than prohibits disclosure in some cases, including some described above, to prevent physical or psychological damage or to enable some final task to be consummated. All of the factors that we recognize sometimes to derange our own moral judgment—inertia, ill-grounded prejudices and generalizations, lack of the courage to confront unpleasant situations, and many more—may operate as powerfully in deranging the views of those from another culture. Their initial sense of what ethics require may, that is, be mistaken, from the point of view of their own norms as well as those of modern, Western, secular culture.

Second, even if a family's judgment of what their culture requires is accurate, we must not presume that a patient like Mrs A will choose, in extremis, to abide by her own cultural norms. Like any immigrant, she may have adopted the norms of broad society, or, acculturated to some lesser degree, she may act according to some hybrid set of values. Concretely, the offering of truth is about her diagnosis; symbolically, it is a process that allows her to declare her own preference regarding which norms shall be respected and how.

A last word is in order about the view implicit in this approach regarding the nature of a bioethical consultation. As these cases illustrate, patients, families, and health-care professionals come to a meeting from different moral worlds, as well as different backgrounds and biographies; and these worlds involve not simply rights and privileges, but duties as well. A successful consultation attempts to clarify on behalf of the different parties their own moral principles and associated moral commitments. It needs to proceed from the premise that all present ultimately share a common goal: the well-being of the patient.

REFERENCES

1. Oken D. What to tell cancer patients: a study of medical attitudes. *JAMA.* 1961;175:1120–1128.
2. Novack DH, Plumer R, Smith RL, Ochitil H, Morrow GR, Bennett JM. Changes in physicians' attitudes toward telling the cancer patient. *JAMA.* 1979; 241:897–900.
3. Welts EP. The Greek family. In: McGoldrick MM, Pearce JK, Giordano J. *Ethnicity and Family Therapy.* New York, NY: Guilford Press; 1982:269–288.
4. Dalla-Vorgia P, Katsouyanni K, Garanis TN, et al. Attitudes of a Mediterranean population to the truth-telling issue. *J Med. Ethics.* 1992;18:67–74.
5. *Cobbs v Grant,* 502 P2d 1 (Cal 1972) (a similar provision for a patient's right to waive being informed was established by the Supreme Court of Canada in *Reibl v Hughes* 2SCR 880 [1980]).
6. Freedman B. The validity of ignorant consent to medical research. *IRB Rev Hum Subjects Res.* 1982;4(2):1–5.
7. The Patient Self Determination Act, sections 4206 and 4751 of the Omnibus Reconciliation Act of 1990, Pub L 101-508.
8. McCloskey E. Between isolation and intrusion: the Patient Self Determination Act. *Law Med Health Care.* 1991;19:80–82.

INFORMED CONSENT

ARATO V. AVEDON

Supreme Court of California, En Banc, 1993

5 Cal. 4th 1172, 23 Cal. Rptr. 2d 131, 858 P. 2d 589

ARABIAN, Justice

A physician's duty to disclose to a patient information material to the decision whether to undergo treatment is the central constituent of the legal doctrine known as "informed consent." In this case, we review the ruling of a divided Court of Appeal that, in recommending a course of chemotherapy and radiation treatment to a patient suffering from a virulent form of cancer, the treating physicians breached their duty to obtain the patient's informed consent by failing to disclose his statistical life expectancy. . . .

I., A

Miklos Arato was a successful 42-year-old electrical contractor and part-time real estate developer when, early in 1980, his internist diagnosed a failing kidney. On July 21, 1980, in the course of surgery to remove the kidney, the operating surgeon detected a tumor on the "tail" or distal portion of Mr. Arato's pancreas. After Mrs. Arato gave her consent, portions of the pancreas were resected, or removed, along with the spleen and the diseased kidney. A follow-up pathological examination of the resected pancreatic tissue confirmed a malignancy. Concerned that the cancer could recur and might have infiltrated adjacent organs, Mr. Arato's surgeon referred him to a group of oncology practitioners for follow-up treatment.

During his initial visit to the oncologists, Mr. Arato filled out a multipage questionnaire routinely given new patients. Among the some 150 questions asked was whether patients "wish[ed] to be told the truth about [their] condition" or whether they wanted the physician to "bear the burden" for them. Mr. Arato checked the box indicating that he wished to be told the truth.

The oncologists discussed with Mr. and Mrs. Arato the advisability of a course of chemotherapy known as "F.A.M.," a treatment employing a combination of drugs which, when used in conjunction with radiation therapy, had shown promise in treating pancreatic cancer in experimental trials. The nature of the discussions between Mr. and Mrs. Arato and the treating physicians, and in particular the scope of the disclosures made to the patient by his doctors, was the subject of conflicting testimony at trial. By their own admission, however, neither the operating surgeon nor the treating oncologists specifically disclosed to the patient or his wife the high statistical mortality rate associated with pancreatic cancer.

Mr. Arato's oncologists determined that a course of F.A.M. chemotherapy was indicated for several reasons. According to their testimony, the high statistical mortality of pancreatic cancer is in part a function of what is by far the most common diagnostic scenario—the discovery of the malignancy well after it has metastasized to distant sites, spreading throughout the patient's body. As noted, in Mr. Arato's case, the tumor was comparatively localized, having been discovered in the tail of the pancreas by chance in the course of surgery to remove the diseased kidney.

Related to the "silent" character of pancreatic cancer is the fact that detection in such an advanced state usually means that the tumor cannot as a practical matter be removed, contributing to the high mortality rate. In Mr. Arato's case, however, the operating surgeon determined that it was possible to excise cleanly the tumorous portion of the pancreas and to leave a margin of about one-half centimeter around the surgical site, a margin that appeared clinically to be clear of cancer cells. Third, the mortality rate is somewhat lower, according to defense testimony, for pancreatic tumors located in the distal part of the organ than for those found in the main body. Finally, then-recent experimental studies on the use of F.A.M. chemotherapy in conjunction with therapeutic radiation treatments had shown promising response rates—on the order of several months of extended life—among pancreatic cancer patients.

Mr. Arato's treating physicians justified not disclosing statistical life expectancy data to their patient on disparate grounds. According to the testimony of his surgeon, Mr. Arato had exhibited great anxiety over his condition, so much so that his surgeon determined that it would have been medically inappropriate to disclose specific mortality rates. The patient's oncologists had a somewhat different explanation. As Dr. Melvin Avedon, his chief oncologist, put it, he believed that cancer patients in Mr. Arato's position "wanted to be told the truth, but did not want a cold shower." Along with the other treating physicians, Dr. Avedon testified that in his opinion the direct and specific disclosure of extremely high mortality rates for malignancies such as pancreatic cancer might effectively deprive a patient of any hope of cure, a medically inadvisable state. Moreover, all of the treating physicians testified that statistical life expectancy data had little predictive value when applied to a particular patient with individualized symptoms, medical history, character traits and other variables.

According to the physicians' testimony, Mr. and Mrs. Arato were told at the outset of the treatment that most victims of pancreatic cancer die of the disease, that Mr. Arato was at "serious" or "great" risk of a recurrence and that, should the cancer return, his condition would be judged incurable. This information was given to the patient and his wife in the context of a series of verbal and behavioral cues designed to invite the patient or family member to follow up with more direct and difficult questions. Such follow-up questions, on the order of "how long do I have to live?," would have signaled to his doctors, according to Dr. Avedon's testimony, the patient's desire and ability to confront the fact of imminent mortality. In the judgment of his chief oncologist, Mr. Arato, although keenly interested in the clinical significance of the most minute symptom, studiously avoided confronting these ultimate issues; according to his doctors, neither Mr. Arato nor his wife ever asked for information concerning his life expectancy in more than 70 visits over a period of a year. Believing that they had disclosed information sufficient to enable him to make an informed decision whether to undergo chemotherapy, Mr. Arato's doctors concluded that their patient had as much information regarding his condition and prognosis as he wished.

Dr. Avedon also testified that he told Mr. Arato that the effectiveness of F.A.M. therapy was unproven in cases such as his, described its principal adverse side effects, and noted that one of the patient's options was not to undergo the treatment. In the event, Mr. Arato consented to the proposed course of chemotherapy and radiation, treatments that are prolonged, difficult and painful for cancer patients. Unfortunately, the treatment proved ineffective in arresting the spread of the malignancy. Although clinical tests showed him to be free of cancer in the several months following the beginning of the F.A.M. treatments, beginning in late March and into April of 1981, the clinical signs took an adverse turn.[1] By late April, the doctors were convinced by the results of additional tests that the cancer had returned and was spreading. They advised the patient of their suspicions and discontinued chemotherapy. On July 25, 1981, a year and four days following surgery, Mr. Arato succumbed to the effects of pancreatic cancer.

B

Not long after his death, Mr. Arato's wife and two children brought this suit against the physicians who had treated their husband and father in his last days, including the surgeon who performed the pancreas resection and the oncologists who had recommended and administered the chemotherapy/radiation treatment. As presented to the jury, the gist of the lawsuit was the claim that in discussing with their patient the advisability of undergoing a course of chemotherapy and radiation, Mr. Arato's doctors had failed to disclose adequately the shortcomings of the proposed treatment in light of the diagnosis, and thus had failed to obtain the patient's informed consent. Specifically, plaintiffs contended that the doctors were aware that, because early detection is difficult and rare, pancreatic cancer is an especially virulent malignancy, one in which only 5 to 10 percent of those afflicted live for as long as five years, and that given the practically incurable nature of the disease, there was little chance Mr. Arato would live more than a short while, even if the proposed treatment proved effective.

Such mortality information, the complaint alleged—especially the statistical morbidity rate of pancreatic cancer—was material to Mr. Arato's decision whether to undergo postoperative treatment; had he known the bleak truth concerning his life expectancy, he would not have undergone the rigors of an unproven therapy, but would have chosen to live out his last days at peace with his wife and children, and arranging his business affairs. Instead, the complaint asserted, in the false hope that radiation and chemotherapy treatments could effect a cure—a hope born of the negligent failure of his physicians to disclose the probability of an early death—Mr. Arato failed to order his affairs in contemplation of his death, an omission that, according to the complaint, led eventually to the failure of his contracting business and to substantial real estate and tax losses following his death.

As the trial neared its conclusion and the court prepared to charge the jury, plaintiffs requested that several special instructions be given relating to the nature and scope of the physician's duty of disclosure. Two proffered instructions in particular are pertinent to this appeal. In the first, plaintiffs asked the trial court to instruct the jury that "A physician has a fiduciary duty to a patient to make a full and fair disclosure to the patient of all facts which materially affect the patient's rights and interests." The second instruction sought by plaintiffs stated that "The scope of the physician's duty to disclose is measured by the amount of knowledge a patient needs in order to make an informed choice. All information material to the patient's decision should be given."

The trial judge declined to give the jury either of the two instructions sought by the plaintiffs. Instead, the court read to the jury a modified version of BAJI No. 6.11, the so-called "reality of consent" instruction drawn from our opinion in *Cobbs* v. *Grant* (1972). . . . As can be seen by a comparison of the two instructions, the texts of which are set out in the margin,[2] the instruction actually given the jury by the trial court substantially recapitulated the wording of BAJI No. 6.11, except for the omission of two brief paragraphs dealing with exceptions to the duty of disclosure and a third paragraph that appears on its face not to have been relevant to the case as it developed at trial.

In addition to the modified version of BAJI No. 6.11, the trial court supplemented its informed consent instruction to the jury with the three special instructions, two requested by plaintiffs and a third offered by defendants, set out below.[3] Finally, with plaintiffs' approval, the trial court gave the jury several generic BAJI instructions dealing with such topics as the general legal duties of physicians and specialists (BAJI Nos. 6.00 & 6.11), the negligence standard of care in medical cases (BAJI Nos. 6.02 & 6.30) and when patient consent is necessary (BAJI No. 6.10).

After concluding its deliberations, the jury returned two special verdicts—on a form approved by plaintiffs' counsel—finding that none of the defendants was negligent in the "medical management" of Mr. Arato, and that defendants "disclosed to Mr. Arato all relevant information which would have enabled him to make an informed decision regarding the proposed treatment to be rendered him." Plaintiffs appealed from the judgment entered on the defense verdict, contending that the trial court erred in refusing to give the jury the special instructions requested by them. As noted, a divided Court of Appeal reversed the judgment of the trial court, and ordered a new trial. We granted defendants' ensuing petition for review and now reverse the judgment of the Court of Appeal.

C

In the Court of Appeal's view, Mr. Arato's doctors had breached the duty to disclose to their patient information material to the decision whether to undergo the radiation and drug therapy. According to the Court of Appeal, because there are so many different cancers, the lethality of which varies dramatically, telling a patient that cancer might recur and would then be incurable, without providing at least some general information concerning the virulence of the particular cancer at issue as reflected in mortality tables, was "meaningless." In addition, the Court of Appeal reasoned that his physicians were under a duty to disclose numerical life expectancy information to Mr. Arato so that he and his wife might take timely measures to minimize or avoid the risks of financial loss resulting from his death. . . .

The fount of the doctrine of informed consent in California is our decision of some 20 years ago in *Cobbs* v. *Grant, supra,* 8 Cal.3d 229, 104 Cal.Rptr. 505, 502 P.2d 1, an opinion by a unanimous court that built on several out-of-state decisions significantly broadening the scope and character of the physician's duty of disclosure in obtaining the patient's consent to treatment.[4] In *Cobbs* v. *Grant,* we not only anchored much of the doctrine of informed consent in a theory of negligence liability, but also laid down four "postulates" as the foundation on which the physician's duty of disclosure rests.

"The first [of these postulates,]" we wrote, "is that patients are generally persons unlearned in the medical sciences and therefore, except in rare cases, courts may safely assume the knowledge of patient and physician are not in parity. The second is that a person of adult years and in sound mind has the right, in the exercise of control over his own body, to determine whether or not to submit to lawful medical treatment.". . .

"The third [postulate,]" we continued, "is that the patient's consent to treatment, to be effective, must be an informed consent. And the fourth is that the patient, being unlearned in medical sciences, has an abject dependence upon and trust in his physician for the information upon which he relies during the decisional process, thus raising an obligation in the physician that transcends arms-length transactions.". . . From these ethical imperatives, we derived the obligation of a treating physician "of reasonable disclosure of the available choices with respect to proposed therapy and of the dangers inherently and potentially involved in each.". . .

II., B

Together with companion decisions in other jurisdictions, *Cobbs* v. *Grant, supra,* . . . is one of the epochal opinions in the legal recognition of the medical patient's protectible interest in autonomous decisionmaking. After more than a generation of experience with the judicially broadened duty of physician disclosure, the accumulated medicolegal comment on the subject of informed consent is both large and discordant. Those critics writing under the banner of "patient autonomy" insist that the practical administration of the doctrine has been thwarted by a failure of judicial nerve and an unremitting hostility to its underlying spirit by the medical profession. Others, equally earnest, assert that the doctrine misapprehends the realities of patient care and enshrines moral ideals in the place of workable rules.

Despite the critical standoff between these extremes of "patient sovereignty" and "medical paternalism," indications are that the *Cobbs*-era decisions helped effect a revolution in attitudes among patients and physicians alike regarding the desirability of frank and open disclosure of relevant medical information.[5] The principal question we must address is whether our holding in *Cobbs* v. *Grant, supra,* . . . as embodied in BAJI No. 6.11, accurately conveys to juries the legal standard under which they assess the evidence in determining the adequacy of the disclosures made by physician to patient in a particular case or whether, as the Court of Appeal here appeared to conclude, the standard instruction should be revised to mandate specific disclosures such as patient life expectancy as revealed by mortality statistics.

In our view, one of the merits of the somewhat abstract formulation of BAJI No. 6.11 is its recognition of the importance of the overall medical context that juries ought to take into account in deciding whether a challenged disclosure was reasonably sufficient to convey to the patient information material to an informed treatment decision. The contexts and clinical settings in which physician and patient interact and exchange information material to therapeutic decisions are so multifarious, the informational needs and degree of dependency of individual patients so various, and the professional relationship itself such an intimate and irreducibly judgment-laden one, that we believe it is unwise to require *as a matter of law* that a particular species of information be disclosed. We agree with the insight in *Salgo, supra,* 154 Cal. App.2d at page 578, 317 P.2d 170, that in administering the doctrine of informed consent, "each patient presents a separate problem, that the patient's mental and emotional condition is important and in certain cases may be crucial, and that in discussing the element of risk a certain amount of discretion must be employed consistent with the full disclosure of facts necessary to an informed consent."

Our opinion in *Cobbs* v. *Grant, supra,* . . . recognized these "common practicalities" of medical treatment which, we said, make the ideal of "full disclosure" a "facile expression[ ]." . . . Eschewing both a "mini-course in medical science" and a duty to discuss "the relatively minor risks inherent in common procedures," we identified the touchstone of the physician's duty of disclosure in the patient's need for "adequate information to enable an intelligent choice," a peculiarly fact-bound assessment which juries are especially wellsuited to make. . . .

This sensitivity to context seems all the more appropriate in the case of life expectancy projections for cancer patients based on statistical samples. Without exception, the testimony of every physician-witness at trial confirmed what is evident even to a nonprofessional: statistical morbidity values derived from the experience of population groups are inherently unreliable and offer little assurance regarding the fate of the individual patient; indeed, to assume that such data are conclusive in themselves smacks of a refusal to explore treatment alternatives and the medical abdication of the patient's well-being. Certainly the jury here heard evidence of articulable grounds for the conclusion that the particular features of Mr. Arato's case distinguished it from the typical population of pancreatic cancer sufferers and their dismal statistical probabilities—a fact plaintiffs [implicitly] acknowledged at trial in conceding that the oncologic referral of Mr. Arato and ensuing chemotherapy were not in themselves medically negligent.

In declining to endorse the mandatory disclosure of life expectancy probabilities, we do not mean to signal a retreat from the patient-based standard of disclosure explicitly adopted in *Cobbs* v. *Grant*. . . . We reaffirm the view taken in *Cobbs* that, because the "weighing of these risks [i.e., those inherent in a proposed procedure] against the individual subjective fears and hopes of the patient is not an expert skill," the test "for determining whether a potential peril must be divulged is its materiality to the patient's decision." . . . In reaffirming the appropriateness of that standard, we can conceive of no trier of fact more suitable than lay jurors to pronounce judgment on those uniquely human and necessarily situational ingredients that contribute to a specific doctor-patient exchange of information relevant to treatment decisions; certainly this is not territory in which appellate courts can usefully issue "bright line" guides.

Rather than mandate the disclosure of specific information as a matter of law, the better rule is to instruct the jury that a physician is under a legal duty to disclose to the patient all material information—that is, "information which the physician knows or should know would be regarded as significant by a reasonable person in the patient's position when deciding to accept or reject a recommended medical procedure"—needed to make an informed decision regarding a proposed treatment. That, of course, is the formulation embodied in BAJI No. 6.11 and the instruction given in this case. Having been properly instructed, the jury returned a defense verdict—on a form approved by plaintiffs' counsel—specifically finding that defendants had "disclosed to Mr. Arato all relevant information which would have enabled him to make an informed decision regarding the proposed treatment to be rendered him."

We decline to intrude further, either on the subtleties of the physician-patient relationship or in the resolution of claims that the physician's duty of disclosure was breached, by requiring the disclosure of information that may or may not be indicated in a given treatment context. Instead, we leave the ultimate judgment as to the factual adequacy of a challenged disclosure to the venerable American jury, operating under legal instructions such as those given here and subject to the persuasive force of trial advocacy.

Here, the evidence was more than sufficient to support the jury's finding that defendants had reasonably disclosed to Mr. Arato information material to his decision whether to undergo the proposed chemotherapy/radiation treatment. There was testimony that Mr. and Mrs. Arato were informed that cancer of the pancreas is usually fatal; of the substantial risk of recurrence, an event that would mean his illness was incurable; of the unproven nature of the F.A.M. treatments and their principal side effects; and of the option of forgoing such treatments. Mr. Arato's doctors also testified that they could not with confidence predict how long the patient might live, notwithstanding statistical mortality tables.

In addition, the jury heard testimony regarding the patient's apparent avoidance of issues bearing upon mortality; Mrs. Arato's testimony that his physicians had assured her husband that he was "clear" of cancer; and the couple's common expectation that he had been "cured," only to learn, suddenly and unexpectedly, that the case was hopeless and life measurable in weeks. The informed consent instructions given the jury to assess this evidence were an accurate statement of the law, and the Court of Appeal in effect invaded the province of the trier of fact in overturning a fairly litigated verdict.

C

In addition to their claim that his physicians were required to disclose statistical life expectancy data to Mr. Arato to enable him to reach an informed treatment decision, plaintiffs also contend that defendants should have disclosed such data because it was material to the patient's *nonmedical* interests, that is, Mr. Arato's business and investment affairs and the potential adverse impact of his death upon them. . . . Plaintiffs contend that since Mr. Arato's contracting and real estate affairs would suffer if he failed to make timely changes in estate planning in contemplation of imminent death, and since these matters are among "his rights and interests," his physicians were under a legal duty to disclose all material facts that might affect them, including statistical life expectancy information. We reject the claim as one founded on a premise that is not recognized in California.

The short answer to plaintiffs' claim is our statement in *Moore, supra,* . . . that a "physician is not the patient's financial adviser." . . . From its inception, the rationale behind the disclosure requirement implementing the doctrine of informed consent has been to protect the patient's freedom to "exercise . . . control over [one's] own body" by directing the course of *medical treatment*. . . . Although an aspect of personal autonomy, the conditions for the exercise of the patient's right of self-decision presuppose a therapeutic focus, a supposition reflected in the text of BAJI No. 6.11 itself. The fact that a physician has "fiducial" obligations which, as the result in *Bowman* illustrates, prohibit misrepresenting the nature of the patient's medical condition, does not mean that he or she is under a duty, the scope of which is undefined, to disclose every contingency that might affect the patient's *nonmedical* "rights and interests." Because plaintiffs' open-ended proposed instruction—that the physician's duty embraces the "disclosure . . . of all facts which materially affect the patient's rights and interests"—failed to reflect the therapeutic limitation inherent in the doctrine of informed consent, it would have been error for the trial judge to give it to the jury.

Finally, plaintiffs make much of the fact that in his initial visit to Dr. Avedon's office, Mr. Arato indicated in a lengthy form he was requested to complete that he "wish[ed] to be told the truth about [his] condition." In effect, they contend that as a result of Mr. Arato's affirmative answer, defendants had an absolute duty to make specific life expectancy disclosures to him. Whether the patient has filled out a questionnaire indicating that he or she wishes to be told the "truth" about his or her condition or not, however, a physician is under a legal duty to obtain the patient's informed consent to any recommended treatment. Although a patient may validly waive the right to be informed, we do not see how a request to be told the "truth" in itself heightens the duty of disclosure imposed on physicians as a matter of law.

III.

The final issue we must resolve concerns the use of expert testimony at trial. As noted, the Court of Appeal concluded that expert testimony offered on behalf of defendants went beyond what was appropriate in support of the so-called "therapeutic exception" to the physician's duty of disclosure, misleading the jury and prejudicing plaintiffs' case. Resolution of this issue requires an understanding of the proper, albeit limited, role of expert testimony in informed consent cases.

Over plaintiffs' objection, the trial court admitted the testimony of two medical experts, Drs. Plotkin and Wellisch, the former a professor of clinical medicine and the latter an expert in the psychological management of cancer patients. Both testified that the standard of medical practice cautioned against disclosing to pancreatic cancer patients specific life expectancy data unless the patient directly requested such information and that, in effect, defendants complied with that standard in not disclosing such information to Mr. Arato under the circumstances. Plaintiffs offered expert medical testimony of their own to counter this evidence; their expert testified that there are a number of indirect and compassionate ways to approach the issue of imminent mortality in dealing with patients with terminal cancer and that the standard of professional practice required that a patient in Mr. Arato's circumstances be given specific numerical life expectancy information.

Plaintiffs now complain that it was error for the trial court to admit expert defense testimony, relying on our statement in *Cobbs* v. *Grant, supra,* . . . that the weighing of the risks accompanying a given therapy "against the individual subjective fears and hopes of the patient is not an expert skill." Plaintiffs fail to distinguish between the two kinds of physician disclosure discussed in *Cobbs.* Our formulation of the scope of the duty of disclosure encompassed "the potential of death or serious harm" known to be inherent in a given procedure and an explanation "in lay terms [of] the complications that might possibly occur." . . . In addition to these disclosures, which we termed the "minimal" ones required of a physician to ensure the patient's informed decision-making, we said that the physician must also reveal to the patient "such additional information as a skilled practitioner of good standing would provide under similar circumstances." . . .

As its verbatim presence in BAJI No. 6.11 testifies, the quoted language, including the reference to the standard of professional practice as the benchmark for measuring the scope of disclosure beyond that implicated by the risks of death or serious harm and the potential for complications, has become an integral part of the legal standard in California for measuring the adequacy of a physician's disclosure in informed consent cases.

In reckoning the scope of disclosure, the physician will for the most part be guided by the patient's decisional needs—or, as we said in *Cobbs* v. *Grant, supra,* "the test for determining whether a potential peril must be divulged is its materiality to the patient's decision." . . . A physician, however, evaluates the patient's decisional needs against a background of professional understanding that includes a knowledge of what information beyond the significant risks associated with a given treatment would be regarded by the medical community as appropriate for disclosure under the circumstances.

It is thus evident that under the formulation we adopted in *Cobbs* v. *Grant, supra,* . . . situations will sometimes arise in which the trier of fact is unable to decide the ultimate issue of the adequacy of a particular disclosure without an understanding of the standard of practice within the relevant medical community. For that reason, in an appropriate case, the testimony of medical experts qualified to offer an opinion regarding what, if any, disclosures—in addition to those relating to *the risk of death or serious injury and significant potential complications posed by consenting to or declining a proposed treatment*—would be made to the patient by a skilled practitioner in the relevant medical community under the circumstances is relevant and admissible. . . .

Because statistical life expectancy data is information that lies outside the significant risks associated with a given treatment, the disclosure of which is mandated by *Cobbs* v. *Grant, supra,* . . . it falls within the scope of the "additional information . . . a skilled practitioner . . . would provide." And since the question of whether a physician should disclose such information turns on the standard of practice within the medical community, the trial court did not err in permitting expert testimony directed at that issue.

CONCLUSION

The judgment of the Court of Appeal is reversed and the cause is remanded with directions to affirm the judgment of the trial court.

LUCAS, C.J., and MOSK, PANELLI, KENNARD, BAXTER and GEORGE, J.J., concur.

NOTES

1. Around this time—on March 12, 1981, according to the record—an article appeared in the Los Angeles Times stating that only 1 percent of males and 2 percent of females diagnosed as having pancreatic cancer live for five years. According to his wife's testimony, Mr. Arato read the Times article and brought it to the attention of his oncologists. One of his oncologists confirmed such a discussion but denied that he told Mr. Arato that the statistics did not apply to his case, as Mrs. Arato testified. Mr. Arato continued to undergo chemotherapy treatment after reading the article and evidently made no changes in his estate planning or business and real estate affairs.
2. The trial judge read to the jury the following instruction:

   "Except as hereinafter explained, it is the duty of the physician to disclose to the patient all material information to enable the patient to make an informed decision regarding proposed treatment. [¶] Material information is information which the physician knows or should know would be regarded as significant by a reasonable person in the patient's position when deciding to accept or reject a recommended medical procedure. To be material a fact must also be one which is not commonly appreciated. [¶] A physician has no duty of disclosure beyond that required of a physician of good standing in the same or similar locality when he or she relied upon facts which would demonstrate to a reasonable person that the disclosure would so seriously upset the patient that the patient would not have been able to rationally weigh the risks of refusing to undergo the recommended treatment. [¶] Even though the patient has consented to a proposed treatment or operation, the failure of the physician to inform the patient as stated in this instruction before obtaining such consent is negligence and renders the physician subject to liability for any damage legally resulting from the failure to disclose or for any injury legally resulting from the treatment if a reasonably prudent person in the patient's position would not have consented to the treatment if he or she had been adequately informed of the likelihood of his [*sic*] premature death."
3. As modified, the following two instructions requested by plaintiffs were read to the jury:

   "The law recognizes that patients are generally persons unlearned in the medical sciences and that the knowledge of the patient and physician are not in parity.

   "The law recognizes that a person of adult years and in sound mind has the right, in the exercise of control over his own body, to determine whether or not to submit to lawful medical treatment."

   The following instruction, modified by the trial court, was given at defendants' request:

   "The doctrine of informed consent imposes upon a physician a duty to disclose relevant information concerning a proposed treatment. However, the doctrine recognizes that the primary duty of a physician is to do what is best for his patient."
4. Influential contemporaneous decisions of other courts include *Canterbury* v. *Spence* (D.C.Cir. 1972) 464 F.2d 772 and *Natanson* v. *Kline* (1960) 186 Kan. 393, 350 P.2d 1093, as well as the much earlier but still powerful opinion by Judge Cardozo in *Schloendorff* v. *Society of New York Hospital* (1914) 211 N.Y. 125, 105 N.E. 92. The origin of the phrase "informed consent" is often attributed to the opinion by Justice Bray in *Salgo* v. *Leland Stanford etc. Bd. Trustees* (1957) 154 Cal.App.2d 560, 578, 317 P.2d 170 (*Salgo*). (See, e.g., Katz, *Informed Consent—A Fairy Tale? Law's Vision* (1977) 39 U.Pitt.L.Rev. 137.) We recently traced the origin and development of the doctrine in American law in *Thor* v. *Superior Court* (1993) 5 Cal.4th 725, 21 Cal. Rptr.2d 357, 855 P.2d 375.
5. According to the report of the Presidential Commission, a survey conducted in 1961 by the Journal of the American Medical Association found that 90 percent of physicians preferred not to inform patients of a diagnosis of cancer; in a follow-up study conducted in 1977, 97 percent of the physicians surveyed said they routinely disclosed cancer diagnoses to patients.

ANTIHYPERTENSIVES AND THE RISK OF TEMPORARY IMPOTENCE: A CASE STUDY IN INFORMED CONSENT

John D. Arras

Dr. Sylvia Kramer pondered what she would tell Robert Williams on his next visit to her primary care clinic. Mr. Williams was an affable 40-year-old African-American, and one of Dr. Kramer's favorite patients. He had recently remarried, and enjoyed telling his doctor about his two young stepdaughters. The problem that brought him to this inner-city clinic was high blood pressure, which was first diagnosed by Dr. Kramer a year ago, during her first year as a resident in family medicine. Mr. Williams's blood pressure had then measured 180/103: not frightening numbers, to be sure, but still very much on the high side of "mild hypertension." If his blood pressure were not lowered, Mr. Williams could anticipate some serious related health problems, such as an increased risk of stroke.

Dr. Kramer's initial recommendation to Mr. Williams was that he attempt to control his weight and blood pressure through a regimen of regular exercise and a sensible diet low in salt and fat. She had recalled one of her mentor's lectures on hypertension: "No need to burden your patients with expensive drugs with side effects when they can solve the problem on their own through good behavior." Although Mr. Williams had achieved some lowering of his blood pressure during the ensuing months, down to 160/95, this improvement still left him in the marginal zone and was, in any case, short-lived. His blood-pressure readings were now consistently elevated. On his last visit, he had expressed some frustration to Dr. Kramer that, try as he might, no amount of exercise or diet seemed to be working.

Given Mr. Williams's lack of progress, Dr. Kramer was considering prescribing a common diuretic, hydrochlorothiazide, as the second line of defense against his hypertension. This particular drug, she knew, has a long history as a cheap and highly effective remedy. The price tag, 5 cents per pill, was particularly attractive to Dr. Kramer, who realized that her clinic patients often had a hard time paying for some of the more "high-tech" and high-priced hypertension medications that had been flooding the market in recent years.

Notwithstanding its relative safety, efficacy, and affordability, this particular drug still posed problems. First, it had a tendency to leech potassium from the body. She could address that problem by prescribing bananas. The second problem, a more serious matter, was a risk of causing impotence in males. The risk was small, however: only about 3 to 5 percent of men who took the pill were likely to be affected, and the impotence was easily reversible. One simply had to stop taking the drug for this side effect to disappear.

Dr. Kramer pondered the question of what "informed consent" should mean in this situation. In particular, she wondered whether she had an obligation to inform Mr. Williams of the risk of temporary impotence when recommending that he start with this diuretic. While this risk was certainly a lot less worrisome than the remote possibility of death attendant upon many medical and surgical procedures, it was still significant. If Mr. Williams, a newlywed, were to experience an unexpected and unexplained episode of sexual dysfunction, he would no doubt be extremely upset and anxious about it. Dr. Kramer, the product of a family-medicine training program committed to the value of patient self-determination, initially felt that she should share all the risks that Mr. Williams would likely consider relevant to his decision. Cost was certainly a factor, but so was his sex life. He should have the right, she reasoned, to make his own trade-offs among competing values. If sexual dysfunction is high on his list of things to avoid, especially at this time in his marriage, he might be willing to pay extra for another drug.

Still somewhat uncomfortable with her conclusion, Dr. Kramer asked the advice of Dr. Robert Black, a senior physician in her program. Dr. Black registered total disbelief upon hearing the resident's plan of action. "Look," he said, "I'm a staunch supporter of patients' rights,

This case study has benefited from helpful discussions with my brother, Ernest Arras, M.D., and from the careful scrutiny of several physician-colleagues at Montefiore Medical Center, including Michael Alderman, Ellen Cohen, Tom McGinn, and Doug Shenson.

autonomy, and all that, but this is just ridiculous. The risk is quite low, entirely reversible, and consider this: if you share this possible side effect with your patient, this little bit of truth is likely to make him extremely anxious about what could happen. You've heard of the Hawthorne effect, haven't you? Telling him about the risk of impotence could actually make Mr. Williams so worried that he would become impotent at your suggestion. I've been practicing medicine for fifteen years, and I've never told a patient about this sort of thing beforehand. If Mr. Williams comes back to you in a couple of weeks complaining about his sex life, you can deal with it then. But in the meantime, don't make a counterproductive fetish of informed consent. Lighten up!"

At this point, Dr. Kramer was truly puzzled. If she were to be entirely honest with her patient, she might end up doing him harm, and all for a very remote and reversible risk. On the other hand, it still bothered her to hide a fact from her patient that she suspected he would consider significant. He was, moreover, a rather shy man, especially about sexual matters. Dr. Kramer was not entirely confident that, should a problem develop, Mr. Williams would feel comfortable talking with a young female physician about his sexual "failure." He might just conclude that it was his or his new wife's fault, not the result of the drug, and live with impaired sexual function for some time.

How should Dr. Kramer resolve her ethical conflict? Should she (a) have a serious discussion with Mr. Williams about the small risk of temporary impotence, (b) casually mention the risk, perhaps using medical jargon, but only in passing along with many other minor risks, (c) withhold information about this particular risk until the patient complained of sexual dysfunction, or (d) withhold the information at first, but inquire specifically at a later date about the patient's sex life?

INFORMED CONSENT—MUST IT REMAIN A FAIRY TALE?

Jay Katz

I. THE PREHISTORY OF INFORMED CONSENT IN MEDICINE

The idea that, prior to any medical intervention, physicians must seek their patients' informed consent was introduced into American law in a brief paragraph in a 1957 state court decision,[1] and then elaborated on in a lengthier opinion in 1960.[2] The emerging legal idea that physicians were from now on obligated to share decisionmaking authority with their patients shocked the medical community, for it constituted a radical break with the silence that had been the hallmark of physician-patient interactions throughout the ages. Thirty-five years are perhaps not long enough for either law or medicine to resolve the tension between legal theory and medical practice, particularly since judges were reluctant to face up to implications of their novel doctrine, preferring instead to remain quite deferential to the practices of the medical profession.

Viewed from the perspective of medical history, the doctrine of informed consent, if taken seriously, constitutes a revolutionary break with customary practice. Thus, I must review, albeit all too briefly, the history of doctor-patient communication. Only then can one appreciate how unprepared the medical profession was to heed these new legal commands. But there is more: Physicians could not easily reject what law had begun to impose on them, because they recognized intuitively that the radical transformation of medicine since the age of medical science made it possible, indeed imperative, for a doctrine of informed consent to emerge.

From *Journal of Contemporary Health Law and Policy,* Vol. 10–67. Used with permission. Deletions approved by the author.

Editors' note: Space limitations have forced us to cut several sections of this article. Many footnotes have been deleted, and the remainder have been renumbered.

Yet, bowing to the doctrine did not mean accepting it. Indeed, physicians could not accept it because, for reasons I shall soon explore, the nature of informed consent has remained in the words of Churchill, "an enigma wrapped in a mystery."

Throughout the ages physicians believed that they should make treatment decisions for their patients. This conviction inheres in the Hippocratic Oath: "I swear by Apollo and Aesculepius [that] I will follow that system of regimen which according to *my* ability and judgment *I* consider for the benefit of *my* patients. . . ."[3] The patient is not mentioned as a person whose ability and judgment deserve consideration. Indeed, in one of the few references to disclosure in the Hippocratic Corpus, physicians are admonished "to [conceal] most things from the patient while attending to him; [to] give necessary orders with cheerfulness and serenity, . . . revealing nothing of the patient's future or present condition."[4] When twenty-five centuries later, in 1847, the American Medical Association promulgated its first Code of Ethics, it equally admonished patients that their "obedience . . . to the prescriptions of [their] physician should be prompt and implicit. [They] should never permit (their] own crude opinions . . . to influence [their] attention to [their physicians]."[5]

The gulf separating doctors from patients seemed unbridgeable both medically and socially. Thus, whenever the Code did not refer to physicians and patients as such, the former were addressed as "gentlemen" and the latter as "fellow creatures." To be sure, caring for patients' medical needs and "abstain[ing] from whatever is deleterious and mischievous"[6] was deeply imbedded in the ethos of Hippocratic medicine. The idea that patients were also "autonomous" human beings, entitled to being partners in decisionmaking, was, until recently, rarely given recognition in the lexicon of medical ethics. The notion that human beings possess individual human rights, deserving of respect, of course, is of recent origin. Yet, it antedates the twentieth century and therefore could have had an impact on the nature and quality of the physician-patient relationship.

It did not. Instead, the conviction that physicians should decide what is best for their patients, and, therefore, that the authority and power to do so should remain vested in them, continued to have a deep hold on the practices of the medical profession. For example, in the early 1950s the influential Harvard sociologist Talcott Parsons, who echoed physicians' views, stated that the physician is a technically competent person whose competence and specific judgments and measures cannot be competently judged by the layman and that the latter must take doctors' judgments and measures on "authority."[7] The necessity for such authority was supported by three claims:

First, *physicians' esoteric knowledge, acquired in the course of arduous training and practical experience, cannot be comprehended by patients.* While it is true that this knowledge, in its totality, is difficult to learn, understand and master, it does not necessarily follow that physicians cannot translate their esoteric knowledge into language that comports with patients' experiences and life goals (i.e., into language that speaks to quality of future life, expressed in words of risks, benefits, alternatives and uncertainties). Perhaps patients can understand this, but physicians have had too little training and experience with, or even more importantly, a commitment to, communicating their "esoteric knowledge" to patients in plain language to permit a conclusive answer as to what patients may comprehend.

Second, *patients, because of their anxieties over being ill and consequent regression to childlike thinking, are incapable of making decisions on their own behalf.* We do not know whether the childlike behavior often displayed by patients is triggered by pain, fear, and illness, or by physicians' authoritarian insistence that good patients comply with doctors' orders, or by doctors' unwillingness to share information with patients. Without providing such information, patients are groping in the dark and their stumbling attempts to ask questions, if made at all, makes them appear more incapable of understanding than they truly are.

We know all too little about the relative contributions which being ill, being kept ignorant, or being considered incompetent make to these regressive manifestations. Thus, physicians' unexamined convictions easily become self-fulfilling prophesies. For example, Eric Cassell has consistently argued that illness robs patients of autonomy and that only subsequent to the act of healing is autonomy restored.[8] While there is some truth to these contentions, they overlook the extent to which doctors can restore autonomy prior to the act of healing by not treating patients as children but as adults whose capacity for remaining authors of their own fate can be sustained and nourished. Cassell's views are reminiscent of Dostoyevsky's Grand Inquisitor who proclaimed that "at the most fearful moments of life," mankind is in need of "miracle, mystery and authority."[9] While, in this modern age, a person's capacity and right to take responsibility for his or her conduct has been given greater recognition than the Grand Inquisitor was inclined to grant, it still does not extend to patients. In the context of illness, physicians are apt to join the Grand Inquisitor at least to the extent of asserting that, while patients, they can only be comforted through subjugation to miracle, mystery and authority.

Third, *physicians' commitment to altruism is a sufficient safeguard for preventing abuses of their professional authority.* While altruism, as a general professional commitment, has served patients well in their encounters with physicians, the kind of protection it does and does not provide has not been examined in any depth. I shall have more to say about this later on. For now, let me only mention one problem: Altruism can only promise that doctors will try to place their patients' medical needs over their own personal needs. Altruism cannot promise that physicians will know, without inquiry, patients' needs. Put another way, patients and doctors do not necessarily have an identity of interest about matters of health and illness. Of course, both seek restoration of health and cure, and whenever such ends are readily attainable by only one route, their interests indeed may coincide.

In many physician-patient encounters, however, cure has many faces and the means selected affect the nature of cure in decisive ways. Thus, since quality of life is shaped decisively by available treatment options (including no treatment), the objectives of health and cure can be pursued in a variety of ways. Consider, for example, differences in value preferences between doctors and patients about longevity versus quality of remaining life. Without inquiry, one cannot presume identity of interest. As the surgeon Nuland cogently observed: "A doctor's altruism notwithstanding, his agenda and value system are not the same as those of the patient. That is the fallacy in the concept of beneficence so cherished by many physicians."[10]

II. THE AGE OF MEDICAL SCIENCE AND INFORMED CONSENT

During the millennia of medical history, and until the beginning of the twentieth century, physicians could not explain to their patients, or—from the perspective of hindsight—to themselves, which of their treatment recommendations were curative and which were not. To be sure, doctors, by careful bedside observation, tried their level best "to abstain from what is deleterious and mischievous," to help if they could, and to be available for comfort during the hours, days or months of suffering. Doing more curatively, however, only became possible with the advent of the age of medical science. The introduction of scientific reasoning into medicine, aided by the results of carefully conducted research, permitted doctors for the first time to discriminate more aptly between knowledge, ignorance and conjecture in their recommendations for or against treatment. Moreover, the spectacular technological advances in the diagnosis and treatment of disease, spawned by medical science, provided patients and doctors with ever-increasing therapeutic options, each having its own particular benefits and risks.

Thus, for the first time in medical history it is possible, even medically and morally imperative, to give patients a voice in medical decisionmaking. It is possible because knowledge and ignorance can be better specified; it is medically imperative because a variety of treatments are available, each of which can bestow great benefits or inflict grievous harm; it is morally imperative because patients, depending on the lifestyle they wish to lead during and after treatment, must be given a choice.

All this seems self-evident. Yet, the physician-patient relationship—the conversations between the two parties—was not altered with the transformation of medical practice during the twentieth century. Indeed, the silence only deepened once laboratory data were inscribed in charts and not in patients' minds, once machines allowed physicians' eyes to gaze not at patients' faces but at the numbers they displayed, once x-rays and electrocardiograms began to speak for patients' suffering rather than their suffering voices.

What captured the medical imagination and found expression in the education of future physicians, was the promise that before too long the diagnosis of patients' diseases would yield objective, scientific data to the point of becoming algorithms. *Treatment,* however, required subjective data from patients and would be influenced by doctors' subjective judgments. This fact was overlooked in the quest for objectivity. Also overlooked was the possibility that greater scientific understanding of the nature of disease and its treatment facilitated better communication with patients. In that respect contemporary Hippocratic practices remained rooted in the past.

III. THE IMPACT OF LAW

The impetus for change in traditional patterns of communication between doctors and patients came not from medicine but from law. In a 1957 California case,[11] and a 1960 Kansas case,[12] judges were astounded and troubled by these undisputed facts: That without any disclosure of risks, new technologies had been employed which promised great benefits but also exposed patients to formidable and uncontrollable harm. In the California case, a patient suffered a permanent paralysis of his lower extremities subsequent to the injection of a dye, sodium urokan, to locate a block in the abdominal aorta. In the Kansas case, a patient suffered severe injuries from cobalt radiation, administered, instead of conventional x-ray treatment, subsequent to a mastectomy for breast cancer. In the latter case, Justice Schroeder attempted to give greater specifications to the informed consent doctrine, first promulgated in the California decision: "To disclose and explain to the patient, in language as simple as necessary, the nature of the ailment, the nature of the proposed treatment, the probability of success or of alternatives, and perhaps the risks of unfortunate results and unforeseen conditions within the body."[13]

From the perspective of improved doctor-patient communication, or better, shared decisionmaking, the fault lines inherent in this American legal doctrine are many:

One: The common law judges who promulgated the doctrine restricted their task to articulating new and more stringent standards of liability whenever physicians withheld material information that patients should know, particularly in light of the harm that the spectacular advances in medical technology could inflict. Thus, the doctrine was limited in scope, designed to specify those minimal disclosure obligations that physicians must fulfill to escape *legal* liability for alleged nondisclosures. Moreover, it was shaped and confined by legal assumptions about the objectives of the laws of evidence and negligence, and by economic philosophies as to who should assume the financial burdens for medical injuries sustained by patients.

Even though the judges based the doctrine on "Anglo-American law['s] . . . premise of thoroughgoing self-determination,"[14] as the Kansas court put it, or on "the root premise . . . fundamental in American jurisprudence that 'every human being of adult years and sound mind has a right to determine what shall be done with his own body,'"[15] as the Circuit Court for the District of Columbia put it in a subsequent opinion, the doctrine was grounded not in battery law (trespass), but in negligence law. The reasons are many. I shall only mention a compelling one: Battery law, based on unauthorized trespass, gives doctors only one defense—that they have made adequate disclosure. Negligence law, on the other hand, permits doctors to invoke many defenses, including "the therapeutic privilege" not to disclose when in their judgment, disclosure may prove harmful to patients' welfare.

[A] recent opinion illustrate[s] the problems identified here.* . . . [T]he Court of Appeal of California, in a groundbreaking opinion, significantly reduced the scope of the therapeutic privilege by requiring that in instances of hopeless prognosis (the most common situation in which the privilege has generally been invoked) the patient be provided with such information by asking, "If not the physician's duty to disclose a terminal illness, then whose?"[16] The duty to disclose prognosis had never before been identified specifically as one of the disclosure obligations in an informed consent opinion.

Thus, the appellate court's ruling constituted an important advance. It established that patients have a right to make decisions not only about the fate of their bodies but about the fate of their lives as well. The California Supreme Court, however, reversed. In doing so, the court made too much of an issue

---

**Editor's note:* The case is *Arato* v. *Avedon,* reprinted on pp. 83–90 of this volume.

raised by the plaintiffs that led the appellate court to hold that doctors must disclose "statistical life expectancy information."[17] To be sure, disclosure of statistical information is a complex problem, but in focusing on that issue, the supreme court's attention was diverted from a more important new disclosure obligation promulgated by the appellate court: the duty to inform patients of their dire prognosis. The supreme court did not comment on that obligation. Indeed, it seemed to reverse the appellate court on this crucial issue by reinforcing the considerable leeway granted physicians to invoke the therapeutic privilege exception to full disclosure: "We decline to intrude further, either on the subtleties of the physician-patient relationship or in the resolution of claims that the physician's duty of disclosure was breached, by requiring the disclosure of information that may or may not be indicated in a given treatment context."[18]

Two: The doctrine of informed consent was not designed to serve as a *medical* blueprint for interactions between physicians and patients. The medical profession still faces the task of fashioning a "doctrine" that comports with its own vision of doctor-patient communication and that is responsive both to the realities of medical practices in an age of science and to the commands of law. . . . Thus, disclosure practices only changed to the extent of physicians disclosing more about the risks of a proposed intervention in order to escape legal liability.

Three: Underlying the legal doctrine there lurks a broader assumption which has neither been given full recognition by judges nor embraced by physicians. The underlying idea is this: That from now on patients and physicians must make decisions jointly, with patients ultimately deciding whether to accede to doctors' recommendations. In *The Cancer Ward,* Solzhenitsyn captured, as only a novelist can, the fears that such an idea engenders. When doctor Ludmilla Afanasyevna was challenged by her patient, Oleg Kostoglotov, about physicians' rights to make unilateral decisions on behalf of patients, Afanasyevna gave a troubled, though unequivocal, answer: "But doctors *are* entitled to the right—doctors above all. Without that right, there'd be no such thing as medicine."[19]

If Afanasyevna is correct, then patients must continue to trust doctors silently. Conversation, to comport with the idea of informed consent, ultimately requires that both parties make decisions jointly and that their views and preferences be treated with respect. Trust, based on blind faith—on passive surrender to oneself or to another—must be distinguished from trust that is earned after having first acknowledged to oneself and then shared with the other what one knows and does not know about the decision to be made. If all of that had been considered by physicians, they would have appreciated that a new model of doctor-patient communication that takes informed consent seriously required a radical break with current medical disclosure practice.

Four: The idea of joint decisionmaking is one thing, and its application in practice another. . . . To translate social policy into *medical* policy is an inordinately difficult task. It requires a reassessment of the limits of medical knowledge in the light of medical uncertainty, a reassessment of professional authority to make decisions for patients in light of the consequences of such conduct for the well-being of patients, and a reassessment of the limits of patients' capacities to assume responsibility for choice in the light of their ignorance about medical matters and their anxieties when ill. Turning now to these problems, I wish to highlight that, in the absence of such reassessments, informed consent will remain a charade, and joint decisionmaking will elude us.

IV. BARRIERS TO JOINT DECISIONMAKING

A. Medical Uncertainty

The longer I reflect about doctor-patient decisionmaking, the more convinced I am that in this modern age of medical science, which for the first time permits sharing with patients the uncertainties of diagnosis, treatment, and prognosis, the problem of uncertainty poses the most formidable obstacle to disclosure and consent. By medical uncertainty I mean to convey what the physician Lewis Thomas observed so eloquently, albeit disturbingly:

> The only valid piece of scientific truth about which I feel totally confident is that we are profoundly ignorant about nature . . . It is this sudden confrontation with the depth and scope of ignorance that represents

> the most significant contribution of twentieth-century science to the human intellect. *We are, at last facing up to it.* In earlier times, we either pretended to understand . . . or ignored the problem, or simply made up stories to fill the gap.[20]

Alvan Feinstein put this in more concrete language: "Clinicians are still uncertain about the best means of treatment for even such routine problems as . . . a fractured hip, a peptic ulcer, a stroke, a myocardial infarction. . . . At a time of potent drugs and formidable surgery, the exact effects of many therapeutic procedures are dubious or shrouded in dissension."[21]

Medical uncertainty constitutes a formidable obstacle to joint decisionmaking for a number of reasons: Sharing uncertainties requires physicians to be more aware of them than they commonly are. They must learn how to communicate them to patients and they must shed their embarrassment over acknowledging the true state of their own and of medicine's art and science. Thus, sharing uncertainties requires a willingness to admit ignorance about benefits and risks; to acknowledge the existence of alternatives, each with its own known and unknown consequences; to eschew one single authoritative recommendation; to consider carefully how to present uncertainty so that patients will not be overwhelmed by the information they will receive; and to explore the crucial question of how much uncertainty physicians themselves can tolerate without compromising their effectiveness as healers. . . .

Moreover, acknowledgement of uncertainty is undermined by the threat that it will undermine doctors' authority and sense of superiority. As Nuland put it, to feel superior to those dependent persons who are the sick, is after all a motivating factor that often influences their choice of medicine as a profession.[22] All of this suggests that implementation of the idea of informed consent is, to begin with, not a patient problem but a physician problem.

B. Patient Incompetence

Earlier, I touched on physicians' convictions that illness and medicine's esoteric knowledge rob patients of the capacity to participate in decision making. Yet we do not know whether this is true. The evidence is compromised by the groping, half-hearted, and misleading attempts to inform patients about uncertainty and other matters which can make doctors' communications so confusing and incomprehensible. If patients then appear stupid and ignorant this should come as no surprise; nor should patients' resigned surrender to this dilemma: "You are the doctor, you decide."

It is equally debatable, as Thomas Duffy has contended, that "[p]aternalism exists in medicine . . . to fulfill a need created by illness."[23] It led him to argue, echoing Cassell, that "obviously autonomy cannot function as the cornerstone of the doctor-patient relationship [since] the impact of disease on personal integrity results in the patient's loss of autonomy. . . . In the doctor-patient relationship, the medical profession should always err on the side of beneficence."[24] If Duffy is correct, however, then informed consent is *ab initio* fatally compromised.

C. Patient Autonomy

Duffy's invocation of beneficence as the guiding principle is deeply rooted in the history of Hippocratic medicine. It finds expression in the ancient maxim: *primum non nocere*, above all do no harm, with "harm" remaining undefined but in practice being defined only as physical harm. Before presenting my views on the controversy over the primacy of autonomy or beneficence, let me briefly define their meaning.

In their authoritative book *Principles of Biomedical Ethics*, Thomas Beauchamp and James Childress defined these principles:

> Autonomy is a form of personal liberty of action where the individual determines his or her own course of action in accordance with a plan chosen by himself or herself. [Respect for individuals as autonomous agents entitles them] to such autonomous determinations without limitation on their liberty being imposed by others.[25]

Beneficence, on the other hand,

> [r]equires not only that we treat persons autonomously and that we refrain from harming them, but also that we contribute to their welfare including their health. [Thus the principle asserts] the duty to help others further their important and legitimate interests . . . to *confer* benefits and actively to prevent and remove harms

> . . . [and] to *balance* possible goods against the possible harms of an action.[26]

Beauchamp and Childress' unequivocal and strong postulate on autonomy contrasts with the ambiguities contained in their postulate on beneficence. What do they mean by "benefits" and "harms" that allow invocation of beneficence? Do they mean only benefits and harms to patients' physical integrity, or to their dignitary integrity as choice-making individuals as well? Furthermore, what degree of discretion and license is permissible in the duty "to balance?" I have problems with balancing unless it is resorted to only as a *rare* exception to respect for autonomy. While human life is, and human interactions are, too complex to make any principle rule absolute, any exceptions must be rigorously justified.

I appreciate that mine is a radical proposal and constitutes a sharp break with Hippocratic practices. If informed consent, however, is ever to be based on the postulate of joint decision making, the obligation "to respect the autonomous choices and actions of others,"[27] as Childress has put it, must be honored. Otherwise, informed consent is reduced to doctors providing more information but leaving decision making itself to the authority of physicians. . . .

VI. THE CURRENT STATE OF PHYSICIAN-PATIENT DECISION MAKING

In his recent book, entitled *How We Die,* Sherwin Nuland, a distinguished surgeon, reflects with profundity and insight on his lifelong interactions with patients. In a chapter on cancer and its treatment he speaks movingly about "death belong-[ing] to the dying and to those who love them."[28] Yet, that privilege is often wrested from them when,

> [d]ecisions about continuation of treatment are influenced by the enthusiasm of the doctors who propose them. Commonly, the most accomplished of the specialists are also the most convinced and unyielding believers in biomedicine's ability to overcome the challenge presented by a pathological process. . . . [W]hat is offered as objective clinical reality is often the subjectivity of a devout disciple of the philosophy that death is an implacable enemy. To such warriors, even a temporary victory justifies the laying waste of the fields in which a dying man has cultivated his life.[29]

Looking back at his work, he concludes that "more than a few of my victories have been Pyrrhic. The suffering was sometimes not worth the success. . . .[H]ad I been able to project myself into the place of the family and the patient, I would have been less often certain that the desperate struggle should be undertaken."[30]

In his view, a surgeon,

> [t]hough he be kind and considerate of the patient he treats . . . allows himself to push his kindness aside because the seduction of The Riddle [the quest for diagnosis and cure] is so strong and the failure to solve it renders him so weak. [Thus, at times he convinces] patients to undergo diagnostic or therapeutic measures at a point in illness so far beyond reason that The Riddle might better have remained unsolved.[31]

Speaking then about the kind of doctor he will seek out when afflicted with a major illness, Nuland does not expect him to "understand my values, my expectations for myself . . . my philosophy of life. *That is not what he is trained for and that is not what he will be good at.*"[32] Doctors can impart information, but "[i]t behooves every patient to study his or her own disease and learn enough about it. [Patients] should no longer expect from so many of our doctors what they cannot give."[33]

Nuland's views, supported by a great many poignant clinical vignettes, sensitively and forthrightly describe the current state of physician-patient decision making, so dominated by physicians' judgments as to what is best. He presents many reasons for this state of affairs. One is based on doctors' "fear of failure:"

> A need to control that exceeds in magnitude what most people would find reasonable. When control is lost, he who requires it is also a bit lost and so deals badly with the consequences of his impotence. In an attempt to maintain control, a doctor, usually without being aware of it, convinces himself that he knows better than the patient what course is proper. He dispenses only as much information as he deems fit, thereby influencing a patient's decision making in ways he does not recognize as self-serving.[34]

I have presented Nuland's observations at some length because they illustrate and support my contentions that joint decisionmaking between doctors and patients still eludes us. My critics had claimed earlier that my work on informed consent was dated because informed consent had become an integral aspect of the practice of medicine. In the paperback edition of *The Silent World of Doctor and Patient,* I argued that they have dismissed too lightly my central arguments:

> [T]hat meaningful collaboration between physicians and patients cannot become a reality until physicians have learned (1) how to treat their patients not as children but as the adults they are; (2) how to distinguish between their ideas of the best treatment and their patients' ideas of what is best; (3) how to acknowledge to their patients (and often to themselves as well) their ignorance and uncertainties about diagnosis, treatment, and prognosis; [and to all this, I now want to add, (4) how to explain to patients the uncertainties inherent in the state of the art and science of medicine which otherwise permits doctors on the basis of their clinical experience to leave unacknowledged that their colleagues on the basis of their clinical experience have different beliefs as to which treatment is best].[35] . . .

The moral authority of physicians will not be undermined by this caring view of interacting with patients. Doctors' authority resides in the medical knowledge they possess, in their capacity to diagnose and treat, in their ability to evaluate what can be diagnosed and what cannot, what is treatable and what is not, and what treatment alternatives to recommend, each with its own risks and benefits and each with its own prognostic implications as to cure, control, morbidity, exacerbation or even death.

The moral authority of physicians resides in knowing better than others the certainties and the uncertainties that accompany diagnosis, treatment, prognosis, health and disease, as well the extent and the limits of their *scientific* knowledge and *scientific* ignorance. Physicians must learn to face up to and acknowledge the tragic limitations of their own professional knowledge, their inability to impart all their insights to all patients, and their own personal incapacities—at times more pronounced than others—to devote themselves fully to the needs of their patients. They must learn not to be unduly embarrassed by their personal and professional ignorance and to trust their patients to react appropriately to such acknowledgment. From all this it follows that ultimately the moral authority of physicians resides in their capacity to sort out *with* patients the choices to be made.

It is in this spirit that duty and caring become interwoven. Bringing these strands together imposes upon physicians the duty to respect patients as persons so that care will encompass allowing patients to live their lives in their own self-willed ways. To let patients follow their own lights is not an abandonment of them. It is a professional duty that, however painful, doctors must obey.

Without fidelity to these new professional duties, true caring will elude physicians. There is much new to be learned about caring that in decades to come will constitute the kind of caring that doctors in the past have wished for but have been unable to dispense, and that patients may have always yearned for. . . .

NOTES

1. *Salgo* v. *Leland Stanford Jr.* Univ. Bd. of Trustees, 317 P.2d 170, 181 (Cal. Dist. Ct. App. 1957).
2. *Natanson* v. *Kline,* 350 P.2d 1093 (Kan. 1960).
3. Hippocrates, *Oath of Hippocrates, in* 1 Hippocrates 299-301 (W.H.S. Jones trans., 1962).
4. 2 Hippocrates 297 (W.H.S. Jones trans., 1962).
5. American Medical Association: Code of Ethics (1847), reprinted in Katz, *The Silent World of Doctor and Patient* 232 (1986).
6. Hippocrates, *supra* note 3, at 301.
7. Talcott Parsons, *The Social System* 464–65 (1951).
8. Eric Cassell, *The Function of Medicine,* Hastings Center Rep., Dec. 1977, at 16, 18.
9. Fyodor Dostoyevsky, *The Brothers Karamazov* 307 (A.P. MacAndrew trans., 1970).
10. Interview with Sherwin Nuland (1993).
11. *Salgo* v. *Leland Stanford Jr.* Univ. Bd. of Trustees, 317 P.2d 170 (Cal. Dist. Ct. App. 1957).
12. *Natanson* v. *Kline,* 350 P.2d 1093 (Kan. 1960).
13. *Id.* at 1106.
14. *Id.* at 1104.
15. *Canterbury* v. *Spence,* 464 F.2d 772, 780 (D.C. Cir. 1972).
16. *Arato* v. *Avedon,* 11 Cal. Rptr. 2d 169, 181 n.19 (Cal. Ct. App. 1992), *vacated,* 858 P.2d 598 (Cal. 1993).
17. *Arato,* 11 Cal. Rptr. 2d at 177.
18. *Arato,* 858 P.2d at 607.
19. Alexander Solzhenitsyn, *The Cancer Ward* 77 (N. Bethell & D. Burg trans., 1969).
20. Lewis Thomas, *The Medusa and the Snail* 73–74 (1979).

21. Alvan R. Feinstein, *Clinical Judgment* 23–24 (1967). Even though written 27 years ago, he has not changed his views. Interview with Alvan R. Feinstein (1994).
22. Interview with Sherwin B. Nuland (1994).
23. Thomas P. Duffy, *Agamemnon's Fate and the Medical Profession*, 9 W. New Eng. L. Rev. 21, 27 (1987).
24. *Id.* at 30.
25. Thomas L. Beauchamp & James F. Childress, *Principles of Biomedical Ethics* 56, 58 (1st ed. 1979).
26. Thomas L. Beauchamp & James F. Childress, *Principles of Biomedical Ethics* 148–49 (2d ed. 1983).
27. James F. Childress, *The Place of Autonomy in Bioethics*, Hastings Center Rep., Jan.–Feb. 1990, at 12, 12–13.
28. Sherwin B. Nuland, *How We Die* 265 (1994).
29. *Id.*
30. *Id.* at 266.
31. *Id.* at 249.
32. *Id.* at 266 (emphasis added).
33. *Id.* at 260.
34. *Id.* at 258.
35. Jay Katz, *supra* note 5, at xi (1986).

TRANSPARENCY: INFORMED CONSENT IN PRIMARY CARE

Howard Brody

While the patient's right to give informed consent to medical treatment is now well-established both in U.S. law and in biomedical ethics, evidence continues to suggest that the concept has been poorly integrated into American medical practice, and that in many instances the needs and desires of patients are not being well met by current policies.[1] It appears that the theory and the practice of informed consent are out of joint in some crucial ways. This is particularly true for primary care settings, a context typically ignored by medical ethics literature, but where the majority of doctor-patient encounters occur. Indeed, some have suggested that the concept of informed consent is virtually foreign to primary care medicine where benign paternalism appropriately reigns and where respect for patient autonomy is almost completely absent.[2]

It is worth asking whether current legal standards for informed consent tend to resolve the problem or to exacerbate it. I will maintain that accepted legal standards, at least in the form commonly employed by courts, send physicians the wrong message about what is expected of them. An alternative standard that would send physicians the correct message, a conversation standard, is probably unworkable legally. As an alternative, I will propose a transparency standard as a compromise that gives physicians a doable task and allows courts to review appropriately. I must begin, however, by briefly identifying some assumptions crucial to the development of this position even though space precludes complete argumentation and documentation.

The Hastings Center Report, Vol. 19, No. 5, Sept/Oct 1989, 5–9. Reprinted with permission.

CRUCIAL ASSUMPTIONS

Informed consent is a meaningful ethical concept only to the extent that it can be realized and promoted within the ongoing practice of good medicine. This need not imply diminished respect for patient autonomy, for there are excellent reasons to regard respect for patient autonomy as a central feature of good medical care. Informed consent, properly understood, must be considered an essential ingredient of good patient care, and a physician who lacks the skills to inform patients appropriately and obtain proper consent should be viewed as lacking essential medical skills necessary for practice. It is not enough to see informed consent as a nonmedical, legalistic exercise designed to promote patient autonomy, one that interrupts the process of medical care.

However, available empirical evidence strongly suggests that this is precisely how physicians currently view informed consent practices. Informed consent is still seen as bureaucratic legalism rather than as part of patient care. Physicians often deny the existence of realistic treatment alternatives, thereby attenuating the perceived need to inform the patient of meaningful options. While patients may be informed, efforts are seldom made to assess accurately the patient's actual need or desire for information, or what the patient then proceeds to do with the information provided. Physicians typically underestimate patients' desire to be informed and overestimate their desire to be involved in decision-making. Physicians may also view informed consent as an empty charade, since they are confident in their abilities to manipulate consent by how they discuss or divulge information.[3]

A third assumption is that there are important differences between the practice of primary care medicine and the tertiary care settings that have been most frequently discussed in the literature on informed consent. The models of informed consent discussed below typically take as the paradigm case something like surgery for breast cancer or the performance of an invasive and risky radiologic procedure. It is assumed that the risks to the patient are significant, and the values placed on alternative forms of treatment are quite weighty. Moreover, it is assumed that the specialist physician performing the procedure probably does a fairly limited number of procedures and thus could be expected to know exhaustively the precise risks, benefits, and alternatives for each.

Primary care medicine, however, fails to fit this model. The primary care physician, instead of performing five or six complicated and risky procedures frequently, may engage in several hundred treatment modalities during an average week of practice. In many cases, risks to the patient are negligible and conflicts over patient values and the goals of treatment or nontreatment are of little consequence. Moreover, in contrast to the tertiary care patient, the typical ambulatory patient is much better able to exercise freedom of choice and somewhat less likely to be intimidated by either the severity of the disease or the expertise of the physician; the opportunities for changing one's mind once treatment has begun are also much greater. Indeed, in primary care, it is much more likely for the full process of informed consent to treatment (such as the beginning and the dose adjustment of an antihypertensive medication) to occur over several office visits rather than at one single point in time.

It might be argued that for all these reasons, the stakes are so low in primary care that it is fully appropriate for informed consent to be interpreted only with regard to the specialized or tertiary care setting. I believe that this is quite incorrect for three reasons. First, good primary care medicine ought to embrace respect for patient autonomy, and if patient autonomy is operationalized in informed consent, properly understood, then it ought to be part and parcel of good primary care. Second, the claim that the primary care physician cannot be expected to obtain the patient's informed consent seems to undermine the idea that informed consent could or ought to be part of the daily practice of medicine. Third, primary care encounters are statistically more common than the highly specialized encounters previously used as models for the concept of informed consent.[4]

ACCEPTED LEGAL STANDARDS

Most of the literature on legal approaches to informed consent addresses the tension between the community practice standard and the reasonable patient standard, with the latter seen as the more satisfactory, emerging legal standard.[5] However, neither standard sends the proper message to the physician about what is expected of her to promote patient autonomy effectively and to serve the informational needs of patients in daily practice.

The community practice standard sends the wrong message because it leaves the door open too wide for physician paternalism. The physician is instructed to behave as other physicians in that specialty behave, regardless of how well or how poorly that behavior serves patients' needs. Certainly, behaving the way other physicians behave is a task we might expect physicians to readily accomplish; unfortunately, the standard fails to inform them of the end toward which the task is aimed.

The reasonable patient standard does a much better job of indicating the centrality of respect for patient autonomy and the desired outcome of the informed consent process, which is revealing the information that a reasonable person would need to make an informed and rational decision. This standard is particularly valuable when modified to include the specific informational and decisional needs of a particular patient.

If certain things were true about the relationship between medicine and law in today's society, the reasonable patient standard would provide acceptable guidance to physicians. One feature would be that physicians esteem the law as a positive force in guiding their practice, rather than as a threat to their well-being that must be handled defensively. Another element would be a prospective consideration by the law of what the physician could reasonably have been expected to do in practice, rather than a retrospective review armed with the foreknowledge that some significant patient harm has already occurred.

Unfortunately, given the present legal climate, the physician is much more likely to get a mixed or an undesirable message from the reasonable patient standard. The message the physician hears from the reasonable patient standard is that one must exhaustively lay out all possible risks as well as benefits and alternatives of the proposed procedure. If one remembers to discuss fifty possible risks, and the patient in a particular case suffers the fifty-first, the physician might subsequently be found liable for incomplete disclosure. Since lawsuits are triggered when patients suffer harm, disclosure of risk becomes relatively more important than disclosure of benefits. Moreover, disclosure of information becomes much more critical than effective patient participation in decisionmaking. Physicians consider it more important to document what they said to the patient than to document how the patient used or thought about that information subsequently.

In specialty practice, many of these concerns can be nicely met by detailed written or videotaped consent documents, which can provide the depth of information required while still putting the benefits and alternatives in proper context. This is workable when one engages in a limited number of procedures and can have a complete document or videotape for each.[6] However, this approach is not feasible for primary care, when the number of procedures may be much more numerous and the time available with each patient may be considerably less. Moreover, it is simply not realistic to expect even the best educated of primary care physicians to rattle off at a moment's notice a detailed list of significant risks attached to any of the many drugs and therapeutic modalities they recommend.

This sets informed consent apart from all other aspects of medical practice in a way that I believe is widely perceived by nonpaternalistic primary care physicians, but which is almost never commented upon in the medical ethics literature. To the physician obtaining informed consent, *you never know when you are finished.* When a primary care physician is told to treat a patient for strep throat or to counsel a person suffering a normal grief reaction from the recent death of a relative, the physician has a good sense of what it means to complete the task at hand. When a physician is told to obtain the patient's informed consent for a medical intervention, the impression is quite different. A list of as many possible risks as can be thought of may still omit some significant ones. A list of all the risks that actually have occurred may still not have dealt with the patient's need to know risks in relation to benefits and alternatives. A description of all benefits, risks, and alternatives may not establish whether the patient has understood the information. If the patient says he understands, the physician has to wonder whether he really understands or whether he is simply saying this to be accommodating. As the law currently *appears* to operate (in the perception of the defensively minded physician), there never comes a point at which you can be certain that you have adequately completed your legal as well as your ethical task.

The point is not simply that physicians are paranoid about the law; more fundamentally, physicians are getting a message that informed consent is very different from any other task they are asked to perform in medicine. If physicians conclude that informed consent is therefore not properly part of medicine at all, but is rather a legalistic and bureaucratic hurdle they must overcome at their own peril, blame cannot be attributed to paternalistic attitudes or lack of respect for patient autonomy.

THE CONVERSATION MODEL

A metaphor employed by Jay Katz, informed consent as conversation, provides an approach to respect for patient autonomy that can be readily integrated within primary care practice.[7] Just as the specific needs of an individual patient for information, or the meaning that patient will attach to the information as it is presented, cannot be known in advance, one cannot always tell in advance how a conversation is going to turn out. One must follow the process along and take one's cues from the unfolding conversation itself. Despite the absence of any formal rules for carrying out or completing a conversation on a specific subject, most people have a good intuitive grasp of what it means for a conversation to be finished, what it means to change the subject in the middle of a conversation, and what it means to later reopen a conversation one had thought was completed when something new has just arisen. Thus, the metaphor suggests that informed consent consists not in a formal process carried out strictly by protocol but in a conversation designed to encourage patient participation in all medical decisions to the extent that the patient wishes to be included. The idea of informed consent as physician-patient conversation could, when properly developed, be a useful analytic tool for ethical issues in informed consent, and could also be a powerful educational tool for highlighting the skills and attitudes that a physician needs to successfully integrate this process within patient care.

If primary care physicians understand informed consent as this sort of conversation process, the idea that exact rules cannot be given for its successful management could cease to be a mystery. Physicians would instead be guided to rely on their own intuitions and communication skills, with careful attention to information received from the patient, to determine when an adequate job had been done in the informed consent process. Moreover, physicians would be encouraged to see informed consent as a genuinely mutual and participatory process, instead of being reduced to the one-way disclosure of information. In effect, informed consent could be demystified, and located within the context of the everyday relationships between physician and patient, albeit with a renewed emphasis on patient participation.[8]

Unfortunately, the conversation metaphor does not lend itself to ready translation into a legal standard for determining whether or not the physician has satisfied her basic responsibilities to the patient. There seems to be an inherently subjective element to conversation that makes it ill-suited as a legal standard for review of controversial cases. A conversation in which one participates is by its nature a very different thing from the same conversation described to an outsider. It is hard to imagine how a jury could be instructed to determine in retrospect whether or not a particular conversation was adequate for its purposes. However, without the possibility for legal review, the message that patient autonomy is an important value and that patients have important rights within primary care would seem to be severely undermined. The question then is whether some of the important strengths of the conversation model can be retained in another model that does allow better guidance.

THE TRANSPARENCY STANDARD

I propose the transparency standard as a means to operationalize the best features of the conversation model in medical practice. According to this standard, adequate informed consent is obtained when a reasonably informed patient is allowed to participate in the medical decision to the extent that patient wishes. In turn, "reasonably informed" consists of two features: (1) the physician discloses the basis on which the proposed treatment, or alternative possible treatments, have been chosen; and (2) the patient is allowed to ask questions suggested by the disclosure of the physician's reasoning, and those questions are answered to the patient's satisfaction.

According to the transparency model, the key to reasonable disclosure is not adherence to existing standards of other practitioners, nor is it adherence to a list of risks that a hypothetical reasonable patient would want to know. Instead, disclosure is adequate when the physician's basic thinking has been rendered transparent to the patient. If the physician arrives at a recommended therapeutic or diagnostic intervention only after carefully examining a list of risks and benefits, then rendering the physician's thinking transparent requires that those risks and benefits be detailed for the patient. If the physician's thinking has not followed that route but has reached its conclusion by other considerations, then what needs to be disclosed to the patient is accordingly different. Essentially, the transparency standard requires the physician to engage in the typical patient-management thought process, only to *do it out loud in language understandable to the patient.*[9]

To see how this might work in practice, consider the following as possible general decision-making strategies that might be used by a primary physician:

1. The intervention, in addition to being presumably low risk, is also routine and automatic. The physician, faced with a case like that presented by the patient, almost always chooses this treatment.
2. The decision is not routine but seems to offer clear benefit with minimal risk.
3. The proposed procedure offers substantial chances for benefit, but also very substantial risks.
4. The proposed intervention offers substantial risks and extremely questionable benefits. Unfortunately, possible alternative courses of action also have high risk and uncertain benefit.

The exact risks entailed by treatment loom much larger in the physician's own thinking in cases 3 and 4 than in cases 1 and 2. The transparency standard would require that physicians at least mention the various risks to patients in scenarios 3 and 4, but would not necessarily require physicians exhaustively to describe risks, unless the patient asked, in scenarios 1 and 2.

The transparency standard seems to offer some considerable advantages for informing physicians what can legitimately be expected of them in the promotion of patient autonomy while carrying out the activities of primary care medicine. We would hope that the well-trained primary care physician generally thinks before acting. On that assumption, the physician can be told exactly when she is finished obtaining informed consent—first, she has to share her thinking with the patient; secondly, she has to encourage and answer questions; and third, she has to discover how participatory he wishes to be and facilitate that level of participation. This seems a much more reasonable task within primary care than an exhaustive listing of often irrelevant risk factors.

There are also considerable advantages for the patient in this approach. The patient retains the right to ask for an exhaustive recital of risks and alternatives. However, the vast majority of patients, in a primary care setting particularly, would wish to supplement a standardized recital of risks and benefits of treatment with some questions like, "Yes, doctor, but what does this really mean for me? What meaning am I supposed to attach to the information that you've just given?" For example, in scenarios 1 and 2, the precise and specific risk probabilities and possibilities are very small considerations in the thinking of the physician, and reciting an exhaustive list of risks would seriously misstate just what the physician was thinking. If the physician did detail a laundry list of risk factors, the patient might very well ask, "Well, doctor, just what should I think about what you have just told me?" and the thoughtful and concerned physician might well reply, "There's certainly a small possibility that one of these bad things will happen to you; but I think the chance is extremely remote and in my own practice I have never seen anything like that occur." The patient is very likely to give much more weight to that statement, putting the risks in perspective, than he is to the listing of risks. And that emphasis corresponds with an understanding of how the physician herself has reached the decision.

The transparency standard should further facilitate and encourage useful questions from patients. If a patient is given a routine list of risks and benefits and then is asked "Do you have any questions?" the response may well be perfunctory and automatic. If the patient is told precisely the grounds on which the physician has made her recommendation, and then asked the same question, the response is much more likely to be individualized and meaningful.

There certainly would be problems in applying the transparency standard in the courtroom, but these do not appear to be materially more difficult than those encountered in applying other standards; moreover, this standard could call attention to more important features in the ethical relationship between physician and patient. Consider the fairly typical case, in which a patient suffers harm from the occurrence of a rare but predictable complication of a procedure, and then claims that he would not have consented had he known about that risk. Under the present "enlightened" court standards, the jury would examine whether a reasonable patient would have needed to know about that risk factor prior to making a decision on the proposed intervention. Under the transparency standard, the question would instead be whether the physician thought about that risk factor as a relevant consideration prior to recommending the course of action to the patient. If the physician did seriously consider that risk factor, but failed to reveal that to the patient, he was in effect making up the patient's mind in advance about what risks were worth accepting. In that situation, the physician could easily be held liable. If, on the other hand, that risk was considered too insignificant to play a role in determining which intervention ought to be performed, the physician may still have rendered his thinking completely transparent to the patient even though that specific risk factor was not mentioned. In this circumstance, the physician would be held to have done an adequate job of disclosing information.[10] A question would still exist as to whether a competent physician ought to have known about that risk factor and ought to have considered it more carefully prior to doing the procedure. But that question raises the issue of negligence, which is where such considerations properly belong, and removes the problem from the context of informed consent. Obviously, the standard of informed consent is misapplied if it is intended by itself to prevent the practice of negligent medicine.

TRANSPARENCY IN MEDICAL PRACTICE

Will adopting a legal standard like transparency change medical practice for the better? Ultimately only empirical research will answer this question. We know almost nothing about the sorts of conversations primary care physicians now have with their patients, or what would happen if these physicians routinely tried harder to share their basic thinking about therapeutic choices. In this setting it is possible to argue that the transparency standard will have deleterious effects. Perhaps the physician's basic thinking will fail to include risk issues that patients, from their perspective, would regard as substantial. Perhaps how physicians think about therapeutic choice will prove to be too idiosyncratic and variable to serve as any sort of standard. Perhaps disclosing basic thinking processes will impede rather than promote optimal patient participation in decisions.

But the transparency standard must be judged, not only against ideal medical practice, but also against the present-day standard and the message it sends to practitioners. I have argued that that message is, "You can protect yourself legally only by guessing all bad outcomes that might occur and warning each patient explicitly that he might suffer any of them." The transparency standard is an attempt to send the message, "You can protect yourself legally by conversing with your patients in a way that promotes their participation in medical decisions, and more specifically by making sure that they see the basic reasoning you used to arrive at the recommended treatment." It seems at least plausible to me that the attempt is worth making.

The reasonable person standard may still be the best way to view informed consent in highly specialized settings where a relatively small number of discrete and potentially risky procedures are the daily order of business. In primary settings, the best ethical advice we can give physicians is to view informed consent as an ongoing process of conversation designed to maximize patient participation after adequately revealing the key facts. Because the conversation metaphor does not by itself suggest measures for later judicial review, a transparency standard, or something like it, may be a reasonable way to operationalize that concept in primary care practice. Some positive side effects of this might be more focus on good diagnostic and therapeutic decisionmaking on the physician's part, since it will be understood that the patient will be made aware of what the physician's reasoning process has been like, and better documentation of management decisions in the patient record. If these occur, then it will be clearer that the standard of informed consent has promoted rather than impeded high quality patient care.

REFERENCES

1. Charles W. Lidz *et al.*, "Barriers to Informed Consent," *Annals of Internal Medicine* 99:4 (1983), 539–43.
2. Tom L. Beauchamp and Laurence McCullough, *Medical Ethics: The Moral Responsibilities of Physicians* (Englewood Cliffs, NJ: Prentice-Hall, 1984).

3. For a concise overview of empirical data about contemporary informed consent practices see Ruth R. Faden and Tom L. Beauchamp, *A History and Theory of Informed Consent* (New York: Oxford University Press, 1986), 98–99 and associated footnotes.
4. For efforts to address ethical aspects of primary care practice, see Ronald J. Christie and Barry Hoffmaster, *Ethical Issues in Family Medicine* (New York: Oxford University Press, 1986); and Harmon L. Smith and Larry R. Churchill, *Professional Ethics and Primary Care Medicine* (Durham, NC: Duke University Press, 1986).
5. Faden and Beauchamp, *A History and Theory of Informed Consent,* 23–49 and 114–50. I have also greatly benefited from an unpublished paper by Margaret Wallace.
6. For a specialty opinion to the contrary, see W. H. Coles *et al.,* "Teaching Informed Consent," in *Further Developments in Assessing Clinical Competence,* Ian R. Hart and Ronald M. Harden, eds. (Montreal: Can-Heal Publications, 1987), 241–70. This paper is interesting in applying to specialty care a model very much like the one I propose for primary care.
7. Jay Katz, *The Silent World of Doctor and Patient* (New York: Free Press, 1984).
8. Howard Brody, *Stories of Sickness* (New Haven: Yale University Press, 1987), 171–181.
9. For an interesting study of physicians' practices on this point, see William C. Wu and Robert A. Pearlman, "Consent in Medical Decisionmaking: The Role of Communication," *Journal of General Internal Medicine* 3:1 (1988), 9–14.
10. A court case that might point the way toward this line of reasoning is *Precourt* v. *Frederick,* 395 Mass. 689 (1985). See William J. Curran, "Informed Consent in Malpractice Cases: A Turn Toward Reality," *New England Journal of Medicine* 314:7 (1986), 429–31.

SECTION 3

CONFLICTING PROFESSIONAL ROLES AND RESPONSIBILITIES

ERRORS IN MEDICINE: NURTURING TRUTHFULNESS

Françoise Baylis

In "When a Physician Harms a Patient by a Medical Error," Finkelstein and colleagues maintain that patients have a right to the truth and that physicians have a corresponding obligation to be truthful. In their view, when an erroneous act or omission results in an adverse outcome for the patient, the physician should truthfully disclose the medical error, offer the patient a sincere apology, and explore the option of financial compensation. In the abstract, this seems reasonable—and some might even argue uncontestable. Why then is it not common practice for physicians to routinely discuss their errors with their patients? In this article, I will critically examine some of the reasons given by physicians for nondisclosure or partial disclosure, and then consider what the medical profession should do to foster more respectful, open, and honest communication about errors with patients.

Reprinted with permission of the author and publisher from *The Journal of Clinical Ethics* 8:4 (1997), pp. 336–340.

WHY DON'T PHYSICIANS DISCUSS MEDICAL ERRORS WITH PATIENTS?

One reason for silence on the part of physicians, as regards not only their own "errors" but those of their colleagues, is genuine uncertainty about whether a particular adverse outcome is the result of an error.

Case 1

A 47-year-old woman is admitted to the gynecology service with suspected ovarian disease. She has a complicated past medical history, including four previous surgical interventions in the lower abdomen and adhesions. She is extremely distressed and very upset over the prospect of another operation. The surgeon considers the options and decides to try laparoscopic surgery as the least traumatic intervention possible. The procedure becomes extremely difficult because of the adhesions and the woman's obesity. The surgeon accidentally nicks the posterior aspect of the bladder. Postoperatively the woman suffers an episode of abdominal sepsis.

In this case there is an unanticipated, unintentional outcome that harms the patient, but is there an error?

Not all harms that result from medical interventions (for example, sepsis, prolonged pain, prolonged hospitalization, additional therapy, permanent disability, death) are due to medical error. For example, some harms are a manifestation of naturally occurring statistical risk. Patients may perceive these harms as errors (especially if the informed-consent process is flawed and the patient does not understand and accept the possibility of an adverse outcome), but these harms are anticipated and predictable for a patient population, and ultimately they are unavoidable.

Medical errors, on the other hand, are avoidable. In general, errors occur when a planned act or omission fails to achieve its intended outcome and this failure has nothing to do with chance or inherent risk. In medicine, errors can happen because a physician doesn't know something she should know, doesn't properly execute a requisite clinical skill, or doesn't bring together the facts of a case in a manner that promotes good judgment. Such errors may be due to circumstances beyond the physician's control, such as unrealistic workloads, stress, and sleep loss. Alternatively, they may be the result of inadvertence, or they may be due to inexperience, ignorance, inability, or impairment.

Determining that a particular unfortunate outcome is the result of an avoidable medical error is not always an easy task. Medical mishaps (including errors) are often multifactorial—in a certain set of circumstances, a sequence or cluster of actions and decisions by different people combine in unfortunate ways that result in unintentional harm. Further, the view that a particular act or omission constitutes a medical error very much depends upon the social, professional, and cultural contexts in which the determination is made. Which is to say that there is an element of subjectivity in naming certain misadventures as errors and in determining levels of culpability. In the case described above it is debatable whether there was error and, if so, whether the error was due to substandard clinical skills or poor judgment in proceeding with laparoscopic instead of conventional surgery.

A second reason why capable, well-meaning physicians are loathe to disclose medical errors to patients is a belief that in many (perhaps most) cases, full disclosure serves no useful purpose—it only increases patients' anxiety and suffering, and contributes to a loss of confidence in the physician in particular and in the profession in general. At least two responses are possible here. First, in some instances, the belief is false—disclosure will not increase anxiety and suffering, nor undermine confidence. Errors can be more or less serious, more or less complex, more or less blameworthy. With minor errors (that is, errors with trivial or limited harmful consequences for patients)—which are the majority of medical errors[1]—increased anxiety and loss of confidence is an unlikely consequence of disclosure. To believe otherwise is to engage in elaborate self-deception, characterizing nondisclosure as "in the best interest" of patients.

Case 2

A four-year-old girl is admitted for investigation of a persisting anemia. There is careful discussion by the healthcare team of the need to plan these investigations well and to take no more blood than necessary. The clinical clerk is left to write the orders after rounds; inadvertently she orders some blood work for this child that was intended for the patient in the next room. When discovered, it is estimated that 10 ccs of blood were taken unnecessarily.

In other instances, as when there are serious errors or a series of minor errors, the concerns about increased anxiety and loss of confidence are accurate. This is not only a likely response, but arguably an appropriate one. Physicians or systems that are prone to serious errors are deserving of skepticism and distrust.

Case 3

A 58-year-old male is admitted for investigation and treatment of persistent hypertension. The junior resident admitting the patient finds a blood pressure of 240/190. He diagnoses this as malignant hypertension and initiates immediate treatment on the ward. A precipitous drop in the patient's blood pressure goes unnoticed in the absence of appropriate monitoring equipment. The man suffers a moderately severe stroke.

While physicians may express concerns about patients' anxiety, suffering, and loss of confidence, in cases with serious adverse consequences for patients, nondisclosure is typically motivated by self-interest or the interests of colleagues (for example, concerns about professional relationships with other physicians, diminished professional reputation owing to a perception of incompetence, fear of disciplinary proceedings or litigation). Efforts to cloak these interests in the "patient's best interest" are, at best, disingenuous.

A third reason why patients are not always truthfully told that there has been a medical error is fear of litigation. Of the many possible reasons given by physicians for nondisclosure, this is likely the most common. Many physicians believe that disclosure of a mistake and an apology will expose them to the risk of legal liability, and they fear not only the possibility of a successful suit but also the process involved (for example, stress and time). This belief, however, is false. Studies have reported that "the absence of explanations, a lack of honesty, [and] the reluctance to apologize," are factors that significantly influence a patient's decision to pursue legal action.[2] As well, physicians' fears are misplaced. Patients usually don't sue decent, capable physicians for their medical errors when the errors are openly discussed with them. Further, while it is reasonably easy for patients to threaten a suit (and for this reason there are many unmeritorious claims), the fact is that few negligently injured patients sue. For example, the recent Harvard Medical Practice Study of New York hospitals found that seven to eight times as many patients suffered negligent injuries as filed malpractice claims.[3] Also, one of the investigators with the Harvard Study who compared hospital files with litigated actions found that fewer than 2 percent of negligent adverse outcomes resulted in claims.[4]

Now in general terms, each of these reasons for less-than-full-disclosure of a medical error—uncertainty regarding the characterization of "error," concern for patients' well-being, and fear of litigation—may account for specific instances of nondisclosure or partial disclosure. They do not in themselves, however, account for the general lack of honesty with patients about medical errors. I want to suggest here that the more encompassing reason for nondisclosure or partial disclosure of medical error is widespread acceptance (if not endorsement) of the practice.

Early in their careers, physicians learn to "manage" medical errors; the coping mechanisms used include denial, discounting, and distancing.[5] Minor errors are typically denied, and this denial may involve negating the concept of error, repressing actual errors, and redefining errors as nonerrors. When the errors are of such magnitude that they cannot be denied, there may be an effort to discount personal responsibility, and externalize blame. And finally, when the physician can no longer deny or discount an error, distancing mechanisms are utilized in which human fallibility and the inevitability of error are embraced in an effort to temper feelings of guilt. At the same time that physicians are socialized into ways of coping with their medical errors, they observe entrenched practice that does not include routine disclosure of medical errors to patients.

In fact, the medical profession, the healthcare institutions in which physicians practice, medical liability insurers, and medical colleagues tolerate, expect, and sometimes actively encourage nondisclosure of medical errors. And so, the physician who discloses an error (and thereby displaces the myth of the infallible physician) must not only risk whatever negative responses may come from the patient (for example, anger, a lawsuit), but she must also risk a loss of personal confidence and self-esteem, diminished professional authority and reputation, as well as a loss of referrals and income. Typically, she risks these consequences alone, and possibly in the face of powerful opposition from colleagues and the profession. In this climate, many physicians who are inclined to be truthful are "led astray by fear or a drive for self-preservation."[6] Truth-telling appears to them to require an act of heroism, the duty to disclose having moved from the realm of the obligatory to the superogatory. This brings me to a discussion of the profession's moral obligations in the face of physicians' silence about medical errors.

In my view, it is not sufficient to shine the moral light on decent, capable physicians and instruct them on their moral duty to disclose their medical errors without, at the same time, attending to the broader social context in which physicians are being directed to be truthful. Such attention suggests that changes to the structure and culture of medicine are needed to empower the capable (yet fallible) physician who is inclined to be truthful. In my view, such changes can be initiated by attending to the reasons for nondisclosure briefly outlined above.

WHAT SHOULD THE PROFESSION DO TO ENCOURAGE HONEST DISCLOSURE OF MEDICAL ERRORS?

First, it is important to provide a collegial and supportive environment in which (possible) medical errors can be discussed openly and honestly with colleagues. Such open discussion could provide a useful forum in which to determine whether an unfortunate outcome is or is not the result of a medical error. In those cases where it is determined that there has been a medical error, helpful suggestions could be made as to ways in which the error could be honestly explained without causing undue anxiety or a loss of confidence. Anecdotally, many physicians report that peer review committees and morbidity and mortality rounds are not always constructive arenas in which to explore errors and plan for their avoidance. Too often the focus is on the attribution of blame, which explains some of the defensiveness frequently exhibited by physicians. Conscientious and competent physicians who are responsible for, or have contributed to, an adverse outcome already experience anguish, guilt, and self-doubt. It is not contempt, but rather support and understanding, that will help them to acknowledge their errors and give them the confidence to discuss these with their patients.

Second, the profession might remind physicians that patients will experience emotions other than (or in addition to) anxiety, if (when) they discover that they have been lied to or misled by their physicians. Truthfulness is a cornerstone of the physician-patient relationship; lying is disrespectful and breeds mistrust and contempt.

Third, the profession might explore ways in which the determination of negligence could be dealt with separately from the issue of compensation. The arguments around comprehensive no-fault medical insurance schemes, where compensation is based on the fact that the patient has suffered an unintended or unexpected injury attributable to medical care (without regard to cause), are too numerous and complex to discuss here. There are important potential advantages, but also significant limitations.[7] The medical profession needs to participate actively in the ongoing process of tort reform with particular attention to what is best for patients, not just physicians.

Finally, attention must be directed toward the profession's obligation to create an environment in which truthfulness with patients regarding medical errors is an expected, common, everyday occurrence. Medicine is not error-free, yet in subtle ways the profession still promotes and reinforces the false belief that physicians are infallible. If the ideal physician is socially constructed as one who doesn't make mistakes, then the real physician who errs may be seen as uniquely fallible. Errors, however, are an "inevitable accompaniment of the human condition, even among conscientious professionals with high standards."[8] More specifically, "mistakes are inevitable in the practice of medicine because of the complexity of medical knowledge, the uncertainty of medical predictions, time pressures, and the need to make decisions despite limited or uncertain knowledge."[9]

The medical profession knows but has yet to accept this reality, as evidenced by the fact that there are all kinds of mechanisms in place to punish and reprimand those who err, but there are few mechanisms to praise and reward those who are truthful with their patients in disclosing their errors. Similarly there is little praise for those who are truthful about the errors of their colleagues. In fact, physicians who dare to report the error(s) of others are usually not revered for "doing the right thing" in the face of serious obstacles, but more typically are cast in the role of traitor.

In closing, the medical profession has a moral obligation to ensure that truth-telling not "fall outside the notion of duty and seem to go beyond it."[10] Truth-telling should not be the mark of the heroic physician, but rather a distinguishing feature of all decent physicians. If the profession is to meet this obligation it cannot continue to tacitly reinforce the status quo, but must strive to make changes that will clearly show physicians that honesty is valued. This will require important changes to both the structure and culture of medicine.

NOTES

1. L.L. Leape, "Error in Medicine," *Journal of the American Medical Association* 272, no. 23 (1994): 1851–57.
2. C. Vincent, M. Young, and A. Philips, "Why Do People Sue Doctors? A Study of Patients and Relatives Taking Legal Action," *Lancet* 343 (1994): 1609–13.
3. Harvard Medical Practice Study Group, *Patients, Doctors, and Lawyers: Medical Injury, Malpractice Litigation, and Patient Compensation in New York* (Cambridge, Mass.: Harvard Medical Practice Study Group, 1990), 6. See also, P.C. Weiler et al., *A Measure of Malpractice* (Cambridge, Mass.: Harvard University Press, 1993), 69–71.
4. T.A. Brennan, "An Empirical Analysis of Accidents and Accident Law: The Case of Medical Malpractice Law," *St. Louis University Law Journal* 36 (1992): 823, at 847.
5. T. Mizrahi, "Managing Medical Mistakes: Ideology, Insularity and Accountibility Among Internists-in-Training," *Social Science and Medicine* 19, no. 2 (1984): 135–46.
6. J.O. Urmson, "Saints and Heroes," in *Moral Concepts*, F. Feinberg, ed. (Oxford, England: Oxford University Press, 1996), 60–73.
7. L.N. Klar, "Tort and No-Fault," *Health Law Review* 5, no. 3 (1997): 2–8; R.E. Astroff, "Show Me the Money! Making the Case for No-Fault Medical Malpractice Insurance," *Health Law Review* 5, no. 3 (1997): 9–17; and "Medical Accidents," in D. Dewees, D. Duff, and M. Trebilcock, *Exploring the Domain of Accident Law. Taking the Facts Seriously* (New York: Oxford University Press, 1996), 95–187.
8. See note 1 above.
9. A.W. Wu et al., "Do House Officers Learn from Their Mistakes?" *Journal of the American Medical Association* 265, no. 16 (1991): 2089–94.
10. See note 6 above.

VITALY TARASOFF ET AL. V. THE REGENTS OF THE UNIVERSITY OF CALIFORNIA ET AL., DEFENDANTS AND RESPONDENTS

551 P.2d 334, 17 Cal.3d 425, Supreme Court of California, In Bank. July 1, 1976.

TOBRINER, Justice.

On October 27, 1969, Prosenjit Poddar killed Tatiana Tarasoff. Plaintiffs, Tatiana's parents, allege that two months earlier Poddar confided his intention to kill Tatiana to Dr. Lawrence Moore, a psychologist employed by the Cowell Memorial Hospital at the University of California at Berkeley. They allege that on Moore's request, the campus police briefly detained Poddar, but released him when he appeared rational. They further claim that Dr. Harvey Powelson, Moore's superior, then directed that no further action be taken to detain Poddar. No one warned plaintiffs of Tatiana's peril.

Plaintiffs can state a cause of action against defendant therapists for negligent failure to protect Tatiana.

The second cause of action can be amended to allege that Tatiana's death proximately resulted from defendants' negligent failure to warn Tatiana or others likely to apprise her of her danger. Plaintiffs contend that as amended, such allegations of negligence and proximate causation, with resulting damages, establish a cause of action. Defendants, however, contend that in the circumstances of the present case they owed no duty of care to Tatiana or her parents and that, in the absence of such duty, they were free to act in careless disregard of Tatiana's life and safety.

In analyzing this issue, we bear in mind that legal duties are not discoverable facts of nature, but merely conclusory expressions that, in cases of a particular type, liability should be imposed for damage done. As stated in *Dillon* v. *Legg:*

> The assertion that liability must . . . be denied because defendant bears no "duty" to plaintiff "begs the essential question—whether the plaintiff's interests are

> entitled to legal protection against the defendant's conduct. . . . [Duty] is not sacrosanct in itself, but only an expression of the sum total of those considerations of policy which lead the law to say that the particular plaintiff is entitled to protection."

In the landmark case of *Rowland* v. *Christian*, Justice Peters recognized that liability should be imposed "for an injury occasioned to another by his want of ordinary care or skill" as expressed in section 1714 of the Civil Code. Thus, Justice Peters, quoting from *Heaven* v. *Pender* stated:

> whenever one person is by circumstances placed in such a position with regard to another . . . that if he did not use ordinary care and skill in his own conduct . . . he would cause danger of injury to the person or property of the other, a duty arises to use ordinary care and skill to avoid such danger.

We depart from "this fundamental principle" only upon the "balancing of a number of considerations"; major ones

> are the foreseeability of harm to the plaintiff, the degree of certainty that the plaintiff suffered injury, the closeness of the connection between the defendant's conduct and the injury suffered, the moral blame attached to the defendant's conduct, the policy of preventing future harm, the extent of the burden to the defendant and consequences to the community of imposing a duty to exercise care with resulting liability for breach, and the availability, cost and prevalence of insurance for the risk involved.

The most important of these considerations in establishing duty is foreseeability. As a general principle, a "defendant owes a duty of care to all persons who are foreseeably endangered by his conduct, with respect to all risks which make the conduct unreasonably dangerous." As we shall explain, however, when the avoidance of foreseeable harm requires a defendant to control the conduct of another person, or to warn of such conduct, the common law has traditionally imposed liability only if the defendant bears some special relationship to the dangerous person or to the potential victim. Since the relationship between a therapist and his patient satisfies this requirement, we need not here decide whether foreseeability alone is sufficient to create a duty to exercise reasonable care to protect a potential victim of another's conduct.

Although, as we have stated above, under the common law, as a general rule, one person owed no duty to control the conduct of another, nor to warn those endangered by such conduct, the courts have carved out an exception to this rule in cases in which the defendant stands in some special relationship to either the person whose conduct needs to be controlled or in a relationship to the foreseeable victim of that conduct. Applying this exception to the present case, we note that a relationship of defendant therapists to either Tatiana or Poddar will suffice to establish a duty of care; as explained in section 315 of the Restatement Second of Torts, a duty of care may arise from either

> (a) a special relation . . . between the actor and the third person which imposes a duty upon the actor to control the third person's conduct, or (b) a special relation . . . between the actor and the other which gives to the other a right of protection.

Although plaintiffs' pleadings assert no special relation between Tatiana and defendant therapists, they establish as between Poddar and defendant therapists the special relation that arises between a patient and his doctor or psychotherapist. Such a relationship may support affirmative duties for the benefit of third persons. Thus, for example, a hospital must exercise reasonable care to control the behavior of a patient which may endanger other persons. A doctor must also warn a patient if the patient's condition or prescribed medication renders certain conduct, such as driving a car, dangerous to others.

Although the California decisions that recognize this duty have involved cases in which the defendant stood in a special relationship both to the victim and to the person whose conduct created the danger, we do not think that the duty should logically be constricted to such situations. Decisions of other jurisdictions hold that the single relationship of a doctor to his patient is sufficient to support the duty to exercise reasonable care to protect others against dangers emanating from the patient's illness. The courts hold that a doctor is liable to persons infected by his patient if he negligently fails to diagnose a contagious disease or, having diagnosed the illness, fails to warn members of the patient's family.

Since it involved a dangerous mental patient, the decision in *Merchants Nat. Bank & Trust Co. of Fargo*

v. *United States* comes closer to the issue. The Veterans Administration arranged for the patient to work on a local farm, but did not inform the farmer of the man's background. The farmer consequently permitted the patient to come and go freely during nonworking hours; the patient borrowed a car, drove to his wife's residence and killed her. Notwithstanding the lack of any "special relationship" between the Veterans Administration and the wife, the court found the Veterans Administration liable for the wrongful death of the wife.

In their summary of the relevant rulings Fleming and Maximov conclude that

> case law should dispel any notion that to impose on the therapists a duty to take precautions for the safety of persons threatened by a patient, where due care so requires, is in any way opposed to contemporary ground rules on the duty relationship. On the contrary, there now seems to be sufficient authority to support the conclusion that by entering into a doctor-patient relationship the therapist becomes sufficiently involved to assume some responsibility for the safety, not only of the patient himself, but also of any third person whom the doctor knows to be threatened by the patient.[1]

Defendants contend, however, that imposition of a duty to exercise reasonable care to protect third persons is unworkable because therapists cannot accurately predict whether or not a patient will resort to violence. In support of this argument amicus representing the American Psychiatric Association and other professional societies cites numerous articles which indicate that therapists, in the present state of the art, are unable reliably to predict violent acts; their forecasts, amicus claims, tend consistently to overpredict violence, and indeed are more often wrong than right. Since predictions of violence are often erroneous, amicus concludes, the courts should not render rulings that predicate the liability of therapists upon the validity of such predictions.

The role of the psychiatrist, who is indeed a practitioner of medicine, and that of the psychologist who performs an allied function, are like that of the physician who must conform to the standards of the profession and who must often make diagnoses and predictions based upon such evaluations. Thus the judgment of the therapist in diagnosing emotional disorders and in predicting whether a patient presents a serious danger of violence is comparable to the judgment which doctors and professionals must regularly render under accepted rules of responsibility.

We recognize the difficulty that a therapist encounters in attempting to forecast whether a patient presents a serious danger of violence. Obviously we do not require that the therapist, in making that determination, render a perfect performance; the therapist need only exercise "that reasonable degree of skill, knowledge, and care ordinarily possessed and exercised by members of [that professional specialty] under similar circumstances." Within the broad range of reasonable practice and treatment in which professional opinion and judgment may differ, the therapist is free to exercise his or her own best judgment without liability; proof, aided by hindsight, that he or she judged wrongly is insufficient to establish negligence.

In the instant case, however, the pleadings do not raise any question as to failure of defendant therapists to predict that Poddar presented a serious danger of violence. On the contrary, the present complaints allege that defendant therapists did in fact predict that Poddar would kill, but were negligent in failing to warn.

Amicus contends, however, that even when a therapist does in fact predict that a patient poses a serious danger of violence to others, the therapist should be absolved of any responsibility for failing to act to protect the potential victim. In our view, however, once a therapist does in fact determine, or under applicable professional standards reasonably should have determined, that a patient poses a serious danger of violence to others, he bears a duty to exercise reasonable care to protect the foreseeable victim of that danger. While the discharge of this duty of due care will necessarily vary with the facts of each case, in each instance the adequacy of the therapist's conduct must be measured against the traditional negligence standard of the rendition of reasonable care under the circumstances. As explained in Fleming and Maximov,

> the ultimate question of resolving the tension between the conflicting interests of patient and potential victim is one of social policy, not professional expertise. . . . In sum, the therapist owes a legal duty not only to his patient, but also to his patient's would-be victim and is subject in both respects to scrutiny by judge and jury. . . .

The risk that unnecessary warnings may be given is a reasonable price to pay for the lives of possible victims that may be saved. We would hesitate to hold that the therapist who is aware that his patient expects to attempt to assassinate the President of the United States would not be obligated to warn the authorities because the therapist cannot predict with accuracy that his patient will commit the crime.

Defendants further argue that free and open communication is essential to psychotherapy; that "Unless a patient . . . is assured that . . . information [revealed by him] can and will be held in utmost confidence, he will be reluctant to make the full disclosure upon which diagnosis and treatment . . . depends." The giving of a warning, defendants contend, constitutes a breach of trust which entails the revelation of confidential communications.

We recognize the public interest in supporting effective treatment of mental illness and in protecting the rights of patients to privacy, and the consequent public importance of safeguarding the confidential character of psychotherapeutic communication. Against this interest, however, we must weigh the public interest in safety from violent assault. The Legislature has undertaken the difficult task of balancing the countervailing concerns. In Evidence Code section 1014, it established a broad rule of privilege to protect confidential communications between patient and psychotherapist. In Evidence Code section 1024, the Legislature created a specific and limited exception to the psychotherapist-patient privilege:

> There is no privilege . . . if the psychotherapist has reasonable cause to believe that the patient is in such mental or emotional condition as to be dangerous to himself or to the person or property of another and that disclosure of the communication is necessary to prevent the threatened danger.

We realize that the open and confidential character of psychotherapeutic dialogue encourages patients to express threats of violence, few of which are ever executed. Certainly a therapist should not be encouraged routinely to reveal such threats; such disclosures could seriously disrupt the patient's relationship with his therapist and with the persons threatened. To the contrary, the therapist's obligations to his patient require that he not disclose a confidence unless such disclosure is necessary to avert danger to others, and even then that he do so discreetly, and in a fashion that would preserve the privacy of his patient to the fullest extent compatible with the prevention of the threatened danger.

The revelation of a communication under the above circumstances is not a breach of trust or a violation of professional ethics; as stated in the Principles of Medical Ethics of the American Medical Association (1957), section 9: "A physician may not reveal the confidence entrusted to him in the course of medical attendance . . . *unless he is required to do so by law or unless it becomes necessary to protect the welfare of the individual or of the community.*" (Emphasis added.) We conclude that the public policy favoring protection of the confidential character of patient-psychotherapist communications must yield to the extent to which disclosure is essential to avert danger to others. The protective privilege ends where the public peril begins.

Our current crowded and computerized society compels the interdependence of its members. In this risk-infested society we can hardly tolerate the further exposure to danger that would result from a concealed knowledge of the therapist that his patient was lethal. If the exercise of reasonable care to protect the threatened victim requires the therapist to warn the endangered party or those who can reasonably be expected to notify him, we see no sufficient societal interest that would protect and justify concealment. The containment of such risks lies in the public interest. For the foregoing reasons, we find that plaintiffs' complaints can be amended to state a cause of action against defendants Moore, Powelson, Gold, and Yandell and against the Regents as their employer, for breach of a duty to exercise reasonable care to protect Tatiana.

CLARK, Justice, dissenting.
Overwhelming policy considerations weigh against imposing a duty on psychotherapists to warn a potential victim against harm. While offering virtually no benefit to society, such a duty will frustrate psychiatric treatment, invade fundamental patient rights and increase violence.

The importance of psychiatric treatment and its need for confidentiality have been recognized by this court. . . .

Assurance of confidentiality is important for three reasons.

DETERRENCE FROM TREATMENT

First, without substantial assurance of confidentiality, those requiring treatment will be deterred from seeking assistance. It remains an unfortunate fact in our society that people seeking psychiatric guidance often tend to become stigmatized. Apprehension of such stigma—apparently increased by the propensity of people considering treatment to see themselves in the worst possible light—creates a well-recognized reluctance to seek aid. This reluctance is alleviated by the psychiatrist's assurance of confidentiality.

FULL DISCLOSURE

Second, the guarantee of confidentiality is essential in eliciting the full disclosure necessary for effective treatment. The psychiatric patient approaches treatment with conscious and unconscious inhibitions against revealing his innermost thoughts. "Every person, however well-motivated, has to overcome resistances to therapeutic exploration. These resistances seek support from every possible source and the possibility of disclosure would easily be employed in the service of resistance." Until a patient can trust his psychiatrist not to violate their confidential relationship," the unconscious psychological control mechanism of repression will prevent the recall of past experiences."[2]

SUCCESSFUL TREATMENT

Third, even if the patient fully discloses his thoughts, assurance that the confidential relationship will not be breached is necessary to maintain his trust in his psychiatrist—the very means by which treatment is effected. "[T]he essence of much psychotherapy is the contribution of trust in the external world and ultimately in the self, modelled upon the trusting relationship established during therapy."[3] Patients will be helped only if they can form a trusting relationship with the psychiatrist. All authorities appear to agree that if the trust relationship cannot be developed because of collusive communication between the psychiatrist and others, treatment will be frustrated.

Given the importance of confidentiality to the practice of psychiatry, it becomes clear the duty to warn imposed by the majority will cripple the use and effectiveness of psychiatry. Many people, potentially violent—yet susceptible to treatment—will be deterred from seeking it; those seeking it will be inhibited from making revelations necessary to effective treatment; and, forcing the psychiatrist to violate the patient's trust will destroy the interpersonal relationship by which treatment is effected.

VIOLENCE AND CIVIL COMMITMENT

By imposing a duty to warn, the majority contributes to the danger to society of violence by the mentally ill and greatly increases the risk of civil commitment—the total deprivation of liberty—of those who should not be confined. The impairment of treatment and risk of improper commitment resulting from the new duty to warn will not be limited to a few patients but will extend to a large number of the mentally ill. Although under existing psychiatric procedures only a relatively few receiving treatment will ever present a risk of violence, the number making threats is huge, and it is the latter group—not just the former—whose treatment will be impaired and whose risk of commitment will be increased.

Both the legal and psychiatric communities recognize that the process of determining potential violence in a patient is far from exact, being fraught with complexity and uncertainty.[4] In fact, precision has not even been attained in predicting who of those having already committed violent acts will again become violent, a task recognized to be of much simpler proportions.

This predictive uncertainty means that the number of disclosures will necessarily be large. As noted above, psychiatric patients are encouraged to discuss all thoughts of violence, and they often express such thoughts. However, unlike this court, the psychiatrist does not enjoy the benefit of overwhelming hindsight in seeing which few, if any, of his patients will ultimately become violent. Now, confronted by the majority's new duty, the psychiatrist must instantaneously calculate potential violence from each patient on each visit. The difficulties researchers have encountered in accurately predicting violence will be heightened for the practicing psychiatrist dealing for brief periods in his office with heretofore nonviolent patients. And, given that the decision not to warn or commit must always be made at the psychiatrist's civil peril, one can expect most doubts will be resolved in favor of the psychiatrist protecting himself.

Neither alternative open to the psychiatrist seeking to protect himself is in the public interest. The warning itself is an impairment of the psychiatrist's ability to treat, depriving many patients of adequate treatment. It is to be expected that after disclosing their threats, a significant number of patients, who would not become violent if treated according to existing practices, will engage in violent conduct as a result of unsuccessful treatment. In short, the majority's duty to warn will not only impair treatment of many who would never become violent, but worse, will result in a net increase in violence.[5]

NOTES

1. Fleming and Maximov, *The Patient or His Victim: The Therapist's Dilemma* (1974) 62 Cal.L.Rev. 1025, 1030.
2. Butler, *Psychotherapy and Griswold: Is Confidentiality a Privilege or a Right?* (1971) 3 Conn.L.Rev. 599, 604.
3. Dawidoff, *The Malpractice of Psychiatrists* (1966) Duke L.J. 696, 704.
4. A shocking illustration of psychotherapists' inability to predict dangerousness, cited by this court in *People* v. *Burnick, supra,* 14 Cal.3d 306, 326–327, fn. 17, 121 Cal.Rptr. 488, 535 P.2d 352, is cited and discussed in Ennis, *Prisoners of Psychiatry: Mental Patients, Psychiatrists, and the Law* (1972): "In a well-known study, psychiatrists predicted that 989 persons were so dangerous that they could not be kept even in civil mental hospitals, but would have to be kept in maximum security hospitals run by the Department of Corrections. Then, because of a United States Supreme Court decision, those persons were transferred to civil hospitals. After a year, the Department of Mental Hygiene reported that one-fifth of them had been discharged to the community, and over half had agreed to remain as voluntary patients. During the year, only 7 of the 989 committed or threatened any act that was sufficiently dangerous to require retransfer to the maximum security hospital. Seven correct predictions out of almost a thousand is not a very impressive record. Other studies, and there are many, have reached the same conclusion: psychiatrists simply cannot predict dangerous behavior." (*Id.* at p. 227.) Equally illustrative studies are collected in Rosenhan, *On Being Sane in Insane Places* (1973) 13 Santa Clara Law. 379, 384; Ennis & Litwack, *Psychiatry and the Presumption of Expertise: Flipping Coins in the Courtroom, supra,* 62 Cal.L.Rev. 693, 750–751.
5. The majority concedes that psychotherapeutic dialogue often results in the patient expressing threats of violence that are rarely executed. (*Ante,* p. 441, p. 27 of 131 Cal.Rptr., p. 347 of 551 P.2d.) The practical problem, of course, lies in ascertaining which threats from which patients will be carried out. As to this problem, the majority is silent. They do, however, caution that a therapist certainly "should not be encouraged routinely to reveal such threats; such disclosures could seriously disrupt the patient's relationships with his therapist and with the persons threatened." (*Id.*)

   Thus, in effect, the majority informs the therapists that they must accurately predict dangerousness—a task recognized as extremely difficult—or face crushing civil liability. The majority's reliance on the traditional standard of care for professionals that "therapist need only exercise 'that reasonable degree of skill, knowledge, and care ordinarily possessed and exercised by members of [that professional specialty] under similar circumstances'" (*ante,* p. 438, p. 25 of 131 Cal.Rptr., p. 345 of 551 P.2d) is seriously misplaced. This standard of care assumes that, to a large extent, the subject matter of the specialty is ascertainable. One clearly ascertainable element in the psychiatric field is that the therapist cannot accurately predict dangerousness, which, in turn, means that the standard is inappropriate for lack of a relevant criterion by which to judge the therapist's decision. The inappropriateness of the standard the majority would have us use is made patent when consideration is given to studies, by several eminent authorities, indicating that "[t]he chances of a second psychiatrist agreeing with the diagnosis of a first psychiatrist 'are barely better than 50–50; or stated differently, there is about as much chance that a different expert would come to some different conclusion as there is that the other would agree.'" (Ennis & Litwack, *Psychiatry and the Presumption of Expertise: Flipping Coins in the Courtroom, supra,* 62 Cal.L.Rev. 693, 701, quoting, Ziskin, Coping With Psychiatric and Psychological Testimony, 126.) The majority's attempt to apply a normative scheme to a profession which must be concerned with problems that balk at standardization is clearly erroneous.

   In any event, an ascertainable standard would not serve to limit psychiatrist disclosure of threats with the resulting impairment of treatment. However compassionate, the psychiatrist hearing the threat remains faced with potential crushing civil liability for a mistaken evaluation of his patient and will be forced to resolve even the slightest doubt in favor of disclosure or commitment.

PLEASE DON'T TELL!

The patient, Carlos R., was a twenty-one-year-old Hispanic male who had suffered gunshot wounds to the abdomen in gang violence. He was uninsured. His stay in the hospital was somewhat shorter than might have been expected, but otherwise unremarkable. It was felt that he could safely complete his recovery at home. Carlos admitted to his attending physician that he was HIV-positive, which was confirmed.

At discharge the attending physician recommended a daily home nursing visit for wound care. However, Medicaid would not fund this nursing visit because a caregiver lived in the home who could adequately provide this care, namely, the patient's twenty-two-year-old sister Consuela, who in fact was willing to accept this burden. Their mother had died almost ten years ago, and Consuela had been a mother to Carlos and their younger sister since then. Carlos had no objection to Consuela's providing this care, but he insisted absolutely that she was not to know his HIV status. He had always been on good terms with Consuela, but she did not know he was actively homosexual. His greatest fear, though, was that his father would learn of his homosexual orientation, which is generally looked upon with great disdain by Hispanics.

Would Carlos's physician be morally justified in breaching patient confidentiality on the grounds that he had a "duty to warn?"

Reproduced with permission of the authors and the publisher from *Hastings Center Report* (November–December 1991): 39–40.

COMMENTARY

Leonard Fleck

If there were a home health nurse to care for this patient, presumably there would be no reason to breach confidentiality since the expectation would be that she would follow universal precautions. Of course, universal precautions could be explained to the patient's sister. In an ideal world this would seem to be a satisfactory response that protects both Carlos's rights and Consuela's welfare. But the world is not ideal.

We know that health professionals, who surely ought to have the knowledge that would motivate them to take universal precautions seriously, often fail to take just such precautions. It is easy to imagine that Consuela could be equally casual or careless, especially when she had not been specifically warned that her brother was HIV-infected. Given this possibility, does the physician have a duty to warn that would justify breaching confidentiality? I shall argue that he may not breach confidentiality but he must be reasonably attentive to Consuela's safety. Ordinarily the conditions that must be met to invoke a duty to warn are: (1) an imminent threat of serious and irreversible harm, (2) no alternative to averting that threat other than this breach of confidentiality, and (3) proportionality between the harm averted by this breach of confidentiality and the harm associated with such a breach. In my judgment, none of these conditions are satisfactorily met.

No one doubts that becoming HIV-infected represents a serious and irreversible harm. But, in reality, is that threat imminent enough to justify breaching confidentiality? If we were talking about two individuals who were going to have intercourse on repeated occasions, then the imminence condition would likely be met. But the patient's sister will be caring for his wound for only a week or two, and wound care does not by itself involve any exchange of body fluids. If we had two-hundred and forty surgeons operating on two-hundred and forty HIV-infected patients, and if each of those surgeons nicked himself while doing surgery, then the likelihood is that only one of them would become HIV-infected. Using this as a reference point, the likelihood of this young woman seroconverting if her intact skin comes into contact with the blood of this patient is very remote at best.

Moreover in this instance there are alternatives. A frank and serious discussion with Consuela about the need for universal precautions, plus monitored, thorough training in correct wound care, fulfills what I would regard as a reasonable duty to warn in these circumstances. Similar instructions ought to be given to Carlos so that he can monitor her performance. He can be reminded that this is a small price for protecting his confidentiality as well as his sister's health. It might also be necessary to provide gloves and other such equipment required to observe universal precautions.

We can imagine easily enough that there might be a lapse in conscientiousness on Consuela's part, that she might come into contact with his blood. But even if this were to happen, the likelihood of her seroconverting is remote at best. This is where proportionality between the harm averted by the breach and the harm associated with it comes in. For if confidentiality were breached and she were informed of his HIV status, this would likely have very serious consequences for Carlos. As a layperson with no professional duty to preserve confidentiality herself, Consuela might inform other family members, which could lead to his being ostracized from the family. And even if she kept the information confidential, she might be too afraid to provide the care for Carlos, who might then end up with no one to care for him.

The right to confidentiality is a right that can be freely waived. The physician could engage Carlos in a frank moral discussion aimed at persuading him that the reasonable and decent thing to do is to inform his sister of his HIV status. Perhaps the physician offers assurances she would be able to keep that information in strict confidence. The patient agrees. Then what happens? It is easy to imagine that Consuela balks at caring for her brother, for fear of infection.

Medicaid would still refuse to pay for home nursing care because a caregiver would still be in the home, albeit a terrified caregiver. Consuela's response may not be rational, but it is possible. If she were to react in this way it would be an easy "out" to say that it was Carlos who freely agreed to the release of the confidential information so now he'll just have to live with those consequences. But the matter is really more complex than that. At the very least the physician would have to apprise Carlos of the fact that his sister might divulge his HIV status to some number of other individuals. But if the physician impresses this possibility on Carlos vividly enough, Carlos might be even more reluctant to self-disclose his HIV status to Consuela. In that case the physician is morally obligated to respect that confidentiality.

COMMENTARY

Marcia Angell

It would be wrong, I believe, to ask this young woman to undertake the nursing care of her brother and not inform her that he is HIV-infected.

The claim of a patient that a doctor hold his secrets in confidence is strong but not absolute. It can be overridden by stronger, competing claims. For example, a doctor would not agree to hold in confidence a diagnosis of rubella, if the patient were planning to be in the presence of a pregnant woman without warning her. Similarly, a doctor would be justified in acting on knowledge that a patient planned to commit a crime. Confidentiality should, of course, be honored when the secret is entirely personal, that is, when it could have no impact on anyone else. On the other hand, when it would pose a major threat to others, the claim of confidentiality must be overridden. Difficulties arise when the competing claims are nearly equal in moral weight.

In this scenario, does Consuela have any claims on the doctor? I believe she does, and that her claims are very compelling. They stem, first, from her right to have information she might consider relevant to her decision to act as her brother's nurse and, second, from the health care system's obligation to warn of a possible risk to her health. I would like to focus first on whether Consuela has a right to information apart from the question of whether there is in fact an appreciable risk. I believe that she has such a right, for three reasons.

First, there is an element of deception in *not* informing Consuela that her brother is HIV-infected. Most people in her situation would want to know if their "patient" were HIV-infected and would presume that they would be told if that were the case. (I suspect that a private nurse hired in a similar situation would expect to be told—and that she would be.) At some level, perhaps unconsciously, Consuela would assume that Carlos did not have HIV infection because no one said that he did. Thus, in keeping Carlos's secret, the doctor implicitly deceives Consuela—not a net moral gain, I think.

Second, Consuela has been pressed to provide nursing care in part because the health system is using her to avoid providing a service it would otherwise be responsible for. This fact, I believe, gives the health care system an additional obligation to her, which includes giving her all the information that might bear on her decision to accept this responsibility. It might be argued that the information about her brother's HIV infection is not relevant, but it is patronizing to make this assumption. She may for any number of reasons, quite apart from the risk of transmission, find it important to know that he is HIV-infected.

Finally, I can't help feeling that this young woman has already been exploited by her family and that the health care system should not collude in doing so again. We are told that since she was twelve, she has acted as "mother" to a brother only one year younger, presumably simply because she is female, since she is no more a mother than he is. Now she is being asked to be a nurse, as well as a mother, again presumably because she is female. In this context, concerns about the sensibilities of the father or about Carlos's fear of them are not very compelling, particularly when they are buttressed by stereotypes about Hispanic families. Furthermore, both his father and his sister will almost certainly learn the truth eventually.

What about the risk of transmission from Carlos to Consuela? Many would—wrongly, I believe—base their arguments solely on this question. Insofar as they did, they would have very little to go on. The truth is that no one knows what the risk would be to Consuela. To my knowledge, there have been no studies that would yield data on the point. Most likely the risk would be extremely small, particularly if there were no blood or pus in the wound, but it would be speculative to say how small. We do know that Consuela has no experience with universal precautions and could not be expected to use them diligently with her brother unless she had some sense of why she might be doing so. In any case, the doctor has no right to decide for this young woman that she should assume a risk, even if he believes it would be remote. That is for her to decide. The only judgment he has a right to make is whether *she* might consider the information that her brother is HIV-infected to be relevant to her decision to nurse him, and I think it is reasonable to assume she might.

There is, I believe, only one ethical way out of this dilemma. The doctor should strongly encourage Carlos to tell his sister that he is HIV-infected or offer to do it for him. She could be asked not to tell their father, and I would see no problem with this. I would have no hesitation in appealing to the fact that Carlos already owes Consuela a great deal. If Carlos insisted that his sister not be told, the doctor should see to it that his nursing needs are met in some other way. In sum, then, I believe the doctor should pass the dilemma to the patient: Carlos can decide to accept Consuela's generosity—in return for which he must tell her he is HIV-infected (or ask the doctor to tell her)—or he can decide not to tell her and do without her nursing care.

DISCLOSING MISATTRIBUTED PATERNITY

Lainie Friedman Ross

INTRODUCTION

Genetic counseling is the process by which individuals are informed about the risks to themselves and/or their offspring of genetic diseases and susceptibilities. The counseling provides information about genetic conditions, their inheritance, short- and long-term implications, and, when relevant, procreative options. To promote "client autonomy," geneticists and genetic counselors emphasize information giving and truth telling. Yet there are situations in which genetic counselors do not disclose pertinent information to all involved parties. The focus of this paper is on one such situation: the case of "non-paternity" or misattributed paternity. In 1990, Dorothy Wertz, John C. Fletcher, and John Mulvihill reported on an international study conducted in 1985–6 in which 1,053 M.D. and Ph.D. geneticists in 18 nations analyzed frequent ethical dilemmas in medical genetics. One case depicted a child with an autosomal recessive disorder for which carrier testing was possible and accurate. Genetic workup revealed that her husband was not the biological father. Of the 677 respondents, 96% believed that "protection of the mother's confidentiality overrode disclosure of true paternity."[1] Of these, 81% said they would tell the woman alone; 13% would tell the couple that they were both genetically responsible, and 2% would ascribe the child's disorder to a new mutation which was unrepeatable. The same question was asked by Deborah Pencarinha, Nora K. Bell, Janice G. Edwards, and Robert G. Best in a 1989 survey of non-doctoral genetic counselors, and their results were even more uniform. Pencarinha *et al.* surveyed 545 counselors. Of the 199 respondents, 98.5% said that they would not disclose misattributed paternity to the male partner in order "to preserve patient confidentiality."[2] Because of their similarity of views, I will refer to both groups when I use the term "counselor."

This practice of the counselors contradicts the recommendations of the President's Commission for the Study of Ethical Problems in Biomedical and Behavioral Research (1983) which studied the question of misattributed paternity. The President's Commission recommended that misattributed paternity be disclosed to both partners.[3] In 1994, however, the Committee on Assessing Genetic Risks of the Institute of Medicine (IOM) recommended that only the woman be informed and that misattributed paternity should not be disclosed to her partner.[4] The IOM's major justification was similar to the rationale given by the genetic counselors: "Genetic testing should not be used in ways that disrupt families."

Editor's note: Some footnotes have been deleted. Students who want to follow up on sources should consult the original article.

Reprinted with permission of the author and publisher from *Bioethics* 10:2 (1996): 114–130.

1. Dorothy Wertz, John C. Fletcher, and John J. Mulvihill, "Medical Geneticists Confront Ethical Dilemmas: Cross-cultural Comparisons among 19 Nations," *American Journal of Human Genetics* 1990; 46; 1202.

2. Deborah F. Pencarinha, Nora K. Bell, Janice G. Edwards, and Robert G. Best, "Ethical Issues in Genetic Counseling: A Comparison of M.S. Counselor and Medical Geneticist Perspectives," in *Journal of Genetic Counseling* 1992; 1(1); 23.

3. President's Commission for the Study of Ethical Problems in Medicine and Biomedical and Behavioral Research, *Screening and counseling for genetic conditions: the ethical, social, and legal implications of genetic screening, counseling, and education programs.* Washington D.C.: U.S. Government Printing Office, 1983, pp. 60–1.

4. Committee on Assessing Genetic Risks, Institute of Medicine, *Assessing Genetic Risks: Implications for Health and Social Policy,* ed. Lori B. Andrews, Jane E. Fullarton, Neil A. Holtzman, and Arno G. Motulsky. Washington D.C.: National Academy Press, 1994. The Committee reiterated this position several times (see pages 6, 23, 38, 70, 100, 127, 163, and 175). Of note is that the Committee did add that there may be "*rare* circumstances that warrant such disclosure (p. 100)," but they did not elaborate about what such circumstances might entail.

In this paper I evaluate and criticize the policy recommended by the IOM and practiced by most counselors in which only the woman is informed about the genetic results of misattributed paternity. I consider whether nondisclosure to either or both partners is consistent with the standards and goals of genetic counselors, and whether the genetic counselor can choose not to disclose this information to the partner based on such concerns as preservation of the family and protection of the woman. I also consider what obligations counselors have to children, a topic ignored to date in the literature.

I THE PRINCIPLES OF GENETIC COUNSELING

Genetic textbooks often cite the rate of misattributed paternity as 10–15%. This number is not based on published evidence. The data that do exist are based on nonrepresentative populations and any extrapolation is problematic. Rather, as the various published studies show, the rate of misattributed paternity is likely to vary between countries, age groups, cultural or ethnic groups, and socioeconomic classes.

Despite the lack of data on how often misattributed paternity occurs, the empirical studies cited above reveal that there is a consensus on how to deal with this occurrence. Both the studies by Wertz *et al.* and Pencarinha *et al.* found that over 95% of counselors would not inform the woman's partner that he is not the biological father.

Given the goals and standards of genetic counseling, the almost unanimous agreement not to disclose misattributed paternity to the male partner is initially surprising. As enumerated by Fraser in 1974, the prime goal of genetic counseling is to promote "client autonomy": to help clients "to understand their options and to choose the course of action which seems most appropriate to them in view of their risk and their family goals and act in accordance with that decision."[5] To achieve client autonomy requires "full disclosure" of information in a "non-directive" manner. Counselors place great emphasis on full disclosure because they realize that different information will have different meaning and different impact on different patients. They also emphasize a non-directive approach in which counselors attempt to give their clients information objectively and allow the clients to come to a decision that is most consonant with their own values and beliefs. The assumption is that all decisions are equally valid. The counselors' goal is to help their clients define what is best for themselves. Genetic counselors pride themselves on helping their clients reach their own decisions and not to impose their own values on their clients.

Who are the clients of the genetic counselor? Consider, first, the scenario in which a couple presents for genetic counseling because their first child has a congenital condition which their pediatrician believes to be genetic. The couple may seek genetic counseling to clarify their child's diagnosis, to understand their future procreative risks, or to undergo prenatal testing and diagnosis. The genetic counselor begins by taking a family history from both the woman and her partner, and when necessary, draws blood from each family member to ascertain the child's diagnosis, its mode of inheritance, and/or its risk of reoccurrence in future children. Genetic tests done on the blood samples provide information about the child, and about each partner as the parent of the child, as individuals, and as a couple. As such, it would seem that both parents and the child are the counselor's clients. Similarly, when a couple presents for in-utero testing of their potential child, both parents and the potential child would seem to be clients even though the procedure is done exclusively on the woman and the fetus. The two cases have morally relevant differences. In the first scenario, each partner has the right to refuse or consent to testing and they make this same decision on behalf of their child. In the second scenario, the woman alone has final authority on whether or not the procedure is performed because prenatal testing requires that she undergo an invasive diagnostic procedure. But in both scenarios, the information that is obtained is relevant to all the parties. As such, information ought to be disclosed to the family. The decision to inform only the woman of unanticipated misattributed paternity implies that the

5. F.C. Fraser, "Genetic Counseling," *American Journal of Human Genetics* 1974; 26: 636–59.

counselor considers the woman alone to be her client, or at least the primary client. This conflicts with the already established counselor-client relationships and the counselor's obligations to *each* of her clients.[6]

If both adult partners seek genetic counseling, then both partners are clients of the genetic counselor. As such, the counselor has a duty to both of them. True disclosure of the findings are relevant to both of them. The purpose of genetic counseling is to disclose as much information as possible to the clients so that they can reach their own decisions. If both the woman and man are clients, then the counselor ought to respect each partner's right to know his or her genetic endowment and the genetic endowment of their child. The decision to conceal misattributed paternity is not consistent with such respect. Rather, the virtually unanimous consensus to disclose misattributed paternity only to the woman implies that counselors consider the woman alone to be their client. While it is and should be the case that pregnant women have ultimate decision making authority over their own body with regard to prenatal testing and whether to continue or terminate a pregnancy, information obtained about the fetus or about a child is not the exclusive property of the woman and the counselor. To argue that only women should be informed is to imply that men are second-class citizens in genetic testing. Non-disclosure shows a lack of respect for the male partner as a person, as a client interested in his own genetic make-up, and as a parent interested in his child's genetic endowment.

Failure to disclose misattributed paternity to the male partner assumes that the woman has a greater interest than her partner in the true genetic explanation of the child's genetic disease. In cases of autosomal recessive diseases, if the partner is the child's biological father, then he is a carrier for the disease and has 50% responsibility for his child's illness. If he is not the biological father, then he is not responsible, but another man is. This is not meant to assign blame, but only to explain the genetic basis of the child's illness and to help the parents make future informed procreative decisions. To deny the partner the knowledge of his true carrier status, or to mislead the partner into believing that his child's illness involved a mutation, is to deny the partner the knowledge of his and/or his child's genetic endowment. If the couple is deciding whether to have another child, the genetic knowledge that a second child is not at risk may be all that is necessary. But what if the parents separate and the partner becomes involved with another woman? He may be reluctant to have more children based on false and incomplete genetic information: genetic information that was supplied by a health care professional. And he may have informed his siblings of his carrier status provoking unnecessary testing or worry on their part.

The decision to conceal misattributed paternity from the partner and to inform the woman confidentially of this finding is contrary to the standards of full-disclosure and non-directiveness. While disclosure of misattributed paternity to the woman empowers her with relevant information regarding her child's parentage based on accurate genetic data and protects and promotes her privacy, it reflects a value judgement as to what each partner ought to know. The unknowing partner is left in the dark as the health care team helps his wife conceal the child's true genetic identity. The male partner's autonomy as an active decision maker is violated because he is denied relevant information.

II DISCLOSURE OF MISATTRIBUTED PATERNITY TO THE MOTHER ALONE

Current practice in genetic counseling supported by the IOM's recent recommendation is to disclose misattributed paternity to the mother alone. The main reason cited in the studies and reiterated by the IOM is the preservation of the family. In this section, I argue that this reason is inappropriate for genetic counselors. The goal of family preservation is a proper goal of marriage and family counselors, not of genetic counselors, particularly when this can only be achieved by deceiving one of her clients. Instead I argue that nondisclosure of misattributed paternity is deceptive and immoral.

6. Judith L. Benkendorf, Nancy P. Callanan, Rose Grobstein, Susan Schmerler, and Kevin T. FitzGerald. "An Explication of the National Society of Genetic Counselors (NSGC) Code of Ethics," *Journal of Genetic Counseling* 1992; 1(1): 31–9.

The surveys' responses and the IOM's recommendation presume that the preservation of the family is a legitimate goal of geneticists and genetic counselors. Genetic counselors are neither trained to be nor hired to be marriage counselors. The decision to withhold sensitive information regarding biology presumes that disclosing misattributed paternity would be detrimental to the family, a claim that has not been empirically proven. It is possible (even probable) that disclosure may be disruptive to the family, but it is also possible that disclosure may give the family an opportunity to confront their problems head-on. Even if it were true that disclosure would disrupt the family, the question still remains whether the counselor should decide not to disclose information in an effort to preserve the family. That may be the counselor's goals; but it may not be the goal of the partners. This may be their opportunity to confront the meaning of their relationship and to decide whether or not to separate. What is best for the couple must be determined by the couple. As such, the counselor's decision not to disclose false paternity is contrary to her emphasis on being non-directive.

If preserving the family is a valid goal of geneticists and genetic counselors, then it is questionable whether the policy of disclosing misattributed paternity to the mother promotes this goal. Consider, for example, one possible scenario of false paternity. Mr. and Mrs. A are married for seven years. Their son, age 5, has cystic fibrosis (CF). They state that the illness has caused great strain on their marriage. They are now reconciled and Mrs. A is pregnant. They want to know if this child has CF. Given the need for genetic linkage testing in CF,[7] the counselor gets blood samples from Mr. and Mrs. A and their older son. The results are inconclusive because Mr. A is not the biological father of their older son. The counselor's disclosure of false paternity to Mrs. A may set back their reconciliation. Even if Mrs. A knew that the child could be her lover's child, she may have convinced herself that her husband is the true father. However if she is informed of the false paternity, she will harbor a secret that could have wide implications on her marriage and on the well-being of the family. This secret knowledge could renew marital tension and discord. She may neglect or abuse the child who is a constant reminder of her past infidelity. As such, it may be better for the marriage if Mrs. A were not informed about the child's true parentage. Disclosure to the mother alone may or may not promote the preservation of the family: its impact will depend on the specific details of the particular family.

7. Cystic Fibrosis is an autosomal recessive illness which means that a child can only be affected if both parents are carriers and pass that gene onto the child. Because there are many mutations for the genes for Cystic Fibrosis, genetic testing can require determining the particular mutation that each parent has. This requires examining the chromosomes of each parent against the child's chromosomes to determine the particular CF genes (linkage testing). In contrast, sickle cell anemia is an autosomal recessive illness which is caused by only one mutation for which direct testing exists. As such, it is unnecessary to link the chromosomes in sickle cell testing.

Consider, further, what it means to fail to disclose misattributed paternity to the woman's partner. Presently, if genetic testing is inconclusive because the putative father is not the biological father, virtually all geneticists and genetic counselors tell the couple that testing was inconclusive. A counselor may fudge the truth and assert that the tests have not been informative with regard to future risk. Alternatively, a counselor may falsely claim that the first child's genetic disease was caused by a rare mutation and that the risk of another affected offspring is negligible. In general, the putative father is never told that he is not the biological father of the affected infant. The woman, however, will be informed about the false paternity in a confidential meeting at a future date and time.

Failure to disclose misattributed paternity to the partner, then, is not merely a lack of full disclosure but requires active deception. The problem with the counselor's decision to actively deceive the partner is that the partner is her client as well. The counselor's action assumes that health care professionals should decide what information is relevant or important to their clients. Traditionally physicians did unilaterally decide whether or not to divulge sensitive information to patients. In the 1960s such practices were questioned and publicly condemned as immoral. The reaction of physicians was a rapid change in disclosure policies. Whereas in the 1950s and 1960s, most physicians did not disclose the diagnosis of cancer to their patients, today such disclosure is commonplace.

Failure to inform the partner of misattributed paternity can also be rejected on deontological grounds: the physician-patient or counselor-client relationship is or should be based on trust and shared decision making. Failure to disclose this information to the male partner prevents him from real participation in decision making. Some men who learn that their children are not biologically their own may want to divorce or separate. Counselors may have legitimate concerns that partners may not want to support a child that they did not sire, but counselors do not have moral responsibility for ensuring the monetary support of children. Rather it is presumptuous for them to think that they are.

The decision to preserve the woman's privacy means that these children will not be informed of their true parentage. How could a child be told that his biological father is not his social father if his social father is not told this as well? Problems may arise, then, if the child's actual biological father has a transmittable genetic illness. Imagine, for example, that the biological father has Huntington's Chorea. If the mother chooses not to inform her child of his true parentage, her son will not know that he is at risk, because as far as he knows, his family history is negative in that regard. He may not learn the truth until after he has sired a family. Likewise, a mother may not choose to tell her daughter that all of her true paternal biological aunts died from breast cancer in their early 30s and that she should undergo mammography beginning at age 20. As genetic diseases become more amenable to treatment, accurate genetic information becomes more relevant to the child's health care.

III NON-DISCLOSURE TO EITHER PARENT

An alternative to the present-day policy of disclosure to the woman alone is a policy in which counselors would not disclose unanticipated misattributed paternity to either parent. Unlike the policy of unilateral disclosure to the woman and unilateral deception of her partner, this can be achieved without using a deception through a policy of "if they don't ask, I won't tell." According to such a policy, the counselors would only divulge that information which the couple specifically requested. Such a policy must be rejected because it is contrary to the educative and resourceful roles to which counselors aspire. Counselors cannot limit their disclosure to information about which their clients directly ask, because part of counseling is to educate clients to know what to ask, and to tell clients what they would have wanted to ask, had they known more genetics.

One rationale for a policy in which neither parent is informed about the finding of misattributed paternity is that the family has not asked about paternity, and the finding is incidental. The family came in to understand their future risk of conceiving an affected child and the finding of false paternity was an incidental finding. Much information is determined in genetic studies, and not all information obtained from genetic testing is revealed as it is the counselor's job to inform the family of genetic risks, not to give them a full degree in genetics. But the information about whether one is or is not a child's biological parent is *never* incidental. Genetic counselors fear the impact of false paternity on marriage precisely because such knowledge is *not* incidental.

If counselors have an obligation to preserve the integrity of their clients' families, then they may decide that family integrity is best achieved if they fail to reveal false paternity to either partner. First, as I argued above, I do not believe that preservation of families is an appropriate goal of genetic counselors. Second, I do not believe that non-disclosure to both parties will necessarily promote family integrity. Recall Mr. and Mrs. A. They may suspect that their first child is not biologically related to Mr. A. They may be embarrassed and decide not to divulge this information freely, but wait and see what the genetic tests reveal. If the counselor were to confirm their suspicion, they may be relieved to learn that Mr. A is not a carrier of the CF gene and that their future progeny are not at risk. If the counselor fails to disclose the false paternity, the couple may undergo an amniocentesis to avoid another child with CF. As such, the non-disclosure results in an unnecessary amniocentesis which risks the woman's and the fetus' health and well-being. This is unacceptable: a counselor *cannot* permit an unnecessary test with known serious risks to prevent a possible but unproven threat to a marriage. In addition, an iatrogenic complication to either the woman or the fetus may cause unanticipated (as well as avoidable) marital discord. Thus, the counselor's attempt to preserve family integrity may backfire. Since counselors do not know the consequences of revealing misattributed paternity, they should not ground their actions on speculative consequences. Rather, counselors must judge the morality of their actions only on the basis of whether their actions comply with their moral duties. Deception is contrary to their obligations to tell the truth and to give their clients accurate information: it cannot be morally justified.

A policy of bilateral non-disclosure is also dangerous because no one in the family knows the true genetic history of their child. This may place the child at risk for knowable, potentially treatable, diseases. Again, imagine that the true biological father has a strong family history of early-onset breast cancer. If the mother knows that her lover and not her husband is the true father, she may encourage her daughter to get breast cancer mammography screening at a much younger age than is generally done in the general population.

A policy of bilateral non-disclosure also leaves the couple at risk for future decisions based on false information. The parents may choose not to have further children based on this inaccurate knowledge. And the parents' siblings may suffer needlessly thinking that they themselves or their children are at risk. Moreover, the decision not to disclose may cause a backlash if the parents learn of the false paternity in another setting (e.g. the child needs a kidney transplant and histocompatibility testing[8] reveals misattributed paternity). What response can the counselor give when both parents converge on her and demand to know what right she had to decide what information they needed?

The failure of a counselor to tell either party of the child's true parentage implies that the counselor believes that the genetic makeup of the clients and their child is not the clients' exclusive property. It implies that the counselor who has analyzed their DNA is the rightful proprietor who can do with it what she wants. Such a claim contradicts the moral and legal standards of disclosure for health care professionals.[9]

If a major goal of genetic counselors is to disclose relevant information to their clients, then the finding of misattributed paternity must be disclosed to both partners because it is relevant to their clients' identity and procreative decisions. Failure to disclose misattributed paternity to either partner leaves the family and the individual members at unnecessary and unjustifiable risk.

IV DISCLOSURE OF MISATTRIBUTED PATERNITY TO BOTH PARENTS

What are the arguments in favor of full disclosure to both parents, particularly the partner who has been routinely overlooked? First, the partner has come to a health professional for information about himself and his child. His genetic background is his, and like all genetic counseling clients, he should be given as much accurate information as possible. It also seems obvious that it is relevant from the partner's perspective to know that the child is not genetically his. Genetic counselors should not speculate as to what the partner will choose to do with this information. To determine that it is better for him not to know detracts from the counselor's main goal of promoting client autonomy.

Another argument in favor of disclosure is the acknowledgement that the relationship is already characterized by deception and this may give the family an opportunity to confront their problems or to redefine the terms of their relationship. While full disclosure may be disruptive to the family, whether this happens and the extent of the disruption will depend on many factors unique to the family which the counselors cannot predict. The family has sought genetic information: it is the geneticist's responsibility to inform them of this as accurately as possible. The information, however, should not be divulged acrimoniously. Rather the information must be given in a sensitive non-judgmental manner that will help to minimize undue harm. The counselor can assess how, when, and in what context to

8. Histocompatibility refers to the compatibility (similarity) of one's immunological status to another. It is genetically determined. A child has 50% histocompatibility with each genetic parent.

9. See, for example, *Canterbury v Spence* 464 F.2d 772 (D.C. Cir. 1972).

divulge this information. She may choose to have a therapist present to enable the family to address their feelings. But ultimately she must inform them of the genetic evidence of misattributed paternity because this is integral to their relationship and identities. This is not to deny that the truth will be painful. But this is true of many medical diagnoses. Outside of the genetic context, it is no longer acceptable for physicians to fail to disclose the true nature of their patients' conditions:[10] the same should be true with genetic information.

Full disclosure to both partners is consonant with the belief that genetic counselors have responsibility to all their competent adult clients. Genetic information is not the counselor's property which she can divulge as she sees fit. It is the property of her clients. Full disclosure empowers the partners so that they can choose how best to use this information. It also makes possible the disclosure of the child's true parentage at some future date.

V OBJECTIONS TO BILATERAL DISCLOSURE

My recommendation of full disclosure to both partners is in conflict with the practices of virtually all geneticists and genetic counselors. Many reviewers were also troubled by my recommendation. The three most common objections to my proposal are that bilateral disclosure: 1. places the woman and child at physical risk; 2. places the woman at psychological risk; and 3. fails to respect the woman's right to privacy. Let me respond to each objection in turn.

First, I do not mean to downplay the *potential* threat to some women and children if misattributed paternity is determined and revealed. But there are no data to support this concern. And in fact, the dominant theme in the family counseling literature is that the woman's behavior has no causal influence on the man's decision to batter, but rather, that the problem lies exclusively in the man.[11]

This is not meant to minimize the serious medical and social issue of domestic violence. Data show that 30% of married American women will experience at least one violent episode in their lifetime and similar data exist in other Western countries. Furthermore 50% of female homicides are perpetrated by male intimates. There are also data to show that abusive men are sexually possessive and jealous. But the relationship of abuse and infidelity has not been extensively examined. In a search of the medical, philosophical and sociological literature between 1975–1995, I was able to locate only two studies which examined this issue. One study found a correlation between wife infidelity and spousal abuse, but it could not prove whether men are abusive because women are unfaithful, or whether women are unfaithful because their partners are abusive. The second reference focused on the more narrow issue of domestic homicide. It stated that men kill their partners more frequently than women kill their partners, and the reasons given for spousal homicides are different. Women invariably kill male partners after years of abuse whereas men kill their female partners for a variety of reasons including revelations of infidelity.

Would my conclusions be different if the data revealed that men became even more aggressive/homicidal upon learning of misattributed paternity? Probably not. Such a finding would underscore the need for policies and programs that educate the public regarding the wide range of information that genetic testing can reveal so that at-risk women would avoid such testing to protect themselves and their children. However, I do not believe it would justify a policy of non-disclosure given that most men do not and would not abuse their partners.

A second concern is the psychological risk that a policy of bilateral disclosure may produce. Imagine that a couple comes in for genetic testing and the counselor explains the wide spectrum of information that genetic testing can and will determine: from extra chromosomes to chromosomal deletions, from false paternity to mistaken identity, from lethal conditions which present in infancy (e.g. Tay Sachs) to those which present in adulthood (e.g. Alzheimer's). Genetic counselors need to help clients decide what information they want to obtain and what information they would rather not have.

10. See, for example, *Arato v. Avedon* 5 Cal. 4th 1172, 23 Cal. Rptr.2d 131, 858 P.2d 598 (1993).

11. See, for example, Douglas Sprenkle, "Wife Abuse Through the Lens of 'Systems Theory,'" *The Counseling Psychologist* 1994: 22(4): 598–602; and Morton Stenchever and Diane Stenchever, "Abuse of Women: An Overview," *Women's Health Issues* 1991; 1(4): 187–192.

If the counselor raises the possibility of unanticipated findings to the couple prior to testing, then the woman is in a bind because it is only her infidelity which can be discovered and revealed: How can the woman, at that point, ask to know the risk of their future children, but not be told about misattributed paternity? Such a request would be an admission of previous infidelity.

One solution would be to better educate the public-at-large regarding what genetic testing can and cannot determine. More specifically, education regarding genetic testing could be emphasized during prenatal care. I would even accept a policy whereby when an appointment for genetic counseling was sought, a counselor would contact the female partner confidentially and inform her in a precounseling session about the potential for misattributed paternity so that she can choose not to undergo testing. This would permit women to decide in an uncoerced non-threatening environment whether or not this is a risk and whether or not this is a risk that they want to confront.

Of course, a decision to back out of testing may still raise suspicions and several readers have argued that my solution does not protect the woman from the psychological risk that revelations about her other sexual relationships may create. How would I resolve the difficulty for her? My response is that it is not my responsibility to do this. The woman, through her voluntary actions, has placed herself in this quandary. If a woman voluntarily has sexual relationships with another man, then her decision should incorporate the risk of discovery both during the affair and afterwards, particularly if a child may be conceived in the process. To argue that women need to be protected by a blanket policy of deception towards their partners suggests that women are not capable of taking responsibility for their actions and their consequences. This suggests that women are not competent to make autonomous decisions regarding sexual relationships (that they are incompetent) and that third-party protection (paternalism) is appropriate and necessary. I reject these conclusions.

Nevertheless, it is true that the risk of disclosure is asymmetrical. The testing can only reveal the woman's infidelities. But conception is also asymmetrical. Only women can be 100% confident of a genetic relationship to the child. As such, gestation is both a privilege and a responsibility. Women need to know that genetic testing can reveal misattributed paternity so that decisions which relate to sexual relationships, reproduction, and genetic counseling are informed. Some women who have had more than one partner may be in denial that these concerns pertain to them, but that does not change the fact that they are responsible for their decisions.

The third objection asks why I perceive disclosure purely as an issue of truth-telling and not as an issue regarding respect for the privacy of the woman. My answer is in the framing of the question. This paper addresses the issue of who has the right to genetic information in the scenario when *both* partners come to the counselor for testing and counseling. My argument is that when both partners are clients of the counselor, they both have the right to the genetic information. In reality, the vast majority of clients are pregnant women, many of whom come alone. In those cases, testing of the woman and the fetus are her decision and her partner does not have any claims to the counselor's disclosures unless she consents to it. But when a couple elects for genetic testing and does not limit the requested information, then the counselor has a moral obligation to disclose the test results to both adult clients.

VI COUNSELOR'S OBLIGATIONS TO THE CHILD

The question of whether the genetic counselor has obligations to reveal misattributed paternity directly to the child is complex. Three reasons to favor disclosure are 1. its role in health care screening, diagnosis, and treatment; 2. its role in procreative decisions, and 3. the importance of genetic identity to one's self-identity. Two reasons to favor nondisclosure are 1. that such knowledge may threaten the parent-child relationship; and 2. that it might threaten the integrity of the family. Which reasons are stronger depend on how one weighs the advantages and disadvantages. Presently, in medical care involving children, parents are empowered to make many decisions on their child's behalf, and to determine what is in their child's best interest, all things considered. In their calculations, parents are allowed to balance the competing and conflicting needs of other family members provided that their decision is not abusive or harmful to the child. While I believe that the genetic counselors have an obligation to the child, I would argue that the counselors should defer to the parents as to when and how the child is to be informed about his true biological identity. Counselors fulfill their obligation by encouraging the parents to disclose the truth about the child's genetic identity to the child when they deem it appropriate. The counselor should also offer to counsel the child directly, but should respect the parents' decision not to reveal false paternity at this time. Likewise, if the child is an infant or otherwise unable to understand the genetic facts, then counseling of the child must be deferred. The counselor should offer to be available at a future time, but he should respect those families who choose to deal with this privately. While the counselor has an obligation to encourage the parents to reveal this information to the child, he or she is not empowered to confront the child, now or in the future, without parental permission. Parents are the guardians of their children. While deceiving one's child regarding his or her genetic identity is morally problematic, to compel parents to tell the truth about genetic parentage is to intrusively interfere into the private family. The counselor's right to interfere in the family is and ought to be limited. It does not and should not extend this far.

VII CONCLUSION

In conclusion, I support the 1983 recommendation of the President's Commission. I believe that the arguments favor disclosure of false paternity to both partners. Men as well as women have a valid interest in knowing the true biological parentage of their legal children. The impact that disclosure of false paternity will have on men, women and families is unknown. Geneticists and genetic counselors must present the data in a responsible yet sensitive way, but the couple ought to be the ultimate arbiter of what to do with their genetic information (including the issue of whether or not to inform the child of his true parentage).

My proposal should not be interpreted to support routine paternity testing or to encourage genetic testing in cases where false paternity is a potential issue. My point is that deception of either adult partner by the counselor is not morally justified and will only further erode the trust which our patients and clients have in the health care profession. The recent recommendation of the Institute of Medicine regarding misattributed paternity is misconceived.

THE HMO PHYSICIAN'S DUTY TO CUT COSTS

William Edwards was 39 when a serious, potentially life-threatening ventricular heart arrhythmia (irregular contractions) was diagnosed during a routine physical examination. The cardiologist first prescribed quinidine, but it failed to bring the arrhythmia under control.

Diisopyramide was successful, but Mr. Edwards complained of severe blurred vision and dry mouth. When the medication was reduced, the side effects disappeared but the arrhythmia returned. At this point the cardiologist decided to combine the diisopyramide with propranolol, a common beta-blocker known to be effective in certain arrhythmias. This controlled the problem, without side effects.

Mr. Edwards continued with this medication regimen for five years until moving to a new town, where he joined a health maintenance organization (HMO). He immediately consulted Dr. Sam Forester, a cardiologist.

Dr. Forester agreed that medication was needed, but he was concerned about diisopyramide, since severe problems had been reported in some patients. Moreover, Mr. Edwards and his original physician had never tried the obvious approach of using propranolol alone.

Both Dr. Forester and Mr. Edwards concluded that there were also risks in shifting to the single drug. Although it was generally safer than diisopyramide and probably should have been tried originally, there was a small chance of a fatal heart attack. On balance, both agreed that the status quo was slightly better for the patient.

Dr. Forester then noticed the financial ledger for Mr. Edwards's care, which included the cost of the medication paid for in full by the HMO. The yearly cost of the diisopyramide was $430; the propranolol cost $26 per year. He realized that even a significant increase in propranolol dosage, something that would involve little risk, would still reduce the HMO's medication bill by about $400.

Should Dr. Forester consider a change in medication, taking into account cost-saving for the HMO, or should he work solely on the basis of the welfare of the patient? If he should take into account the costs to the HMO, should he try to persuade the patient to agree to the change, or should he simply refuse to authorize any further prescriptions for the diisopyramide? Does Mr. Edwards have any moral obligation to take costs to the HMO into account in choosing a medication regimen?

THE DOCTOR'S MASTER

Norman Levinsky

There is increasing pressure on doctors to serve two masters. Physicians in practice are being enjoined to consider society's needs, as well as each patient's needs, in deciding what type and amount of medical care to deliver. Not surprisingly, many government leaders and health planners take this position. More remarkably, important elements of the medical profession are promoting this view.

I would argue the contrary, that physicians are required to do everything that they believe may benefit each patient without regard to costs or other societal considerations. In caring for an individual patient, the doctor must act solely as that patient's advocate, against the apparent interests of society as a whole, if necessary. An analogy can be drawn with the role of a lawyer defending a client against a criminal charge. The attorney is obligated to use all ethical means to defend the client, regardless of the cost of prolonged legal proceedings or even of the possibility that a guilty person may be acquitted through skillful advocacy. Similarly, in the practice of medicine, physicians are obligated to do all that they can for their patients without regard to any costs to society.

Society benefits if it expects its medical practitioners to follow this principle. As Fried[1] has eloquently argued, in any decent, advanced society there are rights in health care, in that "one is entitled to be treated decently, humanely, personally and honestly in the course of medical care. . . ." In such a just society, "the physician who withholds care that it is in his power to give because he judges it is wasteful to provide it to a particular person breaks faith with his patient." A similar position has been stated by Hiatt[2]: "A physician or other provider must do all that is permitted on behalf of his patient. . . . The patient and the physician want no less, and society should settle for no less." A just society must have a group of professionals whose

From *New England Journal of Medicine* 311, no. 24, December 13, 1984: 1573–1575. Reprinted by permission of the publisher.

sole responsibility as health-care practitioners is to their patients as individuals.

The issue is not whether physicians must do everything technically possible for each patient. Rather it is that they should decide how much to do according to what they believe best for that patient, without regard for what is best for society or what it costs. I do not argue, as some have[3], that doctors are obligated to prolong life under all circumstances or that they are required to use their expertise to confer technological immortality on dehumanized bodies. Actual practice is infinitely complex and varied. Caring and experienced doctors will differ about what to do in individual cases. In my opinion, ethical physicians may discontinue life-extending treatment if their decisions are based solely on what they and the patient or his or her surrogate believe to be the patient's best interests. (The legal issues surrounding such decisions are beyond the scope of this paper.) They are not entitled to discontinue treatment on the basis of other considerations, such as cost. This distinction may become blurred if physicians are pressed to balance the needs of their patients with societal needs. The practitioner may make decisions for economic reasons but rationalize them as in the best interests of the individual patient. This phenomenon may be occurring in Britain, where physicians "seem to seek medical justification for decisions forced on them by resource limits. Doctors gradually redefine standards of care so that they can escape the constant recognition that financial limits compel them to do less than their best."[4]

A similar danger lurks if physicians attempt to conserve resources by using probabilities of success or failure to make decisions about the care of individual patients. Estimates of the probable outcome of a clinical condition in a given patient are almost invariably based on "soft data": uncontrolled studies, reports of cases of dubious comparability, or the physician's anecdotal clinical experience—all further devalued by rapidly changing diagnostic and therapeutic techniques. The standard errors of such estimates are undefined but undoubtedly large. Yet leading physicians[5,6] advise doctors to practice probabilistic medicine—i.e., to withhold expensive treatment if the probability of success is low. How is the practitioner to define "low" in everyday practice—2, 5, 10, or 20 percent likelihood of survival with a good quality of life? Even if the dividing line were defined and the requisite precision in estimating outcome could be achieved, the role of the doctor as patient advocate would be subverted by probabilistic practice. This point should not be blurred by using the phrase "hopelessly ill."[5] If there is no hope for a patient, then there is no problem for the doctor in discontinuing treatment. In practice, doctors can rarely be certain who is hopelessly ill. This problem is not resolved by redefining the phrase to exclude consideration of the "rare report of a patient with a similar condition who survived"[5] in deciding whether to continue aggressive treatment. Physicians cannot discharge their responsibility to their individual patients if they try to conserve societal resources by discontinuing treatment on statistical grounds.

An example may indicate the possibilities for disregarding the best interests of a patient in an attempt to conserve societal resources by probabilistic practice. A gerontologist has suggested that we may rapidly be approaching a time when the majority of people will live until the end of a maximal life span to the point of "natural death" at about 85 years of age.[7] Even if the argument is correct as applied to populations, what is the individual doctor to do when caring for a desperately ill 85-year-old patient? Should advanced treatment be withheld, because "high-level medical technology applied at the end of a natural life span epitomizes the absurd?"[7] In terms of probability, the practitioner may be correct in predicting that the patient will not respond to treatment, but how is the physician to know that this person was not destined for a life span of 90 years? On what grounds can the physician withhold maximal treatment?

Another consideration weighs against any dilution of the mandate to doctors to consider solely the needs of their individual patients. Societal decisions about the proper allocation of resources are highly subjective and open to bias. For example, Avorn[8] has argued that cost-benefit analyses in geriatric care tend to turn age discrimination into health policy, because they depend on techniques for quantifying benefits that have a built-in bias against expenditures on health care for the elderly. A large part of the recent increase in overall health-care costs is due to the growing expense of care for older people. Negative attitudes toward aging and the elderly may influence our willingness to meet these costs. Society may encourage physicians to withhold expensive care on the basis of age, even if such care is likely to benefit the individual patient greatly. In Great Britain, persons over age 55 who have end-stage renal disease are steered away from long-term dialysis.[4]

None of the foregoing implies that in caring for individual patients doctors should disregard the escalating cost of medical care. Physicians can help control costs by choosing the most economical ways to deliver optimal care to their patients. They can use the least expensive setting, ambulatory or inpatient, in which first-class care can be given. They can eliminate redundant or useless diagnostic procedures ordered because of habit, deficient knowledge, personal financial gain, or the practice of "defensive medicine" to avoid malpractice judgments.

However, it is society, not the individual practitioner, that must make the decision to limit the availability of effective but expensive types of medical care. Heart and liver transplantation are current cases in point. These are extraordinarily expensive procedures that may prolong a life of "good quality" for some people. Society, through its elected officials, is entitled to decide that the resources required for such programs are better used for other purposes. However, a physician who thinks that his or her patient may benefit from a transplant must make that patient aware of this opinion and assist the patient in obtaining the organ.

The continuous increase in the costs of medical care is a difficult social issue. However, it is not self-evident that expenditures for health care should be limited to any arbitrary percentage of the gross national product, such as the current 11 percent figure. Moreover, if physicians and others make concerted and effective attempts to eliminate health-care expenditures that do not truly benefit patients, it is not a given fact that the proportion of the national wealth devoted to health care will increase indefinitely. It certainly is not self-evident that resources saved by limiting health care will be allocated to other equally worthy programs, such as preventive medicine, health maintenance, or improved nutrition and housing for the needy. In the United States, the societal decision to limit potentially lifesaving health care will not easily be made or enforced—nor should it be, in my opinion. Officials who press for the rationing of medical resources must be prepared for a public outcry, since unlimited availability of useful medical care has been perceived as a right in American society. Governor Lamm of Colorado was recently the target of such a response. Concerned that society cannot afford technological advances such as heart transplants, he quoted favorably a philosopher who believes that it is our societal duty to die. If society decides to ration health care, political leaders must accept responsibility. David Owen, who is both a political leader in Britain and a physician, believes that "it is right for doctors to demand that politicians openly acknowledge the limitations within which medical practice has to operate."[9] I agree and would add that doctors are entitled to lobby vigorously in the political arena for the resources needed for high-quality health care.

Through its democratic processes, American society may well choose to ration medical resources. In that event, physicians as citizens and experts will have a key role in implementing the decision. Their advice will be needed in allocating limited resources to provide the greatest good for the greatest number. As experience in other countries has shown,[4] it may be difficult for doctors to separate their role as citizens and expert advisors from their role in the practice of medicine as unyielding advocates for the health needs of their individual patients. They must strive relentlessly to do so. When practicing medicine, doctors cannot serve two masters. It is to the advantage both of our society and of the individuals it comprises that physicians retain their historic single-mindedness. The doctor's master must be the patient.

NOTES

1. Fried C. Rights and health care—beyond equity and efficiency. *N Engl J Med* 1975; 293:241–5.
2. Hiatt HH. Protecting the medical commons: who is responsible? *N Engl J Med* 1975; 293:235–41.
3. Epstein FH. The role of the physician in the prolongation of life. In: Ingelfinger FJ, Ebert RV, Finland M, Relman AS, eds. *Controversy in internal medicine, II.* Philadelphia: WB Saunders, 1974:103–9.
4. Aaron HJ, Schwartz, WB. *The painful prescription: rationing hospital care.* Washington, D.C.: Brookings Institution, 1984.

5. Wanzer SH, Adelstein SJ, Cranford RE, et al. The physician's responsibility toward hopelessly ill patients. *N Engl J Med* 1984; 310:955–9.
6. Leaf A. The doctor's dilemma—and society's too. *N Engl J Med* 1984; 310:718–21.
7. Fries JF. Aging, natural death, and the compression of morbidity. *N Engl J Med* 1980; 303:130–5.
8. Avorn J. Benefit and cost analysis in geriatric care: turning age discrimination into health policy. *N Engl J Med* 1984; 310:1294–301.
9. Owen D. Medicine, morality and the market. *Can Med Assoc J* 1984; 130:1341–5.

FISCAL SCARCITY AND THE INEVITABILITY OF BEDSIDE BUDGET BALANCING

E. Haavi Morreim

While recognizing that cost containment will profoundly affect health care, many physicians and bioethicists insist that physicians can and should avoid directly compromising their patients' care to save third parties' money. "Physicians are required to do everything they believe may benefit each patient without regard to costs or other societal considerations";[1] "asking physicians to be cost conscious . . . would be asking them to abandon their central commitment to their patients."[2–10] While the physician might assist in creating public or hospital resource policies, and while he sometimes must ration—e.g., where there are too many patients for too few intensive care beds—on this traditional view he must never voluntarily say "no" to his own patient simply to cut costs.

A variant of this traditional view suggests that physicians can ethically participate in cost containment, but only if the health care system as a whole is morally just. A just system must at least assure all citizens a basic minimum of care, and must be "closed." Only if its total resources are fixed can the physician be sure that money saved in the care of one patient will actually help some needier patient, rather than reverting to taxpayers, stockholders, or munitions makers. Unless such criteria are satisfied, the physician may not ethically assist in economic rationing.[11,12]

I will argue that this prescription for aloofness is now untenable. The economic reorganization of health care has introduced a new kind of scarcity, requiring a different sort of rationing than that to which physicians are accustomed. Bedside tradeoffs between one patient's welfare and other parties' competing needs, relatively rare in the past, are now inescapable.

THREE KINDS OF SCARCITY

Prior to the 1980s, limits on health care arose largely through two sources: (1) inadequate access to the health care system, either through the patient's inability to pay for care or through a regional shortage of personnel and facilities,[13] and (2) shortages of specific commodities, such as intensive care beds or hemodialysis units. Arising mainly around new or exotic technologies, serious "commodity scarcities" were otherwise uncommon. Government funding of capital improvements, combined with generous third-party reimbursement practices, generally meant that those who had access to the health care system at all could expect quite a full range of its benefits. Indeed, physicians and other providers had economic incentives not only to ignore costs (except where the patient himself was the payer), but to provide every possible benefit, as

Archives of Internal Medicine 149 (1989): 1012–1015.

retrospective fee-for-service reimbursement rewarded maximal levels of intervention.[14–16]

In recent years, however, a third sort of scarcity has arisen: "fiscal scarcity," a general tightening of health care dollars as government and business, who together pay three-fourths of the nation's health care bill, attempt to gain control over their skyrocketing expenditures. This tightening takes a variety of forms, such as prospective payment, utilization review, preferred provider arrangements, and managed care systems, but collectively signals a fundamental change in the nature of the allocation decisions physicians face.

In commodity scarcity, some discrete item is in limited supply, whether because of natural limits, as in the case of transplant organs, or through sheer cost, as with positron emission tomography. The list of patients needing that resource is usually fairly clear: only those with severe and irreversible hepatic disease are eligible for liver transplant. As a result, the consequences of allocation decisions are equally clear. We know not only the exact identity of those who receive the commodity, but also, reciprocally, the names, or at least the general description, of those who do not. If Mrs. Baker is admitted to the lone available intensive care bed, Mr. Abel, also in need, is not. But Mrs. Jones, recovering from pneumonia on another ward, is unaffected. Equally important, we can also be fairly sure that if one patient is denied the resource, some other needy person will nevertheless benefit. The difficult decision brings at least that consolation.

Because the consequences of commodity allocations are thus fairly clear, so are the trade-offs that must go into those decisions. To distribute transplant organs, we can assemble medical criteria to tell us which patients have the highest probability of living for what length of time, with what functional capacities and deficits.[17] And we can identify some nonmedical values that we can then choose either to include or to ignore. Should a criminal record disqualify one from eligibility for transplant? Should family responsibilities or occupational contributions count? During the early days of hemodialysis, some allocation committees decided that even after excluding, on "medical" grounds, applicants who were more than 40 years old or who suffered from mental illness, a surfeit of remaining candidates did require just such clearly nonmedical considerations.[18,19]

Fiscal scarcity is utterly different. Because every medical decision has its economic cost, literally every medical decision is now subject to scrutiny for its economic as well as its medical wisdom. Suddenly, not this or that item, but all of medicine, is an allocation issue—every laboratory test, every roentgenogram.

Unlike commodity scarcities, the consequences of fiscal allocation decisions are anything but clear. Obviously, the decision to order a $2,000 course of antibiotics rather than a $2 course means that this $2,000 will not be available for alternate use. But beyond that, consequences are amorphous. We cannot possibly name, or even describe generically, who will be denied what as a result of the expenditure. The diminution of funds may constrain future decisions to some degree, although it is rare for any single spending decision to be felt discernibly, even at the level of an individual hospital's finances, let alone at the statewide or national level. The collective impact of many spending decisions does not dictate which sorts of medical care will be constrained for which patients in the future. That is entirely a product of further decision making.

Because the consequences of fiscal allocation decisions cannot be specified, neither can the moral or medical trade-offs be precisely identified. To prescribe a cheaper but slightly less effective antibiotic may or may not affect the patient's outcome at all, and there is no assurance that the money saved will even be used to help other patients rather than be returned to stockholders or taxpayers.[11,12]

GUIDELINES

Commodity and fiscal scarcity can also be distinguished by the sort of criteria that can guide allocation decisions. Because the consequences and trade-offs of commodity decisions are fairly clear, and because decisions are episodic, required only when a particular patient(s) needs a specific item that is in short supply, it is possible to establish fairly explicit criteria, and to apply them fairly rigorously. One can consider whether an alcoholic ought to be denied a liver transplant,[20] and one can formulate a sorting system for allocating intensive care beds[21] or transplant organs.[17]

The decisions of fiscal allocation are not episodic, but chronic. Every decision has its price.

As a result, criteria guiding fiscal allocation must ideally cover every detail of medical care, whether to cull out useless interventions, or, under more stringent circumstances, to eliminate real benefits in some thoughtful, systematic way.

Actually, fiscal efficiency guidelines are now emerging throughout medicine. Many observers argue that physicians are morally obligated to eliminate from their clinical routines those interventions that are of little or no proven value, thereby conserving costs while preserving or even enhancing quality of care.[2,7,22–24] Thus, for example, the American College of Physicians, in collaboration with Blue Cross and Blue Shield, has issued "Diagnostic Testing Guidelines" for such common tests as arterial blood gas analysis, blood cultures, chest roentgenograms, and electrocardiograms. If used as bases on which to deny reimbursement, these guidelines could eventually save up to $10 million per year (James, FE. Blue Cross Plans Coverage Limits on Many Tests. *Wall Street Journal*. April 10, 1987:29). Similarly, many health maintenance organizations have developed guidelines to suggest appropriate uses of hospitalization and sophisticated technologies, while many third-party payers use their own utilization review "cookbooks" to determine which medical interventions warrant reimbursement.

However, such efficiency protocols differ markedly from the kind of rationing criteria we develop for scarce commodities. They will not provide such clear guidance nor, more importantly, will they enable the physician to escape personal involvement in trade-offs between patients' welfare and economic considerations at the bedside. In both formulation and implementation, such guidelines will require some compromises in patient care.

Formulating Guidelines

Those who formulate efficiency protocols must eliminate not just utterly useless practices, but also some interventions of at least marginal value. Although physicians have occasionally been guilty of clear wastefulness as, for instance, admitting patients to the hospital on a Friday for an elective diagnostic workup that cannot begin until Monday, deleting such carelessness surely will not resolve the nation's entire health care challenge.[25] (If it could, then the medical profession would owe the nation a profound apology for triggering an economic crisis through sheer profligacy.)

But once we turn to interventions of marginal value, patient care will inevitably be compromised. Not all patients' care will be impaired, for many will actually be benefitted through reduced iatrogenesis and inconvenience. Nevertheless, to be of marginal benefit is, by definition, to be of some benefit.[14] The benefit may be small, as with palliative treatment of self-limited illness, or it may help only a few patients. Most commonly, marginal interventions reduce diagnostic or therapeutic uncertainty—the extra test to confirm clinical findings, the screening test to detect rare but serious and treatable maladies, the wide-spectrum antibiotic to cover for unidentified organisms.[26–28] In most cases, eliminating such interventions will do no harm. Yet some patients will be deprived of a real benefit, namely those few whose rare disease would have been detected by the now-eliminated diagnostic "zebra-hunt," or whose therapy would have been more effective with more potent agents. We may never know in advance which patients will be harmed and which patients will be helped as efficiency protocols eliminate marginal benefits. But the fact remains that some patients' welfare will have been exchanged for the health of other patients and for the wealth of third parties.

Such trade-offs require important value judgments. The move from "do anything that might help" to "do only what will help" represents a fundamental value shift from "interventionism" to "noninterventionism,"[29] a reversion from modern medicine's technological imperative to its older value, "do no harm." Further, to call a benefit "marginal" is to judge that its value is intrinsically small, or less important than alternative uses of the limited total resources.

This is not to say that physicians should therefore refuse to curb marginal practices. In times of resource scarcity it would be irresponsible to abdicate such essential, albeit difficult, "gray zone" decisions. Our point is only that one cannot "eliminate marginal benefits" without shifting a fundamental value of the profession and compromising at least some patients' care.

Implementing Guidelines

Although they require important value judgments and will inevitably alter quality of care, efficiency protocols can at least be formulated away from the bedside. Unfortunately, physicians' cooperation with cost containment cannot be confined to just this "policy level."[30] Efficiency protocols will not save money until they are implemented at the bedside; and here the physician cannot escape directly saying "no" to his own patients in the name of resource conservation.

Each time an efficiency protocol would suggest suboptimal care for his patient, the physician has several choices. First, he can simply follow the protocol, refraining from any attempt to secure optimal care for his patient. In that case, he will have voluntarily done less than he could for his patient, a clear bedside trade-off.

Alternatively, he could avail himself of the flexibility that is necessarily built into such guidelines. No "cookbook" or computer program, however detailed, could possibly dictate exactly what should be done for each patient. Medical science is too uncertain, and patients too variable, to admit of such crisp determinacy. Any guideline must be tempered by the clinical judgment of a physician who personally knows the patient. Thus, though barium studies of the gastrointestinal tract can normally be safely completed on an outpatient basis, a frail elderly patient may well require inpatient observation. Further, third-party payers and others who apply such guidelines are unlikely to dictate medical decisions outright, lest they increase their own legal risks (*Wickline* v. *State of California*, 228 Cal Rptr 661 [Cal App 2 Dist, 1986]).

Such flexibility means that it is almost always possible for a physician to find some way to justify an exception for his patient any time the guideline might propose suboptimal care. Unfortunately, if the physician makes such an exception for literally every deprivation of even the smallest benefit, he will thwart the efficiency protocol completely. The very point of such guidelines is, after all, to eliminate (marginal) benefits and to distribute the resulting suboptimality of care in the most fair, medically benign way possible. If costs are to be contained, physicians must cooperate, by voluntarily doing less than they might for some of their own patients.

Because this compromise does threaten physicians' traditional fiduciary obligation to promote their own patients' interests above all others',[1] some observers have proposed a third alternative. Others, not the physician, should say "no."[4,8,9] However, although society can and should set basic health resource policies, legislators, bureaucrats, and judges have no business making individual patient care decisions. On another version, clinically knowledgeable hospital administrators or other local laymen would adjudicate requests for care not provided for within the guidelines, or which exceeded some designated threshold of expenditure.[2,3] As the physician pleads his patient's case while others allot or deny benefits, the physician can tell the patient that "they," not he, are rationing care. He maintains unsullied his loyalty to the patient. But at a terrible price.

He is no longer practicing medicine. Although outsiders can plausibly place firm controls, e.g., over the costliest technologies' proliferation and use, such supervision cannot invade the daily details of care. To the extent that others determine which patients will receive how many roentgenograms, which laboratory or radiologic studies, or how many days' hospitalization with what intensity of nursing care, those "others" are literally practicing medicine in the physician's stead, without a license, at that. The physician escapes saying "no" by becoming impotent to say "yes."

Firm guidelines and appeals procedures are initially attractive, perhaps because they are roughly feasible in the allocation of scarce commodities. As we have seen, commodity allocation decisions are episodic, the trade-offs fairly clear, the values often nonmedical, and the verdicts final. But, under fiscal scarcity, all of medicine is at stake. To dictate in advance the permissible economic impact of each health care decision is to dictate the medical decisions themselves, which is an unacceptable intrusion on clinical freedom.

Finally, the physician might try to ignore efficiency protocols and cost considerations altogether. By now this option is sorely tempting. When the physician cooperates with cost containment, he reneges on his fiduciary commitment to serve his patients' interests above all others'. If, on the other hand, he permits outsiders to impose all the economic trade-offs in his patients' care, he has literally abdicated the practice of medicine. Perhaps he should simply ignore cost constraints as best he can, or at least wait until society has put in place a just allocation scheme in which his cooperation will not offend his patients' rights.[11,12]

THE INEVITABILITY OF BEDSIDE RATIONING

Unfortunately, ignoring economics is not an option either. Government and business are determined to control their health care expenditures. And not without justification. Government has other worthy projects to which it owes resources, and business will be less viable in the competitive international marketplace if it cannot control this important cost of production.[15,31,32] But controlling health care expenditures requires controlling spending decisions, and that, in turn, requires the control, or at least cooperation, of physicians, whose medical decisions largely determine health care expenditures.

In some cases, physicians' decisions and options are restricted through *direct controls*, as where a hospital pharmacy's formulary does not carry certain costly drugs, or where the primary care physician must obtain a subspecialist's approval to order an expensive test for his patient. While there is some room for such controls, however, we have already seen that excessive invasion into the daily details of medicine is untenable. Instead, physicians' economic cooperation is more commonly elicited through *incentives*. Whether through such "sticks" as administrators' letters of warning or threats to revoke hospital privileges,[33] or through "carrots" such as bonuses and profit-sharing, physicians are being systematically introduced to the economic consequences of their medical decisions. They are personally, professionally, and financially at risk for the level of care which they choose for their patients.[34]

COMMENT

My conclusion is unsavory, but its logic compelling. No matter how well we trim waste, regardless how efficiently we manage our resources, however generous our health care budget, our finite resources cannot possibly meet the limitless health care needs of the population. Limits necessitate decisions to deny benefits. If the physician has clinical authority to make medical (i.e., spending) decisions, then reciprocally he makes the decisions not to spend. Guidelines can help, but if flexible, they still leave final decisions in the physician's hands. Even where resource controls appear rigid, the physician must still make the decision whether to acquiesce or to challenge them on behalf of each particular patient. The physician remains free in any given case to render maximal care. Yet the requirement to limit the use of resources overall must ultimately translate into individual decisions to refrain from offering particular interventions to particular patients. The physician thus cannot escape reckoning with awkward decisions about when to offer everything and when to comply with the need to do less.

This is not to say that the quality of health care in the United States must decline substantially. Fiscal constraints are not yet dire, and there is still much "fat" to be trimmed from heavy administrative bureaucracy and from clinical routines of care. Further, competition and litigation constantly remind providers to maintain their standards. Neither does fiscal scarcity mean that physicians must now become principally agents of society, or that they must place their patients' interests simply on a par with the myriad of competing considerations. Nor does this constitute moral permission for hasty acquiescence to unpleasant financial or professional pressures, or an endorsement of ad hoc, idiosyncratic economic theorizing at the bedside. Collective research and reflection on optimal resource use is morally, medically, and economically preferable to solo cost-cutting.

Rather, fiscal scarcity means that physicians must now face rationing questions on an altogether different scale than before. Their moral question is no longer whether to participate in cost containment (that would be rather like asking "shall we abide by the law of gravity?"), but how to do so in morally credible ways. Although economic exigencies may force physicians to weigh more carefully the cost of each benefit and the value of the benefit to the patient, they do not require that the physician appraise the value of the patient himself or weigh his benefit to society. The physician can still be his patient's best advocate, even if he is not obligated to provide benefits without limit.

NOTES

1. Levinsky NG. The doctor's master. *N Engl J Med*. 1984;311:1573–1575.
2. Veatch RM. DRGs and the ethical reallocation of resources. *Hastings Cent Rep*. 1986;16:32–40.
3. Veatch RM. *A Theory of Medical Ethics*. New York, NY: Basic Books Inc; 1981.
4. Abrams FR. Patient advocate or secret agent? *JAMA*. 1986;256:1784–1785.
5. Swiryn S. The doctor as gatekeeper. *Arch Intern Med*. 1986;146:1789.
6. Pellegrino E, Thomasma D. *A Philosophical Basis of Medical Practice*. New York, NY: Oxford University Press Inc; 1981.
7. Angell M. Cost containment and the physician. *JAMA*. 1985;254:1203–1207.
8. Hiatt H. Protecting the medical commons: who is responsible? *N Engl J Med*. 1975;293:235–241.
9. Fried C. Rights and health care: beyond equity and efficiency. *N Engl J Med*. 1975;293:241–245.
10. Beauchamp TL, Childress JF. *Principles of Biomedical Ethics*. 2nd ed. New York, NY: Oxford University Press Inc; 1983.
11. Cassel CK. Doctors and allocation decisions: a new role in the new medicare. *J Health Polit Policy Law*. 1985;10:549–564.
12. Daniels N. The ideal advocate and limited resources. *Theor Med*. 1987;8:69:80.
13. Komaroff AL. The doctor, the hospital, and the definition of proper medical practice. In: President's Commission, *Securing Access to Health Care*. Washington, D.C.: U.S. Government Printing Office; 1981;3:225–251.
14. Fuchs VR. The 'rationing' of medical care. *N Engl J Med*. 1984;311:1572–1573.
15. Thurow LC. Learning to say 'no'. *N Engl J Med*. 1984;311:1569–1572.
16. Thurow LC. Medicine versus economics. *N Engl J Med*. 1985;313:611–614.
17. Starzl TE, Hakala TR, Tzak A, et al. A multifactorial system for equitable selection of cadaver kidney recipients. *JAMA*. 1987;257:3073–3075.
18. Sanders D, Dukeminier J Jr. Medical advance and legal lag; hemodialysis and kidney transplantation. *UCLA Law Rev*. 1968;15:367–386.
19. Evans RW. Health care technology and the inevitability of resource allocation and rationing decisions. *JAMA*. 1983;249(pt 2):2208–2219.
20. Flavin DK, Niven RG, Kelsey JE. Alcoholism and orthotopic liver transplantation. *JAMA*. 1988; 259:1546–1547.
21. Engelhardt HT, Rie MA. Intensive care units, scarce resources, and conflicting principles of justice. *JAMA*. 1986;255:1159–1163.
22. Council on Ethical and Judicial Affairs. Recent opinions: economic incentives and levels of care. *JAMA*. 1986;256:224.
23. Wong ET, Lincoln TL. Ready! Fire! . . . Aim! *JAMA*. 1983;250:2510–2513.
24. Egdahl R. Ways for surgeons to increase efficiency of their use of hospitals. *N Engl J Med*. 1983; 309:1184–1187.
25. Schwartz WB. The inevitable failure of current cost-containment strategies. *JAMA*. 1987;257:220–224.
26. Hardison JF. To be complete. *N Engl J Med*. 1979; 300:193–194.
27. Reuben D. Learning diagnostic restraint. *N Engl J Med*. 1984;310:591–593.
28. Baily M. Rationing medical care: processes for defining adequacy. In: Agich GJ, Begley CE, eds. *The Price of Health*. Dordrecht, the Netherlands: D. Reidel Publishing Co; 1986;165–184.
29. Brett AS. Hidden ethical issues in clinical decision analysis. *N Engl J Med*. 1981;305:1150–1153.
30. Brett AS, McCullough LB. When patients request specific interventions. *N Engl J Med*. 1986; 315:1347–1351.
31. Aaron HJ, Schwartz WB. Hospital cost control: a bitter pill to swallow. *Harvard Bus Rev*. 1985; 64:160–167.
32. Board of Trustees. A proposal for financing health care of the elderly. *JAMA*. 1986;256:3379–3382.
33. Hershey N. Fourth-party audit organizations: practical and legal considerations. *Law Med Health Care*. 1986;14:54–65.
34. Egdahl RH, Taft CH. Financial incentives to physicians. *N Engl J Med*. 1986;315:59–61.

WHAT ARE WE TEACHING ABOUT INDIGENT PATIENTS?

Steven H. Miles

An adult woman without health insurance presented to the emergency department of a private, not-for-profit, university hospital. A male acquaintance had assaulted her and had fractured her forearm. After the assault, she impulsively took an overdose of an anticonvulsant, phenytoin. A friend brought her to the emergency department. Because a history of intravenous drug abuse had scarred the patient's peripheral veins, peripheral intravenous access was not possible. An attempt to place a catheter in her subclavian vein led to a pneumothorax and a chest tube. Intravenous access was then obtained through a jugular vein. As the overdose was an emergency, the arm was splinted and she was admitted to the medicine service on which I was the attending physician.

Two days later, she was medically stabilized. The overdose was resolved, the chest tube was pulled. A psychiatrist concluded that the overdose was in response to the stress of the assault rather than because of major depression. A counselor for battered women offered a shelter, follow-up counseling, and assistance in filing a criminal complaint, all of which the patient declined, saying that she could avoid this man. An orthopedic surgeon said the patient's arm required internal fixation to set the fracture but declined to take the patient to surgery because she did not have insurance even though she was eligible for Medicaid, which the surgeon believed would be inadequate reimbursement. When he stood firm on that decision, I spoke with the Chief of Medicine, who took it up with the Chief of Orthopedic Surgery and the hospital lawyer. The surgeons were adamant; the Medicine Department could grant "compassionate" admissions if it so desired, but this placed no obligation on surgical staff.

Reprinted with permission of the author and publisher from *JAMA* (1992) 268:18: 2561–2562.

Editor's note: Most footnotes have been deleted. Students who want to follow up on sources should consult the original article.

Embarrassed, I called the admitting physician at the county hospital to arrange a transfer. Somewhat gruffly, the County physician said that he would not take the patient in transfer. He said that she would be treated, as any other person would, if she presented to their emergency department with a broken arm after we discharged her. I pointed out that this would mean that we would have to remove (and they would have to replace) the central venous catheter whose placement had complicated the patient's stay, and he replied, "Then, get your surgeons to fix her arm."

I told the woman of my ongoing effort to get the fracture set in our hospital. She listened and opined a pessimistic view of my efforts. An hour later, while I was waiting for another call from the hospital attorney, she secretly left the hospital with the central catheter in place. She presented to the county hospital, where the intravenous access was removed and replaced. New radiographs were taken. The fracture was set.

COMMENT

This woman's treatment is neither unusual nor illegal. The hospital honored its legal and moral duty to treat the life-threatening emergency of the overdose. Its staff refused to treat the medically indigent patient when it was legally permissible to do so. The patient abetted the hospital staff's refusal to treat her by leaving the hospital after she concluded that she would not receive care.

Cases like this one are commonly and appropriately presented as anecdotes to illustrate the need for a reform to guarantee universal access to health care. Its delayed treatment and duplicated diagnostic evaluations make it an easy example of the need to reform a complex and inefficient health care system. It is saddening and, to some, infuriating. This kind of officious interpersonal encounter and disrupted medical care for such a clear and simple medical need is not something most readers would lightly tolerate in their own lives.

There is another perspective on this case that should also be highlighted. This case took place in a teaching hospital where it was part of my training of a second-year resident, two interns, and two medical students. They knew the hospital turned indigent patients away from its clinics and emergency department. They were used to the magnified consequences of untreated disease and absent primary care. Even so, they were jarred by the abrupt interruption of this woman's treatment. Surprise quickly turned to accommodation as she became yesterday's news.

This kind of case in teaching hospitals has four adverse consequences for the next generation of physicians.

First, it disrupts the transmission of a professional tradition that recognized the claim of indigent ill persons on the medical profession. The debate about indigent patient care is not new in the United States. What is new is the increasing amount of medical teaching in hospitals that do not have a primary mission of serving the medically indigent. Teaching hospitals used to be places where new physicians observed, learned, and assumed medicine's final obligation to the medically indigent.

Second, teaching young physicians and their patients that physicians may properly put their own advantaged financial interests ahead of their patients' immediate needs fuels cynicism on both sides of the doctor-patient relationship. There are signs that such a cynical redefinition of medical professionalism is becoming more problematic. In the last decade, medical students have become much less inclined to be primarily motivated to seek a meaningful philosophy of life and correspondingly more motivated to become financially very well off. The self-indulgent sense that many house-staff physicians and medical students have of being entitled to a privileged status and income is reinforced when young physicians see their well-off teachers and role models refuse to care for indigent patients. It also may reinforce the stigmatizing, fatalistic attitudes that many house staff have toward poor patients. It may have political consequences as well. Despite physicians' appeals to trust medical professionalism, laws on dumping and physician-owned referral facilities have been enacted. Two thirds of Americans believe that physicians are too interested in making money, and the public is four times as likely as doctors to support limiting physicians' incomes to address the health care cost-access crisis.

Third, teaching students to turn away from indigent patients undermines the broader, ancient message that a physician is bound by "professing" humane kindness (*humanitas*) and compassion (*misericordia*) to those in need. Teaching students that we may turn away from indigent persons may have broad ramifications for the ethos of medicine, for example, to the duty to treat human immunodeficiency virus (HIV)–infected persons. From its inception in the mid-19th century, the American Medical Association (AMA) asserted the doctor's duty to assume the risk of caring for persons with infectious diseases. During the brief pax-antibiotica after World War II, the AMA stressed the doctor's freedom in patient relationships against the encroaching corporatization of health care. In 1986, the AMA suggested that this contractual freedom implied that doctors were not obliged to treat HIV-infected persons. In 1987, the AMA drew on its older, more profound view of the subordination of doctors' privileges to infected persons' needs. Today, a third of doctors, and most orthopedic surgeons, see no duty to care for HIV-infected persons. Fortunately, the ingrained habits of practice with regard to HIV-infected persons are better than the asserted freedom would imply. "Medical altruism" magnifies the efficacy of education about the duty to treat HIV-infected persons. A holistic ethic of medical obligation is endangered when students see their teachers turn away from a poor woman with a broken arm.

Fourth, it diminishes physicians' credibility in the debate about the essential purpose of health care. Schroeder et al[1] have noted that the impressive medical advances have more successfully met the needs of wealthy patients than they have improved the health of our society. Some propose that physicians honor patients' demands for ever more costly, and marginally effective, even futile, treatments out of respect for patient autonomy. When a tertiary care teaching hospital turns away an indigent woman with a broken arm as it honors paying patients' demands for marginally effective care, it

1. Schroeder, SA, Zones, JS, Showstack, JA. Academic medicine as a public trust. *JAMA* 1989;262:803–812.

suggests that "respect for autonomy" refers to the paying customer's privilege rather than to a solemn medical obligation to essential health needs.

ADDRESSING THE NEED

Many physicians recognize that financial constraints on patient care are more than simply a feature of the practice environment but also pose fundamental ethical questions and choices to the profession. Such ethical issues arise as clinicians care for persons with inadequate personal financial resources for needed services, evaluate and transfer indigent patients to other providers, respond to family proxy decision makers who appear to be motivated by what they could gain or lose if treatment is withheld or given, become sensitive to how their own social worth biases influence clinical decisions on behalf of indigent patients, or answer demands for wasteful or inefficient use of medical care. Such issues underlie 10% to 15% of all of the ethical problems that physicians identify in inpatient and outpatient settings. These situations ask physicians to define by practice the profession's view of its virtues and duties with regard to beneficence and justice. In recognizing the ethical issues and in defining the corresponding duties and virtues summoned, many physicians choose to provide thousands of dollars of free and discounted services.

Society and the medical profession are moving toward health care reform even as teaching hospitals mirror our present failure to ensure reliable universal access to basic health care. It would be ironic if this generation of American physicians-in-training were the first to practice in a universal-access health care system after being shown and taught how to turn away from sick people without money. In the United States, physician voluntarism is still the final recourse for medically indigent persons. The voluntary care of indigent persons is not a substitute for health care reform. It is a mitzvah, or good deed, by which doctors are privileged to heal a wound and acknowledge the task and person the profession is accountable to. We cannot afford to cut this class from the education of new physicians.

RECOMMENDED SUPPLEMENTARY READING

GENERAL WORKS

Ahronheim, Judith C.; Moreno, Jonathan D.; and Zuckerman, Connie. *Ethics in Clinical Practice.* 2nd ed. Gaithersburg, MD: Aspen Publishers, Inc., 2000.

Annas, George J. *Standard of Care: The Law of American Bioethics.* Oxford: Oxford University Press, 1993.

Beauchamp, Tom L., and Childress, James F. *Principles of Biomedical Ethics.* 5th ed. New York: Oxford University Press, 2001.

Benjamin, Martin, and Curtis, Joy. *Ethics in Nursing.* New York: Oxford University Press, 1992.

Burt, Robert. *Taking Care of Strangers.* New York: Free Press, 1979.

Campbell, Alastair; Charlesworth, Max; Gillett, Grant; and Jones, Gareth. *Medical Ethics.* New York: Oxford University Press, 1997.

Caplan, Arthur. *If I Were a Rich Man Could I Buy a Pancreas?* Bloomington: Indiana University Press, 1992.

Cassell, Eric. *The Nature of Suffering and the Goals of Medicine.* New York: Oxford University Press, 1991.

Childress, James F. *Practical Reasoning in Bioethics.* Bloomington: Indiana University Press, 1997.

Crigger, Bette-Jane, ed. *Cases in Bioethics.* 3rd ed. New York: St. Martin's Press, 1998.

Downie, R. S., and Calman, Kenneth C. *Healthy Respect: Ethics in Health Care.* New York: Oxford University Press, 1994.

Dubler, Nancy, and Nimmons, David. *Ethics on Call.* New York: Crown, 1992.

Dworkin, Roger B. *Limits: The Role of the Law in Bioethical Decision Making.* Bloomington: Indiana University Press, 1996.

Englehardt, H. Tristram, Jr. *The Foundations of Bioethics.* 2nd ed. New York: Oxford University Press, 1996.

Fried, C. *Medical Experimentation: Personal Integrity and Social Policy.* New York: Elsevier, 1974.

Gert, Bernard; Culver, Charles M.; and Clouser, K. Danner. *Bioethics: A Return To Fundamentals.* New York: Oxford University Press, 1997.

Herbert, Philip. *Doing Right: A Practical Guide for Physicians and Medical Trainees.* New York: Oxford University Press, 1996.

Holms, Helen, and Purdy, Laura, eds. *Feminist Perspectives in Medical Ethics.* Bloomington: Indiana University Press, 1992.

Jonsen, Albert. *The New Medicine and the Old Ethics.* Cambridge, MA: Harvard University Press, 1990.

Kass, Leon. *Toward a More Natural Science.* New York: Free Press, 1985.

Kuhse, Helga, and Singer, Peter. *A Companion to Bioethics.* Oxford: Blackwell Publishers, 1998.

Macklin, Ruth. *Mortal Choices: Bioethics in Today's World.* New York: Pantheon Books, 1987.

May, Thomas. *Bioethics in a Liberal Society: The Political Framework of Bioethics Decision Making.* Baltimore: Johns Hopkins University Press, 2002.

May, William F. *The Patient's Ordeal.* Bloomington: Indiana University Press, 1991.

McGee, Glenn, ed. *Pragmatic Bioethics.* Nashville, TN: Vanderbilt University Press, 1999.

Moreno, Jonathan D. *Deciding Together.* New York: Oxford University Press, 1995.

Polansky, Ronald, and Kuczewski, Mark, eds. *Bioethics: Ancient Themes in Contemporary Issues.* Cambridge, MA: MIT Press, 2000.

Rothman, David J. *Strangers at the Bedside: A History of How Law and Bioethics Transformed Medical Decision Making.* New York: Basic Books, 1991.

Tong, Rosemarie. *Feminist Approaches to Bioethics.* Boulder, CO: Westview Press, 1997.

Veatch, Robert M. *A Theory of Medical Ethics.* New York: Basic Books, 1981.

AUTONOMY, PATERNALISM, AND MEDICAL MODELS

Agich, George J. *Autonomy and Long-Term Care.* Oxford: Oxford University Press, 1993.

Blustein, Jeffrey. "Doing What the Patient Orders: Maintaining Integrity in the Doctor-Patient Relationship." *Bioethics* 7, no. 4 (1993): 289–314.

Bok, Sissela. *Lying.* New York: Pantheon Books, 1978.

———. *Secrets: On the Ethics of Concealment and Revelation.* New York: Pantheon Books, 1982.

———. *Common Values.* University of Missouri Press, 1995.

Brennan, Troy A. *Just Doctoring: Medical Ethics in the Liberal State.* Berkeley: University of California Press, 1991.

Brody, Howard. *The Healer's Power.* New Haven, CT: Yale University Press, 1992.

Churchill, Larry R. "Reviving a Distinctive Medical Ethic." *Hastings Center Report* (May–June 1989): 28–34.

Collopy, Bart J.; Dubler, Nancy; and Zuckerman, Connie. "The Ethics of Home Care: Autonomy and Accommodation." *Hastings Center Report* (special supplement; March–April 1990): 1–16.

Dworkin, Gerald. *The Theory and Practice of Autonomy.* Cambridge, UK: Cambridge University Press, 1988.

Halper, Thomas. "Privacy and Autonomy: From Warren and Brandeis to Roe and Cruzan." *Journal of Medicine and Philosophy* 21, no. 2 (April 1996): 121–135.

"Healthcare Relationships: Ties That Bind." *Cambridge Quarterly of Healthcare Ethics* 3, no. I (Winter 1994): 1–82.

Kant, Immanuel. "On the Supposed Right to Lie from Altruistic Motives." In *Critique of Practical Reason,* trans. L. W. Beck. Chicago: University of Chicago Press, 1949.

Kleinig, John. *Paternalism.* Totowa, NJ: Rowman and Allanheld, 1984.

Kultgen, John. *Autonomy and Intervention: Paternalism in the Caring Life.* New York: Oxford University Press, 1995.

Levi, Benjamin H. *Respecting Patient Autonomy.* Urbana: University of Illinois Press, 1999.

Lidz, Charles; Fischer, Lynn; and Arnold, Robert M. *The Erosion of Autonomy in Long-Term Care.* Oxford: Oxford University Press, 1992.

May, William F. "Code, Covenant, Contract, or Philanthropy." *Hastings Center Report* 5 (December 1975): 29–38.

Pellegrino, Edmund D., and Thomasma, David C. *For the Patient's Good: The Restoration of Beneficence in Health Care.* New York: Oxford University Press, 1988.

Schneider, Carl E. *The Practice of Autonomy: Patients, Doctors, and Medical Decisions.* New York: Oxford University Press, 1998.

Shelp, Earl E., ed. *Virtue and Medicine.* Dordrecht, Holland: D. Reidel Publishing Co., 1985.

Strasser, Mark. "The New Paternalism." *Bioethics* 7, no. 2 (1988): 103–117.

VanDeVeer, Donald. *Paternalistic Intervention: The Moral Bounds of Benevolence.* Princeton, NJ: Princeton University Press, 1986.

Veatch, Robert M. "Models for Medicine in a Revolutionary Age." *Hastings Center Report* 2 (June 1972): 5–7.

INFORMED CONSENT

Appelbaum, Paul S.; Lidz, Charles W.; and Meisel, Alan. *Informed Consent: Legal Theory and Clinical Practice.* New York: Oxford University Press, 1987.

Berg, Jessica; Appelbaum, Paul; Lidz, Charles; and Parker, Lisa. *Informed Consent: Legal Theory and Clinical Practice.* 2nd ed. New York: Oxford University Press, 2001.

Brock, Dan. *Life and Death: Philosophical Essays in Biomedical Ethics.* New York: Cambridge University Press, 1993.

Cassell, Eric J. *Talking with Patients. Vol. 1. The Theory of Doctor-Patient Communication. Vol. 2, Clinical Technique.* Cambridge, MA: MIT Press, 1985.

Faden, Ruth, and Beauchamp, Tom. *A History and Theory of Informed Consent.* New York: Oxford University Press, 1986.

Geller, Gail, et al. "'Decoding' Informed Consent." *Hastings Center Report* (March–April 1997): 28–33.

"In Case of Emergency: No Need for Consent." *Hastings Center Report* (Symposium; January–February, 1997): 7–12.

Katz, Jay. *The Silent World of Doctor and Patient.* New York: Free Press, 1984.

Kuczewski, Mark G. "Reconceiving the Family: The Process of Consent in Medical Decisionmaking." *Hastings Center Report* (March–April, 1996): 30–37.

Marta, Jan. "A Linguistic Model of Informed Consent." *Journal of Medicine and Philosophy* 21, no. 1 (February 1996): 41–60.

President's Commission for the Study of Ethical Problems. *Medicine and Biomedical and Behavioral Research. Making Health Care Decisions: The Ethical and Legal Implications of Informed Consent in the Patient-Practitioner Relationship.* Washington, DC: U.S. Government Printing Office, 1982.

Schuck, Peter H. "Rethinking Informed Consent." *Yale Law Journal* 103 (1994): 899ff.

Veatch, Robert M. "Abandoning Informed Consent." *Hastings Center Report* (March–April 1995): 5–12.

CONFLICTING PROFESSIONAL ROLES AND RESPONSIBILITIES

Agich, George J., ed. *Responsibility in Health Care.* Dordrecht, Holland: D. Reidel Publishing Co., 1982.

Angell, Marcia. "The Doctor as Double Agent." *Kennedy Institute of Ethics Journal* 3, no. 3 (September 1993): 279.

"Conflicts of Interest in Health Care." *American Journal of Law and Medicine* 21, nos. 2 and 3 (1995).

Danis, Marion, and Churchill, Larry. "Autonomy and the Common Weal." *Hastings Center Report* (January–February 1991): 25–31.

"The Ethics of Medical Mistakes: Historical, Legal, and Institutional Perspectives." *Kennedy Institute of Ethics Journal* 11, no. 2 (June 2001).

Fost, Norman. "Ethical Issues in Whistleblowing." *JAMA* 286, no. 5 (Sept. 5, 2001): 1079.

Gray, Bradford H. *The Profit Motive and Patient Care: The Changing Accountability of Doctors and Hospitals.* Cambridge, MA: Harvard University Press, 1991.

———, ed. *For-Profit Enterprise in Health Care.* Washington, DC: National Academy Press, 1986.

"Health Care Capitated Payment Systems." *American Journal of Law and Medicine* 22, nos. 2 and 3 (1996).

Hoy, E. W. "Change and Growth in Managed Care." *Health Affairs,* 10 (Winter 1991): 19.

Kohn, L. T.; Corrigan, J. M.; Donaldson, M. S.; eds. *To Err Is Human: Building a Safer Health System.* Washington, DC: National Academy Press, 2000.

Latham, Stephen R. "Regulation of Managed Care Incentive Payments to Physicians." *American Journal of Law and Medicine* 22, no. 4 (1996): 399–432.

Macklin, Ruth. *The Enemies of Patients.* New York: Oxford University Press, 1993, chapter 7.

Martin, Julia A., and Bjerknes, Lisa K. "The Legal and Ethical Implications of Gag Clauses in Physician Contracts." *American Journal of Law and Medicine* 22, no. 4 (1996): 433–476.

Menzel, Paul T. "Double Agency and the Ethics of Rationing Health Care: A Response to Marcia Angell." *Kennedy Institute of Ethics Journal* 3, no. 3 (1993): 293–302.

Orentlicher, David. "Health Care Reform and the Patient-Physician Relationship." *Health Matrix: Journal of Law-Medicine* 5, no. 1 (1995): 141–180.

Rajendram, Pam R. "Ethical Issues Involved in Disclosing Medical Errors." *JAMA* 286, no. 5 (Sept. 5, 2001): 1078.

Rodwin, Marc A. *Medicine, Money and Morals: Physicians' Conflicts of Interest*. New York: Oxford University Press, 1993.

Rubin, Susan B., and Zoloth, Laurie, eds. *Margin of Error: The Necessity, Inevitability and Ethics of Mistakes in Medicine and Bioethics.* Hagerstown, MD: University Publishing Group, 2000.

Spece, Roy G., Jr.; Shimm, David S.; and Buchanan, Allen E.; eds. *Conflicts of Interest in Clinical Practice and Research.* New York: Oxford University Press, 1996.

Wolf, Susan M. "Health Care Reform and the Future of Physician Ethics." *Hastings Center Report* 24, no. 2 (March–April 1994): 28–41.

Wusthoff, Courtney J. "Medical Mistakes and Disclosure: The Role of the Medical Student," *JAMA* 286, no. 5 (Sept. 5, 2001): 1080–1081.

PART TWO

ALLOCATION, SOCIAL JUSTICE, AND HEALTH POLICY

Even if we believe that all men and women are "created equal," it's hard to deny that we are not equal with regard to health. Some of us, the winners in the "natural lottery," are blessed with good health and live to ripe old age without the meddling of physicians and nurses. Others are born with catastrophic diseases requiring massive amounts of high-technology medicine merely to survive painfully from day to day.

It is also hard to deny that we are not equal with regard to availability of health care. Some are fortunate enough to work for employers who can offer a generous health benefits package or are wealthy enough to either purchase outright all the health care they want or buy enough insurance to cover their needs. Others, the unemployed as well as those who work part-time or for small businesses that cannot afford to offer health benefits, go without health insurance, and many of the poorest members of our population cannot afford adequate nutrition, housing, and clothing, let alone insurance for health care. These losers in the "social lottery"—the working poor, the child in the welfare hotel, the impoverished AIDS patient, the unemployed farmer—often have desperate needs for care that go unmet.

Although attempts have been made to provide a social safety net for the poor, for those poor enough to meet the definition of poverty stipulated by their state-run Medicaid programs, access to health care is often an entitlement in name only. Since most states reimburse only a small fraction of physicians' usual rates, very few of them are willing to treat Medicaid patients. With the notable exception of some extraordinarily devoted physicians, those who do accept such patients are often poorly qualified and offer substandard care in large, impersonal practices featuring "turnstile" medical attention. Hospitals that deal with a predominantly Medicaid population are notoriously understaffed and undersupplied. Patients are regularly subjected to long waiting periods for necessary treatments during which their conditions may badly deteriorate. And these treatments are often delivered through dangerously antiquated technology. At one Brooklyn hospital, a cancer unit's decrepit radiation unit was nicknamed "the killer" due to its tendency to destroy roughly equal portions of both cancerous and healthy tissue. Yet across the street at the university-affiliated hospital, the insured "paying customers" benefited from state-of-the-art technology and care.

Those who are not poor enough to qualify for Medicaid, yet are too poor to afford private health insurance, pose perhaps the greatest challenge both to our nation's emerging health policy and to our collective moral conscience. Numbering roughly forty million people, these uninsured individuals must either go without treatment entirely or obtain care from chaotic emergency rooms. Journalist Laurie Kaye Abraham provides us with a compelling and poignant account of the uninsured,

> Often in advanced stages of treatable disease, with undiagnosed diabetes attacking their kidneys, or even breast tumors large enough to break through their skin. Their conditions certainly are emergencies now but emergencies that . . . did not necessarily have to be. They got so sick waiting, waiting, waiting, because they had no health insurance and did not think they could afford a doctor until they *really* needed one. And even when things went bad enough that they *really* needed one, they still feared they could not afford it—who knows how expensive a doctor's visit will be?—so they stumbled into the emergency room instead. There, the clerks ask if you have insurance but will not draw in their breath when you say you do not, will not ask you to wait while they confer with someone else, will not, cannot, turn you away. (Abraham 1993, 96)

The first section of Part 2 asks how we should think about these inequalities in both the natural and social lotteries. Are they merely instances of misfortune that should elicit pity and perhaps charity, or should we rather view them as injustices calling for rectification? And supposing that health care is a right rather than a privilege, to what kind of health care are we entitled?

Whereas Section 1 applies broad questions of political philosophy to health care, Section 2 examines some of the hard choices forced upon society by the confluence of ever expanding demands for health care, high-cost technology, and the rise of managed care and other cost-constraining strategies. It also examines some of the strategies that have been proposed for making these choices in a way that is fair and fiscally responsible.

Finally, Section 3 takes up two specific instances of broader questions concerning the proper ends of medicine and the important judgments of value that shape our notions of which medical needs ought to receive priority over others. For instance, should decisions about health care allocation take into account the extent to which recipients may have incurred their illness or disease through their own choice of lifestyle? Should judgments of moral character play a role in the allocation of medical resources? What about other important judgments of value that are sometimes invoked to limit access to health services, such as those that structure our traditional concepts of "disease" and "normality"? Together the readings of this section bring the reader back to some of the questions laid out in Section 1 concerning the implications for different conceptions of moral equality on the way we think about the distribution of health and health care in society.

JUSTICE AND HEALTH CARE

A crucial and distressing result of the combined natural and social lotteries is the roughly forty million Americans who remain uninsured and the millions more who remain underinsured. This failure to obtain needed insurance translates into a predictable lack of access to health care. The primary question addressed in Section 1 is whether this lack of access is unjust or merely unfortunate—a failure of charity or a violation of rights. The President's Commission for the Study of Ethical Problems in Medicine and Biomedical and Behavioral Research confronts this question head on in its report, *An Ethical Framework for Access to Health Care*. According to the commission, health care is different from other consumer goods in that it is crucially related to our level of well-being, helping us to ward off pain, suffering, and premature death. Like education, health care is necessary to achieve equal opportunity in society. And health care is freighted with "interpersonal significance." As the philosopher Michael Walzer puts it, failure to obtain needed health care in our society is not merely dangerous; it is also degrading, signaling a lack of full citizenship (Walzer 1983). Given the utter unpredictability of many health care needs and the often huge amounts of money necessary to meet them, the President's Commission concluded that the free market alone cannot be counted on to meet these crucial needs and that society therefore has an obligation to help meet them. The commission insisted, however, that this social obligation is not unlimited; it must be discharged with an eye to the costs and burdens to society in meeting it. Moreover, the fact that society is morally obligated to provide some care does not mean that everyone is entitled to an equal amount of health care or to health care of equal quality. In other words, not all *inequalities* in access to health care constitute *inequities*. As long as everyone is guaranteed access to an acceptable level or, as others have put it, to a "decent level" of health care, society will have lived up to its moral obligation.

Although the President's Commission's approach lacks the rigor of philosophical analysis, it assembles a broad array of cogent arguments in favor of a right to health care. Interestingly, however, the commission self-consciously retreated from the vocabulary of rights in attempting to frame its notion of a social duty, a move that has prompted a good deal of criticism from philosophers (Arras 1984, Bayer 1984). If society has a strong duty to ensure that every citizen has access to at least a decent level of health care, why not conclude that each citizen has a moral right, as opposed to a legal right, against the government to that level of care?

A more focused and philosophical approach to the question can be found in Norman Daniels's work on the connection between "Equal Opportunity and Health Care." Like the President's Commission, Daniels first attempts to explain what is special about health care needs. As opposed to mere preferences we may have for fine wines or top-of-the-line stereo speakers, our health needs are special in that they relate to our ability to function as normal members of our biological species. If our ability to function normally is impaired—for example, because of a broken arm or cancer cells colonizing our bodies—Daniels observes that we will then be unable to enjoy our fair share of what he calls the "normal opportunity range" for our society. In other words, illness prevents us from enjoying the range of opportunities—to be, for instance, an athlete, a businessperson, or a lawyer—to which our natural endowment of talents and skills would have otherwise entitled us. Daniels contends that this lack of equal opportunity will not be viewed as "merely unfortunate" in any society that is committed to providing equal opportunity to its members. Just as we say that children deprived of a decent education are robbed of their right to equal opportunity, so Daniels concludes that people deprived of adequate health care in our society are treated unjustly.

Although Daniels is firmly committed to viewing access to health care as a matter of justice, he too denies that a right to health care would entitle everyone to all the health care that they might want or need. First, our right to health care only covers deviations from normal species functioning, not idiosyncratic desires for nose jobs or "tushy tucks." Second, although health care needs are special compared to goods normally distributed on the free market, they are not so important that society must give them priority over all other needs or go broke trying. Other important interests besides health care—such as needs for good schooling, housing, nutrition, and jobs—must also figure in any robust conception of equal opportunity; so the task for public policy is to weigh and balance all these higher-level interests in fashioning a just *system* that protects equal opportunity. On this view, access to health care is seen as vitally important, but not as so uniquely important that making it available to all threatens to break the societal bank.

In "Class, Health, and Justice," Sarah Marchand, Daniel Wikler, and Bruce Landesman question the way traditional debates about justice and the importance of health focus almost exclusively on whether there is a right to *health care*. As they point out, there is a growing body of evidence that socioeconomic inequalities generate inequalities in health even in wealthy nations with systems of universal access to health care. If inequalities in health persist between socioeconomic classes even in nations with high per capita income rates in which there is universal access to health care, this appears to undermine the idea that health is primarily a factor of individual biology and one's access to health care. Instead, it raises the possibility that social inequalities themselves may influence the health of persons, and if health is indeed special—either because of its close connection to individual welfare, because of the role it plays in determining an individual's opportunity range, or because of some other set of reasons—a focus on the social distribution of *health* may have broader implications for egalitarians than the traditional debate countenances.

The main goal of Marchand, Wikler, and Landesman is to explore these implications in the hope of clarifying two key questions. First, what is the source of the intuitive judgment that it is unfair that members of higher socioeconomic classes tend to live longer, less disease-burdened lives than members of lower classes? Second, what is the appropriate social response to these inequalities, given that they persist in the face of equal access to health care? The answers we give to these questions, they argue, will differ depending on the conception of equality we adopt, and they explore four such conceptions in detail: equity as maximizing the total sum of health for society, equity as equalizing the levels of health between classes, equity as maximizing the health of the lowest socioeconomic class, and equity as priority to the sickest, regardless of class.

Although this is primarily an exploratory paper, simply recognizing the impact of what are sometimes called the "social determinants of health" on the health status of individuals forces liberal egalitarians to rethink some of their most fundamental assumptions about justice and health. Human society is a complex and dynamic system of individual and group interactions mediated by a wide array of social and political institutions. Over time, natural variations in the abilities, goals, and values of these individuals and groups can lead to disparities in wealth and social status. Liberals like Rawls and Daniels can allow a wide range of social and economic inequalities to emerge within society as long as these are not inequalities in basic liberties and as long as the existence of these inequalities works for the betterment of the worst off. If, as Daniels claims, health has special ethical significance because of its impact on individual opportunities, and if, as the public health literature appears to show, those in lower classes lead shorter and more painful lives than those in higher classes, then liberal egalitarians may have to rethink the level of relative socioeconomic inequality that can exist within a just political system.

A very different view of the importance of health and health care is articulated by the philosopher H. Tristram Engelhardt, Jr., who rejects the fundamental assumptions behind such liberal egalitarian theories of health care justice in "Freedom and Moral Diversity." Engelhardt is a self-described postmodernist and libertarian. His postmodernism derives from his conviction that in the modern world there is no one right or canonical answer to the question of what constitutes justice and equality. People from different cultures, religious, or philosophical traditions define these key notions in radically different ways. This is a crucial problem for allocating health care in a pluralistic society, because any scheme for allocating such care must of necessity implicate one or another such vision of justice and the good life. Engelhardt's libertarianism stems from his conviction that free and equal individuals should not be coerced into accepting, much less paying for, the views of others bearing on such basic but ultimately unresolvable questions as the morality of abortion, physician-assisted suicide, the desirability of organ transplants, and the true nature of equality and social justice. In the face of such important and unresolvable questions, libertarians like Engelhardt insist that individuals must remain free from societal or governmental interference to make their own choices about such matters. Thus, although it might be perfectly appropriate, even praiseworthy, for many individuals to band together and pool their extra resources to make health care more available to the poor and unfortunate, libertarians insist that no one should be forced to give away his or her resources for the benefit of others. Access to health care thus remains either a matter of buying and selling on the free market or a matter of charity; failure to access adequate amounts of health care will thus be viewed by libertarians as perhaps unfortunate, but not unjust.

It follows that for Engelhardt the notion of a right to health care is both unfounded and positively dangerous. Unfounded because it must rely on some debatable and not universally endorsed understanding of justice; and dangerous because it would necessarily impinge on the rights and lifestyles of those who embrace other visions of the good life. Although Engelhardt concedes that society might possess a moral warrant to tax its citizens for various purposes, including the provision of some level of health care for its needy citizens, he steadfastly resists the notion that this societal choice is demanded by anyone's corresponding entitlement.

In addition to engaging liberal egalitarian claims, such as those of Daniels and the President's Commission, on the level of political philosophy, Engelhardt offers some practical suggestions for making health care more widely available without foundering on the prohibitions of his postmodern libertarianism. One way to provide greater access to the poor without implicating controversial views of justice and the good life, he contends, would be to establish a voucher system. Given a fund of public monies earmarked for humanitarian purposes, society could distribute health care vouchers to needy individuals who could redeem them at the health system of their choice. Thus, instead of imposing, say, a single view of abortion and euthanasia on all of society, we could leave it up to individuals to cash in their vouchers at avowedly prochoice or prolife health plans as they saw fit. This way, Engelhardt suggests, the poor could obtain expanded access without any accompanying "welfare rights," and without the state imposing a single, "official" morality on everyone.

Engelhardt's approval of taxation for purposes other than maintaining a so-called nightwatchman state consisting solely of police, army, courts, and so forth, appears to deviate from orthodox libertarian doctrine, which views all such taxation as forms of theft and forced labor. Likewise, his claim that individual autonomy must be universally respected in a world of moral diversity would seem to contradict the thoroughgoing relativism of more robust versions of postmodernism. Still, his critique of welfare rights raises important questions bearing on the legitimacy of state health policies and the wisdom of many practical interventions that the partisans of more egalitarian theories cannot ignore.

Whatever the outcome of the argument between liberal egalitarians like Daniels and libertarians like Engelhardt, it remains true that the notion of a right to health, or to some level of health care has only a limited usefulness. Supposing we were to endorse such a right, what would it mean? And how would it help us answer the tough questions facing health policy experts, legislators, and society at large today (Brody 1991)?

At most, as Daniels acknowledges, a right to health care would mean that every citizen had an entitlement to an unspecified amount of health care (a decent minimum) within an overall entitlement to equal opportunity. Since health care needs must ultimately be balanced against other compelling opportunity-related needs, such as nutrition, schooling, and housing, it is impossible to say in the abstract exactly to what kind and amount of health care each person is entitled. Do individuals have a right, for example, to expensive experimental treatments, psychotherapy, organ transplants, AIDS therapies, and so on? The mere stipulation of a right to health care does not appear to be very helpful in coming to grips with these and other crucial questions of health care policy. In each case, we have to ask, How great is the need, how many people will be affected, how likely the harm, how expensive the treatment or diagnostic test, and what are the alternative uses to which our scarce public funds could be put? (see discussion of Section 2 below).

In spite of its manifest limitations in resolving some of the most important and pervasive policy debates in health care, the notion of a right to health or to health care is, we would submit, still very much worth debating. Even though it cannot tell us what level of entitlement is adequate—whether, for example, all AIDS patients are entitled to expensive protease inhibitor therapy—it can tell us whether the inability of forty million people to access decent health insurance is an injustice or merely a large-scale case of bad luck. It might affect the ultimate ability of those millions of people to secure needed health care if we believed society had an obligation, based upon justice, to provide an adequate level of health care for all.

METHODS AND STRATEGIES FOR RATIONING HEALTH CARE

Section 2 takes up some of the vexing allocation problems confronting health policy experts, legislators, and consumers today. The common focus of these policy case studies is the need to make difficult choices in a context of fiscal scarcity (Morreim 1995). If we had unlimited amounts of money, there would be no need to ration health care; but as we all know, money and resources are scarce and health care is expensive, and so we cannot afford to satisfy everyone's preferences and needs for health care. Even if we can reach consensus that there is a right to health care, we must still learn to assign priorities—a tricky business: Who should be saved when all cannot be saved? Which groups of people, and which treatments and diagnostic techniques, should be given highest priority? The articles in this section are intended to give the reader a lively sense of the emerging issues in this area. They are, however, only a small sample of the many complex and difficult questions facing our nation as we struggle to contain health care costs while expanding access to the millions of people whose health needs currently go unmet.

Americans do not like to hear about "rationing" health care. The term conjures up images of tightwad insurance companies or government bureaucrats deciding that some lives are worth less than others. One of the charges that in 1994 helped scuttle the ill-fated Clinton plan for health care reform was the claim that it would necessitate rationing. Well aware of the unpopularity of this notion, the Clinton administration actually forbade its 500 consultants to use the word "rationing" in any correspondence or official documents.

The fact remains, however, that we have always rationed health care in one way or another. By far the most widespread method has also been the most morally suspect: rationing care by ability to pay. But we have also rationed organ transplants, intensive care–unit beds, and other life-sustaining medical treatments. There are, however, important differences between these traditional forms of rationing and what is happening today under managed care. When the poor and uninsured failed to receive needed care, it was usually not the result of an official policy; their inability to access care was the result of structural features of the existing health care system and, therefore, was often treated as though it was a fact of nature. And when patients died of liver or heart failure on a waiting list for an organ transplant, it was usually due to a natural shortage of organs, not to a decision on anyone's part that these lives were simply too expensive to save. So we developed a complicated attitude with regard to rationing: On the one hand, we grew accustomed to the tacit and limited rationing we permitted while fiercely resisting the explicit, publicly imposed rationing, respectively, by doctors on paying customers and by bureaucrats on the poor.

Managed care has changed all this. Operating essentially within closed systems of shared financial resources, managed care organizations (MCOs) must ration health care on a daily basis. Money spent on expensive but marginally effective treatments cannot be used for other purposes within an MCO, so difficult choices must be made. Under this new dispensation, rationing is explicit; it is implemented by physicians at the bedside; it targets insured populations by restricting potentially beneficial services; and it is justified by fiscal scarcity, rather than by natural shortages (Morreim 1995, Eddy 1996). The notion that rationing would be entirely unnecessary if we could only cut the fat by reorganizing our wasteful health care system has been disproven by history and the fact of scarcity. The question now is not, Shall we ration care? but rather, *How* shall we ration, by what principles and processes, and how may we do so without seriously compromising justice and patients' rights?

Setting health care priorities, however, has proven to be a difficult matter. Consider the case of women afflicted with advanced breast cancer for whom standard chemotherapies have failed to effect a remission of the disease. Having exhausted proven medical alternatives, these women frequently seek out investigational or experimental alternatives in the hope of staving off imminent death. Throughout the decade of the nineties, an extremely expensive experimental procedure known as high-dose chemotherapy followed by autologous bone-marrow transplantation (or HDC-ABMT) was thought to hold out tremendous promise as a possible means of helping these desperate women. As philosopher Alex John London explains in "Bone Marrow Transplants for Advanced Breast Cancer: The Story of Christine deMeurers," decisions about providing promising but expensive treatments frequently have to be made when there are no definitive answers about the treatment's efficacy. Costing well over $100,000 per patient, HDC-ABMT was offered at many hospitals and cancer centers to women who saw this highly invasive and onerous treatment as their last best hope of staving off death. Most of these women were relatively young, in their 20s and 30s, and many had families who depended on them. Waiting for the results of rigorous clinical trials to accumulate would have meant foregoing an expensive but promising option. To the managed care companies who were being asked to pay for these costly last-ditch efforts, however, it would not have been a responsible use of scarce resources to spend such large amounts of money without sufficient evidence that HDC-ABMT might succeed where standard therapies had failed.

There is mounting evidence from more recent clinical trials that, in fact, HDC-ABMT is not superior to standard chemotherapy.[1] This information was not available a decade ago, however, and while

1. E. A. Stadtmauer, A. O'Neill, L. J. and Goldstein, P. A., et al., "Conventional-dose chemotherapy compared with high-dose chemotherapy plus autologous hematopoietic stem-cell transplantation for metastatic breast cancer." Philadelphia Bone Marrow Transplant Group. *N Engl J Med* 342, no. 15 (April 13, 2000): 1069–1076.

the results of these trials may dissolve the dilemma about providing access to this particular intervention, there is no shortage of new investigational treatments appearing on the horizon. As a result, we are left with the same general ethical questions, even though they now apply to different investigation treatments. Should insurance providers be forced to pay for promising interventions whose therapeutic merits have yet to be fully measured or vindicated? Is it unconscionably hard-hearted to deny persons a last chance at remission or cure—no matter how remote—merely in order to save money?

Following the narrative of Christine deMeurers, a woman who fought valiant battles against both her MCO and her encroaching terminal breast cancer, Alex John London attempts to put this health policy debate into proper perspective. Rejecting an all-or-nothing perspective on such so-called last-chance therapies, London attempts to focus our attention on the crucial questions we must ask and the procedures we must establish to come to a just and stable resolution of this difficult issue.

The case of experimental bone marrow transplants for women with advanced breast cancer is taken up again by the health policy analyst David M. Eddy, who argues for a form of "cost-effectiveness analysis" in his essay, "The Individual vs. Society: Resolving the Conflict." Following a brief explanation of how our health system has traditionally ignored the true costs of health care, Eddy distinguishes two perspectives on the problem. From one angle, which Eddy calls the "perspective of society," the imperative is to allocate our resources as efficiently as possible among everyone with a claim to them, thereby getting "the most bang for the buck." But from another angle, the perspective of patient-members like Christine deMeurers who know they are sick and have already paid their health insurance premiums, the imperative is to obtain the desired medical care, no matter what the cost.

Eddy makes two important and controversial claims. First, he asserts that the proper perspective from the vantage point of health policy is that of society. When deciding what treatments to fund, MCOs should, Eddy contends, attempt to quantify the respective benefits of various treatments, divide them by their costs, and then opt for those interventions that provide the greatest good for the greatest number of people. Second, Eddy claims that this perspective, with its emphasis on prevention, will often redound to the benefit of everyone. Instead of paying huge amounts of money, for example, to save a few lives with HDC-ABMT, it will work to everyone's advantage to invest instead in breast cancer screening programs that will save more lives at far less cost. Prior to getting sick, all of us would agree to the prevention strategy because with it we have a better chance of not getting advanced cancer in the first place. Thus, although Eddy embraces a utilitarian mode of rationing, he claims that it is consonant with the idea that rationing can best be justified by the choices of patients themselves.

Another way of stating the utilitarian case for cost-effectiveness analysis is to use the language of "quality-adjusted life years," or QALYs. According to the proponents of QALYs, the goal of health policy should be to increase both the length and quality of people's lives. It isn't enough that people should merely live longer; their lives should also be as high in quality as possible. Like good utilitarian consequentialists, these theorists also hold that a particular health improvement should have the same value no matter who receives it, so it should be provided unless its cost prevents a greater improvement from being offered to someone else. In short, like David Eddy, these theorists contend that we should allocate scarce health care resources so as to do the most good for the most people.

As what might be called a health-related utilitarian decision tool, cost-effectiveness analysis is open to many of the traditional criticisms that have been leveled against utilitarian theories more generally (see Introduction). In particular, when cost-effectiveness analysis employs QALYs to make decisions about interpersonal trade-offs it frequently yields outcomes that critics view as unjustly discriminating against the elderly, the disabled, and possibly women and minority groups. At base, the central charge is that, like other versions of the utilitarian calculus, it purchases higher numbers of QALYs in the aggregate of a population by sacrificing equal concern and respect for the dignity and integrity of that population's most vulnerable individuals.

In "Toward a Broader View of Values in Cost-Effectiveness Analysis of Health" Paul Menzel, Marthe R. Gold, Eric Nord, Jose-Louis Pinto-Prades, Jeff Richardson, and Peter Ubel respond to the most trenchant criticisms of cost-effectiveness analysis by reforming the method to incorporate a range of important social values to which more traditional versions were notably unresponsive. For these cautious proponents of cost-effectiveness analysis, flaws in the traditional use of this decision tool can be overcome by a more robust conception of the social values that figure into the calculation of an intervention's "effectiveness." Among their many suggestions, they propose giving special weight to the severity of a person's illness and to lifesaving treatments that stave off death and incorporate what is known as the "rule of rescue" and relativizing QALY scores to the health potential an individual may achieve in light of his or her initial baseline. With these and other suggestions they hope to produce a more sensitive decision tool that can aid policy makers in allocating scarce medical resources without violating some of our deepest intuitions about justice and fairness.

One virtue of these many proposals is that they give an explicit and quantifiable role to considerations of moral equality and a wide array of other important social values. This explicit quantification of social values may also prove something of an obstacle, however, if it requires a social consensus on what may wind up being issues of substantive dispute. If the weights incorporated into such a decision tool are not representative of a deeper social consensus, however, then one might wonder about the legitimacy of the decisions that are arrived at by the use of one system of weights rather than another.

Our apparent inability to reach consensus on such basic but seemingly intractable questions of distributive principles leads Norman Daniels and James Sabin to concentrate on the fairness of our procedures for resolving such knotty questions. In "Last-Chance Therapies and Managed Care," they suggest that if we cannot always agree at the level of principles, then perhaps our best bet is to design various procedural mechanisms that will yield results that are "just enough." Keying on the example of HDC-ABMT for advanced breast cancer, Daniels and Sabin report on a variety of "exemplary practices" recently adopted by managed care plans in the wake of the bad publicity, adverse court decisions, and legislative mandates noted by London. Instead of relying on unilateral denials of care, as in the case of Christine deMeurers, to resolve the tension between the efficient use of resources and the desperate appeals of patients for last-chance therapies, many MCOs are now resorting to such procedural solutions as outside review panels and internal appeals mechanisms that emphasize constructive deliberation and dialogue. By openly experimenting with a variety of such strategies while remaining tolerant of the differing value orientations they represent, Daniels and Sabin hope to "move [us] along a learning curve towards a more patient-centered, cost-effective and ethical health care system." By bringing such tensions and disagreements out into the open where they can be rationally and respectfully discussed among subscribers, patients, physicians, and managers, MCOs will have to acknowledge that such questions are not merely technical and economic, but also deeply political. As London noted, only by dealing with the problems of justly allocating health care through an open and more self-consciously political process can MCOs regain a measure of the trust and legitimacy that they have squandered.

Many of the issues canvassed in this section are centrally relevant to the emerging debate over various proposals to create what is being called a "Patient's Bill of Rights." What is the balance that such legislation should strike between what Eddy calls the perspective of society and the perspective of the individual? Should such legislation attempt to catalog rights to specific services or levels of care, or should it enunciate rights to equal treatment in fair processes of open, public decision making? Whether the era of managed care is over, and what the alternatives are, given the persistent fact of fiscal scarcity and the growing ranks of uninsured, will depend on the answers we give to these questions.

EQUALITY AND THE ENDS OF MEDICINE

In different ways the readings of the previous sections illustrate some of the challenges involved in devising a health care system that treats individuals as moral equals and addresses appropriate health needs without becoming either fiscally profligate or unfairly parsimonious. In Section 1, Marchand, Wikler, and Landesman note the role of broader social factors in influencing the health status of individuals, independently of their access to the health care system. They also note that some of these factors relate to differences in individual lifestyle. Even if we suppose that the notion of equal opportunity generates an entitlement to health care, should this entitlement require an equal standard of care for those who strive to be good stewards of the health they have and for those who squander their prospects for good health through imprudent lifestyle choices? If I am a long-time smoker, is my right to treatment for emphysema or cancer equal to that of my nonsmoking neighbor who eats well and jogs daily? In short, should decisions concerning the allocation of scarce health care resources take into account the virtue or vice of the recipient?

In "Should Alcoholics Compete Equally for Liver Transplantation?" Alvin H. Moss and Mark Siegler raise anew the question of whether "personal desert" should ever figure into our allocation decisions. Ordinarily, our public policies tend not to hold individuals personally responsible for their bad health: lifestyles built around cigarettes or Dunkin' Donuts are generally not thought to be punishable by the withholding of medical treatment. But what if the medical commodity is exceptionally scarce, as is the case with transplantable livers, and the disease in question (end-stage liver failure) is eminently preventable by a change in lifestyle, as is the case (the authors contend) with the disease of alcoholism? Moss and Siegler argue that in the face of extreme scarcity and demonstrable personal responsibility, it is just to give nonalcoholics priority over alcoholics on the list for liver transplants. In short, they argue in this limited context for the principle, "To each according to his or her virtue or vice."

Philosophers Carl Cohen, Martin Benjamin, and others argue in their rebuttal to Moss and Siegler, "Alcoholics and Liver Transplantation," that it is not at all clear that giving livers to reformed alcoholics would be a waste of medical resources. More importantly, they dispute the claim that moral blameworthiness should determine who lives and who dies. If there is no consensus on the true nature of virtue and vice in a pluralistic society, and if such behaviors as smoking and drinking might have some sort of genetic predisposition, we must, they argue, reject the notion that medicine should first inquire into the morality of peoples' habits before deciding whether to treat them.

Any such moralizing of the transplant enterprise would raise thorny questions for policy makers. For example, does the vice in question have to be the cause of the life-threatening condition? If so, why? Furthermore, would we deny a transplant to an alcoholic who had been a documented saint for the greater part of his life? And what about those potential organ recipients who, although not alcoholics, have other problems in the virtue department? Should a liver transplant be offered to a teetotaler who also happens to beat his wife, cheat on his taxes, and abuse children?

The debate over the role that judgments of personal responsibility and merit ought to play in the allocation of scarce medical resources represents a specific instance of a larger set of questions concerning the relevance of the cause of a person's suffering. For Moss and Siegler, the suffering of alcoholics in need of a liver transplant is no less real or important than the suffering of the nonalcoholic transplant candidate. What is important from their perspective, however, is the extent to which the alcoholic is responsible for creating the underlying condition that causes that suffering. As they argue, persons suffering from the same condition may merit differential treatment depending on the causal history of their illness. For Cohen, Benjamin, and others, medicine should not be in the business of making moralistic judgments about the relative worth of persons and their individual responsibility for conditions that no doubt have genetic, physiological, and socioeconomic determinants as well.

Now consider a slightly different case concerning both the role of value judgments in allocating medical care and the relevance of the cause of a person's suffering. In "Growth Hormone Therapy for the Disability of Short Stature" pediatrician David B. Allen challenges what he views as the arbitrary limitations that are placed on access to growth hormone for persons of short stature. Imagine two children, each of very short stature, one whose condition is the result of bad luck in the genetic lottery and the other who is diagnosed with growth hormone deficiency (GHD). Allen challenges the notion that these children ought to be treated differently based on the judgment that GHD is recognized as a disease while chronic short stature is not. Both children suffer equally as a result of their diminutive stature and social norms that reward and revere the tall, and both experience limitations in the range of opportunities available to them as a result of these facts. Why should it matter morally that in one case short stature is caused by something we regard as a disease and in the other case by ancestry and luck, if the suffering and limitations of opportunity are the same in both cases?

Allen's recommendation that growth hormone should be viewed as a treatment for short stature and not for GHD rests, in part, on a recognition that the concepts "disease" and "normal" are themselves value laden and may rely on outdated assumptions about what is within and beyond our control. In "The Genome Project, Individual Differences, and Just Health Care," Norman Daniels takes up this example and attempts to defend the distinction between the treatment of disease and the enhancement of what are otherwise normal abilities or characteristics. Daniels wants to resist what he views as a move toward "equalizing capabilities" because it vastly expands the range of deficiencies in need of correction, resulting in an unattainable social ideal that he fears will undermine the general consensus on the importance of health care as traditionally understood. Daniels plants his feet firmly on the intuition that some health needs are more "urgent" than others and he argues that this intuition is captured by the idea that disease represents a deviation from normal species functioning and that the goal of medicine is to restore individuals to the normal opportunity range that they would have enjoyed had they not be prevented from doing so by what can be publicly recognized as a disease or disability.

Daniels thus recognizes the extent to which the concepts of "disease" and "normality" are value laden and, perhaps, socially constructed. The point of his argument is that, as our ability to control a broader range of our personal traits and characteristics expands, we need to reflect publicly on these values in order to ensure that the most urgent health needs are given priority and that, in trying to correct for every inequality between people we do not wind up creating an even more inequitable health care system. If the test for "urgency" is subjective, relating to the importance that individuals ascribe to some perceived health need, then we risk allowing the health care system to be hijacked by the delicate and the vain whose small breasts, balding head, or chubby chin is the source of profound anguish and personal shame. For Daniels, only a more objective standard rooted in a scientifically informed conception of normal species functioning will yield a conception of "urgency" that is in step with our deeper intuitions about the significance of health and the importance of health care.

JUSTICE, HEALTH CARE, AND HEALTH

AN ETHICAL FRAMEWORK FOR ACCESS TO HEALTH CARE

President's Commission for the Study of Ethical Problems in Medicine and Biomedical and Behavioral Research

The prevention of death and disability, the relief of pain and suffering, the restoration of functioning: these are the aims of health care. Beyond its tangible benefits, health care touches on countless important and in some ways mysterious aspects of personal life that invest it with significant value as a thing in itself. In recognition of these special features, the President's Commission was mandated to study the ethical and legal implications of differences in the availability of health services. In this Report to the President and Congress, the Commission sets forth an ethical standard: access for all to an adequate level of care without the imposition of excessive burdens. It believes that this is the standard against which proposals for legislation and regulation in this field ought to be measured. . . .

Editors' note: Most notes have been deleted. Readers who wish to follow up on sources should consult the original article.

In both their means and their particular objectives, public programs in health care have varied over the years. Some have been aimed at assuring the productivity of the work force, others at protecting particularly vulnerable or deserving groups, still others at manifesting the country's commitment to equality of opportunity. Nonetheless, most programs have rested on a common rationale: to ensure that care be made accessible to a group whose health needs would otherwise not be adequately met.

The consequence of leaving health care solely to market forces—the mechanism by which most things are allocated in American society—is not viewed as acceptable when a significant portion of the population lacks access to health services. Of course, government financing programs, such as Medicare and Medicaid as well as public programs that provide care directly to veterans and the military and through local public hospitals, have greatly improved access to health care. These efforts, coupled with the expanded availability of private health insurance, have resulted in almost 90% of Americans having some form of health insurance coverage. Yet the patchwork of government programs and the uneven availability of private health insurance through the workplace have excluded millions of people. The Surgeon General has stated that "with rising unemployment, the numbers are shifting rapidly. We estimate that from 18 to 25 million Americans—8 to 11 percent of the population—have no health insurance coverage at all." Many of these people lack effective access to health care, and many more who have some form of insurance are unprotected from the severe financial burdens of sickness. . . .

Most Americans believe that because health care is special, access to it raises special ethical concerns. In part, this is because good health is by definition important to well-being. Health care can relieve pain and suffering, restore functioning, and prevent death; it can enhance good health and improve an individual's opportunity to pursue a life plan; and it can provide valuable information about a person's overall health. Beyond its practical importance, the involvement of health care with the most significant and awesome events of life—birth, illness, and death—adds a symbolic aspect to health care: it is special because it signifies not only mutual empathy and caring but the mysterious aspects of curing and healing.

Furthermore, while people have some ability—through choice of life-style and through preventive measures—to influence their health status, many health problems are beyond their control and are therefore undeserved. Besides the burdens of genetics, environment, and chance, individuals become ill because of things they do or fail to do—but it is often difficult for an individual to choose to do otherwise or even to know with enough specificity and confidence what he or she ought to do to remain healthy. Finally, the incidence and severity of ill health is distributed very unevenly among people. Basic needs for housing and food are predictable, but even the most hardworking and prudent person may suddenly be faced with overwhelming needs for health care. Together, these considerations lend weight to the belief that health care is different from most other goods and services. In a society concerned not only with fairness and equality of opportunity but also with the redemptive powers of science, there is a felt obligation to ensure that some level of health services is available to all.

There are many ambiguities, however, about the nature of this societal obligation. What share of health costs should individuals be expected to bear, and what responsibility do they have to use health resources prudently? Is it society's responsibility to ensure that every person receives care or services of as high quality and as great extent as any other individual? Does it require that everyone share opportunities to receive all available care or care of any possible benefit? If not, what level of care is "enough"? And does society's obligation include a responsibility to ensure both that care is available and that its costs will not unduly burden the patient?

The resolution of such issues is made more difficult by the spectre of rising health care costs and expenditures. Americans annually spend over 270 million days in hospitals, make over 550 million visits to physicians' offices, and receive tens of millions of X-rays. Expenditures for health care in 1981 totaled $287 billion—an average of over $1225 for every American. Although the finitude of national resources demands that trade-offs be made between health care and other social goods, there is little agreement about which choices are most acceptable from an ethical standpoint. In this chapter, the Commission attempts to lay an ethical foundation for evaluating both current patterns of access to health care and the policies designed to address remaining problems in the distribution of health care resources. . . .

THE SPECIAL IMPORTANCE OF HEALTH CARE

Although the importance of health care may, at first blush, appear obvious, this assumption is often based on instinct rather than reasoning. Yet it is possible to step back and examine those properties of health care that lead to the ethical conclusion that it ought to be distributed equitably.

Well-Being

Ethical concern about the distribution of health care derives from the special importance of health care in promoting personal well-being by preventing or relieving pain, suffering, and disability and by avoiding loss of life. The fundamental importance of the latter is obvious; pain and suffering are also experiences that people have strong desires to avoid, both because of the intrinsic quality of the experience and because of their effects on the capacity to pursue and achieve other goals and purposes. Similarly, untreated disability can prevent people from leading rewarding and fully active lives.

Health, insofar as it is the absence of pain, suffering, or serious disability, is what has been called a primary good, that is, there is no need to know what a particular person's other ends, preferences, and values are in order to know that health is good for that individual. It generally helps people carry out their life plans, whatever they may happen to be. This is not to say that everyone defines good health in the same way or assigns the same weight or importance to different aspects of being healthy, or to health in comparison with the other goods of life. Yet though people may differ over each of these matters, their disagreement takes place within a framework of basic agreement on the importance of health. Likewise, people differ in their beliefs about the value of health and medical care and their use of it as a means of achieving good health, as well as in their attitudes toward the various benefits and risks of different treatments.

Opportunity

Health care can also broaden a person's range of opportunities, that is, the array of life plans that is reasonable to pursue within the conditions obtaining in society.[1] In the United States equality of opportunity is a widely accepted value that is reflected throughout public policy. The effects that meeting (or failing to meet) people's health needs have on the distribution of opportunity in a society become apparent if diseases are thought of as adverse departures from a normal level of functioning. In this view, health care is that which people need to maintain or restore normal functioning or to compensate for inability to function normally. Health is thus comparable in importance to education in determining the opportunities available to people to pursue different life plans.

Information

The special importance of health care stems in part from its ability to relieve worry and to enable patients to adjust to their situation by supplying reliable information about their health. Most people do not understand the true nature of a health problem when it first develops. Health professionals can then perform the worthwhile function of informing people about their conditions and about the expected prognoses with or without various treatments. Though information sometimes creates concern, often it reassures patients either by ruling out a feared disease or by revealing the self-limiting nature of a condition and, thus, the lack of need for further treatment. Although health care in many situations may thus not be necessary for good physical health, a great deal of relief from unnecessary concern—and even avoidance of pointless or potentially harmful steps—is achieved by health care in the form of expert information provided to worried patients. Even when a prognosis is unfavorable and health professionals have little treatment to offer, accurate information can help patients plan how to cope with their situation.

The Interpersonal Significance of Illness, Birth, and Death

It is no accident that religious organizations have played a major role in the care of the sick and dying and in the process of birth. Since all human beings are vulnerable to disease and all die, health care has a special interpersonal significance: it expresses and nurtures bonds of empathy and compassion. The depth of a society's concern about health care can be seen as a measure of its sense of solidarity in the face of suffering and death. Moreover, health care takes on special meaning because of its role in the beginning of a human being's life as well as the end. In spite of all the advances in the scientific understanding of birth, disease, and death, these profound and universal experiences remain shared mysteries that touch the spiritual side of human nature. For these reasons a society's commitment to health care reflects some of its most basic attitudes about what it is to be a member of the human community.

THE CONCEPT OF EQUITABLE ACCESS TO HEALTH CARE

The special nature of health care helps to explain why it ought to be accessible, in a fair fashion, to all. But if this ethical conclusion is to provide a basis for evaluating current patterns of access to health care and proposed health policies, the meaning of fairness or equity in this context must be clarified. The concept of equitable access needs definition in its two main aspects: the level of care that ought to be available to all and the extent to which burdens can be imposed on those who obtain these services.

Access to What?

"Equitable access" could be interpreted in a number of ways: equality of access, access to whatever an individual needs or would benefit from, or access to an adequate level of care.

Equity as Equality It has been suggested that equity is achieved either when everyone is assured of receiving an equal quantity of health care dollars or when people enjoy equal health. The most common characterization of equity as equality, however, is as providing everyone with the same level of health care. In this view, it follows that if a given level of care is available to one individual it must be available to all. If the initial standard is set high, by reference to the highest level of care presently received, an enormous drain would result on the resources needed to provide other goods. Alternatively, if the standard is set low in order to avoid an excessive use of resources, some beneficial services would have to be withheld from people who wished to purchase them. In other words, no one would be allowed access to more services or services of higher quality than those available to everyone else, even if he or she were willing to pay for those services from his or her personal resources.

As long as significant inequalities in income and wealth persist, inequalities in the use of health care can be expected beyond those created by differences in need. Given people with the same pattern of preferences and equal health care needs, those with greater financial resources will purchase more health care. Conversely, given equal financial resources, the different patterns of health care preferences that typically exist in any population will result in a different use of health services by people with equal health care needs. Trying to prevent such inequalities would require interfering with people's liberty to use their income to purchase an important good like health care while leaving them free to use it for frivolous or inessential ends. Prohibiting people with higher incomes or stronger preferences for health care from purchasing more care than everyone else gets would not be feasible, and would probably result in a black market for health care.

Equity as Access Solely According to Benefit or Need Interpreting equitable access to mean that everyone must receive all health care that is of any benefit to them also has unacceptable implications. Unless health is the only good or resources are unlimited, it would be irrational for a society—as for an individual—to make a commitment to provide whatever health care might be beneficial regardless of cost. Although health care is of special importance, it is surely not all that is important to people. Pushed to an extreme, this criterion might swallow up all of society's resources, since there is virtually no end to the funds that could be devoted to possibly beneficial care for diseases and disabilities and to their prevention.

Equitable access to health care must take into account not only the benefits of care but also the cost in comparison with other goods and services to which those resources might be allocated. Society will reasonably devote some resources to health care but reserve most resources for other goals. This, in turn, will mean that some health services (even of a lifesaving sort) will not be developed or employed because they would produce too few benefits in relation to their costs and to the other ways the resources for them might be used.

It might be argued that the notion of "need" provides a way to limit access to only that care that confers especially important benefits. In this view, equity as access according to need would place less severe demands on social resources than equity according to benefit would. There are, however, difficulties with the notion of need in this context. On the one hand, medical need is often not narrowly defined but refers to any condition for which medical treatment might be effective. Thus, "equity as access according to need" collapses into "access according to whatever is of benefit."

On the other hand, "need" could be even more expansive in scope than "benefit." Philosophical and economic writings do not provide any clear distinction between "needs" and "wants" or "preferences." Since the term means different things to different people, "access according to need" could become "access to any health service a person wants." Conversely, need could be interpreted very narrowly to encompass only a very minimal level of services—for example, those "necessary to prevent death."

Equity as an Adequate Level of Health Care Although neither "everything needed" nor "everything beneficial" nor "everything that anyone else is getting" are defensible ways of understanding equitable access, the special nature of health care dictates that everyone have access to *some* level of care: enough care to achieve sufficient welfare, opportunity, information, and evidence of interpersonal concern to facilitate a reasonably full and satisfying life. That level can be termed "an adequate level of health care." The difficulty of sharpening this amorphous notion into a workable foundation for health policy is a major problem in the United States today. This concept is not new; it is implicit in the public debate over health policy and has manifested itself in the history of public policy in this country. In this chapter, the Commission attempts to demonstrate the value of the concept, to clarify its content, and to apply it to the problems facing health policymakers.

Understanding equitable access to health care to mean that everyone should be able to secure an adequate level of care has several strengths. Because an adequate level of care may be less than "all beneficial care" and because it does not require that all needs be satisfied, it acknowledges the need for setting priorities within health care and signals a clear recognition that society's resources are limited and that there are other goods besides health. Thus, interpreting equity as access to adequate care does not generate an open-ended obligation. One of the chief dangers of interpretations of equity that require virtually unlimited resources for health care is that they encourage the view that equitable access is an impossible ideal. Defining equity as an adequate level of care for all avoids an impossible commitment of resources without falling into the opposite error of abandoning the enterprise of seeking to ensure that health care is in fact available for everyone.

In addition, since providing an adequate level of care is a limited moral requirement, this definition also avoids the unacceptable restriction on individual liberty entailed by the view that equity requires equality. Provided that an adequate level is available to all, those who prefer to use their resources to obtain care that exceeds that level do not offend any ethical principle in doing so. Finally, the concept of adequacy, as the Commission understands it, is society-relative. The content of adequate care will depend upon the overall resources available in a given society, and can take into account a consensus of expectations about what is adequate in a particular society at a particular time in its historical development. This permits the definition of adequacy to be altered as societal resources and expectations change.

With What Burdens?

It is not enough to focus on the care that individuals receive; attention must be paid to the burdens they must bear in order to obtain it—waiting and travel time, the cost and availability of transport, the financial cost of the care itself. Equity requires not only that adequate care be available to all, but also that these burdens not be excessive.

If individuals must travel unreasonably long distances, wait for unreasonably long hours, or spend most of their financial resources to obtain care, some will be deterred from obtaining adequate care, with adverse effects on their health and well-being. Others may bear the burdens, but only at the expense of their ability to meet other important needs. If one of the main reasons for providing adequate care is that health care increases welfare and opportunity, then a system that required large numbers of individuals to forego food, shelter, or educational advancement in order to obtain care would be self-defeating and irrational.

The concept of acceptable burdens in obtaining care, as opposed to excessive ones, parallels in some respects the concept of adequacy. Just as equity does not require equal access, neither must the burdens of obtaining adequate care be equal for all persons. What is crucial is that the variations in burdens fall within an acceptable range. As in determining an adequate level of care, there is no simple formula for ascertaining when the burdens of obtaining care fall within such a range. . . .

A SOCIETAL OBLIGATION

Society has a moral obligation to ensure that everyone has access to adequate care without being subject to excessive burdens. In speaking of a societal obligation the Commission makes reference to society in the broadest sense—the collective American community. The community is made up of individuals, who are in turn members of many other, overlapping groups, both public and private: local, state, regional, and national units; professional and workplace organizations; religious, educational, and charitable organizations; and family, kinship, and ethnic groups. All these entities play a role in discharging societal obligations.

The Commission believes it is important to distinguish between society, in this inclusive sense, and government as one institution among others in society. Thus the recognition of a collective or societal obligation does not imply that government should be the only or even the primary institution involved in the complex enterprise of making health care available. It is the Commission's view that the societal obligation to ensure equitable access for everyone may best be fulfilled in this country by a pluralistic approach that relies upon the coordinated contributions of actions by both the private and public sectors.

Securing equitable access is a societal rather than a merely private or individual responsibility for several reasons. First, while health is of special importance for human beings, health care—especially scientific health care—is a social product requiring the skills and efforts of many individuals; it is not something that individuals can provide for themselves solely through their own efforts. Second, because the need for health care is both unevenly distributed among persons and highly unpredictable and because the cost of securing care may be great, few individuals could secure adequate care without relying on some social mechanism for sharing the costs. Third, if persons generally deserved their health conditions or if the need for health care were fully within the individual's control, the fact that some lack adequate care would not be viewed as an inequity. But differences in health status, and hence differences in health care needs, are largely undeserved because they are, for the most part, not within the individual's control.

Uneven and Unpredictable Health Needs

While requirements for other basic necessities, such as adequate food and shelter, vary among people within a relatively limited range, the need for health care is distributed very unevenly and its occurrence at any particular time is highly unpredictable. One study shows 50% of all hospital billings are for only 13% of the patients, the seriously chronically ill.

Moreover, health care needs may be minor or overwhelming, in their personal as well as financial impact. Some people go through their entire lives seldom requiring health care, while others face medical expenses that would exceed the resources of all but the wealthiest. Moreover, because the need for care cannot be predicted, it is difficult to provide for it by personal savings from income. . . .

WHO SHOULD ENSURE THAT SOCIETY'S OBLIGATION IS MET?

In this country, the chief mechanism by which the cost of health care is spread among individuals is through the purchase of insurance. Another method of distributing health care costs is to rely on acts of charity in which individuals, such as relatives and care givers, and institutions assume responsibility for absorbing some or all of a person's health care expenses. These private forces cannot be expected to achieve equitable access for all, however. States and localities have also played important roles in attempting to secure health care for those in need. To the extent that actions of the market, private charity, and lower levels of government are insufficient in achieving equity, the responsibility rests with Federal government. The actual provision of care may be through arrangements in the private sector as well as through public institutions, such as local hospitals.

Market Mechanisms in Health Care

One means societies employ for meeting needs for goods and services that individuals cannot produce by themselves is the complex legal and economic mechanism known as a market. When health care is distributed through markets, however, an acceptable distribution is not achieved; indeed, given limitations in the way markets work, this result is practically inevitable.

The Inability to Ensure Adequate Care First, many people lack the financial resources to obtain access to adequate care. Since American society encompasses a very wide range in income and wealth, distributing goods and services through markets leads to large differences in their consumption. The variations in need for health care do not, however, match variations in ability to purchase care. The market response to variable risk is insurance. Insurance has long existed for certain calamities—such as fire damage to property—and in the past 30 years, a huge market in health insurance has developed that enables people to share some of the financial risk of ill health. The relevant question for determining equity of access thus becomes: Is everyone able to afford access to adequate care through some combination of insurance and direct payment?

Admittedly, "ability to afford" is an ambiguous concept, given different attitudes toward risk and the importance of health care, and, even more important, possibly insufficient information about the likelihood of ill health and about the possible effects of care. For example, people may want an adequate level of care and may be able to afford to pay for it, but they may lack information about the amount of coverage needed to secure adequate care. As a result, the insurance market may not do a good job of providing plans that actually do protect people adequately. And, of course, some people who can afford to pay for their health care (and who would if they knew they would have to go without it otherwise) fail to make sufficient provisions because they rely on others not being willing to let them suffer. Furthermore, the cost of basic health insurance (which does not even guarantee financial access to adequate care in all cases) is high enough to place it beyond the reach of many families by *any* reasonable standard of affordability. Ironically, those who need the most care will find it most difficult to obtain it, both because their disease or disability impairs their opportunities for accumulating financial resources and because insurers will charge them higher rates. . . .

A Right to Health Care?

Often the issue of equitable access to health care is framed in the language of rights. Some who view health care from the perspective of distributive justice argue that the considerations discussed in this chapter show not only that society has a moral obligation to provide equitable access, but also that every individual has a moral right to such access. The Commission has chosen not to develop the case for achieving equitable access through the assertion of a right to health care. Instead it has sought to frame the issues in terms of the special nature of health care and of society's moral obligation to achieve equity, without taking a position on whether the term "obligation" should be read as entailing a moral right. The Commission reaches this conclusion for several reasons: first, such a right is not legally or constitutionally recognized at the present time; second, it is not a logical corollary of an ethical obligation of the type the Commission has enunciated; and third, it is not necessary as a foundation for appropriate governmental actions to secure adequate health care for all.

Legal Rights Neither the Supreme Court nor any appellate court has found a constitutional right to health or to health care. However, most Federal statutes and many state statutes that fund or regulate health care have been interpreted to provide statutory rights in the form of entitlements for the intended beneficiaries of the program or for members of the group protected by the regulatory authority. . . .

Moral Obligations and Rights The relationship between the concept of a moral right and that of a moral obligation is complex. To say that a person has a moral right to something is always to say that it is that person's due, that is, he or she is morally entitled to it. In contrast, the term "obligation" is used in two different senses. All moral rights imply corresponding obligations, but, depending on the sense of the term that is being used, moral obligations may or may not imply corresponding rights. In the broad sense, to say that society has a moral obligation to do something is to say that it ought morally to do that thing and that failure to do it makes society liable to serious moral criticism. This does not, however, mean that there is a corresponding right. For example, a person may have a moral obligation to help those in need, even though the needy cannot, strictly speaking, demand that person's aid as something they are due.

The government's responsibility for seeing that the obligation to achieve equity is met is independent of the existence of a corresponding moral right to health care. There are many forms of government involvement, such as enforcement of traffic rules or taxation to support national defense, to protect the environment, or to promote biomedical research, that do not presuppose corresponding moral rights but that are nonetheless legitimate and almost universally recognized as such. In a democracy, at least, the people may assign to government the responsibility for seeing that important collective obligations are met, provided that doing so does not violate important moral rights.

As long as the debate over the ethical assessment of patterns of access to health care is carried on simply by the assertion and refutation of a "right to health care," the debate will be incapable of guiding policy. At the very least, the nature of the right must be made clear and competing accounts of it compared and evaluated. Moreover, if claims of rights are to guide policy they must be supported by sound ethical reasoning and the connections between various rights must be systematically developed, especially where rights are potentially in conflict with one another. At present, however, there is a great deal of dispute among competing theories of rights, with most theories being so abstract and inadequately developed that their implications for health care are not obvious. Rather than attempt to adjudicate among competing theories of rights, the Commission has chosen to concentrate on what it believes to be the more important part of the question: What is the nature of the societal obligation, which exists whether or not people can claim a corresponding right to health care, and how should this societal obligation be fulfilled?[2]

MEETING THE SOCIETAL OBLIGATION

How Much Care is Enough?

Before the concept of an adequate level of care can be used as a tool to evaluate patterns of access and efforts to improve equity, it must be fleshed out. Since there is no objective formula for doing this, reasonable people can disagree about whether particular patterns and policies meet the demands of adequacy. The Commission does not attempt to spell out in detail what adequate care should include. Rather it frames the terms in which those who discuss or critique health care issues can consider ethics as well as economics, medical science, and other dimensions.

Characteristics of Adequacy First, the Commission considers it clear that health care can only be judged adequate in relation to an individual's health condition. To begin with a list of techniques or procedures, for example, is not sensible: A CT scan for an accident victim with a serious head injury might be the best way to make a diagnosis essential for the appropriate treatment of that patient; a CT scan for a person with headaches might not be considered essential for adequate care. To focus only on the technique, therefore, rather than on the individual's health and the impact the procedure will have on that individual's welfare and opportunity, would lead to inappropriate policy.

Disagreement will arise about whether the care of some health conditions falls within the demands of adequacy. Most people will agree, however, that some conditions should not be included in the societal obligation to ensure access to adequate care. A relatively uncontroversial example would be changing the shape of a functioning, normal nose or retarding the normal effects of aging (through cosmetic surgery). By the same token, there are some conditions, such as pregnancy, for which care would be regarded as an important component of adequacy. In determining adequacy, it is important to consider how people's welfare, opportunities, and requirements for information and interpersonal caring are affected by their health condition.

Any assessment of adequacy must consider also the types, amounts, and quality of care necessary to respond to each health condition. It is important to emphasize that these questions are implicitly comparative: The standard of adequacy for a condition must reflect the fact that resources used for it will not be available to respond to other conditions. Consequently, the level of care deemed adequate should reflect a reasoned judgment not only about the impact of the condition on the welfare and opportunity of the individual but also about the efficacy and the cost of the care itself in relation to other conditions and the efficacy and cost of the care that is available for them. Since individual cases differ so much, the health care professional and patient must be flexible. Thus adequacy, even in relation to a particular health condition, generally refers to a range of options.

The Relationship of Costs and Benefits The level of care that is available will be determined by the level of resources devoted to producing it. Such allocation should reflect the benefits and costs of the care provided. It should be emphasized that these "benefits," as well as their "costs," should be interpreted broadly, and not restricted only to effects easily quantifiable in monetary terms. Personal benefits include improvements in individuals' functioning and in their quality of life, and the reassurance from worry and the provision of information that are a product of health care. Broader social benefits should be included as well, such as strengthening the sense of community and the belief that no one in serious need of health care will be left without it. Similarly, costs are not merely the funds spent for a treatment but include other less tangible and quantifiable adverse consequences, such as diverting funds away from other socially desirable endeavors including education, welfare, and other social services.

There is no objectively correct value that these various costs and benefits have or that can be discovered by the tools of cost/benefit analysis. Still, such an analysis, as a recent report of the Office of Technology Assessment noted, "can be very helpful to decisionmakers because the process of analysis gives structure to the problem, allows an open consideration of all relevant effects of a decision, and forces the explicit treatment of key assumptions." But the valuation of the various effects of alternative treatments for different conditions rests on people's values and goals, about which individuals will reasonably disagree. In a democracy, the appropriate values to be assigned to the consequences of policies must ultimately be determined by people expressing their values through social and political processes as well as in the marketplace.

Approximating Adequacy The intention of the Commission is to provide a frame of reference for policymakers, not to resolve these complex questions. Nevertheless, it is possible to raise some of the specific issues that should be considered in determining what constitutes adequate care. It is important, for example, to gather accurate information about and compare the costs and effects, both favorable and unfavorable, of various treatment or management options. The options that better serve the goals that make health care of special importance should be assigned a higher value. As already noted, the assessment of costs must take two factors into account: the cost of a proposed option in relation to alternative forms of care that would achieve the same goal of enhancing the welfare and opportunities of the patient, and the cost of each proposed option in terms of foregone opportunities to apply the same resources to social goals other than that of ensuring equitable access.

Furthermore, a reasonable specification of adequate care must reflect an assessment of the relative importance of many different characteristics of a given form of care for a particular condition. Sometimes the problem is posed as: What *amounts* of care and what *quality* of care? Such a formulation reduces a complex problem to only two dimensions, implying that all care can readily be ranked as better or worse. Because two alternative forms of care may vary along a number of dimensions, there may be no consensus among reasonable and informed individuals about which form is of higher overall quality. It is worth bearing in mind that adequacy does not mean the highest possible level of quality or strictly equal quality any more than it requires equal amounts of care; of course, adequacy does require that everyone receive care that meets standards of sound medical practice.

Any combination of arrangements for achieving adequacy will presumably include some health care delivery settings that mainly serve certain groups, such as the poor or those covered by public programs. The fact that patients receive care in different settings or from different providers does not itself show that some are receiving inadequate care. The Commission believes that there is no moral objection to such a system so long as all receive care that is adequate in amount and quality and all patients are treated with concern and respect. . . .

NOTES

1. Norman Daniels, *Health Care Needs and Distributive Justice,* 10 Phil. & Pub. Aff. 146 (1981).
2. Whether the issue of equity is framed in terms of individual rights or societal obligation, it is important to recall that society's moral imperative to achieve equitable access is not an unlimited commitment to provide whatever care, regardless of cost, individuals need or that would be of some benefit to them. Instead, society's obligation is to provide adequate care for everyone. Consequently, if there is a moral right that corresponds to this obligation, it is limited, not open-ended.

EQUAL OPPORTUNITY AND HEALTH CARE

Norman Daniels

A natural place to seek principles of justice for regulating health-care institutions is by examining different general theories of justice. Libertarian, utilitarian, and contractarian theories, for example, each support more general principles governing the distribution of rights, opportunities, and wealth, and these general principles may bear on the specific issue of health care. But there is a difficulty with this strategy. In order to apply such general theories to health care, we need to know what kind of a social good health care is. An analysis of this problem is not provided by general theories of justice. One way to see the problem is to ask whether health-care services, say personal medical services, should be viewed as we view other commodities in our society. Should we allow inequalities in the access to health-care services to vary with whatever economic inequalities are permissible according to more general principles of distributive justice? Or is health care "special" and not to be assimilated with other commodities, like cars or personal computers, whose distribution we allow to be governed by market exchanges among economic unequals?

Is health care special? To answer this question, we must see that not all preferences individuals have—and express, for example, in the marketplace—are of equal moral importance. When we judge the importance to society of meeting someone's preferences we use a restricted measure of well-being. We do not simply ask, how much does the person want something? Or, how happy an individual will be if he gets it? Rather, we are concerned whether the preference is for something that affects well-being in certain fundamental or important ways (cf. Scanlon 1975). Among the kinds of preferences to which we give special weight are those that meet certain important categories of need. Among these important needs are those necessary for maintaining normal functioning for individuals, viewed as members of a natural species. Health-care needs fit this characterization

From *Am I My Parent's Keeper?* by Norman Daniels, Oxford University Press, 1988, pp. 68–73.

of important needs because they are things we need to prevent or cure diseases and disabilities, which are deviations from species-typical functional organization ("normal functioning" for short).

This preference suggests health care may be special in this restricted sense: Health care needs are important to meet because they affect normal functioning. But there is still a gap in our answer: Why give such moral importance to health-care needs merely because they are necessary to preserve normal functioning? Why is preserving normal functioning of special moral importance? The answer lies in the relationship between normal functioning and opportunity, but to make the relationship clear, I must introduce the notion of a normal opportunity range.

The *normal opportunity range* for a given society is the array of life plans reasonable persons in it are likely to construct for themselves. The normal range is thus dependent on key features of the society—its stage of historical development, its level of material wealth and technological development, and even important cultural facts about it. This dependency is one way in which the notion of normal opportunity range is socially relative. Facts about social organization, including the conception of justice regulating its basic institutions, will also determine how that total normal range is distributed in the population. Nevertheless, that issue of distribution aside, normal functioning provides us with one clear parameter affecting the share of the normal range open to a given individual. It is this parameter that the distribution of health care affects.

The share of the normal range open to individuals is also determined in a fundamental way by their talents and skills. Fair equality of opportunity does not require opportunity to be equal for all persons. It requires only that it be equal for persons with similar skills and talents. Thus individual shares of the normal range will not in general be *equal*, even when they are *fair* to the individual. The general principle of fair equality of opportunity does not imply leveling individual differences. Within the general theory of justice, unequal chances of success which derive from unequal talents may be compensated for in other ways. I can now state a fact at the heart of my approach: Impairment of normal functioning through disease and disability restricts individuals' opportunities relative to that portion of the normal range their skills and talents would have made available to them were they healthy. If individuals' fair shares of the normal range are the arrays of life plans they may reasonably choose, given their talents and skills, then disease and disability shrinks their shares from what is fair.

Of course, we also know that skills and talents can be undeveloped or misdeveloped because of social conditions, for example, family background or racist educational practices. So, if we are interested in having individuals enjoy a fair share of the normal opportunity range, we will want to correct for special disadvantages here too, say through compensatory educational or job-training programs. Still, restoring normal functioning through health care has a particular and *limited* effect on an individual's shares of the normal range. It lets them enjoy that portion of the range to which a full array of skills and talents would give them access, assuming that these too are not impaired by special social disadvantages. Again, there is no presumption that we should eliminate or level individual differences: These act as a baseline constraint on the degree to which individuals enjoy the normal range. Only where differences in talents and skills are the results of disease and disability, not merely normal variation, is some effort required to correct for the effects of the "natural lottery."

One conclusion we may draw is that impairment of the normal opportunity range is a (fairly crude) measure of the relative importance of health-care needs, at least at the social or macro level. That is, it will be more important to prevent, cure, or compensate for those disease conditions which involve a greater curtailment of an individual's share of the normal opportunity range. More generally, this relationship between health-care needs and opportunity suggests that the principle that should govern the design of health-care institutions is a principle guaranteeing fair equality of opportunity.

The concept of equality of opportunity is given prominence in Rawls's (1971) theory of justice, and it has also been the subject of extensive critical discussion. I cannot here review the main issues (see Daniels 1985, Chapter 3), nor provide a full justification for the principle of fair equality of opportunity. Instead, I shall settle for a weaker, conditional claim, which suffices for my purposes. Health-care institutions should be among those governed by a principle of fair equality of opportunity, provided two conditions obtain: (1) an acceptable general theory of justice includes a principle that requires basic institutions to guarantee fair equality of opportunity, and (2) the fair equality of opportunity principle acts as a constraint on permissible economic inequalities. In what follows, for the sake of simplicity, I shall ignore these provisos. I urge the fair equality of opportunity principle as an appropriate principle to govern macro decisions about the design of our health-care system. The principle defines, from the perspective of justice, what the moral *function* of the health-care system must be—to help guarantee fair equality of opportunity. This relationship between health care and opportunity is the fundamental insight underlying my approach.

My conditional claim does not depend on the acceptability of any particular general theory of justice, such as Rawls's contractarian theory. A utilitarian theory might suffice, for example, if it were part of an ideal moral code, general compliance with which produced at least as much utility as any alternative code (cf. Brandt 1979). That utilitarian theory could then be extended to health care through the analysis provided by my account. Because Rawls's is the main general theory that has incorporated a fair equality of opportunity principle, I have elsewhere suggested in some detail (Daniels 1985, Chapter 3) how it can be extended, with minor modifications, to incorporate my approach. These details need not distract us here.

The fair equality of opportunity account has several important implications for the issue of access to health care. First, the account is compatible with, though it does not imply, a multitiered health-care system. The basic tier would include health-care services that meet health-care needs, or at least important needs, as judged by their impact on opportunity range. Other tiers might involve the use of health-care services to meet less important needs or other preferences, for example, cosmetic surgery. Second, the basic tier, which we might think of as a "decent basic minimum," is characterized in a principled way, by reference to its impact on opportunity. Third, there should be no obstacles—financial, racial, geographical—to access to the basic tier. (The account is silent about what inequalities are permissible for higher tiers within the system.) Social obligations are focused on the basic tier.

The fair equality of opportunity account also has implications for issues of resource allocation. First, I have already noted that we have a crude criterion—impact on normal opportunity range—for distinguishing the importance of different health-care needs and services. Second, preventive measures that make the distribution of risks of disease more equitable must be given prominence in a just health-care system. Third, the importance of personal medical services, despite what we spend on them, must be weighed against other forms of health care, including preventive and public health measures, personal care and other long-term-care services. A just distribution of health-care services involves weighing the impact of all of these on normal opportunity range. This point has specific implications for the importance of long-term care, but also for the introduction of new high-cost technologies, such as artificial hearts, which deliver a benefit to relatively few individuals at very great cost. We must weigh new technologies against alternatives and judge the overall impact of introducing them on fair equality of opportunity—which gives a slightly new sense to the term "opportunity cost."

This account does not give individuals a basic right to have all of their health-care needs met. Rather, there are social obligations to provide individuals only with those services that are part of the design of a system which, on the whole, protects equal opportunity. If social obligations to provide appropriate health care are not met, then individuals are definitely wronged. Injustice is done to them. Thus, even though decisions have to be made about how best to protect opportunity, these obligations nevertheless are not similar to imperfect duties of beneficence. If I could benefit from your charity, but you instead give charity to someone else, I am not wronged and you have fulfilled your duty of beneficence. But if the just design of a health-care system requires providing a service from which I could benefit, then I am wronged if I do not get it.

The case is similar to individuals who have injustice done to them because they are discriminated against in hiring or promotion practices on a job. In both cases, we can translate the specific sort of injustice done, which involves acts or policies that impair or fail to protect opportunity, into a claim about individual rights. The principle of justice guaranteeing fair equality of opportunity shows that individuals have legitimate claims or rights when their opportunity is impaired in particular ways—against a background of institutions and practices which protect equal opportunity. Health-care rights in this view are thus a species of rights to equal opportunity.

The scope and limits of these rights—the entitlements they actually carry with them—will be relative to certain facts about a given system. For example, a health-care system can protect opportunity only within the limits imposed by resource scarcity and technological development for a given society. We cannot make a direct inference from the fact that an individual has a right to health care to the conclusion that this person is entitled to some specific health-care service, even if the service would meet a health-care need. Rather, the individual is entitled to a specific service only if it is or ought to be part of a system that appropriately protects fair equality of opportunity. . . .

REFERENCES

Brandt, R. 1979. *A Theory of the Good and the Right*. Oxford: Oxford University Press.

Daniels, N. 1985. "Family Responsibility Initiatives and Justice Between Age Groups." *Law, Medicine, and Health Care* 13(4):153–159.

Rawls, J. 1971. *A Theory of Justice*. Cambridge, MA: Harvard University Press.

Scanlon, T. M. 1975. "Preference and Urgency." *Journal of Philosophy* 77(19):655–669.

CLASS, HEALTH, AND JUSTICE

Sarah Marchand, Daniel Wikler, and Bruce Landesman

If living were something that money could buy,
Then the rich would live, and the poor would die.
(Black spiritual, United States)

Perhaps the rich don't buy health, but the outpouring of research documenting class inequalities in health demonstrates that they *do* live longer, and the poor *do* die, in greater numbers at all ages; and the poor are sicker, too (Wilkinson 1996; Kaplan and Lynch 1997). Socioeconomic inequalities in health persist even in the wealthiest countries; they hold true for both treatable and untreatable diseases, and for injuries; and they persist even when differences in risk-taking behavior are taken into account.

Such inequalities in health strike many of us as deeply unjust. But what, precisely, is unjust about them? One's initial response is likely to be that these inequalities demonstrate the need for universal access to health care, and that class inequalities in health must be the result of differences in access to health care services, or in the quality of services received. This body of research shows, however, that class inequalities persist even in countries with universal access to care, where health care resources seem to be distributed justly. The just allocation of health care resources is a challenging task, but class inequalities in health raise broader issues.

A second attempt to locate the injustice in class inequalities in health might find them in the impoverishment of the lowest classes. Surely all but the very poorest countries can avoid exposing a sizable proportion of their populations to avoidable, material deprivation that denies them even a minimally decent standard of living. Insofar as the greater burden of disease associated with lower socioeconomic status is a consequence of material deprivations of this scale, it is unjust. We need no elaborate theory of justice to show that an affluent society's citizens are entitled to have their basic needs met.

This response, however, misses the point of much of the research on the bearing of class on health, which has shown that it is not only the poor

Reprinted with permission of the authors and publisher from *The Milbank Quarterly* 76:3 (1998): 449–467.

whose health suffers as a result of socioeconomic inequality. In rich countries, those at the bottom of the scale may suffer greatly, even though their absolute income is greater than that of the middle classes in less wealthy countries, who may enjoy greater health. Moreover, the richest, even in wealthy countries, enjoy better health and longer life than those in the next position down, even though both income strata are well-to-do by any standard. If class inequalities in health are unjust, these differences also signal a problem of justice quite apart from poverty itself.

The literature on class inequalities in health focuses our attention on a population's *distribution* of health and on the inequalities themselves, whether or not these are linked to poor health care or to poor living standards, the traditional foci of ethical concerns.

We begin with a discussion of the lack of attention to class inequalities in health within the literature of distributive justice. We identify two sources for this neglect: One is a preoccupation with the distribution of health *care* as opposed to the distribution of health. The second is the belief that a concern with class inequalities in health is misplaced because the actual source of injustice is inequality in income and wealth. In this view, the distribution of health may reflect the justice or injustice of the underlying distribution of income and wealth, but it is not an injustice on its own. We defend the thesis that the inequalities in health raise issues of justice independent of both the allocation of health care resources and the general distribution of income and wealth.

In the central section of the paper, we offer four alternative accounts of justice or equity and health. These are not accounts of general theories of justice but, rather, pertain directly to the distribution of health. Only the second of these accounts identifies class inequalities in health as intrinsically unjust. Each of the other three accounts locates the moral problem elsewhere.

We believe each of the four accounts has some plausibility; we mean to open the argument rather than settle it. Questions about the justice of class inequalities in health are ideally answered in the context of a well-formulated general theory of distributive justice. No consensus exists on such a theory, and it is beyond the scope of this article to propose one. Our more modest goal is to place the issue of the nature of the injustice in class inequalities in health in the context of contemporary theories of justice. Our inquiry may also help us to determine when differences over strategies for ameliorating these social inequalities in health stem from differing moral assumptions rather than from disagreements over effectiveness or cost.

For purposes of this discussion, we use the terms "class," "socioeconomic group," and "social stratum" more or less interchangeably. We leave for another occasion the question of whether and how our analysis would be affected by the choice among these social categories.

We close with notes on two further, related topics: first, the implications of the hypothesis that the degree of income inequality in a society affects that society's health, and, second, the problems that personal responsibility for health may bring to any account of justice regarding inequalities in health status.

HEALTH VERSUS HEALTH CARE

Nearly everything philosophers have written on justice and health is confined to issues of the allocation of health *care*. Yet social inequalities in health persist even when health care resources are more equitably distributed. Why, then, have these inequalities not been considered as an issue of distributive justice?

Perhaps some contributors to this literature are simply unaware of important determinants of health, once basic needs have been met, other than biology and health care, leading them to equate the obligation to improve a population's health with the obligation to expand its access to health care. At the same time, there is a growing recognition that some health care may well be too expensive and offer too little benefit to justify inclusion among society's obligations. This is the familiar problem of the "bottomless pit," endlessly swallowing attempts to satisfy all health care needs.

Consider the problem of the bottomless pit as it appears in Kenneth Arrow's (1973) early review of Rawls's *A Theory of Justice* (Rawls 1971). Arrow suggests that "maximin" principles of distributive justice (of which Rawls's principles of justice are an example) cannot escape the problem of the bottomless pit of health care needs. Maximin principles of justice direct us to distribute resources in such a way that the worst position in society (the "minimum" position) is made as well off as possible (the "minimum" position should be "maximized"). Maximin principles are implausible, Arrow argued, when we consider individuals with expensive health care needs as among the occupants of the minimum position. Those with expensive health care needs might require nearly unlimited health care resources, draining the economy and yielding relatively little benefit. Can justice, Arrow asked, plausibly require huge sacrifices of everyone but the worst-off, in order to realize what may be very small benefits for that group?

For many, Arrow's argument suffices to show that we must avoid the notion that we owe people *health*. They conclude that, at most, we owe some fair proportion of health care resources, or perhaps that we have no specific health-related obligations at all. This conclusion, however, does not follow from Arrow's argument. For even if we must exempt expensive health care from maximin principles of justice (to avoid "social hijacking" by expensive needs), we may still be obligated to adopt other social policies—for example, a narrowing of income inequality—under which those in the worst-off position are as well off (and as healthy) as possible.

Other explanations for the focus on health care, rather than health, stem from aspects of the theories of equity or justice themselves and not just their empirical assumptions. In the wake of Rawls's work, philosophers have increasingly turned away from theories of "welfarism" (Dworkin 1981a; Arneson 1989; Cohen 1989). Welfarism is the doctrine that justice (or, for some theorists, morality as a whole) consists in some distribution or other of welfare or "well-being." It states that what matters in questions of morality or justice can only be individuals' welfare. Rejecting welfarism, Rawls proposed that justice is concerned with what he termed "social, primary, goods," such as opportunities, income, and wealth, and not welfare.

One effect of Rawls's influence has been the development of alternatives to welfarism in the form of "resourcist" theories of justice that—as with Rawls's social, primary goods—eschew interpersonal comparisons of welfare in favor of interpersonal comparisons of resources (an exception is Sen's "capabilities," which occupies a zone between resources and welfare (Sen 1980). This shift from welfare to resources can also be described as a shift from outcomes to means; rather than asking what a given bundle of resources can "do" for a person (Sen 1993), or what outcomes he can achieve with it, we ask whether his resource holdings are fair relative to what others have. The claim made by resourcists is that what is fair can be determined without appealing to the concept of welfare.

Health is more easily assimilated to the notion of welfare or outcomes than it is to the notion of means or resources. It is impossible to say, according to resourcist theories, that a particular distribution of health (or of welfare generally) in a given society is just or unjust. From a resourcist perspective, whatever pattern of welfare or health is produced in society by a particular distribution of resources is just, so long as resources are distributed justly.

If these considerations explain why the distribution of health has been ignored in the literature of distributive justice, they do not justify this omission. The factual assumption we mentioned—that health is primarily a function of one's individual biology and of the quality and extent of health care services one receives—is clearly mistaken. For example, health may be affected by the degree of income inequality in a given society, and social policy can usefully address this basic social question. As we come to learn more about the mechanisms by which inequality affects health, other effective social and economic measures may be identified. Arrow's argument about the "bottomless pit" of needy patients does not necessarily have the same force when applied to determinants of health other than expensive, largely futile, acute health care interventions. We discuss other implications of resourcist theories of distributive justice in the next section.

IS HEALTH SPECIAL?

The intuition that it is morally objectionable when people in different income strata have different average life expectancies and health statuses seems to be a fairly robust one. This intuition may not extend to other inequalities, in particular to the fact of income strata themselves and resulting class differences in the standard of living. Health, unlike income and unlike other goods and services, seems special to many of us, in that the case for its equal distribution seems more compelling.

Philosophers and others differ on whether this intuition is rationally defensible. Some egalitarian theories of justice, whether welfarist or resourcist, defend a view diametrically opposed to this intuition. They maintain that justice requires equalizing income and wealth or welfare but that this kind of "global" equality is consistent with inequalities in specific goods, including health. Ronald Dworkin (1981b), a leading egalitarian resourcist theorist, for example, proposes that justice consists in people having the same amount of resources with which to purchase health insurance (he does not discuss other determinants of health); it does not consist in equal health. According to Dworkin, people with equal resources must be allowed to budget their resources as they wish, in light of their differing goals and life plans. Some people will prefer a life of security and purchase as much coverage as they can, leaving little for other things, whereas others will prefer to spend that money on the goods and services they believe will enhance their lives, and so will purchase "bare-bones" coverage.

Although Dworkin's resource egalitarianism is obviously remote from real world inequalities, it illustrates why some believe that there is no "just" distribution of health. We might be tempted to conclude from a theory like Dworkin's that in the real world, where income and wealth are vastly unequal, the basis for our intuition that socioeconomic inequalities in health are unjust is that the inequalities in income and wealth are unjust. We must decide, however, whether it is income inequalities or health inequalities that condemn the other. Perhaps existing inequalities in income and other resources are unjust in part because they produce inequalities in health. For Dworkin, justice requires equalizing income and wealth, irrespective of any consequences for health. If health inequalities are morally wrong sui generis, however, then this may provide a reason for equalizing income and wealth.

In support of the intuition that health is special, and that there can be just or unjust distributions of health, are views that defend different criteria or principles of distribution for various goods (Walzer 1983). Some of these views oppose income inequalities and some do not, but they all maintain that health, as opposed to income and wealth, is regulated by a separate principle of justice (Culyer 1993; Culyer and Wagstaff 1993). One view of this sort is a "specific egalitarianism" that seeks equality in each important good (Tobin 1970). Another approach is to argue that health raises considerations of justice that require its "insulation" from the sphere of the market. Norman Daniels (1985) has argued that health is a requisite of equal opportunity, and thus that health care, like education, should be earmarked for more equal distribution, rather than distributed according to ability and willingness to pay. This is true, according to Daniels, even if individuals' share of society's resources is fair in other respects.

In what follows we present four accounts of equity and health, each presupposing that a society's distribution of health can be prima facia just or unjust. In other words, they presuppose that (1) justice does bear on the issue of a society's distribution of health and that we can formulate goals of an equitable health policy on that basis; but that (2) justice in the sphere of health policy is not justice, all things considered. Only a general theory of distributive justice that addresses the basic social and economic structure of a society can tell us how to balance and weight the various demands of justice, or what to do in cases where they conflict. We do discuss some points of contact between general principles of justice and principles that apply to the domain of health. Although the four accounts of equity and health do treat health as special, we acknowledge that whatever justice demands in that sphere is only provisional and subject to its broader requirements.

EQUITY AND HEALTH: FOUR ALTERNATIVE VIEWS

In the literature documenting the pervasive class differences in health, two goals of health policy are often mentioned: first, that society should seek to maximize the sum total of health of its members, and, second, that society should pursue a policy of equal health between classes. We discuss these two views first. The third and fourth views, also discussed below, revisit "maximin" principles of justice, but they define the minimum position in alternative ways. Importantly, only the second view—that we should attempt to equalize health between classes—reflects the idea that class inequalities in health are intrinsically unjust.

Equity as Maximization

According to the first view, the troubling aspect of richer people's generally longer life span and, on average, healthier lives is the indication that the higher morbidity and mortality of the less well off might be avoidable. Given reasonable assumptions, the better health enjoyed by the upper classes is evidence that the lower classes could also enjoy better health. Data on class differences in health reveal the extent of premature deaths and excess morbidity. What is troubling is that such a "society is less healthy than it could be"; the total sum of health of its members is lower than we might achieve with the right policies in place.

This notion that health policy should aim to produce as much health as possible for a given population seems to be regarded in some quarters as self-evident. A parallel faith in maximization is found in the cost–benefit and cost-effectiveness literature on health care allocation. The premise is borrowed from welfare economics and utilitarianism generally, according to which the goal of social policy should be to maximize the total sum of individual welfare or utilities. That we should maximize health does not follow, however, from the claim that we should maximize welfare; health is only one aspect of welfare, and maximizing welfare may require permitting individuals to strike their own trade-offs between health and other goods, as their values and preferences dictate. Therefore, the view that health policy should aim at maximizing health is the local application of a general principle of justice; it is not derived from the general principle. The view stands or falls on its own merits and not with the general principle. Nonetheless, some of the arguments for and against utilitarianism have their parallels here.

Although maximizing health may be thought of as an imperative of efficiency, philosophers have also given serious attention to maximizing principles as candidates for principles of justice or equity. The fundamental moral assumption of maximizing principles is that we express equal respect for each person by giving her interests the very same weight as others. Behind a maximizing principle is a principle of equality: each person's interests, in this case their health, counts just as much and no more than anyone else's. From this perspective, an improvement in health for the well-off is just as valuable and carries the same moral weight as an improvement in health for the worse-off. Health benefits count equally no matter where they fall. Although a maximizing principle so understood is a theory of distributive justice, it is sometimes said to be a principle of "distributive neutrality" because it directs us to maximize sum total amounts without regard to how that total is distributed.

In the empirical literature on class inequalities in health the goal of maximizing health is sometimes run together with the goal of equalizing health between classes. *The Black Report,* for example, argues that "eliminating social inequalities in health offers the greatest opportunity for achieving overall improvement in the nation's health" (Townsend and Davidson 1982, 200). Similarly, Wilkinson (1996, 16) suggests that our overriding aim should be to "increase the sum total of health of a society" by narrowing health inequalities.

Whether pursuing one of these goals will in fact promote the other simultaneously is an empirical question. Deciding on the goal we should pursue if we must choose between them, however, is an ethical question. There is no reason to think, a priori, that the goal of maximizing health is most efficiently pursued by attempting to narrow class inequalities in health. Even if this proves to be the case, we can ask whether the maximizing view accurately captures the moral concern many share over class inequalities in health.

Our belief is that many people will feel that a maximizing principle fails to explain what is objectionable about the data. It does not entail the view that class inequalities in health are necessarily unjust, and it assigns no special moral urgency to eliminating them. Those who attach importance to eliminating class differences in health for reasons of justice are likely to give priority to policies with that goal, even if they divert energy and resources from other programs devised to increase the sum total of health.

Equity as Equality

The second view proposes that it is unfair *in and of itself* that those of a higher socioeconomic status will, on average, live longer lives, in better health, than those of a lower one.

In support of this view, we might appeal to a principle of the moral equality of persons, as the maximizing view does, but to a different interpretation of that principle. We might argue that treating each person's interests as having the same weight or importance as everyone else's does not imply that improvements in health for the best-off are as valuable as improvements in health for the worst-off. Instead the principle of respect for the moral equality of persons entails the view that people are owed roughly equal prospects for a good life, including prospects for a long and healthy life. Improvements in health for the better-off are therefore not as valuable as improvements in health for the worse-off—and this is true because of, not in spite of, the claim that their interests matter equally from the moral point of view. Because their interests matter equally, we should seek to equalize what is in their interests, like their health.

This view might best capture the common intuition that class inequalities in health are morally wrong. Recall, however, that this intuition does not necessarily extend to comprehensive egalitarianism, defined as the elimination of inequalities in income, wealth, and other resources generally. Can one consistently advocate equality as a principle of distribution for health without committing oneself to an unrestricted principle of equal distribution? The principle underlying egalitarianism in the domain of health would seem to be that justice requires a society in which people have roughly equal prospects for a good life. This principle, however, extends far beyond the domain of health.

It is helpful to return briefly to the issue, raised above, of whether or not health is special in the context of our discussion of the principles of maximizing and equalizing health. Both the maximizing and the equalizing principles are supported by appeals to interpretations of a more fundamental moral principle: the moral equality of people. This "deep" principle, however, gives us no reason to treat health in a distinctive way. Moreover, it offers no reason to believe that class inequalities in health might raise different and more urgent moral concerns than those raised by other kinds of health inequalities, such as the different life expectancy of men and women.

Nevertheless, reasons for counting inequalities in health as unjust can be found within egalitarian theories of justice, and these reasons apply particularly to class inequalities in health. The central claim for egalitarians is that respect for the moral equality of people entails that people should have roughly equal prospects for a good life and that inequalities in those prospects require special moral justification. Equality of life prospects functions as a moral baseline or default position. In some cases, and for certain reasons, deviations from the default position of equality may be morally justified, although each deviation requires a convincing argument. For example, Rawls's theory offers a moral justification for limited inequalities in income and wealth based on the effect of incentives in boosting productivity. Rawls argues that inequalities in the distribution of income and wealth are morally justified if they improve everyone's position (in terms of purchasing power), including the position of the worst-off, from the baseline of equality. Thus a just society, for Rawls, might not be a strictly equal society. This justification for inequality, however, extends to departures from equality only for the goods of income and wealth. Inequality in other goods, like basic rights, opportunities, or health, would have to be morally justified on other grounds.

According to this view, we should conceive of inequalities in income and wealth as special exceptions that we establish to a general principle of equality. In this sense, "class" is special and health is not, but *class* inequalities in health are also special because they are an unjustified consequence of our departure from the moral baseline; health, unlike income and wealth on our assumption, should be regulated by the baseline principle of equality. If the income differences that serve us through their incentive effects also have the undesired effect of burdening the less well-off with disease and premature death, the latter would be an unjust "cost" of the incentives, borne largely by those who least benefited from the resulting economic inequalities.

Perhaps this explains why class inequalities in health may be viewed as impermissible, even in a society that is otherwise just—in particular, a society marked by inequalities in other goods that are morally acceptable. It does not, however, show that only class inequalities in health count as injustices because other inequalities, like those associated with race, may qualify as unjust on other grounds.

Equity as Maximin

A third view on class inequalities in health is that these inequalities are not unjust per se; what is unjust are the low, absolute levels of health of members of society when this can be avoided. Justice, according to this view, is not concerned with people's *relative* position, whether in health, well-being generally, or resources, but rather with their absolute levels. We should feel the same urgency to improve the health of the least advantaged group, even if no one was better off.

Maximin principles of justice reflect this concern: they direct us to maximize the minimum position, regardless of how this affects the gap between the minimum position and other positions. If we define the minimum position in terms of those who have the lowest socioeconomic status and apply maximin in the area of health, then it tells us to maximize the health of the lowest socioeconomic group, regardless of whether this increases or decreases inequalities in health between classes. Thus, society's distribution of health can be assessed as just or unjust only by comparing people's level of health relative to the level that could be achieved under alternative social policies. What matters is not who is doing better than whom, but how well each *could* be doing.

One reason for claiming that justice is concerned with absolute, rather than relative, levels of health is that each of us would prefer a world in which we had more years and better health to a world in which we did not, even if in the first world others lived longer and experienced a better state of health than ours, whereas in the second world their health was equal to ours. Except for "positional goods," we prefer more rather than less for ourselves, even if having more makes us worse off relative to others. Rawls expresses this idea by assuming that principles of justice are chosen by people who are "mutually disinterested"; they care about doing as well for themselves as possible, and they care not at all (they are neither envious or altruistic) about how others are doing.

Moreover, our moral obligations to others seem closely tied to people's absolute position rather than to their relative standing. As Joseph Raz argues:

> What makes us care about various inequalities is not the inequality but the concern identified by the underlying principle. It is the hunger of the hungry, the need of the needy, the suffering of the ill, and so on. The fact that they are worse off in the relevant respect than their neighbors is relevant. But it is relevant not as an independent evil of inequality. Its relevance is in showing that their hunger is greater, their need more pressing, their suffering more hurtful, and therefore our concerns for the hungry, the needy, the suffering, and not our concern for equality, makes us give them priority. (Raz 1986; cited in Parfit 1991)

According to a maximin principle, therefore, we should adopt those social policies under which the lowest socioeconomic class has the highest health possible, but not with the goal of achieving equality. To be sure, policies aimed at improving the health of the worse-off are, in practice, bound to narrow class inequalities in health status. Nonetheless, the motivations behind a policy of equality and a policy of maximin are very different. And only the maximin policy justifies giving priority to the worst-off, as opposed to a focus on all class inequalities in health, including that between the moderately well-off and the rich.

A principle of maximin applied to health raises the same question as the first two principles: why should we maximin health and not welfare or resources more generally? We will not pursue this complicated question here, although we return to it in the next section, where we discuss the effect of degrees of income inequality on health.

There is another problem with a principle of maximin, whether applied to health in particular or to well-being or resources generally. Is it plausible to give absolute priority to improving the health of the worst-off class if those who are next to the worst-off are also doing very badly? And what if even the best-off in a society are also doing miserably, with short life expectancies and poor health? Conversely, a maximin principle looks less appealing when applied to a society in which the most deprived are doing very well, with a generous average life expectancy. These reflections suggest that we intuitively apply some standard of urgency to levels of health that is not captured by maximin's concern only with amounts, rather than what those amounts "mean" for people's lives. If it is true that absolute, rather than relative, levels of health matter, then it is also true that they matter *more* when they are low.

Equity as Priority to the Sickest

Thus far we have discussed principles of (a) maximizing the total sum of health of a society, (b) equalizing levels of health between classes, and (c) maximizing the health of the lowest socioeconomic class. The fourth view takes as its point of departure the criticism of maximin offered above. There we suggested that people intuitively apply some standard of urgency to levels of health and not to the minimum position itself. In Raz's words, we care about the neediness of the needy and about those in the minimum position only in proportion to their neediness. Indeed, the urgency of needs suggests its own minimum position: those who are threatened with the worst harms—who have the shortest life expectancy and most serious diseases and injuries—should count as "the worst-off." Therefore, we should not give priority to the lowest socioeconomic class, but to those with the most urgent needs, regardless of class.

We can bring out the distinctive features of this view by constructing a contrary-to-fact example. Suppose there exists a society in which most members of the upper classes live long, healthy lives, but a small number are stricken with a terrible disease and die young. Few members of this imaginary society's poorest classes escape illness and premature death, but none suffer as badly as the unlucky few in the upper classes. The average health and longevity of the lower classes, then, will be considerably lower than that of the upper classes; but the worst-off *individuals,* at least in respect to their health, will be upper-class. On the fourth view, we should give priority to eliminating and treating the terrible disease of these richer sufferers because they are the worst-off. Such policies that would widen the gap in average health status between the classes would be justified, according to this fourth perspective.

To be plausible, such a principle must claim that the urgency of needs should have relative, not absolute priority (Parfit 1991). The point is not that resources should be expended on the sickest people, without any limitation on the ground of cost or lack of benefit—this is the bottomless pit problem addressed by Arrow. Rather, this view calls for a relative weighting: more urgent needs receive more weight when we balance needs against other factors, including cost and efficacy in our policy decisions. Giving needs relative rather than absolute priority also avoids the objection we raised to maximin: that it ignores the health status of everyone except the worst-off.

This fourth alternative suggests that class inequalities in health are the wrong focus of our concerns. But insofar as urgent needs are much more prevalent among the lowest classes, the real-world effect of such a policy would be to reduce those class inequalities.

INEQUALITY AS A CAUSE OF ILLNESS

According to Wilkinson and others, a society's degree of income inequality is an important determinant of health. While we do not argue for or against Wilkinson's hypothesis, we pause to note its significance for the issue of justice and health inequalities.

As we have discussed above, a maximin principle of justice applied to income and wealth (such as Rawls's "difference principle") may actually require inequalities in those goods should this turn out to increase the shares of those with the smallest allotment (as occurs when a system of incentives produces more wealth that can be shared). The goal is the improvement of the smallest share, or the position of the worst-off, even if to meet this goal we must increase the distance between positions.

Given Wilkinson's hypothesis, a maximin principle of this kind is less appealing when considering its possible consequences for health. If health is correlated with less inequality in income, then a maximin principle applied to income could come at the cost of losses in health. It is impossible to say what the *net* effect of such a policy would be on health. On the one hand, the worst-off, we are to assume, have better purchasing power and a correspondingly higher standard of living. On the other hand, their position relative to others may be worse. Because richer countries seem to be, on average, less healthy than countries that have somewhat less wealth but also less inequality, the tradeoff might well be unfavorable. It is a surprising and unwelcome result that a maximin principle raises this concern.

This consideration suggests a kind of paradox about views of justice that differ over whether relative, as opposed to absolute, positions matter. If justice is concerned with *absolute,* not relative, levels of health, then justice must be concerned with *relative,* rather than absolute, levels of income and wealth.

PERSONAL RESPONSIBILITY FOR HEALTH

One consideration complicating any attempt to locate the source of injustice in class inequalities in health is the notion that people bear some responsibility for their own morbidity and mortality. That much of the illness we suffer from can be traced to "lifestyles" is beyond questioning. Better health habits would do more to keep us alive and healthy than medicine can possibly accomplish. To the extent that differences in health status reflect choices for which individuals bear responsibility, how can these differences be construed as injustices?

Rawls's theory of justice was challenged by the libertarian philosopher Robert Nozick (1974), in part because individual choices would, over time, change any patterns of distribution that a society might establish in the name of distributive justice. Whether the distribution is based on equality, or on maximin, or any other pattern, people's everyday choices are bound to produce a different pattern if they are allowed to trade, give, barter, and squander. Nozick's argument applies also in this consideration of justice and class inequalities in health. Even if we could eliminate, through social policies, those inequalities in health that we consider unjust, the resulting pattern of distribution of health states and life expectancies is likely to be upset as people pursue their very different lifestyles. The pattern that emerges over time may bear little relation to the just pattern that may have once been achieved through deliberate social intervention. Ought we to regard the new pattern as unjust, and thus in need of further intervention and rectification? Or, to the extent that it reflects free and informed choices by those affected, is justice preserved?

If we pursued this analogy in the direction taken by Nozick's critique of Rawls, we might conclude that justice requires no particular pattern of distribution of health states at all—in particular, no reduction of class inequalities in health. But this conclusion would be unwarranted for several reasons: First, much illness and excess mortality does not have a behavioral origin. Second, as we have mentioned, class inequalities in health remain after holding risk-taking behavior constant. Third, and just as important, the central premise of the Nozickian argument—that those engaging in unhealthy lifestyles are responsible for their choices—cannot be taken at face value (Lynch, Kaplan, and Salonen 1997). Some of these "choices" may reflect biological factors that an individual cannot be expected to rein in, such as a familial tendency to obesity. Others result from addictions (even if the original decision to try the addictive drug may have been a free one), or stem from a lack of opportunities to adopt healthier habits.

Moreover, it is not clear that we should hold people responsible for making choices that are normative in their particular social milieu. John Roemer (1995), an economist and philosopher, has argued that unhealthy choices made by large numbers of people in a particular social stratum ought to be regarded as products of that class structure, and the individual should not be held responsible for the risks taken so long as the individual's risk-taking was not greater than others in that same stratum. Whether or not we accept Roemer's thesis (T.M. Scanlon [1995] has commented on its seeming implication that working-class people behave unfreely much of the time), the "lifestyle" argument does not get off the ground unless it is clear that the risky behavior resulting in injury, death, or illness is voluntary. The argument trades on many other questionable premises as well (Wikler 1978).

The concept of personal responsibility for health bears on social policy aimed at class inequalities in health status. One powerful argument in favor of social interventions to ameliorate these inequalities, and indeed for regarding health care as a human right, is that illness and premature death are generally deprivations visited upon people through no fault of their own. For this reason, those who suffer because of bad health are entitled to the sympathy and aid of their fellow citizens (LeGrand 1991). If, however, we are personally responsible for health, and therefore for illness and premature death, then these deprivations cannot be said to have occurred "through no fault of our own" (Culyer and Wagstaff 1993). Such a premise undercuts this powerful altruistic argument and removes some of the fuel for an engine of social change that would seek to eliminate these inequalities.

CONCLUSION

Class inequalities in health are intuitively offensive. The import of research documenting the extent of these differences in health status is clear: if we can do something about them, we should. Nevertheless, we believe that although the serious injustice of these inequalities may be apparent, the precise nature of the injustice is not. We have initiated an analysis of the moral issue, identifying four distinct wrongs that might be thought to lie at the heart of the injustice. Choices among social interventions that target these inequalities might be affected by our view of the particular wrong these policies are designed to correct. Moreover, any attempt to declare an ideal for the distribution of health states must address a number of complicating theoretical considerations, like personal responsibility for health and the selection of health, among all social benefits and elements of human well-being, for equal distribution.

This is an exploratory paper whose modest goal is to point to uncertainties that have not been fully discussed in the burgeoning literature on class inequalities in health. We will present our own view, one that emphasizes absolute gains in health, rather than relative health statuses, on another occasion. Here we argue only that the documentation of class inequalities in health does not in itself identify the source or the nature of the moral problem whose existence they evidently demonstrate.

REFERENCES

Arneson, R. 1989. Equality and Equal Opportunity for Welfare. *Philosophical Studies* 56:77–93.

Arrow, K.J. 1973. Some Ordinalist-Utilitarian Notes on Rawls's Theory of Justice. *Journal of Philosophy* 70(9):245–62.

Cohen, G.A. 1989. On the Currency of Egalitarian Justice. *Ethics* 99:906–44.

Culyer, A.J. 1993. Health, Health Expenditures, and Equity. In *Equity in the Finance and Delivery of Health Care*, eds. E. van Doorslaer, A. Wagstaff, and F.E. Rutten. Oxford: Oxford University Press.

Culyer, A.J., and A. Wagstaff. 1993. Equity and Equality in Health and Health Care. *Journal of Health Economics* 12:431–57.

Daniels, N. 1985. *Just Health Care*. Cambridge: Cambridge University Press.

Dworkin, R. 1981a. What is Equality? Part 1: Equality of Welfare. *Philosophy and Public Affairs* 10(3):185–246.

———. 1981b. What is Equality? Part 2: Equality of Resources. *Philosophy and Public Affairs* 10(4):283–345.

Kaplan, G.A., and J.W. Lynch. 1997. Whither Studies on the Socioeconomic Foundations of Population Health? *American Journal of Public Health* 87:1409–11.

LeGrand, J. 1991. *Equity and Choice*. London: HarperCollins.

Lynch, J.W, G.A. Kaplan, and J.T. Salonen. 1997. Why Do Poor People Behave Poorly? Variation in Adult Health Behaviors and Psychosocial Characteristics by Stages of the Socioeconomic Lifecourse. *Social Science and Medicine* 44:809–19.

Nozick, R. 1974. *Anarchy, State, and Utopia*. New York: Basic Books.

Parfit, D. 1991. Equality or Priority? Lawrence: University of Kansas Libraries.

Rawls, J. 1971. *A Theory of Justice*. Cambridge: Harvard University Press.

Raz, J. 1986. *The Morality of Freedom*. Oxford: Oxford University Press.

Roemer, J. 1995. Equality and Responsibility. *Boston Review* 22 (2).

Scanlon, T.M. 1995. A Good Start. *Boston Review* 22 (2).

Sen, A. 1980. Equality of What? In *Tanner Lectures on Human Values*, ed. S.M. McMurrin. Cambridge: Cambridge University Press.

———. 1993. Capability and Well-Being. In *The Quality of Life*, eds. M.C. Nussbaum and A. Sen. Oxford: Clarendon Press.

Tobin, J. 1970. On Limiting the Domain of Inequality. *Journal of Law and Economics* 13:263–78.

Townsend, P., and N. Davidson. Eds. 1982. *Inequalities in Health: The Black Report*. Harmondsworth, U.K.: Penguin.

Walzer, M. 1983. *Spheres of Justice*. New York: Basic Books.

Wikler, D. 1978. Persuasion and Coercion for Health: Ethical Issues in Government Efforts to Change Life-Styles. *Milbank Memorial Fund Quarterly/Health and Society* 56:303–38.

Wilkinson, R. 1996. *Unhealthy Societies: The Afflictions of Inequality*. London: Routledge.

FREEDOM AND MORAL DIVERSITY: THE MORAL FAILURES OF HEALTH CARE IN THE WELFARE STATE

H. Tristram Engelhardt, Jr.

I. AN INTRODUCTION: BEYOND EQUALITY

In his 1993 health-care reform proposal, Bill Clinton offered health care as a civil right. If his proposal had been accepted, all Americans would have been guaranteed a basic package of health care. At the same time, they would have been forbidden to provide or purchase better basic health care, as a cost of participating in a national system to which they were compelled to contribute. A welfare entitlement would have been created and an egalitarian ethos enforced.[1] This essay will address why such egalitarian proposals are morally unjustifiable, both in terms of the establishment of a uniform health-care welfare right, and in terms of the egalitarian constraints these proposals impose against the use of private resources in the purchase of better-quality basic health care, not to mention luxury care.

In framing health-care welfare policy, one must address people's fears of being impoverished while at risk of death and suffering when medicine can offer a benefit. Simultaneously, one must confront significantly different understandings of the appropriate use of medicine, the claims of justice, and the meaning of equality. Any approach to providing health care for those who cannot afford it must come to terms with the substantial disagreements that separate individuals and communities regarding provision of health care by the state. In addition, the attempt to frame a uniform policy must confront the nonegalitarian consequences of human freedom. To be free is to make choices that have nonegalitarian results.

I shall argue that our disagreements about equality, fairness, and justice have a depth similar to that of our disagreements about contraception, abortion, third-party-assisted reproduction, and physician-assisted suicide, in that they are not resolvable in general secular moral terms. The lesson of the post-modern era is that there are as many secular accounts of equality, justice, and fairness as there are religious groups, sects, and cults.[2] There is no principled basis for choosing a particular content-full account as canonical. As a consequence, establishing a particular content-full notion of equality, fairness, and justice in health care is the secular equivalent of establishing, for a secular national health-care system, the Roman Catholic proscriptions regarding contraception: it would be morally arbitrary and without secular moral justification. Consequently, there are robust secular moral limitations on the establishment of particular views of equality, limitations resulting from the centrality of human persons as the source of secular moral authority. There are good grounds for holding that current health-care policies, such as those embodied in Medicare, which forbid recipients from paying more for better basic care from participating physicians while coercing them to contribute to this program, are immoral. I argue in this essay that welfare rights in health care, if they are to be established, should be recognized as the creations of limited governmental insurance policies and not as expressions of foundational rights to health care or claims of equality or fairness.[3]

II. MEDICAL WELFARE: TEMPTATIONS AND DISAGREEMENTS IN THE FACE OF FINITUDE

Health care claims attention because of the dramatic ways in which medicine and the biomedical sciences address our finitude, vulnerability, and

---

From *Social Philosophy and Policy*, Vol. 14, No. 2, Summer 1997, 180–196. Reprinted with permission from Cambridge University Press.

Editors' note: Some notes have been deleted. Readers who wish to follow up on sources should consult the original article.

mortality. Political support for the governmental provision of health care often involves the view that to deny someone health care is to deny him or her protection against suffering, disease, disability, and death. The suppressed premise is that such a denial would be unfair. This view has difficulties. First, one must show how and why needs generate rights. Second, unlike food, clothing, and shelter, which can be provided at relatively minimal costs while still being sufficient for health and life, health care frequently confronts disabilities, diseases, disorders, and threats of death that cannot be overcome even with maximum medical efforts and the costs they involve. Often, illness can be cured only in part, suffering ameliorated only to some extent, disabilities remedied only to some degree, and death postponed only for a short time. In many cases, no matter how much one does, more resources could have been invested with some benefit for some recipients or possible recipients of health care. Just as ever more resources could be invested in avoiding accidental injuries and deaths by improving workplace safety, or invested in diminishing highway deaths by licensing only those cars that have front and side air bags as well as the front-end collision protection available in luxury cars, so, too, in medicine more resources could always be invested in preventive and curative endeavors without ever being fully successful against our finite, vulnerable, and mortal condition. Death and suffering are inescapable, so that we must decide what finite effort we should make to postpone death and avoid some suffering. We must ask whether there is secular moral authority coercively to impose one particular approach and whether it may be an egalitarian one.

The human condition itself conspires against discovering a generally convincing understanding of what should count as a basic adequate package of health-care services. First, there is the problem that medical knowledge is limited and probabilistic. Practicing medicine requires accepting that all life is a gamble, that medicine is a part of life, and that therefore health-care professionals must gamble with the suffering, disability, and death of all whom they treat. Moreover, resources that one might use to improve knowledge and technology are themselves limited. On the one hand, there is not enough money to avoid all suffering, disability, and death. On the other hand, there is not enough knowledge to know with certainty when particular interventions will succeed or fail. As a result, given the finitude of resources and the indefinite range of threats to well-being and life, investments in protection against suffering, disability, and death must take into account probabilities of success and failure. Investments must be limited and one must gamble.

To gamble, one must be willing to lose. Suppose that, as a matter of public policy, one has decided that in order to make good use of resources, one will not provide resources to the poor for a particular intervention—even when it might offer some protection against suffering, disability, and death—because the costs, probability of failure, and/or likely poor quality of results outweigh the possible benefits. In such a case, one must be willing to allow people to experience suffering, disability, and death when the resources are not available. One must also confront the circumstance that those with sufficient resources will purchase protection against death and suffering which is not available to all. In short, since ever more resources could always be invested in health care with some positive benefit, one faces two especially troubling policy questions: (1) May a basic, less-than-optimal package of health care be established for the poor? (2) May individuals, communities, and organizations use their own funds and energies to secure for themselves even better basic protection, as well as supplementary protection, against death and suffering? If secular morality (a) cannot reveal a content-full canonical morality that requires an egalitarian health-care policy, but (b) rather reveals that individuals are the source of secular moral authority, then one will need to endorse a national health-care policy that accepts both moral diversity and inequality.

III. BAD LUCK, UNFAIRNESS, AND INEQUALITY

If the authority of persons over themselves is morally legitimate, then individuals will, through their free choices, set limits to the realization of government-endorsed visions of the good and of human flourishing. Among the goods with which freedom will collide are those of equality and long life. To be free in any way that allows one to pursue particular goods or goals despite risks of death or disability is to be free to place oneself at risk of needing additional health care. To be free in any way that allows the acquisition of wealth as well as the giving and receiving of funds, valuables, and labor is to be free in ways that produce inequalities in opportunity and outcome. If the authority of governments is derived from the free consent of citizens, then citizens can freely limit governmental authority by withholding consent. Freedom brings into question the plausibility of a uniform and equal basic health-care entitlement. Insofar as people are free and have their own resources, some will take greater risks than others and some will purchase better protection than many can afford. Beyond that, one faces other persistent inequalities and a significant diversity of views about how one should respond to inequalities.

All will die, though some will die in their youth and others will live long lives. Inequality in health is, for many, especially vexing, since it involves significant differences in suffering and length of life. Still, differences in health status are not, on average, dramatically related to the level of access to high-cost health care. Cross-national comparative data concerning health-care investments and life expectancies suggest that differences in access to high-technology medicine pale in importance when compared to differences attributable to gender, income, and genetic luck. Women outlive men, the rich outlive the poor, and high-status individuals tend to outlive low-status individuals. For example, in the United Kingdom men and women in 1991 had life expectancies at birth of 73.2 and 78.8 years, respectively, while those in the United States had life expectancies of 72.0 and 78.9 years, respectively, though the United Kingdom invested $1,151 per person for health care, 7.1 percent of its gross domestic product, in comparison with the United States, which invested $3,094 per person, 13.6 percent of its gross domestic product. At age 80, the life expectancy was 6.3 years for men and 8.3 years for women in the United Kingdom, versus 7.2 years for men and 9.1 years for women in the United States. Though the differences in resource investment for health care likely express themselves in these differences in life expectancies at age 80, in absolute terms the differences due to gender still outweighed the differences between the two systems.

Given these data, a national health-care policy which focused on equality in mortality outcomes would most plausibly direct energies toward developing new ways to address the health needs of men and toward preventing pediatric deaths. Indeed, for egalitarians concerned with equality in life expectancies, a cross-national examination of life-expectancy outcomes by gender would seem to mandate a major commitment to the increased study of diseases of men, an increase in the representation of men in research protocols, and the development of better treatments for life-threatening conditions facing men. Such egalitarians would also favor the prevention of pediatric deaths over improvements in geriatric medicine, because of the robust inequalities in life presented, say, in the comparison between having a life span of twelve years versus one of seventy-two years. If one invokes an expository device such as John Rawls's original position,* one can easily imagine a characterization of the contractors such that they would regard those dying young as the least well-off, and would therefore direct energies against pediatric life-threatening conditions before directing resources to geriatric care, other than perhaps comfort care. A somewhat similar case can be made for directing medical research toward diseases afflicting the poor and persons of low status. In short, a dedicated pursuit of equality in mortality expectations should give priority to medical research and treatment development for men, children, the poor, and persons of low status.

Not all will agree with this approach, either in detail or in its foundations. Since we do not share one concrete morality, the very energies which direct our concerns toward medical issues separate us into disagreeing communities of moral commitment. Disputes regarding bioethics and health-care policy cut to the moral quick regarding equality, not only because individuals and communities differ with respect to the weight assigned to equality interests, but also because of the moral ambiguity of the term itself. If one is to develop an egalitarian policy, one must establish the importance and compelling moral authority of a particular form or understanding of equality. The difficulty is that our understandings of the importance of equality differ substantially.

**Editors' note:* See the Introduction.

To appreciate the force of these differences, one might imagine three worlds. The first world has ten people in it, each with six units of goodness or utility. In a second world there are nine people with six units of goodness or utility and one person with ten units. If one is on principle an egalitarian of outcomes, one will regard the second world as worse than the first, even though no one is worse off and the total amount of utility or goodness is greater. If one is morally concerned to rectify the inequalities of the second world, one will incline to what can be characterized as an egalitarianism of envy. That is, one will want all persons to be made equal, even when some have more without dispossessing those who have less. This attitude toward equality can be understood as a form of envy in the sense of an endorsed discontent with the good fortune of others, holding unequalizing good fortune to be unfair, even if it is not at the expense of others. Inequality in and of itself is regarded as a circumstance to be rectified in preference to and in priority over other goods or right-making conditions. Finally, one can consider a third world with nine people with six units of goodness or utility and one person with only one unit. If one wishes to improve the lot of the tenth person as cheaply and efficiently as possible, not because the person's share is unequal, but because that person lacks important goods and satisfactions, one can be characterized as endorsing an egalitarianism of altruism. One is not, in principle, concerned that some have more. Instead, one has sympathy for those who, in having less, lack a good.[4]

How one regards the inequalities presented in the descriptions of these three worlds is important for assessing how one regards inequalities in health care and elsewhere. This is especially significant for health-care policy, given that major differences in per-capita investments in health care across nations do not lead to dramatic differences in mortality expectations, once one has achieved a rather modest level of investment (e.g., Greece does very well with $452 of health care per person).[5] One must look to other considerations for the special place of equality in debates regarding health-care policy. Perhaps the special place given to equality in health care depends on (1) the ways in which medicine is felt to bear on our finitude, in particular, on the postponement of death and the blunting of suffering, as well as (2) the difficulties of steadfastly refusing to commit communal funds to rescue persons with expensive health needs, even when (a) some individuals with disposable resources may decide to have themselves treated when they have such needs, and (b) individuals without the funds demand such treatment. If one is to set limits on public health-care expenditures when it has been decided that the costs of such interventions on average outweigh the benefits, while recognizing the authority of persons to make choices about themselves and to use their resources as they wish, one must commit oneself to opposing high-cost last-minute state attempts at medical rescue for the poor and one must accept inequalities in access to health care.

Even if one were resolved to set egalitarian limits on health-care expenditures, one would still be confronted with a diversity of equalities. One would need a basis in principle for choosing among: an equality of opportunity in using one's own resources to pursue one's own health-care goals; an equality of opportunity supported by governmental funds in the acquisition of health care; an equality of opportunity supported by governmental funds and by proscriptions against unbalancing this equality by private purchases.[6] If one pursued an equality of outcome rather than an equality of opportunity, one would need to choose among: an equality of outcome supported by research and treatment directed toward avoiding the premature death of men, children, etc.; an equality of outcome directed toward equalizing the likelihood of suffering, including the use of nonvoluntary euthanasia; an equality of outcome directed toward equalizing wealth, etc. One would also need a basis for choosing among conflicting views of governmental authority that could be invoked in the coercive realization of a particular ethos of health-care delivery. Does the government have the moral authority only to ensure that the provision of health care will be honest and nonfraudulent? Does the government also have the moral authority to ensure that everyone receives the health care that the government deems to be appropriate? Does the government have the secular moral authority to forbid the rich from leaving the country in order to purchase better health care abroad?

At stake also are conflicting views of what it is for the state to own the resources which politicians might wish to redistribute for egalitarian purposes, and what it is for individuals and groups to have holdings independently of the state. For example, does one own resources because one has produced them or has been given those resources by those who have produced them? Or does one only own resources if such entitlements conform to a governmentally endorsed understanding of a desirable or right distribution of resources? For that matter, why are communal claims to possess resources advantaged over those made by individuals? In addition, one must decide what counts as just, fair, right, and good. For example, do needs generate rights, so that if resources are not available to meet health-care needs, such a state of affairs is unfair? Or are some outcomes simply unfortunate without being unfair? For instance, if certain screening programs can decrease the risk of developing cancer, does such protection against possible death count as a need that generates a right to a service for which others have a moral obligation to pay? Or is the nonprovision of such a service unfortunate, but not unfair? Or, if one's admission to a critical-care unit will convey a small chance of survival at a very high cost, does one have a need for health care that generates a right to the resources of others in order to purchase such critical care? Or is the nonavailability of such resources, save for the rich, simply unfortunate, not unfair?

There are, in addition, substantive disagreements regarding how to understand the relationship among individuals, communities, societies, and states. These disagreements are functions of different accounts of how one should characterize the communal, societal, and/or political space within which individuals find different kinds of morally authoritative structures. For example, should welfare, in the sense of group-provided insurance against losses in the natural and social lotteries,[7] be provided at the level of the state for all citizens, or instead at the level of particular communities and associations? One might envisage such provision occurring not just through companies, but also through religious and ideological groups. A number of these could transcend national boundaries, such as, perhaps, a worldwide Vaticare health-care welfare system for Roman Catholics, with the payment for care denominated in Vatican lira. Past history indicates that such approaches can succeed quite well even when they are unassociated with a particular religious or moral vision. In our contemporary postmodern world of deep disagreements regarding appropriate moral understandings of health care, such associations offer the opportunity of maintaining moral and religious integrity within structures committed to a particular vision of health care. Under such an arrangement, one will need to tolerate others' doing evil within their own associations; yet when associations (rather than governments) are the social structures which embody content-full moralities, one can distance oneself as a citizen from such undertakings and avoid immediate collaboration with what one recognizes as wrong.

IV. HEALTH-CARE WELFARE PROVISION: WHY IT IS SO INTRUSIVE AND PROBLEMATIC

The provision of health care as a basic uniform civil right is more intrusive than any other element of the welfare state: health care dramatically touches all the important passages of life, from reproduction and birth to suffering and death. The commitment to a particular package of services brings with it a particular interpretation of the significance of reproduction, birth, health, suffering, death, and equality (e.g., it involves specific positions regarding artificial insemination by donors, prenatal diagnosis with the possibility of selective abortion, physician-assisted suicide, voluntary active euthanasia, and unequal access to better basic health care). A uniform welfare right to health care involves endorsing and establishing one among a number of competing concrete moralities of life, death, and equality. Because of this tie to morally controversial interventions, the establishment of uniform, universal health-care welfare rights directly or indirectly involves citizens, patients, physicians, nurses, and others in receiving or providing health care in a health-care system which they may find morally opprobrious.

Since all elements of personal behavior have some impact on the likelihood of disease, disability, and death, the establishment of a uniform, encompassing health-care welfare system involves the risk of medically politicizing all elements of personal conduct. For example, how should one regard a person who smokes heavily? Does a smoker irresponsibly expose the nation's health-care system to unnecessary costs? Or is such an individual a superpatriot, supporting the long-term fiscal solvency of the government? That is, should one consider such an individual a cost-saver, taking into account not only the costs of health care for smoking-related illnesses, but also the Social Security obligations (which would increase if the person were to live a more wholesome, longer life), possible long-term Medicare costs (which would be incurred if the individual adopted wholesome, nonsmoking behaviors, and thus lived to be eligible), and possible long-term Medicaid costs (which would rise if the individual adopted wholesome, nonsmoking behaviors, lived longer, and developed Alzheimer's, etc.)? Should one also consider the affluence and therefore increased life expectancies that may result from wealth generated from the tobacco industry? Who burdens whom, and under what circumstances, depends on who pays as well as on the freedom of individuals to agree to engage in certain behaviors and to accept the consequences involved.

An encompassing health-care welfare entitlement does not merely tend to impose a particular vision of morality, human flourishing, and responsible risk-taking; it also tends to constrain the free choice of those with disposable resources. The notion of a guaranteed basic benefit package can take on a coercive character, so that individuals are not allowed to purchase better basic care but may only purchase additional care which is not provided through the guaranteed benefit package. For example, after being compelled by state force to contribute to a Medicare system, so-called beneficiaries may not offer more money for a covered service in order to gain access to a premier physician. Current Medicare law forbids Medicare patients from rewarding their physicians and health-care providers for better basic service. Nor may they legally offer to pay more for a longer, more careful provision of the basic services covered under Medicare. Once covered by Medicare for physician services, for example, they may not volunteer to pay five times the reimbursement schedule (i.e., have Medicare pay its fee and they pay four times that in addition) for a house call by a distinguished internist. In short, their resources are devalued by a system to which they are compelled to contribute and which will then not allow them to benefit from their required contributions if they wish to purchase better basic care. Substantive, coercively imposed health-care policies come into tension with the free and peaceable choices of individuals (e.g., the patient who might wish to purchase better basic care from a willing physician, while still receiving Medicare benefits which that patient has been compelled to fund).

Health-care welfare rights are, for all these reasons, problematic. The framing of health-care policy requires (1) gambling with human life, (2) accepting unavoidable inequalities in morbidity and mortality, (3) recognizing multiple and competing notions of equality in health care, and (4) acknowledging the intrusiveness of health-care rights if they bring with them particular moral visions of reproduction, suffering, and death. It also requires (5) appreciating the dangers of imposing a particular medicalized view of lifestyles in the service of health policy, and (6) noting the temptation to restrict free choices in order to achieve what is taken to be, on some particular understanding, a suitable level of efficiency or equity, while (7) confronting the diversity of our moral visions.

V. WHY THE MORAL DISPUTES WILL NOT GO AWAY, WHY WE ARE NOT ONE MORAL COMMUNITY WHEN IT COMES TO MATTERS OF HEALTH-CARE WELFARE PROVISION, AND WHY A PARTICULAR SUBSTANTIVE MORAL VISION OF FAIRNESS MAY NOT BE IMPOSED ON ALL

It is not merely a matter of fact or of sociological circumstance that we possess diverse understandings of the significance of reproduction, birth, disability, suffering, and death, as well as diverse understandings of how one ought to gamble in the face of finitude or how one ought to take account of our inequalities and disparate misfortunes with respect to death and suffering. The crucial point is that we do not possess the basis for resolving such controversies in terms of a content-full morality. The goal of demonstrating that we are one secular moral community—such that we ought to agree as a matter of justice, fairness, or moral probity regarding an all-encompassing health-care welfare system—is elusive. Rather than uniting citizens in a single moral community, the attempt to develop a uniform, encompassing health-care welfare right, as a matter of principle, and not only as a matter of fact, reveals our moral differences concerning the meaning and importance of equality, as well as our differences concerning the proper understanding of reproduction, suffering, and death.

The difficulty in resolving our moral controversies is foundational: one must already possess particular background moral premises, together with rules of moral evidence and inference, in order to resolve a moral controversy by sound rational argument. One needs a perspective from which one can make a morally authoritative choice among competing visions of the right and the good. An appeal to moral intuitions will not suffice. One's own moral intuitions will conflict with other moral intuitions. An appeal to ever-higher levels of moral intuition will not be decisive either, for further disagreements and appeals can in principle be extended indefinitely. Nor will an appeal to a consensus be any more successful. It will simply raise a number of questions: How does any particular consensus confer moral authority? How extensive must a consensus be to confer such authority? And from whom does such authority derive? (The appeal to consensus appears to invoke a secular version of a claim for the divine authority of majorities: *vox populi, vox Dei.*) In short, how much of a majority authorizes what use of force and why? In order to establish policy, one must know which substantive account of the right and/or the good is authoritative. However, the higher-level perspective from which one would make such a choice must itself be informed by an understanding of the right and/or the good.

Imagine that one agrees that a society—through public policy in general, and in health-care policy in particular—should attempt to maximize liberty, equality, prosperity, and security. To calculate and compare the consequences of alternative approaches, one must already know how to compare liberty, equality, prosperity, and security. The comparative consequences of competing approaches cannot be assessed simply by an appeal to consequences. One must already have an independent morality allowing one to compare the different kinds of outcomes at stake, namely, liberty consequences, equality consequences, prosperity consequences, and security consequences. Nor will attempting to maximize the preferences of citizens determine which health policy has the best consequences. One must first know how to compare impassioned versus rational preferences. One must know how, if at all, one is to revise or correct preferences. In addition, one will need to know God's discount rate for preference satisfaction over time; that is, one must have an absolute standard or must know whether each person's own standard should be used, whatever it might be, in the moment the person attempts the discounting. Nor will it do to appeal to a disinterested observer, a hypothetical chooser, or a set of hypothetical contractors. If such are truly disinterested, they will have no moral sense and will be unable to make a principled choice. To make a principled choice, they must already be informed by a particular moral sense or thin theory of the good. But of course, the choice of the correct moral sense or thin theory of the good is what is at stake. The same difficulty can be recapitulated for any account of moral rationality or of the decision-theoretic resolution of disputes. In order morally to assess behavior or policy, one must appeal to a standard. To use a standard, however, one must know which standard is morally canonical. The result is that a canonical content-full moral vision can be established as binding by sound rational argument only by begging the question. To choose with moral authority, one must already have authoritative normative guidance. The question is: "Which (and whose) guidance?"

Postmodernity as an epistemological predicament, not merely as a sociological fact, is the recognition that, outside of a revelation of a canonical standard, one cannot authoritatively choose among content-full understandings of moral probity, justice, or fairness without begging the question or engaging in an infinite regress. In order to show how a conclusion is warranted, one must always ask whose moral rationality, which sense of justice, is being invoked. At the same time, one must recognize that there are numerous competing moral accounts or narratives. As we have seen, there are numerous and competing understandings of the importance and significance of equality. In such a circumstance, if all do not listen to God, so as to find revealed to them the canonical content-full notion of moral probity, fairness, justice, and equality, and if all attempts by sound rational argument to establish the canonical content-full account of moral probity, justice, and fairness beg the question, then one can arrive at moral authority when individuals meet as moral strangers, not by drawing authority either from God or from reason, but only from the permission of those who participate. Moral authority will not be the authority of God or reason, but of consent, agreement, or permission. General secular moral authority is thus best construed as authorization.[8] The practice of deriving moral authority from permission makes possible a sparse practice of secular morality that does not presume any particular content-full view of the right or the good.

In such circumstances, permission or the authority it provides becomes the source of moral authority without any endorsement of permission as either good or bad. The securing of permission provides authority even when it does not provide motivation (permission does secure secular moral authority for the appropriate, albeit limited, use of state coercion, which can motivate compliance with the practice of deriving authority from permission). The point is that it is possible to secure a justification for state coercion and to determine which instances of coercion carry secular moral authority. The question is not "What will motivate moral action?" (though this issue is important), or "What level of moral disagreement makes governance difficult or impossible?" (or, for that matter, "What strategies by governments support public peace or effective governance?"). The question is, rather, "Under what circumstances can those ruling claim secular moral authority, so that those who disobey laws are not only at risk of being punished, but also at risk of being blameworthy?" Acting with permission offers a sparse, right-making condition for the collaboration of individuals who do not share a common understanding of what God demands or what moral rationality requires, but who claim an authority for their common endeavors.

Secular morality is procedural, and its legitimacy is limited by the consent of those who participate in common endeavors. Consequently, the paradigm moral activities of secular morality are the free market, contract formation, and the establishment of limited democracies.

In particular, democracies will have only that secular moral authority which can be derived either from the actual consent of all their members or from the practice of never using persons without their permission. The result will be that one will at most be able to justify the material equivalent of Robert Nozick's ultraminimal state. The point is that, in the absence of a canonical, content-full secular morality, (1) health-care policy must derive its authority from the consent of the governed, (2) not from a prior understanding of justice, fairness, or equality, and (3) may not be all-encompassing, because the scope of its authority is limited by the limits of the consent of those involved. One will need to create policy instead of attempting to discover guidance in secular morality. One must proceed not by an appeal to a canonical, content-full understanding of the right or the good, but by an appeal to the permission of those involved. There will be no way to discover the correct balance among the various undertakings to which a community could direct its resources (e.g., how one should use common funds when faced with the claims of partisans of whooping cranes versus those of aged humans). As a consequence, limited democracies will be obliged to leave space so that individuals and communities can peaceably pursue their own visions of human flourishing and of appropriate health care. Still, if the state has legitimately acquired common resources, it is at liberty to create limited policy answers. One can explore many of the secular moral limits in health-care policy without attending to the general secular moral limits on state authority, by assuming that the state possesses legitimately acquired funds.[9]

VI. TAKING MORAL DIVERSITY AND LIMITED DEMOCRACY SERIOUSLY

The concern to establish health-care welfare provision is encumbered by a cluster of moral difficulties tied to the inability to establish, by sound rational argument, a canonical morality regarding equality in access, not to mention regarding such important issues as third-party-assisted reproduction, abortion, physician-assisted suicide, and euthanasia. Though there is, on the part of many, a strong desire to establish an encompassing and equal right to health care, there are even stronger grounds for recognizing the morally problematic character of this desire. The substantial and significant differences in moral vision concerning matters of equality—and concerning the appropriate ways to regard reproduction, birth, suffering, and death—make any uniform, governmentally imposed right to health care highly morally problematic. Such an imposition would involve the secular equivalent of establishing a particular religious morality. If we do not share a common understanding of equality, fairness, and justice, and if there is in principle no way through sound rational argument to determine which understanding of justice, fairness, and equality should guide governmental undertakings, and if, in addition, health care is particularly intrusive and morally troubling when it brings with it a content-full moral understanding of reproduction, birth, suffering, and death, then the provision of any general protection against morbidity and mortality is best offered as a limited insurance against losses in the natural and social lotteries.

These considerations argue against any particular universally mandated set of health-care services and in favor of the equivalent of a voucher for the poor, which would allow the purchase of health care from various morally different health-care delivery networks. The limits of secular moral authority require acquiescing in the creation of health-care networks and associations providing morally different forms of basic health care. The only restrictions that may be imposed with secular moral authority will involve the guarantee that participants in the various health-care networks join freely in the particular medical moralities they choose.

In order to establish a limited welfare right to health care without going aground on diverse visions of moral probity and justice, secular health-care provision for the indigent may not be justified in terms of a particular account of equality, fairness, or justice, nor may it establish a particular medical morality regarding reproduction, suffering, and death. The use of vouchers could avoid much of this difficulty if such vouchers could be applied to different alternative, basic menus of service. Different communities or associations with different moral visions could then establish morally competing health-care systems into which individuals could enter for basic services using such vouchers. Better yet would be a policy that avoided even the necessity of establishing basic menus of service and instead allowed the use of health-care purchase accounts to which funds could be provided for the poor to use in purchasing basic medical services.

Under such circumstances, the government would provide basic health-care protection against morbidity and mortality for the indigent without imposing a content-full morality. Medical needs could be both defined and addressed in a range of significantly different terms. In a truly free and limited democracy, competing health-care systems could come into existence to take advantage of the availability of the health-care vouchers (as well as the availability of payments from private insurers and direct payments from patients). For the sake of illustration, one could imagine two systems, one supported by Roman Catholics and another by New Age agnostics. The first would not offer artificial insemination by donors, prenatal diagnosis and abortion, or physician-assisted suicide and euthanasia. It would provide limitations on health-care expenditures in terms of religious understandings of the appropriate line between proportionate and disproportionate care, that is, between ordinary and extraordinary care. This line would vary with the social status of the individual (i.e., it would be *proportionem status*). In addition, religiously attentive hospice and comfort care would be offered to all.

In contrast, the system appealing to agnostic New-Agers would offer artificial insemination for unmarried women, prenatal diagnosis and selective abortion, and specially discounted treatment with an agreement to be euthanatized under certain conditions when health care is unlikely to provide a significant extension of life with an acceptable quality. Hospice care would be tied to effective and painless euthanasia. A voucher system or health-care purchase account that took moral diversity seriously would allow individuals to avoid interventions they recognized as morally inappropriate and to purchase in their stead those they saw as acceptable (or to select care so as to achieve a savings of funds). The result would be a policy that provided basic protection against health-care needs without establishing one view of equality and medical moral probity as dominant over the others.

The data indicate that such a basic welfare package would afford significant mortality protection. If individuals were left free to choose particular packages of basic health care (offered within particular medical moralities and constrained only by the free consent of the participants), then help could be provided for the poor while avoiding the significant moral costs of generally imposing one of the many secular medical moralities at the expense of the others. Such an approach to health-care policy would require accepting our finitude, including the limits of governmental moral authority, while acknowledging our moral diversity.

NOTES

1. The White House Domestic Policy Council, *The President's Health Security Plan* (New York: Times Books, 1993), presents a robustly egalitarian blueprint for health-care policy. In its "Ethical Foundations of Health Reform," the Clinton plan rejects a tiered system: "The system should avoid the creation of a tiered system providing care based only on differences of need, not individual or group characteristics" (p. 11). When the plan recommends that a new federal criminal statute be enacted prohibiting "the payment of bribes, gratuities or other inducements to administrators and employees of health plans, health alliances or state health care agencies" (p. 199), the goal is *inter alia* to proscribe payment to physicians for better basic care. The implications and the stated purpose of the plan are egalitarian.
2. I take it that the postmodern era is characterized by the circumstance, as a matter of sociological fact, (1) that all people do not share the same moral narrative or account, and (2) that this moral diversity is apparent and widely recognized. Moreover, as a matter of our epistemological condition, (3) there is no way to establish in purely secular terms the correct moral narrative or account without begging the question or engaging in an infinite regress, and (4) this is also widely recognized.
3. See also H. Tristram Engelhardt, Jr., *Bioethics and Secular Humanism: The Search for a Common Morality* (Philadelphia: Trinity Press International, 1991), esp. pp. 130–38.
4. One might interpret the so-called Oregon proposal as driven by an egalitarianism of altruism. Oregon proposed limiting the range of health-care resources available to Medicaid recipients so that all the poor could be covered. The proposal was that all the poor should be insured, although (1) Medicaid recipients would not receive the same level of health care as previously, and (2) the affluent would be able to purchase better basic care, as well as luxury care (i. e., there would be a tiered provision of health care with a limited package for the poor and with the affluent left free to purchase whatever they wished and could afford).
5. Schieber, Poullier, and Greenwald, "Health System Performance."
6. Norman Daniels provides a justification of an egalitarian approach to health care that, in the service of equality of opportunity, advances arguments for proscribing the purchase of better basic diagnostic and therapeutic interventions. See Norman Daniels, *Just Health Care* (New York: Cambridge University Press, 1985). Daniels was among the advisory members of the White House Task Force on National Health Reform, which developed President Clinton's 1993 health-care reform proposal.
7. The term "natural and social lotteries" identifies the natural and social forces that advantage and disadvantage individuals irrespective of their deserts: some live long and healthy lives, while others contract serious diseases and die young (examples of the natural lottery); some inherit fortunes, while others are born destitute (examples of the social lottery).
8. Moral constraints do exist within secular morality; they are derived from the right-making character of appeals to permission as the only source of authority in secular public policy. Even if all do not listen to God, and if reason cannot disclose a canonical content-full moral vision, one can still derive authority from common agreement, that is, from permission. See Engelhardt, *The Foundations of Bioethics*, 2nd ed. (New York: Oxford University Press, 1996), pp. 135–88.
9. I do not here explore the considerable difficulties faced in providing a general secular moral justification for taxation. Instead, attention is directed to how one ought to proceed in using common resources, presuming that they can be acquired legitimately. For my treatment of issues bearing on the legitimacy of taxation, see *The Foundations of Bioethics*, pp. 154–80.

METHODS AND STRATEGIES FOR RATIONING HEALTH CARE

BONE MARROW TRANSPLANTS FOR ADVANCED BREAST CANCER: THE STORY OF CHRISTINE DEMEURERS

Alex John London

It was a frightening discovery.[1] At 32, Christine deMeurers was an active woman with a husband, two children, and a new job as a school teacher. It was 1992 and in the heat of late August the deMeurers were unprepared for the turn their lives were about to take. Christine had been at her new job for less than two months when she found a small lump in her left breast. A visit to her physician and some tests revealed that her worst fears were true; Christine had breast cancer.

The reality of her situation hit like a thunderclap. The speed with which breast cancer is treated can mean the difference between life and death, and the deMeurers knew it. Moving as quickly as possible, Christine underwent a radical mastectomy, radiation therapy, and a course of chemotherapy which ended in March of 1993. By May it was clear that her cancer had spread and Christine was told she had Stage IV metastatic breast cancer.

Like many Americans, the deMeurers received their health insurance through their employer, and like a growing number of people in this country they were members of a managed care plan. Christine had recently been hired to teach at the same school in Elsinore, California, where her husband had been teaching since 1989, and they had each signed up for the least expensive of the three health plans their school offered, Health Net of Woodland Hills, California.

There is no reason to think that the deMeurers were unhappy with the treatment Christine had received from Health Net by the end of March 1993. Although it had not stopped the spread of her cancer, Christine had received prompt and aggressive treatment for a disease that affects 1 of every 9 American women and is the second leading cause of cancer deaths among women. At the end of these first months of 1993, Christine had exhausted the standard therapies that were available at the time, and it looked as though her cancer would soon overtake her.

Yet Christine's oncologist, Dr. Mahesh Gupta, offered hope. He suggested that Christine might be a candidate for a new procedure known as high-dose chemotherapy with autologous bone marrow transplant, or HDC/ABMT. Although the use of this procedure on women with Stage IV breast cancer was new and its efficacy largely unknown, HDC/ABMT was already accepted as a successful treatment of many non-solid forms of cancer such as Hodgkins disease and leukemia. The theory behind the procedure is simple. There is a direct correlation between the dose of chemotherapy a patient receives and its effect on the targeted cancer. The problem, however, is that there is a natural limit to the amount of these toxic agents the body can endure. In HDC/ABMT physicians remove stem cells from a patient's bone marrow, purify them of cancer cells, and then freeze them for later use. Patients are then exposed to near lethal doses of chemotherapy, up to 10 times the normal level. In addition to killing cancer cells, however, such concentrated amounts of these potent chemicals inevitably kill much of the patient's remaining bone marrow. So after receiving this high dose of chemotherapy the harvested and purified stem cells are transplanted back into the patient. There was, nevertheless, very little information and certainly no consensus among experts as to the efficacy of this procedure on solid tumors like Christine's.

Nevertheless, Dr. Gupta assured Christine that there were still options available, and in a breach of Health Net policy he referred her directly to a colleague at the Scripps Clinic in nearby La Jolla. Dissatisfied with their reception there, the deMeurers flew to Denver where Christine was evaluated by Dr. Roy B. Jones at the University of Colorado. Unlike their reception at Scripps, the deMeurers found a welcome ally in Dr. Jones who examined Christine on June 8, 1993 and told her that she might benefit from the HDC/ABMT procedure. It was a ray of hope in a very dark period of their lives.

On the same day that Christine was being examined by Dr. Jones, however, Health Net formally decided not to pay for the procedure on the grounds that the treatment "is not uniformly accepted as proven and effective for the treatment of metastatic breast cancer." The treatment was excluded under the so-called "investigational clause" in the Health Net contract. The deMeurers were crushed, but undaunted. Together they decided to try to obtain the new procedure any way they could, and they began taking every step possible. Christine secured permission to see a new oncologist who agreed with Dr. Jones' assessment of her situation and agreed to refer her to UCLA medical center. At the same time they began trying to raise the $100,000 it would take to pay for the procedure, and they hired a lawyer to write a formal appeal to Health Net's decision on Christine's behalf.

On June 25, Christine met with Dr. John Glaspy at the UCLA medical center who spelled out the risks involved with the procedure itself, the three months it would take to recover from the severity of the chemotherapy, and the rather steep price tag it entailed. Dr. Glaspy was himself a cautious proponent of the use of HDC/ABMT on women with Stage IV breast cancer, even though a 1992 review article by the respected health policy expert Dr. David Eddy had concluded that there were no data to support the claim that this procedure was in any way superior to the standard dose of chemotherapy when treating women with metastatic breast cancer.[2] Cautious but optimistic, Dr. Glaspy said that he would perform the procedure if that was what they wanted. The deMeurers readily accepted.

What Dr. Glaspy did not know, what the deMeurers had purposefully made sure he would not know, was that Christine was a member of the Health Net plan. Wary of the influence that they suspected Health Net administrators had already exerted on the course of Christine's care, the deMeurers had decided to present themselves to Dr. Glaspy as paying customers rather than as members of a managed care plan. Ironically, this also prevented the deMeurers from finding out that Dr. Glaspy was a member of the Health Net committee which earlier that year had voted to deny coverage for bone marrow transplants to patients with Stage IV breast cancer.

Soon after their visit to UCLA, the deMeurers learned that Health Net had rejected their appeal. Preliminary tests at UCLA had shown that Christine's cancer had responded to initial doses of chemotherapy, but it was also quickly becoming clear that they would be unable to raise such a substantial amount of money on their own. So the deMeurers authorized their attorney to file for an injunction to force Health Net to pay for treatment and they enlisted Dr. Glaspy's help. The revelation that Christine was a member of Health Net put Dr. Glaspy in a terrible position. As a member of Health Net's transplantation committee, he had advocated covering HDC/ABMT for metastatic breast cancer. But in the end he had agreed with the committee's consensus to exclude it from coverage. Committed to advocating for his patient's interests, on September 13 Dr. Glaspy wrote to Health Net in support of Christine's injunction, "As a physician representing Christine, I have a responsibility to represent her interests and to help her achieve her goals in her health care." Exactly one week later, however, at the request of Health Net lawyers, he submitted a second, much less sanguine statement to Health Net concluding "This procedure is of unproven efficacy in the treatment of metastatic breast cancer, and the results of clinical trials to date are not sufficient to establish beyond doubt that it is superior to standard dose chemotherapy."

The deMeurers felt betrayed and alone. The second letter from Dr. Glaspy only strengthened their resentment of Health Net and their distrust of its doctors. Dr. Glaspy was also painfully aware of the blow he had dealt to the deMeurer's trust. But he was also aware of the dissatisfaction his first letter had caused at Health Net, especially in light of the fact that he was a member of the committee that voted not to cover this procedure. Health Net was upset that a member of its own committee was actively trying to thwart the very regulations he had helped to design, and the phone calls of Health Net officials to Dr. Glaspy's boss, Dr. Dennis Slamon, revealed the depth of the company's dissatisfaction.

In an attempt to salvage as much of the medical center's relationship with the deMeurers and with Health Net as possible, Dr. Slamon arrived at a compromise. He decided that UCLA would absorb the costs of Christine's procedure, thus relieving Health Net of any obligation to pay and enabling Christine to receive the health care she so desperately wanted. On September 23, 1993 Christine was admitted to UCLA to begin the first phase of treatment. According to her husband, she experienced four disease-free months after recovering from the severe chemotherapy, but by the Spring of 1994 she was ill again and on March 10, 1995 Christine deMeurers succumbed to her cancer.

The story of Christine deMeurers is not typical of most people's experience with managed care, but because it is such an extreme case it casts some of the most serious problems facing the American health care system into stark relief. It is the story of a family coping with a terrible disease and unifying around the common cause of exhausting every possible treatment option. It is also the story of a woman who must not only battle cancer, but must also struggle with her insurance company for the treatment she so desperately wants. Similarly, Christine's story illustrates the way physicians have found themselves trapped between two worlds of health care. In Dr. Glaspy we see the old fee-for-service system and the new medicine under managed care clashing in its most palpable form. In these ways, Christine's story is a miniature portrait of the way we think about health care in America and the problems we are facing as the cost of care outstrips our collective ability to pay for it.

After World War II, medical research in the United States flourished, and the marriage of increased research funding with top-flight science gave birth to a formidable array of new therapeutic drugs and devices that enabled physicians to conquer injuries and diseases in a way that would have been unthinkable only years earlier. As amazing as the feats such advances were making possible, however, was the price tag that came with them. The nation's health care expenditures began to climb sharply in the post-war years, and by 1976 General Motors announced that it was spending more money on the health care of its workers than on steel. As the decade drew to a close there was a collective recognition on the part of the corporate sector that something had to be done to keep the cost of health care from hemorrhaging out of control.[3]

Because most Americans receive their health insurance through their employers, the corporate sector was coming to see the high cost of their employees' benefits as a threat to their ability to remain competitive. The choice seemed terrible but unavoidable. How long before industry would have to choose between competitive viability and employee health care? It was in response to this dilemma that managed care companies like Health Net arose with the mandate of stemming the swiftly rising tide of health care costs.

In an important way, the rise of managed care and our reaction to the way it has tried to carry out its mandate illustrates the fundamentally paradoxical relationship that Americans have to medicine in general and to their health care providers in particular. On the one hand, we embrace the values of frugality and fiscal sensibility which lead us to protest against the dizzying rate at which health care costs have been rising. At the same time, we will not tolerate receiving anything less than the latest, most sophisticated health care.[4] We don't want to see restrictions put on our liberty when it comes to being able to seek out and obtain the latest and most advanced medical procedures from the most well-trained providers, yet we also bristle at the restrictions on our liberty that come in the form of the higher taxes, product prices, or insurance premiums that inevitably result from the exercise of this freedom.

In the story of Christine deMeurers we have a concrete and powerful illustration of the way these conflicting values can intersect in the lives of the most vulnerable people. Christine represents the way we have come to look to the frontiers of medicine in the face of the ravages of sickness and disease. Here is a young, productive woman with a life of her own, a family, children, who is also dying from a terrible disease. When the standard modalities of treatment are exhausted, she looks to the frontiers of medical science and places her hopes in a relatively untested procedure of questionable therapeutic value for the chance to live out some portion of her remaining months free of disease. With no other medical options and without the resources to secure this chance for herself, she looks to a third party to cover the expenses and make it possible.

Debate over the benefit that receiving HDC/ABMT had for Christine deMeurers is still mixed. The officials at Health Net stick by their initial decision to deny coverage and Dr. Glaspy admits that Christine would probably have lived longer without the treatment. Clinical trials to test the efficacy of the procedure are under way in a number of cities across the country, but there is still no consensus on whether HDC/ABMT is more effective than standard chemotherapy for women with metastatic breast cancer. For Alan deMeurers, however, the procedure was worth it. It allowed his wife to live a better quality of life for a few short months and to spend one final Christmas with him and their two children. Even if Dr. Glaspy is right, it is the quality of the life Christine led for those four months that matters most to her husband, not simply the length of time she remained alive.

The public reaction to cases like Christine's has mostly been one of outrage. The media was critical of the influence Health Net officials exerted on the medical decisions of the program's physicians, and juries were eager to teach the plan's plutocratic administrators a lesson. In 1993 Health Net lost a lawsuit filed by Jim Fox, the husband of Nelene Fox, a Health Net subscriber who had been denied HDC/ABMT for her Stage IV breast cancer on the grounds that it was experimental and investigational. The jury awarded Nelene's estate $12 million in actual damages and $77 million in punitive damages, although Health Net later agreed to pay only $5 million in exchange for their right to appeal the verdict. Nevertheless, the members of the jury were eager to send a message to health care companies. "You cannot substitute profits for good-quality health care," one juror was quoted as saying.

The Fox verdict precipitated a rash of similar judgments on behalf of women who had been denied coverage for HDC/ABMT for advanced breast cancer, and in 1995 a California arbitration board awarded one million dollars to the estate of Christine deMeurers on the ground that phone calls which Health Net officials had placed to Christine's physicians at various stages in her treatment had exerted undue influence on the doctor-patient relationship. In addition to a fury of litigation, these cases have given rise to legislation in a number of states requiring insurers to pay for HDC/ABMT for women with metastatic breast cancer. The result of these suits and of state congressional action has been to free up patients' access to specialists and to procedures which their insurance providers would otherwise have excluded as investigational or experimental. Yet, amidst the lurid details of some of the questionable activities on the part of officers at Health Net and other HMOs, and in the rush to right what look like injustices that were being perpetrated against the women who were denied access to HDC/ABMT, we seem to have lost sight of the difficult but enduring questions at the very heart of this issue. Should we, should the government or insurance companies, pay for people's access to procedures of this nature? Should we pay for costly medical procedures of unknown therapeutic benefit when there are people struggling to get access to a host of genuinely effective therapies? Are four disease-free months in the life of a terminally ill person worth the $100,000 to $200,000 it takes to secure them? Could this money be better spent somewhere else? If we do not draw the line on medical expenses in front of cases like this, then where do we draw it?

In the wake of cases like those of the deMeurers and the Foxes, we have struggled with these questions in a very piecemeal and largely inchoate way. On the one hand, the judiciary has consistently sided with plaintiffs in these cases, making it very clear that those with the resources to make themselves heard and with voices articulate enough to make their case compelling can receive access to these sorts of therapies while the less articulate and less well-off cannot. On the other hand, as of the end of 1995 at least seven states had mandated coverage for HDC/ABMT for breast cancer although such mandates do not necessarily apply to all forms of insurance providers, and it is rare that such mandates are formulated around a coherent set of health care goals.[5]

The patchwork of judicial and legislative decisions rendered in response to these cases amounts to a de facto way of answering the difficult questions posed a moment ago. But surely this is no way to deal with such important and fundamental issues of public policy. The system may provide greater access for some, but in a way that seems arbitrary at best and inequitable or unjust at worst. We may benefit from the psychological comforts of avoiding some very public, "tragic choices," but this is very likely the illusory comfort of the fine new garments the Emperor is wearing.[6] We have to ask ourselves whether we have responded to these cases in such a way as to make the system more just, or whether we haven't simply shifted the burden of injustice off of those who are most capable of defending themselves onto those who are least able to do so.

By acquiescing to the de facto practice that has emerged for dealing with these cases, we have done ourselves, our health care providers, and our third-party payers a terrible disservice. We have left unanswered important questions about which kinds of medical interventions we should be in the business of helping people obtain. We have left the insurance industry without substantive guidelines by which to determine the kinds of interventions they need to cover and the kinds they may need to exclude. This in turn perpetuates a system of disclosure on the part of insurers which keeps subscribers largely in the dark as to the nature of excluded therapies, the methods used for making such determinations, and the process by which the subscriber can influence these guidelines or appeal such decisions. This may have provided litigious subscribers with the power to obtain exotic medical interventions, but the system in which this kind of arbitrary power exists seems to work against our common commitment to reducing health care costs and to spreading the burdens of doing so evenly among the members of society. To that extent, the maintenance of this piecemeal way of creating public policy works against many of our own explicit and publicly held commitments to fairness and fiscal responsibility.

This leaves subscribers with the unenviable feeling of being trapped in an unfriendly system that has been imposed on them from above. In the absence of some form of communal conversation about these difficult and enduring questions, we will make little headway against the antagonistic and largely adversarial relationship developing between patients, their insurance providers, and the health care workers who are increasingly asked to facilitate the very different aims of these two parties.[7] We need to ask ourselves why so many of these cases wound up in the judicial system. Would subscribers who were given a more active role in the creation of policy guidelines or in the decision-making process of their insurance provider feel the need to take their claims to court? How can we facilitate a more active role for subscribers? Similarly, are there ways we could improve the system so that subscribers whose claims have been denied can appeal their decision and feel that their needs are receiving legitimate and sincere consideration? Would subscribers be as eager to litigate if they felt their claims had received fair consideration in an equitable review process? Would lawsuits have as much merit if insurance companies could point to such a process of appeal?

By giving subscribers a more active role in the formation of the guidelines that govern their care, insurance providers will give their subscribers a stake in making sure such guidelines are both fair and effective. It will also reassure subscribers that they are being treated as ends in themselves and not as mere means. But in order to accomplish these goals we are going to have to improve the way that insurance providers disclose information to their subscribers, and this means that providers and subscribers alike are going to have to deliberate together on how to answer some very important questions. In the case of HDC/ABMT this means that we are going to have to ask whether women with advanced breast cancer should receive coverage for this procedure, and if not, why not.

Health Net, like most managed care companies, denied coverage for HDC/ABMT on the grounds that it was investigational or experimental. The rationale behind this move was simple. First, insurers could make a strong case that there is only an obligation to pay for therapies that are proven to have some therapeutic benefit. The case for this normative claim looks especially strong when we add the premise that there are not even enough resources to cover everyone's access to proven therapies. Second, with this argument on the table the claim that a drug or a procedure is experimental looks more like a straightforward descriptive claim than it does a controversial normative judgment. So excluding an intervention as experimental allowed the insurance provider to maintain the appearance of making coverage decisions without having to make delicate and controversial judgments about the monetary value of the length and quality of human life. Finally, this general attitude toward experimental treatments was perfectly consistent with the public's view of human experimentation in the wake of scandals such as Willowbrook, Tuskegee, and the Jewish Chronic Disease Hospital case.* That is, the denial of access to experimental drugs and procedures fit nicely with the public's view that such things were usually dangerous and to be avoided.

In the 1980s, however, social attitudes towards experimental treatments started to change as patients dying of AIDS began to clamor for access to the experimental drugs and devices which were being held up in what they came to view as a paternalistic system of federal oversight. In the 1980s experimental drugs and procedures came to be seen, not as dangerous things to which no one wanted to be subjected, but rather as the last desperate hope for dying patients. This shift in attitude put pressure on the normative claim that people should not receive access to experimental drugs, but it also brought into question the notion that labeling something as experimental was a purely descriptive and non-normative claim.

Time and again the insurance industry's claim that HDC/ABMT was experimental was challenged by lawyers and physicians. What makes a drug or procedure experimental? Is it the fact that it is not a part of the established medical practice? But medicine is a notoriously recalcitrant social practice and it can take some time for innovative and effective procedures to be widely adopted. This raises the question of whose medical practice we are talking about. Are we concerned with the standard practices of the larger medical community or only of the most knowledgeable experts? Lawyers had no problem finding expert oncologists to testify about the number of their colleagues who were performing HDC/ABMT on women with advanced breast cancer at some of the most prestigious medical institutions in the world. So if this was the criterion for something's being "experimental," HDC/ABMT didn't seem to fit the bill. Perhaps then something is experimental when it has not received FDA approval. But many of the drugs and procedures involved in HDC/ABMT had received FDA approval for other uses, and there are many drugs and procedures that are used effectively for purposes for which they were not initially approved. Also, FDA approval often requires that a procedure's efficacy be shown in a randomized clinical trial, but there are difficult moral problems associated with conducting this kind of trial on a procedure of this sort.

As a result, in case after case, judges and juries told managed care companies that the experimental

*_Editor's note:_ See Part 5, Section 1.

exclusion clause in their subscriber contract did not apply to HDC/ABMT for advanced breast cancer. But these judgments were based on the inadequate definitions offered by the managed care companies. They should not be taken as speaking to the underlying question of whether this is the sort of treatment third parties should be financing. If policy holders and their providers are going to have an open and productive debate about this question, then they are going to have to ask frank questions about the kinds of health care goals they are willing to support and to what degree. Undoubtedly this is going to require each of us to look at the giant pink elephant standing in the middle of the room: How much money are we willing to spend to improve the quality of a terminally ill patient's life for a few months given the other kinds of health care needs our plan must meet?

The questions raised by cases like that of Christine deMeurers are often perceived as instances of the familiar and intractable conflict between consequentialist concerns about money and utility and deontic concerns for the dignity of persons. Although they can easily be understood along these lines, it is important to see that this is not the only or necessarily the best way to think about them. It is true that a careful look at the historical record will show that at the time, many of these cases may have in fact been about a straightforward conflict between money and autonomy. But this might simply be evidence for the inadequacy of this way of structuring the problem rather than for the claim that this is the only way to structure it.

One thing seems clear. To the extent that plan members are forced to submit to policies which they themselves have not either helped to shape or voluntarily chosen, people will continue to feel that someone else has put a price on the length and quality of their lives, and this will continue to foster feelings of antagonism and resentment.[8] To the extent that plan members can actively participate in shaping the policies which govern their treatment or choose their plan based on the policies that best reflect their conception of the value of health care, the restrictions placed on their care will represent an extension of their own autonomy. To that extent they will represent people's considered judgments about the way their needs should be met given the fact of fiscal scarcity and the need to distribute the benefits and burdens of health care fairly amongst the members of the plan. Considerations of costs and benefits may be important factors which shape these decisions, but in the end the moral legitimacy of these decisions will be based on the fact that the resulting policies are the product of the autonomous and considered judgments of the very people they are meant to cover.

In the end, the story of Christine deMeurers confronts us with two basic and interconnected problems. First, how should we answer the difficult questions with which this case confronts us? Second, how can we make sure that there are not more cases like this? How can we ensure that there are structures in place which will facilitate our ability to deliberate about these questions together, and which will reflect the conclusions that such deliberations reach? How can we shape the practices and procedures of our health care system in a way that will facilitate and accommodate this increased interaction between providers, subscribers, and health care workers? We should not shrink from making these difficult decisions together or from the recognition that some of these choices may be tragic, so long as we can maintain the conviction that the decisions we make are fair and that the system we create is more just than the one we have now.

NOTES

1. The details presented here about Christine deMeurers' battle with breast cancer and her HMO have been taken from published accounts by Erik Larson, "The Soul of an HMO," *Time Magazine* (January 22, 1996) and George Anders, *Health Against Wealth* (New York: Houghton Mifflin Company, 1996), chapter seven.
2. David Eddy, "High Dose Chemotherapy with Autologous Bone Marrow Transplantation for the Treatment of Metastatic Breast Cancer," *Journal of Clinical Oncology* 1992, 10(4):657–670.
3. For a more detailed account of the rise of managed care see E. Haavi Morreim, *Balancing Act: The New Medical Ethics of Medicine's New Economics* (Washington, D.C.: Georgetown University Press, 1995) pp. 8–17 and George Anders, *Health Against Wealth* op cit.
4. For a trenchant criticism of the conflicting views Americans have about health and health care see Daniel Callahan, *What Kind of Life* (Washington, D.C.: Georgetown University Press, 1994).

5. Reinhard Priester, Karen G. Gervais and Dorothy E. Vawter, *Improving Coverage for Unproven Health Care Interventions* (Minnesota Center for Health Care Ethics, August, 1996), p. 5.
6. For the view that we should avoid the appearance of making tragic choices, even when the choices themselves are unavoidable, see Guido Calabresi and Philip Bobbitt, *Tragic Choices* (New York: W. W. Norton and Company, 1978).
7. For an analysis of the way the interests of these three parties can conflict and some suggestions for managing these conflicts see my "Thrasymachus and Managed Care: How Not to Think About the Craft of Medicine" in Ronald Polansky and Mark Kuczewski, eds. *Bioethics: Ancient Themes in Contemporary Issues.* (Cambridge: MIT Press, 2000).
8. For a view of the importance of subscriber consent within a managed care plan, see Paul T. Menzel, *Strong Medicine* (New York: Oxford University Press, 1990). For the importance of being able to select a plan that coheres with one's vision of the role of health care in one's life, see Ezekiel J. Emanuel, *The Ends of Human Life* (Cambridge: Harvard University Press, 1991).

THE INDIVIDUAL VS. SOCIETY: RESOLVING THE CONFLICT

David M. Eddy

An individual can be in conflict with society whenever the individual uses a disproportionate amount of a health care service without paying for it.[1] This either forces others to cover the cost of replacing the service or, if the cost is not repaid and the service is not replaced, deprives others of the benefits of the service. The first causes others financial harm. The second causes harm to their health. In either case, the "others" are what we call "society."

If the individual is incapable of paying, and if the service is considered essential,[2] then the use of such a service is considered acceptable; it is viewed as part of society's obligation to individuals in need. However, as the individual's ability to pay increases, as the benefit provided by the service decreases, and as the cost of the service increases, the conflict grows.

THE SOURCE OF THE CONFLICT

The potential for conflict arises because in health care, unlike most other sectors of our economy, our country has evolved elaborate mechanisms to spread the high financial costs of medical care. The most obvious mechanism is private health insurance, but Social Security taxes for Medicare, taxes for Medicaid, health maintenance organizations, corporate health plans, and charities are other examples. All these mechanisms have a common feature—the pooling of resources. Individuals pay funds into the pool according to a variety of formulas, and individuals—sometimes the same ones, sometimes others—draw funds from the pool when the need arises.

This pooling of resources has the desirable effects of averaging out what each individual has to pay for health care and greatly reducing the possibility of a disastrous bill. But along with this benefit comes a liability. The pool connects actions of individuals in a way that creates the potential for conflict among them. Ideally, each individual will draw from the pool only his or her "fair share" of resources. In an ideal insurance program, the fair share is determined by Mother Nature; the events that determine which individuals will withdraw from the pool and how much they will withdraw are beyond the individual's control. An example is an earthquake. In health care, however, individuals and their physicians have substantial control over how much individuals withdraw from the pool. If

From *Journal of the American Medical Association*, Vol. 265, 2399–2401, 2405–2406.

an individual draws more than his or her fair share, then other people will either have to replenish the pool or go without the benefits of the lost services.

WHAT IS A FAIR SHARE?

If the line between a fair share and an unfair share were clear, individuals could be prevented fairly easily from drawing an unfair or inequitable share. Unfortunately, in the context of health care, the concept of fairness or equity is complex and difficult to implement. In health care, "equitable" cannot mean an equal amount of services. Different people have different needs depending on whether they are healthy or sick, the type and severity of their disease, and other factors. In the context of health care, a preferable definition of *equitable* is that services should be used in such a way that the services received by each individual should provide them with approximately equal amounts of benefit per unit of resource consumed. Thus, an equitable distribution means equal yield or, more colloquially, equal "bang for the buck." This definition has the desirable property that, if followed, it will use the available resources to yield the greatest total benefit.

The idea is most easily understood through examples. It would not be equitable to use a magnetic resonance imaging test on a person with classic history and symptoms of a stress headache instead of on a person suspected of having a tumor; or to tie up prenatal services by giving a few women monthly ultrasound examinations to keep as mementos, while other women receive no prenatal care at all; or to let a Medicaid budget be drained by a patient who is brain dead from a gunshot wound and on life support, while scores of other patients with good prognoses go untreated. Put in terms of some measure of effectiveness, such as life expectancy, it would be inequitable to give one person a service that adds 10 days of life expectancy at a cost of $1000 while another person fails to receive a service that would have gained 100 days for the same $1000. Whenever an individual uses services in a way that provides relatively low yield, the potential for conflict exists. Others will either have to pay more money to compensate for the inefficiency or will have to go without the services that went elsewhere.

TWO PERSPECTIVES

If all choices in health care took the form just described, the conflict between an individual and society would probably never arise. When a decision maker faces a limited resource and must determine which of two options yields the greater benefit from the resource, either the choice will be obvious or it will not make much difference. However, most medical decisions do not take this form. Instead of facing a limited resource and being asked to pick which patient would benefit the most from the resource, most decision makers, especially practitioners, face a patient and must decide which services to provide to that patient. For this type of decision, the connection between individuals is less obvious, and it is more difficult to appreciate that trying to maximize care for a particular patient will affect the financial or health outcomes of other people.

To understand the conflict between the individual and society, it is helpful to distinguish the two perspectives. In one, which is often called the public health or societal perspective, the decision maker sees a resource and wants to allocate it as efficiently as possible across patients. In the other, which might be called the patients' perspective, the decision maker sees an individual patient and wants to choose resources to optimize that patient's care. Both decision makers have the same goal of providing the best possible health care to the people they serve. However, because they see different people in different settings and make decisions in different directions, the strategies they propose are often in conflict.

TWO POSITIONS

The two perspectives roughly correspond to the two positions each of us can be in with respect to a health care service.[3] We are in one position (the "first position") when we do not yet have a health problem that would need the service and are deciding whether to buy coverage for the service. We are in another position (the "second position") when we have a disease, we know much more about what services we want, and this year's bills have already been paid. With admitted simplification, society is people when they are in the first position, whereas patients are people when they are in the second position. The conflict arises because what is best for us when we are in one position is not necessarily best for us when we are in the other position.[1]

THE CONFLICT

Unfortunately, when decisions are made from the patient's perspective, it is more difficult for the decision maker to determine when an individual is getting a disproportionate share of resources. First, from the patient's perspective, with its narrow focus on one person, it is not obvious that the level of care given to one person will affect the health and economic outcomes of other people. But even when this is appreciated, practitioners and patients can easily depersonalize the other people as "society," an insurance company, or the government, forgetting that these entities are really other patients, premium payers, and taxpayers. Some practitioners even see it as their duty to try to capture a disproportionate share of services for their patients. They perceive themselves as having an ethical responsibility to place the needs of their individual patients above the ill-defined needs of society, to serve as their patients' advocates in a battle with society. Any concern that their patients might receive an unfair share can be rationalized by assuming that if all practitioners look out for other patients with equal vigor, everything will work out fine.

There are several problems with this reasoning. One is that, in fact, we do not maximize the care of all individuals evenly. Some receive large amounts of resources, with little expectation of benefit, while others get far fewer resources even though the yield would have been much greater. The discrepancies affect not only the uninsured who draw from the pool only for urgent care, but also people who ostensibly have full insurance coverage. The discrepancies can occur because of such factors as geography, place of treatment (eg, a research center vs a community hospital), availability of resources, variations in providers' opinions about the outcomes of particular interventions, aggressiveness of the patient, aggressiveness of the physician, recent court cases or news articles, and the strength of a lobby for a particular disease. A second problem is that attempts to maximize every patient's care are likely to drive costs beyond the point that the people who will eventually pay the bill are willing to pay. But an even more impressive problem is that decisions from the perspective of the patients, where the attention is directed toward individuals after they seek care, do not maximize the health of even those individuals.

AN ILLUSTRATION

[I have elsewhere] illustrated these problems with a purposely simplified example of a hypothetical corporation that offered to 1000 of its 50-year-old female employees two options. One option would cover breast cancer screening from age 50 to 65 years; the other would cover high-dose chemotherapy with autologous bone marrow transplantation (HDC-ABMT) for women who develop metastatic breast cancer. To a woman in the first position (and from the public health perspective), breast cancer screening would reduce her chance of dying of breast cancer by about 0.7 percentage points (from 3.57% to 2.88%), increase her life expectancy by about 44 days, and cost her about $1200. To the same woman, coverage of HDC-ABMT would decrease her chance of dying of breast cancer by about 0.03 percentage points (from 3.57% to 3.54%), increase her life expectancy by about 2.5 days, and cost her about $1500. (The estimates for HDC-ABMT assume that the treatment has a 5% cure rate, which has not actually been demonstrated. The implications of other assumptions can be calculated proportionately. For example, a cure rate of 15% would imply a decrease in probability of dying of 0.09 percentage points and an increase in life expectancy of 7.5 days.) When applied to the 1000 women in the corporation, the first option would prevent about seven breast cancer deaths, add about 120 person-years of life, and cost about $1.2 million. The second option would prevent, at best, one death, would add about 7 person-years of life, and would cost about $1.5 million. Thus, from the first position, the public health perspective, or society's point of view, option 1 provides considerably greater benefit at lower cost and is the preferred program. However, from the perspective of an individual patient who has terminal breast cancer (the second position), a program that covers HDC-ABMT is preferable.

WHY NOT DO BOTH?

How can the conflict be resolved? In addition to highlighting the conflict, this example illustrates several approaches that might be used to try to resolve it. The most obvious question is, "Why not cover both screening and high-dose chemotherapy?"

That is a possibility. Its merits depend on whether women find the additional benefits to be worth the costs. To appreciate the issues, imagine that you are a 50-year-old average-risk woman employed by the corporation. From your point of view, the options appear as shown in Table 1.

Compared with option 1, are you willing to pay about $1100 more to buy option 3 ($2303 − $1195 = $1108), which will reduce your chance of dying of breast cancer by an additional 0.02 percentage points (from 2.88% to 2.86%) and add 2 days of life expectancy? Think hard and understand that if you choose option 3 you will actually have to pay the money; you will not be allowed to pass the cost off to someone else. If you and your coworkers truly prefer option 3, then indeed the solution to the conflict is to cover both screening and HDC-ABMT. This resolves the conflict because although you will be covered for HDC-ABMT, which draws a resource from the pool, you will be paying enough money into the pool to replace the expected cost. Thus, one way to resolve the conflict is to ask people if they are willing to pay for the additional services, and if they are, respect their wishes.

Now suppose you and your coworkers do not think that the benefits of adding HDC-ABMT to screening are worth the cost. Three remaining approaches might be tried to resolve the conflict. One is for the company to give you no choice—it might unilaterally create and bill you for a program that provides coverage for both screening and HDC-ABMT, even though you would rather keep the money than have coverage for HDC-ABMT. This approach, which might be called the "do-it-anyway" approach, does eliminate the health side of the conflict because it covers the service and replenishes the fund. However, this approach does not address the financial side of the conflict; you and your colleagues will be forced to pay for something you did not consider to be worth its costs. The do-it-anyway approach only converts the effect of the conflict from a health harm to a financial harm.

A second approach is to make option 3 an employee benefit and pass the costs on to consumers of the corporation's products. Call this the "pass-the-buck" approach. If you are an employee of the corporation, you should like this approach; it gives you a benefit at no cost. The fact that the benefit is not worth the cost is moot as far as you are concerned because you do not have to pay the cost. However, this approach is obviously unfair to the consumers of the product. Not only will they have to pay for a benefit they will never get—the benefit will go to you and your coworkers—but they will be paying for a benefit that the recipients themselves (you) determined was not worth its cost. Consumers might tolerate this for one company and one coverage policy because the costs would be highly diluted. But if this were to become the general method for resolving the conflict between the individual and society, everyone would use it, the costs of all products (and Social Security taxes and income taxes) would be affected, and the total burden on consumers would be huge. Furthermore, this approach boomerangs; you will end up paying for other peoples' health benefits. For example, when you buy a car, about $700 of your money goes to pay for other peoples' health

TABLE 1

Health and Economic Outcomes of Three Health Plans From the Perspective of a 50-Year-Old Asymptomatic Average-Risk Woman*

	Baseline	Option 1, screen	Option 2, HDC-ABMT	Option 3, both
Probability of getting breast cancer, %	8.22	8.22	8.22	8.22
Probability of dying of breast cancer, %	3.57	2.88	3.54	2.86
Increase in life expectancy, days	0	44	2.5	46
Cost, $†	0	1195	1506	2303

*Calculations performed on CAN*TROL.[4] Screen indicates screening of women between the ages of 50 and 65 years for breast cancer, and HDC-ABMT, high-dose chemotherapy with autologous bone marrow transplantation to age 65 years.
†Present value of costs, discounted to age 50 years at 5%.

benefits (Walter B. Maher, Chrysler Corporation, written communication, March 4, 1991). Every year, one way or another, every household in the country pays about $7000 for somebody's health care (calculated by dividing the total expenditures for health care by the number of households). Like the previous approach, this one does not solve the conflict between the individual and society; it only hides it better by spreading the financial burden to a larger number of people.

The third approach is to respect your wishes when you say you are not willing to pay for option 3. If you decide that the health benefits of covering HDC-ABMT are not as important to you as the money required to buy that coverage, this approach would take you at your word, not bill you for the cost of HDC-ABMT, and not cover the cost of HDC-ABMT if you should get metastatic breast cancer. This approach, which might be called the "patient choice" approach, is consistent with rationing by patient choice.[5] It resolves the conflict because it does not ask anyone else to pay the cost of a service you yourself were unwilling to pay for. The drawback to this approach is that if you should develop metastatic breast cancer, HDC-ABMT would not be covered. You could change your mind in the sense that you would not be forbidden from getting HDC-ABMT, but you would have to pay for it yourself, in full. You might end up regretting this decision, but that is not a conflict between you and society; it is a choice you made for yourself. You would be in conflict with society only if you tried to demand coverage for the HDC-ABMT, even though you declined to buy it when you had the chance.

An important conclusion of this exercise is that all the approaches that resolved the conflict are based on the same principle—let people decide what they are willing to pay for, respect those decisions, and adhere to those decisions. Notice that this principle would also allow you to choose none of the options. That is, if you look at Table 1 and decide that not even the benefits of option 1 are worth its cost, this principle would say that neither screening nor HDC-ABMT should be covered. This principle is difficult to apply for a variety of practical reasons, such as incomplete information about the relative merits of interventions, variations in peoples' preferences, and the interposition of third-party payment. Nonetheless, the principle must be understood if practical methods are to be developed to implement it.

The only remaining question is, when should people be asked to make their decisions—when they are in the first position or the second? To determine the guideline for treating breast cancer, should we show Table 1 to women before they get breast cancer, or should we show women who have metastatic breast cancer a modified table that indicates no benefit for screening?

WHICH POSITION IS "CORRECT?"

Both positions are real and have important things to say about the use of health care resources. When resolving the conflict between the individual and society, however, there are several reasons to give precedence to decisions made in the first position. One is that a person in the first position can look into the future to anticipate what he or she would want when he or she reaches the second position. In contrast, once a person reaches the second position, it is too late to fulfill the desires of the first position, at least with respect to that disease. Thus, the first position includes the second, but not vice versa.

But a more impressive reason is that by any aggregate measure of health care quality, such as morbidity rates, mortality rates, life expectancy, measures of health status, or quality-adjusted life-years, and for any specified level of resources, choices made from the first position can always provide as high a quality of care as choices made from the second position and can often provide a higher quality of care. This means that if guidelines are systematically defined from the first position (the public health perspective) more people will live longer, with higher quality, at lower cost than if guidelines are defined from the second position (the patient's perspective). Policies designed from the first position provide greater good for the greater number.

These statements are true because people in the first position always have more options from which to choose. Any option available to the second position is also available to the first position, but there are often options available to the first position that are not available to the second position. To the extent that the additional options available to the first position offer greater benefit and/or lower cost than the options available to the second position, decisions made from the first position will result in a higher quality of care and/or lower cost. In the example, individuals in the first position could choose from any of the options in Table 1. But by the time a person reaches the second position, the only viable option is option 2. Option 1, which would have provided more benefit at lower cost, is no longer available.

One might wonder if guidelines defined from the first position can always provide benefits and costs that are at least as good as guidelines from the second position, are there any advantages to making guidelines from the second position? Choices made from the second position have two main virtues. First, they give the appearance that everything that possibly can be done for an individual patient is being done. I use the word *appearance* because, in fact, while everything will have been done for a patient after he or she gets a disease, everything will not have been done for that person if the person's entire lifetime is considered. Nonetheless, if option 2 or 3 is chosen rather than option 1, neither patients nor physicians will have to face the emotional anguish of knowing that some potentially beneficial treatment was available but not covered.

The second virtue is closely related to the first. Patients in the second position tend to be much more visible than people in the first position. To the extent that other people who are unrelated to the patient (call them onlookers) place value on attempts to maximize care for an identified individual as opposed to unidentified people, setting policies from the second position can provide the onlookers with vicarious benefit. Memorable examples are a little girl who falls in a well or even whales trapped in Alaskan ice. The vicarious benefit onlookers derive from attempts to save identified individuals offsets at least some of the harm caused by spending large amounts of money that could have yielded greater benefit if used in other ways.

However, both of these virtues can be incorporated in decisions made from the first position. To address the first, add a line to the balance sheet to register the fact that if a woman chooses option 1 but ends up developing breast cancer, she will suffer the anguish of not having HDC-ABMT covered (Table 2). People should think hard about this additional outcome when making their choices because, under the patient-choice approach, they must live with the decision.

To address the second benefit, the pertinent question is whether the amount of vicarious benefit

TABLE 2

Health and Economic Outcomes of Three Health Plans From the Perspective of a 50-Year-Old Asymptomatic Average-Risk Woman*

	Baseline	Option 1 screen	Option 2 HDC-ABMT	Option 3 both
Probability of getting breast cancer, %	8.22	8.22	8.22	8.22
Probability of dying of breast cancer, %	3.57	2.88	3.54	2.86
Increase in life expectancy, days	0	44	2.5	46
Probability of suffering the anguish of not having HDC-ABMT covered, %	…	3.57	0	0
Cost, $†	0	1195	1506	2303

*Calculations performed on CAN*TROL.[4] Screen indicates screening of women between the ages of 50 and 65 years for breast cancer, and HDC-ABMT, high-dose chemotherapy with autologous bone marrow transplantation to age 65 years.
†Present value of costs, discounted to age 50 years at 5%.

received by the onlookers is sufficient to outweigh the harm that results from the inefficient use of resources. The amount of such benefit will depend on the nature and visibility of the particular case. Whether right or wrong, live television coverage of attempts to rescue a 5-year-old girl from a well will provide more vicarious benefit than newspaper coverage of a 50-year-old woman fighting with an insurance company for an investigational breast cancer treatment, which in turn will provide more vicarious benefit than hearing about a homeless person who needs better nutrition. To incorporate this feature of a guideline, each option should be studied for the potential of vicarious benefit; a helpful measure is its "newsworthiness."

WHAT HAPPENS NOW?

Our current practices tend to accentuate rather than resolve the conflict. We have little idea of the level of services for which people are willing to pay, we make most decisions from the second position, and we use the pass-the-buck approach to pay for those decisions. The lack of systematic information about the relative benefits and harms of many interventions, and about peoples' preferences for benefits, harms, and costs, deprives us of the anchor we need to determine the total size of the pool, or to determine what constitutes a fair share of services. Most decisions that reflect the second position are not the result of any careful analysis or public debate but simply a consequence of the fact that the great majority of the encounters between individuals and the health care system occur when patients are in the second position. As for paying for services, we have raised the pass-the-buck approach to a fine art. For example, not only do employees get health benefits covered by their employers, who pass them on to consumers, but employees do not have to pay taxes on the benefits as income, the employers can deduct the costs as a business expense, and the government can pass all the lost tax revenues on to future generations through budget deficits. The fact that most decisions are made from the second position and reflect the patient's perspective produces just what we would expect: Most patients want everything possible and expect somebody else to pay for it. Practitioners undoubtedly sense that many of the services they provide are excessive, but their responses vary widely, with some discouraging their use, some staying neutral, and some encouraging them.

Thus, to a great extent the current "solution" to the conflict between the individual and society today is for individuals to try to extract as much from society as possible. We are in a tailspin: individual patients drive up costs, which are passed on to other people, who try to recover their "fair share" by overusing services when their turn comes around.

WHAT IS THE SOLUTION?

Because of the magnitude and complexity of the problem, resolving the conflict will be extremely difficult. To begin, it is helpful to describe what we want to achieve and then try to get closer to that goal than we are now. Ideally, we would have good information about the benefits, harms, and costs of services, about the level of health care for which people are willing to pay, and, correspondingly, about the level of resources that should be made available for health care. Ideally there would be some agreed-on measure of benefit per resource that would serve as a threshold for deciding when coverage of a particular service is fair. When the yield of a service is below the threshold, physicians and patients would voluntarily restrain themselves from seeking coverage for that service from the pool. Conversely, if a particular service has a high yield but is underused, steps would be taken to stimulate that service.

Many problems will prevent us from reaching this ideal. They include lack of good information about the health and economic outcomes of many activities; the fact that the outcomes of a service depend on the specific indications for which it is used (which means there will be few simple guidelines); the lack of a tradition of asking patients their preferences; the fact that preferences are highly personal and variable (which means there will be few single correct answers); and the fact that physicians and patients have strong incentives to maximize services after patients seek care.

Despite these problems, it is certainly possible to improve on our current approach. The first step is to recognize the problem. Physicians and patients must understand that when they attempt to maximize care from the patient's perspective, they might not only be in conflict with society, but they might well be fostering guidelines that are not even in their own long-term interest. Everyone must also understand that behind the abstract label of society are real people; when individuals receive a disproportionate amount of services at the expense of society, they harm the health and finances of other people just like themselves.

The second step is to learn more about the benefits, harms, and costs of the most important interventions and about what people want from the health care system. We should pick two to three dozen representative health problems that span the most important diseases and types of activities, estimate their benefits, harms, and costs, and ask people whether the benefits and harms are worth the costs, using the type of questions described elsewhere.[3] This exercise would provide essential information about whether we are currently spending too much or too little on health care and would provide the threshold that determines the fair share to be covered from pooled resources. The recent programs of the Agency for Health Care Policy and Research are an important step in this direction. The third step is to identify some services that, on the basis of clinical judgment and common sense are suspected to be overused or underused, estimate their health and economic outcomes, and ask people if they are worth their costs. While uncertainty and variability will limit our progress, we can achieve some success by analyzing the extremes. The last steps are to incorporate what we learn into practice policies and then to adhere to those guidelines.

Because it involves human behavior and self-control, the last step will be the most difficult and will require great leadership from practitioners. Medicine has a long tradition of trying to maximize care for individual patients, a tradition not only based on compassion, but strongly reinforced by medical education, pressure from patients, families, the press, the courts, and professional and financial incentives. But the act of pooling resources across individuals requires that that tradition be modified. In return for gaining the benefits derived from sharing costs, individuals must also accept some responsibilities and limitations. A responsibility is to respect others who contribute to the pool. A limitation is to not withdraw from it an unfair share.

NOTES

1. Eddy DM. The individual vs society: is there a conflict? *JAMA.* 1991;265:1446, 1449–1450.
2. Eddy DM. What care is essential? What services are basic? *JAMA.* 1991;265:782, 786–788.
3. Eddy DM. Connecting value and costs: Whom do we ask, and what do we ask them? *JAMA.* 1990;264: 1737–1739.
4. Eddy DM. A computer-based model for designing cancer control strategies. *NCI Monogr.* 1986;2:75–82.
5. Eddy DM. Rationing by patient choice. *JAMA.* 1991; 265:105–108.

TOWARD A BROADER VIEW OF VALUES IN COST-EFFECTIVENESS ANALYSIS OF HEALTH

Paul Menzel, Marthe R. Gold, Erik Nord, Jose-Louis Pinto-Prades, Jeff Richardson, and Peter Ubel

The promise of cost-effectiveness analysis in health care is that it allows policymakers to compare what at first blush are apples and oranges. CEA purports to show how much health benefit is likely to be produced by very different investments. It attempts to express the effectiveness of health care interventions and programs in common units of health-related value, such as "quality adjusted life years"

(QALYs), that allow the benefits of various treatments to be quantified on the same scale of measurement.

The work CEA can do is indeed remarkable. It can take programs with qualitatively very different outcomes—life-saving dialysis and quality-enhancing hip replacements, for example—and inform us of their costs in relation to their *comparable* effects—their QALYs. This ability to compare disparate effects is one of several respects in which CEA is the child of utilitarian welfare economics. In that larger discipline too, a huge range of values gets collected into one common and measurable notion, "utility." Moreover, welfare economics' conception of "value to society" is typically built up out of individuals' utilities, combined in some way. In all of these respects—its one scale of value, its quantifying of that value, and its combining of individual pieces of value into aggregate wholes for society—conventional health economics is just what one would expect of a specialty within economics.

How does CEA in health care obtain its single metric of value for comparing widely different effects? Typically three factors are incorporated. The first, and by far the most conceptually complex, is the size of the quality improvement that treatment produces: the saving of life and its maintenance at a certain level. This change is expressed as a savings or improvement of *health-related quality of life*. Call it the "size of treatment effect." It is here that mortality and morbidity are compared and combined. Death is assigned the value 0, full health the value 1.0, and all other health states better than death are arrayed in between, from most to least severe, on the basis of responses that interview subjects give to certain questions. Various types of questions are used to elicit opinions about quality of life. In "time trade-off" questions, for example, respondents may be asked how many of an anticipated twenty remaining years of their lives they would be willing to sacrifice in order to obtain the complete cure of a specified health condition. Suppose that on average their answer is four—that is, 20 percent of their remaining time. Then they have rated the quality of life in that state of health at 0.8, a 20 percent reduction from 1.0.

The second factor used to construct comparable units of value is the duration of that health improvement, and the third factor is the number of persons receiving it. Conventional CEA simply multiplies these factors: the size of treatment effect is multiplied by both the duration of that benefit and the number of beneficiaries. For example, if hip replacements generally raise recipients' health-related quality of life from 0.8 to 0.98, effectively last 10 years, and cost $18,000 each, they typically produce 1.8 QALYs at a cost of $10,000 per QALY. If a year of inpatient hemodialysis typically costs $32,000 and saves a life of 0.8 health-related quality, it produces 0.8 QALYs at a cost per QALY of $40,000. If the medical demand for these two procedures were not being met, these numbers suggest that it would be better to invest in additional hip replacements rather than in expanded dialysis.

The quantified effects used in CEA are classic expressions of a form of "utility"—what might be called "health-related utility." While CEA is technically a descriptive analysis because it does not actually tell decisionmakers to maximize health-related utilities, it reveals which categories of health care investments will maximize them. Utilitarianism is its philosophical parent. Thus it is not surprising that conventional CEA provokes many of the same ethical objections that plague utilitarianism in general: that it gives inadequate attention to the individual person and too much to the aggregate good, and that it is insensitive to issues of distributive justice involving the least advantaged. One might, of course, simply dismiss CEA because of the weaknesses of the utilitarian philosophy that it reflects. One might also continue to use it while becoming pointedly aware of its limitations. We will urge, however, an alternative: to examine specific values that conventional CEA fails to incorporate with an eye toward reforming the methodology of CEA itself.

Prominent among the factors that conventional CEA currently disregards or underestimates when assessing a treatment are the initial severity of the illness, any unique value of lifesaving or other

---

Paul Menzel, Marthe R. Gold, Erik Nord, Jose-Luis Pinto-Prades, Jeff Richardson, and Peter Ubel, "Toward a Broader View of Values in Cost-Effectiveness Analysis in Health," *Hastings Center Report* 29, no. 3 (1999): 7–15.

Editor's note: Most footnotes have been deleted. Students who want to follow up on sources should consult the original article.

treatment in the face of death, the fact that patients' limited potential for increased health may be a long-term identifying characteristic of their lives, and age (not the effect of age on the duration of the health improvement, but age itself). Because of these oversights, recommendations emerging from CEA can stand starkly at odds with the values of justice and nondiscrimination. This exposes CEA not only to ethical but also to political attack—what politician wants to defend policies that expose individuals to injustice in the name of an impersonal, aggregate good?

Thus the central proposal we make in this paper: that CEA should explore how social values might be better incorporated into the "effectiveness" side of economic analysis. Several of the values we will discuss have already been noted—and a few pursued—in the CEA literature. The U.S. Public Health Service Panel on Cost-Effectiveness in Medicine, for example, explicitly noted the special attention that should be given to the severity of a patient's initial condition. Our goal is to pursue the analysis of such values more explicitly and methodically, as well as to suggest the systematic inclusion of such factors in CEA itself.

Although some of the factors we discuss may affect so-called "individual utility," they are mainly relevant to "societal value." In societal value, the focus is explicitly on interpersonal trade-offs—decisions about what services to provide among the wide array of possible services that often affect different groups of people. It is such trade-offs that motivate and figure centrally in the large-scale use of CEA for allocating preventive or acute care services at the "budget" or "coverage" level for large populations, as distinct from the "admission" or "bedside" level, where many feel that interpersonal trade-offs should not be dealt with numerically.

These matters inevitably constitute a delicate conversation between two separate perspectives, economics and bioethics, each with markedly different sets of analytical tools. It is vital that bridges be built between them. No field reckons more directly with "nasty" and value-loaded trade-offs than health economics. And while bioethics has seldom shown much awareness of the realities of scarce financial resources, it wrestles openly with multiple values and the tensions among them. Philosophically inclined bioethicists should not shun the discipline of economics, and economists should become accustomed to wrestling with challenges to their allegedly limited evaluative horizons.

THREE NEGLECTED ETHICAL FACTORS

Some aspects of treatment are such that omitting them from allocative decisionmaking is ethically objectionable. This is a more demanding notion than the simple claim that such aspects involve overlooked "preferences" or unexamined "values." For the omission of a factor to be ethically objectionable, one has to be able to articulate some argument for the preferences it generates, not merely point out that people hold those preferences.

Let us call such independently supported values "ethical factors." Admittedly, the line between societal values that are ethical factors and those that are not is not firm. A good moral argument can be made that it is paternalistic or antidemocratic to ignore *any* of a population's preferences about allocation of health care (assuming that those preferences are not irrational or ethically objectionable, as when they reflect discriminatory attitudes). If so, CEA ought to incorporate all the societal values that we discuss, not only the ethical factors. Nonetheless, three values seem to stand out as factors that CEA really ought not to neglect.

Severity of Illness

Conventional CEA takes the severity of illness into account only insofar as it is one of two variables that determine the size of treatment effect—the difference between initial and post-treatment health. Conventional CEA does not accord any weight to the severity of illness per se. But the evidence suggests that people often wish to give greater priority to treatment of those who are worse off, above and beyond the priority it already has within CEA.

For example, in a study of 150 Norwegian politicians accountable for health policy at the county level, subjects were asked to decide whether to provide treatments that would offer "a little" help for a severe illness, or treatments that would ameliorate a moderate illness "considerably." They had three choices: divide resources evenly between the two illnesses and their treatments, allocate most to treatment of the severe illness, or allocate most to treatment of the moderate illness. Nearly half (45 percent) chose equal division, and 37 percent gave priority to the severe illness. Only 11 percent gave priority to the moderate illness.

The key to severity's ethical relevance is that, inherently, treating the more severely ill is helping those who are in greater need, and our society gives a fundamental general priority to helping "the worst off"—those whose life prospects make them the most disadvantaged. Also, we reduce inequality if we give priority to patients with more severe illness. If two treatments can raise one person's health-related quality of life from 0.5 to 0.9 and that of another from 0.3 to 0.6, treating the less severe illness leaves the two individuals with respective health-related quality of life values of 0.3 and 0.9, while treating the more severe illness leaves them much closer together, at 0.5 and 0.6.

The empirical data suggesting an independent concern for severity thus appear to have an ethical basis. To be sure, critics might challenge the data. Perhaps the study respondents accorded extra priority to treating the most severely ill not because they saw them as more ill, but because they believed that their health improvement would be greater. But it would be dogmatic for health economists simply to insist on this explanation. And, in fact, one study conveyed quite clearly that the more severely ill were receiving a smaller benefit, yet it still yielded a distinct preference for treating the more severe illnesses.

Lifesaving and Treatment in the Face of Death

The most severe illnesses, of course, put people face-to-face with death. The belief that when identifiable patients face a great risk of avoidable death they have a unique claim on resources has been called the "rule of rescue." Rooted in the Kantian tradition of considering the individual as an ultimate "end-in-itself," this rule resists the usual quantitative aggregation of economic analysis. Conventional CEA has conducted its business as if the rule could be ignored—or at least as if it were not the sort of factor that CEA could account for.

This stance damages the credibility of health economics. As David Hadorn has argued, "any plan to distribute health care services must take [the rule of rescue] . . . into account if the plan is to be acceptable to society."[1] There is ample evidence that our society will devote considerable effort and resources to avert the death of identified people—to save the girl down the well, astronauts in space, sailors lost at sea, and so on. Public policy reflects the rule as well. In Oregon, for example, all lifesaving services were placed in a separate high-priority category in the state's Medicaid rationing list. And several studies provide corroborating evidence that people place a special value on care in the face of death, at least when the care has a plausible prospect of success.

A relatively simple thought experiment illustrates the intuitive power of lifesaving's value. Imagine two groups of patients stricken with a life-threatening illness. Those in the first group were previously in full health and can be returned to full health with treatment. Those in the second group have paraplegia, which will be unaffected by treatment of their life-threatening condition. Both, if treated, will live the same number of additional years. Assume that the health-related quality of life of paraplegia is 0.8, as calculated from "time trade-off" responses from people who actually are paraplegic. Conventional CEA would then recommend saving those in the first group, who can be returned to full health, before saving an equal number in the second group. It would recommend shifting priority to those with paraplegia only if the number of lives saved there at similar cost was at least 20 percent greater than the number of people returned to normal health. Yet few among us, reflecting seriously on the value of continuing to live, believe that it is less important to save the lives of people with paraplegia than the lives of those who are fully mobile. The value of lifesaving appears to overwhelm the influence of the differences in health-related quality of life on which conventional CEA focuses.

This example also reveals that lifesaving and other treatment in the face of death pose particular concerns about discrimination against those who are disabled or chronically ill. In conventional economic analysis, the value of saving lives can be influenced by whose lives, and of what quality, they are. Those who are disabled or chronically ill will of course resist any such influence on valuations, and for good reason. Suppose, again, that the disabled person has ranked her individual quality of life at 0.8. This willingness to accept a 20 percent shorter remaining life in order to be cured from a permanent disability does not in any way indicate that she thought her life, in relation to the prospect of death, any less valuable and important than the life of a fully healthy person. One number can have two meanings, but we cannot assume that it does; here, in fact, the 0.8 that expresses a willingness to trade time within a life does not constitute a comparative judgment about the value of different individuals' lives.

This point about the potential for discrimination in conventional CEA must not be overstated. The lifesaving interventions or programs assessed in CEA rarely pertain selectively to a disabling condition such as paraplegia, so that discrimination against those who are chronically ill or disabled may be far less common in the actual use of CEA than one would surmise from studying its theoretical model. Still, it is not a sufficient defense of conventional CEA to argue that, serendipitously, disabled patients rarely have life-threatening diseases or conditions requiring separate lifesaving treatments. First, such separate diseases and treatments can and do occur—an example is HIV, for which there are HIV-specific medications. Second, rationing can indeed occur by categories of patients within the scope of a single treatment, not just by entire treatments. For example, patients with chronic pulmonary disease might be poorer candidates for coronary artery bypass grafts than patients with normal lungs, and they could therefore be excluded from such surgery in carefully crafted practice guidelines. Third, an allocation model's potential for discrimination against those who are disabled is hardly rendered irrelevant by the probable realities of its use. It is enough that conceptually the model's implications are sharply at odds with society's values about discrimination.

The special value of treatment in the face of death actually pertains to more than lifesaving services. It is present, for example, in widespread attitudes toward hospice and other non-lifesaving terminal care. Putting up with severe pain for a six-month period when one expects to live for many years is one thing; having to put up with it at the end of one's life is another. People generally, not just patients facing death, have a special concern that life not end in pain. Thus palliative measures for patients with terminal conditions produce an extra value not possessed by palliative measures provided to other patients, even when the palliation is of nominally equal effectiveness.

In claiming that conventional CEA underestimates the value of care in the face of death, we are by no means agreeing with those who would consider the value of life absolute. People are, in fact, perfectly and knowledgeably willing to trade some lifesaving interventions for other health services. Yet at the same time, the value that public opinion places on care in the face of death appears to be inadequately captured by conventional CEA.

Level of Health Potential

The societal value of priority for more severe illnesses focuses independently on a patient's starting point, as distinct from the size of treatment effect. The end point can also have an independent relevance, not accounted for in calculating the size of the treatment effect. Most people are reluctant to place at a disadvantage patients who are already burdened with a lower potential for overall health. We shall call this consideration the "level of potential" factor.

This value is probably one factor in the preference for not denying lifesaving treatment to people with paraplegia in the example discussed above. But consider a broader, non-lifesaving case; suppose that treatment can improve the health-related quality of life of one group of people from 0.6 to 0.8 and that of another from 0.6 to 1.0, and that the first group's end point of 0.8 represents its members' maximum prospective health potential. Should we really regard the second group's treatment effect as having twice the value of the first's? Treatment "fully cures" those in both groups, at least within the perspective of the possibilities available to them. Their health potential defines, in significant part, the lives they can lead. Since a life with that potential is the best life that they ever will have, it is plausible to think that for those with the limited potential, reaching their 0.8 level counts as notably more than half the value of the other group's improvement from 0.6 to full health.

The essential ethical claim here is that where people are "located" in life in relation to their maximum realistic potential is an important factor in resource allocation. In part this may be a function of our aversion to inequality: if we give priority to treating those who can be returned to full health, the gap is the difference between 1.0 and 0.6, while if we treat those with the limited potential, the gap is only the difference between 0.8 and 0.6. With more empirical research, other moral elements besides aversion to inequality may come to light as involved in the societal preference for compensating for the downward pressure of low end-state potential in net "effectiveness."

The study of Norwegian politicians mentioned above also provides suggestive empirical support for the importance of the level of potential factor. The respondents were given another dilemma. Two illnesses, both equally common and involving the same degree of suffering, have treatments that are equally costly. The best treatment of illness A helps patients a little, and the best treatment of illness B helps a lot. With an increase in funding that can cover treatment for only one set of patients, not for both groups, respondents were asked to choose between two different allocations: either allocate most of the increase to treatments for illness B, since the effects are greater, or divide the increase evenly between the two groups, on the ground that they are equally entitled to treatment. Almost half (48 percent) chose the second, more egalitarian view, while 24 percent chose the first.

Admittedly, the currently available data about public preferences do not unequivocally confirm that a limited level of health potential is an important societal value. Nonetheless, they appear to conflict with the way health potential is considered in conventional CEA. Moreover, the ethical argument for giving special consideration to a limited long-term health potential can be powerfully articulated.

OTHER VALUES

Severity of illness, care in the face of death, and limited health potential may be the factors most clearly connected to the distribution of health care, and therefore the most important to add to CEA, but they are not the only relevant considerations. There is a range of values that an expanded model of CEA might include.

Conventional CEA views societal benefit as directly proportional to the gain in health utility produced by treatment, and views this, in turn, as a linear function of the average improvement in health-related quality of life and the number of people benefited by such outcomes. At least two factors may qualify this simple linear relationship between numbers of people and total value.

Maintenance of Hope

Suppose we can allocate resources either to a program that will yield a certain benefit to a great number of people, or to one that generates the same benefit but for a smaller number. Suppose too that while fewer benefit, the number of people treated remains the same. That is, the second treatment is effective less often. The efficient allocation—as judged by conventional CEA—would be to devote all of the resources to the first program. Several studies reveal, however, that many people wish to preserve the hope of treatment for everyone, and that to accomplish this, they are willing to devote some resources to those in the "inefficient" treatment category. Were those public preferences to be heeded, a smaller number would be helped, at no higher average level of benefit than a larger number could have been.

Assurance of Treatment

There is also evidence that many people prefer ensuring that everyone in a disease or treatment category is entitled to treatment, even when it would be more efficient to provide the treatment to only some in the category. They consider it inequitable to exclude some from treatment that most receive. Moreover, incomplete coverage within a category may give rise to feelings of uncertainty—feelings that are themselves disutilities, though not focused on health benefit.

Maintenance of hope and assurance of treatment have an interesting relationship. They appear at opposite ends of a spectrum in which the percentage of patients treated in an illness category moves from 0 to 100. Maintenance of hope creates an especially

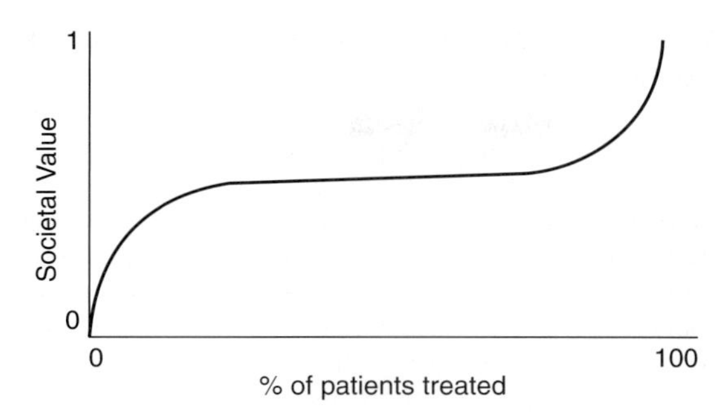

FIGURE 1

great benefit as the first patients are treated. Assurance of treatment creates a disproportionate benefit at the other end of the spectrum, as a program approaches full coverage. (See Figure 1.) If these two factors both bear up under further empirical investigation, aggregate value will turn out to be a nonlinear function of the probability that a person in the medically appropriate population will receive treatment.

The implication is that to maintain hope we might provide inefficient services to a few patients in some illness categories rather than to none at all, as long as they were selected by a sufficiently fair procedure. In other cases we might offer a treatment to everyone in an illness category despite the diminished odds of cost-effective outcomes for those added at the margin. In either case, we will have gone against the outcome-efficiency orientation of conventional economic analysis.

Considerably more study is needed before we would urge that maintenance of hope and assurance of treatment be included in CEA. Such research should be undertaken, however, for the available evidence already suggests that the practice of treating total value as directly proportional to the number of people effectively treated does not satisfactorily reflect our societal values.

Duration Discounting

Conventional CEA takes duration into account in a strictly proportionate fashion. It multiplies the value of one year's worth of a treatment effect by the number of years for which the effect lasts, then discounts the value obtained in each year past the first in order to obtain its present value. The reason for "time preference discounting," as it is called, is that people prefer near-term benefits to long-term benefits; if two values are the same but one is longer term, the long-term value counts for less in the present.

Empirical studies, however, suggest that at least in health care people adopt a different and more marked pattern of discounting—different perhaps when people evaluate the duration of different treatment options in their own lives, and very likely when they consider duration in the context of interpersonal comparisons. In interpersonal comparisons, for example, respondents in Australia thought that saving ten people for ten years each would be equivalent to saving seven people for twenty years each. That is, it took 140 years accumulated in twenty-year spans to equal in value 100 years accumulated in ten-year spans.

There are at least three possible reasons people might adopt such a pattern. First, at the level of individual utility, a "quantity effect" may obtain that is similar to diminishing marginal utility generally: because of the benefits already achieved, the last year of life in a ten-year span is not seen to be as valuable as any one of the earlier years (or certainly not the first). At the level of societal value, people may have an aversion to inequality that leads them to value duration less than proportionately. Assuming that two people are roughly of the same age, it seems more equitable to extend their lives for ten years each than to extend one person's life for twenty. Or, again at the level of societal value, the level of potential factor may be associated with duration; the ten-year extension, in contrast to the twenty-year extension, will accrue to patients who have a shorter potential life span.

Regardless of which explanations are supported by future research, it appears safe to say that to capture society's values adequately, CEA will need to discount the value of longer spans of life or health more than it already does. To determine exactly how, health economists need to embark on a wide range of studies of duration, keeping pure time preference of the individual distinct from the other elements that may arise in social values. Perhaps such research will also reveal the relative importance of these different elements in the way people discount long-term health benefits. Moreover, not only the size of the total discount but the ethical arguments for its use need to be investigated and debated. One possible outcome of such research is that we will come to accept discounting for some benefits but reject it for others.

Age

While duration is directly accounted for in conventional CEA (even if incorrectly), the related factor of age is not directly taken into account at all. Indirectly, of course, it is, as treatments for those who are relatively elderly often produce benefits of shorter duration than treatments for those who are relatively young, thereby making treatments of young persons productive of more life-years than treatments of elderly persons. In addition to this indirect effect of age, however, there is evidence that the way age itself figures into health care allocation preferences is at odds with conventional CEA. Many would probably say that more than one seventy-year-old would have to be saved for ten years to equal the value of saving one thirty-year-old for ten years. Moreover, this preference persists when one rids respondents of any implicit presumptions that the quality of life between seventy and eighty must be lower than that between thirty and forty.

The primary moral basis for this preference for young persons is undoubtedly linked to our belief that the distribution of benefits should be egalitarian. Just as those who are most severely ill should be treated first, even when their benefit from treatment may be smaller, so also the young should be treated first, even when their gain is smaller, so that they obtain a fairer and more equal chance of living a long life. There may, of course, be societies in which reverence for the elderly overrides these egalitarian considerations, and in those contexts, allocations recommended by conventional CEA would be in line with public preferences. For societies that do not have a strong differential reverence for the elderly, however, conventional CEA is likely to yield what seem to be inappropriate results. Of course, it may be that the societal values that contradict conventional CEA treatment are "ageist." And perhaps, in fact, the societal issues are so contentious that empirical investigation will show little in the way of a predominant social preference for according greater priority to the young than is already indirectly built into CEA. But more research is warranted.

WHOM TO ASK

Undoubtedly there are other factors typically omitted from CEA that people consider relevant to interpersonal social value. Among the candidates: personal responsibility, citizenship and nationality, compensation for those who are disadvantaged in other ways than via their health, health effects on others, non-health effects on others, and the degree of either personal or community control thought to be preserved by a given program. Without more empirical data or more persuasive ethical justification, however, we do not recommend that they be placed on the research agenda of items that might be included in a more sophisticated CEA.

A more pressing question, and a long-standing practical and ethical controversy within CEA, concerns whom should be asked to rate individual health-related quality of life. Should a condition be rated only by those who have or have had it, or should the general public have the final say? In quantifying an improvement in health-related quality of life, conventional CEA has primarily and appropriately focused not on any objective health increment that would be difficult to construe as value, but on the subjective value or utility of the gain. Often, though, CEA has then proceeded to measure that subjective value—here at the level of individual utility—in ways that do not include people who have had the condition. This raises ethical doubts about whether CEA adequately reflects the perspective of those primarily affected by the policies it influences.

It is not uncommon for patients' ratings of their own health-related quality of life—especially those by chronically ill patients—to be higher than others' ratings of the same health states. And although some studies show little systematic difference in patients' and nonpatients' ratings, in no studies are patients' ratings lower than nonpatients'. Thus the balance of current evidence points toward a difference. And since CEA claims to measure the value of the real effects of health care, unless patients lack the capacity to express these judgments, what would justify asking anyone else to judge the value of their treatments? Even if provided with a rich description of the condition, why would others be better judges of the value of life with that condition than those who have actually lived with it?

We suggest that including societal values along with individual health utilities presents the opportunity for an ethically more adequate resolution of this whom-to-ask issue. A strong case can be made for eliciting societal values from representatives of the general public, but preference input about societal values needs to be kept distinct from input about individual utility and health-related quality of life ratings. This implies—or at least suggests—a two-part model for CEA. In the first part, individual utilities would be elicited from patients and ex-patients. In the second part, interpersonal trade-off preferences, based in part on knowledge of affected people's individual utilities, would be elicited from representatives of the community. Once the community representatives' input about societal value is secure, the case for asking patients and ex-patients about individual utility becomes stronger. Were this to be accepted practice, CEA could more adequately respond to the objection that it has not considered the values of individuals affected by allocation policies.

Undoubtedly other matters, both practical and theoretical, complicate this thorny issue. The question needs to stay open. Our claim here is only that distinguishing social value from individual health utility changes the larger context in which the whom-to-ask debate takes place. At the level of "societal value," focused on interpersonal trade-offs, the prima facie ethical case favors consulting representative people in the overall group or society. One reason is the "insurance principle": if people determine the final value of insured services only after they know of their particular need for these services, they may inflate that value so as to take advantage of others in the society, by forcing them to provide the financial resources for the services. This argument provides little justification for eliciting health-related quality of life ratings from community representatives, however. When measuring individual utility, the prima facie ethical case favors asking patients and ex-patients the questions from which tables of health-related quality of life ratings are constructed.

One should not underestimate the importance for CEA of crafting a morally sound position on this question. One of the strongest responses that a society can make to people who are disadvantaged by a social policy is to note that they (or people relevantly similar to them) had a major role in the decision-making process that led to the policy. The implications for the use of CEA are not hard to see. If, in the process of discerning relevant values, CEA has queried people who can reasonably be construed to represent those who are disadvantaged by an allocation, a ready response to critics is available. If such people have not been queried, the results will be harder to defend, especially in a political context.

Since the societal values that we urge CEA to attempt incorporating would seem to be properly elicited from the general population, and since prima facie it seems best to elicit health-related quality of life ratings from current or former patients wherever possible, those who wish to elicit even health-related quality of life ratings from the general public shoulder the burden of proof.

A BROADENING OF VIEWS

Despite the clear recognition in economic theory that individual utility may be affected by the well-being of others, many economists pay little attention to the fact in practice. Perhaps it is unsurprising, then, that they pay even less attention to the possibility that social welfare involves values that cannot be explained by individual utilities, however these are combined. We do not by any means believe that individual utilities are irrelevant, but we do claim that their almost exclusive emphasis in much applied economic research is not justified in the health sector.

Economists' relative disregard of distributive issues is often rationalized on the ground that maximizing the value of output leaves open the possibility of redistributing income in such a way that no one will be worse off and some will remain better off, and that it is then the responsibility of governments to take care of this subsequent distribution. As has been recognized by virtually all health economists, however, it is often not possible to redistribute health, or to compensate for health care allocations through the distribution of other goods. It is difficult to compensate someone who died because one program received priority over another.

Largely because of such difficulties, interpersonal decisions about health care should certainly not be aimed solely—perhaps not even primarily—at maximizing individual utilities. If societal values are not taken into account at the start, serious ethical questions about fairness and discrimination go unaddressed.

Some will undoubtedly maintain that it would be best to leave societal values entirely out of the CEA enterprise, to relegate quantitative analysis to the very limited task of conveying information about individual utilities. Economist Alan Williams, however, has correctly argued that the great deficiency of that approach is that it leaves considerations of equity floating without any conception of how important they should be. If left floating, then they either get used as trump cards, without regard to what amount of individual health utility is sacrificed for them, or they are simply ignored, on the ground that "there is no way of establishing what bearing, if any, those [equity] principles actually had upon the [decisionmaking outcomes]. . . . [If ignored,] it is tempting to conclude that the rhetoric [of equity] is not matched by any real commitment to do anything effective. . . . The quest for greater quantification of equity considerations seems worth pursuing on those grounds alone, despite the hostility it is likely to engender from those who mistakenly equate precision with lack of humanity."

CEA in health care should broaden its conception of the array of values that might be accounted for in the "effectiveness" side of its ledger, adding societal values to the mix. If and when empirical research and ethical analysis of selected societal values reveals them to be clear, quantifiable, of sufficient societal importance, and not irrational or ethically discriminatory, the structure of CEA should be adjusted to allow for their inclusion. To be sure, any such modification of CEA's structure must be pursued carefully so that we do not create an illusion of specificity and importance not justified by what we actually know of societal preferences and their ethical foundations. Nevertheless, it is time for health economics to recognize the relevance of these values and the ethical issues to which they speak. It is also time for bioethicists to assist with the considerable task of discerning them in as precise and usable a form as possible.

REFERENCES

1. David Hadorn, "Setting Health Care Priorities in Oregon: Cost-Effectiveness Meets the Rule of Rescue," *JAMA* 265 (1991): 2218–25.

LAST-CHANCE THERAPIES AND MANAGED CARE: PLURALISM, FAIR PROCEDURES, AND LEGITIMACY

Norman Daniels and James Sabin

I. COVERAGE FOR UNPROVEN LAST-CHANCE THERAPIES

The most difficult and explosive responsibility for any health care system is deciding whether patients with life-threatening illnesses will receive insurance coverage for unproven treatments they believe may make the difference between life and death.

Potentially life-saving treatments with proven efficacy and safety (proven net benefit) and quack treatments for which there is no scientific rationale, rarely pose major problems about insurance coverage. In a country as wealthy as the United States, effective last-chance treatments without alternatives generally are and should be covered virtually all the time. When shared resources from cooperative schemes are involved, as in public or private insurance, rather than individuals paying with their own resources, quack treatments will and should virtually never be covered, even if the patient or doctor passionately believe in the purported cure.

The difficult practical and ethical challenges come from promising but unproven last-chance treatments, for which we use high-dose chemotherapy with autologous bone marrow transplant (ABMT) for advanced breast cancer as our key example.[1] Not covering treatments that ultimately prove to be effective lets curable patients die prematurely, and even if a treatment ultimately proves to be ineffective, not covering it may create the impression that critically ill patients are being abandoned in their moment of need. Covering treatments that ultimately prove to be ineffective or harmful reduces the quantity and quality of the patient's remaining life, wastes substantial resources, and undermines clinical research. These are the moral stakes in the decision.

There are also other costs and risks in these decisions. Denials of coverage for seriously ill people are highly visible. Even health plans that use impeccable science and patient-centered deliberation while trying to hold the traditional, contractually-specified line against unproven therapies risk horrendous publicity, expensive litigation, and legislative mandates requiring coverage.

We shall later see (in Section II) that there is room for reasonable people to disagree about how to weigh the conflicting values and principles in these cases. There is no convincing, principled argument or social consensus for determining the relative importance of (1) giving some (how much?) priority to meeting the *urgent claims* of patients in last-chance situations, (2) providing *stewardship* of collective resources, (3) producing the public good of *scientific knowledge* about the effectiveness of unproven therapies, and (4) respecting *patient autonomy* through collaborative decision making about risks and benefits.

We can try to gloss over the ethical uncertainties in these cases by pretending that terms like "investigational," "experimental," and "medical necessity" tell us what to do. These terms, however, explain little and dodge the genuine ethical dilemmas. Without extensive explanation of the reasoning process they will not—and should not—satisfy the public or the courts. The ethical challenges posed by unproven but promising last-chance technologies are not helped at all by the language of current medical insurance benefit contracts. They are also made harder to solve by the climate of distrust that surrounds insurers, including managed care organizations (MCOs) of all types. Why should the public accept as *legitimate* decisions made by MCOs that limit access to "unproven" last-chance therapies, especially if some responsible clinicians and their patients believe them to be effective?

In a three-year research project involving collaboration with a number of leading managed care organizations, we have been investigating, through a series of policy case studies, how insurers and health plans make coverage decisions about the adoption and application of new technologies.[2] In this policy discussion, we report on some very promising "exemplary practices" we have observed for managing last-chance therapies. We believe it would be premature to try to choose among these "exemplary practices." Because of the deep moral disagreement about the underlying issues, it would be wise for society to experiment with several promising strategies in order to learn more over time about how well they work and how morally acceptable they seem in light of actual practice.

Before describing the moral disagreement in more detail in Section III, we shall begin with some background about the scientific and societal context in which the practices we describe have been developed. In Section IV, we describe the "exemplary practices" in more detail, showing how the differences among them might be mapped onto different moral views about the weight we should assign various relevant considerations. In Section V, we return to the issue of the legitimacy of MCO decisions, suggesting how some of these practices could meet more general conditions for establishing legitimacy. In Section VI, we discuss a consequence of our view that we should experiment with a variety of fair procedures, namely that we may have to learn to tolerate what looks like violations of a formal requirement of justice. Finally, in the concluding section, we suggest ways in which the different "exemplary practices" can provide valuable lessons about coming to grips with limits in the domain of health care.

II. A BRIEF SOCIAL HISTORY

By 1989, and definitely by 1990, patients with advanced breast cancer, with the support of some clinicians, began to seek coverage for admittedly experimental use of ABMT from MCOs, including our collaborating sites. Analogues to this treatment had proven effective for some lymphatic cancers, and there was some scientific rationale for extending the treatment to solid tumors. Despite the enthusiasm of the clinicians, and the desperate belief of the breast cancer patients, many of whom were well-organized and informed, there was at the time no hard clinical evidence, and especially no controlled trials, that showed an advantage to the risky treatment over standard treatments.

During this period in the early 1990s, technology assessment of the therapy was undertaken at a number of our collaborating MCOs and by the Medical Advisory Panel (MAP) of the Blue Cross/Blue Shield (BC/BS) Technology Evaluation Center (TEC).[3] The National Cancer Institute authorized four randomized clinical trials for ABMT in advanced breast cancer in 1991 (with support from TEC), but these results would not be available for some time. There were no published controlled clinical trials until the Bezwoda et al. study in 1995.[4] Early evaluations of this technology had to be based on weaker forms of evidence. Between 1991 and 1994, several MCOs (as well as the Oregon Health Services Commission) decided that the technology was not ready for standard coverage, based on this early evidence regarding safety and efficacy. (As early as 1990, one of our collaborating sites, Health Partners, provided coverage under "alternative funding" for participation in clinical trials.) Similarly, early evaluations by the MAP found that there was inadequate evidence of efficacy or net benefit for ABMT for advanced breast cancer.

It was not until February 1996 that the BC/BS Medical Advisory Panel (MAP) finally decided that the therapy did meet its criteria for status as a noninvestigational technology. At its February 1996 meeting, the MAP evaluated evidence from the only published study of a randomized clinical trial (Bezwoda et al. 1995), as well as evidence from ongoing studies. The discussion suggested that the published study could not support conclusions about the greater efficacy of the therapy over standard treatments used in the U.S., but the MAP voted that its criteria were met.[5] A consideration of the identical evidence in June 1996 by California State Blue Shield led to the decision that the MAP criteria were not yet satisfied.[6] Several MCOs that had undertaken similar technology assessments also continued to believe, as of mid-1996, that there was insufficient evidence to show that the therapy met reasonable criteria of safety and efficacy for advanced breast cancer in comparison to standard treatments—even if it had by then become nearly "standard" therapy.

Like HIV patients desperate to try "promising" drugs prior to full FDA testing, however, breast cancer patients in the early 1990s demanded that they be allowed to decide whether the risks were worth taking.[7] The "gatekeeper" here, however, was not the FDA, charged with keeping unsafe pharmaceuticals off the market, but insurers, who, by contract, had no obligation to provide coverage for "investigational" treatments. When some MCOs, with adequate, evidence-based reason on their side, insisted the therapy was still "investigational" and "unproven," and might even prove worse than standard therapies, patients pursued both litigation and legislation, and the media "exposed" the denials. As early as 1991, *60 Minutes* featured a story about Aetna declining coverage for ABMT for breast cancer. In California in 1993, the estate of Nelene Fox won an $89 million suit against Health Net, which had originally denied coverage, then provided it. The suit charged the delay cost Fox her life. This suit cast a pall over traditional procedures for assessing the status of last-chance therapies.

Throughout the early 1990s, many insurers were providing coverage for patients participating in approved clinical trials. Unfortunately, this coverage seemed "arbitrary and capricious" according to an important study in the *New England Journal of Medicine,* which said coverage was not correlated with pretreatment clinical characteristics of the patients, the design or phase of the study, or the response to induction therapy.[8] That study showed that as many as three out of four patients seeking coverage for participation in a trial were granted it, and another half of those who threatened legal action when initially denied also received coverage. Activism clearly paid off for patients seeking treatment.

Responding to well-organized and highly visible advocates for these women, some state legislatures mandated coverage as early as 1994 and 1995, despite protests, for example in Minnesota and Massachusetts, that the mandates would make it impossible to continue proper clinical trials aimed at finding out if the procedure was truly superior to standard therapy. In other states, though legislative mandates were not passed, lawsuits in effect compelled coverage, since large punitive damages were imposed where coverage was denied or delayed. The resulting legal climate made it too risky and costly to deny what was still an unproven therapy.

Some insurers responded earlier than others to the handwriting on the wall, reading the message that traditional efforts to manage last-chance therapies by "holding the line" against investigational treatments were not working. Following the *60 Minutes* expose in 1991, Aetna, under the initiative of William McGivney, introduced a procedure in which an independent panel would be invoked when patients wanted a last-chance treatment that internal review denied coverage for (see Section IV for more detailed discussion). The same approach was adopted by Kaiser of Northern California in 1993. Other approaches were introduced in the same period, including Oregon Blue Cross Blue Shield's (1994) use of a transplant coordinator to manage the coverage of clinical trials for unproven last-chance therapies. In 1996, Health Partners introduced a special process for evaluating "promising therapies" that fall in the space between clearly investigational and standard treatment. It is this "new wave" of approaches that is the focus of our discussion in subsequent sections.

Before turning to the details of these newer approaches, we want to make three points. First, the social climate—including well-organized women's groups, a crusading media, committed practitioners, suspicious courts, and opportunistic legislators—clearly made the standard "technology assessment" approach to holding the line against coverage for last-chance "investigational" therapies untenable. Second, the legal and political interventions also had the effect of making it more difficult to find out if high-dose chemotherapy with stem cell support actually worked for advanced breast cancer. Although some MCOs decided to provide coverage for clinical trials, others (for example Harvard Community Health Plan, in an evaluation just before the Massachusetts mandate in 1994) were ethically uneasy about insisting on participation in trials, where patients would not always get the experimental regimen. The effect of compelling coverage meant that enrollment in NIH sponsored clinical trials was slowed. The public intervention through the courts and legislatures thus had the effect of frustrating another publicly supported goal in health care, namely, to make the system more efficient by pushing it to adopt "outcomes-based" medicine.

Third, the challenge to limit-setting by MCOs has its international analogues in publicly administered and financed health care systems that offer universal coverage. Even where public agencies might be thought to be a more "legitimate" locus for limit-setting decisions, a similar moral challenge is made. The suggestion is that "bureaucratic" decisions driven too much by "budget limitations" ignore the fact of urgent need in these cases, that is, that the moral priorities of decision makers are inappropriate. It would take us too far afield to discuss the similarities and differences between these cases (e.g., in England, Norway, and New Zealand) and those in the U.S., but it is important to see that the moral dimension of these issues arises across differences in institutional design, financing, national culture, and even incentives. We return to this issue briefly in Section V.

III. MORAL DISAGREEMENT AND ACCESS TO LAST-CHANCE THERAPIES

Reasonable people disagree about the best way to manage access to last-chance therapies because they disagree about the relative importance of several values or principles that come into conflict in these cases. In a pluralist society, where the underlying disagreement may involve conflicts among more comprehensive and systematic moral views, this means there is no one way of managing last-chance therapies that all agree is morally superior. In effect, we may have to learn to live with alternative best practices, not agreement on one approach, even if, as we shall see in Section V, this raises a challenge to one aspect of our traditional thinking about fairness and justice.

The general and difficult moral problem that all health plans must solve is how to meet the diverse needs of the insured population under reasonable resource constraints. This problem involves balancing population-centered concerns against patient-centered ones. Promising but unproven last-chance treatments evoke the general problem especially sharply since so much is at stake for the individual patients while at the same time the proposed treatments are often quite costly.

The major population-centered concerns are the prudent use of shared resources ("stewardship") and the promotion of public goods, such as knowledge about safety and efficacy produced through clinical trials. Those who emphasize these concerns will prefer policies under which collective resources would only be used for last-chance treatments that meet a threshold of established net benefit, and unproven therapies, if paid for at all, would only be covered in the context of controlled clinical trials, including randomized controlled trials in which a patient might receive a placebo or the standard treatment.

The key patient-centered concerns include: giving proper attention to patient needs, especially urgent needs as in the last-chance situations; avoiding harm, including the psychological harm that can arise from adversarialism; and managing uncertainties and risks through collaborative treatment planning. Those who emphasize these concerns will prefer policies for last-chance treatments that create a much lower standard of evidence that must be met for a treatment to be offered to a patient and that allow patients and their clinicians more leeway in judging the relative weight of risks and benefits. They are less likely to promote policies that would require patients to enter controlled trials, since they have no assurance in those trials of receiving the desired treatment.

Reasonable people will differ, however, in the degree to which they want to trade population-centered values in favor of patient-centered ones because of the urgency of the situation. There is no higher-level agreement on how much weight to give to the competing values or principles. Careful deliberation may resolve some of the conflicts, for often our views are not systematically considered, but it is unlikely to eliminate all of them. In many cases, the disagreement about weights may reflect significant differences in comprehensive moral views that people hold. For example, some "communitarians" will give more weight to guardianship of collective resources and the maximization of health benefits for a community that is cooperating to share resources. Classic liberals will give more weight to respect for individual autonomy. "Communitarians" and "liberals" will recognize the relevance of the reasons to which the other gives priority, since in other contexts, these factors also count as reasons for them in their thinking about how to solve the general problem of meeting needs under resource constraints. But the disagreement about weights or priorities will probably persist.

This disagreement about weights will then lead people to have different views about the acceptability of different ways of managing last-chance therapies. In the next section, we draw on our empirical study of decision making about coverage in MCOs to describe in more detail a set of "exemplary practices" regarding promising but unproven last-chance therapies. Our point is to show how they can be thought to reflect these different judgments about how to weigh competing values. We do not try to show that any one is best, since we know of no persuasive argument to that conclusion. Rather, we present each as a reasonable, good-faith effort to solve the problem.

IV. SOME EXEMPLARY PRACTICES IN MANAGING LAST-CHANCE THERAPIES

We begin with the earliest approach to managing last-chance therapies, the terminal illness program William McGivney started at Aetna in 1991. This program, used primarily in an indemnity insurance context, served as Aetna's *modus operandi* until the end of 1996 after Aetna purchased and merged with U.S. Healthcare. It was later adapted for use in an MCO setting by Northern California Kaiser Permanente and eventually became the model for the 1996 Friedman-Knowles legislation in California.

In the Aetna program, when medical directors in the field received a request for an unproven but promising last-chance cancer treatment that was not covered under established company policy, they referred the request to the home office at Hartford, where a consulting oncologist reviewed the clinical situation. A key feature of the program was that the home-office oncologist was only empowered to *approve* requests. If the consulting oncologist believed the request did not represent reasonable clinical practice for the particular patient, the case was automatically referred outside the company for independent review by the Medical Care Ombudsman Program in Bethesda, Maryland.

The Ombudsman Program, which was founded by Grace Monaco in 1991, provides independent expert opinion about appropriate treatment in serious but ambiguous clinical situations. On a timetable which can be as short as 24 hours, the Ombudsman Program will put together a panel of 2–3 experts with no affiliation to the insurer or the provider of the proposed treatment, to assess whether the proposed treatment has any scientific rationale for the particular patient. This is not a technology assessment of the new technology but an expert clinical assessment of the *potential value of the technology for a particular patient*. Typically, at least one of the experts is prepared to testify in court if the case should come to litigation.

Aetna did not restrict its own consulting oncologist from rendering negative coverage decisions because the consultant lacked competence. Any time that specialized technical expertise was needed, Aetna could have hired additional consultants at less cost to itself than using the Ombudsman Program. The problem Aetna was trying to solve with its terminal illness program was one of *trust*, not lack of technical expertise. The fact and appearance of "conflict of interest" was removed: if Aetna would say no only if an independent consultant said no, then the "no" should not be construed as a cost-driven decision. In circumstances of life-threatening illness and ambiguous information, the patient's trust in the decision-making process can be the difference between peace and outrage, or acceptance versus litigation.

In 1993, the Northern California region of Kaiser Permanente took the program that Aetna had developed in a primarily *indemnity* insurance context and adapted it for its own 3600 physician *prepaid group practice HMO*. Kaiser's experience helps us understand the mechanism through which Aetna's innovative way of addressing the patient's concern about the insurer's potential conflict of interest helps the decision-making process.[9]

Like Aetna, Northern California Kaiser Permanente decided to let patients in last-chance situations know that they could go outside of Kaiser for an independent opinion from the Ombudsman Program if they were not satisfied with the internal decision-making process. This was a controversial step for Kaiser to take. Some Kaiser doctors worried that allowing automatic appeal outside the HMO would diminish the group's ability to manage care rationally and feared that the program itself might be very costly.

What actually happened was exactly the opposite of what was feared. From 1994–1996, only 6 of the 2.5 million northern California members asked for referral to the Ombudsman program. When the patients' concerns about insurer trustworthiness and potential conflict of interest were addressed in advance by the option of going outside of Kaiser for independent consultation, patients and families were much readier to enter into a reflective dialogue with their Kaiser physicians about what treatment approach really made sense for them.

The Aetna-Kaiser "last-chance" policy might simply be dismissed as a cost-benefit calculation made by the MCO. Put cynically, it is better to pay for a few treatments than face lawsuits, any one of which would be more costly than a bunch of treatments. But it also can be defended—and is by some MCOs that adopt it—on more explicitly moral grounds that connect its adoption with our earlier discussion.

The policy can be defended morally in this way. It recognizes the fundamental importance in a medical system of "shared decision making" between patients and clinicians about risk taking. If an unproven last-chance therapy is viewed by some acknowledged experts as the most appropriate treatment for the patient, and if the patient understands the risks as presented by parties on all sides, then organizations have no better option than to rely on the informed decision of the patient and her clinician. This is not the same as saying that a patient can be granted just any last wish regarding treatment: there must be some basis in evidence and expert view that the therapy is not quackery. In the external review model, that expert view is provided by the independent panel. Under those conditions, simply refusing to provide coverage fails to acknowledge the obligation not to impose paternalistically a plan's own judgment about acceptable risks and benefits on the choices of desperately ill patients with few options. To be sure, the role of the MCO as a guardian of shared resources is reduced, but this is defensible in light of both the urgency of the patients' needs, and the special importance, in light of the uncertainty and the severity of need, of promoting a climate of shared decision making. Indeed, a proponent of this view might even say that the decision to hold to a hard-line denial is so likely to lead to a waste of resources in the legal and political climate that actually surrounds MCOs that the more efficient way to respect resources is to adopt the more lenient strategy toward last-chance therapies.

The Aetna-Kaiser approach has been embodied in new legislation. Under the Friedman-Knowles Experimental Treatment Act, passed by the California legislature in 1996, the kind of independent consultation process that Aetna and Kaiser Northern California have piloted will become mandatory for all California insurers starting July 1, 1998. The provisions of the bill are quite detailed, but the basic concept is simple. If a patient with a condition that has no effective therapy and is likely to cause death within two years is denied coverage for a new treatment that has some scientific promise, an independent expert review of the decision must be offered.

What is so important about the Friedman-Knowles bill is the effort to use legislation to influence the quality of the decision-making process without making any attempt to mandate what the decisions themselves should be. The bill does not mandate any specific treatments as so many states have done and continue to do. Rather, it mandates an organizational decision-making process designed to reduce fears about conflict of interest and increase deliberative reflection and clarity about the reasons for coverage decisions. (We note that in August 1997, the California Legislature considered legislation that takes a step backwards—toward mandating coverage for ABMT for breast cancer. Some proponents of the legislation say it eliminates "inequities" in coverage, since state employee benefits mandate ABMT but other insurers do not, an issue we return to in Section VI; critics say the state should not be making these disease-specific sorts of coverage decisions.)

Oregon Blue Cross Blue Shield has developed an approach to unproven bone marrow transplant regimens that reflects a slightly different moral framework. In 1993, in the aftermath of the *Fox* v. *Health Net* case, Oregon Blue Cross Blue Shield created a new, full-time role of transplant coordinator. The transplant coordinator is a clinically experienced nurse whose job is to work directly with patients and families, transplant programs, employers, and the Oregon Blue Cross Blue Shield benefit systems to create mutually satisfactory individualized treatment plans.

Whereas Aetna and Kaiser use the option for independent review outside of the organization to allay patient concerns about conflict of interest and promote collaboration, Oregon Blue Cross Blue Shield's distinctive approach is an unusually open and accountable process of deliberation and reason-giving and an especially strong emphasis on supporting scientific treatment evaluation. Instead of the infamous "gag rule," the Oregon program has developed what might be called a "let's talk it over openly and at great length rule!"

In ethics classes at medical, nursing, and business schools we try to teach students to identify the key facts and values in a situation and to develop options to advance the most important values that apply. This is what the Blue Cross transplant coordinator does every day, except she does it in circumstances of time pressure and high emotion, not in a classroom. When we interviewed her for our research project, we told her that her role seemed to be ⅓ nurse clinician, ⅓ nurse manager, and ⅓ ethics professor.

Here are the kinds of things the transplant coordinator says in dealing with the multiple stakeholders in the decision-making process:

- To a confused and frightened patient: "Do you have this article about the treatment? Have you read this other one? I'm going to be at the library this afternoon—why don't you come and meet me there and we can go over the information together?"
- To explain the importance of consistency to a wealthy patient: "Just because you're a VIP who

lives in the West Hills, you don't really want to make me treat you any differently than the person who comes to clean your house, do you?"

- To an employer who wants Blue Cross to cover an employee for a treatment that has no scientific justification: "But it's not based on sound science. Do you want to do the same thing for all the other women in your employee group? And even if you do, what will you tell their sisters who can't have the treatment? We want to be able to support scientific research that's going to answer the question."
- And, to a provider who is asking the insurer to cover an unproven treatment: "Then build your case to us, make your proposal so that when we make this decision, we can have sound rationale for a similar case on the next patient that you or someone else may send to us."

These comments illustrate the kind of deliberative dialogue that will have to happen hundreds of thousands and perhaps millions of times for doctors, patients, health plans, and society to move along a learning curve towards a more patient-centered, cost-effective, and ethical health care system.

The Oregon Blue Cross process, like the Aetna-Kaiser, places its ultimate emphasis on encouraging open deliberation between patient, clinician, and, in this case, coordinator. When we asked the coordinator how she was able to achieve trust with patients without the promise of an external, independent review, as in the Aetna-Kaiser approach, she said that she would view an instance of a patient going to external review as a failure on her part to have engaged the patient in the kind of deliberative give and take that her approach requires. The promise of external review, she feared, could lure patients away from the need to engage in deliberation with her.

Although deliberation and shared decision making were the key goals, Oregon Blue Cross Blue Shield has another priority as well—supporting clinically important research. If a promising but unproven last-chance treatment is available in a scientifically valid clinical trial, the plan will cover it. The coordinator claimed that as of our visit in June, 1996, no patients had resorted to litigation, and a significant number decided that the unproven treatments they initially requested were, after careful thinking, not really what they wanted.

In contrast to the Aetna-Kaiser approach, Oregon Blue Cross Blue Shield appears to put more emphasis on redirecting its stewardship responsibility toward supporting research. At the same time, since outright denial of unproven therapies was much less likely than in a traditional "hold the line" approach, it became possible to involve the patient in shared decision making.

In 1996, Health Partners, a prominent HMO in Minnesota, began to develop a special policy regarding "promising" but still unproven therapies. For selected "promising treatments," Health Partners will provide coverage even though the technology still falls into the category of "investigational" and would traditionally be excluded from coverage by contract language. The rationale for singling out the category of "promising treatments" is to introduce consistent policy about a particular technology, thereby avoiding case-by-case responses to individual requests.

Although this approach clearly relaxes the traditional hard line about stewardship, it keeps the health plan in control of what counts as "promising." Compared to the case-by-case decision-making by Aetna, Kaiser of Northern California, and Oregon Blue Cross Blue Shield, the Health Partners approach appears to place more emphasis on the organization's stewardship role. It remains to be seen whether the approach of offering greater consistency technology-by-technology at the cost of less flexibility in deciding individual cases leads to more or less conflict and litigation.

V. LEGITIMACY AND FAIRNESS

MCOs operate in a social climate of distrust. The vigorous effort at cost containment initiated by large employers (and the government) has largely been invisible to the public. Instead, managed care organizations have taken the heat for cost containment and system change. In this climate of distrust, the issue of legitimacy arises in a sharp form: why should patients or clinicians who think they are being denied medically appropriate treatments, even unproven last-chance therapies, accept as legitimate the decisions of MCOs? More to the point, under what conditions should the public come to view these decisions as legitimate?

Elsewhere,[10] we have argued that if the following four conditions were met, MCOs would take a large step toward earning legitimacy, at least over time:

1. Decisions regarding coverage for new technologies (and other limit-setting decisions) and their rationales must be publicly accessible.
2. The rationales for coverage decisions should aim to provide a *reasonable* construal of how the organization should provide "value for money" in meeting the varied health needs of a defined population under reasonable resource constraints. Specifically, a construal will be "reasonable" if it appeals to reasons and principles that are accepted as relevant by people who are disposed to finding terms of cooperation that are mutually justifiable.
3. There is a mechanism for challenge and dispute resolution regarding limit-setting decisions, including the opportunity for revising decisions in light of further evidence or arguments.
4. There is either voluntary or public regulation of the process to ensure that conditions 1–3 are met.

These four conditions capture at least the central necessary elements of a solution to the legitimacy and fairness problems for coverage decisions about new treatments. Condition 1 requires openness or publicity, that is, clarity about the reasons for decisions. Condition 2 involves some constraints on the kinds of reasons that can play a role in the rationale: it recognizes the fundamental interest all parties have to finding a justification all can accept as reasonable. Conditions 3 and 4 provide mechanisms for connecting deliberation and decisions within MCOs to a broader deliberative process, that is, for making them accountable to the results of a wider deliberation about what fairness requires.[11]

The procedures for managing last-chance therapies discussed in the previous section can meet these conditions. The first point to note is that the rationale for a plan's adopting one procedure rather than another should itself be made public, as Condition 1 requires. In such a rationale, giving more weight to responsibility for stewardship (as perhaps in the "promising-therapy" strategy) than another strategy does is the type of reason that meets Condition 2; so does the opposite weighting. Our main point in the discussion in the previous section is that each of the exemplary strategies could be defended publicly with reasons that meet these legitimacy conditions. What varies among these procedures is not the appeal to inappropriate reasons but the different weights reasonable people might give to relevant reasons.

In their implementation, any of these procedures should meet the conditions as well. For example, in the procedure followed by Oregon Blue Cross Blue Shield in managing patients who may be left out of available clinical trials, there is an effort to engage the patient in reason-giving of exactly the sort required by Condition 2. Similarly, the results of previous deliberations about particular cases could be made publicly available (still respecting confidentiality), so they were accessible to other patients seeking to develop claims about coverage in their cases. In effect, a kind of case law should emerge that governs the operation of the MCO and is accessible to patients and clinicians. Similarly, the kind of deliberation engaged in by the external ombudsman program used by Aetna and Kaiser, and now mandated by California law, could also meet the publicity conditions and the restrictions on types of reason-giving.

We noted earlier that the legitimacy problem in the U.S. has its analogue in publicly administered systems. In other countries, even where public commissions have been established to approve "principles" for priority-setting and limit-setting in those systems, the agencies that make actual decisions often keep their results quiet, perhaps implicit in quietly made budget decisions, and fail to meet the conditions we articulate. We believe compliance with these conditions would contribute to establishing greater legitimacy for hard choices made in those systems as well.

VI. FORMAL VS. PROCEDURAL JUSTICE

There may not be just one best or fairest way to manage last-chance therapies. At least, reasonable people may not agree on what the best procedure is, and in light of that disagreement, we should experiment with a family of "best practices," or so we have argued. There is a troubling implication of this view that some may view as a fatal objection. We see it not as a flaw in our approach but as a manifestation of an unavoidable moral uncertainty, which we must learn to respect and to live with.

Here is the problem. Suppose we have two patients, Groucho and Harpo, who are indistinguishable with regard to the relevant features of their cases. Both make the same claim that they need a particular high-dose chemotherapy with stem cell support for their advanced cancers. Let us suppose that this treatment has not yet been shown to provide a net benefit for the condition, which is in any case fatal on standard treatments. Groucho belongs to BestHealth and Harpo to GreatCare, two responsible MCOs that manage last-chance therapies in different ways. For the sake of specificity, suppose BestHealth uses a version of the external appeal procedure (like Aetna or Kaiser) and that GreatCare covers people in clinical trials if they meet the protocols or can make a reasonable case that they should be so covered (like Oregon Blue Cross Blue Shield). Suppose finally that Groucho is denied the transplant but that Harpo is given it. When Groucho hears about Harpo, should we agree if he complains that one of them has been treated unfairly?

Groucho claims that a fundamental principle of justice has been violated, the *formal* principle that like cases be treated similarly. If his case is just like Harpo's in all relevant ways, then they should either both get the treatment or neither should. The formal principle does not tell us how both should be treated, only that they should be treated similarly. Specifically, if there are *reasons* why Harpo should get the treatment, Groucho insists, then they apply equally to him, and he should receive it as well.

Groucho's complaint that a formal principle of justice is violated actually turns on there being a substantive reason or principle that grounds the decision to treat Harpo. To see this point, consider this variation on the case: in both MCOs, a coin is flipped about whether to give the treatment. Groucho loses and Harpo wins. When Groucho complains that like cases are being treated dissimilarly, we can now say to him, "The cases are unlike: there was a coin toss, and you lost and he won." There is no violation of the formal principle if there is a non-reason-based procedure used to distinguish the cases, as there is in the case of a coin toss. Alternatively, we can construe this as a case in which a principle is appealed to and uniformly applied, namely the principle that winners but not losers of coin-tosses (or other random processes) will get the treatment.

Neither BestHealth nor GreatCare flips coins, however. Within their different procedures, each encourages the giving of reasons and the deliberation about cases in light of reasons. We presuppose that the difference in their procedures for managing these cases rests on a difference in the ways the two organizations weight certain values, i.e., the values of urgency, stewardship, and shared decision-making with patients. Suppose further that we are right to claim there is no argument we all can accept that shows that one weighting (and thus one procedure) is clearly morally more justifiable than the other. That weighting, and thus the choice of fair procedure, is itself the focus of reasonable disagreement.

Generally, when there is a violation of the formal principle of justice, we are challenged to evaluate the weight attributed to a reason or principle that was applied in one case but not the other. We are asked to find a difference in the cases, that is, to show that they were not really similar in all relevant ways, or to affirm the uniform application of that reason or principle or of some alternative principle. But in the condition of moral pluralism we face, we have no candidate principle that purports to enjoy "our" endorsement independently of the fair procedure we are employing. A reason that may seem compelling or decisive in one process may not have that force in another. To be sure, we are not flipping coins in either case. We are deliberating carefully in a reason-driven and reason-giving way. But the weight given reasons in each setting is a reasonable reflection of other moral disagreements and moral uncertainty—the very uncertainty about what counts as a just outcome that compels us to adopt a procedural approach to fair outcomes. Groucho can be told this: Harpo was given the treatment because his plan reasoned about his case differently than your plan, and both ways of reasoning are relevant and arguably fair.

How tolerable would a system be if it produced situations in which a Groucho and Harpo were treated differently? We might think it makes a difference how centralized or decentralized a system is. In a decentralized system such as ours, for example, it may be difficult to require that insurance schemes use one rather than another procedurally fair way of deliberating about cases (though legislation such as the Friedman-Knowles Experimental Treatment Act imposes uniformity, at least at one stage of decision making). On what basis should the choice between procedures and weightings be made? Can we show a superior outcome to insisting on one such process rather than another? Without such a compelling regulatory reason, we might have trouble justifying public regulation requiring just one form of managing last-chance cases.

Despite the decentralization in our health care system, however, our courts arguably can impose a kind of unifying framework. Groucho might sue BestHealth, saying that not only does he want the treatment, and not only does some clinician he prefers say it is appropriate, but GreatCare has given the treatment to someone just like him. In practice, the courts could make unworkable an effort to experiment with different fair procedures to see what their advantages and disadvantages really are. On the other hand, what has often carried the day in actual suits on these matters is a demonstration of a lack of fair process and a kind of arbitrariness within an organization. If each of the fair procedures constitutes a reasonable defense against that sort of claim, then the courts might welcome an effort to rely more directly on fair procedures applied within plans. An analogy here would be the way in which the courts have welcomed decision making by ethics committees in hospitals as a preferable route to having these kinds of cases continuously adjudicated in the courts.

Would it be a compelling regulatory reason that we find differential treatment unacceptable and have to avoid it, if only by insisting on uniform process by convention? That might be true in a decentralized system, but it seems even more likely to be true in a national health care system. In the U.K., for example, it might seem more troubling that Groucho did not get his transplant in London but Harpo got his in Manchester. Here too, however, there might be disagreements among *meaningful political units,* the districts, about what constituted the "best" procedure. If that is true, then there might be even more reason to tolerate variation than there is in the U.S., where people are grouped into insurance schemes, not meaningful political units that have ways of selecting their procedures in a democratic fashion.

How acceptable differential treatment would be seems to depend, then, on whether a persuasive political rationale for uniformity can be developed. In a decentralized system, the political rationale would have to be sufficient to override the presumption that "private" insurers have the authority to select from among a set of comparably fair procedures. Of course, the political rationale might simply be that the legal system would not allow differential treatment; but that too remains to be seen.

In a national health care system, the political rationale for uniformity would have to show that differential treatment among districts was less acceptable than giving them the autonomy to select their own procedures. If meaningful political units, like districts, felt strongly enough about their choices of procedures, the costs of uniformity might be too high. For the problem we are facing, then, it remains unclear how unacceptable it would be for Harpo to get a last chance when Groucho does not.

VII. CONCLUSIONS

Making decisions and policies about payment for promising but unproven last-chance therapies presents the most difficult moral and clinical policy challenge a health care system can face. Important values, all of which command respect and attention, inevitably come into conflict in these difficult situations, especially (1) giving some (how much?) priority to meeting the *urgent claims* of patients in last-chance situations, (2) providing *stewardship* of collective resources, (3) producing the public good of *scientific knowledge* about the effectiveness of unproven therapies, and (4) respecting *patient autonomy* through collaborative decision making about risks and benefits.

General principles of distributive justice do not tell us how to weigh the relative claims of these competing considerations. Nevertheless, the insurers and MCOs whose programs we describe have developed procedures for making decisions and policies that can be defended on the basis of justifiable—although different—weights they give to the different values. In our decentralized, competitive system—largely in response to political and legal pressures patients and clinicians have focused on these plans—an important social experiment has emerged. Different procedural "solutions" to the problem of limit setting in the case of new technologies are being developed and honed in practice. What can we learn from the experiment?

If we as a society can tolerate the inevitable differences in decisions and policies that the different configurations of values will create, we will have an opportunity to learn from the dialectic between principles and practice. We will see more clearly through a legacy of specific decisions and their outcomes just what the moral and nonmoral benefits and costs of the different approaches are. What we learn will help us refine our notions of fair procedure and in turn help us produce better solutions to the general problem of limit-setting in health care that all societies are struggling with. In the last 20–30 years, we have learned much and seen important changes in how individual clinicians and patients negotiate the difficult issues of clinical planning in the context of threats to life itself. If we have enough societal fortitude, and a modicum of strong political leadership, close study of the experiences generated by the kinds of programs we have described can help us do the same at the level of social policy.

NOTES

1. We distinguish the case of promising but unproven last-chance therapies from the case of treatments that professionals decide are futile. In futility cases, the judgment of the professional is that there will be harm to the patient, or there is at least clear evidence that there will be no benefit. The patient or family might disagree, perhaps because they seek miracles or perhaps because they view mere physiological functioning as a benefit. Here there is a conflict between stewardship and the somewhat confusing notion of patient "autonomy." The conflict eases if we restrict the plausible core of patient autonomy to a (positive) right to participate in decisions about treatment and a (negative) right to refuse treatment, and we distinguish that core from an (implausible) "entitlement" to have whatever treatment one desires, which involves unrestricted claims on resources held by others. There is also a conflict between paternalism (in the form of a legitimate concern to avoid doing harm) and a patient's or family's judgment about what counts as a benefit. These are interesting issues, but this kind of case is marked by clear professional judgment rooted in considerable *certainty about the evidence.* In the last-chance cases we are concerned with, it is professional *uncertainty*, not certainty, that is key.
2. Case studies completed to date include, Sabin, J., Daniels, N., 1997a. "How MCOs deliberated about coverage for lung volume reduction surgery: A Focal Case Study," (unpublished manuscript), and Wilkinson, S., Sabin, J., and Daniels, N. 1997. "How MCOs decided to cover pallidotomy for advanced Parkinson's Disease: A Focal Case Study," (unpublished manuscript). See also Daniels, N. and Sabin, J. 1997. "Limits to Health Care: Fair Procedures, Democratic Deliberation, and the Legitimacy Problem for Insurers," *Philosophy and Public Affairs* 26, no. 4 (Fall 1997): 303–350.
3. Other technology assessment centers not affiliated with MCOs, such as ECRI, also undertook evaluations.
4. Bezwoda, W.R., Seymour, L., Dansey, R.D., "High-dose Chemotherapy with Hematopoietic Rescue as Primary Treatment for Metastatic Breast Cancer: A Randomized Trial." 1995. *J Clin Oncol* 13:2483–89.
5. The MAP criteria are as follows:

   (1) The technology must have final approval from the appropriate government regulatory body.
   (2) The scientific evidence must permit conclusions concerning the effect of the technology on health outcomes.
   (3) The technology must improve the net health outcome.
   (4) The technology must be as beneficial as any established alternative.
   (5) The improvement must be attainable outside the investigational settings.

   The South African study (Bezwoda et al. 1995) used as its control a regimen of standard chemotherapy that was inferior in outcomes to the conventional therapy that would standardly be available in the U.S. and elsewhere. Showing that high-dose chemotherapy was superior to a conventional regimen that itself was far inferior to conventional therapy commonly in use should not persuade us of the superior efficacy of the high-dose regimen.
6. The California Blue Shield evaluation took place in a public setting, the only such open technology assessment process that we know of aside from Oregon

Health Resources Commission. At its discussion, the panel seemed comfortable supporting its conclusion only after it was assured that no one actually wanting the high-dose chemotherapy was unable to get it, despite its investigational status.

7. See Norman Daniels, *Seeking Fair Treatment: From the AIDS Epidemic to National Health Care Reform*, New York: Oxford University Press, 1995, Chapter 6.
8. Peters, W.P., and Rogers, M.C. 1994. "Variation in Approval by Insurance Companies for Coverage of Autologous Bone Marrow Transplantion for Breast Cancer," *NEJM* 330:7:473–7.
9. Beebe, D.B., Rosenfeld, A.B., Collins, N.: "An Approach to Decisions about Coverage of Investigational Treatments." *HMO Practice* 11(2): 65–67, 1997 (June).
10. See Daniels and Sabin, "Limits to Health Care: Fair Procedures, Democratic Deliberation, and the Legitimacy Problem for Insurers," *Philosophy and Public Affairs* 26, no. 4 (Fall 1997): 303–350.
11. These conditions were developed independently but fit reasonably well with the principles of publicity, reciprocity, and accountability governing democratic deliberation cited by Amy Gutmann and Dennis Thompson, *Democracy and Disagreement* (Cambridge: Harvard University Press, 1996). For reservations about their account, see Norman Daniels, "Enabling Democratic Deliberation," Pacific Division of the American Philosophical Association, March, 1997.

EQUALITY AND THE ENDS OF MEDICINE

SHOULD ALCOHOLICS COMPETE EQUALLY FOR LIVER TRANSPLANTATION?

Alvin H. Moss and Mark Siegler

Until recently, liver transplantation for patients with alcohol-related end-stage liver disease (ARESLD) was not considered a treatment option. Most physicians in the transplant community did not recommend it because of initial poor results in this population and because of a predicted high recidivism rate that would preclude long-term survival. In 1988, however, Starzl and colleagues reported one-year survival rates for patients with ARESLD comparable to results in patients with other causes of end-stage liver disease (ESLD). Although the patients in the Pittsburgh series may represent a carefully selected population, the question is no longer, Can we perform transplants in patients with alcoholic liver disease and obtain acceptable results? But, Should we? This question is particularly timely since the Health Care Financing Administration (HCFA) has recommended that Medicare coverage for liver transplantation be offered to patients with alcoholic cirrhosis who are abstinent. The HCFA proposes that the same eligibility criteria be used for patients with ARESLD as are used for patients with other causes of ESLD, such as primary biliary cirrhosis and sclerosing cholangitis.

From *Journal of the American Medical Association* Vol. 265, 1296–1298.

Editors' note: All notes have been deleted. Readers who wish to follow up on sources should consult the original article.

SHOULD PATIENTS WITH ARESLD RECEIVE TRANSPLANTS?

At first glance, this question seems simple to answer. Generally, in medicine, a therapy is used if it works and saves lives. But the circumstances of liver transplantation differ from those of most other lifesaving therapies, including long-term mechanical ventilation and dialysis, in three important respects:

Nonrenewable Resource

First, although most lifesaving therapies are expensive, liver transplantation uses a nonrenewable, absolutely scarce resource—a donor liver. In contrast to patients with end-stage renal disease, who may receive either a transplant or dialysis therapy, every patient with ESLD who does not receive a liver transplant will die. This dire, absolute scarcity of donor livers would be greatly exacerbated by including patients with ARESLD as potential candidates for liver transplantation. In 1985, 63,737 deaths due to hepatic disease occurred in the United States, at least 36,000 of which were related to alcoholism, but fewer than 1000 liver transplants were performed. Although patients with ARESLD represent more than 50 percent of the patients with ESLD, patients with ARESLD account for less than 10 percent of those receiving transplants (*New York Times*, April 3, 1990:B6 [col 1]). If patients with ARESLD were accepted for liver transplantation on an equal basis, as suggested by the HCFA, there would potentially be more than 30,000 additional candidates each year. (No data exist to indicate how many patients in the late stages of ARESLD would meet transplantation eligibility criteria.) In 1987, only 1182 liver transplants were performed; in 1989, fewer than 2000 were done. Even if all donor livers available were given to patients with ARESLD, it would not be feasible to provide transplants for even a small fraction of them. Thus, the dire, absolute nature of donor liver scarcity mandates that distribution be based on unusually rigorous standards—standards not required for the allocation of most other resources such as dialysis machines and ventilators, both of which are only *relatively* scarce.

Comparison with Cardiac Transplantation

Second, although a similarly dire, absolute scarcity of donor hearts exists for cardiac transplantation, the allocational decisions for cardiac transplantation differ from those for liver transplantation. In liver transplantation, ARESLD causes more than 50 percent of the cases of ESLD; in cardiac transplantation, however, no one predominant disease or contributory factor is responsible. Even for patients with end-stage ischemic heart disease who smoked or who failed to adhere to dietary regimens, it is rarely clear that one particular behavior caused the disease. Also, unlike our proposed consideration for liver transplantation, a history of alcohol abuse is considered a contraindication and is a common reason for a patient with heart disease to be denied cardiac transplantation. Thus, the allocational decisions for heart transplantation differ from those for liver transplantation in two ways: determining a cause for end-stage heart disease is less certain, and patients with a history of alcoholism are usually rejected from heart transplant programs.

Expensive Technology

Third, a unique aspect of liver transplantation is that it is an expensive technology that has become a target of cost containment in health care. It is, therefore, essential to maintain the approbation and support of the public so that organs continue to be donated under appropriate clinical circumstances—even in spite of the high cost of transplantation.

General Guideline Proposed

In view of the distinctive circumstances surrounding liver transplantation, we propose as a general guideline that patients with ARESLD should not compete equally with other candidates for liver transplantation. We are *not* suggesting that patients with ARESLD should *never* receive liver transplants. Rather, we propose that a priority ranking be established for the use of this dire, absolutely scarce societal resource and that patients with ARESLD be lower on the list than others with ESLD.

OBJECTIONS TO PROPOSAL

We realize that our proposal may meet with two immediate objections: (1) Some may argue that since alcoholism is a disease, patients with ARESLD should be considered equally for liver transplantation. (2) Some will question why patients with

ARESLD should be singled out for discrimination, when the medical profession treats many patients who engage in behavior that causes their diseases. We will discuss these objections in turn.

Alcoholism: How Is It Similar to and Different from Other Diseases?

We do not dispute the reclassification of alcoholism as a disease. Both hereditary and environmental factors contribute to alcoholism, and physiological, biochemical, and genetic markers have been associated with increased susceptibility. Identifying alcoholism as a disease enables physicians to approach it as they do other medical problems and to differentiate it from bad habits, crimes, or moral weaknesses. More important, identifying alcoholism as a disease also legitimizes medical interventions to treat it.

Alcoholism is a chronic disease, for which treatment is available and effective. More than 1.43 million patients were treated in 5586 alcohol treatment units in the 12-month period ending October 30, 1987. One comprehensive review concluded that more than two thirds of patients who accept therapy improve. Another cited four studies in which at least 54 percent of patients were abstinent a minimum of one year after treatment. A recent study of alcohol-impaired physicians reported a 100 percent abstinence rate an average of 33.4 months after therapy was initiated. In this study, physician-patients rated Alcoholics Anonymous, the largest organization of recovering alcoholics in the world, as the most important component of their therapy.

Like other chronic diseases—such as type I diabetes mellitus, which requires the patient to administer insulin over a lifetime—alcoholism requires the patient to assume responsibility for participating in continuous treatment. Two key elements are required to successfully treat alcoholism: the patient must accept his or her diagnosis and must assume responsibility for treatment. The high success rates of some alcoholism treatment programs indicate that many patients can accept responsibility for their treatment. ARESLD, one of the sequelae of alcoholism, results from 10 to 20 years of heavy alcohol consumption. The risk of ARESLD increases with the amount of alcohol consumed and with the duration of heavy consumption. In view of the quantity of alcohol consumed, the years, even decades, required to develop ARESLD, and the availability of effective alcohol treatment, attributing personal responsibility for ARESLD to the patient seems all the more justified. We believe, therefore, that even though alcoholism is a chronic disease, alcoholics should be held responsible for seeking and obtaining treatment that could prevent the development of late-stage complications such as ARESLD. Our view is consistent with that of Alcoholics Anonymous: alcoholics are responsible for undertaking a program for recovery that will keep their disease of alcoholism in remission.

Are We Discriminating Against Alcoholics?

Why should patients with ARESLD be singled out when a large number of patients have health problems that can be attributed to so-called voluntary health-risk behavior? Such patients include smokers with chronic lung disease; obese people who develop type II diabetes; some individuals who test positive for the human immunodeficiency virus; individuals with multiple behavioral risk factors (inattention to blood pressure, cholesterol, diet, and exercise) who develop coronary artery disease; and people such as skiers, motorcyclists, and football players who sustain activity-related injuries. We believe that the health care system should respond based on the actual medical needs of patients rather than on the factors (e.g., genetic, infectious, or behavioral) that cause the problem. We also believe that individuals should bear some responsibility—such as increased insurance premiums—for medical problems associated with voluntary choices. The critical distinguishing factor for treatment of ARESLD is the scarcity of the resource needed to treat it. The resources needed to treat most of these other conditions are only moderately or relatively scarce, and patients with these diseases or injuries can receive a share of the resources (i.e., money, personnel, and medication) roughly equivalent to their need. In contrast, there are insufficient donor livers to sustain the lives of all with ESLD who are in need. This difference permits us to make some discriminating choices—or to establish priorities—in selecting candidates for liver transplantation based on notions of fairness. In addition, this reasoning

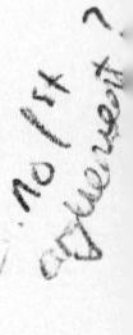

enables us to offer patients with alcohol-related medical and surgical problems their fair share of relatively scarce resources, such as blood products, surgical care, and intensive care beds, while still maintaining that their claim on donor livers is less compelling than the claims of others.

REASONS PATIENTS WITH ARESLD SHOULD HAVE A LOWER PRIORITY ON TRANSPLANT WAITING LISTS

Two arguments support our proposal. The first argument is a moral one based on considerations of fairness. The second one is based on policy considerations and examines whether public support of liver transplantation can be maintained if, as a result of a first-come, first-served approach, patients with ARESLD receive more than half the available donor livers. Finally, we will consider further research necessary to determine which patients with ARESLD should be candidates for transplantation, albeit with a lower priority.

Fairness

Given a tragic shortage of donor livers, what is the fair or just way to allocate them? We suggest that patients who develop ESLD through no fault of their own (e.g., those with congenital biliary atresia or primary biliary cirrhosis) should have a higher priority in receiving a liver transplant than those whose liver disease results from failure to obtain treatment for alcoholism. In view of the dire, absolute scarcity of donor livers, we believe it is fair to hold people responsible for their choices, including decisions to refuse alcoholism treatment, and to allocate organs on this basis.

It is unfortunate but not unfair to make this distinction. When not enough donor livers are available for all who need one, choices have to be made, and they should be founded on one or more proposed principles of fairness for distributing scarce resources. We shall consider four that are particularly relevant:

- *To each, an equal share of treatment.*
- *To each, similar treatment for similar cases.*
- *To each, treatment according to personal effort.*
- *To each, treatment according to ability to pay.*

It is not possible to give each patient with ESLD an *equal share*, or, in this case, a functioning liver. The problem created by the absolute scarcity of donor livers is that of inequality; some receive livers while others do not. But what is fair need not be equal. Although a first-come, first-served approach has been suggested to provide each patient with an equal chance, we believe it is fairer to give a child dying of biliary atresia an opportunity for a *first* normal liver than it is to give a patient with ARESLD who was born with a normal liver a *second* one.

Because the goal of providing each person with an equal share of health care sometimes collides with the realities of finite medical resources, the principle of *similar treatment for similar cases* has been found to be helpful. Outka stated it this way: "If we accept the case for equal access, but if we simply cannot, physically cannot, treat all who are in need, it seems more just to discriminate by virtue of categories of illness, rather than between rich ill and poor ill." This principle is derived from the principle of formal justice, which, roughly stated, says that people who are equal in relevant respects should be treated equally and that people who are unequal in relevant respects should be treated differently. We believe that patients with ARESLD are unequal in a relevant respect to others with ESLD, since their liver failure was preventable; therefore, it is acceptable to treat them differently.

Our view also relies on the principle of, *To each, treatment according to personal effort.* Although alcoholics cannot be held responsible for their disease, once their condition has been diagnosed they can be held responsible for seeking treatment and for preventing the complication of ARESLD. The standard of personal effort and responsibility we propose for alcoholics is the same as that held by Alcoholics Anonymous. We are not suggesting that some lives and behaviors have greater value than others—an approach used and appropriately repudiated when dialysis machines were in short supply. But we are holding people responsible for their personal effort.

Health policymakers have predicted that this principle will assume greater importance in the future. In the context of scarce health care resources, Blank foresees a reevaluation of our health care priorities, with a shift toward individual responsibility and a renewed emphasis on the individual's obligation to society to maximize one's health.

Similarly, more than a decade ago, Knowles observed that prevention of disease requires effort. He envisioned that the next major advances in the health of the American people would be determined by what individuals are willing to do for themselves.

To each, treatment according to ability to pay has also been used as a principle of distributive justice. Since alcoholism is prevalent in all socioeconomic strata, it is not discrimination against the poor to deny liver transplantation to patients with alcoholic liver disease. In fact, we believe that poor patients with ARESLD have a stronger claim for a donor liver than rich patients, precisely because many alcohol treatment programs are not available to patients lacking in substantial private resources or health insurance. Ironically, it is precisely this group of poor and uninsured patients who are most likely not to be eligible to receive a liver transplant because of their inability to pay. We agree with Outka's view of fairness that would discriminate according to categories of illness rather than according to wealth.

Policy Considerations Regarding Public Support for Liver Transplantation

Today, the main health policy concerns involve issues of financing, distributive justice, and rationing medical care. Because of the many deficiencies in the U.S. health care system—in maternal and child health, in the unmet needs of the elderly, and in the millions of Americans without health insurance—an increasing number of commentators are drawing attention to the trade-offs between basic health care for the many and expensive, albeit lifesaving, care for the few.

Because of its high unit cost, liver transplantation is often at the center of these discussions, as it has been in Oregon, where the legislature voted to eliminate Medicaid reimbursement for all transplants except kidneys and corneas. In this era of health care cost containment, a sense of limits is emerging and allocational choices are being made. Oregon has already shown that elected officials and the public are prepared to face these issues.

In our democracy, it is appropriate that community mores and values be regarded seriously when deciding the most appropriate use of a scarce and nonrenewable organ symbolized as a "Gift of Life." As if to underscore this point, the report of the Task Force on Organ Transplantation recommended that each donated organ be considered a national resource for the public good and that the public must participate in decisions on how to use this resource to best serve the public's interests.

Much of the initial success in securing public and political approval for liver transplantation was achieved by focusing media and political attention not on adults but on children dying of ESLD. The public may not support transplantation for patients with ARESLD in the same way that they have endorsed this procedure for babies born with biliary atresia. This assertion is bolstered not only by the events in Oregon but also by the results of a Louis Harris and Associates national survey, which showed that lifesaving therapy for premature infants or for patients with cancer was given the highest health care priority by the public and that lifesaving therapy for patients with alcoholic liver disease was given the lowest. In this poll, the public's view of health care priorities was shared by leadership groups also polled: physicians, nurses, employers, and politicians.

Just because a majority of the public holds these views does not mean that they are right, but the moral intuition of the public, which is also shared by its leaders, reflects community values that must be seriously considered. Also indicative of community values are organizations such as Mothers Against Drunk Driving, Students Against Drunk Driving, corporate employee assistance programs, and school student assistance programs. Their existence signals that many believe that a person's behavior can be modified so that the consequences of behavior such as alcoholism can be prevented. Thus, giving donor livers to patients with ARESLD on an equal basis with other patients who have ESLD might lead to a decline in public support for liver transplantation.

SHOULD ANY ALCOHOLICS BE CONSIDERED FOR TRANSPLANTATION? NEED FOR FURTHER RESEARCH

Our proposal for giving lower priority for liver transplantation to patients with ARESLD does not completely rule out transplantation for this group. Patients with ARESLD who had not previously been offered therapy and who are now abstinent could be acceptable candidates. In addition, patients lower on the waiting list, such as patients with ARESLD who have been treated and are now abstinent, might be eligible for a donor liver in some regions because of the increased availability of donor organs there. Even if only because of these possible conditions for transplantation, further research is needed to determine which patients with ARESLD would have the best outcomes after liver transplantation.

Transplant programs have been reluctant to provide transplants to alcoholics because of concern about one unfavorable outcome: a high recidivism rate. Although the overall recidivism rate for the Pittsburgh patients was only 11.5 percent, in the group of patients who had been abstinent less than 6 months it was 43 percent. Also, compared with the entire group in which one-year survival was 74 percent, the survival rate in this subgroup was lower, at 64 percent.

In the recently proposed Medicare criteria for coverage of liver transplantation, the HCFA acknowledged that the decision to insure patients with alcoholic cirrhosis "may be considered controversial by some." As if to counter possible objections, the HCFA listed requirements for patients with alcoholic cirrhosis: patients must meet the transplant center's requirement for abstinence prior to liver transplantation and have documented evidence of sufficient social support to ensure both recovery from alcoholism and compliance with the regimen of immunosuppressive medication.

Further research should answer lingering questions about liver transplantation for ARESLD patients: Which characteristics of a patient with ARESLD can predict a successful outcome? How long is abstinence necessary to qualify for transplantation? What type of a social support system must a patient have to ensure good results? These questions are being addressed. Until the answers are known, we propose that further transplantation for patients with ARESLD be limited to abstinent patients who had not previously been offered alcoholism treatment and to abstinent treated patients in regions of increased donor liver availability, and that it be carried out as part of prospective research protocols at a few centers skilled in transplantation and alcohol research.

COMMENT

Should patients with ARESLD compete equally for liver transplants? In a setting in which there is a dire, absolute scarcity of donor livers, we believe the answer is no. Considerations of fairness suggest that a first-come, first-served approach for liver transplantation is not the most just approach. Although this decision is difficult, it is only fair that patients who have not assumed equal responsibility for maintaining their health or for accepting treatment for a chronic disease should be treated differently. Considerations of public values and mores suggest that the public may not support liver transplantation if patients with ARESLD routinely receive more than half of the available donor livers. We conclude that since not all can live, priorities must be established and that patients with ARESLD should be given a lower priority for liver transplantation than others with ESLD.

ALCOHOLICS AND LIVER TRANSPLANTATION

Carl Cohen, Martin Benjamin, and the Ethics and Social Impact Committee of the Transplant and Health Policy Center, Ann Arbor, Michigan

Alcoholic cirrhosis of the liver—severe scarring due to the heavy use of alcohol—is by far the major cause of end-stage liver disease. For persons so afflicted, life may depend on receiving a new transplanted liver. The number of alcoholics in the United States needing new livers is great, but the supply of available livers for transplantation is small. *Should those whose end-stage liver disease was caused by alcohol abuse be categorically excluded from candidacy for liver transplantation?* This question, partly medical and partly moral, must now be confronted forthrightly. Many lives are at stake.

Reasons of two kinds underlie a widespread unwillingness to transplant livers into alcoholics: First, there is a common conviction—explicit or tacit—that alcoholics are morally blameworthy, their condition the result of their own misconduct, and that such blameworthiness disqualifies alcoholics in unavoidable competition for organs with others equally sick but blameless. Second, there is a common belief that because of their habits, alcoholics will not exhibit satisfactory survival rates after transplantation, and that, therefore, good stewardship of a scarce lifesaving resource requires that alcoholics not be considered for liver transplantation. We examine both of these arguments.

THE MORAL ARGUMENT

A widespread condemnation of drunkenness and a revulsion for drunks lie at the heart of this public policy issue. Alcoholic cirrhosis—unlike other causes of end-stage liver disease—is brought on by a person's conduct, by heavy drinking. Yet if the dispute here were only about whether to treat someone who is seriously ill because of personal conduct, we would not say—as we do not in cases of other serious diseases resulting from personal conduct—that such conduct disqualifies a person from receiving desperately needed medical attention. Accident victims injured because they were not wearing seat belts are treated without hesitation; reformed smokers who become coronary bypass candidates partly because they disregarded their physicians' advice about tobacco, diet, and exercise are not turned away because of their bad habits. But new livers are a scarce resource, and transplanting a liver into an alcoholic may, therefore, result in death for a competing candidate whose liver disease was wholly beyond his or her control. Thus we seem driven, in this case unlike in others, to reflect on the weight given to the patient's personal conduct. And heavy drinking—unlike smoking, or overeating, or failing to wear a seat belt—is widely regarded as morally wrong.

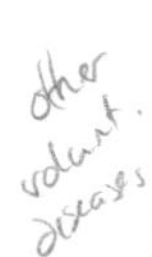

Many contend that alcoholism is not a moral failing but a disease. Some authorities have recently reaffirmed this position, asserting that alcoholism is "best regarded as a chronic disease." But this claim cannot be firmly established and is far from universally believed. Whether alcoholism is indeed a disease, or a moral failing, or both, remains a disputed matter surrounded by intense controversy.

Even if it is true that alcoholics suffer from a somatic disorder, many people will argue that this disorder results in deadly liver disease only when coupled with a weakness of will—a weakness for which part of the blame must fall on the alcoholic. This consideration underlies the conviction that the alcoholic needing a transplanted liver, unlike a nonalcoholic competing for the same liver, is at least partly responsible for his or her need. Therefore, some conclude, the alcoholic's personal failing is rightly considered in deciding upon his or her entitlement to this very scarce resource.

Is this argument sound? We think it is not. Whether alcoholism is a moral failing, in whole or in part, remains uncertain. But even if we suppose that it is, it does not follow that we are justified in categorically denying liver transplants to those alcoholics suffering from endstage cirrhosis. We could rightly preclude alcoholics from transplantation only if we assume that qualification for a new organ requires some level of moral virtue or is canceled by some level of moral vice. But there is absolutely no agreement—and there is likely to be none—about what constitutes moral virtue and vice and what rewards and penalties they deserve. The assumption that undergirds the moral argument for precluding alcoholics is thus unacceptable. Moreover; even if we could agree (which, in fact, we cannot) upon the kind of misconduct we would be looking for, the fair weighting of such a consideration would entail highly intrusive investigations into patients' moral habits—investigations universally thought repugnant. Moral evaluation is wisely and rightly excluded from all deliberations of who should be treated and how.

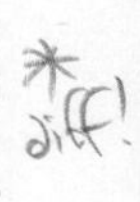

From *Journal of the American Medical Association* Vol. 265, 1299–1301.

Editors' note: All notes have been deleted. Readers who wish to follow up on sources should consult the original article.

Indeed, we do exclude it. We do not seek to determine whether a particular transplant candidate is an abusive parent or a dutiful daughter; whether candidates cheat on their income taxes or their spouses; or whether potential recipients pay their parking tickets or routinely lie when they think it is in their best interests. We refrain from considering such judgments for several good reasons: (1) We have genuine and well-grounded doubts about comparative degrees of voluntariness and, therefore, *cannot pass judgment fairly.* (2) Even if we could assess degrees of voluntariness reliably, we *cannot know what penalties different degrees of misconduct deserve.* (3) *Judgments of this kind could not be made consistently in our medical system*—and a fundamental requirement of a fair system in allocating scarce resources is that it treat all in need of certain goods on the same standard, without unfair discrimination by group.

If alcoholics should be penalized because of their moral fault, then all others who are equally at fault in causing their own medical needs should be similarly penalized. To accomplish this, we would have to make vigorous and sustained efforts to find out whose conduct has been morally weak or sinful and to what degree. That inquiry, as a condition for medical care or for the receipt of goods in short supply, we certainly will not and should not undertake.

The unfairness of such moral judgments is compounded by other accidental factors that render moral assessment especially difficult in connection with alcoholism and liver disease. Some drinkers have a greater predisposition for alcohol abuse than others. And for some who drink to excess, the predisposition to cirrhosis is also greater; many grossly intemperate drinkers do not suffer grievously from liver disease. On the other hand, alcohol consumption that might be considered moderate for some may cause serious liver disease in others. It turns out, in fact, that the disastrous consequences of even low levels of alcohol consumption may be much more common in women than in men. Therefore, penalizing cirrhotics by denying them transplant candidacy would have the effect of holding some groups arbitrarily to a higher standard than others and would probably hold women to a higher standard of conduct than men.

Moral judgments that eliminate alcoholics from candidacy thus prove unfair and unacceptable. The alleged (but disputed) moral misconduct of alcoholics with end-stage liver disease does not justify categorically excluding them as candidates for liver transplantation.

MEDICAL ARGUMENT

Reluctance to use available livers in treating alcoholics is due in some part to the conviction that, because alcoholics would do poorly after transplant as a result of their bad habits, good stewardship of organs in short supply requires that alcoholics be excluded from consideration.

This argument also fails, for two reasons: First, it fails because the premise—that the outcome for alcoholics will invariably be poor relative to other groups—is at least doubtful and probably false. Second, it fails because, even if the premise were true, it could serve as a good reason to exclude alcoholics only if it were an equally good reason to exclude other groups having a prognosis equally bad or worse. But equally low survival rates have not excluded other groups; fairness therefore requires that this group not be categorically excluded either.

In fact, the data regarding the post-transplant histories of alcoholics are not yet reliable. Evidence gathered in 1984 indicated that the 1-year survival rate for patients with alcoholic cirrhosis was well below the survival rate for other recipients of liver transplants, excluding those with cancer. But a 1988 report, with a larger (but still small) sample number, shows remarkably good results in alcoholics receiving transplants: 1-year survival is 73.2%—and of 35 carefully selected (and possibly non-representative) alcoholics who received transplants and lived 6 months or longer, only two relapsed into alcohol abuse. Liver transplantation, it would appear, can be a very sobering experience. Whether this group continues to do as well as a comparable group of non-alcoholic liver recipients remains uncertain. But the data, although not supporting the broad inclusion of alcoholics, do suggest that medical considerations do not now justify categorically excluding alcoholics from liver transplantation.

A history of alcoholism is of great concern when considering liver transplantation, not only because of the impact of alcohol abuse upon the entire system of the recipient, but also because the life of an alcoholic tends to be beset by general disorder.

Returning to heavy drinking could ruin a new liver, although probably not for years. But relapse into heavy drinking would quite likely entail the inability to maintain the routine of multiple medication, daily or twice-daily, essential for immunosuppression and survival. As a class, alcoholic cirrhotics may therefore prove to have substantially lower survival rates after receiving transplants. All such matters should be weighed, of course. But none of them gives any solid reason to exclude alcoholics from consideration categorically.

Moreover, even if survival rates for alcoholics selected were much lower than normal—a supposition now in substantial doubt—what could fairly be concluded from such data? Do we exclude from transplant candidacy members of other groups known to have low survival rates? In fact we do not. Other things being equal, we may prefer not to transplant organs in short supply into patients afflicted, say, with liver cell cancer, knowing that such cancer recurs not long after a new liver is implanted. Yet in some individual cases we do it. Similarly, some transplant recipients have other malignant neoplasms or other conditions that suggest low survival probability. Such matters are weighed in selecting recipients, but they are insufficient grounds to categorically exclude an entire group. This shows that the argument for excluding alcoholics based on survival probability rates alone is simply not just.

THE ARGUMENTS DISTINGUISHED

In fact, the exclusion of alcoholics from transplant candidacy probably results from an intermingling, perhaps at times a confusion, of the moral and medical arguments. But if the moral argument indeed does not apply, no combination of it with probable survival rates can make it applicable. Survival data, carefully collected and analyzed, deserve to be weighed in selecting candidates. These data do not come close to precluding alcoholics from consideration. Judgments of blameworthiness, which ought to be excluded generally, certainly should be excluded when weighing the impact of those survival rates. Some people with a strong antipathy to alcohol abuse and abusers may, without realizing it, be relying on assumed unfavorable data to support a fixed moral judgment. The arguments must be untangled. Actual results with transplanted alcoholics must be considered without regard to moral antipathies.

The upshot is inescapable: there are no good grounds at present—moral or medical—to disqualify a patient with end-stage liver disease from consideration for liver transplantation simply because of a history of heavy drinking.

SCREENING AND SELECTION OF LIVER TRANSPLANT CANDIDATES

In the initial evaluation of candidates for any form of transplantation, the central questions are whether patients (1) are sick enough to need a new organ and (2) enjoy a high enough probability of benefiting from this limited resource. At this stage the criteria should be non-comparative. Even the initial screening of patients must, however, be done individually and with great care.

The screening process for those suffering from alcoholic cirrhosis must be especially rigorous—not for moral reasons, but because of factors affecting survival, which are themselves influenced by a history of heavy drinking—and even more by its resumption. Responsible stewardship of scarce organs requires that the screening for candidacy take into consideration the manifold impact of heavy drinking on long-term transplant success. Cardiovascular problems brought on by alcoholism and other systematic contraindications must be looked for. Psychiatric and social evaluation is also in order, to determine whether patients understand and have come to terms with their condition and whether they have the social support essential for continuing immunosuppression and follow-up care.

Precisely which factors should be weighed in this screening process have not been firmly established. Some physicians have proposed a specified period of alcohol abstinence as an "objective" criterion for selection—but the data supporting such a criterion are far from conclusive, and the use of this criterion to exclude a prospective recipient is at present medically and morally arbitrary.

Indeed, one important consequence of overcoming the strong presumption against considering alcoholics for liver transplantation is the research opportunity it presents and the encouragement it gives to the quest for more reliable predictors of medical success. As that search continues, some defensible guidelines for case-by-case determination have been devised, based on factors associated with sustained recovery from alcoholism and other considerations related to liver transplantation success in general. Such guidelines appropriately include (1) refined diagnosis by those trained in the treatment of alcoholism, (2) acknowledgment by the patient of a serious drinking problem, (3) social and familial stability, and (4) other factors experimentally associated with long-term sobriety.

The experimental use of guidelines like these, and their gradual refinement over time, may lead to more reliable and more generally applicable predictors. But those more refined predictors will never be developed until prejudices against considering alcoholics for liver transplantation are overcome.

Patients who are sick because of alleged self-abuse ought not be grouped for discriminatory treatment—unless we are prepared to develop a detailed calculus of just deserts for health care based on good conduct. Lack of sympathy for those who bring serious disease upon themselves is understandable, but the temptation to institutionalize that emotional response must be tempered by our inability to apply such considerations justly and by our duty *not* to apply them unjustly. In the end, some patients with alcoholic cirrhosis may be judged, after careful evaluation, as good risks for a liver transplant.

OBJECTION AND REPLY

Providing alcoholics with transplants may present a special "political" problem for transplant centers. The public perception of alcoholics is generally negative. The already low rate of organ donation, it may be argued, will fall even lower when it becomes known that donated organs are going to alcoholics. Financial support from legislatures may also suffer. One can imagine the effect on transplantation if the public were to learn that the liver of a teenager killed by a drunken driver had been transplanted into an alcoholic patient. If selecting even a few alcoholics as transplant candidates reduces the number of lives saved overall, might that not be good reason to preclude alcoholics categorically?

No. The fear is understandable, but excluding alcoholics cannot be rationally defended on that basis. Irresponsible conduct attributable to alcohol abuse should not be defended. No excuses should be made for the deplorable consequences of drunken behavior, from highway slaughter to familial neglect and abuse. But alcoholism must be distinguished from those consequences; not all alcoholics are morally irresponsible, vicious, or neglectful drunks. If there is a general failure to make this distinction, we must strive to overcome that failure, not pander to it.

Public confidence in medical practice in general, and in organ transplantation in particular, depends on the scientific validity and moral integrity of the policies adopted. Sound policies will prove publicly defensible. Shaping present health care policy on the basis of distorted public perceptions or prejudices will, in the long run, do more harm than good to the process and to the reputation of all concerned.

Approximately one in every 10 Americans is a heavy drinker, and approximately one family in every three has at least one member at risk for alcoholic cirrhosis. The care of alcoholics and the just treatment of them when their lives are at stake are matters a democratic polity may therefore be expected to act on with concern and reasonable judgment over the long run. The allocation of organs in short supply does present vexing moral problems; if thoughtless or shallow moralizing would cause some to respond very negatively to transplanting livers into alcoholic cirrhotics, that cannot serve as good reason to make such moralizing the measure of public policy.

We have argued that there is now no good reason, either moral or medical, to preclude alcoholics categorically from consideration for liver transplantation. We further conclude that it would therefore be unjust to implement that categorical preclusion simply because others might respond negatively if we do not.

GROWTH HORMONE THERAPY FOR THE DISABILITY OF SHORT STATURE

David B. Allen

INTRODUCTION AND CONCEPTUAL GUIDELINES

Limited availability of human growth hormone (GH) once provided a barrier to expanding its use beyond children who were unequivocally GH deficient (GHD). By necessity, strict arbitrary criteria were established to identify classic GHD children entitled to GH. Today, increased availability of recombinant DNA-derived GH has allowed investigation of its growth-promoting effect in short children who do not fit traditional definitions of GHD. Increased supply has created increased demand: more than twice as many children received GH therapy in 1989 and 1990 than in 1985 and 1986 at an average annual cost per child of $10,000.

Advantages conferred by increased height in social, economic, professional, and political realms of Western society are well-documented. Stigmatization and discrimination are shared by *all* extremely short children, whether GHD or not. *If* GH is shown to have growth-promoting effects in non-GHD children and *if* treatment of such children can be accomplished without toxicity, then what ethical criteria should determine entitlement to long-term, invasive, and (currently) expensive therapy? Would it be justified to restrict access to GH based on the diagnosis of GHD? And whatever the indication for GH therapy, to what attained height should GH therapy be considered an entitlement?

Answering these questions requires rethinking of the medical indications for GH therapy. Toward the goal of achieving both controlled but fair access to GH, the following conceptual guidelines are proposed: (1) GH be viewed as a treatment for the disability of short stature (SS) and not for the diagnosis of GHD; (2) GH-responsiveness, not GHD, be the central criterion for GH treatment; and (3) entitlement to (and reimbursement for) GH therapy be guided by the degree of disability and the degree of GH-responsiveness rather than by a child's diagnosis.

THE CONTINUUM OF GROWTH HORMONE SECRETION: DISEASE, POTENTIAL, AND HANDICAP

The once clear boundary between GHD and GH sufficiency has become blurred. Traditional criteria for the diagnosis of GHD do not identify all children who are GH-responsive. A continuum of "inadequate" GH secretion likely spans classic and partially GHD children, children with delayed growth and puberty, and other poorly growing short children who pass provocative tests but still secrete less GH than their peers. Furthermore, GH *augmentation* therapy in short children with no detectable abnormalities of GH secretion increases growth velocity and, if given for sufficient time prior to puberty, may increase eventual adult height.

Arguments emphasizing proven GHD as the primary criterion for GH therapy are often rooted in notions of disease, handicap, or potential. The treatment of disease, "an abnormal condition of an organism that impairs normal physiologic functioning" (*American Heritage Dictionary,* 1985), is one function of medicine. One might argue that GH therapy be confined to those with the "disease" of GHD. Restoration of hormonal equilibrium by supplementing deficient or suppressing excessive levels of hormones is a justifiable, time-honored principle in endocrinology. The GHD child is viewed

---

Reprinted with permission of the author and publisher. From *Access to Treatment With Human Growth Hormone: Medical, Ethical, and Social Issues.* Supplement to *Growth, Genetics, and Hormones,* Vol. 8 (Supp. 1): 70–73, May 1992.

Editor's note: All footnotes have been deleted. Students who want to follow up on sources should consult the original article.

as more entitled to therapy because something has been taken away that needs to be restored. The American Academy of Pediatrics statement recommending GH therapy only for GHD children concludes with the old adage, "If it ain't broke, don't fix it." But what exactly is "broke" when it comes to SS and GH therapy? This view ignores both the likely, though yet unrecognized, physiologic "defects" that lead to genetic SS and its accompanying psychosocial impairment. Both GHD and non-GHD short children, if they have a disease at all, have the disease of SS.

If the legitimate function of medicine includes the alleviation of handicap, "a disadvantage or deficiency, especially a physical or mental disability that prevents or restricts normal achievement," then the short child's well-being is viewed in the context of his or her interaction with the environment. GH therapy is justified by recognition that extreme SS interferes with normal activities such as driving a car and reaching shelves, as well as competition for jobs, schools, incomes, and mates. After all, preventing handicapping SS is the primary impetus for treating GHD children. Other beneficial physiologic effects occur with GH therapy, but these are of secondary importance. Growth rate and final adult height are the measures by which we judge therapeutic success. Whether burdens associated with SS of a given degree qualify for designation as a handicap is not the central question. The point is that short children of equal height have the same handicap regardless of the cause.

The concept of potential is also invoked to distinguish treatment of GHD and non-GHD children. For some, a GHD child with parents of normal height is "meant," by virtue of genetic endowment, to be taller than the child with familial SS. He or she is entitled to treatment with GH until a height appropriate for the genetic endowment is attained. GH supplementation of the familial short child who appears to be GH-sufficient is "tampering with nature" and outside the proper province of medicine. But this analysis fails, since both children (given an equal height prognosis) are equally unlucky, one by virtue of having GHD and the other by virtue of having short parents. For both, attaining maximum adult height requires "tampering with nature" by providing exogenous GH.

EQUITABLE RESTRICTION OF GROWTH HORMONE THERAPY

While concepts of disease, handicap, and potential do not distinguish GHD from GH-responsive children with regard to entitlement to GH therapy, it does not follow that *all* GH-responsive short children are entitled to therapy. Resolving that question requires consideration of balancing benefits and risks and asking further questions about allocation of health-care resources.

Response to GH is not an "all or none" phenomenon. GHD children are likely to be *more* responsive than non-GHD children, justifying their preferential treatment as a class. Possible GH toxicity in non-GHD children, while apparently rare, still requires further study. Risks of psychosocial stigmatization also require careful consideration; short, otherwise normal children exposed to injections to promote growth may conclude (with some accuracy) that their bodies are unacceptable in the eyes of their parents and physicians. Statistically significant increments in final adult height may not actually improve psychosocial adaptation, failing a primary objective of GH therapy. Finally, unrestricted access to GH would shift the bell-shaped curve of height upward without changing the handicap for those at the lower percentiles in competing for social, professional, and athletic status.

Assuming that clinical trials of GH in non-GHD children show efficacy with acceptable risk, how might access to GH therapy be equitably restricted? First, the goals in treating SS must be clarified. If the goal is to achieve each child's maximum height potential, GH therapy would (ethically) need to be offered to any potentially responsive short child. Providing GH therapy only to those with documented GHD and treating them until maximal adult stature is reached would be unfair to equally short, non-GHD children who could grow with GH supplementation. On the other hand, if the goal is to alleviate the disability of extreme SS (from any cause), GH-responsive short children should have equal access to treatment until they reach a height no longer considered a handicap.

This latter goal, bringing short children into the normal opportunity range for height, coincides with society's duty to provide basic needs to its citizens. There is no duty to provide the *very best* opportunity for all, and an insistence on equal access to GH by those who have already achieved a normal final height compromises this goal. To improve opportunities for those truly disabled by height, GH must be selectively available to them. The challenge is to define this group, and to apply criteria of disability consistently in deciding when to commence and when to *discontinue therapy*. The diagnosis of GHD should not be rewarded with unlimited access to GH while access is denied to equally handicapped non-GHD but potentially GH-responsive children.

TOWARD RESPONSIBLE USE OF GROWTH HORMONE

Any definition of "handicapping height" would be arbitrary, but the difficulty in defining boundaries precisely should not be an obstacle to making distinctions. Decisions about treatment are always based on probability, not certainty. While current methods for height prediction remain suboptimal, *some* determination of a height considered a handicap needs to be made if GH allocation in the future is to be both controlled and fair.

Emphasizing degree of disability and GH-responsiveness as selection criteria for therapy equitably fulfills reasonable goals of growth-promoting therapy. Children disadvantaged by stature, regardless of pathogenesis, would be brought closer to or within the normal opportunity range for height. The attainment of maximum height potential would not be a valid treatment goal, and the use of GH to make normal-statured children taller would be opposed. The normal range of height would not be altered, but rather the disparity between percentiles—for example, between the 0.1th and 1st percentiles would be lessened. By restricting GH therapy to those seeking only to achieve the normal opportunity range for height, we would not exploit the perception that taller is better.

Widespread distribution of GH has been deterred in part by high drug prices and concern about toxicity. Assuming efficacy of GH in increasing final adult height, the relevant question is not how much should be spent on GHD versus non-GHD children but rather how should health-care resources be responsibly and fairly expended on the treatment of SS in general. Resources for this endeavor may in fact be limited, but treatment of severely SS individuals can still be approached with *consistency*. If our goal is to help (all) children attain a height closer to the normal opportunity range, the cause of the SS really should not matter. The central question about allocation of GH is this: To what maximum height should any GH-treated child be entitled to receive private or public support?

Moreover, the crisis in GH allocation will expand not with its failures but with its successes, and not as the cost of therapy rises but as it falls. These impediments, which may be resolved soon, have distracted attention from the issue of responsible use of GH. What we can do with GH therapy is not necessarily what we *should* do. We who prescribe GH should now ask how we would respond if families who do not require insurance reimbursement strongly request GH therapy. Without guidelines for restriction based arbitrarily on likely final adult height, access to treatment would increasingly reflect ability to pay, providing yet another societal advantage to those already well-off. Rather, a consistent goal of growth-promoting therapy should be to lessen the burden for those who are so short as to be handicapped; that is, to provide GH therapy to those disabled by height only until a height within the normal opportunity range is attained. Consideration of degree of disability, rather than diagnosis, both when commencing and when discontinuing GH therapy, will most responsibly contain an expanding cohort of candidates for GH treatment.

The physician's duty to respond to the needs of each child does not necessarily extend to parental aspirations or hopes for the child. In an era of plentiful GH, child advocacy requires consideration of the needs of all children, bringing as many as possible into the normal opportunity range of height without deliberately trying to make some taller than others. The paradox of GH therapy is that no policy regarding its use will ever eliminate the 1st percentile. GH cannot replace parental love and nurturing of a child, regardless of the child's height. Prudent use of GH will recognize these limitations, encouraging physicians to respond to concerns about SS more often with counseling than with injections.

THE GENOME PROJECT, INDIVIDUAL DIFFERENCES, AND JUST HEALTH CARE

Norman Daniels

The mapping of the human genome is likely to have important implications for the just distribution of health care services. Some of these implications will be the result of the new medical technologies that will be developed once we learn more about the human genome. Despite their likely importance, I will not speculate about them in what follows, nor will I comment on the way they add to the burden we already have in deciding how to disseminate and ration new technologies under conditions of resource scarcity. Instead, I want to focus on the fact that the mapping of the genome will give us specific, new *information about individual variation.* This information can be used in good and bad, fair and unfair ways, and it raises, or rather refocuses, important questions about how we should distribute health care resources. . . .

. . . [C]an we defend the distinction between medical therapies that *treat* and those that *enhance* in the face of new genetic information that allows us to pinpoint the genetic contributors to traits we want to alter? Imagine, for example, that we will come to identify particular genes or patterns of genes that contribute to making people very short. (I say "imagine" advisedly, since all interesting traits are highly heterogeneous; in what follows, we indulge in some of the fanciful expectations advanced by human genome proponents.) These genes do not represent pathology of the usual sort; for example, they do not lead to growth hormone deficiency. But being able to look at the microstructure underlying the "normal" distribution of height may produce strong pressures to identify a new class of "bad genes" and to suggest that people who have those genes now have a claim on others to assist them in changing their traits. These questions thus have vast implications for resource allocation. . . . [T]hey also take us deep into political philosophy. What we are really asking is which inequalities among people give rise to claims on others and which are matters of individual responsibility. . . .

CAN WE RETAIN THE TREATMENT VERSUS ENHANCEMENT DISTINCTION?

We have social obligations to treat disease and disability because of their impact on opportunity, and so we should not accept the barriers to access that follow from standard underwriting practices. Are these obligations limited to treating disease and disability? Or does any condition that creates an inequality in opportunity for welfare or advantage among individuals give rise to claims on others? In rejecting the argument from actuarial fairness, we countered an attack from the right on our social obligations to treat disease and disability. I want to consider now an attack from the left on the way I have formulated these obligations. The attack rests on the view that our egalitarian concerns require us to eliminate inequalities among people that arise from many conditions other than disease and disability. In effect, it is a demand for a more radical version of equality of opportunity. In the context of health care, the attack takes the form of a challenge to the distinction between treatment and enhancement.

I suggested earlier that the genome project may provide us with information that will erode the distinction we often draw between uses of medical technology for treatment of disease and disability and uses that enhance human appearance or performance. This distinction is closely connected to the frequently used, but poorly understood,

From Timothy F. Murphy and Marc A. Lappé, eds., *Justice and the Human Genome Project*. Berkeley: University of California Press, 1994. Edited and reprinted with permission.

Editor's note: Most footnotes have been deleted. Students who want to follow up on sources should consult the original article.

concept of "medical necessity." Many public and private insurance schemes in the United States (and Canada) claim to provide only medically necessary services: many services that involve only enhancement (such as "cosmetic" surgery) are thus excluded from coverage on these grounds. I shall suggest in what follows that the treatment versus enhancement distinction does have a moral justification, at least relative to a *standard* way of thinking about equality of opportunity. The genetic information about human variation provided by the genome project may make that distinction seem more arbitrary, and to the extent that it does, it poses a challenge to the standard model and the use to which I have put it in thinking about justice and health care. Of course, this is not a conceptually novel threat; viewed from the perspective of the attack from the left, the distinction and the standard model it depends on already seem arbitrary. But the new information may heighten the appearance of moral arbitrariness, and that is the reason for discussing the issue here.

Many medical technologies, new and old, can alter people in ways they desire to be changed. When do we have a social obligation to ensure that such preferences are met? Do rights to health care include entitlements to have those preferences met, resources permitting? What should insurance cover?

The most inclusive answer to these questions would be that we have such obligations whenever someone desires to eliminate an unwanted physical or mental condition. This would allow "subjective" preferences to place enormous demands on resources, making everyone hostage to the extravagant tastes of everyone else. Since we generally do not believe it is medicine's task to make everyone equally happy, we reject this view and its implication that we should have to pay for liposuction or face lifts. Instead, we think obligations arise only when medical treatments address more important problems. The stance we thus take about medicine is compatible with rejecting, as Rawls and Dworkin do, a broad form of egalitarianism that would require us to ensure the equal welfare or happiness of all individuals.

A less inclusive answer would be that we have obligations to provide medical care whenever people desire to eliminate conditions that put them at some disadvantage. The notion of disadvantage is meant to be objective, including some forms of suffering as well as the competitive disadvantages that result from the lack of capabilities, such as marketable talents or skills. This view has some initial moral appeal when the disadvantages are not our fault or the (even unlucky) result of our prior choices. Our egalitarian inclinations may incline us to think we owe something toward eliminating them. If we adopt such a radical view—the left position I referred to earlier—we may have to assign medicine a much greater role as a social equalizer than we now assign it. At least currently, it is not medicine's task to make everyone an equal competitor, wherever possible eliminating all inequalities in the distribution of talents and skills or other capabilities.

A more modest answer, one that tends to match a wide range of our practices, including our insurance practices, is that we have obligations to provide services whenever someone desires that a medical *need* be met. Generally, this is taken to mean that the service involves *treatment of a disease or disability,* where disease and disability are seen as departures from species-typical normal functional organization or functioning. Characterizing medical need in this way implies a contrast between uses of medical services that *treat* disease (or disability) conditions and uses that merely *enhance* human performance or appearance. Enhancement does not meet a medical need even where the service may correct for a competitive disadvantage that does not result from prior choices. Accordingly, medicine has the role of making people *normal* competitors, not *equal* competitors; this role fits, I shall claim, with the standard model for thinking about equality of opportunity.

Despite its wide appeal, the distinction between treatment and enhancement may seem arbitrary in light of hard cases such as these:

> Johnny is a short 11-year-old boy with documented GH [growth hormone] deficiency resulting from a brain tumor. His parents are of average height. His predicted adult height without GH treatment is approximately 160 cm (5 feet 3 inches).
>
> Billy is a short 11-year-old boy with normal GH secretion according to current testing methods. However, his parents are extremely short, and he has a predicted adult height of 160 cm (5 feet 3 inches).[1]

These cases make the distinction seem arbitrary for several reasons. First, Johnny and Billy will suffer disadvantage equally if they are not treated. There is no reason to think the difference in the underlying causes of their shortness will lead people to treat them in ways that make one happier or more advantaged than the other. Second, although Johnny is short because of dysfunction whereas Billy is short because of his (normal) genotype, both are short through no choice or fault of their own. The shortness is in both cases the result of a biological "natural lottery." Both thus seem to suffer undeserved disadvantages. Third, Billy's preference for greater height, just like Johnny's, is a preference that most people hold; it is not peculiar, idiosyncratic, or extravagant. Indeed, it is a response to a social prejudice, "heightism." The prejudice is what we should condemn, not the fact that they both form an "expensive taste" in reaction to it.

Cases such as these raise the following question: does the concept of disease underlying the treatment versus enhancement distinction force us to treat relevantly similar cases in dissimilar ways? Are we violating the old Aristotelian requirement that justice requires treating like cases similarly? Is dissimilar treatment unfair or unjust?

Despite the challenge of hard cases, the treatment versus enhancement distinction should play a role in deciding what obligations we have to provide medical services. To show that this distinction is not arbitrary from the viewpoint of justice, despite the hard cases, I shall argue that it fits better than do alternatives with what I call the *standard model* for thinking about equality of opportunity. Of course, the standard model may itself be indefensible, a point I will return to shortly. First, though, I want to show that the standard model helps specify a reasonable limit on the central task of health care.

Earlier I noted that disease and disability restrict the range of opportunities open to an individual. Health care services maintain, restore, and compensate for losses of function that result from disease and disability. They thus restore people to the range of capabilities they *could be expected to have had* without disease or disability, given their allotment of talents and skills. Our *standard model* for thinking about equality of opportunity thus depends on *taking as a given the fact that talents and skills and other capabilities are not distributed equally* among people. Some people are better at some things than others. Accordingly, we ensure people *fair* equality of opportunity if we judge them by their capabilities while ignoring "morally irrelevant" traits such as sex or race when we place people in schools, jobs, and offices. Often, however, we must correct for cases in which capabilities have been misdeveloped through racist, sexist, or other discriminatory practices. Similarly, by preventing or treating disease and disability, we can correct for impairment of the capabilities people would otherwise have. The standard model does not call for eliminating differences in normal capabilities in general, let alone through medical enhancement.

This limitation of the standard model can appear arbitrary. As I noted earlier, our capabilities are themselves the result of a natural and social lottery, and we do not "deserve" them. We just are fortunate or unfortunate in having them. We can mitigate this underlying arbitrariness somewhat as follows. Those who are better endowed with marketable capabilities are likely to enjoy more goods such as income, wealth, and power. If we constrain inequalities in these goods so that those who are worst off do as well as possible, considering all alternatives, then social cooperation will work to the benefit of all. Still, this constraint does not eliminate all inequalities in the individual capabilities or in the resulting opportunities individuals enjoy, especially since we are enjoined to judge people by their capabilities and not by their "morally irrelevant" traits such as sex or race. If our egalitarian concerns require that we strive to give people equal capabilities, wherever technologically feasible, then we should not settle for mitigating the effects of the normal distribution of capabilities, as proponents of the standard model of equality of opportunity would have it. Rejecting the standard model pushes us toward equalizing all differences in capabilities; from that perspective, the distinction between treatment and enhancement has no point, at least where enhancement is aimed at equalizing capabilities.

Information from the genome project might make the distinction between disease (including genetic disease) and the normal distribution of capabilities seem more arbitrary. Suppose we learn that some particular pattern of genes explains the extreme shortness of Billy, the child who was not deficient in growth hormone. That is, we learn just which "losing numbers" in the natural lottery placed Billy in the bottom one percent of the normal distribution for height. Identifying these genes may then tempt us to think of them as "bad" ones: they lead to Billy's unhappiness or disadvantage in a "heightist" world. We will then be sorely tempted to think of them very much on the model of genetic defects or diseases, especially if they work through mechanisms that have some analogy to pathological defects. In other words, we will be tempted to medicalize what we have hitherto considered normal. What, after all, allows us to treat the "bad genes" differently from genes that lead to growth hormone deficiency or to receptor insensitivity to growth hormone? If we can remedy the effects of these genes with growth hormone treatment or other treatments, including genetic tampering, we might think it quite arbitrary to maintain the treatment versus enhancement distinction.

I want to offer several points as a limited defense of the standard model and the treatment versus enhancement distinction. Both versions of equality of opportunity, the standard model and the more radical one that requires equalizing capabilities, seem to appeal to the same underlying intuition—that advantages and disadvantages resulting from the natural lottery are not themselves deserved. But they use the intuition differently. The standard model suggests we mitigate the effects of normally distributed capabilities through restrictions on other inequalities we allow. Since some inequality in capabilities is a fact of life, the task is to mitigate their effects while adopting principles that let everyone benefit from social cooperation. The criticism from the left rests far more weight on the underlying intuition: it says that wherever possible we must actually try to reduce variance in the distribution of capabilities, equalizing them wherever possible. I believe that the standard model better captures our actual concerns about equality than the more radical version. (Of course, our actual concerns may be too limited, so this is not a conclusive argument.)

Some supporting evidence for this point derives from our moral beliefs and practices concerning health care. We regard medical services as meeting *urgent needs* when they are aimed at restoring or maintaining "normal functioning." Our consensus about where to draw the line focuses on eliminating disease and disability. We already have many technologies that can enhance functioning for individuals, even giving them advantages (such as beauty or athletic performance) they previously did not have. But we generally resist assimilating these cases of enhancement to cases of treatment because we do not see them as meeting important needs. Although these enhancing services alter traits that may be the results of a natural lottery, they involve optimizing capabilities that are not departures from normal functional organization or functioning.

Of course, what makes the case of Billy and Johnny problematic is that they both suffer equal disadvantage as a result of the natural lottery (and social prejudice). But there is justification for adhering to a distinction that captures and sustains social agreement on important matters, even if the distinction seems arbitrary in isolated hard cases. The line between treatment and enhancement is generally uncontroversial and ascertainable through publicly accepted methods, such as those of the biomedical sciences. Being able to draw a line in this way allows us to refer counterfactually in a relatively clear and objective way to the range of opportunities a person *would have had* in the absence of disease and disability; it facilitates public agreement. Because of these virtues, not every hard case counts as a counterexample that warrants overturning the distinction.

The "equal capabilities" approach, bolstered by new information from the genome project, is likely to undermine agreement on the importance of meeting medical needs. According to it, we would now have many more such needs, for much of what we now take to be normal would become conditions in need of rectification. Since we are far less likely to think that it is "urgent" to correct the effects of these newly labeled "bad genes," shifting away from the standard model is likely to undermine consensus on the moral importance of health care.

Will it be possible to hold the line? Some relief may come from a more careful attempt to examine the distinction between genetic disease and normal variation. This may enable us to offer a theoretical justification, coming out of the biological sciences, for a baseline distinction. It is important to note that I am not trying to save the appeal to a natural baseline here because there is something magical or metaphysically basic about it. Nor am I violating Hume's injunction against deriving "ought" from "is." Rather, the natural baseline both facilitates and reflects moral agreement about the urgency of medical care. I also believe there is moral justification for limiting in some ways the task involved in protecting equality of opportunity, otherwise it will be discredited as too demanding an ideal. If, however, no theoretical justification is forthcoming that lets us distinguish "bad" (or nonoptimal) genes from genetic disease, then we will have to give more complex justifications for drawing the line between cases in which we have obligations to provide services and those in which we do not. My claim is simply that it will be harder to reach consensus on these justifications without the ability to appeal to a natural baseline, however imperfectly drawn.

I have been offering reasons not to expand our goals in protecting equality of opportunity from the more limited ones of the standard model to the more encompassing one of equalizing capabilities. Nevertheless, our obligations to provide medical services need not derive solely from the concerns about equality of opportunity that I have argued are central. For example, I think we have compelling reasons for providing public funding of nontherapeutic abortions that go beyond their importance for preventive health care. Similarly, suppose an inexpensive treatment became available for improving cognitive capabilities in childhood; administering it would greatly enhance the results of education, close the gap between poor but "normal" students and others, and contribute greatly to social productivity. We might then have compelling reasons to seek enhancement in this way, even if they differ from our standard justification for the importance of health care. Of course, we already have excellent reasons for putting more resources into education, yet we do not, despite the fact that our failure to do so results in misdeveloped talents and skills along race and class lines. . . .

NOTES

1. D. B. Allen and N. C. Fost, "Growth Hormone Therapy for Short Stature: Panacea or Pandora's Box?" *Journal of Pediatrics* 117:1(1990): 16–21.

RECOMMENDED SUPPLEMENTARY READING

GENERAL WORKS

Abraham, Laurie K. *Mama Might Be Better Off Dead: The Failure of Health Care in Urban America.* Chicago: University of Chicago Press, 1993.

Agich, George J., and Begley, Charles E., eds. *The Price of Health.* Boston: D. Reidel Publishing Co., 1986.

Annas, George J. *Standard of Care: The Law of American Bioethics.* Oxford: Oxford University Press, 1993.

Beauchamp, Dan E. *The Health of the Republic: Epidemics, Medicine, and Moralism as Challenges to Democracy.* Philadelphia, PA: Temple University Press, 1988.

Brock, Dan W. *Life and Death: Philosophical Essays in Biomedical Ethics.* New York: Cambridge University Press, 1993.

Cates, Diana Fritz, and Lauritzen, Paul. *Medicine and the Ethics of Care.* Washington, DC: Georgetown University Press, 1993.

Daniels, Norman. *Just Health Care.* Cambridge: Cambridge University Press, 1985.

———. *Seeking Fair Treatment: From the AIDS Epidemic to National Health Care Reform.* New York: Oxford University Press, 1995.

Daniels, Norman; Light, Donald W.; and Caplan, Ronald L. *Benchmarks of Fairness for Health Care Reform.* New York: Oxford University Press, 1996.

Dougherty, Charles. *Back to Reform: Values, Markets, and the Health Care System.* New York: Oxford University Press, 1996.

Emanuel, Ezekiel. *The Ends of Human Life: Medical Ethics in a Liberal Polity.* Cambridge, MA: Harvard University Press, 1991.

Hall, Mark A. *Making Medical Spending Decisions: The Law, Ethics, and Economics of Rationing Mechanisms.* New York: Oxford University Press, 1996.

Light, Donald, and Hughes, David. *Sociological Perspectives on Health Care Rationing.* Oxford, MA: Blackwell Publishers, 2001.

Loewy, Erich H., and Loewy, Roberta Springer, eds. *Changing Health Care Systems from Ethical, Economic, and Cross Cultural Perspectives.* New York: Kluwer Academic Publishers, 2001.

Morreim, E. Haavi. *Balancing Act: The New Medical Ethics of Medicine's New Economics.* Washington, DC: Georgetown University Press, 1995.

President's Commission for the Study of Ethical Problems in Medicine and Biomedical and Behavioral Research. *Securing Access to Health Care.* Washington, DC: U.S. Government Printing Office, 1983.

Zoloth, Laurie. *Health Care and the Ethics of Encounter: A Jewish Discussion of Social Justice.* Chapel Hill: University of North Carolina Press, 1999.

JUSTICE, HEALTH CARE, AND HEALTH

Arras, John. "Retreat from the Right to Health Care: The President's Commission and Access to Health Care." *Cardozo Law Review* 6 (1984): 321–345.

Bayer, Ronald. "Ethics, Politics, and Access to Health Care: A Critical Analysis of the President's Commission." *Cardozo Law Review* 6 (1984): 303–320.

Brock, Dan; Buchanan, Allan; Daniels, Norman; and Wikler, Daniel. *From Chance to Choice: Genetics and Justice.* New York: Cambridge University Press, 2000.

Brody, Baruch. "Why the Right to Health Care Is Not a Useful Concept for Policy Debates." In *Rights to Health Care,* edited by T. J. Bole III and W. B. Bondeson. The Netherlands: Kluwer Academic Publishers, 1991.

Buchanan, Allen. "Equal Opportunity and Genetic Intervention," *Social Philosophy and Policy* 12, no. 2 (Summer 1995): 105–135.

Callahan, Daniel. *What Kind of Life: The Limits of Medical Progress.* New York: Simon & Schuster, 1990.

Daniels, Norman. *Seeking Fair Treatment: The Lesson of AIDS for National Health Care.* New York: Oxford University Press, 1995.

Daniels, Norman, and Sabin, James E. *Setting Limits Fairly: Can We Learn to Share Medical Resources?* New York: Oxford University Press, 2002.

Daniels, Norman; Kennedy, Bruce; and Kawachi, Ichiro. *Is Inequality Bad for Our Health?* Boston: Beacon Press, 2000.

Evans, Robert G. "Health Care as a Threat to Health: Defense, Opulence, and the Social Environment." *Daedalus* 123 no. 4 (Fall 1994): 21–43.

Evans, Timothy; Whitehead, Margaret; Diderichsen, Finn; Bhuiya, Abbas; and Wirth, Meg; eds. *Challenging Inequities in Health: From Ethics to Action.* New York: Oxford University Press, 2001.

Gutmann, Amy. "For and Against Equal Access to Health Care." *Milbank Quarterly* 59 (Fall 1981): 542–560.

Marmot, M. G., and Wilkinson, Richard G., eds. *Social Determinants of Health.* New York: Oxford University Press, 1999.

Morreim, E. Haavi. *Holding Health Care Accountable: Law and the New Medical Marketplace.* New York: Oxford University Press, 2001.

Murphy, Timothy F., and Lappé, Marc A., eds. *Justice and the Human Genome Project.* Berkeley: University of California Press, 1994.

Veatch, Robert M. *The Foundations of Justice: Why the Retarded and the Rest of Us Have Claims to Equality.* New York: Oxford University Press, 1986.

Walzer, Michael. *Spheres of Justice: A Defense of Pluralism and Equality.* New York: Basic Books, 1983.

METHODS AND STRATEGIES FOR RATIONING HEALTH CARE

Aaron, Henry J., and Schwartz, William B. *The Painful Prescription: Rationing Health Care.* Washington, DC: Brookings Institution, 1984.

Blank, Robert H. *The Price of Life: The Future of American Health Care.* New York: Columbia University Press, 1997.

Churchill, Larry R. *Rationing Health Care in America: Perceptions and Principles of Justice.* Notre Dame, IN: University of Notre Dame Press, 1987.

Daniels, Norman. "Rationing Fairly: Programmatic Considerations." *Bioethics* 7, nos. 2–3 (1993): 224–233.

Daniels, Norman, et al. "Meeting the Challenges of Justice and Rationing." *Hastings Center Report* 24, no. 4 (July–August 1994): 27–42.

Daniels, Norman, and Sabin, James. "Limits to Health Care: Fair Procedures, Democratic Deliberation, and the Legitimacy Problem for Insurers." *Philosophy and Public Affairs* 26, no. 4 (Fall 1997): 303–350.

———. "High-Dose Chemotherapy with Autologous Bone Marrow Transplantation for the Treatment of Metastatic Breast Cancer." *Journal of Clinical Oncology* 10, no. 4 (1992): 657–670.

Eddy, David M. *Clinical Decision Making: From Theory to Practice.* Sudbury, MA: Jones and Bartlett, 1996.

Hall, Mark A. *Making Medical Spending Decisions: The Law, Ethics, and Economics of Rationing Mechanisms.* New York: Oxford University Press, 1997.

Kamm, Frances M. *Morality, Mortality: Death and Whom to Save from It.* Oxford: Oxford University Press, 1993.

"The Law and Policy of Health Care Rationing: Models and Accountability." *University of Pennsylvania Law Review* 140, no. 5 (May 1992): 1505–1998.

Light, Donald, and Hughes, David, eds. *Sociological Perspectives on Health Care Rationing.* Oxford: Blackwell Publishers, 2001.

Mann, Jonathan M. *Health and Human Rights: A Reader.* New York: Routledge, 1999.

"Managed Care Systems: Emerging Health Issues from an Ethics Perspective." *Journal of Law, Medicine and Ethics* 23, no. 3 (symposium 1995).

Menzel, Paul T. *Medical Costs, Moral Choices.* New Haven, CT: Yale University Press, 1983.

———. *Strong Medicine: The Ethical Rationing of Medical Care.* New York: Oxford University Press, 1990.

Nelson, James Lindemann. "Measured Fairness, Situated Justice: Feminist Reflections on Health Care Rationing." *Kennedy Institute of Ethics Journal* 6 (1996): 53–68.

Nord, Erik. *Cost-Value Analysis in Health Care: Making Sense Out of QALYs.* New York: Cambridge University Press, 1999.

Pongrace, Paul Earl, III. "HDC/ABMT Experimental Treatment or Cure-All? (Ask the Insurance Companies)." *The Journal of Pharmacy & Law* 2, no. 2 (1994): 329–356.

Priester, Reinhard; Gervais, Karen G.; and Vawter, Dorothy E. *Improving Coverage for Unproven Health Care Interventions.* Minneapolis: Minnesota Center for Health Care Ethics, 1996.

Ubel, Peter A. *Pricing Life: Why It's Time for Health Care Rationing.* Cambridge, MA: MIT Press, 1999.

Wikler, Daniel. "Ethics and Rationing: 'Whether,' 'How,' or 'How Much'?" *Journal of the American Geriatrics Society* 40, no. 4 (1992): 398–403.

Wong, Kenman L. *Medicine and the Marketplace: The Moral Dimensions of Managed Care.* Notre Dame, IN: University of Notre Dame Press, 1998.

EQUALITY AND THE ENDS OF MEDICINE

Allen, David, and Fost, Norman, eds. "Access to Treatment with Human Growth Hormone: Medical, Ethical, and Social Issues." *Growth, Genetics and Hormones* 8 (May 1992): 1–77.

Binstock, Robert H., and Post, Stephen G., eds. *Too Old for Health Care? Controversies in Medicine, Law, Economics and Ethics.* Baltimore: Johns Hopkins University Press, 1991.

Breggin, P. *Talking Back to Prozac.* New York: St. Martin's Press, 1994.

Callahan, Daniel. *Setting Limits.* New York: Simon & Schuster, 1987.

Canterbury, R. J., and Lloyd, E. "Smart Drugs: Implications of Student Use." *Journal of Primary Prevention* 14 (1994): 197–207.

Daniels, Norman. *Am I My Parents' Keeper?* New York: Oxford University Press, 1987.

Davis, Kathy. *Reshaping the Female Body: The Dilemma of Cosmetic Surgery.* New York: Routledge, 1995.

Dean, W.; Morgenthaler, J.; and Fawkes, S. *Smart Drugs II: The Next Generation.* Menlo Park, CA: Health Freedom Publications, 1993.

Elliott, Carl. "Hedgehogs and Hermaphrodites: Toward a More Anthropological Bioethics." In *Philosophy of Medicine and Bioethics: A Twenty-Year Retrospective and Critical Appraisal,* edited by R. Carson and C. Burns. Dordrecht, The Netherlands: Kluwer Academic Publishers, 1997.

Gardner, William. "Can Human Genetic Enhancement Be Prohibited?" *Journal of Medicine and Philosophy* 20 (1995): 65–84.

Holtug, Nils. "Does Justice Require Genetic Enhancements?" *Journal of Medical Ethics* 25 (1997): 137–143.

Homer, Paul, and Holstein, Martha, eds. *A Good Old Age? The Paradox of Setting Limits.* New York: Simon & Schuster, 1990.

Jecker, Nancy S. "Age-Based Rationing and Women." *Journal of the American Medical Association* 266, no. 21 (December 4, 1991): 3012–3015.

———, ed. *Aging and Ethics: Philosophical Problems in Gerontology.* Clifton, NJ: Humana Press, 1991.

Jorgensen, O. L., and Christiansen, Jens L. "Growth Hormone Therapy—Brave New Senescence: GH in Adults." *Lancet* 341 (1993): 1247–1248.

Kramer, Peter D. *Listening to Prozac.* New York: Viking, 1993.

Parens, Erik, ed. *Enhancing Human Traits: Conceptual Complexities and Ethical Implications.* Washington, DC: Georgetown University Press, 1998.

Resnik, David B. "Genetic Engineering and Social Justice: A Rawlsian Approach." *Social Theory and Practice* 23, no. 3 (Fall 1997): 427–448.

White, Gladys. "Human Growth Hormone: The Dilemma of Expanded Use in Children." *Kennedy Institute of Ethics Journal* 3, no. 4 (December 1993): 401.

PART THREE

DEFINING DEATH, FORGOING LIFE-SUSTAINING TREATMENT, AND EUTHANASIA

Death remains as inevitable as always, yet somehow today it seems harder to achieve. In the past, diseases such as pneumonia, formerly called "the old man's friend," led to a speedy and fairly gentle death. Today such infections can be treated, and many of the more rapid causes of death can be staved off. Thus, the benefits of medical advances bring with them burdens, and here the burden is the possibility of a lingering death, surrounded not by loved ones in the home, but by medical hardware in an intensive-care unit.

Indeed, it is now possible to sustain individuals for years in a "persistent vegetative state," a state in which they do not feel, think, or have any awareness of their surroundings. Some would argue that someone who lacks a capacity for *any* conscious activity is not, in any meaningful ethical sense, alive. This raises the first issue of this chapter: How do we define death?

THE DEFINITION OF DEATH

Most scholars accept that to analyze the concept of "death," you need first to agree on its definition, then formulate a measurable criterion to show that the definition has been fulfilled, and finally develop a series of clinical tests to show that the criterion has been satisfied. The definition of "death" might seem straightforward, since "death" is a nontechnical word that is used widely and correctly. Someone is dead when he or she is no longer living; death is the end and absence of life. However, developments in medical technology over the last few decades, as well as reflective scholarship on those developments, have called into question, not only the clinical tests for determining when an individual has died, but also what the tests should measure (the criterion of death) and even our understanding of what death is (its definition).

Before the development of high-technology forms of life support—in particular, the respirator—death was pretty straightforward. People were dead when they stopped breathing and their hearts stopped beating. The traditional criterion of death, then, is the cessation of heart-lung, or cardiopulmonary, function. And the clinical test for determining the cessation of cardiopulmonary function might be as simple as putting a mirror in front of the patient's mouth to see if he or she was still breathing, or listening for a heartbeat. Today, however, people whose respiration and heartbeat have ceased can be resuscitated, and their breathing can be artificially maintained; and when this is done, the heart can continue to beat even in the absence of any input from the brain. Hence, a patient with an intact heart can be maintained on a respirator even when his or her brain functions have ceased entirely.

This new state of affairs created the need for rethinking death. In 1968, an ad hoc committee of the Harvard Medical School, chaired by Henry K. Beecher,* issued a report recommending that patients on life support, whose brain function had completely and irreversibly ceased, be declared dead and then removed from the respirator. Beecher favored brain-based, or neurological, criteria for diagnosing death, not primarily to resolve conceptual uncertainties about the meaning of death, but to solve several practical problems stemming from new technologies, including organ transplantation and the prevention of waste of medical resources (Pernick 1999). Organs that remain in a patient's dead body quickly deteriorate and become unusable. Transplant surgeons needed to remove organs quickly without risking accusations of murder. In addition, Beecher wanted to end the futile waste of scarce and expensive medical resources, such as respirators, on patients who could no longer benefit from them.

By the late 1970s, the issue of providing futile care and prolonging dying, epitomized by the case of Karen Quinlan (see "Advance Directives," p. 250), gave further impetus to the shift to neurological criteria for diagnosing death. Quinlan herself did not meet the criteria of the whole brain-death, recommended by the Harvard committee, since her brain stem continued to function. She was not brain dead, but rather alive in a persistent vegetative state (PVS), a state in which the capacity for thought and feeling, or for conscious awareness of any kind, has been permanently lost. Nevertheless, in the case of both PVS and brain-dead patients, the continued use of life support appeared futile and wasteful to many people, and emphasized the need for a shift to neurological criteria for diagnosing death.

Two main schools of thought have emerged regarding neurological criteria of death. One is the whole-brain criterion, advocated by the Harvard report. The Harvard criteria specified that death required the termination of all functions of the whole brain, both conscious and reflexive activities. The other approach is the higher-brain criterion. It maintains that death occurs when there is the permanent loss of consciousness. Since consciousness has its seat in the cerebral cortex, the individual is dead when the cortex or higher-brain irreversibly loses function, even if there is brain stem activity.

The whole-brain criterion was adopted by the influential President's Commission for the Study of Ethical Problems in Medicine and Biomedical and Behavioral Research. A selection from the Commission's 1981 report, *Defining Death,* is the first reading in Section 1. Unlike the Harvard Committee, the President's Commission explicitly grounds its whole-brain criterion in a rejection of a "higher-brain" definition of death, which it regards as too radical, too far from the ordinary conception of death. In rejecting the "neocortical death" or "higher brain death" proposal, the Commission argues that whole-brain death is not, as one might think, a wholly new concept of death. Rather, the Commission suggests, it is simply that artificial ventilation has made the traditional cardiopulmonary indicators of death invalid for a set of patients, and brain death substitutes new diagnostic measures for them.

According to the Commission, then, the *concept* of death remains the same, whatever the *criteria* for determining death are taken to be. If this is right, then even the term "brain dead" is misleading: after all, we do not say that someone diagnosed as dead according to traditional cardiopulmonary criteria is "heart dead" or "lung dead." Moreover, if someone who is "brain dead" is really dead, it is a mistake to say (as newspapers sometimes do) that the patient was declared "brain dead" on a certain day and "died" on a subsequent day. But is the confusion, which exists among medical specialists and bioethicists as much as among laypeople, merely verbal confusion as we adjust to new criteria for death? Or is brain death something distinct from death as it is commonly understood?

It might seem that the definition of "death" is a matter for science, in particular, biology. Certainly, science has a role to play in our understanding of death, for example, in determining the most reliable criteria of death. However, the issue is not simply which criteria most reliably mark the irreversible

---

**Editor's note:* Beecher, a respected anesthesiologist, is the author of a 1966 article in the *New England Journal of Medicine* that called attention to a number of experimental studies that had put patients at risk and were done without informed consent. See Part 5, Experimentation on Human Subjects.

loss of life. Rather, our understanding of what constitutes human death depends on our understanding of what it is to be a human being. As one commentator has put it, "The ensuing controversy between advocates of whole-brain and higher-brain criteria for diagnosing brain death often reflected a conceptual contest over whether mental activity or bodily integration constitute the essence of human life" (Pernick 1999). This conceptual contest is primarily a philosophical, not a scientific, question. If we think of the human being primarily as an *organism,* and if we take the brain to be the organ that coordinates and unifies the organism's biological functioning, then the whole-brain theory might provide the best account of death, for the organism dies when the entire brain permanently ceases functioning. But if we think of the human being primarily as a *person,* and if we think that the person is gone when the capacities for awareness, thought, and social interaction are permanently lost, then the higher-brain criterion might be considered the better view. Thus, the concept of death, while undoubtedly partly biological, is also metaphysical and evaluative. Moreover, death traditionally has had medical, social, and legal consequences. It marks the point at which medical treatment can be unilaterally withdrawn (that is, without consent), organs harvested (with appropriate consent), property disposed of, the body buried or cremated, the surviving spouse can remarry, and so forth. If death is an ethically and legally significant boundary, after which it is permissible to do things that it is not permissible to do before, then we need a moral argument for where this boundary should be drawn.

In "The Impending Collapse of the Whole-Brain Definition of Death," Robert M. Veatch tries to provide such a moral argument. He opts for a higher-brain-oriented definition of death because he believes that the essence of a human being is integration of a mind and a body. Under such a definition, patients with irreversible loss of consciousness, such as patients in a persistent vegetative state (PVS), as well as anencephalic babies, who are born without a cerebral cortex, would be considered dead. Veatch begins by arguing that the whole-brain definition of death has become obsolete. No one really believes anymore that literally all functions of the entire brain must be irreversibly lost for an individual to be dead, for individual, isolated brain cells can live even though integrated supercellular brain function is destroyed. Moreover, small amounts of electrical activity can be recorded on an EEG (electroencephalogram), even when the brain is permanently nonfunctioning. Adherents of the whole-brain theory explain that these sorts of brain activity should be ignored in determining brain death because such activity does not contribute to the functioning of the organism as a whole. However, Veatch thinks that once whole-brain theorists make this response, they are well on the way to the higher-brain-oriented approach he favors.

An advantage of the higher-brain approach is that it solves the practical problems of futile treatment and organ retrieval. At the same time, its critics point out the danger of a "slippery slope." If PVS patients and anencephalic babies are dead, and thus potential organ donors, what about infants with other devastating impairments, such as hydranencephalic infants, whose cerebral hemispheres have been largely or entirely destroyed in utero by infection? What about senile elderly patients with only marginal consciousness? Veatch thinks that the higher-brain-oriented approach is not susceptible to slippery-slope arguments because, unlike the whole-brain approach, it has a principle for determining death: a living human being exists when, and only when, the capacities for organic (bodily) and mental function are present together in a single human entity. However, it is far from clear how to interpret "the capacities for organic and mental function." And even if that issue is settled, there remains considerable controversy about the application of the principle itself; whether, for example, anencephalics totally lack awareness, and whether human beings with other disorders also lack a capacity for mental function (Shinnar and Arras 1989; Capron 1987; Shewmon et al. 1989).

Veatch agrees with those who think that the debate about which criteria to use for determining death is a conceptual and moral debate. The debate about the definition of death is actually a debate about the moral status of human beings, a debate about when humans should be treated as full members of the moral community. However, recognizing that we are unlikely to get uniformity on this issue in a pluralistic society, Veatch supports (within limits) conscience clauses that would permit individuals to choose their own definition of death based on their religious and philosophical convictions.

The higher-brain approach favored by Veatch is not, at present, anywhere accepted as law or public policy. All fifty states have adopted the whole-brain criterion for brain death. Nevertheless, scholars are increasingly becoming skeptical of the conceptual foundations of the whole-brain approach, with some advocating a return to traditional cardiorespiratory criteria of death (Truog 1997). Others think that the problem is not the whole-brain criterion, but the assumption that there is a single definition or criterion of death appropriate for all purposes. This approach is represented here by Baruch A. Brody, in the article, "How Much of the Brain Must Be Dead?"

Like Veatch, Brody agrees that the whole-brain criterion—the irreversible cessation of all of the integrative functions of the brain—is untenable because many patients diagnosed as brain dead in fact retain some brain functions, including truly integrative functions, such as neurohormonal regulation. But whereas Veatch uses such evidence to lend support to a higher-brain approach, Brody suggests that the problem lies with the idea of a precise time of death, an idea that once made sense when the points in the process of dying were always close in time. Now that medicine can (and sometimes has good reason to) sustain some of the body's functions when others have stopped, it becomes impossible to pick a single moment at which death occurs. Death is not an event, but a chain of events. The organism is fully alive before the chain of events occurs, fully dead when it ends, but neither dead nor fully alive during its process. "Death is a process in a world governed by fuzzy logic," Brody states.

Nor do we need to choose a moment at which an organism is "really" dead to know when it is appropriate to terminate treatment, retrieve organs, or bury or cremate the body. Instead, Brody suggests, we should uncouple the determination of death from its medical, legal, social, and religious consequences. Life support can be withdrawn when the cerebral cortex becomes permanently nonfunctioning, since at that point there is no longer a person who can be benefited by medical treatment. Ending life support at this point is justified as the appropriate stewardship of social resources. (Brody would make an exception in those rare cases where the full costs of continued care were paid for by the patient or family.) Organs can be harvested at the stage when the organism can no longer breathe on its own. Brody notes that this is current practice, but stresses that the justification is not some criterion of death justified by some definition of death: "Instead, we argued for it on the grounds that it preserves the proper balance between trying to maximize the supply of organs to save lives and trying to preserve public support for organ transplantation by not harvesting organs in cases that would be socially unacceptable." Finally, we should wait for asystole (complete absence of electrical activity in the heart) which usually occurs after all support ends. This would respect the feelings of family members without having any negative effects regarding unilateral withdrawal of life support or harvesting of organs.

Defenders of the whole-brain criterion deny that the problems with brain death represent fatal flaws for producing a coherent concept linking the definition, criterion, and tests of death. While admitting that all of the brain's functions do not cease when the medical tests for brain death are satisfied, they believe it is possible to distinguish between the brain's functions, and to define death as the permanent cessation of the critical functions of the organism as a whole (Bernat 1999). James Bernat argues that the uncoupling of the social and legal consequences of death from a definition and criterion of death could have morally undesirable results, such as the removal of individuals from life support being dependent on the family's finances. Finally, Brody's reason given for waiting for asystole before burying or cremating PVS patients from whom life-sustaining treatment has been stopped is respect for family sentiments. "What Brody does not point out," Bernat comments, "is that family sentiments oppose burying or cremating a spontaneously breathing and heart-beating PVS patient because it is obvious to families and to everyone else that spontaneously breathing and moving PVS patients are not dead." However, the consensus that such patients are not dead might be seen as a reasonable constraint on policy options, rather than a reason to reject a sociocultural approach to death.

One of the fundamental challenges for bioethics today is to decide when to terminate treatment for patients who are, by present definitions, alive. Competent patients have a well-established, common-law right to refuse even life-sustaining medical treatment. As articulated by the eminent judge, Benjamin Cardozo, in a rightly celebrated formulation, "Every adult human being of adult years and sound mind has a right to determine what shall be done with his own body. . . ." But what exactly do we mean by a "sound mind," and how are we to distinguish sound minds from unsound minds?

DECISIONAL CAPACITY AND THE RIGHT TO REFUSE TREATMENT

Although most patients either clearly possess or clearly lack the capacity for autonomous decision making, a significant portion fall into a troublesome gray area between competence and incompetence.* In Section 2, the factual and conceptual difficulties involved in determining competency are well illustrated in the case of Mary Northern, a stubborn 72-year-old woman suffering from gangrene of both feet. Although Ms. Northern's physicians insisted that surgical amputation of her feet was required to save her life, she adamantly refused to grant them permission to operate. Contrary to the opinion of her physicians, she maintained that her feet were improving and that surgery was thus unnecessary. While her physicians characterized her refusal as irrational, a court-appointed guardian remarked on her good memory and overall coherence and intelligence. Her physicians found her to be "psychotic" with regard to discussions about her feet, but her guardian concluded that she was of "sound mind." Mary Northern's own testimony, delivered from her bed in an intensive-care unit, supported both conclusions. Who was right? More importantly, what do we mean by "competency," and what standards of decision-making capacity should be imposed on patients like Mary Northern?

According to Allen Buchanan and Dan W. Brock in "Deciding for Others: Competency," competency ought to be understood not as a global attribute, but rather as a "decision-relative" concept. In other words, persons should be thought of as competent to do this or that, or to make this or that decision. Obviously, the same patient might thus be competent to refuse an easily explainable procedure but incompetent to manage her own complex finances. In addition, Buchanan and Brock argue that our concept of competency encompasses not merely an assessment of the patient's actual psychological capacities, but also a complex societal weighting of the values of well-being and autonomy. Noting that our task is to avoid two diametrically opposed kinds of error—stripping capable patients of the autonomy or allowing impaired patients to make foolish and self-destructive decisions—Buchanan and Brock contend that our standard of competency must be *decided* rather than merely *discovered*. Contrary to those who argue for some minimal standard of competency in every case or judge a patient's choice according to some objective canon of normalcy, Buchanan and Brock focus our attention on the quality of the patient's process of reasoning and on the risks and benefits posed by the decision. In Mary Northern's case, for example, a situation involving a life-or-death decision by a woman of questionable competence, they would have insisted that the patient meet a high standard of decision-making capacity. We leave it to readers to decide whether this "sliding-scale" approach masks ethically problematic, paternalistic judgments as objective medical or psychiatric competency determinations; or whether it correctly avoids attributing autonomy to all conscious patients, regardless of cognitive impairment, whose decisions may be manifestly against their own best interests.

Some refusals of treatment cause consternation among physicians not because there is genuine doubt about the ability of the patient to understand his or her condition, treatment alternatives, possible outcomes, and the like, but rather because the patient's refusal seems patently irrational. Must all treatment refusals be honored, or only those that meet certain standards of rationality, legal competence, or professional medical ethics? Must doctors honor the refusal of any legally competent patient, no matter how irrational the choice

**Editor's note:* Strictly speaking, "competence" is a legal term. Thus understood, only judges have the authority to declare a patient "incompetent." In the less formal context of this book, however, we define "competency" as the capacity for autonomous decision making.

might seem? What if sound medical practice offers a high probability of curing an otherwise fatal condition—should our medical ethic condone such self-destructive treatment refusals? Is the paternalistic imposition of therapy against the patient's will ever justified?

These questions converge in this section's case study. A freak accident left Don Cowart with severe burns on over 65 percent of his body. Despite the severity of his injuries, he was clearly competent, and he repeatedly asked to be allowed to die. Don's doctor at first dismissed his patient's pleas to stop treatment as the typical response of burn victims to the pain of their wounds and treatment. In time, however, he discussed Don's wish to die with Don, his mother, and his lawyer. Should Don have been allowed to discontinue his painful daily treatments in order to go home and die? Should his mother and lawyer have been able to block his treatment refusal? And is the ultimate outcome of Cowart's life—completing a law degree, passing the bar, and setting up a small practice—relevant to whether he should have been allowed to die?

ADVANCE DIRECTIVES

In our discussion of Section 1, we considered the proposal that permanently unconscious individuals should be considered dead. This would remove the problem of making medical decisions on their behalf, since dead people do not get medical attention. This is one advantage of the higher-brain conception of death, but higher-brain theory is, as we saw, still quite controversial. Moreover, there are many patients who are incapacitated because of temporary unconsciousness, and many others who are permanently incapacitated, although not completely unconscious. Someone must make medical decisions for such patients, hence the problem of proxy decision making, which we explore in Section 3. If one individual is to be given life-or-death authority over another, on what basis should such a proxy make a decision?

The first, and still very important, legal decision in this area involved Karen Ann Quinlan, who slipped into a coma in April 1975. When it became clear that she was in a persistent vegetative state, her parents sought to have her respirator removed. Her doctors refused, and her parents took the case to court. The court found that Karen, were she competent, would have had a right to refuse treatment, and held that Karen's guardian could assert that right on Karen's behalf, provided that she would have wanted it exercised in such circumstances. The problem was that Karen had never specified what she would want done—she was, after all, a healthy 21-year-old prior to her sudden loss of consciousness. Despite this lack of evidence for implementing the standard that has come to be known as "the substituted judgment test," the court favored the right of Karen's family to make the decision to refuse her treatment. It stated that if *their* decision was that Karen would have wanted treatment stopped, they could exercise Karen's right of privacy. The court found such a choice permissible based on the medical prognosis—Karen had lost all chance of returning to a sapient, cognitive existence—and suggested that hospitals set up "ethics committees" to oversee such decisions and, in particular, confirm the prognoses.

The *Quinlan* case prompted the enactment of the nation's first living-will statute, California's Natural Death Act, in 1976. A living will is a document executed by a competent adult that directs medical treatment in the event of his or her future incapacitation. The California statute is very narrow. It allows the removal of life-sustaining treatment only after the patient has been diagnosed with a terminal illness that will cause death imminently. "Thus," as George J. Annas notes in "The Health Care Proxy and the Living Will," even though this statute was inspired by her story, it would not have helped Quinlan, because she was not terminally ill." Indeed, she continued to live for another ten years after being taken off the respirator.

A second landmark case involved another young woman, Nancy Cruzan, who entered a persistent vegetative state, in this case, as a result of a car accident in 1983. Like Karen Quinlan, Nancy Cruzan did not die when removed from the respirator, but continued to breathe on her own and was placed on a feeding tube. After four years, when it became apparent that her condition would not change, her father attempted to have the feeding tube removed so that she could die. Nancy's parents were granted permission by a Missouri trial court to terminate her artificial nutrition and hydration, but the Missouri Supreme Court reversed the decision on the grounds that there was not "clear and convincing evidence" that she would have wanted the feeding tube removed. On June 25, 1990, the U.S. Supreme Court upheld, by a 5–4 decision, the judgment of the Missouri Supreme Court. This was the first so-called right-to-die case to reach the U.S. Supreme Court.

The Court made two notable claims in *Cruzan*. First, it rejected the view that there is a moral or legal difference between taking someone off a respirator and removing a feeding tube. The Court said that in this context they are both forms of medical treatment, and both can be rejected. Second, the Court upheld Missouri's right to use the most stringent standard—the clear and convincing evidence standard—in determining whether life-prolonging treatment may be removed from incompetents. The Court did not say that this standard *must* be used, only that there is nothing in the Constitution that prevents a state from applying this test.

At this point, other people came forward who had known Nancy Cruzan by her married name of Davis and so did not connect her with the case until they heard the details from the media. They had worked with her in a program for handicapped children, where she had stated repeatedly that she would not want to be force fed or kept alive on a machine. The Cruzans returned to court with this testimony in October 1990, and this time Missouri's attorney general and Ms. Cruzan's court-appointed guardian *ad litem* did not object to the Cruzans' request. The judge who had originally said that the tube could be removed repeated his findings of three years before. The tube was removed and, twelve days later, on December 26, 1990, Nancy Cruzan died.

Living wills are intended to provide "clear and convincing" evidence of what the person "would have wanted," thus providing a basis for proxy decision making. However, relatively few people (fewer than 10 percent of Americans) make living wills. Moreover, according to Annas, virtually all living-will statutes suffer from four major shortcomings: they are applicable only to those who are "terminally ill" (thus inapplicable to PVS patients who can survive for years); they limit the types of treatment that can be refused, usually allowing refusal only of "artificial" or "extraordinary" therapies; they make no provision for the designation of a decision maker to act on the person's behalf; and there is no penalty if health care providers do not honor these documents. Another problem with living wills is that it is extremely difficult to foresee every medical problem and possible treatment that might arise. Living wills also require physicians to make treatment decisions based on their interpretation of the document, rather than on a discussion of the treatment options with a person acting on the patient's behalf.

The cases presented by Stuart J. Eisendrath and Albert R. Jonsen in "The Living Will: Help or Hindrance?" provide dramatic illustrations of these problems. For example, in Case 1, Mrs. T specified in a living will that if she should have a severe and disabling stroke, she wanted to be allowed to die if there was "no reasonable expectation of her recovery from physical or mental disability." The case highlights the vague nature of such phrases, and the difficulty of determining what a "reasonable expectation" is and what should count as "recovery."

A solution to the problems of foresight and interpretation is to replace living wills with durable-power-of-attorney forms, which would name a "health care proxy" or "surrogate" empowered to make medical decisions for the incapacitated person. Every state already has a durable-power-of-attorney law; however, the current trend is for states to enact additional proxy laws that deal specifically with health care. These laws authorize a proxy to make any decisions that the patient would have made if he or she were still competent. These decisions must prove consistent with the wishes of the patient, if known, or they must prove otherwise consistent with the patient's best interests.

Many people find the "clear and convincing" standard imposed in *Cruzan* and other cases far too stringent, especially in the case of individuals who are permanently and irreversibly unconscious. Such critics may ask whether life is of any benefit or value to someone who cannot hear, feel, think, or be aware of anything. A much more difficult decision arises in the case of minimally conscious patients, for they may get some benefit out of their lives, severely limited though they are. Some argue that a family, based on its intimate knowledge of the person over a lifetime, should have the right to terminate life support for a severely demented relative. However, in many cases it is extremely difficult even for family members to know what the patient would have wanted.

Even if it is possible to ascertain what the patient would have wanted when he or she was competent, should this be the deciding factor? That is, should treatment decisions be made on the basis of the preferences and values of the once-competent individual, or on the basis of the interests of the patient as he or she is now? This issue is sharply highlighted in the scenarios by Norman L. Cantor ("Testing the Limits of Prospective Autonomy: Five Scenarios") and in Section 4, "Choosing for Others."

CHOOSING FOR OTHERS

Admitting the limitations of the substituted judgment standard raises a serious problem: On what grounds does a proxy decide for an incompetent? *In the Matter of Claire C. Conroy,* a highly influential case decided by the same court that decided *Quinlan,* attempts to answer this. *Conroy* holds that when the subjective test is inapplicable, a patient's family can still terminate treatment if they meet an objective standard: if they can prove that the burdens of the patient's life clearly and markedly outweigh the benefits. The *Conroy* majority says these burdens should be measured in terms of physical pain and suffering, thus rendering the objective test very stringent. Justice Handler, in his partial dissent, would allow the benefits/burdens assessment to encompass more than physical pain, considering personal privacy, dignity, and bodily integrity as well. The point of disagreement between the majority and dissenting opinions is a crucial one: it can be seen as the difference between authorizing quality-of-life assessments limited to relatively objective factors such as pain, and authorizing quality-of-life assessments that include a variety of factors bearing upon the quality of someone's life.

In "The Severely Demented, Minimally Functional Patient," John D. Arras reiterates the difficulties of determining what an incompetent person "would have wanted." Pulling out a feeding tube may indicate either a preference for death, or only irritation caused by the tube. Previous independence and avoidance of doctors may or may not mean that the patient would prefer death to being sustained by tube feedings. Given the problems with a subjective standard, it may seem that an objective best-interests standard is the appropriate test. However, the best-interests standard is not always applicable. For example, it is untenable for PVS patients who *have* no interests in the ordinary sense of the term. A best-interests standard would require that treatment always continue, given the very slight possibility of recovery or misdiagnosis and the absence of pain or other burdens—a result Arras terms "paradoxical," since if anyone's life need not be maintained, surely PVS patients are at the top of the list. For PVS patients, a decision in favor of nontreatment should be based not on an objective weighing of benefits and burdens to the patient—since PVS patients cannot be benefited or burdened—but rather on a judgment that the patient has ceased to be a "person" in any meaningful sense.

Decision making is very different for marginally or moderately functional individuals who can think, feel, and relate to others. Even if such patients are incapable of rational decision making, they nevertheless are clearly persons with interests that can be either advanced or frustrated by their caregivers. These patients are, Arras says, entitled to a "patient-centered best-interests" medical analysis. However, applying a best-interests analysis to minimally functional patients, such as Arras's Mrs. Smith, is problematic. It is difficult to determine either the benefits or the burdens of continued existence in her condition. Nevertheless, Arras maintains that it is highly doubtful that the burdens of Mrs. Smith's life "clearly and markedly" outweigh the benefits; thus, a literal application of the *Conroy* formula would lead to the conclusion that the G-tube should be surgically implanted. The trouble with this conclusion is that it appears to leave out something important: namely, the patient's probable feelings about privacy, dependency, dignity, and bodily integrity. To focus solely on physical pain is to reduce Mrs. Smith "from the full-fledged person that she once was to a mere physical repository of pleasures and pains."

Considerations of this sort led Justice Handler to his eloquent dissent in *Conroy.* Arras notes, however, that Handler's dissent is also problematic. If we consider only Mrs. Smith's *present interests,* then these are indeed reduced to sensations of pleasure and pain. In her present state, she is not bothered by a lack of dignity or bodily integrity. If we consider the interests of the formerly competent Mrs. Smith, it is possible that she would have been appalled at being kept alive in her present condition. The trouble is that we cannot know this, since she left behind neither an advance directive nor a pattern of analogous choices that clearly demonstrate what she would have wanted under her present circumstances. Thus, the ambiguities of substituted judgment lead to the adoption of an objective best-interests standard, while the deficiencies of the objective standard—with its narrow focus on pain to the exclusion of other important values—send us back to the substituted judgment test. To get us out of this dilemma, Arras opts for a procedural solution, one that allows families or other trustworthy surrogates to make treatment decisions—including removing feeding tubes—for severely demented patients as they see fit, unless their decisions clearly violate the patient's best interests.

Opposed to Arras's "quality of life" approach is the statement from the U.S. Bishops' Pro-Life Committee, entitled "Nutrition and Hydration: Moral and Pastoral Reflections." It enumerates some basic principles of the Catholic moral tradition that apply to decisions about medically assisted nutrition and hydration. In a careful and nuanced discussion, the Bishops affirm their opposition to the deliberate taking of life, even permanently unconscious life, while at the same time they express support for the view that one is not obliged to prolong the life of a dying person by every possible means.

These issues continue to be debated in the courts as *In re the Conservatorship of the Person of Robert Wendland,* a recent California case, demonstrates. Wendland suffered profound brain injuries in a truck accident in 1993. After being unconscious for sixteen months, he regained some degree of consciousness; exactly how much was vigorously disputed by the parties. (It is also unclear whether he recovered from a persistent vegetative state, as Wesley J. Smith maintains, or never was in one.) If Wendland had appointed his wife, Rose, as his agent to make health care decisions on his behalf, California law would have allowed her to refuse treatment, including life-prolonging treatment, on his behalf. Like most people, however, Robert Wendland did not have a living will nor had he appointed a health care proxy. The legal issue, then, was whether Rose, as court-appointed conservator, could authorize the withholding of life-sustaining treatment, and on what basis. The relevant California statute, Probate Code section 2355, stated that a court-appointed conservator has "exclusive authority to give consent" for medical treatment as he or she "in good faith based on medical advice determines to be necessary. . . ." The California Supreme Court struck down the statute in part, because it agreed with Robert's mother, Florence, that it failed to give constitutionally adequate protection to incompetent patients. This was the first time that a state supreme court partially struck down (or amended) a statute that expressly permitted the kind of treatment refusal that Rose made. The California Supreme Court ruled that conservators who want to withdraw life-sustaining treatment from a conscious conservatee must provide clear and convincing evidence that the conservatee would have wanted to die or that removing the feeding tube would be in the patient's best interests.

Wendland is important for several reasons. First, it draws a very bright line between the permanent vegetative state and all states in which the patient has any consciousness, and requires that termination of life-support treatment for non-PVS patients be governed by the clear and convincing evidence standard. Interestingly, both commentators in Section 4 oppose making this distinction, albeit for very different reasons. Lawrence Nelson thinks that requiring clear and convincing evidence in order to remove life-sustaining treatment from minimally conscious, but non-PVS, patients imposes an impossibly high standard on family members, while Wesley J. Smith thinks that requiring a less stringent standard for PVS patients discriminates against the permanently unconscious.

Second, *Wendland* did not touch the legal authority of surrogates or agents appointed by a competent adult to refuse life-prolonging treatment. It is only court-appointed conservators who must demonstrate clear and convincing evidence of the patient's wishes or best interests before authorizing the withholding of life-prolonging treatment from conscious patients. This distinction has left unclear the legal authority to make medical decisions of close family members who are neither patient-appointed surrogates nor court-appointed conservators. Since the overwhelming majority of persons in this country do not execute a written advance directive, most families would fall into this group. Nelson points out that the *Wendland* decision gives family members in California "a strong (albeit perverse in light of the opinion's own reasoning) incentive *not* to seek conservatorship authority over medical decisions."

Third, *Wendland* is important because it is the first major right-to-die case which has attracted the attention not only of pro-life organizations, but disability rights advocates as well. The disability rights groups—which did not file amici briefs in *Quinlan* or *Conroy*—are now pushing for judicial rules that would make it harder to stop life-sustaining treatment on those they see as "disabled." Those on the other side, including several medical organizations, many health providers, and forty-three individual bioethicists, view such rules as merely prolonging the inevitable deaths of severely brain-injured patients. Readers will have to decide for themselves whether *Wendland* subjects incompetent patients to burdensome treatment which does not benefit them, and which they would refuse if they were able, as Nelson suggests, or whether, as Smith claims, it erects "a significant and important legal bulwark protecting the lives of many cognitively disabled people."

The *Wendland* case raises an issue touched on by both Arras and Cantor: whether treatment decisions should be made on the basis of the interests of the once-competent patient, or only on the basis of the interests of the individual as he or she is now. Rebecca S. Dresser and John A. Robertson opt for basing treatment decisions on the actual interests of the incompetent patient in "Quality of Life and Non-Treatment Decisions for Incompetent Patients." They criticize "the orthodox judicial approach," as enunciated in *Quinlan,* as both conceptually flawed and dangerous. In the orthodox approach, incompetent patients have the same right to refuse treatment as do competent ones, a right that may be exercised on their behalf by surrogates, or proxies. The proxy is to determine what the incompetent patient would have chosen, either by relying on advance directives or by using substituted judgment. The orthodox approach ostensibly promotes patient self-determination, protects individuals from overtreatment, recognizes a central role for family discretion, and avoids troublesome quality-of-life determinations. However, Dresser and Robertson fault the orthodox approach on all these counts. The first issue, the autonomy of incompetent patients, cannot be respected because autonomy is literally a characteristic that belongs only to patients capable of making their own choices. Also, it is wrong to assume that the incompetent patient's prior preferences indicate the patient's current interests. Competent individuals have interests in work, family, friendships, and hobbies. They may feel that life without the possibility of pursuing these interests would be no longer worth living. However, severely demented individuals no longer have these interests. A life that may seem demeaning to a competent individual may still be of value to the incompetent patient. Why should the values and preferences of the person, while competent, prevail over the interests of the incompetent person? This is unlike the situation of a person making an ordinary will, since the testator no longer has interests after he or she is dead. By contrast, the maker of a living will may be authorizing decisions that are contrary to his or her own best interests.

The orthodox approach is dangerous, according to Dresser and Robertson, because it is likely to lead to undertreatment. They discuss several cases, including *Spring* and *Hier,* in which courts authorized nontreatment for elderly incompetent patients based on substituted judgment. Use of this standard "opens the door to nontreatment of nursing home residents and other severely debilitated persons" based on what others think they would have wanted. Instead, Dresser and Robertson recommend that such decisions be based on the patients' actual interests. Such an approach requires a forthright consideration of quality of life. If the patient is permanently unconscious, then treatment is not warranted, because, in their view, some capacity to interact with the environment must be present for life to be of value to an individual. Moreover, when the patient has no interest in continued existence, then the family's burdens and financial costs may be taken into account. Treatment might also be withheld from barely conscious patients on the grounds that their lives are not of value to them. Like Arras, Dresser and Robertson would allow families to request nontreatment for minimally conscious individuals, not because the patient would prefer nontreatment, but rather on the grounds that such life does not clearly confer a genuine benefit. However, as the commentaries on *Wendland* illustrate, people can differ dramatically on what kinds of life constitute a benefit. Wesley J. Smith would argue that letting minimally conscious or even permanently unconscious individuals die because others view their lives as having little worth violates the right to life. For those who maintain that continued existence is always in patients' best interests, a current interests approach that allows for the removal of life-prolonging treatment is no more likely to prevent undertreatment for nursing home residents and other severely debilitated persons than a substituted judgment approach.

Nancy K. Rhoden attempts to answer the question posed by Dresser and Robertson in "The Limits of Legal Objectivity": Why should the values and preferences of the once-competent person take precedence over the interests of the incompetent person? Her answer is that respect for persons requires us to adhere to the express and implicit wishes of individuals when they were competent. She says "It is at least one, if not an overriding, component of treating persons with respect that we view them as they view themselves. If we are to do this, we must not ignore their prior choices and values." Applying this approach to the *Conroy* case, Rhoden suggests that the objective test strips the individual of his or her uniqueness and personality. She reminds us that Claire Conroy was not "just anyone; she was a specific human being—Aunt Claire." While we can, and should, make quality-of-life assessments from a present-oriented perspective for individuals who were never competent (infants and severely retarded people), something is wrong, Rhoden argues, when we treat formerly competent patients as if they were never competent. She acknowledges that paying attention to advance directives and prior values does give primacy to the competent person, but this is not inexplicable or unjustifiable: "[I]t is, after all, competent persons who have the considered moral values, life plans, and treatment preferences that underlie our respect."

Rhoden also argues that the objective test endangers all of our choices, because any of us could become suddenly incapacitated. In the objective current interests approach, a competent patient's "right" to refuse treatment will be upheld only for the time he remains competent. If he has a stroke that renders him incompetent, treatment decisions will be made on the basis of his present interests. Rhoden says, "Taken to an extreme, this could mean that a Jehovah's Witness could refuse a blood transfusion until he 'bled out,' after which he could be transfused."

EUTHANASIA AND PHYSICIAN-ASSISTED SUICIDE (PAS)

Whether life is always worthwhile, or whether there are times when death is preferable to life, is an issue that has become more pressing in recent years. One reason for the growing importance of this issue is the ability of modern medicine to keep people alive who would have died in earlier medical eras. The elongation of dying through modern medical technology has raised the issue of euthanasia even more persistently than in the past. "Euthanasia" (literally, a "beautiful death") means an easy or painless death, but has come to stand for deliberately bringing about such a death through action or inaction. On the one hand, euthanasia would appear to be antithetical to all that medical practice stands for (indeed, the Hippocratic oath specifically enjoins inducing death, even if the patient requests it). On the other hand, if the purpose of medicine is not simply to prevent death but to alleviate suffering, then perhaps euthanasia is not entirely foreign to good, ethical medical practice. Indeed, it has been practiced openly by physicians for several years in the Netherlands, with the acceptance of the country's highest court and a broad majority of physicians and the populace. In 2001, euthanasia became fully legal in the Netherlands, provided specific guidelines are met.

Another reason for the recent attention to euthanasia, suicide, and physician-assisted suicide (PAS) is the AIDS epidemic. Many people with AIDS want the solace of knowing that they will be able to end their lives before either the pain becomes unbearable or they become demented. However, suicide is not always easily accomplished. According to a New York doctor with a large AIDS practice, "the reality is that most people with AIDS have very strong cardiovascular systems. Taking overdoses of most common prescription pills is not going to kill you" ("AIDS Patients Seek Solace in Suicide but Many Find Pain and Uncertainty," *New*

York Times, Tuesday, 14 June 1994, C6). Also, people can develop a tolerance for morphine. A botched suicide attempt may leave a person alive, but without any brain function. When doctors are involved, things are less likely to go wrong. For this reason, many doctors say they favor changing laws that currently prohibit them from legally assisting in suicides of people with terminal illnesses; other doctors, however, still say they have qualms about assisted suicide, even in the case of AIDS.

There are two distinctions of fundamental importance to the moral assessment of euthanasia. The first is between active euthanasia (deliberately *bringing death about* through some action, such as administering a lethal injection) and passive euthanasia (deliberately *allowing death to occur* through some form of inaction, such as refraining from performing corrective surgery). Often this distinction has been characterized as the difference between "killing" and "letting die." A second distinction is made between voluntary euthanasia (actively requested by the patient) and nonvoluntary euthanasia, in which the patient (for example, a PVS patient) lacks the capacity to consent. Writers on the topic disagree as to whether all forms of euthanasia are permissible, or only some forms. Most people would agree that the voluntary/nonvoluntary distinction is at least relevant to, if not decisive in determining, the permissibility of euthanasia; some still maintain, however, that the distinction between active and passive euthanasia—if it can be coherently drawn at all—has no moral relevance (Steinbock and Norcross, 1994).

Legally, nevertheless, there is an important difference between actively causing someone's death and allowing him or her—even deliberately—to die. Liability for allowing to die depends on the relation between the "victim" and the one who allows him or her to die. A doctor who stops treatment at the request of a patient is unlikely to be liable for the patient's death, as long as the doctor acts within the bounds of accepted medical practice. Indeed, a doctor who continues treating a competent patient who has refused treatment is theoretically liable for battery (although few, if any, doctors have ever been successfully sued for treating without consent). Killing a patient, even at his or her request, is quite another matter. Assisting a suicide is a crime in most jurisdictions. In recent years, California and Washington have attempted initiatives to legalize doctor-assisted suicide; neither state succeeded. In 1994, Oregon became the only state to legalize PAS. Under the state's Death with Dignity Act, a terminally ill patient may be given a prescription for lethal drugs if two doctors agree the person has less than six months to live and is mentally competent to make the decision to end his or her life. Opponents sought to repeal the act, but this attempt was rejected by the voters, with a greater margin than had passed the original act, in November 1997. In the first four years of legalization, about 90 people have died after ingesting medications received under the act. Many more have obtained lethal prescriptions but have died of natural causes before taking the drugs.

One of the few jurisdictions where there was no law, until recently, against assisting a suicide was Michigan. For this reason, the controversial Dr. Jack Kevorkian chose Michigan as the place to perform several "medicides," as he calls them, using the "suicide machine" he invented for the purpose. Michigan quickly moved to pass a statute making assisted suicide a crime so that Dr. Kevorkian could be charged the next time he helped someone to die. However, on May 2, 1994, a Detroit jury acquitted Dr. Jack Kevorkian of charges that he had violated Michigan's law barring assisted suicide. Comments from jurors made it clear that the jury regarded Dr. Kevorkian as justified in helping terminally ill patients to die. As of this writing, Dr. Kevorkian has helped approximately 100 individuals to die.

Dr. Timothy E. Quill, the first author in Section 5 ("Death and Dignity: A Case of Individualized Decision Making"), prescribed barbiturates for his longtime patient, Diane, who requested them to kill herself in order to avoid a lingering, painful (or drugged) death from leukemia. Many commentators have contrasted Dr. Quill with Dr. Kevorkian. Dr. Kevorkian is a retired pathologist; Dr. Quill a practicing internist. Dr. Kevorkian has helped about 100 people to die; Dr. Quill only 1. Dr. Kevorkian does not know the individuals he helps to die, neither the details of their medical conditions nor their psychological states. Dr. Quill knew Diane very well, and met regularly with her over several months after she requested the barbiturates. Clearly, Dr. Quill is a conscientious, compassionate physician who had the deepest concern for his patient's well-being and the deepest respect for her choices. Having said that, did Dr. Quill do the right thing? And should such behavior be sanctioned by law?

During 1996, two federal appeals courts held that state laws criminalizing assisted suicide violated the Fourteenth Amendment to the United States Constitution. In June, 1997, the Supreme Court reversed the decisions in both *Washington* v. *Glucksberg* and *Vacco* v. *Quill*, holding that there is no constitutional right to physician-assisted suicide. This has settled (for the time being) the constitutional question. However, the moral and legal debate over whether one has a right to die is far from over. The Court decision, most legal commentators said, simply returns the question to the states. However, the ability of states to make their own decisions regarding physician-assisted suicide has been challenged. On November 6, 2001, Attorney General John Ashcroft, declaring that assisted suicide is *not* a "legitimate medical purpose" for prescribing or dispensing medication, authorized federal drug agents to revoke the license of any doctor who prescribes lethal drugs, even one acting within all terms of the Oregon law. Ashcroft's action illustrates a tension between the constitutional doctrine of federal supremacy and the principle of states' rights. Although conservatives generally support the rights of states to make their own decisions on most policy matters, social and religious conservatives have long sought to undermine or even abolish the Oregon law, holding that any official sanction of suicide is immoral. Oregon officials said they would go to court to try to block the order, and "even those who said they were personally opposed to physician-assisted suicide, generally responded with outrage to an action in the nation's capital that so clearly undercut the expressed will of the states' voters" (Sam Howe Verhovek, "Federal Agents Are Directed to Stop Physicians Who Assist Suicides," *New York Times*, Wednesday, November 7, 2001, A20). A temporary restraining order, blocking Ashcroft's move, was granted by a federal judge in November 2001, enabling doctors to continue prescribing lethal medication under the terms of the law. On April 17, 2002, Federal District Court Judge Robert R. Jones confirmed the temporary restraining order. In a decision sharply critical of Ashcroft, Judge Jones called his directive an attempt by opponents of Oregon's law "to get through the administrative door what they could not get through the Congressional door" and said that there is no indication in any federal statute, including the drug law, "that Congress delegated to federal prosecutors the authority to define what constitutes legitimate *medical* practices" (Adam Liptak, "Judge Blocks U.S. Bid to Ban Suicide Law," *New York Times*, April 18, 2002, A16).

The case in favor of assisted suicide is made by six well-known moral philosophers in the "The Philosophers' Brief," the third article in Section 5. The basis of their position is the general moral principle that every competent person has the right to make momentous personal decisions about life's value, including decisions about when life ceases to be worth living. At the same time, the authors acknowledge that people may make such momentous decisions impulsively or out of depression, and that the state has the right to adopt safeguards to ensure that a patient's decision for suicide is informed, competent, and free. The philosophers address the risk that legalizing PAS might jeopardize vulnerable patients, and they conclude that such patients might be better, rather than less, well protected if assisted suicide were legalized with appropriate safeguards.

In "Physician-Assisted Suicide: A Tragic View," John D. Arras lays out the pros and cons of legalizing PAS. Although Arras is "deeply sympathetic to the central values motivating the push for PAS and euthanasia," he ultimately concludes that the social risks of legalization outweigh the benefits. While there may be individual cases in which assisted suicide is the best choice, it does not follow that legalizing PAS is the wisest social policy. A better approach would be to improve radically the palliative care terminally ill patients receive. "At the end of this long and arduous process," Arras writes, "when we finally have an equitable, effective, and compassionate health care system in place . . . , then we might well want to reopen the discussion of PAS and active euthanasia."

Margaret Battin has updated her article, "Euthanasia: The Way We Do It, The Way They Do It," for the sixth edition, providing a cross-cultural comparison of assistance in dying in the Netherlands, Germany, and the United States, as well as in countries whose policies are to some extent patterned after them: Belgium, Switzerland, Australia, Canada, and the United Kingdom. In the Netherlands, voluntary active euthanasia, while until recently prohibited by statute, has nevertheless been legally tolerated, provided the physician meets a rigorous set of guidelines. Euthanasia and assisted suicide are infrequently chosen, but are a "conspicuous option in terminal illness."

The painful history of Nazism in Germany, and the killing of mentally and physically handicapped patients (which led eventually to the Holocaust), has resulted in Germany's rejection of physician participation in causing death. "Euthanasia is viewed as always wrong, and the Germans view the Dutch as stepping out on a dangerously slippery slope," writes Battin. At the same time, assisted suicide is not a violation of the law, and the German Society for Humane Dying publishes a booklet listing drugs available by prescription, together with the specific dosages necessary for producing a certain, painless death. However, the removal of physicians from participating in assisted suicide means that decisions for suicide are not necessarily medically evaluated, either to confirm the patient's diagnosis or prognosis, or to rule out treatable depression as the motivating factor.

The United States differs from both the Netherlands and Germany in significant ways. Unlike all the countries discussed here—not only the Netherlands and Germany, but also Belgium, Switzerland, Canada, Australia, and the United Kingdom—we have no national health insurance, and cost increasingly plays a role in health care decisions. Battin, who generally supports physician aid-in-dying for the reasons given in "The Philosophers' Brief," briefly examines the ways in which some safeguards function in different societies and concludes that PAS is a better alternative in the United States than euthanasia, given our cultural context, because PAS grants physicians a measure of control while it leaves the fundamental decision up to the patients themselves.

Forty years ago, in an influential article criticizing proposed "mercy-killing" legislation, Yale Kamisar warned against giving the choice of euthanasia to gravely ill patients, saying:

> Will we not sweep up, in the process, some who are not really tired of life, but think others are tired of them; some who do not really want to die, but who feel they should not live on, because to do so when there looms the legal alternative of euthanasia is to do a selfish or a cowardly act? Will not some feel an obligation to have themselves "eliminated" in order that funds allocated for their terminal care might be better used by their families or, financial worries aside, in order to relieve their families of the emotional strain involved? (Kamisar, 1958)

Most defenders of PAS try to argue that, with proper safeguards, Kamisar's fears will not materialize. By contrast, in what may be the most provocative article in this collection ("Is There a Duty to Die?"), John Hardwig suggests that there can be a moral obligation (not merely a right) to choose death. The basis of this obligation is the burden imposed on family members who care for sick and dying patients. It might seem that Hardwig is using a consequentialist analysis to derive a duty to die. In fact, his reasoning owes at least as much to Kantian ethics as to utilitarianism, for he says, "To think that my loved ones must bear whatever burdens my illness, debility, or dying process might impose upon them is to reduce them to means to my well-being. And that would be immoral." We leave it to the reader to decide whether Hardwig's claim of a duty to die is a moral advance, or, as Felicia Ackerman argues in " 'For Now I Have My Death': The 'Duty to Die' versus the Duty to Help the Ill Stay Alive," a reflection of "our society's bias against and systematic devaluation of the old and ill."

THE DEFINITION OF DEATH

DEFINING DEATH*

President's Commission for the Study of Ethical Problems in Medicine and Biomedical and Behavioral Research

WHY UPDATE DEATH?

For most of the past several centuries, the medical determination of death was very close to the popular one. If a person fell unconscious or was found so, someone (often but not always a physician) would feel for the pulse, listen for breathing, hold a mirror before the nose to test for condensation, and look to see if the pupils were fixed. Although these criteria have been used to determine death since antiquity, they have not always been universally accepted.

Developing Confidence in the Heart-Lung Criteria

In the eighteenth century, macabre tales of "corpses" reviving during funerals and exhumed skeletons found to have clawed at coffin lids led to widespread fear of premature burial. Coffins were developed with elaborate escape mechanisms and speaking tubes to the world above . . . , mortuaries employed guards to monitor the newly dead for signs of life, and legislatures passed laws requiring a delay before burial.

The medical press also paid a great deal of attention to the matter. In *The Uncertainty of the Signs of Death and the Danger of Precipitate Interments* in 1740, Jean-Jacques Winslow advanced the thesis that putrefaction was the only sure sign of death. In the years following, many physicians published articles agreeing with him. This position had, however, notable logistic and public health disadvantages. It also disparaged, sometimes with unfair vigor, the skills of physicians as diagnosticians of

---

From the President's Commission for the Study of Ethical Problems in Medicine and Biomedical and Behavioral Research, *Defining Death: A Report on the Medical, Legal and Ethical Issues in the Determination of Death*, Washington, D.C.: U.S. Government Printing Office, 1981, 12–20, 31–43.

Editors' note: The notes have been omitted. Readers who wish to follow up on sources should consult the original article.

death. In reply, the French surgeon Louis published in 1752 his influential *Letters on the Certainty of the Signs of Death*. The debate dissipated in the nineteenth century because of the gradual improvement in the competence of physicians and a concomitant increase in the public's confidence in them.

Physicians actively sought to develop this competence. They even held contests encouraging the search for a cluster of signs—rather than a single infallible sign—for the diagnosis of death. One sign did, however, achieve prominence. The invention of the stethoscope in the mid–nineteenth century enabled physicians to detect heartbeat with heightened sensitivity. The use of this instrument by a well-trained physician, together with other clinical measures, laid to rest public fears of premature burial. The twentieth century brought even more sophisticated technological means to determine death, particularly the electrocardiograph (EKG), which is more sensitive than the stethoscope in detecting cardiac functioning.

The Interrelationships of Brain, Heart, and Lung Functions

The brain has three general anatomic divisions: the cerebrum, with its outer shell called the cortex; the cerebellum; and the brainstem, composed of the midbrain, the pons, and the medulla oblongata. . . . Traditionally, the cerebrum has been referred to as the "higher brain" because it has primary control of consciousness, thought, memory, and feeling. The brainstem has been called the "lower brain," since it controls spontaneous, vegetative functions such as swallowing, yawning, and sleep-wake cycles. It is important to note that these generalizations are not entirely accurate. Neuroscientists generally agree that such "higher brain" functions as cognition or consciousness probably are not mediated strictly by the cerebral cortex; rather, they probably result from complex interrelations between brainstem and cortex.

Respiration is controlled in the brainstem, particularly the medulla. . . . Neural impulses originating in the respiratory centers of the medulla stimulate the diaphragm and intercostal muscles, which cause the lungs to fill with air. Ordinarily, these respiratory centers adjust the rate of breathing to maintain the correct levels of carbon dioxide and oxygen. In certain circumstances, such as heavy exercise, sighing, coughing, or sneezing, other areas of the brain modulate the activities of the respiratory centers or even briefly take direct control of respiration.

Destruction of the brain's respiratory center stops respiration, which in turn deprives the heart of needed oxygen, causing it too to cease functioning. The traditional signs of life—respiration and heartbeat—disappear: the person is dead. The "vital signs" traditionally used in diagnosing death thus reflect the direct interdependence of respiration, circulation, and the brain.

The artificial respirator and concomitant life-support systems have changed this simple picture. Normally, respiration ceases when the functions of the diaphragm and intercostal muscles are impaired. This results from direct injury to the muscles or (more commonly) because the neural impulses between the brain and these muscles are interrupted. However, an artificial respirator (also called a ventilator) can be used to compensate for the inability of the thoracic muscles to fill the lungs with air. Some of these machines use negative pressure to expand the chest wall (in which case they are called "iron lungs"); others use positive pressure to push air into the lungs. The respirators are equipped with devices to regulate the rate and depth of "breathing," which are normally controlled by the respiratory centers in the medulla. The machines cannot compensate entirely for the defective neural connections since they cannot regulate blood gas levels precisely. But, provided that the lungs themselves have not been extensively damaged, gas exchange can continue and appropriate levels of oxygen and carbon dioxide can be maintained in the circulating blood.

Unlike the respiratory system, which depends on the neural impulses from the brain, the heart can pump blood without external control. Impulses from brain centers modulate the inherent rate and force of the heartbeat but are not required for the heart to contract at a level of function that is ordinarily adequate. Thus, when artificial respiration provides adequate oxygenation and associated medical treatments regulate essential plasma components and blood pressure, an intact heart will continue to beat, despite loss of brain functions. At present, however, no machine can take over the functions of the heart except for a very limited time and in limited circumstances (e.g., a heart-lung machine used during surgery). Therefore, when a severe injury to the heart or major blood vessels prevents the circulation of the crucial blood supply to the brain, the loss of brain functioning is inevitable because no oxygen reaches the brain.

Loss of Various Brain Functions

The most frequent causes of irreversible loss of functions of the whole brain are (1) direct trauma to the head, such as from a motor vehicle accident or a gunshot wound, (2) massive spontaneous hemorrhage into the brain as a result of ruptured aneurysm or complications of high blood pressure, and (3) anoxic damage from cardiac or respiratory arrest or severely reduced blood pressure.

Many of these severe injuries to the brain cause an accumulation of fluid and swelling in the brain tissue, a condition called cerebral edema. In severe cases of edema, the pressure within the closed cavity increases until it exceeds the systolic blood pressure, resulting in a total loss of blood flow to both the upper and lower portions of the brain. If deprived of blood flow for at least 10 to 15 minutes, the brain, including the brainstem, will completely cease functioning. Other pathophysiologic mechanisms also result in a progressive and, ultimately, complete cessation of intracranial circulation.

Once deprived of adequate supplies of oxygen and glucose, brain neurons will irreversibly lose all activity and ability to function. In adults, oxygen and/or glucose deprivation for more than a few minutes causes some neuron loss. Thus, even in the absence of direct trauma and edema, brain functions can be lost if circulation to the brain is impaired. If blood flow is cut off, brain tissues completely self-digest (autolyze) over the ensuing days.

When the brain lacks all functions, consciousness is, of course, lost. While some spinal reflexes often persist in such bodies (since circulation to the spine is separate from that of the brain), all reflexes controlled by the brainstem as well as cognitive, affective, and integrating functions are absent. Respiration and circulation in these bodies may be generated by a ventilator together with intensive medical management. In adults who have experienced irreversible cessation of the functions of the entire brain, this mechanically generated functioning can continue only a limited time because the heart usually stops beating within two to ten days. (An infant or small child who has lost all brain functions will typically suffer cardiac arrest within several weeks, although respiration and heartbeat can sometimes be maintained even longer.)

Less severe injury to the brain can cause mild to profound damage to the cortex, lower cerebral structures, cerebellum, brainstem, or some combination thereof. The cerebrum, especially the cerebral cortex, is more easily injured by loss of blood flow or oxygen than is the brainstem. A 4 to 6 minute loss of blood flow—caused by, for example, cardiac arrest—typically damages the cerebral cortex permanently, while the relatively more resistant brainstem may continue to function.

When brainstem functions remain, but the major components of the cerebrum are irreversibly destroyed, the patient is in what is usually called a "persistent vegetative state" or "persistent noncognitive state." Such persons may exhibit spontaneous, involuntary movements such as yawns or facial grimaces, their eyes may be open, and they may be capable of breathing without assistance. Without higher brain functions, however, any apparent wakefulness does not represent awareness of self or environment (thus, the condition is often described as "awake but unaware"). The case of Karen Ann Quinlan has made this condition familiar to the general public. With necessary medical and nursing care—including feeding through intravenous or nasogastric tubes, and antibiotics for recurrent pulmonary infections—such patients can survive months or years, often without a respirator. (The longest survival exceeded 37 years.)

Conclusion: The Need for Reliable Policy

Medical interventions can often provide great benefit in avoiding irreversible harm to a patient's injured heart, lungs, or brain by carrying a patient through a period of acute need. These techniques have, however, thrown new light on the interrelationship of these crucial organ systems. This has created complex issues for public policy as well.

For medical and legal purposes, partial brain impairment must be distinguished from complete and irreversible loss of brain functions or "whole brain death." The President's Commission regards the cessation of the vital functions of the entire brain—and not merely portions thereof, such as those responsible for cognitive functions—as the only proper neurologic basis for declaring death. This conclusion accords with the overwhelming consensus of medical and legal experts and the public.

Present attention to the "definition" of death is part of a process of development in social attitudes and legal rules stimulated by the unfolding of biomedical knowledge. In the nineteenth century increasing knowledge and practical skill made the public confident that death could be diagnosed reliably using cardiopulmonary criteria. The question now is whether, when medical intervention may be responsible for a patient's respiration and circulation, there are other equally reliable ways to diagnose death.

The Commission recognizes that it is often difficult to determine the severity of a patient's injuries, especially in the first few days of intensive care following a cardiac arrest, head trauma, or other similar event. Responsible public policy in this area requires that physicians be able to distinguish reliably those patients who have died from those whose injuries are less severe or are reversible. . . .

Understanding the "Meaning" of Death

It now seems clear that a medical consensus about clinical practices and their scientific basis has emerged: certain states of brain activity and inactivity, together with their neurophysiological consequences, can be reliably detected and used to diagnose death. To the medical community, a sound basis exists for declaring death even in the presence of mechanically assisted "vital signs." Yet before recommending that public policy reflect this medical consensus, the Commission wished to know whether the scientific viewpoint was consistent with the concepts of "being dead" or "death" as they are commonly understood in our society. These questions have been addressed by philosophers and theologians, who have provided several formulations.

The Commission believes that its policy conclusions . . . including the [Uniform Determination of Death Act] must accurately reflect the social meaning of death and not constitute a mere legal fiction. The Commission has not found it necessary to resolve all of the differences among the leading concepts of death because these views all yield interpretations consistent with the recommended statute.

Three major formulations of the meaning of death were presented to the Commission: one focused upon the functions of the whole brain, one upon the functions of the cerebral hemispheres, and one upon non-brain functions. Each of these formulations (and its variants) is presented and evaluated.

The "Whole Brain" Formulations

One characteristic of living things which is absent in the dead is the body's capacity to organize and regulate itself. In animals, the neural apparatus is the dominant locus of these functions. In higher animals and man, regulation of both maintenance of the internal environment (homeostasis) and interaction with the external environment occurs primarily within the cranium.

External threats, such as heat or infection, or internal ones, such as liver failure or endogenous lung disease, can stress the body enough to overwhelm its ability to maintain organization and regulation. If the stress passes a certain level, the organism as a whole is defeated and death occurs.

This process and its denouement are understood in two major ways. Although they are sometimes stated as alternative formulations of a "whole brain definition" of death, they are actually mirror images of each other. The Commission has found them to be complementary; together they enrich one's understanding of the "definition." The first focuses on the integrated functioning of the body's major organ systems, while recognizing the centrality of the whole brain, since it is neither revivable nor replaceable. The other identifies the functioning of the whole brain as the hallmark of life because the brain is the regulator of the body's integration. The two conceptions are subject to similar criticisms and have similar implications for policy.

The Concepts The functioning of many organs—such as the liver, kidneys, and skin—and their integration is "vital" to individual health in the sense that if any one ceases and that function is not restored or artificially replaced, the organism as a whole cannot long survive. All elements in the system are mutually interdependent, so that the loss of any part leads to the breakdown of the whole, and eventually, to the cessation of functions in every part.

Three organs—the heart, lungs, and brain—assume special significance, however, because their interrelationship is very close and the irreversible cessation of any one very quickly stops the other two and consequently halts the integrated functioning of the organism as a whole. Because they were easily measured, circulation and respiration were traditionally the basic "vital signs." But breathing and heartbeat are not life itself. They are simply used as signs—as one window for viewing a deeper and more complex reality: a triangle of interrelated systems with the brain at its apex. As the biomedical scientists who appeared before the Commission made clear, the traditional means of diagnosing death actually detected an irreversible cessation of integrated functioning among the interdependent bodily systems. When artificial means of support mask this loss of integration as measured by the old methods, brain-oriented criteria and tests provide a new window on the same phenomenon.

On this view, death is that moment at which the body's physiological system ceases to constitute an integrated whole. Even if life continues in individual cells or organs, life of the organism as a whole requires complex integration, and without the latter, a person cannot properly be regarded as alive.

This distinction between systemic, integrated functioning and physiological activity in cells or individual organs is important for two reasons. First, a person is considered dead under this concept even if oxygenation and metabolism persist in some cells or organs. There would be no need to wait until all metabolism had ceased in every body part before recognizing that death has occurred.

More importantly, this concept would reduce the significance of continued respiration and heartbeat for the definition of death. This view holds that continued breathing and circulation are not in themselves tantamount to life. Since life is a matter of integrating the functioning of major organ systems, breathing and circulation are necessary but not sufficient to establish that an individual is alive. When an individual's breathing and circulation lack neurologic integration, he or she is dead.

The alternative "whole brain" explanation of death differs from the one just described primarily in the vigor of its insistence that the traditional "vital signs" of heartbeat and respiration were merely surrogate signs with no significance in themselves. On this view, the heart and lungs are not important as basic prerequisites to continued life but rather because the irreversible cessation of their functions shows that the brain had ceased functioning. Other signs customarily employed by physicians in diagnosing death, such as unresponsiveness and absence of pupillary light response, are also indicative of loss of the functions of the whole brain.

This view gives the brain primacy not merely as the sponsor of consciousness (since even unconscious persons may be alive), but also as the complex organizer and regulator of bodily functions. (Indeed, the "regulatory" role of the brain in the organism can be understood in terms of thermodynamics and information theory.) Only the brain can direct the entire organism. Artificial support for the heart and lungs, which is required only when the brain can no longer control them, cannot maintain the usual synchronized integration of the body. Now that other traditional indicators of cessation of brain functions (*i.e.*, absence of breathing), can be obscured by medical interventions, one needs, according to this view, some new standards for determining death—that is, more reliable tests for the complete cessation of brain functions.

Critique Both of these "whole brain" formulations—the "integrated functions" and the "primary organ" views—are subject to several criticisms. Since both of these conceptions of death give an important place to the integrating or regulating capacity of the whole brain, it can be asked whether that characteristic is as distinctive as they would suggest. Other organ systems are also required for life to continue—for example, the skin to conserve fluid, the liver to detoxify the blood.

The view that the brain's functions are more central to "life" than those of the skin, the liver, and so on, is admittedly arbitrary in the sense of representing a choice. The view is not, however, arbitrary in the sense of lacking reasons. As discussed previously, the centrality accorded the brain reflects both its overarching role as "regulator" or "integrator" of other bodily systems and the immediate and devastating consequences of its loss for the organism as a whole. Furthermore, the Commission believes that this choice overwhelmingly reflects the views of experts and the lay public alike.

A more significant criticism shares the view that life consists of the coordinated functioning of the various bodily systems, in which process the whole brain plays a crucial role. At the same time, it notes that in some adult patients lacking all brain functions it is possible through intensive support to achieve constant temperature, metabolism, waste disposal, blood pressure, and other conditions typical of living organisms and not found in dead ones. Even with extraordinary medical care, these functions cannot be sustained indefinitely—typically, no longer than several days—but it is argued that this shows only that patients with nonfunctional brains are dying, not that they are dead. In this view, the respirator, drugs, and other resources of the modern intensive-care unit collectively substitute for the lower brain, just as a pump used in cardiac surgery takes over the heart's function.

The criticism rests, however, on a premise about the role of artificial support vis-à-vis the brainstem which the Commission believes is mistaken or at best incomplete. While the respirator and its associated medical techniques do substitute for the functions of the intercostal muscles and the diaphragm, which without neuronal stimulation from the brain cannot function spontaneously, they cannot replace the myriad functions of the brainstem or of the rest of the brain. The startling contrast between bodies lacking *all* brain functions and patients with intact brainstems (despite severe neocortical damage) manifests this. The former lie with fixed pupils, motionless except for the chest movements produced by their respirators. The latter cannot only breathe, metabolize, maintain temperature and blood pressure, and so forth, *on their own* but also sigh, yawn, track light with their eyes, and react to pain or reflex stimulation.

It is not easy to discern precisely what it is about patients in this latter group that makes them alive while those in the other category are not. It is in part that in the case of the first category (*i.e.*, absence of all brain functions) when the mask created by the artificial medical support is stripped away what remains is not an integrated organism but "merely a group of artificially maintained subsystems." Sometimes, of course, an artificial substitute can forge the link that restores the organism as a whole to unified functioning. Heart or kidney transplants, kidney dialysis, or an iron lung used to replace physically impaired breathing ability in a polio victim, for example, restore the integrated functioning of the organism as they replace the failed function of a part. Contrast such situations, however, with the hypothetical of a decapitated body treated so as to prevent the outpouring of blood and to generate respiration: continuation of bodily functions in that case would not have restored the requisites of human life.

The living differ from the dead in many ways. The dead do not think, interact, autoregulate, or maintain organic identity through time, for example. Not all the living can always do *all* of these activities, however; nor is there one single characteristic (*e.g.*, breathing, yawning, etc.) the loss of which signifies death. Rather, what is missing in the dead is a cluster of attributes, all of which form part of an organism's responsiveness to its internal and external environment.

While it is valuable to test public policies against basic conceptions of death, philosophical refinement beyond a certain point may not be necessary. The task undertaken in this Report is to provide and defend a statutory standard for determining that a human being has died. In setting forth the standards recommended in this Report, the Commission has used "whole brain" terms to clarify the understanding of death that enjoys near-universal acceptance in our society. The Commission finds that the "whole brain" formulations give resonance and depth to the biomedical and epidemiological data presented in [a part of the study not reproduced here]. Further effort to search for a conceptual "definition" of death is not required for the purpose of public policy because, separately or together, the "whole brain" formulations provide a theory that is sufficiently precise, concise, and widely acceptable.

Policy Consequences Those holding to the "whole brain" view—and this view seems at least implicit in most of the testimony and writing reviewed by the Commission—believe that when respirators are in use, respiration and circulation lose significance for the diagnosis of death. In a body without a functioning brain, these two functions, it is argued, become mere artifacts of the mechanical life supports. The lungs breathe and the heart circulates blood only because the respirator (and attendant medical interventions) cause them to do so, not because of any comprehensive integrated functioning. This is "breathing" and "circulation" only in an analogous sense: the function and its results are similar, but the source, cause, and purpose are different between those individuals with and those without functioning brains.

For patients who are not artificially maintained, breathing and heartbeat were, and are, reliable signs either of systemic integration and/or of continued brain functioning (depending on which approach one takes to the "whole brain" concept). To regard breathing and respiration as having diagnostic significance when the brain of a respirator-supported patient has ceased functioning, however, is to forget the basic reasoning behind their use in individuals who are not artificially maintained.

Although similar in most respects, the two approaches to "whole brain death" could have slightly different policy consequences. The "primary organ" view would be satisfied with a statute that contained only a single standard—the irreversible cessation of all functions of the entire brain. Nevertheless, as a practical matter, the view is also compatible with a statute establishing irreversible cessation of respiration and circulation as an alternative standard, since it is inherent in this view that the loss of spontaneous breathing and heartbeat are surrogates for the loss of brain functions.

The "integrated functions" view would lead one to a "definition" of death recognizing that collapse of the organism as a whole can be diagnosed through the loss of brain functions as well as through loss of cardiopulmonary functions. The latter functions would remain an explicit part of the policy statement because their irreversible loss will continue to provide an independent and wholly reliable basis for determining that death has occurred when respirators and related means of support are *not* employed.

The two "whole brain" formulations thus differ only modestly. And even conceptual disagreements have a context; the context of the present one is the need to clarify and update the "definition" of death in order to allow principled decisions to be made about the status of comatose respirator-supported patients. The explicit recognition of both standards—cardiopulmonary and whole brain—solves that problem fully. In addition, since it requires only a modest reformulation of the generally accepted view, it accounts for the importance traditionally accorded to heartbeat and respiration, the "vital signs" which will continue to be the grounds for determining death in the overwhelming majority of cases for the foreseeable future. Hence the Commission, drawing on the aspects that the two formulations share and on the ways in which they each add to an understanding of the "meaning" of death, concludes that public policy should recognize both cardiopulmonary and brain-based standards for declaring death.

The "Higher Brain" Formulations

When all brain processes cease, the patient loses two important sets of functions. One set encompasses the integrating and coordinating functions, carried out principally but not exclusively by the cerebellum and brainstem. The other set includes the psychological functions which make consciousness, thought, and feeling possible. These latter functions are located primarily but not exclusively in the cerebrum, especially the neocortex. The two "higher brain" formulations of brain-oriented definitions of death discussed here are premised on the fact that loss of cerebral functions strips the patient of his psychological capacities and properties.

A patient whose brain has permanently stopped functioning will, by definition, have lost those brain functions which sponsor consciousness, feeling, and thought. Thus the higher brain rationales support classifying as dead bodies which meet "whole brain" standards, as discussed in the preceding section. The converse is not true, however. If there are parts of the brain which have no role in sponsoring consciousness, the higher brain formulation would regard their continued functioning as compatible with death.

The Concepts Philosophers and theologians have attempted to describe the attributes a living being must have to be a person. "Personhood" consists of the complex of activities (or of capacities to engage in them) such as thinking, reasoning, feeling, and human intercourse which make the human different from, or superior to, animals or things. One higher brain formulation would define death as the loss of what is essential to a person. Those advocating the personhood definition often relate these characteristics to brain functioning. Without brain activity, people are incapable of these essential activities. A breathing body, the argument goes, is not in itself a person; and, without functioning brains, patients are merely breathing bodies. Hence personhood ends when the brain suffers irreversible loss of function.

For other philosophers, a certain concept of "personal identity" supports a brain-oriented definition of death. According to this argument, a patient literally ceases to exist as an individual when his or her brain ceases functioning, even if the patient's body is biologically alive. Actual decapitation creates a similar situation: the body might continue to function for a short time, but it would no longer be the "same" person. The persistent identity of a person as an individual from one moment to the next is taken to be dependent on the continuation of certain mental processes which arise from brain functioning. When the brain processes cease (whether due to decapitation or to "brain death") the person's identity also lapses. The mere continuation of biological activity in the body is irrelevant to the determination of death, it is argued, because after the brain has ceased functioning the body is no longer identical with the person.

Critique Theoretical and practical objections to these arguments led the Commission to rely on them only as confirmatory of other views in formulating a definition of death. First, crucial to the personhood argument is acceptance of one particular concept of those things that are essential to being a person, while there is no general agreement on this very fundamental point among philosophers, much less physicians or the general public. Opinions about what is essential to personhood vary greatly from person to person in our society—to say nothing of intercultural variations.

The argument from personal identity does not rely on any particular conception of personhood, but it does require assent to a single solution to the philosophical problem of identity. Again, this problem has persisted for centuries despite the best attempts by philosophers to solve it. Regardless of the scholarly merits of the various philosophical solutions, their abstract technicality makes them less useful to public policy.

Further, applying either of these arguments in practice would give rise to additional important problems. Severely senile patients, for example, might not clearly be persons, let alone ones with continuing personal identities; the same might be true of the severely retarded. Any argument that classified these individuals as dead would not meet with public acceptance.

Equally problematic for the "higher brain" formulations, patients in whom only the neocortex or subcortical areas have been damaged may retain or regain spontaneous respiration and circulation. Karen Quinlan is a well-known example of a person who apparently suffered permanent damage to the higher centers of the brain but whose lower brain continues to function. Five years after being removed from the respirator that supported her breathing for nearly a year, she remains in a persistent vegetative state but with heart and lungs that function without mechanical assistance.* Yet the implication of the personhood and personal identity arguments is that Karen Quinlan, who retains brainstem function and breathes spontaneously, is just as dead as a corpse in the traditional sense. The Commission rejects this conclusion and the further implication that such patients could be buried or otherwise treated as dead persons.

Policy Consequences In order to be incorporated in public policy, a conceptual formulation of death has to be amenable to clear articulation. At present, neither basic neurophysiology nor medical technique suffices to translate the "higher brain" formulation into policy. First, as was discussed in [a part of the study not reproduced here], it is not known which portions of the brain are responsible for cognition and consciousness; what little is known points to substantial interconnections among the brainstem, subcortical structures, and the neocortex. Thus, the "higher brain" may well exist only as a metaphorical concept, not in reality. Second, even when the sites of certain aspects of consciousness

*_Editors' note:_ Karen Quinlan died on June 11, 1985.

can be found, their cessation often cannot be assessed with the certainty that would be required in applying a statutory definition.

Even were these difficulties to be overcome, the adoption of a higher brain "definition" would depart radically from the traditional standards. As already observed, the new standard would assign no significance to spontaneous breathing and heartbeat. Indeed, it would imply that the existing cardiopulmonary definition had been in error all along, even before the advent of respirators and other life-sustaining technology.

In contrast to this, the position taken by the Commission is deliberately conservative. The statutory proposal presented in [the Uniform Determination of Death Act] offers legal recognition for new diagnostic measures of death, but does not ask for acceptance of a wholly new concept of death. On a matter so fundamental to a society's sense of itself—touching deeply held personal and religious beliefs—and so final for the individuals involved, one would desire much greater consensus than now exists before taking the major step of radically revising the concept of death.

Finally, patients declared dead pursuant to the statute recommended by the Commission would be also considered dead by those who believe that a body without higher brain functions is dead. Thus, all the arguments reviewed thus far are in agreement that irreversible cessation of *all* brain functioning is sufficient to determine death of the organism.

The Non-Brain Formulations

The Concepts The various physiological concepts of death so far discussed rely in some fashion on brain functioning. By contrast, a literal reading of the traditional cardiopulmonary criteria would require cessation of the flow of bodily "fluids," including air and blood, for death to be declared. This standard is meant to apply whether or not these flows coincide with any other bodily processes, neurological or otherwise. Its support derives from interpretations of religious literature and cultural practices of certain religious and ethnic groups, including some Orthodox Jews and Native Americans.

Another theological formulation of death is, by contrast, not necessarily related to any physiologic phenomenon. The view is traditional in many faiths that death occurs the moment the soul leaves the body. Whether this happens when the patient loses psychological capacities, loses all brain functions, or at some other point, varies according to the teachings of each faith and according to particular interpretations of the scriptures recognized as authoritative.

Critique The conclusions of the "bodily fluids" view lack a physiologic basis in modern biomedicine. While this view accords with the traditional criteria of death, as noted above, it does not necessarily carry over to the new conditions of the intensive care unit—which are what prompt the reexamination of the definition of death. The flow of bodily fluids could conceivably be maintained by machines in the absence of almost all other life processes; the result would be viewed by most as a perfused corpse, totally unresponsive to its environment.

Although the argument concerning the soul could be interpreted as providing a standard for secular action, those who adhere to the concept today apparently acknowledge the need for a more public and verifiable standard of death. Indeed, a statute incorporating a brain-based standard is accepted by theologians of all backgrounds.

Policy Consequences The Commission does not regard itself as a competent or appropriate forum for theological interpretation. Nevertheless, it has sought to propose policies consistent with as many as possible of the diverse religious tenets and practices in our society.

The statute set forth in the UDDA [Uniform Determination of Death Act] does not appear to conflict with the view that the soul leaves the body at death. It provides standards by which death can be determined to have occurred, but it does not prevent a person from believing on religious grounds that the soul leaves the body at a point other than that established as marking death for legal and medical purposes.

The concept of death based upon the flow of bodily fluids cannot be completely reconciled with the proposed statute. The statute is partially consistent with the "fluids" formulation in that both would regard as dead a body with no respiration and circulation. As noted previously, the overwhelming majority of patients, now and for the foreseeable future, will be diagnosed on such basis. Under the statute, however, physicians would declare dead those bodies in which respiration and circulation continued *solely* as a result of artificial maintenance, in the absence of all brain functions. Nonetheless, people who believe that the continued flow of fluids in such patients means they are alive would not be forced by the statute to abandon those beliefs nor to change their religious conduct. While the recommended statute may cause changes in medical and legal behavior, the Commission urges those acting under the statute to apply it with sensitivity to the emotional and religious needs of those for whom the new standards mark a departure from traditional practice. Determinations of death must be made in a consistent and evenhanded fashion, but the statute does not preclude flexibility in responding to individual circumstances after determination has been made.

THE IMPENDING COLLAPSE OF THE WHOLE-BRAIN DEFINITION OF DEATH

Robert M. Veatch

For many years there has been lingering doubt, at least among theorists, that the currently fashionable "whole brain–oriented" definition of death has things exactly right. I myself have long resisted the term "brain death" and will use it only in quotation marks to indicate the still common, if ambiguous, usage. The term is ambiguous because it fails to distinguish between the biological claim that the brain is dead and the social/legal/moral claim that the individual as a whole is dead because the brain is dead. An even greater problem with the term arises from the lingering doubt that individuals with dead brains are really dead. Hence, even physicians are sometimes heard to say that the patient "suffered brain death" one day and "died" the following day. It is better to say that he "died" on the first day, the day the brain was determined to be dead, and that the cadaver's other bodily functions ceased the following day. For these reasons I insist on speaking of persons with dead brains as individuals who are dead, not merely persons who are "brain dead."

The presently accepted standard definition, the Uniform Determination of Death Act, specifies that an individual is dead who has sustained "irreversible cessation of all functions of the entire brain, including the brain stem."[1] It also provides an alternative definition specifying that an individual is also dead who has sustained "irreversible cessation of circulatory and respiratory functions." The President's Commission for the Study of Ethical Problems in Medicine and Biomedical and Behavioral Research made clear, however, that circulatory and respiratory function loss are important only as indirect indicators that the brain has been permanently destroyed (p. 74).

DOUBTS ABOUT THE WHOLE BRAIN–ORIENTED DEFINITION

It is increasingly apparent, however, that this consensus is coming apart. As long ago as the early 1970s some of us doubted that literally the entire brain had to be dead for the individual as a whole to be dead.[2]

Hastings Center Report Vol. 23, No. 4, 1993, 18–24.

From the early years it was known, at least among neurologists and theorists who read the literature, that individual, isolated brain cells could be perfused and continue to live even though integrated supercellular brain function had been destroyed. When the uniform definition of death said *all functions of the entire brain* must be dead, there was a gentleman's agreement that cellular-level functions did not count. The President's Commission recognized this, positing that "cellular activity alone is irrelevant" (p. 75). This willingness to write off cellular-level functions is more controversial than it may appear. After all, the law currently does not grant a dispensation to ignore cellular-level functions, no matter how plausible that may be. Keep in mind that critics of soon-to-be-developed higher brain definitions of death would need to emphasize that the model statute called for loss of *all* functions.

By 1977 an analogous problem arose regarding electrical activity. The report of a multicenter study that was funded by the National Institutes of Neurological Diseases and Stroke found that all of the functions it considered important could be lost irreversibly while very small (2 microvolt) electrical potentials could still be obtained on EEG. These were not artifact but real electrical activity from brain cells. Nevertheless, the committee concluded that there could be "electrocerebral silence" and therefore the brain could be considered "dead" even though these small electrical charges could be recorded.[3]

It is possible that the members of the committee believed that these were the result of nothing more than cellular-level functions, so that the same reasoning that permitted the President's Commission to write off little functions as unimportant would apply. However, no evidence was presented that these electrical potentials were arising exclusively from cellular-level functions. It could well be that the reasoning in this report expanded the existing view that cellular functions did not count to the view that some minor supercellular functions could be ignored as long as they were small.

More recently the neurologist James Bernat, a defender of the whole brain–oriented definition of death, has acknowledged that:

> the bedside clinical examination is not sufficiently sensitive to exclude the possibility that small nests of brain cells may have survived . . . and that their continued functioning, although not contributing significantly to the functioning of the organism as a whole, can be measured by laboratory techniques. Because these isolated nests of neurons no longer contribute to the functioning of the organism as a whole, their continued functioning is now irrelevant to the dead organism.[4]

The idea that functions of "isolated nests of neurons" can remain when an individual is declared dead based on whole brain–oriented criteria certainly stretches the plain words of the law that requires, without qualification, that *all functions of the entire brain* must be gone. That exceptions can be granted by individual private citizens based on their personal judgments about which functions are "contributing significantly" certainly challenges the integrity of the idea that the whole brain must be dead for the individual as a whole to be dead.

There is still another problem for those who favor what can now be called the "whole-brain definition of death." It is not altogether clear that the "death of the brain" is to be equated with the "irreversible loss of function." At least one paper appears to hold out not only for loss of function but also for destruction of anatomical structure.[5] Thus we are left with a severely nuanced and qualified whole brain–oriented definition of death. For it to hold as applied in the 1990s, one must assume that function rather than structure is irreversibly destroyed and that not only can certain cellular-level functions and microvolt-level electrical functions be ignored as "insignificant," but also certain "nests of cells" and associated supercellular-level functions can as well.

By the time the whole brain–oriented definition of death is so qualified, it can hardly be referring to the death of the whole brain any longer. What is particularly troublesome is that private citizens—neurologists, philosophers, theologians, and public commentators—seem to be determining just which brain functions are insignificant.

THE HIGHER BRAIN–ORIENTED ALTERNATIVE

The problem is exacerbated when one reviews the early "brain death" literature. Writers trying to make the case for a brain-based definition of death over a heart-based one invariably pointed out that certain functions were irreversibly lost when the brain was gone. Then, implicitly or explicitly, they made the moral/philosophical/religious claim that individuals who have irreversibly lost these key functions should be treated as dead.

While this function-based defense of a brain-oriented definition of death served the day well, some of us realized that the critical functions cited were not randomly distributed throughout the brain. For instance, Henry Beecher, the chair of the Harvard Ad Hoc Committee, identified the following functions as critical: "the individual's personality, his conscious life, his uniqueness, his capacity for remembering, judging, reasoning, acting, enjoying, worrying, and so on."[6]

Of course, all these functions are known to require the cerebrum. If these are the important functions, the obvious question is why any lower brain functions would signal the presence of a living individual. This gave rise to what is now best called the *higher brain–oriented definition of death*: that one is dead when there is irreversible loss of all "higher" brain functions.[7] At first this was referred to as a cerebral or a cortical definition of death, but it seems clear that just as some brain stem functions may be deemed insignificant, likewise, some functions in the cerebrum may be as well. Moreover, it is not clear that the functions of the kind Beecher listed are always necessarily localized in the cerebrum or the cerebral cortex. At least in theory someday we may be able to build an artificial neurological organ that could replace some functions of the cerebrum. Someone who was thinking, feeling, reasoning, and carrying on a conversation through the use of an artificial brain would surely be recognized as alive even if the cerebrum that it had replaced was long since completely dead. I have preferred the purposely ambiguous term "higher brain function," as a way to make clear that the key philosophical issue is which of the many brain functions are really important.

Although that way of putting the question may offend the defenders of the more traditional whole-brain definition of death, once they have made the move of excluding the cellular, electrical, and supercellular functions they consider "insignificant," they are hardly in a position to complain about the project of sorting functions into important and unimportant ones.

CRITICISMS OF THE HIGHER BRAIN FORMULATIONS

Several defenders of the whole brain–oriented concept have claimed that defining death in terms of loss of certain significant brain functions involves a change in the concept of death. This, however, rests on the implausible claim of Alex Capron, the executive director of the President's Commission, that the move from a heart-oriented to a whole brain–oriented definition of death is not a change in concept at all, but merely the recognition of new diagnostic measures for the traditional concept of death (p. 41). It is very doubtful, however, that the move to a whole brain–oriented concept of death is any less of a fundamental change in concept than movement to a higher brain–oriented one. From the beginning of the debate many people with beating hearts and dead brains would have been alive under the traditional concept of death focusing on fluid flow, but are clearly dead based on a then-newer whole brain–oriented concept. Most understood this as a significant change in concept. In any case, even if there is a greater change in moving to a definition of death that identifies certain functions of the brain as significant, the mere fact that it is a conceptual change should not count against it. Surely, the critical question is which concept is right, not which concept squares with traditional views.

A second major charge against the higher brain–oriented formulations has been that we are unable to measure precisely the irreversible loss of these higher functions based on current neurophysiological techniques (p. 40). By contrast it has been assumed that the irreversible loss of all functions of the entire brain is measurable based on current techniques.

Although laypeople generally do not realize it, the measurement of death based on any concept can never be 100 percent accurate. The greatest error rates have certainly been with the heart-oriented concepts of death. Many patients have been falsely determined to have irreversibly lost heart functions. In earlier days we simply did not have the capacity to measure precisely. Even today there may be no reason to determine precisely whether the heart could be restarted in the case of a terminally ill, elderly patient who is ready to die.

There is even newly found ambiguity in the notion of irreversibility.[8] We are moving rapidly toward the day when organs for transplant will be obtained from non-heart-beating cadavers who have been determined to be dead based on heart function loss. It will be important for death to be pronounced as quickly as possible after the heart function has been found irreversibly lost. It is not clear, however, whether death should be pronounced when the heart has permanently stopped (say, following a decision based on an advance directive to withdraw a ventilator), but could be started again. In the minutes when it could be started, but will not be because the patient has refused resuscitation, can we say that the individual is dead?

Likewise, it is increasingly clear that we must acknowledge some, admittedly very small, risk of error in measuring the irreversible loss of all functions of the entire brain. Alan Shewmon has argued that the determination of the death of the entire brain cannot be made with as great a certainty as some neurologists would claim.[9] Some neurologists have persisted in claiming that brains are dead (or have irreversibly lost all function) even though electrical function still remains.[10] Clearly, brains with electrical function must have some living tissues; claims these brains are dead must rest on the assumption that remaining functions are insignificant.

None of this should imply that the death of the brain cannot be measured with great accuracy. But it is wrong to assume that similar or greater levels of accuracy cannot be obtained in measuring the irreversible loss of key higher functions, including consciousness. The literature on the persistent vegetative state repeatedly claims that we can know with great accuracy that consciousness is irreversibly lost.[11] The AMA's Councils on Scientific Affairs and Ethical and Judicial Affairs have concluded that the diagnosis can be made with an error rate of less than one in a thousand.[12] In fact the President's Commission itself said that "the Commission was assured that physicians with experience in this area can reliably determine that some patients' loss of consciousness is permanent."[13]

Even if we could not presently measure accurately the loss of key higher functions such as consciousness, that would have a bearing only on the clinical implementation of the higher brain–oriented definition, not the validity of the concept itself. Defenders of the higher brain formulation might continue to use the now old-fashioned measures of loss of all function, but only because of the assurance that if all functions are lost, the higher functions certainly are. Such a conservative policy would leave open the question of whether we could someday measure the loss of higher functions accurately enough to use the measures clinically.

Still another criticism is the claim that any higher brain formulation would rely on a concept of personhood or personal identity that is philosophically controversial (pp. 38–39). Personhood theories are notoriously controversial. It is simply wrong, however, to claim that any higher brain–oriented concept of death is based on either personhood or personal identity theories. I, for one, have acknowledged the possibility that there are living human beings who do not satisfy the various concepts of personhood. As long as the law is only discussing whether someone is a living individual, the personhood debate is irrelevant.

Perhaps the most serious charge against the higher brain–oriented formulations is that they are susceptible to the so-called slippery slope argument.[14] Once one yields on the insistence that all functions of the entire brain must be irreversibly gone before an individual is considered dead, there seems to be no stopping the slide of eliminating functions considered insignificant. The argument posits that once totally and permanently unconscious individuals who have some other brain functions (such as brain stem reflexes) remaining are considered dead, someone will propose that those with only marginal consciousness similarly lack significant function and soon all manner of functionally compromised humans will be defined as dead. Since being labeled dead is normally an indicator that certain moral and legal rights cease, such a slide toward considering increasing numbers of marginally functional humans as dead would be morally horrific.

But is the slippery slope argument plausible? In its most significant form, such an argument involves a claim that the same principle underlying one apparently tolerable judgment also entails other, clearly unacceptable judgments. For example, imagine we were trying to determine whether the elderly could be excluded from access to certain health care services based on the utilitarian principle of choosing the course that produced the maximum aggregate good for society. The slippery slope argument might be used to show that the same principle entails implications presumed clearly unacceptable, such as excluding health care from the socially unproductive. To the extent that one is certain that the empirical assumptions are correct (for example, that the utilitarian principle does entail excluding care from the unproductive) and one is confident that such an outcome would be morally unacceptable, then one might attempt to use slippery slope arguments to challenge the proposal to withhold health care from the elderly. The same principle used to support one policy also entails other policies that are clearly unacceptable.

The slippery slope argument is valid insofar as it shows that the principle used to support one policy under consideration entails clearly unacceptable implications when applied to different situations. In principle, there is no difference between the small, potentially tolerable move and the more dramatic, unacceptable move. However, as applied to the definition of death debate, the slippery slope argument can actually be used to show that the whole brain–oriented definition of death is less defensible than the higher brain–oriented one.

As we have seen, the whole brain–oriented definition of death rests on the claim that irreversible loss of all functions of the entire brain is necessary and sufficient for an individual to be dead. That, in effect, means drawing a sharp line between the top of the spinal cord and the base of the brain (i.e., the bottom of the brain stem). But is there any principled reason why one would draw a line at that point?

In the early years of the definition of death debate, the claim was made that an individual was dead when the central nervous system no longer retained the capacity for integration. It was soon discovered, however, that this could be taken to imply that one was "alive" as long as some spinal cord function remained. That was counterintuitive (and also made it more difficult to obtain organs for transplant). Hence, very early on it was agreed that simple reflexes of the spinal cord did not count as an indicator of life. Presumably the principle was that reflex arcs that do not integrate significant bodily functions are to be ignored.

But why then do brain stem reflexes mediated through the base of the brain stem count? By the same principle, if spinal reflexes can be ignored, it would seem that some brain stem reflexes might be as well. An effort to show that brain stem reflexes are more integrative of bodily function is doomed to fail. At most there are gradual, imperceptible gradations in complexity between the reflexes of the first cervical vertebra and those of the base of the brain stem. Some spinal reflexes that trigger extension of the foot while the contralateral arm is withdrawn certainly cover larger distances.

Whatever principle could be used to exclude the spinal reflexes surely can exclude some brain stem reflexes as well. We have seen that the defenders of the whole brain–oriented position admit as much when they start excluding cellular-level functions and electrical functions. Certainly, those who exclude "nests of cells" in the brain as insignificant have abandoned the whole-brain position and are already sliding along the slippery slope.

By contrast the defenders of the higher brain–oriented definition of death can articulate a principle that avoids such slipperiness. Suppose, for example, they rely on classical Judeo-Christian notions that the human is essentially the integration of the mind and body and that the existence of one without the other is not sufficient to constitute a living human being. Such a principle provides a bright line that would clearly distinguish the total and irreversible loss of consciousness from serious but not total mental impairments.

Likewise, the integration of mind and body provides a firm basis for telling which functions of nests of brain cells count as significant. It avoids the hopeless task of trying to show why brain stem reflexes count more than spinal ones or trying to show exactly how many cells must be in a nest before it is significant. There is no subjective assessment of different bodily functions, no quibble about how much integration there must be for the organism to function as a whole. The principle is simple. It relies on qualitative considerations: when, and only when, there is the capacity for organic (bodily) and mental function present together in a single human entity is there a living human being. That, I would suggest, is the philosophical basis for the higher brain–oriented definition of death. It avoids the slippery slope on which the defenders of the whole brain–oriented position have found themselves; it, and only it, provides a principled reason for avoiding the slippery slope.

CONSCIENCE CLAUSES

There is one final development that signals the demise of the whole brain–oriented definition of death as the single basis for declaring death. It should be clear by now that the definition of death debate is actually a debate over the moral status of human beings. It is a debate over when humans should be treated as full members of the human community. When humans are living, full moral and legal human rights accrue. Saying people are alive is simply shorthand for saying that they are bearers of such rights. That is why the definition of death debate is so important. It is also why, in principle, there is no scientific way in which the debate can be resolved. The determination of who is alive—who has full moral standing as a member of the human community—is fundamentally a moral, philosophical, or religious determination, not a scientific one.

In a pluralistic society, we are not likely to reach agreement on such moral questions, which is why no one definition of death has carried the day thus far. When one realizes that there are many variants on each of the three major definitions of death, each of which has some group of adherents, it seems unlikely that any one position is likely to gain even a majority anytime soon. For example, defense of the higher brain–oriented position stands or falls on the claim that the essence of the human being is the integration of a mind and a body, a position reflecting religious and philosophical assumptions that are not beyond dispute. (Other defenders of the higher brain position, for example, are more Manichaean, holding that only the mind is important; they apparently are committed to a view that a human memory transferred to a computer with a capacity to continue mental function would still have all the essential ingredients of humanness and that the same living human being continues to live on the computer hard drive.) These are disputes not likely to be resolved soon.

As a society we have a method for dealing with fundamental disputes in religion and philosophy. We tolerate diversity and affirm the right of conscience to hold minority beliefs as long as actions based on those beliefs do not cause insurmountable problems for the rest of society. That is precisely what in 1976 I proposed doing in the dispute over the definition of death.[15] I proposed a definition of death with a conscience clause that would permit individuals to choose their own definition of death based on their religious and philosophical convictions. I did not say at the time, but should have, that the choices would have to be restricted to those that avoid violating the rights of others and avoid creating insurmountable social problems for the rest of society. For example, I assume that people would not be able to pick a definition that required society to treat them as dead even though they retained cardiac, respiratory, mental, and neurological integrating functions. Likewise, I assume that people would not be permitted to pick a definition that would insist that they be treated as alive when all these functions were absent. There are minimal public health considerations that would set limits on the choices available, but certainly the three major options would be tolerable: heart-, whole brain–, and higher brain–oriented definitions.

The state of New Jersey has gone part of the way recently by adopting a law with a conscience clause that would permit religious objectors to designate in advance that a heart-oriented definition should be used in pronouncing their deaths.[16] Since it is now widely accepted that anyone can write an advance directive mandating withdrawal of life support once one is permanently unconscious, any persons who favor a higher brain–oriented definition of death already have the legal right to make choices that end up with them dead in anyone's sense of the term very shortly after they had lost higher brain functions. Permitting them to designate that they be called dead when they are permanently unconscious changes very little.

There is a litany of worries over conscience clauses that defenders of the whole brain–oriented definitions cite. They worry about life insurance paying off at different times, depending on which definition is chosen, and about homicide charges being dependent on such choices, but these are already with us when people are permitted to use advance directives to control the timing of their deaths. They worry about health insurance costs, but for those who choose a higher brain–oriented formulation the only implication is lower costs. For those who choose a heart-oriented definition potentially higher health insurance costs could result, but that position is held only by a small minority, and it is technically so difficult to maintain a beating heart in someone whose brain is dead that the costs will probably not be significant. If they were, the problem could be addressed by clarifying that standard health insurance would not cover the medical costs for maintaining someone who is "alive with a dead brain." None of these problems has arisen in New Jersey, and none is likely to arise. In short, there is no reason to suspect that the use of a conscience clause will result in social chaos—only in greater respect for minority religious and philosophical views that would otherwise be suppressed by the tyranny of the majority. For convenience it would probably be prudent to adopt a single "default definition" favored by a majority; it would make little difference which definition is used as long as the minority who had strong preference for an alternative had the right to designate in advance its choice of another definition. As with surrogate decision making for terminal care and the procurement of cadaver organs, I think it would be reasonable for the next of kin to have the right of surrogate decision making in the case of minors or mentally incompetent individuals who had not expressed a preference while competent.

CRAFTING NEW PUBLIC LAW

Changing current law to conform to these suggestions will be complex and should be done with deliberate speed, but it should be done. Two changes would be needed in the current definition of death: (1) incorporating the higher brain function notion and (2) incorporating some form of the conscience clause.

Present law makes persons dead when they have lost all functions of the entire brain. It is uniformly agreed that the law should incorporate only this basic concept of death, not the precise criteria or tests needed to determine that the whole brain is dead. That is left up to the consensus of neurological experts.

All that would be needed to shift to a higher brain formulation is a change in the wording of the law to replace "all functions of the entire brain" with some relevant, more limited alternative. There are at least three options: references to higher brain functions, cerebral functions, or consciousness. While we could simply change the wording to read that an individual is dead when there is irreversible cessation of all higher brain functions, that poses a serious problem. We are now suffering from the problems created by the vagueness of the referring to "all functions of the entire brain." Even though referring to "all higher brain functions" would be conceptually correct, it would be even more ambiguous. It would lack needed specificity.

This specificity could be achieved by referring to irreversible loss of cerebral functions, but we have already suggested two problems with that wording. Just as we now know there are some isolated functions of the whole brain that should be discounted, so there are probably some isolated cerebral functions that most would not want to count either. For example, if, hypothetically, an isolated "nest" of cerebral motor neurons were perfused so that if stimulated the body could twitch, that would be a cerebral function, but not a significant one for determining life any more than a brain stem reflex is. Second, in theory some really significant functions such as consciousness might someday be maintainable even without a cerebrum—if, for example, a computer could function as an artificial center for consciousness. The term "cerebral function" adds specificity but is not satisfactory.

The language that seems best if integration of mind and body is what is critical is "irreversible cessation of the capacity for consciousness." That is, after all, what the defenders of the higher brain formulations really have in mind. (If someone were to claim that some other "higher" function is critical, that alternative could simply be plugged in.) As is the case now, the specifics of the criteria and tests for measuring irreversible loss of capacity for consciousness would be left up to the consensus of neurological expertise, even though measuring irreversible loss of capacity for a brain function such as consciousness involves fundamentally nonscientific value judgments. If the community of neurological expertise claims that irreversible loss of consciousness cannot be measured, so be it. We will at least have clarified the concept and set the stage for the day when it can be measured with sufficient accuracy. We have noted, however, that neurologists presently claim they can in fact measure irreversible loss of consciousness accurately.

A second significant change in the definition of death would be required to incorporate the conscience clause. It would permit individuals, while competent, to execute documents choosing alternative definitions of death that are, within reason, not threatening to significant interests of others. While the New Jersey law permits only the alternative of a heart-oriented definition, my proposal, assuming irreversible loss of consciousness were the default definition, would permit choosing either heart-oriented or whole brain–oriented definitions as alternatives.

The New Jersey law presently permits only competent adults to execute such conscience clauses. This, of course, excludes the possibility of parents choosing alternative definitions for their children. I had long ago proposed that, just as legal surrogates have the right to make medical treatment decisions for their wards provided that these decisions are within reason, so they should be permitted to choose alternative definitions of death provided the individual had never expressed a preference. This would, for example, permit Orthodox Jewish parents to require that the state continue to treat their child as alive even though he or she had suffered irreversible loss of consciousness or of total brain function. (Whether the state also requires insurers to continue paying for support of these individuals deemed living is a separate policy issue.) While the New Jersey law tolerates only variation with an explicitly religious basis, I would favor variation based on any conscientiously formulated position.

As a shortcut the law could state that patients who had clearly irreversibly lost consciousness because heart and lung function had stopped could continue to be pronounced dead based on criteria measuring heart and lung function. That this was simply an alternative means for measuring permanent loss of consciousness would have to be set out more clearly than in the present Uniform Determination of Death Act. I see no reason to continue including the alternative measurement in the legal definition. I would simply allow it to fall under the criteria to be articulated by the consensus of experts. This leads to a proposal for a new definition of death, which would read as follows:

> An individual who has sustained irreversible loss of consciousness is dead. A determination of death must be made in accordance with accepted medical standards.
>
> However, no individual shall be considered dead based on irreversible loss of consciousness if he or she, while competent, has explicitly asked to be pronounced dead based on irreversible cessation of all functions of the entire brain or based on irreversible cessation of circulatory and respiratory functions.
>
> Unless an individual has, while competent, selected one of these definitions of death, the legal guardian or next of kin (in that order) may do so. The definition selected by the individual, legal guardian, or next of kin shall serve as the definition of death for all legal purposes.

If one favored only the shift to consciousness as a definition of death without the conscience clause, only paragraph one would be necessary. One could also craft a similar definition using the whole brain–oriented definition of death as the default definition. Some have proposed an additional paragraph prohibiting a physician with a conflict of interest (such as an interest in the organs of the deceased) from pronouncing death. I am not convinced that paragraph is needed, however.

A PRINCIPLED REASON FOR DRAWING THE LINE

It has been puzzling why what at first seemed like a rather minor debate over when a human was dead should have persisted as long as it has. Many thought the definition of death debate was a technical argument that would be resolved in favor of the more fashionable, scientific, and progressive brain-oriented definition as soon as the old romantics attached to the heart died off. It is now clear that something much more complex and more fundamental is at stake. We have been fighting over the question of who has moral standing as a full member of the human moral community, a matter that forces on us some of the most basic questions of human existence: the relation of mind and body, the rights of religious and philosophical minorities, and the meaning of life itself.

I am not certain whether some version of the higher brain–oriented definition of death will be adopted in any legal jurisdiction anytime soon, but

I am convinced that the now old-fashioned whole brain–oriented definition of death is becoming less and less plausible as we realize that no one really believes that literally all functions of the entire brain must be irreversibly lost for an individual to be dead. Unless there is some public consensus expressed in state or federal law conveying agreement upon exactly which brain functions are insignificant, we will all be vulnerable to a slippery slope in which private practitioners choose for themselves exactly where from the top of the cerebrum to caudal end of the spinal cord to draw the line. There is no principled reason to draw it exactly between the base of the brain and the top of the spine. Better that we have a principled reason for drawing it. To me, the principle is that for human life to be present—that is, for the human to be treated as a member in full standing of the human moral community—there must be integrated functioning of mind and body. That means some version of a higher brain–oriented formulation.

NOTES

1. President's Commission for the Study of Ethical Problems in Medicine and Biomedical and Behavioral Research, *Defining Death: Medical, Legal and Ethical Issues in the Definition of Death* (Washington, D.C.: U.S. Government Printing Office, 1981), p. 2. Page numbers for subsequent citations are in the text.
2. Robert M. Veatch, "The Whole-Brain-Oriented Concept of Death: An Outmoded Philosophical Formulation," *Journal of Thanatology* 3 (1975): 13–30.
3. Earl A. Walker et al., "An Appraisal of the Criteria of Cerebral Death: A Summary Statement," *JAMA* 237 (1977): 982–86, at 983.
4. James L. Bernat, "How Much of the Brain Must Die on Brain Death?" *Journal of Clinical Ethics* 3, no. 1 (1992): 21–26, at 25.
5. Paul A. Byrne, Sean O'Reilly, and Paul M. Quay, "Brain Death: An Opposing Viewpoint," *JAMA* 242 (1979): 1985–90.
6. Cited in Robert M. Veatch, *Death, Dying, and the Biological Revolution* (New Haven: Yale University Press, 1976), p. 38.
7. Robert M. Veatch, "Whole-Brain, Neocortical, and Higher Brain Related Concepts," in *Death: Beyond Whole-Brain Criteria*, ed. Richard M. Zaner (Dordrecht, Holland: D. Reidel Publishing Company, 1988), pp. 171–86.
8. David J. Cole, "The Reversibility of Death," *Journal of Medical Ethics* 18 (1992): 26–30.
9. Alan D. Shewmon, "Caution in the Definition and Diagnosis of Infant Brain Death," in *Medical Ethics: A Guide for Health Professionals*, ed. John F. Monagle and David C. Thomasma (Rockville, Md.: Aspen Publishers, 1988), pp. 38–57.
10. Stephen Ashwal and Sanford Schneider, "Failure of Electroencephalography to Diagnose Brain Death in Comatose Patients," *Annals of Neurology* 6 (1979): 512–17.
11. Ronald B. Cranford and Harmon L. Smith, "Some Critical Distinctions between Brain Death and the Persistent Vegetative State," *Ethics in Science and Medicine* 6 (Winter 1979): 199–209; Phiroze L. Hansotia, "Persistent Vegetative State," *Archives of Neurology* 42 (1985): 1048–52.
12. Council on Scientific Affairs and Council on Ethical and Judicial Affairs, "Persistent Vegetative State and the Decision to Withdraw or Withhold Life Support," *JAMA* 263 (1990): 426–30, at 428.
13. President's Commission for the Study of Ethical Problems in Medicine and Biomedical and Behavioral Research, *Deciding to Forego Life-Sustaining Treatment: Ethical, Medical, and Legal Issues in Treatment Decisions* (Washington, D.C.: U.S. Government Printing Office, 1983), p. 177.
14. Bernat, "How Much of the Brain Must Die on Brain Death?" pp. 21–26.
15. Veatch, *Death, Dying, and the Biological Revolution*, pp. 72–76.
16. New Jersey Declaration of Death Act (1991), *New Jersey Statutes Annotated*, Title 26, 6A-1 to 6A-8.

HOW MUCH OF THE BRAIN MUST BE DEAD?

Baruch A. Brody

The proponents of the standard criterion of brain death (death occurs at that point in time when there is an irreversible cessation of functioning of the entire brain) encounter difficulties in reconciling it with the definition (irreversible loss of integrative functioning) and the clinical tests (no stem reflexes, no respiratory efforts, no responsiveness) normally associated with that criterion. The solution to this problem is neither to defend the standard criterion by modifying the tests or the definition nor to look for another criterion based on another definition and to employ other tests that confirm the satisfaction of that criterion. Rather, one should recognize that (1) criteria of death postulate a particular point as an answer to a series of questions, (2) death is a process rather than an event that occurs at a particular point in time, and (3) the answers to these different questions are to be found at different points in the process, so that no one point can be picked as the moment of death. Rather than seeking a point in the process to serve as the criterion of death and as an answer to these questions, one should choose different points in the process as appropriate answers to the different questions.

Halevy and I made these arguments in a 1993 paper.[1] This chapter expands on that position. In the first section, "Restating the Problem," I briefly review our evidence of the difficulties faced in reconciling the tests, the criterion, and the underlying definition. Under "Possible Responses," I amplify our criticisms of several suggestions that have been made in response to these difficulties, including the suggestion that advances in neurology might provide better tests that would resolve the difficulties. In the final section, "The Halevy-Brody Response," I explain our theory and use it to evaluate the current debate about procuring organs from anencephalics.

First, however, I want to make it clear that part of the intellectual background to our 1993 paper is the acceptance of the fundamental insight of fuzzy logic, namely, that the world does not easily divide itself into sets and their complements. Death and its complementary property life determine mutually exclusive but not jointly exhaustive sets. Although no organism can fully belong to both sets, organisms can be in many conditions (the very conditions that have created the debates about death) during which they do not fully belong to either. That is why you cannot find the answers to the questions by finding the right moment in the process to serve as the moment for belonging to the set of the dead. Death is a fuzzy set.

RESTATING THE PROBLEM

To understand the difficulties Halevy and I raised, one needs to remember that the whole-brain criterion of death, with its associated clinical tests, is put forward on the basis of a definition that provides its rationale. According to the definition, the organism is alive only when its functioning is integrated. Given that both the cortex and the stem play central roles in the integration of the functioning of the organism, the organism dies only when all of these integrative functions of all of the parts of the brain irreversibly cease. This is the criterion of death. The clinical tests (such as those for responsiveness/voluntary movements and apnea) test for the presence of these integrative functions.

Both the cortical criterion of death and the cardiorespiratory criterion of death are also based upon definitions that provide their rationales. According to the cortical definition, life requires the functioning of a person. Given that the cortex is the physiological location for functions (such as consciousness, thought, and feeling) that are essential

Editor's note: Many footnotes have been deleted. Students who want to follow up on sources should consult the original article.

Reprinted with permission of the author and publisher from Stuart J. Youngner, Robert M. Arnold, and Rene Schapiro, eds., *The Definition of Death: Contemporary Controversies*. Baltimore: The Johns Hopkins University Press, 1999.

for the existence of a person, death occurs when the cortex irreversibly loses the capacity for those functions. According to the cardiorespiratory definition, the organism is alive only when the vital "bodily fluids"—air and blood—continue to flow through the organism. Given that this flow requires respiration and circulation, the organism dies when those two functions cease.

For each of these definitions, there are, of course, problems either with the definition or with the relation between the definition and its associated criterion. Parts of the body other than the brain help integrate the organism's functioning, so why does the first definition lead to the criterion of the cessation of the integrative functions of only the brain? Is it sufficient for death, as the second definition maintains, that the person has stopped functioning, or must other functions also cease before death has occurred? If the flow of the "vital fluids" is maintained artificially, is the organism still alive according to the third definition, especially if the organism is conscious and capable of responding and moving spontaneously? I shall return to aspects of these problems below. What I want to note for now is that adherents of these three competing criteria have recognized the importance of there being justifying definitions for the criteria; without such a definition, all that you have is an arbitrarily chosen criterion. This point is central for understanding the difficulties raised in our paper.

Halevy and I called attention to the fact that there are organisms who satisfy all of the standard clinical tests for whole-brain death but who have not lost all of the integrative functions of the brain. The most important example is neurohormonal regulation. The presence of this residual neurohormonal regulation in a significant percentage of organisms who satisfy the usual tests for brain death and whose respiration and circulation are being maintained artificially (usually to allow for the possibility of organ donation) is well documented. Most crucially, this regulation is just as much and as important an example of the integrative functioning of the brain as is the brain's control of respiration or of responsive movements. Given the definition behind the whole-brain criterion, this functioning of the brain should have to cease before the criterion is really met. As the usual tests do not ensure this, they are inadequate as tests for the satisfaction of the criterion *given the definition that supposedly justifies that criterion.*

In the article in the *Annals of Internal Medicine,* Halevy and I also call attention to two other functions of the brain that do not necessarily cease when the normal clinical tests are met: (1) continued functioning of the auditory pathways as evidenced by brainstem evoked potentials and (2) continued cortical functioning as evidenced by EEG readings. I would today put less emphasis on them. To begin with, the latter is present only in very special cases and the extent of the former is not clearly known. Second, and more important, while they constitute brain functions, it is not clear that either integrates the functioning of the entire organism. If not, then both should be irrelevant to the death of the organism. According to the definition that supposedly justifies the whole-brain criterion, only the integrative functioning of the brain must irreversibly cease before the organism dies, so these functions may not count.

Halevy and I emphasized these other two functions to illustrate another problem. Patients who meet the normal clinical tests for brain death may not satisfy the criterion used by the President's commission and embodied in the law, the "irreversible cessation of all functions of the brain." These examples are very relevant to illustrate the dissonance between the clinical tests and that legal criterion. The point I am making here is that they may not be relevant to illustrating the dissonance between the clinical tests and the whole-brain criterion justified by the associated definition, a criterion that refers only to the cessation of *integrative* functions.

In short, our difficulty may be stated as follows: (1) the true whole-brain criterion of death is that the organism dies when all of the integrative functioning of the entire brain ceases; (2) when the normal clinical tests are met, at least one form of integrative functioning of the brain, neurohormonal regulation, has often not ceased, and there may be other forms of integrative functioning that have not ceased; (3) there is, therefore, an incongruity between the normal clinical tests and the whole-brain criterion as understood in light of the definition that justifies it.

POSSIBLE RESPONSES

Given the above argument, one can identify a series of possible responses: (1) The incongruity between tests and criterion exists, but we should not worry about it because it occurs in only a few cases or because it makes no difference, as current practice works well. (2) These residual functions are either not integrative functioning or not integrative functioning of the right type, so there is really no incongruity between tests and criterion. (3) There is an incongruity between tests and criterion which cannot be ignored, and we should resolve it by improving the tests employed through advances in neurology. (4) There is an incongruity between the clinical tests and the criterion which cannot be ignored, and we should resolve it by adopting some other criterion based on some other justifying definition. (5) The incongruity is indicative of a fundamental problem that is best resolved by giving up on the search for a single criterion of death that answers all of the questions that a criterion of death is traditionally understood as answering. This last response is the conclusion Halevy and I adopted.

Should we worry about the incongruity, since it occurs in only a few cases? The claim that it occurs in only a few cases is mistaken. If, of course, organisms are declared dead on the basis of the usual tests and removed from life support, neurohormonal regulation (and many other functions of the organism) will soon cease. But that may show only that taking dependent living organisms off life support soon produces death. The crucial question about the extent of the incongruity is how often these functions are still occurring when the usual tests are first met and before the organism is taken off life support. The data cited in our 1993 paper show that this occurs in a significant percentage of cases.

Should we worry about the incongruity even if it occurs in many cases, since the use of the current tests works well? It all depends upon what you mean by "the tests work well." They certainly have enabled the organ procurement programs to harvest a significant number of additional organs by declaring death on the basis of the tests without waiting for neurohormonal regulation to cease. They also have enabled physicians to discontinue life support in many cases where the families insisted on doing everything so long as death had not occurred. The need to respect that family preference stops when death is pronounced on the basis of the current tests, even when neurohormonal regulation has not ceased. But does that mean that the tests have worked well? Not if the organisms in question still are alive, as they are according to the current criterion when regulation has not yet ceased. If they are still alive, the use of the current tests has in many cases resulted in killings to harvest organs and in discontinuing life support by misleading families about when death has occurred. It is hard to understand why that should be described as working well. I suggest below that the claim that the current tests work well can be reconstructed to make some sense once one drops, as Halevy and I have advocated, the search for a criterion of death. But until one does so, the incongruity means that the current tests are not working well.

Are the residual functions integrative functions or integrative functions of the right type? Bernat has suggested that they are not:

> However, in some cases, a critical number of neurons have been destroyed but a few continue to function in isolation. For example, some unequivocally whole-brain-dead patients continue to manifest rudimentary but recordable electroencephalographic activity or hypothalamic neuroendocrine activity sufficient to prevent diabetes insipidus. Because these isolated nests of independently operating neurons no longer contribute critically to the functions of the organism as a whole, their continued activity remains consistent with the whole-brain criterion of death.[2] (569)

I am not convinced by this objection. Although it is true that the residual cortical activity is separated from the functioning of the organism as a whole and is in that sense an isolated nest of operating neurons, this is just not true of the neurohormonal regulation that, by definition, is integrated with the functioning of the rest of the organism. Another residual functioning that Bernat does not mention, intact auditory pathways, is harder to classify, although it is certainly not a clear-cut example of purely isolated nests of operating neurons. That is why I said above that, for the purposes of this chapter, the residual neurohormonal functioning deserves the most attention. It is without any doubt residual integrative functioning of the very sort that is supposed to mean that the patient is still alive, according to the justifying definition that lies behind the whole-brain criterion of death. This last point also serves as a criticism of Pallis's recent response to our argument:

> What is the *philosophical* significance, for instance, of a given TSH level detected a specified number of hours after a clinical diagnosis of brain death? . . . A "concept" which "dares not speak its name" in fact often lurks behind most such "challenges." It is that death on neurological grounds should mean but one thing: the irreversible loss of function of the totality of the intracranial contents . . . This is advanced without specification of the functions, the loss of which would demarcate the living from the dead. This approach hardly warrants being described as a "philosophical" concept of death.[3] (21)

The relevant functions are, of course, the brain's integrative functions, and the level of thyroid-stimulating hormone (TSH) is evidence that some of them are still intact. None of this requires, of course, that all of the intracranial contents should have stopped functioning.

I confess that I am surprised by Dr. Bernat's response. After all, his 1981 paper with Culver and Gert is a landmark paper precisely because it clarified for the first time the justifying definition of continued integrative functioning ("functioning of the organism as a whole") as lying behind the whole-brain criterion.[4] In that paper, the first example of the functioning of the organism as a whole is neuroendocrine control (390). Why, then, does Bernat now describe it as a purely isolated nest of operating neurons?

Isn't the obvious response to modify the clinical tests so that the criterion of the irreversible cessation of the integrative functioning of the entire brain is satisfied when the new set of tests is met? Couldn't we test for neurohormonal regulation and (if we were concerned about it as integrative functioning) for intact auditory and visual pathways? In fact, the use of such tests has been suggested by various authors. There is, however, a major problem, which Halevy and I noted, with this suggestion. Data from the transplant community which has studied this question to determine whether hormone replacement should be part of the management of potential donors, suggest that hormonal levels due to residual neurohormonal functioning may remain intact for more than 72 hours. These are some of the best data available. They include patients where angiography indicated a complete cessation of intracranial blood flow, indicating the presence of a dual blood supply.

Consequently, the adoption of these new tests would mean a serious challenge to the transplant community in maintaining both the viability of organs and the willingness of families to donate. There could be a significant loss of organs. Moreover, putting aside the transplantation setting, maintaining organisms on life support until the new tests are met, when the families insist that everything be done until death occurs, can be very expensive, so we should not rush to add additional tests.

There is a crucial difference between the criticism of this response and the criticism of the other responses. The problem with the first three responses is that they fail on intellectual grounds. The justification for the brain-death criterion means that the functions which remain and are the source of the dissonance cannot be disregarded if one wants to maintain intellectual honesty. The problem with the fourth response is that it fails on practical grounds. We want to be able to harvest organs and to disconnect life support unilaterally long before the suggested new tests are satisfied. Some might suggest that this is irrelevant. If we want theoretical soundness, we must pay the practical prices. One of the merits of the proposal Halevy and I put forward is that it offers the opportunity to be both theoretically sound and practical. I will return to this point below.

Perhaps the best response is to modify the criterion of death and the justifying definition. Three versions of this response are found in the literature: (1) Adopt as the criterion of death the permanent cessation of respiratory activity or the permanent cessation of cardiac as well as respiratory activity (the two options most advocated in the debate in the Orthodox Jewish community about brain death and organ transplantation). (2) Adopt as the criterion of death the permanent cessation of respiratory activity and of consciousness (Pallis's brainstem criterion).[3] (3) Adopt as the criterion of death the permanent cessation of consciousness (the higher-brain criterion).

There is more to be said about each of these suggestions than is possible in this chapter, so I will confine myself to just a few observations. (1) The adoption of the view that death requires the irreversible cessation of both cardiac and respiratory functioning may mean a significant and expensive prolongation of the dying process as well as the end of organ transplantation as we know it. A strong futility policy might avoid the former, while a modification of the Pittsburgh protocol might preserve some transplantation. Unless we have powerful intellectual reasons for preserving that criterion, other than adherence to the traditional definition, it is a poor suggestion on practical grounds. (2) Neither a purely respiratory criterion nor a combined respiratory/consciousness criterion lends itself to a justifying definition. The former criterion involves only one of the traditional vital "bodily fluids," and it is hard to see why one is to be preferred to the other. The latter criterion comes from two very different definitions, and it is hard to see why the two criteria should be combined. Pallis points out quite correctly that they are "embedded in coherent historical and cultural matrices" (21). However, the fact that each is embedded in a coherent matrix does not ensure that their combination is embedded in a coherent matrix. (3) The suggestion that we adopt a higher-brain criterion for the death of the person, based upon the definition that the person dies when the cognitive and affective functioning required to be a person ceases, makes a lot of sense when discussing the death of the person. But are we only looking for an account of the death of the person? Perhaps we really want an account that encompasses the death of the full organism? We certainly seem to want that type of account before burial or cremation.

THE HALEVY-BRODY RESPONSE

Our response to the incongruity begins by recognizing that the death of the organism is a process rather than an event. Consider the organism that suffers damage to its brain so that it is no longer conscious and can no longer engage in responsive or voluntary movements. At some later stage, it loses the capacity to breathe on its own so that its respiration must be supported artificially. At a later stage, its capacity to regulate hormonal levels stops. Somewhere during this time period, its auditory pathways stop functioning. Finally, its heart stops beating. Is it really meaningful to suppose that the organism died at some specific point in this process? Isn't it more reasonable to say that the search for a criterion of death (a specific moment) made sense when these points were always close in time to each other because medicine lacked the capacity to protect some of the functions when the others had stopped, but no longer makes sense today when medicine can, and sometimes has good reasons to, keep some of the functions going for longer periods? Isn't it more reasonable to say that the organism was fully alive before the chain of events began, is fully dead by the end of the chain of events, and is neither during the process. Fuzzy logic enables us to say that in a precise fashion.

But don't we have to identify a specific point of time at which the organism died? Aren't there important questions which need to be answered and can only be answered by identifying the precise point in the process at which the organism died? These questions include when life support can unilaterally (without patient or surrogate concurrence) be withdrawn, when organs can be harvested, and when the organism can be buried or cremated. Perhaps not. While traditionally it has been thought that the way to answer these questions is to find that precise moment of death, perhaps that is the mistake. Perhaps these questions need to be examined and answered each on its own, with the answer to one question (some point in the process) not necessarily being the answer to the other questions. That is the heart of Halevy's and my proposal.

In our paper, we suggested that life support could in these cases be unilaterally withdrawn when the organism no longer composes a person because the cortex no longer functions. We emphasized that allowing for this unilateral withdrawal would constitute an appropriate stewardship of social resources. Elsewhere, I have argued that even those moral and religious traditions that place great emphasis on the value of the life of human organisms can accept such appeals to stewardship. Notice, by the way, that such an argument would not apply to those *rare* cases where the resources of the patient or family paid for the full costs of the continued care.

In our paper, Halevy and I suggested that organs could be harvested at that stage in the process after the loss of cortical functioning when the organism can no longer breathe on its own. This, of course, corresponds to current practice. We defended it, however, not by adopting some criterion of death justified by some definition of death. Instead, we argued for it on the grounds that it preserves the proper balance between trying to maximize the supply of organs to save lives and trying to preserve public support for organ transplantation by not harvesting organs in cases that would be socially unacceptable.

This approach offers, I believe, a basis for evaluating AMA approval—later withdrawn—of harvesting organs from still-breathing anencephalics, allowing for a reasoned consideration of their proposal while rejecting their justification of it. The AMA continues to accept the current criterion of death, with its implication that such anencephalics are still alive. They also recognize that harvesting organs means, on their own assumptions, killing the anencephalic organism, although they avoid using that word, preferring to talk instead about "sacrificing" it. To justify their conclusion, they argue that anencephalics, who have never and who never will experience consciousness, can be killed because they have no interest in being alive and there are no compelling social interests in preserving their life. This argument succeeds only if one is willing to change deontological constraints ("thou shall not kill living human organisms") into teleological rules ("killing human organisms is wrong when their interests or social interests are harmed"). The implications of this are very disturbing.

I respectfully suggest that the Council on Ethical and Judicial Affairs adopted this change without even arguing for it because the council, following much of the recent bioethical literature, does not understand deontological constraints. Things would be very different if they argued that anencephalics are in that class of in-between organisms that are neither fully alive nor fully dead. Then, they might argue that the deontological constraints do not apply to them and that we should settle the question by balancing the benefits of additional organs (needed, e.g., by other newborns with hypoplastic left hearts) against the risks to public acceptance of organ procurement if the public does not see anencephalics as being in this in-between category. That, I submit, could be the basis for a reasoned discussion of the AMA proposal, one following the framework presented in our paper.

There is, however, one further complication that must, I now believe, be taken into account. In our article and in the analysis just presented, the assumption is that the deontological constraint against killing human organisms applies only to those who are fully alive; once the organism is in the in-between range, we need only consider the policy trade-off. But is that assumption necessarily true? What happens to deontological constraints in a world of fuzzy sets? This additional issue will require a reasoned discussion, although the contours of the discussion are at the moment quite unclear.

What about burying or cremating the organism? Here, we suggested, maximum leeway could be given to respecting family sentiments by waiting for asystole, which usually occurs soon after all support ends. We can adopt that approach, saying that, on the basis of the traditional definition, the organism is fully dead only at that point, because that does not require us to wait for asystole before withdrawing life support unilaterally or harvesting organs.

In conclusion, then, our response answers the three questions in ways that are both theoretically defensible and practically useful. It is able to do so only because it does not answer them by adopting a consonant definition, criterion, and test of death. The dissonance we identified makes that impossible in a world that also needs to harvest organs and control health care expenditures. It is able to do so, instead, because it recognizes the implications of the fact that death is a process in a world governed by fuzzy logic.

REFERENCES

1. Halevy A, Brody B. Brain death: Reconciling definitions, criteria, and tests. *Ann Intern Med* 1993; 119:519–25.
2. Bernat JL. Brain death occurs only with destruction of the cerebral hemispheres and the brain stem. *Arch Neurol* 1992; 49:569–70.
3. Pallis C. Further thoughts on brainstem death. *Anaesth Intensive Care* 1995; 23:20–23.
4. Bernat JL, Culver CM, Gert B. On the criterion and definition of death. *Ann Intern Med* 1981; 94:389–94.

DECISIONAL CAPACITY AND THE RIGHT TO REFUSE TREATMENT

STATE OF TENNESSEE DEPARTMENT OF HUMAN SERVICES V. MARY C. NORTHERN

Court of Appeals of Tennessee, Middle Section, Feb. 7, 1978

On January 24, 1978, the Tennessee Department of Human Services filed this suit alleging that Mary C. Northern was 72 years old, with no available help from relatives; that Miss Northern resided alone under unsatisfactory conditions as a result of which she had been admitted to and was a patient in Nashville General Hospital; that the patient suffered from gangrene of both feet which required the removal of her feet to save her life; that the patient lacked the capacity to appreciate her condition or to consent to necessary surgery.

Attached to the complaint are identical letters from Drs. Amos D. Tackett and R. Benton Adkins, which read as follows:

> Mrs. Mary Northern is a patient under our care at Nashville General Hospital. She has gangrene of both feet probably secondary to frostbite and then thermal burning of the feet. She has developed infection along with the gangrene of her feet. This is placing her life in danger. Mrs. Northern does not understand the severity or consequences of her disease process and does not appear to understand that failure to amputate the feet at this time would probably result in her death. It is our recommendation as the physicians in charge of her case, that she undergo amputation of both feet as soon as possible.

On January 24, 1978, the Chancellor appointed a guardian ad litem to defend the cause and to receive service of process pursuant to Rule 4.04(2) T.R.C.P. On January 25, 1978, the guardian ad litem answered as follows:

> The Respondent, by and through her guardian ad litem, states as follows:
>
> 1. She is 72 years of age and a resident of Davidson County, Tennessee.

Editors' note: The suit was filed under the state "Protective Services for the Elderly" Act, which permits a court to appoint a guardian for the purposes of consent to medical treatment if an elderly person is in imminent danger of death without treatment and lacks capacity to consent to it.

2. She is presently in the intensive care unit of General Hospital, Nashville, Tennessee, because of gangrenous condition in her two feet.
3. She feels very strongly that her present physical condition is improving, and that she will recover without the necessity of surgery.
4. She is in possession of a good memory and recall, responds accurately to questions asked her, is coherent and intelligent in her conversation, and is of sound mind.
5. She is aware that the Tennessee Department of Human Services has filed this complaint, knows the nature of the complaint, and does not wish for her feet to be amputated.

. . .

On January 26, 1978, there was filed in this cause a letter from Dr. John J. Griffin, reporting that he found the patient to be generally lucid and sane, but concluding:

> Nonetheless, I believe that she is functioning on a psychotic level with respect to ideas concerning her gangrenous feet. She tends to believe that her feet are black because of soot or dirt. She does not believe her physicians about the serious infection. There is an adamant belief that her feet will heal without surgery, and she refused to even consider the possibility that amputation is necessary to save her life. There is no desire to die, yet her judgment concerning recovery is markedly impaired. If she appreciated the seriousness of her condition, heard her physicians' opinions, and concluded against an operation, then I would believe she understood and could decide for herself. But my impression is that she does not appreciate the dangers to her life. I conclude that she is incompetent to decide this issue. A corollary to this denial is seen in her unwillingness to consider any future plans. Here again I believe she was utilizing a psychotic mechanism of denial.
>
> This is a schizoid woman who has been urged by everyone to have surgery. Having been self-sufficient previously (albeit a marginal adjustment), she is continuing to decide alone. The risks with surgery are great and her lifestyle has been permanently disrupted. If she has surgery there is a tremendous danger for physical and psychological complications. The chances for a post-operative psychosis are immense, yet the surgeons believe an operation is necessary to save her life. I would advise delaying surgery (if feasible) for a few days in order to attempt some work for strengthening her psychologically. Even if she does not consent to the operation after that time, however, I believe she is incompetent to make the decision.

On January 28, 1978, this Court entered an order reciting the following:

> From all of the above the Court finds:
>
> 1. That the respondent is not now in 'imminent danger of death' in the extreme sense of the words, but that her present condition is such that 'imminent danger of death' may reasonably be expected during her continued hospitalization.
> 2. That both feet of respondent are severely necrotic and affected by wet gangrene, an infection which probably will result in death unless properly treated by amputation of the feet.
> 3. That the probability of respondent's survival without amputation is from 5 percent to 10 percent and the probability of survival after amputation is about 50 percent, with possible severe psychotic results.
> 4. That, with or without amputation, the prognosis of respondent's condition is poor.
> 5. That respondent is an intelligent, lucid, communicative, and articulate individual who does not accept the fact of the serious condition of her feet and is unwilling to discuss the seriousness of such condition or its fatal potentiality.
> 6. That, because of her inability or unwillingness to recognize the actual condition of her feet which is clearly observable by her, she is incompetent to make a rational decision as to the amputation of her feet.
> 7. That respondent has no wish to die, but is unable or unwilling to recognize an obvious condition which will probably result in her death if untreated.
>
> This Court is therefore of the opinion that a responsible individual should be named with authority to consent to amputation of respondent's feet when urgently recommended in writing by respondent's physicians because of the development of (symptoms) indicating an emergency and severe imminence of death.

. . .

> [Appellant's first assignment of error states:]
>
> Such actions by the Court were injurious to the appellant because they deprived her of her right to make her own decisions—regardless as to whether death might be a probable consequence—as to whether she was willing to surrender control of her own person and life.

This controversy arises from the fact that Miss Northern's attending physicians have determined that all of the soft tissue of her feet has been killed by frostbite, that said dead tissue has become infected with gangrene, and that the feet must be removed to prevent loss of life from spreading of gangrene and its effects to the entire body. Miss Northern has refused to consent to the surgery.

The physicians have determined, and the Chancellor and this Court have found, that Miss Northern's life is critically endangered; that she is mentally incapable of comprehending the facts which constitute that danger; and that she is, to that extent, incompetent, thereby justifying State action to preserve her life.

As will be observed from the bill of exceptions, a member of this Court asked Miss Northern if she would prefer to die rather than lose her feet, and her answer was "possibly." This is the most definitive expression of her desires in this record.

The patient has *not* expressed a desire to die. She evidences a strong desire to live and an equally strong desire to keep her dead feet. She refuses to make a choice.

If the patient would assume and exercise her rightful control over her own destiny by stating that she prefers death to the loss of her feet, her wish would be respected. The doctors so testified; this Court so informed her; and this Court now reiterates its commitment to this principle.

The appellant has filed three supplemental assignments of error, of which the first is:

> 1. The statute, T.C.A. §§ 14-2301, *et seq.*, is impermissibly vague; and, therefore, void and unconstitutional. The two phrases used in the statute, 'imminent danger of death' and 'capacity to consent' have not been defined in the statute nor is the Court given any assistance to determine when either standard has been met in the legal context, rather than a medical context.

In the judgment of this Court, the words "imminent danger of death" are no more vague than is consistent with the nature of the subject matter.

. . .

The words, "imminent danger of death" mean conditions calculated to and capable of producing within a short period of time a reasonably strong probability of resultant cessation of life if such conditions are not removed or alleviated. Such is undoubtedly the legislative intent of the words.

"Imminent danger of death" should be reasonably interpreted to carry out the purposes of the statute. For an authorization to mildly encroach upon the freedom of the individual, a relatively mild imminence or danger of death may suffice. On the other hand, the authorization of a drastic encroachment upon personal freedom and bodily integrity would require a correspondingly severe imminence of death.

In the present case, the Chancellor was not called upon to act until the imminence of death was moderately severe. By the time of the hearing before this Court, the imminence of death had lessened somewhat but remained real and appreciable. Accordingly this Court, recognizing a present real and appreciable imminence of death, made provision for drastic emergency measures to be taken only in event of severe and urgent imminence of death.

Appellant also complains of vagueness of the meaning of "capacity to consent." Capacity means mental ability to make a rational decision, which includes the ability to perceive, to appreciate all relevant facts, and to reach a rational judgment upon such facts.

Capacity is not necessarily synonymous with sanity. A blind person may be perfectly capable of observing the shape of small articles by handling them, but not capable of observing the shape of a cloud in the sky.

A person may have "capacity" as to some matters and may lack "capacity" as to others.

In 44 C.J.S. Insane Persons § 2, pp. 17, 18, partial insanity is defined as follows:

> *Partial insanity*. Although it is hard to define the invisible line that divides perfect and partial insanity, the law recognizes a state of mind called 'partial insanity,' that is, insanity on a particular subject only, sometimes denominating it 'insane delusion' or 'monomania.' The use of the term, however, has been criticized. Partial insanity has been said to be the derangement of one or more of the faculties of the mind, which prevents freedom of action. Ordinarily it is confined to a particular subject, the person being sane on every other. The degree of insanity, as partial or total, is to be measured by the extent and number of the delusions existing in the mind of the person in question. . . .

In the present case, this Court has found the patient to be lucid and apparently of sound mind generally. However, on the subjects of death and amputation of her feet, her comprehension is blocked, blinded, or dimmed to the extent that she is incapable of recognizing facts which would be obvious to a person of normal perception.

For example, in the presence of this Court, the patient looked at her feet and refused to recognize the obvious fact that the flesh was dead, black, shriveled, rotting, and stinking.

The record also discloses that the patient refuses to consider the eventuality of death which is, or ought to be, obvious in the face of such dire bodily deterioration.

As described by the doctors and observed by this Court, the patient wants to live and keep her dead feet, too, and refuses to consider the impossibility of such a desire. In order to avoid the unpleasant experience of facing death and/or loss of feet, her mind or emotions have resorted to the device of denying the unpleasant reality so that, to the patient, the unpleasant reality does not exist. This is the "delusion" which renders the patient incapable of making a rational decision as to whether to undergo surgery to save her life or to forgo surgery and forfeit her life.

The physicians speak of probabilities of death without amputation as 90 to 95 percent and the probability of death with surgery as 50–50 (1 in 2). Such probabilities are not facts, but the existence and expression of such opinions are facts which the patient is unwilling or unable to recognize or discuss.

If, as repeatedly stated, this patient could and would give evidence of a comprehension of the facts of her condition and could and would express her unequivocal desire in the face of such comprehended facts, then her decision, however unreasonable to others, would be accepted and honored by the Courts and by her doctors. The difficulty is that she cannot or will not comprehend the facts.

The first supplemental assignment of error is respectfully overruled.

The second supplemental assignment of error is as follows:

> 2. The Chancellor erred by denying the Appellant her rights to substantive and procedural due process. The entire legal proceedings involved in this case and on appeal are unprecedented; the order of the Chancellor granting the appeal but refusing the automatic stay of thirty days allowed by the Rules is one example of the procedural wrongs which was not in accordance with the established legal practice, and contrary to the expected procedure to be followed. The proposed amputation will not only permanently deprive the Appellant of her two limbs, but most likely will significantly and irreparably alter her personality for the worse, and make her mentally and physically dependent upon the State.

Whatever the propriety or impropriety of the action of the Chancellor in attempting to effectuate his action in spite of the appeal, the error, if any, has been rendered harmless by the action of this Court, after appeal, in reviewing and modifying his actions.

This Court does not recognize that it has been guilty of any improper deviation from correct procedure. The gravity of the condition of the patient and the resultant emergency in time required the unusual action of the Court under § 27-327 T.C.A. and the unusual acceleration of hearings and actions taken.

This Court is painfully and acutely aware of the possible tragic results of amputation. According to the doctors, the patient has only a 50 percent chance of surviving the surgery; and, if she survives, she will never be able to walk and may suffer severe mental and emotional problems.

On the other hand, the doctors testified, and this Court finds, that the patient's chances of survival without amputation are from 5 percent to 10 percent—a rather remote and fragile chance. Moreover, as testified by the doctors and found by this Court, even if the patient should survive without amputation, she will never walk because the dead flesh will fall off the bones of her feet leaving only bare bones.

> IT IS, THEREFORE, ORDERED, ADJUDGED AND DECREED that
>
> 1. Mary C. Northern is in imminent danger of death if she does not receive surgical amputation of her lower extremities and she lacks the capacity to consent or refuse consent for such surgery.
> 2. That Honorable Horace Bass, Commissioner of Human Services of the State of Tennessee or his successor in office is hereby designated and authorized to act for and on behalf of said Mary C. Northern in consenting to surgical amputation of her lower extremities and of exercising such custodial supervision as is necessarily incident thereto

> at any time that Drs. Amos D. Tackett and R. Benton Adkins join in signing a written certificate that Mary C. Northern's condition has developed to such a critical stage as to demand immediate amputation to save her life. The previous order of this Court is likewise so modified.

As modified, the order of the Chancellor is affirmed. The cause is remanded for further appropriate proceedings.

. . .

Modified, Affirmed, and Remanded.*

*On May 1, 1978, Mary Northern died in a Nashville hospital as a result of a clot from the gangrenous tissue migrating through the bloodstream to a vital organ. Because of complications rendering surgery more dangerous, the proposed surgery was never performed.

TRANSCRIPT OF PROCEEDINGS: TESTIMONY OF MARY C. NORTHERN

January 28, 1978

Testimony of Mary Northern: [The following interview took place at the bedside of Mary Northern in the Intensive Care Unit of the Nashville General Hospital. Present were Judge Todd, Judge Drowota, and the Reverend Palmer Sorrow, a friend and frequent visitor of the patient. Eds.]

Judge Todd: Now, Mrs. Mary, you know that there have been some proceedings in court about you, and that's the reason why the judges are here. And we wanted to see you and talk to you.

Miss Northern: Yes.

Judge Todd: And give you a chance to talk to us.

Miss Northern: Yeah.

Judge Todd: I understand that you had a little problem of getting too cold out there at your house.

Miss Northern: Yes.

Judge Todd: That's right.

Miss Northern: Yes. Well, now, it's a point of this, the swelling of my foot was—was very dangerous looking.

Judge Todd: Yes ma'am.

Miss Northern: And so that's what caused most of the trouble, and the—it's starting to go down. Give it a chance, it is starting to go down, and it's almost . . . Well, these—these ankles and the—along on these legs have gone down wonderfully.

Judge Todd: Yes, now, Mrs. Mary, these doctors have been talking to us at great length about the condition of your feet.

Mr. Sorrow: I think it's okay.

Miss Northern: Okay.

Judge Todd: —and they tell us this about your feet. Now, mind you . . . we don't know whether it's so or not, but I want you to know what they have told us. . . . They tell us that your feet have been frostbitten before, and that they got well.

Miss Northern: Yes.

Judge Todd: What they tell us, that your feet were frostbitten a great deal worse this time than they were . . . before.

Miss Northern: Yes.

Judge Todd: And they tell us this,—now I am going to say some things to you that might be a little uncomfortable, but I want—I don't believe these doctors have told it to you just like they told it to us.

Miss Northern: Yeah.

Judge Todd: So I want to give it to you just like they have given it to us. They tell us that this time every bit of the flesh on your two feet is completely dead.

Miss Northern: I know—No, it isn't, it will revive.

Judge Todd: I understand.

Miss Northern: Four or five days ago it started to go down.

Judge Todd: All right. Now they tell us this, that when you came in . . . here that your feet were swollen. . . . And they tell us that the swelling has gone down.

Miss Northern: Yes.

Judge Todd: But they tell us that your feet are shriveling up like a dead person's feet—

Miss Northern: Unh-unh.

Judge Todd: —rather than a live person's feet.

Miss Northern: No, no. . . . I can get and walk all the way down to the shopping places.

Judge Todd: Now they tell us—We questioned them very, very thoroughly about this thing, and they tell us that you can move your toes. And then I asked them how could a person move his toes if his foot was dead? You see? And here's what they tell us. They tell us that the ligaments that move the toes . . . are dead, but they are still just like strings,—

Miss Northern: Yeah.

Judge Todd: —and that the muscles that move the toes are up here where they are still alive, and therefore a dead foot can move its toes.

Miss Northern: Well, they are not going to—they are not going to take my legs away. They are not going to take my legs away from me, you understand this?

Judge Todd: Yes, ma'am.

Miss Northern: And they are not going to—I think it's rather silly, because they all—all of em have gotten viable.

Judge Todd: Yes, ma'am. Yes, ma'am. Now here is the thing that disturbs us. The doctors tell us that you have a very heavy infection which they are keeping in control by antibiotics, but that your temperature has started to rise, that you have a hundred and one temperature . . . which indicates that the infection is increasing. And we questioned them very closely now, we have been a long time—

Miss Northern: You understand they are going to do it. Now, does this have something to do with the Metropolitan Government, has it not? Well, the Metropolitan Government can't take anything—do me this way, you know?

Judge Todd: Yes, sir. Now, here is what I want to present to you. You are a very intelligent woman for your age. I want to compliment you on that, you really are. I said you were like my mother, but you do circles around my mother as far as talking and thinking.

Now, you are educated, and you know this business of "if," and I want to ask you an "if" question. If your feet, the flesh of your feet, really is dead, and if you have one chance in ten of living without surgery, that it is, if—if the feet are left on, that nine chances to one that you will not live, it will kill you,—

Miss Northern: I am not going to have—

Judge Todd: —would you still say, "I want that one chance?"

Miss Northern: Well, of course,—

Judge Todd: Ma'am?

Miss Northern: —this is not going to do anything like this. All—All of these thing,—

Judge Todd: Yes, ma'am.

Miss Northern: —and my feet have gone down.

Judge Todd: Yes, ma'am.

Miss Northern: My ankles are—

Judge Todd: Yes, ma'am. Now, let me ask you one more question.

Miss Northern: I am not going to—Let me tell you something. I am not going to argue any more with you, because I know you have a multiple of opinions.

Judge Todd: No, I haven't formed any opinions, that's the reason I came up to talk to you. I haven't decided.

Miss Northern: It's an opinion you formed, and I am not going to let you tell me—

Judge Todd: I am just telling you what they told me. Now let me ask you one more little thing.

If the time comes that this infection gets so bad that you are practically unconscious and can't talk to anybody, would you then be willing for the doctors to go ahead and do what they think should be done? . . .

Mr. Sorrow: That's an "if"—That's an "if" question.

Judge Todd: "If."

Miss Northern: I think that's an understandable idea.

Judge Todd: Yes, ma'am.

Miss Northern: An amongst your—your own opinion former—opinion former.

Judge Todd: Yes. Now, if the time comes that you are so sick that you can't make the decision, are you willing for the doctors to make the decision for you then?

Miss Northern: Well, I think that that's an unreasonable way to look at it because you want an opinion.

Judge Todd: Yes, ma'am.

Miss Northern: And you see, that's—that—Groundhog Day and the—all the weather and everything else, now, it's an opinion.

Judge Todd: Judge, is there anything you would like to ask?

Judge Drowota: Well, I have the same questions, though, with the "if." And as Reverend Sorrow has said, if in fact at some day there is a feeling that—and you are unconscious and we can't ask you—

Mr. Sorrow: It's a question of whether to let you die.

Judge Drowota: —should we let you die, or would you rather live your life without your feet?

Miss Northern: I am giving my feet a chance to get well.

Mr. Sorrow: Right, right. Okay. Let's say we have given it a chance to get well, and if the infection didn't get out of your system and you became unconscious, he is saying, would you rather—

Miss Northern: I am not making any further . . . statement.

Judge Todd: In other words, you are not willing to admit that you might get unconscious?

Miss Northern: No.

Judge Todd: I see. All right.

Miss Northern: You are pretty handsome; it's rather nice to have all you handsome men come at you this morning.

Mr. Sorrow: Can they look at your feet?

Miss Northern: No, no. Can you see me?

Judge Todd: I think maybe you better see your feet.

Miss Northern: You know where they are? . . . They are there.

Judge Todd: I need to ask you this, Miss Mary. . . . When have you seen your feet?

Mr. Sorrow: Have you seen them recently? Have they let you see your feet real close?

Miss Northern: They let me see my feet. I can see my feet.

Judge Todd: When did you see them, do you remember?

Miss Northern: I seen them two or three times. Don't look at the feet. Let's don't look at the feet.

Judge Todd: I tell you what let's do.

Miss Northern: Don't look at the feet.

Judge Todd: Let's don't look at the feet. I tell you what let's do. . . . Let's you and I look at them together at the same time and see what we can.

Miss Northern: They are down there.

Judge Todd: I want you to look at them with me. Would you do it?

Miss Northern: Isn't—I just don't understand, it's sadism about it. I can't understand it.

A Nurse: Let's all look at your feet.

Miss Northern: Okay. All right, General.

A Nurse: All of us together. Let's get your gown down. There we go. Now—

Miss Northern: That's all peeling off of that. It's all getting well. It's all going down.

Judge Drowota: Do you have feeling in your feet?

Miss Northern: Oh, yes, they were knocking all around, and they're banging up against this thing and everything.

Mr. Sorrow: Can you feel it when you do that?

Miss Northern: Yeah.

Mr. Sorrow: Is there feeling?

Miss Northern: Yeah. . . .

Judge Todd: —Would you—would you just bear with us just for one more thing?

Miss Northern: You want to establish your point.

Judge Todd: No, we don't. I am asking you—

Miss Northern: You got your points all in writing and established it, according to your own—

Judge Todd: Yes, ma'am. If the time comes that you have to choose between losing your feet and dying, would you rather just go ahead and die than lose your feet? If that time comes?

Miss Northern: It's possible—It's possible only if I—Just forget it. I—You are making me sick talking.

Judge Todd: I know. I know. And I am sorry. Would you be willing to say to me that you just don't want to live if you can't have your feet? Is that the way you feel?

Miss Northern: I don't understand why it's so important to you people, why it's so important. . . .

Judge Todd: Mrs. Mary, you see a judge has to see both sides of the thing, and these people have come and told us something, and now we want you to tell us what you want to tell us so we can decide.

Miss Northern: A billion of you have been here.

Judge Todd: I understand. And that's the reason we came out to see you, so we could let you—

Miss Northern: I don't want to discuss it any more. I made my point.

Judge Todd: I believe, Mrs. Mary, that you have made your point that you would rather—that you don't want to live if you can't have your feet; isn't that about it?

Miss Northern: That's possible. . . . It's possible to see it that way, to have that opinion. I don't want you all to change your opinion.

Judge Todd: No. I want you to tell me if you really feel that way. Tell me because I want to know it. I want to consider how you feel.

Judge Drowota: Or if you would rather live and have your feet. I mean, without your feet. See, you have got me confused, Miss Mary.

Judge Todd: She wants to live and have her feet.

Mr. Sorrow: That's exactly what she wants.

Miss Northern: This is ridiculous. I am tired. And ridiculous, you know it is.

Mr. Sorrow: I think they are trying to look at your side of it and understand how you feel, and, of course, somebody else in your position, we don't know what we would do, and so I guess they are saying so many people have told these judges so much they want to see Miss Mary and say, "How do you feel, how do you feel?"

Miss Northern: It's gotten a little roll.

Mr. Sorrow: Like a snowball.

Miss Northern: This is—Let's leave it alone. Let's leave it alone. And you keep your opinions. I am through with it.

Judge Todd: I wish I could be through with it. Let me leave you with a little thought, Miss Mary.

Miss Northern: All right. . . .

Judge Todd: Did you ever read the Sermon on the Mount?

Miss Northern: Yes.

Judge Todd: You remember one thing the Good Lord said?

Miss Northern: What?

Judge Todd: If thy eye offend thee,—

Miss Northern: Oh, yes, take the eye out.

Judge Todd: —cast it out. If thy hand offend you, cut it off. Now, if and when your feet begin to offend you, maybe, maybe, you will remember that little verse.

Miss Northern: I thank you.

DECIDING FOR OTHERS: COMPETENCY

Allen Buchanan and Dan W. Brock

COMPETENCE AND INCOMPETENCE

Discussions of competence have often been hampered by a failure to distinguish carefully among the following questions:

- What is the appropriate *concept* of competence?
- Given an analysis of the appropriate concept of competence, what *standard* (or standards) of competence must be met if an individual is to be judged to be competent?
- What are the most reliable *operational measures* for ascertaining whether a given standard of competence is met?
- *Who* ought to make a determination of competence?
- What *sorts of institutional arrangements* are needed to assure that determinations of competence are made in an accurate and responsible way?

Each of these questions will be addressed separately. This section—which is concerned with the theoretical underpinnings of determinations of

From *Milbank Quarterly,* 64:2, 1986, 67–80. Reprinted with permission from Blackwell Publishers.

Editor's note: References have been cut. Readers wishing to follow up sources should consult the original article.

competence—will concentrate on the first three questions. The last two, which raise more practical and concrete concerns, can only be addressed in detail after the ethical framework has been laid out and the realities of current practices have been described.

THE CONCEPT OF COMPETENCE

Competence as Decision-Relative

The statement that a particular individual is (or is not) competent is incomplete. Competence is always competence *for some task*—competence *to do something*. The concern here is with competence to perform the task of making a decision. Hence, competence is to be understood as *decision-making capacity*. But the notion of decision-making capacity is itself incomplete until the nature of the choice as well as the conditions under which it is to be made are specified. Thus competence is decision-relative, not global. A person may be competent to make a particular decision at a particular time, under certain circumstances, but incompetent to make another decision, or even the same decision under different conditions. A competency determination, then, is a determination of a particular person's capacity to perform a particular decision-making task at a particular time and under specified conditions.

Any individual may be competent to perform some tasks (e.g., drive a car), but not others (e.g., solve differential equations). The tasks relevant to this article vary substantially, and include making decisions about medical treatment, entering into contracts, deciding whether to continue to live on one's own in an unsupervised setting, and so forth. It is true, of course, that for some individuals, decision-making capacity is entirely lacking (for instance, when the individual is permanently unconscious), but these are the unproblematic cases.

Decision-making tasks vary substantially in the capacities they require for performance at an appropriate level of adequacy. For example, even restricted to medical treatment decisions, there is substantial variation in the complexity of information that is relevant to a particular treatment decision and that, consequently, must be understood by the decision maker. There is, therefore, variation in what might be called the *objective demands* of the task in question—here, the level of abilities to understand, reason, and decide about the options in question. But there is also variation of several sorts in a subject's ability to meet the demands of a particular decision. Many factors that diminish or eliminate competence altogether vary over time in their presence or severity in a particular person. For example, the effects of dementia on a person's cognitive capacities is at some stages commonly not constant, particularly in cases of borderline competence. Instead, mental confusion may come and go; periods of great confusion are sometimes followed by comparative lucidity.

In other cases, the environment and the behavior of others may affect the relative level of decision-making competence. For example, side effects of medications often impair competence, but a change of medication may reduce those effects. Behavior of others may create stresses for a person that diminish decision-making capacities, but that behavior can often be altered, or the situations in which it occurs can be avoided. Further, cognitive functioning can sometimes be enhanced by familiar surroundings and diminished by unfamiliar ones. A person may be competent to make a decision about whether to have an elective surgical procedure if the choice is presented in the familiar surroundings of home by someone known and trusted, but may be incompetent to make that same choice in what is found to be the intimidating, confusing, and unfamiliar environment of a hospital.

Factors such as these mean that even for a given decision, a person's competence may vary over time, and so be intermittent. The values that support the right of the competent person to participate in health care decisions also require that caretakers utilize periods of lucidity when they occur. Sometimes the emergency nature of the situation will not permit this, but it is no doubt possible to involve intermittently competent persons in decision making substantially more than is done at present. Sometimes, with opportune timing or other appropriate measures (such as medications), the intermittently competent person may be able to be involved in decision making at a time when he or she is clearly competent. Often, however, the person either consistently remains in, or can only be brought to, a state of borderline competence for the decision at hand. These borderline cases of questionable competence require more careful analysis of and clarity about the nature of the competency determination. They also illustrate the need for greater sophistication on the part of medical care providers and others about physical and mental problems that frequently affect the elderly.

Capacities Needed for Competence

What capacities are necessary for a person competently to decide about such matters as health care, living arrangements, financial affairs, and so forth? As already noted, the demands of these different decisions will vary, but it is nevertheless possible to generalize about the necessary abilities. Two may be distinguished: the capacity for communication and understanding, and the capacity for reasoning and deliberation. Although these capacities are not entirely distinct, significant deficiencies in any of them can result in diminished decision-making competence. A third important element of competence is that the individual must have a set of values or conception of the good.

1 Under *communication and understanding* are included the various capacities that allow a person to take part in the process of becoming informed on and expressing a choice about a given decision. These include the ability to communicate and the possession of various linguistic, conceptual, and cognitive abilities necessary for an understanding of the particular information relevant to the decision at hand. The relevant cognitive abilities, in particular, are often impaired by disease processes to which the elderly are especially subject, including most obviously various forms of dementia, but also aphasia due to stroke and, in some cases, reduced intellectual performance associated with depression (pseudodementia). Even where cognitive function is only minimally impaired, ability to express desires and beliefs may be greatly diminished or absent (as in some patients with amyotrophic lateral sclerosis).

2 Understanding also requires the ability to appreciate the nature and meaning of potential alternatives—what it would be and "feel" like to be in possible future states and to undergo various experiences. In young children this is often prevented by the lack of sufficient life experience. In the case of elderly persons facing diseases with progressive and extremely debilitating deterioration, it is hindered by people's generally limited ability to understand a kind of experience radically different from their own and by the inability of severely impaired individuals to communicate the character of their own experience to others. Major psychological blocks—such as fear, denial, and depression—can also significantly impair the appreciation of information about an unwanted or dreaded alternative. In general, communication and understanding require the capacities to receive, process, and make available for use the information relevant to particular decisions.

3 Competence also requires *capacities for reasoning and deliberation*. These include capacities to draw inferences about the consequences of making a certain choice and to compare alternative outcomes based on how they further one's good or promote one's ends. Some capacity to employ rudimentary probabilistic reasoning about uncertain outcomes will commonly be necessary, as well as the capacity to give due consideration to potential future outcomes in a present decision. Reasoning and deliberation obviously make use of both capacities mentioned earlier: understanding the information and applying the decision maker's values.

4 Finally, a competent decision maker also requires a *set of values or conception of what is good* that is reasonably consistent and stable. This is needed in order to be able to evaluate particular outcomes as benefits or harms, goods or evils, and to assign different relative weight or importance to them. Often what will be needed is the capacity to decide on the import and relative weight to be accorded different values, since that may not have been fully determined before a particular choice must be made. Competence does not require a fully consistent set of goals, much less a detailed "life plan" to cover all contingencies. Sufficient internal consistency and stability over time in the values relative to a particular decision, however, are needed to yield a decision outcome. Although values change over time and although ambivalence is inevitable in the difficult choices faced by many persons of questionable competence concerning their medical care, living arrangements, and personal affairs, sufficient value stability is needed to permit, at the very least, a decision that can be stated and adhered

to over the course of its discussion, initiation, and implementation.

Competence as a Threshold Concept, Not a Comparative One

Decision-making competence, and the skills and capacities necessary to it, is one of the three components in standard analyses of the requirements for informed consent in health care decision making. The informed-consent doctrine requires the free and informed consent of a competent patient to medical procedures that are to be performed. The idea underlying this doctrine is that of a patient deciding, in consultation with a physician, what health care, if any, will best serve the patient's aims and needs. If the decision is not voluntary, but instead coerced or manipulated, it will likely serve another's ends or another's view of the patient's good, not the patient's own view, and will, in a significant sense, originate with another and not the patient. If the appropriate information is not provided to the individual in a form the patient can understand, the patient will not be able to ascertain how available alternatives might serve his or her aims. Finally, if the patient is not competent, either the individual will be unable to decide at all or the decision-making process will be seriously flawed.

Sometimes incompetence will be uncontroversially complete, as with patients who are in a persistent vegetative state or who are in a very advanced state of dementia, unable to communicate coherently at all. Often, however, defects in the capacities and skills noted above as necessary to competence will be partial and a matter of degree, just as whether a patient's decision is voluntary or involuntary, informed or uninformed, is also often a matter of degree. Does this mean that competence itself should be thought of as sometimes partial and possessed in different degrees? It is certainly the case that persons are commonly thought of and said to be more or less competent to perform many tasks, not just decision making. Nevertheless, because of the role competency determinations play in health care generally, and in the legal process in particular, it is important to resist the notion that persons can be determined to be more or less competent, or competent to some degree. The difficulty with taking literally the notion that competence is a matter of degree can be seen clearly by looking at the function of the competency determination within the practice of informed consent for health care, or within other areas of the law in which it plays a role, such as conservatorship or guardianship for financial affairs.

That function is, first and foremost, to sort persons into two classes: (1) those whose voluntary decisions (about their health care, financial affairs, and so on) must be respected by others and accepted as binding, and (2) those whose decisions, even if uncoerced, will be set aside and for whom others will be designated as surrogate decision makers. The function of the competency determination, then, is to make an "all or nothing" classification of persons with regard to their competence to make particular decisions, not to make "matter of degree" findings about their decision-making capacities and skills. Persons are judged, both in the law and more informally in health care settings, to be either competent or incompetent to make a particular decision—even though the underlying capacities and skills forming the basis of that judgment are possessed in different degrees. Competence, then, is in this sense a threshold concept, not a comparative one.

The foregoing makes clear that the crucial question in the competency determination is *how* defective an individual's capacities and skills to make a particular decision must be for the individual to be found incompetent to make that decision, so that a surrogate decision maker becomes necessary. In keeping with the primary objective of this article, the analysis of that question focuses on medical decisions. Here, the familiar doctrine of informed consent provides considerable guidance.

The central purpose of assessing competence is to determine whether a patient may assert his or her right to decide to accept or refuse a particular medical procedure, or whether that right shall be transferred to a surrogate. We must, therefore, ask what values are at stake in whether people are allowed to make such decisions for themselves. The informed-consent doctrine assigns the decision-making right to patients themselves; but what fundamental values are served by the practice of informed consent? In the literature dealing with informed consent, many different answers—and ways of formulating answers—to that question have been proposed, but we believe the most important values at stake are: (1) promoting and protecting the patient's well-being, and (2) respecting the patient's self-determination. It is in examining the effect of these two values that the answer to the proper standard of decision-making competence will be found.

STANDARDS OF COMPETENCE: UNDERLYING VALUES

Promotion of Individual Well-Being

There is a long tradition in medicine that the physician's first and most important commitment should be to serve the well-being of the patient. The more recent doctrine of informed consent is consistent with that tradition, if it is assumed that, at least in general, competent individuals are better judges of their own good than others are. The doctrine recognizes that while the physician commonly brings to the physician-patient encounter medical training that the patient lacks, the patient brings knowledge that the physician lacks: knowledge of particular subjective aims and values that are likely to be affected by whatever decision is made.

As medicine's arsenal of possible interventions has dramatically expanded in recent decades, alternative treatments (and the alternative of no treatment) now routinely promise different mixes of benefits and risks to the patient. Moreover, since health is only one value among many, and is assigned different importance by different persons, there is commonly no one single intervention for a particular condition that is best for everyone. Which, if any, intervention best serves a particular patient's well-being will depend in part on that patient's aims and values. Health care decision making thus usually ought to be a joint undertaking between physician and patient, since each brings knowledge and experience that the other lacks, yet that is necessary for decisions that will best serve the patient's well-being.

In the exercise of their right to give informed consent, then, patients often decide in ways that they believe will best promote their own well-being as they conceive it. As is well known, and as physicians are frequently quick to point out, however, the complexity of many treatment decisions—together with the stresses of illness with its attendant fear, anxiety, dependency, and regression, not to mention the physical effects of illness itself—means that a patient's ordinary decision-making abilities are often significantly diminished. Thus, a patient's treatment choices may fail to serve his or her good or well-being, even as that person conceives it. Although one important value requiring patient participation in their own health care decision making is the promotion of patient well-being, that same value sometimes also requires persons to be protected from the harmful consequences to them of their own choices.

Respect for Individual Self-Determination

The other principal value underlying the informed-consent doctrine is respect for a patient's self-determination, understood here as a person's interest in making important decisions about his or her own life. Although often conceived in the law under the right to privacy, the leading legal decisions in the informed-consent tradition appeal fundamentally to the right of individual self-determination. No attempt will be made here to analyze the complex of ideas giving context to the concept of individual self-determination, nor of the various values that support its importance. But it is essential to underline that many persons commonly want to make important decisions about their life for themselves, and that desire is in part independent of whether they believe that they are always in a position to make the best choice. Even when we believe that others may be able to decide for us better than we ourselves can, we sometimes prefer to decide for ourselves so as to be in charge of and responsible for our lives.

The interest in self-determination should not be overstated, however. People often wish to make such decisions for themselves simply because they believe that, at least in most cases, they are in a better position to decide what is best for themselves than others are. Thus, when in a particular case others are demonstrably in a better position to decide for us than we ourselves are, a part, but not all, of our interest in deciding for ourselves is absent.

Conflict Between the Values of Self-Determination and Well-Being

Because people's interest in making important decisions for themselves is not based solely on their concern for their own well-being, these two values of patient well-being and self-determination can sometimes conflict. Some people may appear to decide in ways that are contrary to their own best interests or well-being, even as determined by their own settled conception of their good, and others may be unable to convince them of their mistake. In other cases, others may know little of a person's own settled values, and the person may simply be deciding in a manner sharply in conflict with how most reasonable persons would decide. It may be difficult or even impossible to determine, however, whether this conflict is simply the result of a difference in values between this individual and most reasonable persons (for example, a difference in the weights assigned to various goods), or whether it results from some failure of the patient to assess correctly what will best serve his or her own interests or good.

In the conflict between the values of self-determination and patient well-being, a tradeoff between avoiding two kinds of errors should be sought. The first error is that of failing to protect a person from the harmful consequences of his or her decision when the decision is the result of serious defects in the capacity to decide. The second error is failing to permit someone to make a decision and turning the decision over to another, when the patient is able to make the decision him or herself. With a stricter or higher standard for competence, more people will be found incompetent, and the first error will be minimized at the cost of increasing the second sort of error. With a looser or more minimal standard for competence, fewer persons will be found incompetent, and the second sort of error is more likely to be minimized at the cost of increasing the first.

Evidence regarding a person's competence to make a particular decision is often uncertain, incomplete, and conflicting. Thus, no conceivable set of procedures and standards for judging competence could guarantee the elimination of all error. Instead, the challenge is to strike the appropriate balance and thereby minimize the incidence of either of the errors noted above. No set of procedures will guarantee that all and only the incompetent are judged to be incompetent.

But procedures and standards for competence are not merely inevitably imperfect. They are inevitably *controversial* as well. In the determination of competence, there is disagreement not only about which procedures will minimize errors, but also about the proper standard that the procedures should be designed to approximate. The core of the controversy derives from the different values that different persons assign to protecting individuals' well-being as against respecting their self-determination. We believe there is no uniquely "correct" answer to the relative weight that should be assigned to these two values, and in any event it is simply a fact that different persons do assign them different weight.

DECIDING ON STANDARDS OF COMPETENCE

Focusing only on the two values of patient well-being and self-determination is an oversimplification. Because other values are at stake, room for controversy about the proper standard of competence increases. For example, also important to the appropriate standard of competence is the value of maintaining public confidence in the integrity of the medical profession, so as to protect and foster the trust necessary to physician-patient relationships that function well.

The standard of competence, then, cannot be discovered. There is no reason to believe that there is one and only one optimal tradeoff to be struck between the competing values of well-being and self-determination, nor, hence, any one uniquely correct level of capacity at which to set the threshold of competence—even for a particular decision under specified circumstances. In this sense, setting a standard for competence is a value choice, not a scientific or factual matter. Nevertheless, the choice need not be and should not be arbitrary. Instead, it should be grounded in (1) a reflective appreciation of the values in question, (2) a clear understanding of the goals that the determination of competence is to serve, and (3) an accurate prediction of the practical consequences of setting the threshold at this level rather than elsewhere.

People may disagree on exactly where the threshold should be set not only because they assign different weights to the values of self-determination and well-being, but also because they make different estimates of the probability that others will err in trying to promote a person's interests. Unanimous agreement on an optimal standard is not necessary, however, for workable social arrangements for determining competence, any more than it is for determining who may vote or who may drive an automobile.

Different Standards of Competence

A number of different standards of competence have been identified and supported in the literature, though statutory and case law provide little help in articulating precise standards. It is not feasible to discuss here all the alternatives that have been proposed. Instead, the range of alternatives will be delineated and the difficulties of the main standards will be examined.

No single standard is adequate for all medical treatment decisions, much less so for decisions about living arrangements, financial affairs, participation in research, and so forth. It was argued above that a standard of competence must set a balance between the two principal values at stake in health care decision making: promoting and protecting the patient's well-being while respecting the patient's self-determination.

An example of a minimal standard of competence is that the patient merely be able to express a preference. This standard respects every expressed choice of a patient, and so is not, in fact, a criterion of *competent* choice at all. It entirely disregards whether defects or mistakes are present in the reasoning process leading to the choice, whether the choice is in accord with the patient's conception of his or her good, and whether the choice would be harmful to the patient. It thus fails to provide any protection for patient well-being, and it is insensitive to the way the value of self-determination itself varies with differences in people's capacities to choose in accordance with their conceptions of their own good.

At the other extreme are standards that look to the *content* or *outcome* of the decision, for example, the standard that the choice be a reasonable one, or be what other reasonable or rational persons would choose. On this view, failure of the patient's choice to match some such allegedly objective standard of choice entails that it is an incompetent choice. Such a standard maximally protects patient well-being—according to the standard's conception of well-being—but fails adequately to respect patient self-determination.

At bottom, a person's interest in self-determination is his or her interest in defining, revising over time, and pursuing his or her own particular conception of the good life. There are serious risks associated with any purportedly objective standard for the correct decision—the standard may ignore the patient's own distinctive conception of the good and may involve the substitution of another's conception of what is best for the patient. Moreover, even such a standard's claim to protect maximally a patient's well-being is only as strong as the objective account of a person's well-being on which the standard rests.

The issue is theoretically complex and controversial, but any standard of individual well-being that does not ultimately rest on an individual's own informed preferences is both problematic in theory and subject to intolerable abuse in practice. Thus, a standard that judges competence by comparing the content of a patient's decision to some objective standard for the correct decision may fail even to protect appropriately a patient's well-being. An adequate standard of competence will focus primarily not on the content of the patient's decision, but on the *process* of reasoning that leads up to that decision.

While an adequate competency evaluation and standard focuses on the patient's understanding and reasoning, rather than upon the particular decision that issues from them, the key issue remains. What level of reasoning is required for the patient to be competent? In other words, how well must the patient understand and reason to be competent? How much can understanding be limited or reasoning be defective and still be compatible with competence? It is important to emphasize another question faced by those evaluating competence. How certain must those persons evaluating competence be about how well the patient has understood and reasoned in coming to a decision? This last question is important because it is common in cases of marginal or questionable competence for there to be a significant degree of uncertainty about the patient's decision-making process that can never be eliminated.

Relation of the Standard of Competence to Expected Harms and Benefits

Because the competency evaluation requires setting a balance between the two values of respecting patients' rights to decide for themselves and protecting them from the harmful consequences of their own choices, it should be clear that no single standard of competence—no single answer to the questions above—can be adequate. That is simply because the degree of expected harm from choices made at a given level of understanding and reasoning can vary from virtually none to the most serious, including major disability or death.

There is an important implication of this view that the standard of competence ought to vary with the expected harms or benefits to the patient of acting in accordance with a choice—namely, that just because a patient is competent to consent to a treatment, it does not follow that the patient is competent to refuse it, and vice versa. For example, consent to a low-risk life-saving procedure by an otherwise healthy individual should require a minimal level of competence, but refusal of that same procedure by such an individual should require the highest level of competence.

Because the appropriate level of competence properly required for a particular decision must be adjusted to the consequences of acting on that decision, no single standard of decision-making competence is adequate. Instead, the level of competence appropriately required for decision making varies along a full range from low/minimal to high/maximal. Table 1 illustrates this variation.

The presumed net balance of expected benefits and risks of patient choice in comparison with other alternatives refers to the physician's assessment of the expected effects in achieving the goals of prolonging life, preventing injury and disability, and relieving suffering from a particular treatment option as against its risks of harm. The table indicates that the relevant comparison is with other available alternatives, and the degree to which the net benefit/risk balance of the alternative chosen is better or worse than that for other treatment options. It should be noted that a choice might

TABLE 1

Decision-Making Competence and Patient Well-Being

Presumed net balance of expected benefits and risks of patient choice in comparison with other alternatives	Level of decision-making competence required	Grounds for believing patient's choice best promotes/protects own well-being
Net balance substantially better than for possible alternatives.	Low/minimal	Principally the benefit/risk assessment made by others.
Net balance roughly comparable to that of other alternatives.	Moderate/median	Roughly equally from the benefit/risk assessment made by others and from the patient's decision that the chosen alternative best fits patient's conception of own good.
Net balance substantially worse than for another alternative or alternatives.	High/maximal	Principally from patient's decision that the chosen alternative best fits own conception of own good.

properly require only low/minimal competence, although its expected risks exceeded its expected benefits, because all other available alternatives had substantially worse expected risk/benefit ratios.

Table 1 also indicates, for each level of competence, the grounds for believing that a patient's own choice best promotes his or her well-being. This brings out an important point. For all patient choices, other people responsible for deciding whether those choices should be respected should have grounds for believing that the choice, if it is to be honored, is reasonably in accord with the patient's good and does reasonably protect or promote the patient's well-being (though the choice need not, of course, *maximize* the patient's interests). When the patient's level of decision-making competence is only at the low/minimal level, the grounds derive only minimally from the fact that the patient has chosen the option in question; they principally stem from others' positive assessment of the choice's expected effects for life and health.

At the other extreme, when the expected effects of the patient's choice for life and health appear to be substantially worse than available alternatives, the requirement of a high/maximal level of competence provides grounds for relying on the patient's decision as itself establishing that the choice best fits the patient's good (his or her own particular aims and ends). That highest level of competence is required to rebut the presumption that if the choice seems not best to promote life and health, then that choice is not, in fact, reasonably related to the patient's interests.

When the expected effects for life and health of the patient's choice are approximately comparable to those of alternatives, a moderate/median level of competence is sufficient to provide reasonable grounds that the choice promotes the patient's good and that his or her well-being is adequately protected. It is also reasonable to assume that as the level of competence increases (from minimal to maximal), the value or importance of respecting the patient's self-determination increases as well, since a part of the value of self-determination rests on the assumption that persons will secure their good when they choose for themselves. As competence increases, the likelihood of this happening increases.

Thus, according to the concept of competence endorsed here, a particular individual's decision-making capacity at a given time may be sufficient for making a decision to refuse a diagnostic procedure when forgoing the procedure does not carry a significant risk, although it would not necessarily be sufficient for refusing a surgical procedure that would correct a life-threatening condition. The greater the risk—where risk is a function of the severity of the expected harm and the probability of its occurrence—the greater the level of communication, understanding, and reasoning skills required for competence to make that decision. It is not always true, however, that if a person is competent to make one decision, then he or she is competent to make another decision so long as it involves equal risk. Even if this risk is the same, one decision may be more complex, and hence require a higher level of capacity for understanding options and reasoning about consequences.

Relation of Refusal of Treatment to Determination of Incompetence

A common criticism of the way physicians actually practice is that patients' competence is rarely questioned until they refuse to consent to a physician's recommendation for treatment. It is no doubt true that patients' competence when they accept physicians' treatment recommendations should be questioned more often than it now is, because consent without understanding provides little basis for believing the choice is best for the patient, and because the physician's judgment about what is medically best is fallible. Nevertheless, treatment refusal does reasonably raise the question of a patient's competence in a way that acceptance of recommended treatment does not. It is a reasonable assumption that physicians' treatment recommendations are more often than not in the interests of their patients. Consequently, it is a reasonable presumption—though rebuttable in any particular instance—that a treatment refusal is contrary to the patient's interest. Exploration of the reasons for the patient's response, including determination of whether the decision was a competent one, are appropriate—though reassessment of the recommendation is often appropriate as well.

It is essential to distinguish here, however, between grounds for calling a patient's competence into question and grounds for a finding of incompetence. Treatment refusal does reasonably serve to trigger a competency evaluation. On the other hand, a disagreement with the physician's recommendation or refusal of a treatment recommendation is no basis whatsoever for a finding of incompetence. This conclusion follows from the premise noted earlier that the competency evaluation, as well as evidence in support of a finding of incompetence, should address the *process* of understanding and reasoning of the patient, *not* the *content* of a decision.

Another essential distinction is between two quite different types of treatment refusal: a refusal of all the treatment options offered, and refusing the one treatment that the physician believes to be best while accepting an alternative treatment that lies within the range of medically sound options. If there is more than one medically sound treatment option—in the sense that competent medical judgment is divided as to which of two or more treatments would be optimal—then the patient's refusal to accept the option that the physician believes is optimal should not even raise the question of the patient's competence, much less entail a finding of incompetence, at least so long as the option the patient chooses lies within the range of medically sound options.

CONTRAST WITH FIXED MINIMUM THRESHOLD CONCEPTION OF COMPETENCE

Before elaborating the implications of this analysis for operational measurements of competence, it will be useful to contrast it with a widely held alternative conception that has been implicitly rejected here. According to this other conception—which may be called the "fixed minimal capacity" view—competence is *not* decision-relative. The simplest version of this view holds that a person is competent if he or she possesses the relevant decision-making capacities at some specified level, regardless of whether the decision to be made is risky or nonrisky, and regardless of whether the information to be understood or the consequences to be reasoned through are simple or complex. This concept of competence might also be called the "minimal threshold status concept," since the idea is that if a person's decision-making capacities meet or exceed the specified threshold, then the status of being a *competent individual* is to be ascribed to that person. According to this view, competence is an attribute of persons dependent solely on the level of decision-making capacities they possess (though these may vary, of course, from day to day or even from hour to hour, depending upon the effects of disease, medications, emotional states, and so on).

In contrast, according to the conception of competence espoused here, competence is a *relational* property. Whether a person is competent to make a given decision depends not only upon that person's own capacities but also upon certain features of the decision—including risk and information requirements. There are at least five points in favor of this approach.

First, a concept that allows a raising or lowering of the standard for decision-making capacities depending upon the risks of the decision in question is clearly more consonant with the way people actually make informal competency determinations in areas of judgment in which they have the greatest confidence and in which there is the most consensus. For example, you may decide that your 5-year-old child is competent to choose between a hamburger and a hotdog for lunch, but you would not think the child competent to make a decision about how to invest a large sum of money. This is because the risk in the latter case is greater, and the information required for reasoning about the relevant consequences of the options is much more complex. It is worth emphasizing that incompetence due to developmental immaturity, as in the case of a child, is in many respects quite different from the increasing incompetence due to a degenerative disease such as Alzheimer's. These and other cases of incompetence do have in common, however, the relevance of the degree of risk for determining the appropriate level of competence.

Second, the decision-relative concept of competence also receives indirect support from the doctrine of informed consent. The more risky the decision a patient must make, and the more complex the array of possible benefits and burdens, the greater the amount of information that must be provided and the higher the standard of understanding required on the part of the patient. For extremely low-risk procedures, with a clear and substantial benefit and an extremely small probability of significant harm, the information that must be provided to the patient is correspondingly less.

Third, perhaps the most important reason for preferring the decision-relative concept of competence is that it better coheres with our basic legal framework in two distinct respects. First, in its treatment of minors, the law has already tacitly adopted the decision-relative concept and rejected the minimum threshold concept. The courts as well as legislatures now recognize that a child can be competent to make some decisions but not others—that competence is not an all-or-nothing status—and that features of the decision itself (including risk) are relevant factors in determining whether the child is competent to make that decision. This approach is increasingly popular, and is utilized in, for example, "limited conservatorships," where some decision-making authority is expressly left with the conservatee.

In addition, the law in this country has, in general, steadfastly refused to recognize a right to interfere with a *competent* patient's voluntary choice on purely paternalistic grounds—that is, solely to prevent harms or to secure benefits for the competent patient him or herself. Instead, the law makes a finding of incompetence a necessary condition for justified paternalism. According to the decision-relative concept of competence, the greater the potential harm to the individual, the higher the standard of competence. From this it follows that a finding of incompetence is more likely in precisely those instances in which the case for paternalism is strongest—cases in which great harm can be easily avoided by taking the decision out of the individual's hands. Thus, the concept of competence favored here allows paternalism in situations in which the case for paternalism seems strongest, while at the same time preserving the law's fundamental tenet that, in general, people may be treated paternalistically only when they are incompetent to make their own decisions.

The fourth reason for preferring the decision-relative concept of competence is that it allows a finding of incompetence for a particular decision to be limited to that decision, and so it is not equivalent to a change in the person's overall status as a decision maker. Consequently, the decision-relative concept of competence contains a built-in safeguard to allay the fear that paternalism—even if justified in a particular case considered in isolation—is likely to spill over into other areas, eventually robbing the individual of all sovereignty over his or her own life. Further, any finding of incompetence is likely to evoke strong psychological reactions from some patients because to be labeled as "an incompetent" is to be returned to a childlike status. By making it clear that incompetence is decision-relative and hence may be limited to certain areas, the concept of competence used here can at least minimize the potentially devastating assault on self-esteem that a finding of incompetence represents to some individuals.

Finally, the decision-relative concept of competence has another clear advantage over the minimum threshold concept: It allows a better balance between the competing values of self-determination and well-being that are to be served by a determination of competence. The alternative concept, on its most plausible interpretation, also represents a balancing of these fundamental values, but in a cruder fashion (Brock 1983). Setting a minimal threshold of decision-making capacities represents a choice about the proper balance of tradeoff between respect for self-determination and concern for well-being, but it does so on the basis of an extremely sweeping, unqualified generalization—about the probability that unacceptable levels of harm will occur if individuals are left free to choose—over an indefinitely large number of highly diverse potential decisions.

But as indicated earlier, decisions can vary enormously in their information requirements, in the reasoning ability needed to draw inferences about relevant consequences, and in the magnitude of risk involved. Hence, any such sweeping generalization will be very precarious. If the generalization errs in one direction—by underestimating the overall harm that would befall individuals if the threshold for competence were set at one level—then the minimal threshold of decision-making capacities will be set so low that many people who are judged competent will make disastrous choices. If the generalization errs in the other direction—by overestimating the harm that would result if the threshold were set at a particular level—then many people will be interfered with for no good reason. Thus, regardless of where the minimal threshold is set, it seems likely that it will provide either too much protection or too little. The decision-relative concept of competence avoids relying upon such crude generalizations about harm and permits a finer balance to be struck between the goods of protecting well-being and respecting self-determination.

A CHRONICLE: DAX'S CASE AS IT HAPPENED

Keith Burton

. . . The story of Don Cowart is remarkable in some ways but commonplace in others. A man's wish to die is rather extraordinary in and of itself; but the pattern of events that shapes such a wish often is woven of the fabric of life's everyday occurrences. Such is the case with Cowart.

Ray and Ada Cowart moved their family from the Rio Grande Valley to the small East Texas town of Henderson in the sixties. Ray prospered over the years as a rancher and real estate agent. Ada became a teacher in the Henderson school district. Their three children—Don, Jim, and Beth—were no different from other kids reared in a close-knit community. In fact, they were ordinary people living ordinary lives.

"Donny Boy," as he came to be called by his father, was popular in school and excelled in athletics. He was captain of his high school football team and performed in rodeos. He liked to take risks, a trait that often dismayed his mother. It was risk taking that would later lure him to skydiving, surfing, and other sports of chance.

Don Cowart left Henderson in 1966 to attend the University of Texas at Austin. He had planned to return home at his graduation three years later to join his father in business; however, when notified of his military draft selection, Cowart instead elected to join the U.S. Air Force. He became a pilot and served in Vietnam. He married a high school sweetheart in 1972, but they divorced eight months later. In May 1973 he was discharged from active duty and returned to Henderson, where he began working with his father in real estate.

July 23, 1973, seemed no different to Cowart from any other Wednesday. It was hot and sultry as the afternoon sun slipped low along the pine trees in the countryside near Henderson. Ray and Don had driven out to a ranch to look over some property being offered for sale by the owner. They parked their car on a bridge over a dry creek and took off by foot. They talked and laughed together as they surveyed points of interest on the land. Their business completed, the Cowarts then returned to their car to go home for dinner.

The accident happened with no warning. The Cowart men had returned to their car but had not been able to start the engine. Ray had lifted the hood and removed the air cleaner from the engine. He primed the carburetor by hand and instructed Don to try the ignition. Several tries failed. It seemed to Don that the battery was near exhaustion. A final attempt proved fateful, however, as a blue flame shot from the carburetor and ignited a terrible explosion and fire.

Ray Cowart was hurled into heavy underbrush by the force of the explosion. The blast rocked the car and showered window glass over Don's body. Around them, the fireball spread quickly, consuming pine trees and the scrub vegetation in the area. Don reacted quickly. He climbed from the burning car and began running toward the woods. But he was forced to stop by a fear that he would become entangled in the underbrush and slowly burn to death.

Don wheeled about and decided to chance the dirt road on which they had driven in. He ran through three walls of fire, emerged into a clearing, then fell to the ground and rolled his body to extinguish the flames. He got back to his feet and resumed running in search of help for his father.

It all seemed dreamlike. Don noticed his vision was blurred as though swimming under water. His eyes had been badly burned. Now the pain was coming in waves, and he knew it was real. He kept running.

Loud voices filtered through the woods. Don collapsed at the roadside as help arrived. He heard the footsteps of a man and then the exclamation, "Oh, my God!" when a farmer found him. Don sent the man after his father and lay wondering how badly he was burned. When the man returned, Don asked him to bring a gun—a gun he would use to kill himself. The farmer refused.

In shock, Don assumed he and his father had caused the explosion by igniting gasoline from the car's engine. Later he would learn that the explosion actually had been caused by a leaking propane gas transmission line in the area where they had parked. It was a freak event. A pocket of propane gas had formed in the dry creek bed. When the carburetor flamed up, it had ignited the gas.

From *Dax's Case: Essays in Medical Ethics and Human Meaning*, edited by Lonnie D. Kliever, Southern Methodist University Press, 1989. Reprinted with permission.

Rescuers took the Cowart men to a hospital in nearby Kilgore. There, a decision was made to transport them by ambulance to a special burn unit at Dallas's Parkland Hospital. Ray Cowart died en route to Dallas. Don Cowart remembers incredible pain, his begging for pain medication, and the paramedic's refusal to administer drugs prior to their arrival in Dallas. By this time, Ada Cowart, too, was on her way to Dallas. She had returned home first to pack several changes of clothes. The radio had said the men were badly hurt. She didn't expect to return to Henderson any time soon.

Even as the ambulance sped the 140 miles from Kilgore to Dallas, Don Cowart's treatment regimen had begun. By telephone, Dr. Charles Baxter, head of Parkland's burn unit, had directed fluid therapies to help in preventing shock to vital organs. On examination in Dallas, Baxter found Cowart had severe burns over 65 percent of his body. His face suffered third-degree burns and both eyes were severely damaged. His ears and hands were also deeply burned. Fluid therapies continued and were aided by several other measures: the insertion of an intertracheal tube to control the airway, catheters placed in every body opening, treatment with antibiotics, cleansing the wounds with antibacterial drugs, and tetanus prophylaxis. Heavy doses of narcotics were given for the pain.

In the early days of Don's 232-day hospitalization at Parkland, doctors could not predict whether he would survive. It was touch and go for many weeks. Ada Cowart felt helpless; she could do little more than sit in the waiting area outside the intensive care unit with relatives of other burn victims, where she prayed and hoped for the best. Doctors permitted only short visits with her son. Don had given his mother power of attorney in the Parkland emergency room, and she in turn deferred to the medical professionals on treatment decisions.

For Cowart, there were countless whirlpool tankings in solutions to cleanse his wounds, procedures to remove dead tissue, grafts to protect living tissue, the amputation of badly charred fingers from both hands and the removal of his right eye. The damaged left eye was sewn shut. And there was terrible pain.

Through it all, Don had remained constant in his view that he did not want to live. His demands to die had started with the farmer at the accident site. They had continued at the Kilgore hospital, in the ambulance, and now at Parkland. He didn't want treatment that would extend his misery and he made this known to his mother and family, Dr. Charles Baxter, a nurse named Leslie Kerr, longtime friend Art Rousseau, attorney Rex Houston, and many others.

Baxter remained undaunted by Don's pleas to stop treatment, dismissing them at first as the typical response of burn victims to the pain of their wounds and treatment. In time, however, he openly discussed Cowart's wish to die with Don, his mother, and his lawyer, considering all the medical and legal ramifications. Failing to get Ada Cowart's and Rex Houston's consent to the withdrawal of treatment, Baxter continued to deliver it.

For her part, Ada Cowart understood her son's pain and anguish. She was haunted, nonetheless, by these thoughts: What if treatment were ceased and Don changed his mind in a near-death state? Would it be too late? Furthermore, her religious beliefs simply made mercy killing or suicide deplorable options. These religious constraints were reinforced by her fear that her son had not yet made his "peace with God."

Rex Houston also had mixed feelings about Don's wishes. On the one hand, he sympathized with Cowart's condition—being unable to so much as take medication to end his life without the assistance of others. On the other hand, it was Houston's duty to reach a favorable resolution of a lawsuit filed against the pipeline owners for Ray Cowart's death and for Don Cowart's disability. With regard to the latter, he needed a living plaintiff to achieve the best damage award for the Cowart family. Moreover, Houston believed that such an award would provide the financial means necessary for Don Cowart's ultimate rehabilitation. He therefore encouraged Cowart to see the legal proceedings through.

In February 1974, the lawsuit was settled out of court—one day prior to trial. Almost immediately, Don's demands to die quickened. There had been talk before with Art Rousseau of getting a gun. Don had asked Leslie Kerr if she would help him by injecting an overdose of medication. Now Cowart even talked with Houston about helping him get to a window of his sixth-floor hospital room, where presumably he would leap to his death. All listened but none agreed to help.

On March 12, 1974, Don was discharged from Parkland. He, his family, and his doctors agreed that his condition had improved sufficiently to warrant his transfer to the Texas Institute for Research and Rehabilitation in Houston. Nine months removed from his medical residency, Dr. Robert Meier of TIRR found Cowart to be a passive recipient of medical care, although the philosophy of treatment in this rehabilitation center encouraged patient involvement in treatment decisions. Previously Don had no say in his care; now he would be offered choices in his own treatment.

All seemed to go well during the first three weeks of his stay, until Cowart realized the pain he had endured might continue indefinitely, thanks to a careless comment by a resident plastic surgeon that his treatment would be years in completion. Faced with that prospect, Cowart refused treatment for his open burn areas and stopped taking food and water. In a matter of days, Cowart's medical condition deteriorated rapidly. Finding his patient in serious condition, Dr. Meier was deeply perplexed about what to do next. He believed it his duty to help Cowart achieve the highest measure of rehabilitation, but he was not inclined to force upon the patient care he did not wish to receive. Faced with this dilemma, he called for a meeting with Ada Cowart and Rex Houston to discuss with Don the future course of his treatment.

Ada Cowart was outraged by Don's condition. She had been discouraged from staying with her son at TIRR, and in her absence his burns had worsened. He was again near death, due to his refusal of whirlpool tankings and dressing changes. It was agreed in the meeting that Cowart would be transferred to the burn unit of John Sealy Hospital of the University of Texas Medical Branch in Galveston, where his injuries could again be treated by burn specialists.

On April 15, 1974, Don was admitted to the Galveston hospital, in chronic distress from infected wounds, poor nutrition, and severe depression. His right elbow and right wrist were locked tight. The stubs of his fingers on both hands were encased in grotesque skin "mittens." There was practically no skin on his legs. His right eye socket and closed left eye oozed infection. And excruciating pain remained his constant nemesis.

Active wound care was initiated immediately and further skin grafts were advised by Dr. Duane Larson to heal the open wounds on Cowart's chest, legs, and arms. But Cowart bitterly protested the daily tankings and refused to consent to surgery. One night he even crawled out of bed, hoping to throw himself through the window to his death, but he was discovered on the floor and returned to bed.

Frustrated by Cowart's behavior, Dr. Larson consulted Dr. Robert White of psychiatric services for an evaluation of Don's mental competency. White remembers being puzzled by Cowart: Was he a man who tolerated discomfort poorly or perhaps was profoundly depressed? Or was this an extraordinary man who had undergone such an incredible ordeal that he was frustrated beyond normal limits? White concluded, and a colleague confirmed, that Cowart was certainly not mentally incompetent. In fact, he was so impressed with the clarity of Cowart's expressed wish to die that he asked permission to do a videotape interview for classroom use in presenting the medical, ethical, and legal problems surrounding such cases. That filmed interview, which White entitled Please Let Me Die, *eventually became a classic on patient rights in the field of medical ethics.*

Having been declared mentally competent, Cowart still found it difficult to gain control over his treatment. He and his mother argued constantly over treatment procedures. Rex Houston helped get changes in his wound care but turned a deaf ear to Cowart's plea to go home to die from his wounds or to take his own life. In desperation, Cowart turned to other family members for assistance in securing legal representation, but without success. Finally, with White's help, Cowart reached an attorney who had represented Jehovah's Witnesses attempting to refuse medical treatment, but he was not optimistic that a lawsuit would free him from the hospital.

Rebuffed on every hand, Cowart reluctantly became more cooperative. White secured changes in Don's pain medication before and after the daily tankings, making treatments more bearable. Psychotherapy and medication helped improve his overall outlook by relieving his depression and improving his sleep. Encouraged that he might still regain sight in his left eye, Don more or less accepted his daily wound care and even agreed to surgical skin grafts early in June 1974. By July 15, his physical condition had improved enough to allow him to transfer out of the burn unit of the John Sealy Hospital to the psychiatric unit of the Jennie Sealy Hospital in the University of Texas Medical Branch under White's direct care while his wounds continued to heal.

Amid these changes there were still periodic conflicts between Cowart and those around him over his confinement in the hospital. There were reiterated demands to die and protests against treatment. A particularly explosive encounter between Cowart and Larson occurred on the day preceding his second and last major surgical procedure in the Galveston hospital. Cowart had agreed to undergo surgery to free up his hands, but the night before he changed his mind. The next morning, Larson angrily confronted Cowart with the challenge that, if he really wanted to die, he would agree to the surgery that would enable him to leave the hospital and go home where he could take his own life if he wished. Anxious to do exactly that, Cowart consented to the surgery, which was performed on July 31.

Don Cowart's stormy stay at Galveston finally ended on September 19, 1974. He had been hospitalized for a total of fourteen months, but at last he was going home. His prognosis upon dismissal was listed simply as "guarded."

Cowart was glad to be back in Henderson. The little things counted the most—sleeping in his own bed, listening to music, visiting with friends. But it was different for him than before the accident. He was totally blind, his left eye having failed to recover. His hands and arms remained useless. He was badly scarred. A dropped foot now required that someone assist him in walking. Some of his burn sites still were not healed.

Everything he did required the help of others. Someone had to feed him, bathe him, and help with personal functions. The days seemed endless. He tried to find peace in sleep, but even this dark release was impossible without drugs. While he couldn't see himself, Don knew his appearance drew whispers and stares in restaurants.

He had his tapes, talking books, television, and CB radio. He could use his sense of hearing, though not as well as before due to the explosion and burns. And he could think. For a while, he could see in his mind's eye the memories of earlier times. Then the memories started to fade.

Ada Cowart had lost much, but she never lost her religious faith. There had been times when even she had admitted that maybe it would have been best if Don had died with her husband. She reconciled her doubt with the thought that no mother can give up the life of a son. Ada never gave up hope that Don could find new faith in God.

Homecoming brought peace for a time. As Don's early excitement for returning home gave way to deep depression and despair, however, conflict returned to their lives. They argued about how he could occupy himself, how he dressed, his personal habits, and his future. Frustration led to a veiled suicide attempt, Don stealing away from the house during the night to try throwing himself in the path of trucks hauling clay to a brick plant. The police found him and brought him home quietly.

For the next five years, Cowart lived in a shadow world of painful rehabilitation, chronic boredom, and failed relationships. His difficulties were not for want of trying. With Rex Houston's encouragement and assistance he tried pursuing a law degree. Fortunately, his legal settlement with the pipeline company provided the financial means for the nursing care and tutorial assistance which would be required because of his massive handicaps.

Cowart tested out his abilities as a blind student in two undergraduate courses at the University of Texas in Austin during the fall of 1975. He spent the spring at home in Henderson preparing for the tests that were required for admission to law school. In the summer of 1976, he enrolled for a part-time course load in Baylor University's School of Law.

Don handled his studies at Baylor in fine fashion despite his handicaps, but the strain was tremendous. He was forced to live with other people, his independence was limited, and his sleep problems persisted. When a special relationship with a woman ended abruptly in the spring of 1977, his life caved in. He tried to commit suicide by taking an overdose of pain and sleep medications, but he was discovered in time to have his stomach pumped at the hospital emergency room. He had trouble picking up his studies again, so he dropped out before the spring quarter was completed.

Cowart returned home defeated and discouraged, living with his mother for the next half year. He resumed his studies at Baylor in the spring of 1978, only to drop out again before he had completed the third quarter in the fall of 1979. He again retreated to his mother's home, filled with doubts that he would ever be able to pass the bar. By the spring of 1980, he was ready for another try at schooling, this time in a graduate program in building construction of Texas A&M University. Once again, the old patterns of sleepless nights and boring days got the best of him and he made a half hearted effort at slashing his wrists with a razor blade.

Looking back, Cowart saw his futile efforts to take his own life as a bitter human comedy. The doctors in Galveston had encouraged him to accept treatment that would free him of hospitalization and permit him to end his life, if that was his wish. But he found it difficult to find a way of killing himself without bringing further misery on himself—brain damage or further hospitalization. Ironically, he realized that he was no more successful in ending his life than in making his life work.

As a last resort, Cowart contacted White for help and was voluntarily readmitted under White's care to the Jennie Sealy Hospital on April 12, 1980. During his month-long stay, he met with White for psychotherapy treatments daily. Even more important, his sleep problems were finally resolved by weaning him away from the heavy sleep medications that he had taken for years. Cowart describes that experience as being like "coming out of a fog." For the first time since his harrowing burn treatment ordeal, his sleep became normal and his depression lifted.

It was during this stay that I met Don Cowart and we began early discussions of a film that would eventually come to be known as Dax's Case. *I still call him Don because that is how I know him, but he legally changed his name to Dax in the summer of 1982. Some commentators on the film speculate that this change of name reflects some personal metamorphosis that Cowart went through during his lengthy rehabilitation period. But Cowart offers a simpler explanation. As a blind man with impaired hearing, he often found himself responding to comments addressed to others bearing the name of Don. I accepted his reasons for changing his name but asked him not to think the poorer of me for persisting in calling him Don.*

It would be easy to believe that Dax's Case, *more than five years in the making, served as a crucible for Don Cowart's rehabilitation. During this time, new hope and independence came into his life. He started a mail-order specialty foods business in Henderson using his creative powers. He moved into his own house. He became an articulate spokesperson for "the right to die" under auspices of Concern for Dying. And he married a former high school classmate in February 1983.*

There is always another chapter, however. Even now, Don's life continues to shift. His first venture in business did not succeed financially. His second marriage ended unhappily. Amid failure has also come achievement. He returned to law school at Texas Tech University in Lubbock, where he completed his law degree in May and passed the bar in the summer of 1986. He set up a small law practice in Henderson and has recently taken in his first partner. He continues to represent his views on patient rights at educational symposiums and public forums. In time, he hopes to become a specialist in personal injury cases.

COMMENTARY

Robert B. White

Donald's wish seemed in great measure logical and rational; as my psychiatric duties brought me to know him well, I could not escape the thought that if I were in his position I would feel as he did. I asked two other psychiatric colleagues to see the patient, and they came to the same conclusion. *Should his demand to die be respected?* I found myself in sympathy with his wish to put an end to his pathetic plight. On the other hand, the burden on his mother would be unthinkable if he left the hospital, and none of us who were responsible for his care could bring ourselves to say, "You're discharged; go home and die."

Another question occurred to me as I watched this blind, maimed, and totally helpless man defy and baffle everyone: could his adamant stand be the only way available for him to regain his independence after such a prolonged period of helplessness and total dependence?

Consequently, I decided to assist him in the one area where he did want help—obtaining legal assistance. He obviously had the right to legal recourse, and I told him I would help him obtain it. I also told him that I and the other doctors involved could not accede immediately to his demand to leave; we could not participate in his suicide. Furthermore, he was, I said, in no condition to leave unless his mother took him home, and that was an unfair burden to place on her. I urged him to have the surgery; then, when he was able to be up and about, he

---

Hastings Center Report, July 1975, 9–10.

could take his own life if he wished without forcing others to arrange his death.

But Donald remained adamant, and the patient, his attorney, and I had several conferences. Finally, the attorney reluctantly agreed to represent the patient in court. The patient and I agreed that if the court ruled that he had the right to refuse further treatment, the life-sustaining daily trips to the Hubbard tank and all his other life-sustaining treatment would be stopped. If he wished, he could remain in the hospital in order to be kept as free of pain as possible until he died.

Had Donald been burned a few years ago, before our increasingly exquisite medical and surgical technology became available, none of the moral, humanitarian, medical, or legal questions his case raised would have had time to occur; he would simply have died. But Donald lived, and never lost his courage or tenacity. He has imposed upon us the responsibility to explore the questions he has asked. On one occasion Donald put the matter very bluntly: "What gives a physician the right to keep alive a patient who wants to die?"

As we increase our ability to sustain life in a wrecked body we must find ways to assess the wishes of the person in that body as accurately as we assess the viability of his organs. We can no longer blindly hold to our instinctive tendency to regard death as an adversary to be defeated at any price. Nor must we accept immediately and at face value a patient's demand to be allowed to die. That demand may often be his only way to assert his will in the face of our unyielding determination to defeat death. The problem is relatively simple when brain death has occurred or when a patient refuses surgery for cancer. But what of the patient who has entered willingly on a prolonged and difficult course of treatment, and then, at the point at which he will obviously survive if the treatment is continued, decides that he does not want further treatment because he cannot tolerate the kind of future life that his injuries or illness will impose upon him?

The outcome of Donald's case does not resolve these questions but it should add to the depth of our reflections. Having won his point, having asserted his will, having thus found a way to counteract his months of total helplessness, Donald suddenly agreed to continue the treatment and to have the surgery on his hands. He remained in the hospital for five more months until medically ready to return home. In the six months since he left, Donald has regained a considerable measure of self-sufficiency. Although still blind, he will soon have surgery on his eye, and it is hoped some degree of useful vision will be restored. He feeds himself, can walk as far as half a mile, and has become an enthusiastic operator of a citizen's band radio. When I told him of my wish to publish this case report, he agreed, and stated that he had been thinking of writing a paper about his remarkable experiences.

COMMENTARY

H. Tristram Engelhardt, Jr.

This case raises a fundamental moral issue: how can one treat another person as free while still looking out for his best interests (even over his objections)? The issue is one of the bounds and legitimacy of paternalism. Paternalistic interventions are fairly commonplace in society: motorcyclists are required to wear helmets, no one may sell himself into slavery, etc. In such cases society chooses to intervene to maintain the moral agency of individuals so that their agency will not be terminated in death or in slavery. Society chooses in the purported best interest (i.e., to preserve the condition of self-determination itself—freedom) of the would-be reckless motorcyclist or slave. Or, in the paradigmatic case of paternalism, the choice by parents for their children is justifiable in that at a future time as adults, the children will say that their parents chose in their best interests (as opposed to the parents simply using their children for their own interests). That is, the paternalism involved in surrogate consent can be justified if the individual himself cannot choose, and one chooses in that individual's best interests so that if that person were (or is in the future) able to choose, he or she would (will) agree with the choice that has been made in his or her behalf.

Thus, one can justify treating a burned patient when first admitted even if that person protested: one might argue that the individual was not able to choose freely because of the pain and serious impact of the circumstances, and that by treating initially one gave the individual a reasonable chance to choose freely in the future. One would interpret the patient to be temporarily incompetent and have someone decide in his behalf. But once that initial time has passed, and once the patient is reasonably able to choose, should one respect a patient's request to refuse lifesaving therapy even if one has good reason to believe that later the patient might change his or her mind? This is the problem that this case presents.

Yet, what are the alternatives which are morally open: (1) to compel treatment, (2) at once to cease treatment, or (3) to convince the patient to persist, but if the patient does not agree, then to stop therapy. Simply to compel treatment is not to acknowledge the patient as a free agent (i.e., to vitiate the concept of *consent* itself), and simply to stop therapy at once may abandon the patient to the exigencies of unjustified despair. The third alternative recognizes the two values to be preserved in this situation: the freedom of the patient and the physician's commitment to preserve the life of persons.

But in the end, individuals, when able, must be allowed to decide their own destiny, even that of death. When the patient decides that the future quality of life open to him is not worth the investment of pain and suffering to attain that future quality of life, that is a decision proper to the patient. Such is the case *even if* one had good reasons to believe that once the patient attained that future state he would be content to live; one would have unjustifiably forced an investment of pain that was not agreed to. Of course, there are no easy answers. Physicians should not abandon patients when momentary pain overwhelms them; physicians should seek to gain consent for therapy. But when the patient who is able to give free consent does not, the moral issue is over. A society that will allow persons to climb dangerous mountains or do dare-devil stunts with cars has no consistent grounds for paternalistic intervention here. Further, unlike the case of the motorcyclist or the would-be slave, in this case one would force unchosen pain and suffering on another in the name of their best interests, but in circumstances where their best interests are far from clear. That is, even if such paternalistic intervention may be justifiable in some cases (an issue which

---

Hastings Center Report, June 1975, 9–10.

Author's note: This article explores the sparse secular morality that can bind moral strangers, not the thick morality that should guide all persons in their choices regarding dying and death. The first is not adequate for a good death.

is different from the paternalism of surrogate decision-making, and which I will not contest at this point), it is dubious here, for the patient's choice is not a capricious risking on the basis of free action, but a deliberate choice to avoid considerable hardship. Further, it is a uniquely intimate choice concerning the quality of life: the amount of pain which is worth suffering for a goal. Moreover, it is, unlike the would-be slave's choice, a choice which affirms freedom on a substantial point—the quality of one's life.

In short, one must be willing, as a price for recognizing the freedom of others, to live with the consequences of that freedom: some persons will make choices that they would regret were they to live longer. But humans are not only free beings, but temporal beings, and the freedom that is actual is that of the present. Competent adults should be allowed to make tragic decisions, if nowhere else, at least concerning what quality of life justifies the pain and suffering of continued living. It is not medicine's responsibility to prevent tragedies by denying freedom, for that would be the greater tragedy.

ADVANCE DIRECTIVES

THE LIVING WILL: HELP OR HINDRANCE?

Stuart J. Eisendrath and Albert R. Jonsen

Physicians are accustomed to handing their patients written instructions that prescribe a certain form of medical care, usually a medication. They are not accustomed to receiving from their patients written instructions that prescribe how they, the physicians, are to provide, or not provide, medical care. Yet the living will is just such a document, and it is appearing in the offices of physicians. It is one manifestation of the increasingly strong affirmation that patients should have substantial control over their medical care.

As a legal doctrine and an ethical imperative, informed consent has become the central feature of that affirmation. Although often difficult to achieve and sometimes lightly treated, informed consent has become a standard of good practice and is, in principle, hardly controversial. Its obverse—"informed refusal"—is much more controversial. Although strong legal grounds and persuasive ethical justifications support the refusal of medical care by patients, the occasions of such refusal are frequently disruptive and disturbing. The living will has even more potential for such disruption and disturbance, since it is a refusal in writing rather than viva voce. Argument rages in the literature of medical ethics about the circumstances in which a refusal should itself be refused; anxiety and uncertainty appear in the clinical setting. Psychiatric consultants, legal advisors, and ethicists are summoned.

The living will is a statement that directs the physicians to act in certain ways during the terminal phase of the patient's illness when he may no longer be mentally competent. The physician is instructed not to take measures that would prolong the life of the patient. This form of instruction was devised in 1969 by the Euthanasia Educational Council, now known as "Concern for Dying." This document was intended to be "a simple, reasonable

Journal of American Medical Association, Vol. 249:15, 1983, 2054–2058.

statement of the belief in the right of the dying to die and not to be kept alive by artificial and heroic measures."[1] Within six years of its appearance, more than a half million copies had been distributed, frequently by churches and senior citizens groups. Different formulations of the living will have since appeared. Persons sometimes will write a living will in their own words.

The functions of the living will are multiple. The foremost idea has been to allow the patient maximal autonomy in deciding the extent of the medical interventions he would want for himself in the future should he become incompetent. Signing the living will before medical interventions, when the patient is healthy and of sound mind, presumably gives that individual control over the end of his life. Not only does such a device provide the patient autonomy, but it can also reduce futile pain and suffering. It may also assist the physician and the patient's family in the onerous and heartrending task of making decisions about the measure of care for the dying patient. Finally, as Bok suggests, it may lift the burden of choice from dying persons at a time when they have neither the strength nor will to worry about alternative forms of care. These many benefits contribute to the growing popularity of directions concerning care at the end of life.[2]

"Living will" is a phrase that sounds contradictory to persons trained in the law: a "will" is a document whose terms are to be executed after the death of the testator. The living will directs actions before the death of the testator that will usually hasten that death. When the living will first appeared, its standing was highly questionable. Not only was it a peculiar sort of "will," but its terms might direct acts that could be construed as illegal, and its language, which contains such words as *extraordinary* and *heroic*, was vague. Doubts might be cast on its authenticity and on the persistence of the testator's intention at the time the will is to be executed.[3]

Acknowledging the legal questions about the living will, legislators in several states who were sympathetic with the purpose of such a document attempted to create a device with a more solid legal basis. Spearheaded by Walter Sackett, a physician legislator in Florida, legislative efforts were unsuccessful until the California Natural Death Act, sponsored by Senator Barry Keene of California, was signed by Governor Jerry Brown in 1976. At present, ten states have passed similar legislation (Arkansas, California, Idaho, Kansas, New Mexico, North Carolina, Oregon, Texas, and Washington). Inevitably, passage of such legislation is accompanied by controversy. At the extremes, proponents of mercy killing are pitted against right-to-life advocates. In the center, physicians object that laws are unnecessary and intrusive; patients argue their rights are ignored without legislation.[4] Some thoughtful commentators worry that when such laws are passed, patients who have signed and witnessed living wills will be maintained alive for unreasonable periods of time because of physicians' fear of malpractice.[5]

The California law is strictly drawn. It requires the patient to sign a document in which the words are prescribed exactly in the law. This document directs the physician to refrain from life-sustaining procedures when "in the judgment of the attending physician, death is imminent whether or not such procedures are utilized." The letter of the law seems to make the Act irrelevant for many clinical situations where it might be expected to be helpful.[6] However, the letter of the law does not seem to deter physicians. A survey of 275 physicians showed that few of them were familiar with the precise provisions of the Act. At the same time, two thirds of the respondents said they had patients who had signed the Act and two thirds said the Act had made a difference in their clinical decisions about those patients.[7] Another survey reported that California physicians who were familiar with the Act considered its principal value to lie less in having a legal directive than in the opportunity it provided to discuss appropriate care during terminal illness while the patient was still alert and competent.[8]

Whether a patient presents a legally sanctioned document or an unofficial living will to the physician, questions of interpretation are certain to arise. If the physician and patient can discuss together the document's wishes and intentions, agreement can be reached about the extent and nature of care during terminal illness. It is, of course, highly desirable that such common agreement be reached. However, the living will or its legal counterpart may appear in the clinical situation after the patient has ceased to be an active participant. Either it may be given to the physician at an earlier time, without its intent ever being clarified, or relatives may produce it during the course of a serious illness. Difficulties of interpretation can then become extreme. Even those physicians who sincerely desire to follow their patients' wishes may be uncertain how to do so. Case 1 illustrates this problem. In contrast, case 2 demonstrates that the presence of a living will can facilitate clinical decision (as it is intended to do).

REPORT OF CASES

Case 1 Mrs T. was a 65-year-old woman who was admitted to the vascular surgery service for evaluation of an asymptomatic carotid bruit. The bruit had been discovered on a routine physical examination when the patient had seen her personal physician with a fracture of her right humerus, which had occurred while playing golf. Arteriography disclosed a high-grade stenosis of her left carotid, and a thromboendarterectomy was suggested as a prophylactic procedure to prevent a disabling stroke. The patient consented to the operation but stated to a house officer before the procedure that she had signed a living will four years earlier, shortly after her husband had died of a lingering illness. The patient reaffirmed on the day before surgery that she wished the living will to be carried out should she experience a severe and disabling stroke as a sequela of the surgery. She knew that a stroke was a possibility from the surgery, since several months earlier a friend of hers had had a severe stroke after an endarterectomy. She stated that she felt life was worth living only if she could be healthy and independent.

She presented the following living will (The Concern for Dying format) to the house officer:

> To my family, my physician, my lawyer, and to any medical facility in whose care I happen to be, or to any individual who may become responsible for my health and welfare or affairs. Death is as much a reality as birth, maturity, and old age. It is the one certainty of life. If the time comes when I, Mrs T., can no longer take part in decisions for my own future, let this statement stand as an expression of my wishes while I am of sound mind. If a situation should arise in which there is no reasonable expectation of my recovery from physical or mental disability, I request that I be allowed to die and not be kept alive by artificial means or heroic measures. I do not fear death itself as much as the indignities of deterioration, dependence, and hopeless pain. I therefore ask that medications be mercifully administered to me to alleviate suffering, even though this may hasten the moment of death. This request is made after careful consideration. I hope that you who care for me will feel morally bound to follow its mandate. I recognize that this appears to place a heavy responsibility upon you, but it is with the intention of relieving you of such responsibility and of placing it upon myself, in accordance with my strong convictions, that this statement is made. Signed (by the patient).

The patient underwent surgery, which was uneventful. She awoke and had full neurological functioning. Approximately 30 minutes later, however, she began to experience progressive right-sided weakness and a neurological picture compatible with a dense stroke in the distribution of the left middle cerebral artery. She was taken back to the operating room and reexplored, and an extensive clot formation was removed from her carotid artery.

After this reoperation, the patient continued to have a profound neurological deficit manifested by right-sided paresis and responsiveness to deep pain only. She was transferred from the recovery room to the Intensive Care Unit and received assisted ventilation. The patient's lack of responsiveness persisted for several days, and it appeared that she might be left with a permanent, profound neurological impairment. Added to this, aspiration pneumonia developed. It was decided that a tracheostomy should be done to control her ventilation over a long term. This procedure was performed electively. Certain staff members raised the question, "Why are we doing this to this lady? Wasn't her living will specific in spelling out what she didn't want to have happen?" In answer to this question, her attending physicians stated that one week after her stroke, it was impossible to tell how much function the patient would regain: "We must continue acute care, hoping for the best at this point." Others questioned this approach, stating that if they persisted, the patient would end up trapped in a poorly functioning body, unable even to take her own life should she desire to do so. As a previously vigorous woman, this is precisely what she did not want, they asserted. The patient's respiratory status improved considerably with antibiotic treatment, and she was transferred to the vascular surgery floor.

At this point, the patient's brother questioned the patient's attending physician about the appropriateness of continuing medical treatment. He suggested, with the most sincere intention, that the patient be sedated and, in essence, be allowed to die. In a letter to the patient's attending surgeon, the brother referred to her living will and implied that he might begin litigation if the patient was allowed to continue living in this neurologically impaired state. Nonetheless, the nurses persisted in encouraging the patient to make rehabilitative efforts. An ethics consultation was requested.

A medical ethics committee exists at this institution. It is used for consultation in difficult cases, and, while neither binding nor having legal force, its advice is usually found helpful.[9,10] The medical ethics committee gathered information. The patient's neurological status was meticulously reviewed. Neurology consultants could not be definitive in stating the patient's prognosis for recovery, stating that it would take several months for the ultimate prognosis to become certain. As part of the ethics consultation, a psychiatric consultation was obtained to clarify the patient's current level of competence to make decisions as well as to estimate the validity of her previously signed living will. The psychiatrist found the patient to be globally aphasic and unable to communicate by any means. From history gathered from the patient's family, however, it became clear that she had never had any psychiatric disorder, nor was there any family history of such. It was also apparent that the patient's decision to sign a living will had not been the result of any discernible psychiatric illness, e.g. a depressive suicidal wish.

On the basis of information provided by neurology and psychiatric consultants, the medical ethics committee suggested to the attending physician that the living will not be acted on at this point in time. The committee suggested that respiratory support not be withdrawn and there be no authorization of an order not to resuscitate the patient if she developed cardiopulmonary arrest. The reason for this conclusion was the uncertainty of the prognosis. It was simply impossible, on the basis of the medical evidence, to predict to what extent the conditions stated in the living will ("deterioration, dependence, and hopeless pain") would become manifest. In view of the psychiatric evidence and the history, the will could be taken as a valid expression of the patient's wishes, but, at the same time, the conditions envisioned by those wishes could not be reliably predicted. Thus, the will should not determine the clinical decisions, at least until the picture about future levels of function became more certain. This conclusion ran the risk, of course, of leaving this woman alive in the condition which she wanted to avoid. Faced with this dilemma, the ethics consultants followed the venerable rule of thumb, "in cases of doubt, favor life."[11] It should be noted that if the patient had presented a California Natural Death Act Directive, the condition required by this law, "imminent death whether or not treatment is provided," would certainly not be fulfilled, making the directive inoperative according to its strict letter.

Ten days after her transfer to the vascular surgery floor, the patient became capable of written and verbal communication. The tracheostomy was capped, and she began speaking short phrases and was able to understand verbal and written questions and instructions. In a few days, her ability to speak increased remarkably. This improvement occurred approximately three weeks after the onset of her stroke. Improvement continued at a dramatic rate, and within a week, plans were made to discharge the patient to a rehabilitation center. Before leaving the medical center, the patient was asked about having signed the living will and her views of her recent medical care. She responded by saying that the living will was "a good thing in certain conditions." She did not feel, however, that she herself had been in a condition in which such a document should have been invoked. She stated, "I didn't want to be a vegetable."

This statement highlighted the quandary that the staff had found themselves in several weeks earlier. What had the patient meant in her living will when she used the term "no reasonable expectation of my recovery from physical or mental disability?" Who would define what the term "reasonable" would mean? Who would define what the term "recovery" would mean? Had the patient meant by her recovery that she should be in a condition in which she'd be able to play her usual game of golf or move around in a wheelchair? What level of disability was the patient describing in her living will? At the patient's discharge, the staff felt satisfied that they had not misinterpreted the patient's desires from her living will document. Almost universally, they believed that they had carried out the most appropriate medical treatment for this patient.

As a postscript to this case, several months after the patient's discharge, the patient's brother wrote a note to the medical and nursing staff who had treated the patient. In his note, he stated that both he and the patient were glad that the staff had stood firm in providing the patient with maximal therapeutic efforts in the face of his demands for reduced care. He described her progress in her rehabilitation efforts. He thanked the staff for being "so helpful" during the critical decision-making period.

Case 2 Mrs Z. was a 55-year-old woman who was a foreign language teacher. She was admitted to the Intensive Care Unit with an aspiration pneumonia, which was believed caused by a diminished gag reflex secondary to her 20-year history of multiple sclerosis. For several days, the patient received appropriate antibiotic therapy, and her pneumonia cleared. The patient seemed to be at continuous risk for a recurrence of aspiration, since her diminished gag reflex was presumably caused by irreversible nerve damage.

The question of what preventive measures could be used was explored by staff members. One member suggested oversewing the patient's epiglottis to prevent recurrent aspirations. This procedure would require a permanent tracheostomy, and the patient would lose laryngeal speech capability. This intervention would have profound implications for this patient, because she had been grossly debilitated by the years of multiple sclerosis and was confined to a bed at home. Her only interaction with friends involved speech. She was an articulate and highly educated person. Her major pastime was as a foreign language tutor for university students. Thus, the loss of verbal communication would have a major and unique impact on this patient. In presenting the option of permanent tracheostomy *v* the possibility of recurrent aspiration pneumonia, it was pointed out to the patient that she had essentially no pulmonary reserve and that future episodes of aspiration would almost certainly be fatal. She stated that she would rather die than be unable to speak.

In discussing the options with the patient, the attending physicians were unclear how well she comprehended the decision before her. They obtained a psychiatric consultation to evaluate the patient's mental status and competence to make this major decision. In reviewing the history, the psychiatric consultant found that the patient had been hospitalized for urinary tract infections six weeks before the current hospitalization. At that time, a psychiatric consultation had been obtained, since the patient had been noted to be "hallucinating and paranoid." Antipsychotic medication had been recommended but never administered. In evaluating the patient's current mental status, the psychiatrist found her to be guarded in her responses and uncooperative with formal cognitive testing. It appeared that the patient might have a mild organic brain syndrome. Although there was no clear-cut evidence of any psychosis, it was difficult to determine whether the patient fully understood the implications of the choices she was to make regarding her medical care. At this point, the patient's sole surviving sister came from a distant city. The sister brought forth the following living will, which the patient had signed four years earlier:

> TO WHOM THIS MAY CONCERN: The undersigned hereby directs all doctors and hospitals that she does not wish to be kept alive artificially, in the event that the outcome and prognosis is such that undersigned will not be able to lead a useful life, and with the prognosis as such, in the opinion of competent medical practitioners, that the medical treatment being rendered is just prolonging life without the possibility of reasonable recovery. Signed (by the patient).

According to the sister, the patient had clarified to her that a "useful life" meant the ability to relate to others meaningfully by verbal communication. From the sister's description, it was clear that the patient was mentally lucid at the time she had signed this document. With this information, it was much easier for the attending physician to rest with the patient's decision not to have a tracheostomy. Although she seemed to have a general understanding of what the tracheostomy would mean, the living will supported the idea that the patient would not want to be kept alive in the condition in which she would exist indefinitely but be unable to speak—her criteria for a useful life.

In this case, the living will substantially helped the staff to make a reasonable decision that they felt comfortable with. The patient did not receive a tracheostomy and was transferred to a rehabilitation facility for further treatment. Should she aspirate again, her probable death would be the result of a decision she herself had participated in both by word and by living will. Several months after the transfer, she remained in the same medical condition.

COMMENT

It is clear legally and ethically that a competent patient's refusal of treatment should be honored. The living will is an attempt to carry the patient's wishes into the time when the patient is no longer able to be a spokesman on his or her behalf. Yet the first case raises many of the difficulties inherent in implementing a living will. Although one of the living will's main purposes is to promote patient autonomy, this case illustrates how difficult it can be to achieve this in the clinical setting. The medical staff had a difficult time deciding on the proper treatment of this patient, not because they wished to impose their will on her, but rather because they could not interpret exactly what her desires would be given her medical condition. Her living will was not specific enough to assist the medical staff in attempting to fulfill her desires. Although her document used terms like "a reasonable expectation of recovery," these terms are open to a variety of interpretations. The ambiguity allows the staff to project their own attitudes and feelings onto a given statement, setting the stage for conflict and controversy.[12]

In Mrs T.'s case, for example, some of the staff members believed a great injustice was being done when the patient was given a tracheostomy tube, stating that Mrs T.'s living will spoke against such procedures. Medical indications for the tracheostomy, and, indeed, for rehabilitative care after her neurological insult, were clear. Nonetheless, the split in the staff's response to the patient's document made the pursuit of clinically appropriate treatment controversial. Projection of staff's attitudes is not uncommon in critically ill patients. This phenomenon has been well described in the psychiatric consultation literature.[13,14] Conflicting attitudes were aired in the discussion of the patient's treatment, because the staff had to guess at what the specific conditions were that the patient alluded to in her document.

Hindrance of staff management highlights one of the drawbacks of a living will, i.e., in cases where it is most needed—for example, when the patient's communication is grossly if not totally impaired, then the living will can become a source of confusion because of variably interpretable phrases included in the document.

In contrast to the first case, the second case illustrates how a living will can be extremely helpful. In this case, the document signed by the patient alleviated the burden of decision making for the family and attending physicians. This case differed considerably from the first in that the prognosis was much more certain (although less favorable). In addition, the patient appeared to have a reasonable idea of what decision she was making by signing this document, since she had lived with the disabling effects of multiple sclerosis for approximately 15 years.

There is little question in this case of the patient having full control of her faculties at the time she signed the will, which was several years before hospitalization. Even though during her current hospitalization there was uncertainty as to her ability to comprehend fully the medical decisions facing her, it did seem that she had a general understanding of what her options were. That impression was greatly enhanced when her sister brought in the supporting document. It should be noted that if the physicians had determined that the surgery was the most appropriate treatment and they regarded the patient as incompetent, a judicial authorization would have been a prerequisite.

The second case was also clearer than the first in that the possible long-term outcomes were more sharply defined, i.e., the value of the surgical procedure to oversew the patient's epiglottis had the definite outcome of ensuring the prolongation of her life, whereas, the failure to do so carried the serious risk of reaspiration and almost certain death. For this patient, the ability to speak was critical for her desire to continue living.

These two cases point out the advantages and disadvantages of the living will in a clinical situation. The advantages are that patients' autonomy can be honored with greater certainty, unacceptable pain and suffering avoided, and physicians absolved from doing what might be medically possible but personally, to patient and physician, undesirable. The disadvantages arise from the lack of specificity in written documents and the uncertainty of prognosis. These disadvantages can be alleviated in part if physicians undertake to clarify the patient's intention by detailed conversation in advance of the situation when the terms of the will must be interpreted. In the first case, the patient presented the living will to the anesthesiology resident the night before the surgery. The resident accepted it, put it in the record, but did not discuss it. In the second case, the physicians, with the help of the patient's sister, were able to interpret the patient's intentions, but it would have been desirable for the patient herself to discuss the matter with her physician (which she had not) during the long course of her illness.

The presence of a relative or friend who can be relied on to interpret faithfully and honestly the patient's wishes is invaluable. While such people have no legal standing as a surrogate, their advice can be helpful and should be readily accepted unless there is some suspicion of bias. One attempt has been made to provide, by legislative means, standing for a person appointed by the patient, but it failed to pass.[15] Even without such standing, a patient who writes a living will might be advised to indicate in the document those persons who might serve as its interpreter. Naturally, physicians should be aware of the law regarding proxy decisions for incompetent patients that prevail in the jurisdiction in which they practice.[16]

Whenever possible, a frank discussion of the terms of the living will is always advisable. It may happen that such a discussion leads the physician to judge that the restrictions placed on clinical discretion are unacceptable. If this were to happen, the physician would be obliged to inform the patient that he or she cannot fulfill the conditions of the living will in good conscience. Should the patient insist, it would be necessary to withdraw from the case after timely notice and referral.

Some physicians might find the living will contrary to their personal ethic;[11] others might have religious objections to its terms. Catholic physicians should not be troubled, since their moral theology permits withdrawing from "extraordinary treatments" at the patient's request; however, some Catholic physicians might find objections to what they consider an antilife tone.[17] Orthodox Jewish physicians are more likely to find the living will objectionable on this ground.[18] However, most religious doctrines, as well as the current common opinion in medical ethics, justify the living will in principle. The difficulties lie largely in its application, as we have tried to show in this article.

In the absence of opportunities for clarification by discussion, the living will can be, at best, one piece of evidence among others about the patient's wishes. It needs to be weighed, along with medical indications, estimates of future quality of life, and other expressions of the patient's preferences contributed by friends and family, in reaching a suitable clinical decision.[19] The living will, despite its difficulties, should always be taken seriously as an expression of the patient's autonomy. Although it might not be decisive in certain circumstances, it is always deserving of consideration.

NOTES

1. Bass AN: Euthanasia to date. *Vassar Qtrly* 1975, p 72.
2. Bok S: Personal directions for care at the end of life. *N Engl J Med* 1976;295:367–369.
3. Keene B: Can we make the Natural Death Act a better law? Read before the California Medical Association annual scientific assembly, San Francisco, March 19, 1978.
4. Garland M: The right to die in California. *Hastings Cent Rep* 1976;6:5–7.
5. Lebacqz K: Against the California Natural Death Act. *Hastings Cent Rep* 1977;7:14–15.
6. Jonsen AR: Dying right in California: The Natural Death Act. *Clin Res* 1978;26:55–60.
7. Redleaf D, Schmitt S: Natural Death Act study: Some surprising results. *Santa Clara Med Soc Bull* Jan 1979.
8. Klutch M: Survey results after one year's experience with the Natural Death Act. *West J Med* 1978;128: 329–330.
9. Veatch RM: Hospital ethics committees: Is there a role? *Hastings Cent Rep* 1977;6:22–25.
10. Levine C: Hospital ethics committees: A guarded prognosis. *Hastings Cent Rep* 1977;7:25–27.
11. Epstein F: The role of the physician in the prolongation of life, in Ingelfinger FJ, Relman AS, Finland M (eds): *Controversy in Internal Medicine II.* Philadelphia, WB Saunders Co, 1974, pp 103–109.
12. Jackson DL, Youngner S: Patient autonomy and "death with dignity." *N Engl J Med* 1979;301:404–408.
13. Eisendrath SJ, Dunkel J: Psychological issues in intensive care unit staff. *Heart Lung* 1979;8:751–758.
14. McCartny JR: Refusal of treatment: Suicide or competent choice? *Gen Hosp Psychiatry* 1979;1:338–344.

15. Relman AS: Michigan's sensible "living will." *N Engl J Med* 1979;300:1270–1271.
16. Meyers DW: *Medico-Legal Implications of Death and Dying*. San Francisco, Bancroft-Whitney Co, 1981.
17. Hellegers AE, Wakin E: Is the right to die wrong? *US Catholic* 1978;43:13–17.
18. Horowitz E: The California Natural Death Act and us. *Sh'ma* 1977;7:93–103.
19. Jonsen AR, Siegler M, Winslade WJ: *Clinical Ethics*. New York, Macmillan Publishing Co, 1982.

THE HEALTH CARE PROXY AND THE LIVING WILL

George J. Annas

American medicine is awash in forms: insurance forms, disability forms, informed-consent forms, and forms for various examinations, to name just a few. Forms can help make the practice of medicine more efficient, but they can also make it more routinized, impersonal, and bureaucratic. Congress and the President have decreed that beginning December 1, 1991, all hospitals, nursing facilities, hospice programs, and health maintenance organizations that serve Medicare or Medicaid patients must provide all their new adult patients with written information describing the patients' rights under state law to make decisions about medical care, including their right to execute a living will or durable power of attorney. New forms will be routinely added to the practice of medicine. Their purpose is to help implement a right that has been universally recognized: the right to refuse any and all medical interventions, even life-sustaining interventions. The challenge is to use these forms to foster communication between doctor and patient, as well as respect for the patient's autonomy.

New England Journal of Medicine 324, No. 17, April 25, 1991: 1210–1213.

Editor's note: The notes have been omitted. Readers wishing to follow up on sources should consult the original article.

HISTORICAL CONTEXT

The term "living will" was coined by Luis Kutner in 1969 to describe a document in which a competent adult sets forth directions regarding medical treatment in the event of his or her future incapacitation. The document is a will in the sense that it spells out the person's directions. It is "living" because it takes effect before death. Public interest in this document has always been high, and a national organization, Concern for Dying, has devoted most of its resources for the past 20 years to educating the public and professionals about the living will. A sister organization, Society for the Right to Die (which has merged with Concern for Dying to form the National Council for Death and Dying), simultaneously devoted its primary efforts to encouraging states to pass legislation giving formal legal recognition to the living will.

In 1976 the country's attention focused on the case of Karen Ann Quinlan, a young woman in a persistent vegetative state, and her parents' attempts to have her ventilator removed so she could die a natural death. The New Jersey Supreme Court granted the parents' petition and held that an "ethics committee" could grant all parties concerned legal immunity for their actions. The court did this because it believed that it was the fear of legal liability that prevented Quinlan's physicians from honoring her parents' request. Her story prompted the enactment of the nation's first living-will statute, California's Natural Death Act, in 1976.

The California statute is very narrow. A legally enforceable declaration can be executed only 14 days or more after a person is diagnosed as having a terminal illness, defined as one that will cause the patient's death "imminently," whether or not life-sustaining procedures are continued. Thus, even though this statute was inspired by her story, it would not have helped Quinlan, because she was not terminally ill.

By 1991, more than 40 states had enacted living-will statutes. All these laws provide immunity to physicians and other health care professionals who follow the patient's wishes as expressed in a living will. Virtually all of them also suffer from four major shortcomings, however: they are applicable only to those who are "terminally ill"; they limit the types of treatment that can be refused, usually to "artificial" or "extraordinary" therapies; they make no provision for the person to designate another person to make decisions on his or her behalf, or set forth the criteria for such decisions; and there is no penalty if health care providers do not honor these documents.

ADDRESSING THE LIMITATIONS OF THE LIVING WILL

These problems led to calls for second-generation legislation on the living will. Other shortcomings were also noted. Living wills require a person to predict accurately his or her final illness or injury and what medical interventions might be available to postpone death, and living wills require physicians to make decisions on the basis of their interpretation of a document, rather than a discussion of the treatment options with a person acting on behalf of the patient. The proposed solution to these problems was not to modify the living will but to replace it with another form, one assigning a durable power of attorney to a designated person (known, in this context, as appointing a health care proxy). The person named in the document (also called the health care proxy) is variously known as the attorney, the agent, the surrogate, or the proxy—four terms that are synonyms in this context.

Every state has a durable-power-of-attorney law that permits persons to designate someone to make decisions for them if they become incapacitated. Although these statutes were enacted primarily to permit the agent to make financial decisions, no court has ever invalidated a durable power of attorney specifically designed to enable the designated person to make health care decisions. In the recent *Cruzan* case—in which Nancy Cruzan's parents, basing their attempt on their daughter's previous statements, sought to have her tube feeding discontinued after she had been left in a persistent vegetative state by an automobile accident—Justice Sandra Day O'Connor advised citizens to employ this device. In her concurring opinion, O'Connor observed that the decision in *Cruzan* "does not preclude a future determination that the Constitution requires the States to implement the decisions of a duly appointed surrogate." The *Cruzan* case itself, which involved facts essentially identical to those in *Quinlan*, gave impetus to the concept of a health care proxy, just as the *Quinlan* case had previously increased interest in the living will. Physicians are legally and ethically bound to respect the directions of a patient set forth in a living will, but living wills are limited because no one can accurately foretell the future, and interpretation may be difficult. Attempts to make the living will less ambiguous by developing comprehensive checklists with alternative scenarios may be too confusing and abstract to be useful to either patients or heath care providers, although opinions on this differ.

THE MOVE TO DESIGNATE HEALTH CARE PROXIES

Although new laws are not necessary in any state (because of existing laws regarding the assignment of a durable power of attorney), the current trend in the United States is for states to enact additional proxy laws that specifically deal with health care. Such laws generally specify the information that must be included in the proxy form and the standards on which treatment decisions must be based and grant good-faith immunity for all involved in carrying out the treatment decision. Two of the best-written proxy laws have recently become effective in New York (in January 1991) and Massachusetts (in December 1990). The New York law is based on a recommendation of the New York State Task Force on Life and the Law, and that group's statement of its rationale is still the best introduction to the concept of the health care proxy. The Massachusetts proxy law is largely modeled on the New York law.

The heart of both laws (and all proxy laws) is the same: to enable a competent adult (the "principal") to choose another person (the "proxy" or "agent") to make treatment decisions for him or her if he or she becomes incompetent to make them. The agent has the same authority to make decisions that the patient would have if he or she were still competent. Instead of having to decipher a document, the physician is able to discuss treatment options with a person who has the legal authority to grant or withhold consent on behalf of the patient. The manner in which the agent must exercise this authority is also crucial. The agent must make decisions that are consistent with the wishes of the patient, if these are known, and otherwise that are consistent with the patient's best interests.

Proxy laws also permit the principal to limit the authority of the agent in the document (for example, by not granting authority to refuse cardiopulmonary resuscitation or tube feeding), but the more limitations the principal puts on the agent, the more the document appointing a health care proxy resembles a living will. In addition, because every limitation is subject to interpretation, the likelihood that a dispute will arise about the meaning of the document is increased. One compromise is to give the agent blanket authority to make decisions and to detail one's values and wishes with as much precision as possible in a private letter to the agent. The agent could use this letter when it was relevant to the actual decision and keep it private when it was not relevant.

IMPLEMENTING LAWS REGARDING HEALTH CARE PROXIES

The goal of appointing a proxy is to simplify the process of making decisions and to make it more likely that the patient's wishes will be followed—not to complicate existing problems. If hospitals and hospital lawyers cooperate, this goal will be attained, because the vast majority of physicians will welcome the ability to discuss treatment options with a person, chosen by the patient, who has the legal authority to give or withhold consent. Hospitals can help their patients by making a simple proxy form available, by educating their medical, nursing, and social-service staffs about the laws governing health care proxies, and by supporting decisions made by the agents. Hospitals can impede the process of making good decisions, however, if they concentrate on the paperwork rather than on the way in which decisions are made. Some Massachusetts attorneys, for example, have already drafted a 13-page, singlespaced proxy form that is all but unintelligible to nonlawyers. Others have begun to explore and to catalogue all the reasons why physicians and hospitals might want to seek judicial review before honoring the decision of a health care agent. Neither of these strategies is constructive. The use of complex forms and obstructive strategies makes it likely that treatment decisions will actually be made by the hospital's lawyers and the agent's lawyers, not by the agent and the physician. If this happens, the trend to designating a health care agent will be frustratingly counterproductive, since, instead of encouraging a focus on the patient and the patient's wishes, where it belongs, the new proxy forms will add another layer of bureaucracy and another outsider to the decision process.

The most useful form for both patients and providers is a simple one-page document that sets forth all necessary information in easily comprehensible language. [A] one-page form, which is easily understood and meets all the requirements of the new Massachusetts proxy law (as well as those of the New York law) was developed by a broad-based task force made up of representatives of all the major health care organizations in the state, including the Massachusetts Medical Society, the Massachusetts Hospital Association, the Massachusetts Nurses Association, the Massachusetts Federation of Nursing Homes, and also the Massachusetts Department of Public Health, as well as the Massachusetts Executive Office of Elder Affairs and the Massachusetts Bar Association. This model form (available in bulk from Massachusetts Health Decisions, 101 Tremont St., No. 600, Boston, MA 02108), which also includes instructions and spaces for the optional signatures of the agent and an alternate (naming an alternate is not required), will be distributed across the state. The degree of cooperation in its development was virtually unprecedented and may provide a model for future efforts.

ADDING TO THE DOCUMENT DESIGNATING A PROXY

Perhaps out of concern for efficiency, some commentators have advocated combining an organ-donor form with the form designating a health care proxy. This is a serious error for at least two reasons. First, much effort has been expended over the past 20 years to separate the issues of organ donation and treatment decisions in the public's mind, since the main reason people do not sign organ-donor cards is that they believe doctors might "do something to me before I'm really dead." Tying organ donation to treatment refusals that might lead to death only heightens this concern and is likely to lead people to use neither form. Second, the proxy form takes effect when the patient becomes incompetent; in contrast, the organ-donor form takes effect only on the patient's death. The health care agent can have nothing to say about organ donation, because the agent can make only treatment decisions, an authority that dies with the patient. Organ donation is laudable, but it is not related to the designation of a health care agent, and the principal should authorize donation on a separate form designed for that purpose. Organ-donor forms may teach another lesson as well. No physician in the United States will honor an organ-donor form over the objections of the patient's family. Similarly, physicians have difficulty honoring a patient's living will over the family's objections. Because it identifies a person with legal authority to talk with the physician, the health care proxy is likely to be a more effective mechanism to implement the patient's wishes.

It should be stressed that forms naming a health care proxy do not substantively change existing law; they merely make it procedurally easier for a person to designate an agent who is authorized to make whatever health care decisions the person could legally make if competent, and they give health care providers legal immunity for honoring such decisions. The patient can, for example, give the agent the authority to refuse any and all medical care, but the agent has no more legal authority than the principal to insist on assisted suicide or to demand a lethal injection. The naming of an agent also solves the problem of a dispute among family members concerning treatment, since the agent has the legal and ethical right and responsibility to make the decision. When a long-lost relative arrives and demands that "everything be done or I'll sue," the physician can refer that person to the agent, rather than try to achieve a consensus.

LIMITS OF THE CONCEPT OF THE HEALTH CARE PROXY

Only competent adults who actually execute a document can name a health care agent. Since fewer than 10 percent of Americans have either living wills or organ-donor cards, few may use this mechanism. It has no application to children, the mentally retarded, or others unable to appreciate the nature and consequences of their decisions. Treatment decisions for these groups will continue to be governed by the vague "best interests" standard, which is the functional equivalent of "reasonable medical care," "appropriate medical care," or "indicated medical care." The document will also be of limited use in the emergency department, although in rare cases the health care agent may arrive with the principal and there may be time for consultation and informed consent before a specific intervention is tried. Nor will the document solve problems of futility. Physicians will retain the right not to offer treatment that is contraindicated, useless, or futile.

THE RESPONSIBILITY OF PHYSICIANS

I have encouraged members of both the Boston Bar Association and the Massachusetts Bar Association to make health care–proxy forms available to the public and their clients free of charge as a public service. Many have agreed. It will also be useful to the public if physicians make such forms available to their patients and encourage them to fill them out. Physicians may also be more comfortable about relying on the decisions of the designated agent if patients are willing to discuss their choice of agent with the physician, although this is not a requirement. Any form that is used must be written in language that both patients and health care providers can easily understand; the form need not be written by a lawyer and should not require a lawyer to interpret.

Like soldiers in past wars, Americans serving in the Persian Gulf wrote their wills. This time, however, many also wrote living wills or executed durable powers of attorney. As one reporter observed, "In the process, the soldiers had to clarify ambiguous personal relationships, chart out their children's lives, and, in some cases, confront their own mortality for the first time." Designating a health care agent gives us all the opportunity to confront our mortality and to determine who among our friends and relatives we want to make treatment decisions on our behalf when we are unable to make them ourselves. A clear focus on these substantive issues, rather than on forms or formalities, could help patients feel more secure that their wishes regarding medical treatment will be respected, and could help health care professionals be more secure that the treatment decisions made for incompetent patients actually reflect the patients' wishes. These are certainly worthy goals.

TESTING THE LIMITS OF PROSPECTIVE AUTONOMY: FIVE SCENARIOS

Norman L. Cantor

Several examples will help crystallize the potential tension between an advance directive and the contemporaneous interests of an incompetent patient. In the following scenarios, assume that all patients were fifty years old at the time of making an advance directive and that the critical medical decisions are confronted five years later. Assume also that no evidence exists that the patient changed his or her mind or wavered in resolve between preparation of the advance directive and losing competence.

Scenario 1: Person A, a Jehovah's Witness, prescribes in an advance directive that blood transfusions should not be administered regardless of the life-saving potential of such medical intervention. She is aware of the life and death implications of this religiously motivated instruction. Later, A becomes prematurely senile and incompetent. Still later, the senile patient develops bleeding ulcers which demand blood transfusions. With a blood transfusion, she will survive and continue to live as a "pleasantly senile" person for a number of years. The senile A no longer has recollection of, or interest in, religion; however, she remained an avid Jehovah's Witness up until the time of incompetency. Should the attending physician administer a life-saving blood transfusion?

Scenario 2: Person B believes both that life should be preserved to the maximum extent possible and that suffering is preordained and carries redemptive value in an afterlife. B prepares an advance directive in which all possible life-extending medical intervention is requested and all pain relief is rejected. At the time of the preparation of the directive, B has a conversation with a physician in which the physician explicitly warns B that many terminal illnesses entail excruciating pain. Despite that admonition, B directs that all means to preserve life be utilized and that analgesics be omitted. Subsequently, B suffers from cancer, which both affects his brain, rendering him incompetent, and causes him to suffer excruciating pain. Further medical treatment such as radiation or chemotherapy will extend B's life, but will not itself relieve the pain or cause any remission in which competence would

From *Advance Directives and the Pursuit of Death with Dignity* by Norman L. Cantor, Indiana University Press, 1993. Reprinted with permission from the publisher.

return. Should the attending physician sedate the patient, or cease the life-prolonging medical intervention, or both?

Scenario 3: Person C is an individual with chronic heart problems. Physicians have informed C that at some stage he will need a heart transplant in order to survive. C prepares an advance directive stating that if he becomes incompetent and survival becomes dependent on a heart transplant, then such a transplant should be rejected because of its expense. C prefers to leave a substantial monetary legacy to his children. Later, C becomes prematurely senile and incompetent. Still later, C's heart deteriorates and a heart transplant becomes necessary to preserve C's life. With the transplant, C will very likely continue to live for three to five years. Without it, C will die within a few months. The transplant will cost $100,000 and is not covered by any insurance or government benefit program. C's estate totals $100,000. Should a life-extending heart transplant be performed?

Scenario 4: Person D is a health-care professional sensitive to society's needs for organ and tissue donations. In her advance directive, D provides that if she should become incompetent but remain physically healthy, then she wishes to donate a kidney and bone marrow to needy recipients. Later, D is afflicted with Alzheimer's disease and reaches a point of profound dementia. Needy recipients for kidney and bone marrow transplants have been located. The prospective transplant operations will pose only a slight risk to D and entail only mild pain. At the same time, the now incompetent D has no recollection of her prior instruction and no appreciation of the altruism involved in donating an organ or tissue. She will derive no contemporaneous gain from the contemplated operations. Should the transplants be performed in accord with D's advance directive?

Scenario 5: Person E is a sociology professor known for her intellectual sharpness. E takes enormous pride in that intellectual acuity. E drafts an advance directive prescribing that if she should become mentally impaired and incompetent to the point where she can no longer read and comprehend a sociology text, then all life-preserving medical intervention should be withheld. When reminded by her spouse about the potential for happiness in an incompetent state, E replies that she deems significant mental dysfunction to be degrading and personally distasteful. For her, such a debilitated existence is a fate worse than death. Later, E suffers a serious stroke which renders her permanently incompetent and incapable of reading or performing intellectual tasks. E is also unable to swallow and is therefore dependent on artificial nutrition. At the same time, E does not appear to be in any pain and seems to derive some pleasure from listening to music. Should the life-preserving nasogastric tube be continued?

In each of the above situations, people have issued advance directives which effectuate their personal values and concepts of dignity. Yet implementation of those prior instructions conflict in some measure with the contemporaneous interests or well-being of the incompetent persona. Can the advance directive prevail? Does prospective autonomy encompass the prerogative to impact negatively on the incompetent persona?

CHOOSING FOR OTHERS

IN THE MATTER OF CLAIRE C. CONROY

Supreme Court of New Jersey. 98 N.J. 321, 486 A. 2d 1209, decided Jan. 17, 1985

SCHREIBER, J.

At issue here are the circumstances under which life-sustaining treatment may be withheld or withdrawn from incompetent, institutionalized, elderly patients suffering from severe and permanent mental and physical impairments and a limited life expectancy.

Plaintiff, Thomas C. Whittemore, nephew and guardian of Claire Conroy, an incompetent, sought permission to remove a nasogastric feeding tube, the primary conduit for nutrients, from his ward, an eighty-four-year-old bedridden woman with serious and irreversible physical and mental impairments, who resided in a nursing home. John J. Delaney, Jr., Conroy's guardian *ad litem*, opposed the guardian's petition. The trial court granted the guardian permission to remove the tube, and the Appellate Division reversed. . . .

At the time of trial, Ms. Conroy was no longer ambulatory and was confined to bed, unable to move from a semi-fetal position. She suffered from arteriosclerotic heart disease, hypertension, and diabetes mellitus; her left leg was gangrenous to her knee; she had several necrotic decubitus ulcers (bed sores) on her left foot, leg, and hip; an eye problem required irrigation; she had a urinary catheter in place and could not control her bowels; she could not speak; and her ability to swallow was very limited. On the other hand, she interacted with her environment in some limited ways: she could move her head, neck, hands, and arms to a minor extent; she was able to scratch herself, and had pulled at her bandages, tube, and catheter; she moaned occasionally when moved or fed through the tube, or when her bandages were changed; her eyes sometimes followed individuals in the room; her facial expressions were different when she was awake from when she was asleep; and she smiled on occasion when her hair was combed, or when she received a comforting rub.

Editors' note: Case has been shortened and most legal references have been omitted.

Dr. Kazemi and Dr. Davidoff, a specialist in internal medicine who observed Ms. Conroy before testifying as an expert on behalf of the guardian, testified that Ms. Conroy was not brain dead, comatose, or in a chronic vegetative state. They stated, however, that her intellectual capacity was very limited, and that her mental condition probably would never improve. Dr. Davidoff characterized her as awake, but said that she was severely demented, was unable to respond to verbal stimuli, and, as far as he could tell, had no higher functioning or consciousness. Dr. Kazemi, in contrast, said that although she was confused and unaware, "she responds somehow."

The medical testimony was inconclusive as to whether, or to what extent, Ms. Conroy was capable of experiencing pain. Dr. Kazemi thought that Ms. Conroy might have experienced some degree of pain from her severely contracted limbs, or that the contractures were a reaction to pain, but that she did not necessarily suffer pain from the sores on her legs. According to Dr. Davidoff, it was unclear whether Ms. Conroy's feeding tube caused her pain, and it was "an open question whether she [felt] pain" at all; however, it was possible that she was experiencing a great deal of pain. Dr. Davidoff further testified that she responded to noxious or painful stimuli by moaning. The trial court determined that the testimony of a neurologist who had examined Ms. Conroy would not be necessary, since it believed that it had sufficient evidence about her medical condition on which to base a decision.

Both doctors testified that if the nasogastric tube were removed, Ms. Conroy would die of dehydration in about a week. Dr. Davidoff believed that the resulting thirst could be painful but that Ms. Conroy would become unconscious long before she died. Dr. Kazemi concurred that such a death would be painful. . . .

Ms. Conroy's only surviving blood relative was her nephew, the guardian, Thomas Whittemore. He had known her for over fifty years, had visited her approximately once a week for four or five years prior to her commitment to the nursing home, and had continued to visit her regularly at the nursing home for some time. The record contained additional evidence about the nephew's and aunt's financial situations and the history of their relationship. Based on the details of that record, there was no question that the nephew had good intentions and had no real conflict of interest due to possible inheritance when he sought permission to remove the tube.

Mr. Whittemore testified that Ms. Conroy feared and avoided doctors and that, to the best of his knowledge, she had never visited a doctor until she became incompetent in 1979. He said that on the couple of occasions that Ms. Conroy had pneumonia, "[y]ou couldn't bring a doctor in," and his wife, a registered nurse, would "try to get her through whatever she had." He added that once, when his wife took Ms. Conroy to the hospital emergency room, "as foggy as she was she snapped out of it, she would not sign herself in, and she would have signed herself out immediately." According to the nephew, "[a]ll [Ms. Conroy and her sisters] wanted was to . . . have their bills paid and die in their own house." He also stated that he had refused to consent to the amputation of her gangrenous leg in 1982 and that he now sought removal of the nasogastric tube because, in his opinion, she would have refused the amputation and "would not have allowed [the nasogastric tube] to be inserted in the first place."

. . .

The trial court decided to permit removal of the tube. It reasoned that the focus of inquiry should be whether life has become impossibly and permanently burdensome to the patient. If so, the court held, prolonging life becomes pointless and perhaps cruel. It determined that removal of the tube would lead to death by starvation and dehydration within a few days, and that the death might be painful. Nevertheless, it found that Ms. Conroy's intellectual functioning had been permanently reduced to a very primitive level, that her life had become impossibly and permanently burdensome, and that removal of the feeding tube should therefore be permitted.

The guardian *ad litem* appealed. While the appeal was pending, Ms. Conroy died with the nasogastric tube intact. Nevertheless, the Appellate Division decided to resolve the meritorious issues, finding that they were of significant public importance and that this type of case was capable of repetition but would evade review because the patients involved frequently die during litigation.

. . .

The Appellate Division . . . held that the right to terminate life-sustaining treatment based on a guardian's judgment was limited to incurable and terminally ill patients who are brain dead, irreversibly comatose, or vegetative, and who would gain no medical benefit from continued treatment. As an alternative ground for its decision, it held that a guardian's decision may never be used to withhold nourishment, as opposed to the treatment or attempted curing of a disease, from an incompetent patient who is not comatose, brain dead, or vegetative, and whose death is not irreversibly imminent. Depriving a patient of a basic necessity of life, such as food, under those circumstances, the court stated, would hasten death rather than simply allow the illness to take its natural course. The court concluded that withdrawal of Ms. Conroy's nasogastric tube would be tantamount to killing her—not simply letting her die—and that such active euthanasia was ethically impermissible. The Appellate Division therefore reversed the trial court's judgment.

We granted the guardian's petition for certification, despite Ms. Conroy's death, since we agree with the Appellate Division that the matter is of substantial importance and is capable of repetition but evades review. . . .

I

This case requires us to determine the circumstances under which life-sustaining treatment may be withheld or withdrawn from an elderly nursing-home resident who is suffering from serious and permanent mental and physical impairments, who will probably die within approximately one year even with the treatment, and who, though formerly competent, is now incompetent to make decisions about her life-sustaining treatment and is unlikely to regain such competence. . . .

The *Quinlan* decision dealt with a special category of patients: those in a chronic, persistent vegetative or comatose state. In a footnote, the opinion left open the question whether the principles it enunciated might be applicable to incompetent patients in "other types of terminal medical situations . . . , not necessarily involving the hopeless loss of cognitive or sapient life." We now are faced with one such situation: that of elderly, formerly competent nursing-home residents who, unlike Karen Quinlan, are awake and conscious and can interact with their environment to a limited extent, but whose mental and physical functioning is severely and permanently impaired and whose life expectancy, even with the treatment, is relatively short. The capacities of such people, while significantly diminished, are not as limited as those of irreversibly comatose persons, and their deaths, while no longer distant, may not be imminent. Large numbers of aged, chronically ill, institutionalized persons fall within this general category.

Such people (like newborns, mentally retarded persons, permanently comatose individuals, and members of other groups with which this case does not deal) are unable to speak for themselves on life-and-death issues concerning their medical care. This does not mean, however, that they lack a right to self-determination. The right of an adult who, like Claire Conroy, was once competent, to determine the course of her medical treatment remains intact even when she is no longer able to assert that right or to appreciate its effectuation. As one commentator has noted:

> Even if the patient becomes too insensate to appreciate the honoring of his or her choice, self-determination is important. After all, law respects testamentary dispositions even if the testator never views his gift being bestowed. [Cantor, 30 *Rutgers L.Rev.* at 259.] . . .
>
> Any other view would permit obliteration of an incompetent's panoply of rights merely because the patient could no longer sense the violation of those rights. [*Id.* at 252.]

Since the condition of an incompetent patient makes it impossible to ascertain definitively his present desires, a third party acting on the patient's behalf often cannot say with confidence that his treatment decision for the patient will further rather than frustrate the patient's right to control his body. Nevertheless, the goal of decision-making for incompetent patients should be to determine and effectuate, insofar as possible, the decision that the patient would have made if competent. Ideally, both aspects of the patient's right to bodily integrity—the right to consent to medical intervention and the right to refuse it—should be respected.

In light of these rights and concerns, we hold that life-sustaining treatment may be withheld or withdrawn from an incompetent patient when it is clear that the particular patient would have refused the treatment under the circumstances involved. The standard we are enunciating is a subjective one, consistent with the notion that the right that we are seeking to effectuate is a very personal right to control one's own life. The question is not what a reasonable or average person would have chosen to do under the circumstances but what the particular patient would have done if able to choose for himself.

The patient may have expressed, in one or more ways, an intent not to have life-sustaining medical intervention. Such an intent might be embodied in a written document, or "living will," stating the person's desire not to have certain types of life-sustaining treatment administered under certain circumstances. It might also be evidenced in an oral directive that the patient gave to a family member, friend, or health care provider. It might consist of a durable power of attorney or appointment of a proxy authorizing a particular person to make the decisions on the patient's behalf if he is no longer capable of making them for himself. It might take the form of reactions that the patient voiced regarding medical treatment administered to others. *See, e.g., Storar*, 52 *N.Y.*2d 363, 420 *N.E.*2d 64, 438 *N.Y.S.*2d 266 (withdrawal of respirator was justified as an effectuation of patient's stated wishes when patient, as member of Catholic religious order, had stated more than once in formal discussions concerning the moral implications of the *Quinlan* case, most recently two months before he suffered cardiac arrest that left him in an irreversible coma, that he would not want extraordinary means used to keep him alive under similar circumstances). It might also be deduced from a person's religious beliefs and the tenets of that religion, or from the patient's consistent pattern of conduct with respect to prior decisions about his own medical care. Of course, dealing with the matter in advance in some sort of thoughtful and explicit way is best for all concerned.

Any of the above types of evidence, and any other information bearing on the person's intent, may be appropriate aids in determining what course of treatment the patient would have wished to pursue. In this respect, we now believe that we were in error in *Quinlan*, to disregard evidence of statements that Ms. Quinlan made to friends concerning artificial prolongation of the lives of others who were terminally ill. Such evidence is certainly relevant to shed light on whether the patient would have consented to the treatment if competent to make the decision.

Although all evidence tending to demonstrate a person's intent with respect to medical treatment should properly be considered by either surrogate decision-makers, or by a court in the event of any judicial proceedings, the probative value of such evidence may vary depending on the remoteness, consistency, and thoughtfulness of the prior statements or actions and the maturity of the person at the time of the statements or acts. Thus, for example, an offhand remark about not wanting to live under certain circumstances made by a person when young and in the peak of health would not in itself constitute clear proof twenty years later that he would want life-sustaining treatment withheld under those circumstances. In contrast, a carefully considered position, especially if written, that a person had maintained over a number of years or that he had acted upon in comparable circumstances might be clear evidence of his intent.

Another factor that would affect the probative value of a person's prior statements of intent would be their specificity. Of course, no one can predict with accuracy the precise circumstances with which he ultimately might be faced. Nevertheless, any details about the level of impaired functioning and the forms of medical treatment that one would find tolerable should be incorporated into advance directives to enhance their later usefulness as evidence.

Medical evidence bearing on the patient's condition, treatment, and prognosis, like evidence of the patient's wishes, is an essential prerequisite to decision-making under the subjective test. The medical evidence must establish that the patient fits within the Claire Conroy pattern: an elderly, incompetent nursing-home resident with severe and permanent mental and physical impairments and a life expectancy of approximately one year or less. In addition, since the goal is to effectuate the patient's right of informed consent, the surrogate decision-maker must have at least as much medical information upon which to base his decision about what the patient would have chosen as one would expect a competent patient to have before consenting to or rejecting treatment. Such information might include evidence about the patient's present level of physical, sensory, emotional, and cognitive functioning; the degree of physical pain resulting from the medical condition, treatment, and termination of treatment, respectively; the degree of humiliation, dependence, and loss of dignity probably resulting from the condition and treatment; the life expectancy and prognosis for recovery with and without treatment; the various treatment options; and the risks, side effects, and benefits of each of those options. Particular care should be taken not to base a decision on a premature diagnosis or prognosis.

We recognize that for some incompetent patients it might be impossible to be clearly satisfied as to the patient's intent either to accept or reject the life-sustaining treatment. Many people may have spoken of their desires in general or casual terms, or, indeed, never considered or resolved the issue at all. In such cases, a surrogate decision-maker cannot presume that treatment decisions made by a third party on the patient's behalf will further the patient's right to self-determination, since effectuating another person's right to self-determination presupposes that the substitute decision-maker knows what the person would have wanted. Thus, in the absence of adequate proof of the patient's wishes, it is naive to pretend that the right to self-determination serves as the basis for substituted decision-making.

We hesitate, however, to foreclose the possibility of humane actions, which may involve termination of life-sustaining treatment, for persons who never clearly expressed their desires about life-sustaining treatment but who are now suffering a prolonged and painful death. An incompetent, like a minor child, is a ward of the state, and the state's *parens patriae* power supports the authority of its courts to allow decisions to be made for an incompetent that serve the incompetent's best interests, even if the person's wishes cannot be clearly established. This authority permits the state to authorize guardians to withhold or withdraw life-sustaining treatment from an incompetent patient if it is manifest that such action would further the patient's best interests in a narrow sense of the phrase, even though the subjective test that we articulated above may not be satisfied. We therefore hold that life-sustaining treatment may also be withheld or withdrawn from a patient in Claire Conroy's situation if either of two "best interests" tests—a limited-objective or a pure-objective test—is satisfied.

Under the limited-objective test, life-sustaining treatment may be withheld or withdrawn from a patient in Claire Conroy's situation when there is some trustworthy evidence that the patient would have refused the treatment, and the decision-maker is satisfied that it is clear that the burdens of the patient's continued life with the treatment outweigh the benefits of that life for him. By this we mean that the patient is suffering, and will continue to suffer throughout the expected duration of his life, unavoidable pain, and that the net burdens of his prolonged life (the pain and suffering of his life with the treatment less the amount and duration of pain that the patient would likely experience if the treatment were withdrawn) markedly outweigh any physical pleasure, emotional enjoyment, or intellectual satisfaction that the patient may still be able to derive from life. This limited-objective standard permits the termination of treatment for a patient who had not unequivocally expressed his desires before becoming incompetent, when it is clear that the treatment in question would merely prolong the patient's suffering.

Medical evidence will be essential to establish that the burdens of the treatment to the patient in terms of pain and suffering outweigh the benefits that the patient is experiencing. The medical evidence should make it clear that the treatment would merely prolong the patient's suffering and not provide him with any net benefit. Information is particularly important with respect to the degree, expected duration, and constancy of pain with and without treatment, and the possibility that the pain could be reduced by drugs or other means short of terminating the life-sustaining treatment. The same types of medical evidence that are relevant to the subjective analysis, such as the patient's life expectancy, prognosis, level of functioning, degree of humiliation and dependency, and treatment options, should also be considered.

This limited-objective test also requires some trustworthy evidence that the patient would have wanted the treatment terminated. This evidence could take any one or more of the various forms appropriate to prove the patient's intent under the subjective test. Evidence that, taken as a whole, would be too vague, casual, or remote to constitute the clear proof of the patient's subjective intent that is necessary to satisfy the subjective test—for example, informally expressed reactions to other people's medical conditions and treatment—might be sufficient to satisfy this prong of the limited-objective test.

In the absence of trustworthy evidence, or indeed any evidence at all, that the patient would have declined the treatment, life-sustaining treatment may still be withheld or withdrawn from a formerly competent person like Claire Conroy if a third, pure-objective test is satisfied. Under that test, as under the limited-objective test, the net burdens of the patient's life with the treatment should clearly and markedly outweigh the benefits that the patient derives from life. Further, the recurring, unavoidable, and severe pain of the patient's life with the treatment should be such that the effect of administering life-sustaining treatment would be inhumane. Subjective evidence that the patient would not have wanted the treatment is not necessary under this pure-objective standard. Nevertheless, even in the context of severe pain, life-sustaining treatment should not be withdrawn from an incompetent patient who had previously expressed a wish to be kept alive in spite of any pain that he might experience.

Although we are condoning a restricted evaluation of the nature of a patient's life in terms of pain, suffering, and possible enjoyment under the limited-objective and pure-objective tests, we expressly decline to authorize decision-making based on assessments of the personal worth or social utility of another's life, or the value of that life to others. We do not believe that it would be appropriate for a court to designate a person with the authority to determine that someone else's life is not worth living simply because, to that person, the patient's "quality of life" or value to society seems negligible. The mere fact that a patient's functioning is limited or his prognosis dim does not mean that he is not enjoying what remains of his life or that it is in his best interests to die. But see *President's Commission Report*, at 135 (endorsing termination of treatment whenever the surrogate decision-maker in his discretion believes it is in the patient's best interests, defined broadly to "take into account such factors as the relief of suffering, the preservation or restoration of functioning, and the quality as well as the extent of life sustained"). More wide-ranging powers to make decisions about other people's lives, in our view, would create an intolerable risk for socially isolated and defenseless people suffering from physical or mental handicaps.

We are aware that it will frequently be difficult to conclude that the evidence is sufficient to justify termination of treatment under either of the "best interests" tests that we have described. Often, it is unclear whether and to what extent a patient such as Claire Conroy is capable of, or is in fact, experiencing pain. Similarly, medical experts are often unable to determine with any degree of certainty the extent of a nonverbal person's intellectual functioning or the depth of his emotional life. When the evidence is insufficient to satisfy either the limited-objective or pure-objective standard, however, we cannot justify the termination of life-sustaining treatment as clearly furthering the best interests of a patient like Ms. Conroy.

The surrogate decision-maker should exercise extreme caution in determining the patient's intent and in evaluating medical evidence of the patient's pain and possible enjoyment, and should not approve withholding or withdrawing life-sustaining treatment unless he is manifestly satisfied that one of the three tests that we have outlined has been met. When evidence of a person's wishes or physical or mental condition is equivocal, it is best to err, if at all, in favor of preserving life. . . .

II

We emphasize that in making decisions whether to administer life-sustaining treatment to patients such as Claire Conroy, the primary focus should be the patient's desires and experience of pain and enjoyment—not the type of treatment involved.

Thus, we reject the distinction that some have made between actively hastening death by terminating treatment and passively allowing a person to die of a disease as one of limited use in a legal analysis of such a decision-making situation.

Characterizing conduct as active or passive is often an elusive notion, even outside the context of medical decision-making.

> Saint Anselm of Canterbury was fond of citing the trickiness of the distinction between "to do" (*facere*) and "not to do" (*non facere*). In answer to the question "What's he doing?" we say "He's just sitting there" (positive), really meaning something negative: "He's not doing anything at all." [*D. Walton*, at 234 (footnote omitted).]

The distinction is particularly nebulous, however, in the context of decisions whether to withhold or withdraw life-sustaining treatment. In a case like that of Claire Conroy, for example, would a physician who discontinued nasogastric feeding be actively causing her death by removing her primary source of nutrients, or would he merely be omitting to continue the artificial form of treatment, thus passively allowing her medical condition, which includes her inability to swallow, to take its natural course? The ambiguity inherent in this distinction is further heightened when one performs an act within an overall plan of nonintervention, such as when a doctor writes an order not to resuscitate a patient.

> Consequently, merely determining whether what was done involved a fatal act or omission does not establish whether it was morally acceptable. . . . [In fact, a]ctive steps to terminate life-sustaining interventions may be permitted, indeed required, by the patient's authority to forego therapy even when such steps lead to death. [*President's Commission Report*, at 67, 72.]

For a similar reason, we also reject any distinction between withholding and withdrawing life-sustaining treatment. Some commentators have suggested that discontinuing life-sustaining treatment once it has been commenced is morally more problematic than merely failing to begin the treatment. Discontinuing life-sustaining treatment, to some, is an "active" taking of life, as opposed to the more "passive" act of omitting the treatment in the first instance. In the words of one writer, "[T]he difference between taking away that which one has come to count on as normal support for life and not instituting therapy when a new crisis begins . . . fits nicely a basic moral distinction throughout life—we are not morally obligated to help another person, but we are morally obligated not to interfere with his life-sustaining routines."

This distinction is more psychologically compelling than logically sound. As mentioned above, the line between active and passive conduct in the context of medical decisions is far too nebulous to constitute a principled basis for decision-making. Whether necessary treatment is withheld at the outset or withdrawn later on, the consequence—the patient's death—is the same. Moreover, from a policy standpoint, it might well be unwise to forbid persons from discontinuing a treatment under circumstances in which the treatment could permissibly be withheld. Such a rule could discourage families and doctors from even attempting certain types of care and could thereby force them into hasty and premature decisions to allow a patient to die.

Some commentators, as indeed did the Appellate Division here, have made yet a fourth distinction, between the termination of artificial feedings and the termination of other forms of life-sustaining medical treatment. According to the Appellate Division:

> If, as here, the patient is not comatose and does not face imminent and inevitable death, nourishment accomplishes the substantial benefit of sustaining life until the illness takes its natural course. Under such circumstances nourishment always will be an essential element of ordinary care which physicians are ethically obligated to provide. [190 *N.J.Super.* at 473, 464, A.2d 303.]

Certainly, feeding has an emotional significance. As infants we could breathe without assistance, but we were dependent on others for our lifeline of nourishment. Even more, feeding is an expression of nurturing and caring, certainly for infants and children, and in many cases for adults as well.

Once one enters the realm of complex, high-technology medical care, it is hard to shed the "emotional symbolism" of food. However, artificial feedings such as nasogastric tubes, gastrostomies, and intravenous infusions are significantly different from bottle-feeding or spoon-feeding—they are medical procedures with inherent risks and possible side effects, instituted by skilled health-care providers to compensate for impaired physical functioning. Analytically, artificial feeding by means of a nasogastric tube or intravenous infusion can be seen as equivalent to artificial breathing by means of a respirator. Both prolong life through mechanical means when the body is no longer able to perform a vital bodily function on its own.

Furthermore, while nasogastric feeding and other medical procedures to ensure nutrition and hydration are usually well tolerated, they are not free from risks or burdens; they have complications that are sometimes serious and distressing to the patient.

Nasogastric tubes may lead to pneumonia, cause irritation and discomfort, and require arm restraints for an incompetent patient. The volume of fluid needed to carry nutrients itself is sometimes harmful.

Finally, dehydration may well not be distressing or painful to a dying patient. For patients who are unable to sense hunger and thirst, withholding of feeding devices such as nasogastric tubes may not result in more pain than the termination of any other medical treatment. Indeed, it has been observed that patients near death who are not receiving nourishment may be more comfortable than patients in comparable conditions who are being fed and hydrated artificially. Thus, it cannot be assumed that it will always be beneficial for an incompetent patient to receive artificial feeding or harmful for him not to receive it.

Under the analysis articulated above, withdrawal or withholding of artificial feeding, like any other medical treatment, would be permissible if there is sufficient proof to satisfy the subjective, limited-objective, or pure-objective test. A competent patient has the right to decline any medical treatment, including artificial feeding, and should retain that right when and if he becomes incompetent. In addition, in the case of an incompetent patient who has given little or no trustworthy indication of an intent to decline treatment and for whom it becomes necessary to engage in balancing under the limited-objective or pure-objective test, the pain and invasiveness of an artificial feeding device, and the pain of withdrawing that device, should be treated just like the results of administering or withholding any other medical treatment.

III

The decision-making procedure for comatose, vegetative patients suggested in *Quinlan*, namely, the concurrence of the guardian, family, attending physician, and hospital prognosis committee, is not entirely appropriate for patients such as Claire Conroy, who are confined to nursing homes. . . .

Because of the special vulnerability of mentally and physically impaired, elderly persons in nursing homes and the potential for abuse with unsupervised institutional decision-making in such homes, life-sustaining treatment should not be withdrawn or withheld from a nursing-home resident like Claire Conroy in the absence of a guardian's decision, made in accordance with the procedure outlined below, that the elements of the subjective, limited-objective, or pure-objective test have been satisfied. A necessary prerequisite to surrogate decision-making is a judicial determination that the patient is incompetent to make the decision for himself and designation of a guardian for the incompetent patient if he does not already have one.

As noted above, the guardian will resolve the issues in these matters and make the ultimate decision with such concurrences as we have required. Ordinarily, court involvement will be limited to the determination of incompetency, and the appointment of a guardian unless a personal guardian has been previously appointed, who will determine whether the standards we have prescribed have been satisfied. The record in this case did not satisfy those standards. The evidence that Claire Conroy would have refused the treatment, although sufficient to meet the lower showing of intent required under the limited-objective test, was certainly not the "clear" showing of intent contemplated under the subjective test. More information should, if possible, have been obtained by the guardian with respect to Ms. Conroy's intent. What were her ethical, moral, and religious beliefs? She did try to refuse initial hospitalization, and indeed had "scorned medicine." However, she allowed her nephew's wife, a registered nurse, to care for her during several illnesses. It was not clear whether Ms. Conroy permitted the niece to administer any drugs or other forms of medical treatment to her during these illnesses. Although it may often prove difficult, and at times impossible, to ascertain a person's wishes, the Conroy case illustrates the sources to which the guardian might turn. For example, in more than eight decades of life in the same house, it is possible that she revealed to persons other than her nephew her feelings regarding medical treatment, other values, and her goals in life. Some promising avenues for such an inquiry about her personal values included her response to the illnesses and deaths of her sisters and others, and her statements with respect to not wanting to be in a nursing home.

Moreover, there was insufficient information concerning the benefits and burdens of Ms. Conroy's life to satisfy either the limited-objective or pure-objective test. Although the treating doctor and the guardian's expert testified as to Claire Conroy's condition, neither testified conclusively as to whether she was in pain or was capable of experiencing pain or thirst. There was medical agreement that removal of the tube would have caused pain during the period of approximately one week that would have elapsed before her death, or at least until she were to lapse into a coma. On the other hand, there was little, if any, evidence of the discomfort, suffering, and pain she would endure if she continued to be fed and medicated through the tube during her remaining life—contemplated to be up to one year. Apparently her feedings sometimes occasioned moaning, but it remains unclear whether these were reflex responses or expressions of discomfort. Moreover, although she tried to remove the tube, it is not clear that this was intentional, and there was little evidence that she was in distress. Her treating physician also offered contradictory views as to whether the contractures of her legs caused pain or whether, indeed, they might be the result of pain, without offering any evidence on that issue. The trial court rejected as superfluous the offer to present as an expert witness a neurologist, who might have been able to explain what Ms. Conroy's reactions to the environment indicated about her perception of pain.

The evidence was also unclear with respect to Ms. Conroy's capacity to feel pleasure, another issue as to which the information supplied by a neurologist might have been helpful. What was known of her awareness of the world? Although Ms. Conroy had some ability to smile and scratch, the relationship of these activities to external stimuli apparently was quite variable.

The trial transcript reveals no exploration of the discomfort and risks that attend nasogastric feedings. A casual mention by the nurse/administrator of the need to restrain the patient to prevent the removal of the tube was not followed by an assessment of the detrimental impact, if any, of those restraints. Alternative modalities, including gastrostomies, intravenous feeding, subcutaneous or intramuscular hydration, or some combination, were not investigated. Neither of the expert witnesses presented empirical evidence regarding the treatment options for such a patient.

It can be seen that the evidence at trial was inadequate to satisfy the subjective, the limited-objective, or the pure-objective standard that we have set forth. Were Claire Conroy still alive, the guardian would have been required to explore these issues prior to reaching any decision. Guardians—and courts, if they are involved—should act cautiously and deliberately in deciding these cases. The consequences are most serious—life or death. . . .

The judgment of the Appellate Division is reversed. In light of Ms. Conroy's death, we do not remand the matter for further proceedings.

HANDLER, J., concurring in part and dissenting in part. . . .

In my opinion, the Court's objective tests too narrowly define the interests of people like Miss Conroy. While the basic standard purports to account for several concerns, it ultimately focuses on pain as the critical factor. The presence of significant pain in effect becomes the sole measure of such a person's best interests. "Pain" thus eclipses a whole cluster of other human values that have a proper place in the subtle weighing that will ultimately determine how life should end.

The Court's concentration on pain as the exclusive criterion in reaching the life-or-death decision in reality transmutes the best-interests determination into an exercise of avoidance and nullification rather than confrontation and fulfillment. In most cases the pain criterion will dictate that the decision be one not to withdraw life-prolonging treatment and not to allow death to occur naturally. First, pain will not be an operative factor in a great many cases. "[P]resently available drugs and techniques allow pain to be reduced to a level acceptable to virtually every patient, usually without unacceptable sedation." *President's Commission Report*, at 50–51. *See id.* at 19 n. 19 *citing* Saunders, "Current Views on Pain Relief and Terminal Care," in *The Therapy of Pain* 215 (Swerdlow, ed. 1981) (a hospice reports complete control of pain in over 99% of its dying patients). Further, as was true in Miss Conroy's case, health care providers frequently encounter difficulty in evaluating the degree of pain experienced by a patient. Finally, "[o]nly a minority of patients—fewer than half of those with malignancies, for example—have substantial problems with pain. . . ." *President's Commission Report*, at 278. Thus, in a great many cases, the pain test will become an absolute bar to the withdrawal of life-support therapy.

The pain requirement, as applied by the Court in its objective tests, effectively negates other highly relevant considerations that should appropriately bear on the decision to maintain or to withdraw life-prolonging treatment. The pain standard may dictate the decision to prolong life despite the presence of other factors that reasonably militate in favor of the termination of such procedures to allow a natural death. The exclusive pain criterion denies relief to that class of people who, at the very end of life, might strongly disapprove of an artificially extended existence in spite of the absence of pain. Thus, some people abhor dependence on others as much, or more, than they fear pain. Other individuals value personal privacy and dignity, and prize independence from others when their personal needs and bodily functions are involved. Finally, the ideal of bodily integrity may become more important than simply prolonging life at its most rudimentary level. Persons, like Miss Conroy, "may well have wished to avoid . . . '[t]he ultimate horror [not of] death but the possibility of being maintained in limbo, in a sterile room, by machines controlled by strangers.'" *In re Torres*, 357 N.W.2d at 340, quoting Steel, "The Right to Die: New Options in California," 93 *Christian Century* [July–Dec. 1976].

Clearly, a decision to focus exclusively on pain as the single criterion ignores and devalues other important ideals regarding life and death. Consequently, a pain standard cannot serve as an indirect proxy for additional and significant concerns that may bear on the decision to forgo life-prolonging treatments. . . .

I would therefore have the Court adopt a test that does not rely exclusively on pain as the ultimately determinative criterion. Rather, the standard should consist of an array of factors to be medically established and then evaluated by the decision-maker both singly and collectively to reach a balance that will justify the determination to withdraw or to continue life-prolonging treatment. The withdrawal of life-prolonging treatment from an unconscious or comatose, terminally ill individual near death, whose personal views concerning life-ending treatment cannot be ascertained, should be governed by such a standard.

Several important criteria bear on this critical determination. The person should be terminally ill and facing imminent death. There should also be present the permanent loss of conscious thought processes in the form of a comatose state or profound unconsciousness. Further, there should be the irreparable failure of at least one major and essential bodily organ or system. Obviously the presence or absence of significant pain is highly relevant.

In addition, the person's general physical condition must be of great concern. Progressive, irreversible, extensive, and extreme physical deterioration, such as ulcers, lesions, gangrene, infection, incontinence, and the like, which frequently afflict the bedridden, terminally ill, should be considered in the formulation of an appropriate standard. The medical and nursing treatment of individuals in *extremis* and suffering from these conditions entails the constant and extensive handling and manipulation of the body. At some point, such a course of treatment upon the insensate patient is bound to touch the sensibilities of even the most detached observer. Eventually, pervasive bodily intrusions, even for the best motives, will arouse feelings akin to humiliation and mortification for the helpless patient. When cherished values of human dignity and personal privacy, which belong to every person living or dying, are sufficiently transgressed by what is being done to the individual, we should be ready to say: enough.

In my view, our understanding as to how life should end must be infused with the fundamental human moral values that serve us while we live. As we have faced life, so should we be able to face death. When an individual's personal philosophy or moral values cannot otherwise be brought to bear to resolve the dilemma of whether to live or die, then factors that generally and normally shape basic human moral values should be taken into account. These factors should be assessed reasonably and fairly from the patient's perspective. They should be weighed and balanced by an appropriate, responsible surrogate decision-maker in reaching the final awesome decision whether to withdraw life-prolonging treatment from the unfortunate and hapless patient. I believe that a decision informed by these considerations would be conducive to the humane, dignified, and decent ending of life.

THE SEVERELY DEMENTED, MINIMALLY FUNCTIONAL PATIENT: AN ETHICAL ANALYSIS

John D. Arras

Mrs. Smith, an 85-year-old resident of a nursing home, was transferred to the hospital for treatment of pneumonia. Although she has responded well to antibiotic therapy, her overall condition and prognosis remain grim. For the past 3 years her mental state has been steadily deteriorating due to a series of strokes which have finally rendered her severely demented. She is now nonambulatory, incapable of sitting up in bed, and uncommunicative most of the time. When she does talk, her speech is completely incoherent and repetitive. Mrs. Smith shows no signs of recognizing or remembering her family and primary caregivers. The nurses in charge of her care assert that she appears to experience pleasure only when her hair is combed or her back rubbed.

During her recovery from the pneumonia, Mrs. Smith began to have problems with swallowing food. Following a precipitous decline in her caloric intake, her son and daughter (the only involved family members) consented to the placement of a nasogastric tube. Mrs. Smith continually pulled out the tube, however, and continues to resist efforts to reinsert it.

The health care team faces difficult choices regarding Mrs. Smith's care. Foremost among them is whether her physicians should surgically insert a gastrostomy tube in spite of her aversive behavior. Mrs. Smith has neither left behind a living will nor has she indicated to family or friends at the nursing home what her preferences would be regarding life-sustaining care in this sort of circumstance. Both her son and daughter have stated that she would nevertheless not have wanted a gastrostomy tube inserted and would, if she could presently decide, prefer an earlier death to being sustained indefinitely in the twilight of her minimally functional condition. In defense of this claim, they note that she has always been a very active, independent person who avoided doctors whenever possible.

PROBING THE PATIENT'S SUBJECTIVITY

The first order of business in deciding for incompetent patients is to inquire, whenever possible, what the patient would want were she presently able to communicate. In the absence of a designated proxy or living will that speaks with rare precision about which modes of treatment are to be forgone under which circumstances, this task is more difficult than many commentators and jurists would have us think. The case before us yields two distinct sources of revelation bearing on the patient's putative subjective wishes regarding the present decision. As we

From *Journal of the American Geriatrics Society* 36 (1988): 938–944. Reprinted with permission.

shall see, neither provides evidence sufficiently compelling for us to conclude with moral certitude that she would not allow the insertion of a G-tube.

Extrapolating from the Patient's Prior Values

First, we have the testimony of family members who claim that the patient's character traits of independence and aloofness from physicians point to the conclusion that she would not want to be sustained by a G-tube. Although this claim may well be *plausible* and at least *consistent* with Mrs. Smith's previously held attitudes and behaviors, it would require a great leap of both faith and logic to conclude that evidence of this sort *entails* a negative decision on life-sustaining treatment. As several commentators have pointed out, there is a great difference between the degree of respect owed to a patient's *actual choices*, even choices made prior to the advent of incompetency, and to his or her preferences or tastes.[1–4] It is one thing to have negative attitudes toward aggressive life support, but it is quite another to actually refuse it in your own case. By doing so, a person *commits* himself or herself to a particular course of action and it is this commitment, rather than mere attitudes or generalized preferences abstracted from the particular details of choosing situations, that commands especially stringent respect.

Even if someone's generalized views about life, dependency, and doctors deserve the status of right claims, which they do not, they usually do not yield unequivocal answers to treatment dilemmas. Supposing that Mrs. Smith was indeed fiercely independent and skeptical of the medical profession, does this necessarily mean that she would prefer death to her present "twilight state" sustained by tube feedings? Conversely, if Mrs. Smith were an exceptionally dependent sort of person who actively sought and followed the advice of physicians, would that mean that she would presently prefer an indefinite extension of her barely conscious existence to an early death? Although such character traits indisputably have *some* evidentiary value, they appear to be compatible with a range of possible responses.[4] In Mrs. Smith's case, it is certainly *plausible* that she would decline the insertion of a G-tube, but that is not the only plausible interpretation. For all we know, she might have been content, were she miraculously lucid and communicative for an instant, to accede to the operation rather than go peacefully into that dark night. The question for Mrs. Smith's caregivers, then—and we shall explore this point more fully later on—is not whether her loved ones have provided a uniquely correct extrapolation of her previous values to her present situation, for in most cases that will simply be an unattainable goal; rather, the question is whether their plausible invocations of her values and character traits should be given the benefit of the doubt.

The Evidentiary Value of Aversive Behavior

Mrs. Smith has been constantly pulling out her nasogastric tube and waving off the attentions of her caregivers. What are we to make of this behavior? In contrast to the patient's previous preferences and attitudes, which are ill-matched in their generality to the concreteness of the present situation, Mrs. Smith's aversive behavior at least has the advantage of being contemporaneous. She is extubating herself right here and now. According to Daniel Callahan,[5] a philosopher who generally sees no justification for terminating food and fluids in severely demented patients, such behavior constitutes a "clear signal" mandating withdrawal of the tube.

But a clear signal of what? It is crucial to remember at this juncture that Mrs. Smith is severely demented and completely incompetent. Even though her aversive behavior occurs in the present, it is the behavior of a woman who has completely lost her rational capacity. She cannot even recognize her family, let alone engage in sophisticated deliberations bearing on the respective benefits and burdens of continued tube feeding in her minimally functional state versus an earlier death. Aphasic but otherwise competent patients might be able to send clear signals under such circumstances, but not Mrs. Smith, whose behavior appears to be freighted with a variety of possible meanings.

It is possible that her tube-pulling represents a firm and fixed present desire to forgo aggressive life-sustaining treatments in favor of an early death. It is also possible that it signals some kind of deeply sedimented personal desire manifested in spite of her present incompetence. But it is equally possible that her aversive behavior is nothing more than an elemental reflex signaling only her transient irritation from the tube. Nasogastric tubes *are* bothersome and sometimes painful intrusions, and one need not entertain sophisticated benefit-burden calculations to wish merely to be rid of such noxious stimuli. Thus, the interpretive options range from deeply intentional options for death in the face of minimally functional existence to reflexes of an almost exclusively physiological nature.

Mrs. Smith's "signal" is thus anything but clear, and this is a significant fact for her caregivers to ponder. While aversive behavior expressive of deeply sedimented personal values should be accorded the same degree of respect allotted to general character traits and attitudes, aversive reflexes to unpleasant stimuli should command little, if any, deference from surrogate decision-makers. Small children extubate themselves all the time, but no one would view such actions as a "clear signal" of a wish to die. The real problem facing Mrs. Smith's physicians is that they have no reliable way of discerning the "real meaning" behind her ongoing resistance to feeding tubes. It would certainly help if Mrs. Smith had been known to shun tube feeding even while she was competent, for that would at least provide some plausible evidence connecting her presently aversive behavior to sedimented preferences. But in the absence of such a record, the meaning of her "rejection" remains profoundly unclear.

Given the inconclusiveness of this inquiry into the patient's previous attitudes and present behavior, her caregivers might reasonably shift their focus of attention away from the patient's elusive subjectivity and toward a more objective assessment of her "best interests."

THE BEST-INTERESTS STANDARD

In the absence of reliable indicators of the patient's actual or hypothetical preferences, courts and commentators recommend an inquiry into the best interests of the patient.[6,7] What course of action (or inaction) will bring about the best overall result for the patient? Rather than finding this "objective" path an easier route to the correct decision, caregivers attempting to apply such a test to the case of a severely demented, minimally functional patient such as Mrs. Smith will immediately confront a series of equally perplexing questions. What will be the actual impact of placing a G-tube on Mrs. Smith's well-being? What definition of the good will ground their assessments of her best interests? And, given her low level of functioning, is it quite accurate even to describe Mrs. Smith as a full-fledged "person" with actual, discernable interests? Since these exceedingly difficult questions lack intuitively obvious answers, perhaps the best way to proceed is to examine categories of patients on either side of Mrs. Smith on the continuum of incompetency, categories that do yield fairly firm moral intuitions, and then attempt to locate a proper response to her case by means of "moral triangulation." Needless to say, the clarity and distinctness of these idealized categories often become somewhat blurred in real clinical situations, but there is still considerable theoretical value in discussing our responses to clear-cut cases.

Patients in Persistent Vegetative States

What if, instead of being minimally functional, Mrs. Smith were completely nonfunctional? (We shall call this hypothetical patient Mrs. Jones.) What if, instead of slowly declining into a twilight of consciousness, she were to have experienced a protracted period of anoxia that consigned her to a persistently vegetative condition? Although still alive, Mrs. Jones would subsist on brain-stem activity alone, her neocortex—the physical substratum of her capacity for consciousness—having been completely destroyed. She would thus persist in countless sleep-wake cycles, unable to connect with the world and with her past through conscious awareness, unable to plan or hope for better circumstances, unable even to perceive pleasure or pain. What rights, if any, would Mrs. Jones have, and what duties would be owed her by caregivers?

If we were to apply straightforwardly the best-interests test to the case of Mrs. Jones, we would be hard-pressed to discover actual interests that could be meaningfully imputed to her. Lacking consciousness, she lacks a conception of herself as a moral agent with real interests in continued life and in the pursuit of her own vision of the good. Lacking the ability to experience pleasure and pain, she cannot be physically benefitted or harmed.[8] Indeed, as several commentators have pointed out, her only remaining interest in staying alive is based on the miniscule possibility that she has been misdiagnosed and could possibly regain some degree of consciousness in the future.[9] Apart from that slimmest of chances, she has no interests that might be assessed through a best-interests test.

If we seek a solution to the problem of Mrs. Jones in an examination of her best interests, we discover the paradoxical result that her best interests will probably be served by further treatment. True, except for the possibility of misdiagnosis, she cannot be benefitted in any way by continued existence, but her lack of capacity for conscious experience renders her equally incapable of being harmed by further treatments and the extension of her life. Thus, we cannot say, as the best-interests test would appear to require, that Mrs. Jones is being excessively burdened by her treatments or that she would be "better-off dead." This result is indeed paradoxical, because if anyone's life need not be maintained, one would think that patients in persistently vegetative conditions must be at the top of the list.

Given the vanishingly small likelihood of misdiagnosis, especially after the passage of several weeks, I would argue that it is ethically appropriate to treat all PVS patients as though they had no interests either for or against treatment. Since continued medical interventions cannot realistically be thought to benefit them in any way, since caregivers cannot realistically be thought to have duties toward patients who cannot be helped or harmed, and since such treatments entail considerable costs—including the expenditure of huge sums of money, the time and energy of caregivers, and emotional strains on survivors—they may be ethically forgone.

The important lesson here is that although a rigorously patient-centered best-interests test might be ethically appropriate in most cases involving incompetent patients, it cannot be meaningfully applied when the patient under consideration lacks all fundamentally human capacities. In cases such as this, a judgment in favor of nontreatment must be based not on an objective weighing of benefits and burdens to the patient—for such patients are capable of neither benefit nor burden—but rather upon a judgment that the patient has ceased to be a "person" in any meaningful moral sense. Once this determination has been made, it is then ethically permissible to consider the financial and emotional impact of continued treatment upon other interested parties.[10] Certainly some families will, for religious or other personal reasons, continue to request life-sustaining treatments for their persistently vegetative relations; but others would be acting ethically to request the termination of all medical care, including artificially administered food and fluids.

Marginally Functional Patients

On the other side of Mrs. Smith are those patients who might usefully be described as "marginally functional." Mr. Black, for example, is a 90-year-old man presenting with rectal bleeding and suspected colon cancer who refuses a laparotomy to confirm the diagnosis. "I have lived a good life," he says, "and I don't want any surgery." His daughter, to whom he appears very close, concurs with his decision. Although Mr. Black appears on the surface to be sufficiently competent to make this decision, subsequent examinations by liaison psychiatrists reveal a glaring absence of short-term memory and significant confusion about his medical diagnosis and surroundings. He is described as "pleasantly demented."

Although patients like Mr. Black are strictly speaking incapable of rational decision-making most or all of the time, they differ from Mrs. Jones in their ability to reason, albeit rather poorly, in their ability to relate to other persons, and in their capacities to experience emotions, pain, and pleasure. Notwithstanding their inability to make most health care decisions, these patients are clearly "persons" with a multitude of interests that can be advanced or frustrated by their caregivers. In spite of their deficits and relatively low quality of life, such moderately functional patients have every right to a patient-centered best-interests analysis. While invasive, painful, and risky surgery may or may not eventually be deemed to be in Mr. Black's best interests, his capacities for experiencing the world are sufficiently intact to rule out any thought of forgoing other sorts of life-sustaining therapies, such as artificial nutrition and hydration.

The Minimally Functional Patient

Returning now to the example of Mrs. Smith, we find her to fall squarely between the permanently vegetative and moderately functional patient. Like the totally nonfunctional, vegetative patient, she is so demented that she lacks most of the criteria of "moral personhood."[11] Unfortunately, she appears to have been reduced to a mere shell of her former self. She can no longer reason, communicate (except in the most rudimentary, reflexive manner), relate to her family, or experience manifestations of love. Indeed, it is doubtful that she can be accurately described as a self-conscious, moral agent whose identity through time is cemented by the bonds of memory. There is, in cases such as this where the psychological glue of memory has given out, simply no enduring "self" there.[12] Formerly a self-conscious moral agent with a well-defined idea of the good, hopes and plans for the future, Mrs. Smith has been reduced to a mere locus of transient sensations. As philosopher James Rachels[13] puts it, she continues to have biological life, but her *biographical* life has come to an end.

On the other hand, Mrs. Smith resembles Mr. Black at least in her possession of some conscious life, albeit on a very low level, and in her ability to experience pleasure, pain, and perhaps some rudimentary emotions. Although she is not a "person" in the strict sense, she does have some interests. Insofar as she is open to pleasure and pain, she has a definite interest in experiencing the former and avoiding the latter. How might a "best-interests" test be applied to someone like Mrs. Smith?

Better-Off Dead? In order to justify the termination of food and fluids under a best-interests test, decision-makers would have to show that the burdens of a patient's life with the proposed treatment would clearly and markedly outweigh whatever benefits she might derive from continued life.[7] In other words, they would have to show that the patient would be "better-off dead."

The most influential formulation of this best-interests test, the majority opinion in the Conroy case, requires not merely that the burdens of life clearly outweigh the benefits, but also that further treatment would be inhumane due to the presence of severe and uncontrollable pain.[7] The court's motivation in establishing such a strict standard is not hard to grasp. While people might disagree about the desirability of persisting in a minimally functional condition, severe and intractable pain is presumably something that just about everyone would prefer to avoid. It is this nearly universal sentiment that death would be preferable to a life of unmitigated pain and suffering that gives this test an air of "objectivity," as opposed to the subjectivity of tests based upon the patient's past preferences.

How then would this strict formula apply to Mrs. Smith? As we have seen, there isn't much to place in the "benefits" column. No longer able to take food by mouth or to interact meaningfully with her family and caregivers, it appears that Mrs. Smith experiences few pleasures apart from an occasional rub or combing. The only possible benefit to be derived from further treatment would appear to be the indefinite continuation of this twilight existence. And although the patient might conceivably derive some pleasure merely from lying in bed and dwelling in her alien world, it is highly doubtful that such a patient—bereft of memory, a sense of continuing selfhood, hopes, and plans—could possibly have an interest in, or be benefitted by, *continued* existence.

Given Mrs. Smith's low level of existence, it is equally difficult to discern the burdens of continued treatment. To be sure, she will experience some degree of pain and discomfort from the surgical insertion of a G-tube, but this pain will not approximate the kind of prolonged, severe, and intractable pain required by the Conroy best-interests formula.

Another possible source of pain and suffering would be the forcible imposition of medical treatment against the wishes of the incompetent patient. Even incompetent patients can have strong preferences for or against treatment or diagnostic procedures, and even if these preferences are not well grounded in medical reality or in the patient's previously authentic value system, forcible treatment will often be experienced as a painful and humiliating violation. Although this kind of coercion need not be thought of as a violation of the patient's autonomy, which may have already been destroyed by dementia, the pain, humiliation, distrust, and hostility it engenders must nevertheless be counted in any best-interests calculation. In some cases, Mr. Black's for example, the negative consequences of forcing treatment may not be worth the gains.

In Mrs. Smith's case, however, the side effects of coercive treatment are likely to be nonexistent. As we have already seen, her aversive reaction to NG tube feeding could just as easily be ascribed to immediate physical discomfort as to some deep-seated desire to die through the refusal of life-sustaining treatment. Mrs. Smith is probably too demented at this point to have preferences about tube feedings or to acknowledge the forcible imposition of surgery over against her aversive behavior. It is highly unlikely, then, that she would experience the insertion of a G-tube as a violation of her wishes (no matter how distorted) or as a painful humiliation.

In the absence of any persistent and severe pain underlying her condition, it would appear highly doubtful that the burdens of Mrs. Smith's continued existence clearly and markedly outweigh the benefits, even when the benefits approach zero. A literal reading and application of the Conroy formula would thus lead to the conclusion that the G-tube should be surgically implanted and that she should be maintained indefinitely with artificial nutrition and hydration.

Limitations of the Best-Interests Standard Not everyone will be satisfied with this result. Those who believe that quality of life should never affect treatment decisions will no doubt applaud this conclusion, but others might well think that something important has been left out of our deliberations. Judge Handler,[7] the lone dissenter in *Conroy*, identifies this missing factor as a legitimate concern for the patient's probable feelings about broader issues, such as privacy, dependency, dignity, and bodily integrity. By focusing the entire best-interests discussion upon the narrow issue of pain, we tend to reduce the patient from the full-fledged person that she once was to the status of a mere physical repository of pleasures and pains. Is this crudely hedonistic notion of the good an adequate or desirable measure of humane treatment decisions for minimally functional patients? Should we simply ignore the patient's probable responses to such abject dependency and daily violations of dignity?

Although Judge Handler's dissent eloquently pinpoints a major shortcoming of the *Conroy* best-interests formula, it is problematical in its own right. Specifically, it is unclear how Judge Handler's concerns for these larger issues of privacy and dignity might be grafted onto the *Conroy* best-interests formula. That test, let us recall, attempts to ascertain the *present* best interests of patients; it asks about the present and future benefits and burdens likely to be experienced by the patient. The obvious problem for Judge Handler's proposed enlargement of this formula is that severely demented, minimally functional patients like Mrs. Smith are presently incapable of experiencing what more functional patients would describe as insults to their privacy, dignity, and physical integrity. Although it is quite possible that the formerly competent Mrs. Smith would have been appalled at the loss of dignity entailed by her present situation, the present Mrs. Smith knows nothing of dignitary insults or violations of privacy. She is so demented that she cannot be affected, one way or the other, by solicitude for her present responses to these larger, humanistic issues.

In order to vindicate Judge Handler's concerns, we will have to reintroduce them at the stage of our inquiry into the patient's prior preferences (i.e., the substituted judgment test). Under that test, we would have to show that Mrs. Smith would have clearly viewed continued treatment under these circumstances as an indignity, and that she would have preferred an early death to the insertion of a G-tube. The problem with this move is that, as we have already seen, Mrs. Smith left behind neither a precise advance directive nor a pattern of analogous choices that clearly demonstrate what she would have wanted under present circumstances. Indeed, our earlier failure to provide this sort of clear evidence mandated our present effort to find a solution in terms of Mrs. Smith's best interests.

So we have come full circle. Our inability to satisfy a rigorous substituted judgment test required us to search for a solution in terms of Mrs. Smith's best interests. But the best-interests test, at least as articulated in *Conroy*, led to an unacceptably narrow focus on pain that excluded important values. Mrs. Smith's present lack of capacity to appreciate such values finally led us back again to the substituted judgment test. Clearly, something has gone wrong here.

A PROCEDURAL SOLUTION

According to lawyer-bioethicist Nancy Rhoden,[4] the problem lies not in our inability to come up with better evidence of a patient's wishes or level of pain and suffering, but rather in the questions we are asking. She argues convincingly that both the substituted judgment and best-interests tests set the standard of evidence far too high. By requiring *clear and convincing* evidence either that a patient's prior values would dictate the withdrawal of life-sustaining treatment or that the burdens of a patient's life outweigh the benefits, these tests establish a standard that cannot realistically be met by the kinds of evidence we are likely to have at our disposal. As we have seen, in the absence of a carefully drafted living will, a durable power of attorney, or severe and intractable pain, it will rarely be *clear* either that a patient would have refused treatment or that death is in her best interests. Given the usual evidentiary materials at hand, in most cases the best we can do is conclude that forgoing treatment is *probably* what the patient would have wanted, or that death is *likely* to be in the patient's best interests, although we will never know for sure in either case.

To be sure, there are some easy cases where a patient's best interests are clearly and perceptibly being violated. For example, greedy relatives might request the termination of treatment that could realistically return the patient to a good quality of life; or guilt-ridden relatives might press for full resuscitative measures on a moribund patient riddled with metastatic cancer. But apart from such clear-cut cases of unmistakable undertreatment and overtreatment, most of the truly problematical cases (like Mrs. Smith's) fall into a vast gray area between these extremes where the patient's best interests will remain unclear and largely inscrutable. Our problem, then, is that we have been asking questions for which there exist, in most of the hard cases at least, no clearly correct answers.

Rhoden's solution, in which I concur, is to bypass this substantive impasse with a procedural solution. Taking her cue from the President's Commission report[6] addressed to the problem of severely impaired newborns, she argues that when a proposed course of action falls into the gray area of uncertainty, involved and well-intentioned family members should have discretion to decide as they see fit. Presumably, they will invoke precisely the same kinds of evidence bearing on the patient's value system, religious affiliation, quality of life, and the potential benefits and burdens of treatment, but they would not be held to a standard of evidence requiring that their choice be uniquely correct.

To be sure, many caring and well-meaning family members will also want to weigh the impact of continued treatment upon themselves and the family unit. Sometimes the ongoing provision of care and treatment to severely demented patients like Mrs. Smith can impose great burdens, both financial and emotional, upon families. I believe that such concerns are for the most part inevitable and that they often subtly color treatment decisions even when officially banished under the auspices of the usual ethical-legal standards. This is to be expected and should not give us grounds for concern so long as the case originally falls within the gray area of ethical ambiguity, and so long as the interests of family do not *clearly* violate the best interests of the patient.

The correct question for us, then, is not whether forgoing treatment is clearly the right answer, but rather whether Mrs. Smith's case falls into the problematical gray area. If it does, then the decision of a trustworthy surrogate should prevail over objections from caregivers, unless the latter can show a clear violation of best interests. Since a case must exhibit considerable ethical ambiguity to fall into this gray zone in the first place, we should expect that well-meaning and ethically sensitive people will reach different conclusions about the care of such patients. The opinions of trustworthy surrogates should be given priority simply because they are usually in the best position to assess the prior wishes and best interests of incompetent patients, and because their familial and emotional bonding to patients usually gives them a greater claim than members of the health care team.[6]

What, then, are the boundaries of the gray area? When is a case sufficiently ambiguous to warrant our trust in surrogate decision-making? We can begin with a reassertion of the *Conroy* case's best-interests formula. If a patient's capacity for benefitting from continued life appears to be eclipsed by the constant presence of severe and intractable pain, then the case falls either in the gray area or the clear-cut zone of nontreatment. I would add that this imbalance of burdens over benefits need not be conclusively proven by clear and convincing evidence. It should be sufficient merely for the surrogate to make a strong case that the burdens are disproportionate to the benefits. In Mrs. Smith's case, however, no such claim can be made.

In the absence of severe pain, we must ask whether the patient is genuinely capable of benefitting from continued existence. Does she recognize and interact with other persons, including her family and caregivers? Does she have a sufficiently intact self to conceive of the future and to care about what happens in it? If the answers to these questions are negative, even if the patient is capable of some rudimentary physical pleasures, I would argue that the patient has no real interest in either continued life or the administration of life-sustaining treatments and thus falls squarely into the gray area.

Mrs. Smith fits this profile. She is so demented that she cannot recognize family or caregivers. Her memory is so depleted, and her sense of self so fractured, that she cannot be said to have genuinely human interests.

Since the boundaries of this morally ambiguous zone will inevitably correspond to the limits of societal toleration, it will often be helpful to ask what most reasonable people would want for themselves in this circumstance. Although this question is generally not allowed in more patient-centered inquiries into the patient's prior preferences or best interests, it should be allowable here, where we are merely trying to determine whether a case is sufficiently morally problematic to fit into the gray zone. If we ask the question with regard to Mrs. Smith, I think that the overwhelming majority of persons would say that they would rather die than continue to live in such a physically, emotionally, and socially impoverished state.

Another useful clue is to ask how we would have responded to Mrs. Smith's death from lack of adequate nutrition had it occurred prior to the advent of artificial feeding. No doubt there would have been the inevitable sadness associated with the death of any human being, but there would have been no shock, no outrage, no sense of tragedy, nor even any feeling that death had deprived her of any real benefits. The predominant response to such a death would most likely have been relief, both for the sake of the patient and for her loved ones.

In such cases, the only apparent rationale for the imposition of life-sustaining technologies is that since they exist, they must be used. And the more they are used, the more pervasive their presence in hospital and long-term care facilities, the more their expanded use assumes the necessity of a moral imperative. But it is precisely here, in cases such as Mrs. Smith's, that we must pause to ask about the proper uses of such technologies. If they do nothing to further the real interests of patients, if all they do is to prolong the biological existence of patients whose biographical lives have long since come to an end, then biomedical technologies assume the status of idols—i.e., inanimate objects worshipped by the human beings who created them, objects that return to dominate us rather than serving our purposes.

NOTES

1. Dworkin R: Autonomy and the Demented Self. *Milbank Quarterly* 64: supp. 2, 4–16, 1986.
2. Buchanan A, Brock DW: Deciding for Others. *Milbank Quarterly* 64:supp. 2, 71, 1986.
3. Dresser R: Life, Death, and Incompetent Patients: Conceptual Infirmities and Hidden Values in the Law. *Arizona Law Review* 28: 376–379, 1986.
4. Rhoden NK: Litigating Life and Death. *Harvard Law Review* 102: 2, 375–446, Dec. 1988.
5. Callahan D: *Setting Limits: Medical Goals in an Aging Society*. New York, Simon & Schuster, 1987, p. 192.
6. President's Commission for the Study of Ethical Problems in Medicine and Biomedical and Behavioral Research: Deciding to Forego Life Sustaining Treatment. Washington, D.C., U.S. Government Printing Office, 1983, p. 134 ff.
7. In re Conroy, 98 N.J. 321, 486 A.2d 1209 (1985).
8. Cranford RE: The Persistent Vegetative State: The Medical Reality (Getting the Facts Straight). *Hastings Cent Rep* 18:27–32, Feb./Mar. 1988.
9. Feinberg J: The Rights of Animals and Unborn Generations, in *Rights, Justice, and the Bounds of Liberty*.

Princeton, Princeton University Press, 1980, pp. 176–177.

10. Arras JD: Quality of Life in Neonatal Ethics: Beyond Denial and Evasion, in Weil WB, Benjamin M, (eds): *Ethical Issues at the Outset of Life*. Boston, Blackwell, 1987, pp. 151–186.
11. Engelhardt HT: *The Foundations of Bioethics*. New York, Oxford University Press, 1986.
12. Brock DW: Justice and the Severely Demented Elderly. *J Med Philos* 13:1, 73–99, Feb. 1988.
13. Rachels J: *The End of Life*. New York, Oxford University Press, 1986.

NUTRITION AND HYDRATION: MORAL AND PASTORAL REFLECTIONS

U.S. Bishops' Pro-Life Committee

INTRODUCTION

Modern medical technology seems to confront us with many questions not faced even a decade ago. Corresponding changes in medical practice have benefited many, but have also prompted fears by some that they will be aggressively treated against their will or denied the kind of care that is their due as human persons with inherent dignity. Current debates about life-sustaining treatment suggest that our society's moral reflection is having difficulty keeping pace with its technological progress.

A religious view of life has an important contribution to make to these modern debates. Our Catholic tradition has developed a rich body of thought on these questions, which affirms a duty to preserve human life but recognizes limits to that duty.

Our first goal in making this statement is to reaffirm some basic principles of our moral tradition, to assist Catholics and others in making treatment decisions in accord with respect for God's gift of life.

These principles do not provide clear and final answers to all moral questions that arise as individuals make difficult decisions. Catholic theologians may differ on how best to apply moral principles to some questions not explicitly resolved by the church's teaching authority. Likewise, we understand that those who must make serious healthcare decisions for themselves or for others face a complexity of issues, circumstances, thoughts and emotions in each unique case.

This is the case with some questions involving the medically assisted provision of nutrition and hydration to helpless patients—those who are seriously ill, disabled or persistently unconscious. These questions have been made more urgent by widely publicized court cases and the public debate to which they have given rise.

Our second purpose in issuing this statement, then, is to provide some clarification of the moral issues involved in decisions about medically assisted nutrition and hydration. We are fully aware that such guidance is not necessarily final, because there are many unresolved medical and ethical questions related to these issues and the continuing development of medical technology will necessitate ongoing reflection. But these decisions already confront patients, families and health-care personnel every day. They arise whenever competent patients make decisions about medically assisted nutrition and

Editors' note: The article has been edited and all footnotes omitted. Readers wishing to follow up on sources should consult the original article.

hydration for their own present situation, when they consider signing an advance directive such as a "living will" or health-care proxy document, and when families or other proxy decision-makers make decisions about those entrusted to their care. We offer guidance to those who, facing these issues, might be confused by opinions that at times threaten to deny the inherent dignity of human life. We therefore address our reflections first to those who share our Judeo-Christian traditions, and secondly to others concerned about the dignity and value of human life who seek guidance in making their own moral decisions.

MORAL PRINCIPLES

The Judeo-Christian moral tradition celebrates life as the gift of a loving God and respects the life of each human being because each is made in the image and likeness of God. As Christians we also believe we are redeemed by Christ and called to share eternal life with him. From these roots the Catholic tradition has developed a distinctive approach to fostering and sustaining human life. Our church views life as a sacred trust, a gift over which we are given stewardship and not absolute dominion. The church thus opposes all direct attacks on innocent life. As conscientious stewards we have a duty to preserve life, while recognizing certain limits to that duty:

(1) Because human life is the foundation for all other human goods, it has a special value and significance. Life is "the first right of the human person" and "the condition of all the others."

(2) All crimes against life, including "euthanasia or willful suicide," must be opposed. Euthanasia is "an action or an omission which of itself or by intention causes death, in order that all suffering may in this way be eliminated." Its terms of reference are to be found "in the intention of the will and in the methods used." Thus defined, euthanasia is an attack on life which no one has a right to make or request, and which no government or other human authority can legitimately recommend or permit. Although individual guilt may be reduced or absent because of suffering or emotional factors that cloud the conscience, this does not change the objective wrongfulness of the act. It should also be recognized that an apparent plea for death may really be a plea for help and love.

(3) Suffering is a fact of human life, and has special significance for the Christian as an opportunity to share in Christ's redemptive suffering. Nevertheless there is nothing wrong in trying to relieve someone's suffering; in fact it is a positive good to do so, as long as one does not intentionally cause death or interfere with other moral and religious duties.

(4) Everyone has the duty to care for his or her own life and health and to seek necessary medical care from others, but this does not mean that all possible remedies must be used in all circumstances. One is not obliged to use either "extraordinary" means or "disproportionate" means of preserving life—that is, means which are understood as offering no reasonable hope of benefit or as involving excessive burdens. Decisions regarding such means are complex, and should ordinarily be made by the patient in consultation with his or her family chaplain or pastor and physician when that is possible.

(5) In the final stage of dying one is not obliged to prolong the life of a patient by every possible means: "When inevitable death is imminent in spite of the means used, it is permitted in conscience to take the decision to refuse forms of treatment that would only secure a precarious and burdensome prolongation of life, so long as the normal care due to the sick person in similar cases is not interrupted."

(6) While affirming life as a gift of God, the church recognizes that death is unavoidable and that it can open the door to eternal life. Thus, "without in any way hastening the hour of death," the dying person should accept its reality and prepare for it emotionally and spiritually.

(7) Decisions regarding human life must respect the demands of justice, viewing each human being as our neighbor and avoiding all

discrimination based on age or dependency. A human being has "a unique dignity and an independent value, from the moment of conception and in every stage of development, whatever his or her physical condition." In particular, "the disabled person (whether the disability be the result of a congenital handicap, chronic illness or accident, or from mental or physical deficiency, and whatever the severity of the disability) is a fully human subject, with the corresponding innate, sacred and inviolable rights." First among these is "the fundamental and inalienable right to life."

(8) The dignity and value of the human person, which lie at the foundation of the church's teaching on the right to life, also provide a basis for any just social order. Not only to become more Christian, but to become more truly human, society should protect the right to life through its laws and other policies.

While these principles grow out of a specific religious tradition, they appeal to a common respect for the dignity of the human person. We commend them to all people of good will.

QUESTIONS ABOUT MEDICALLY ASSISTED NUTRITION AND HYDRATION

In what follows we apply these well-established moral principles to the difficult issue of providing medically assisted nutrition and hydration to persons who are seriously ill, disabled or persistently unconscious. We recognize the complexity involved in applying these principles to individual cases and acknowledge that, at this time and on this particular issue, our applications do not have the same authority as the principles themselves.

1. IS THE WITHHOLDING OR WITHDRAWING OF MEDICALLY ASSISTED NUTRITION AND HYDRATION ALWAYS A DIRECT KILLING?

In answering this question one should avoid two extremes.

First, it is wrong to say that this could not be a matter of killing simply because it involves an omission rather than a positive action. In fact a deliberate omission may be an effective and certain way to kill, especially to kill someone weakened by illness. Catholic teaching condemns as euthanasia "an action or an omission which of itself or by intention causes death, in order that all suffering may in this way be eliminated." Thus "euthanasia includes not only active mercy killing but also the omission of treatment when the purpose of the omission is to kill the patient."

Second, we should not assume that all or most decisions to withhold or withdraw medically assisted nutrition and hydration are attempts to cause death. To be sure, any patient will die if all nutrition and hydration are withheld. But sometimes other causes are at work—for example, the patient may be imminently dying, whether feeding takes place or not, from an already existing terminal condition. At other times, although the shortening of the patient's life is one foreseeable result of an omission, the real purpose of the omission was to relieve the patient of a particular procedure that was of limited usefulness to the patient or unreasonably burdensome for the patient and the patient's family or caregivers. This kind of decision should not be equated with a decision to kill or with suicide.

The harsh reality is that some who propose withdrawal of nutrition and hydration from certain patients do directly intend to bring about a patient's death and would even prefer a change in the law to allow for what they see as more "quick and painless" means to cause death. In other words, nutrition and hydration (whether orally administered or medically assisted) are sometimes withdrawn not because a patient is dying, but precisely because a patient is not dying (or not dying quickly) and someone believes it would be better if he or she did, generally because the patient is perceived as having an unacceptably low "quality of life" or as imposing burdens on others.

When deciding whether to withhold or withdraw medically assisted nutrition and hydration, or other forms of life support, we are called by our moral tradition to ask ourselves: What will my decision do for this patient? And what am I trying to achieve by doing it? We must be sure that it is not our intent to cause the patient's death—either for its own sake or as a means to achieving some other goal such as the relief of suffering.

2. IS MEDICALLY ASSISTED NUTRITION AND HYDRATION A FORM OF "TREATMENT" OR "CARE"?

Catholic teaching provides that a person in the final stages of dying need not accept "forms of treatment that would only secure a precarious and burdensome prolongation of life," but should still receive "the normal care due to the sick person in similar cases." . . . But the teaching of the church has not resolved the question whether medically assisted nutrition and hydration should always be seen as a form of normal care.

Almost everyone agrees that oral feeding, when it can be accepted and assimilated by a patient, is a form of care owed to all helpless people. . . . But our obligations become less clear when adequate nutrition and hydration require the skills of trained medical personnel and the use of technologies that may be perceived as very burdensome—that is, as intrusive, painful or repugnant. Such factors vary from one type of feeding procedure to another, and from one patient to another, making it difficult to classify all feeding procedures as either "care" or "treatment."

Perhaps this dilemma should be viewed in a broader context. Even medical "treatments" are morally obligatory when they are "ordinary" means—that is, if they provide a reasonable hope of benefit and do not involve excessive burdens. Therefore we believe people should make decisions in light of a simple and fundamental insight: Out of respect for the dignity of the human person we are obliged to preserve our own lives and help others preserve theirs, by the use of means that have a reasonable hope of sustaining life without imposing unreasonable burdens on those we seek to help, that is, on the patient and his or her family and community.

We must therefore address the question of benefits and burdens next, recognizing that a full moral analysis is only possible when one knows the effects of a given procedure on a particular patient.

3. WHAT ARE THE BENEFITS OF MEDICALLY ASSISTED NUTRITION AND HYDRATION?

. . .

Nutrition and hydration, whether provided in the usual way or with medical assistance . . . benefit patients in several ways. First, for all patients who can assimilate them, suitable food and fluids sustain life, and providing them normally expresses loving concern and solidarity with the helpless. Second, for patients being treated with the hope of a cure, appropriate food and fluids are an important element of sound health care. Third, even for patients who are imminently dying and incurable, food and fluids can prevent the suffering that may arise from dehydration, hunger and thirst.

. . . But sometimes even food and fluids are no longer effective in providing this benefit because a patient has entered the final stage of a terminal condition. At such times we should make the dying person as comfortable as possible and provide nursing care and proper hygiene as well as companionship and appropriate spiritual aid. Such a person may lose all desire for food and drink and even be unable to ingest them. Initiating medically assisted feeding or intravenous fluids in this case may increase the patient's discomfort while providing no real benefit; ice chips or sips of water may instead be appropriate to provide comfort and counteract the adverse effects of dehydration. Even in the case of the imminently dying patient, of course, any action or omission that of itself or by intention causes death is to be absolutely rejected. . . .

4. WHAT ARE THE BURDENS OF MEDICALLY ASSISTED NUTRITION AND HYDRATION?

. . .

The risks and objective complications of medically assisted nutrition and hydration will depend on the procedure used and the condition of the patient. In a given case a feeding procedure may become harmful or even life-threatening. . . .

If the risks and burdens of a particular feeding procedure are deemed serious enough to warrant withdrawing it, we should not automatically deprive the patient of all nutrition and hydration but should ask whether another procedure is feasible that would be less burdensome. We say this because some helpless patients, including some in a "persistent vegetative state," receive tube feedings not because they cannot swallow food at all but because tube feeding is less costly and difficult for health-care personnel. . . .

Many people see feeding tubes as frightening or even as bodily violations. Assessments of such burdens are necessarily subjective; they should not be dismissed on that account, but we offer some practical cautions to help prevent abuse.

First, in keeping with our moral teaching against the intentional causing of death by omission, one should distinguish between repugnance to a particular procedure and repugnance to life itself. The latter may occur when a patient views a life of helplessness and dependency on others as itself a heavy burden, leading him or her to wish or even to pray for death. Especially in our achievement-oriented society, the burden of living in such a condition may seem to outweigh any possible benefit of medical treatment and even lead a person to despair. But we should not assume that the burdens in such a case always outweigh the benefits; for the sufferer, given good counseling and spiritual support, may be brought again to appreciate the precious gift of life.

Second, our tradition recognizes that when treatment decisions are made, "account will have to be taken of the reasonable wishes of the patient and the patient's family, as also of the advice of the doctors who are specially competent in the matter." . . .

Third, we should not assume that a feeding procedure is inherently repugnant to all patients without specific evidence. In contrast to Americans' general distaste for the idea of being supported by "tubes and machines," some studies indicate surprisingly favorable views of medically assisted nutrition and hydration among patients and families with actual experience of such procedures. . . .

While some balk at the idea, in principle cost can be a valid factor in decisions about life support. For example, money spent on expensive treatment for one family member may be money otherwise needed for food, housing and other necessities for the rest of the family. Here, also, we offer some cautions. . . . Even for altruistic reasons a patient should not directly intend his or her own death by malnutrition or dehydration, but may accept an earlier death as a consequence of his or her refusal of an unreasonably expensive treatment.

. . . Individual decisions about medically assisted nutrition and hydration should [not] be determined by macroeconomic concerns such as national budget priorities and the high cost of health care. These social problems are serious, but it is by no means established that they require depriving chronically ill and helpless patients of effective and easily tolerated measures that they need to survive.

Third, tube feeding alone is generally not very expensive and may cost no more than oral feeding. What is seen by many as a grave financial and emotional burden on caregivers is the total long-term care of severely debilitated patients, who may survive for many years with no life support except medically assisted nutrition and hydration and nursing care. . . .

In the context of official church teaching, it is not yet clear to what extent we may assess the burden of a patient's total care rather than the burden of a particular treatment when we seek to refuse "burdensome" life support. On a practical level, those seeking to make good decisions might assure themselves of their own intentions by asking: Does my decision aim at relieving the patient of a particularly grave burden imposed by medically assisted nutrition and hydration? Or does it aim to avoid the total burden of caring for the patient? If so, does it achieve this aim by deliberately bringing about his or her death?

Rather than leaving families to confront such dilemmas alone, society and government should improve their assistance to families whose financial and emotional resources are strained by long-term care of loved ones.

5. WHAT ROLE SHOULD "QUALITY OF LIFE" PLAY IN OUR DECISIONS?

Financial and emotional burdens are willingly endured by most families to raise their children or to care for mentally aware but weak and elderly family members. It is sometimes argued that we need not endure comparable burdens to feed and care for persons with severe mental and physical disabilities, because their low "quality of life" makes it unnecessary or pointless to preserve their lives.

But this argument—even when it seems motivated by a humanitarian concern to reduce suffering and hardship—ignores the equal dignity and sanctity of all human life. Its key assumption—that people with disabilities necessarily enjoy life less than others or lack the potential to lead meaningful lives—is also mistaken. Where suffering does exist, society's response should not be to neglect or eliminate the lives of people with disabilities, but to help correct their inadequate living conditions. Very often the worst threat to a good "quality of life" for these people is not the disability itself, but the prejudicial attitudes of others—attitudes based on the idea that a life with serious disabilities is not worth living.

This being said, our moral tradition allows for three ways in which the "quality of life" of a seriously ill patient is relevant to treatment decisions:

(1) Consistent with respect for the inherent sanctity of life, we should relieve needless suffering and support morally acceptable ways of improving each patient's quality of life.
(2) One may legitimately refuse a treatment because it would itself create an impairment imposing new serious burdens or risks on the patient. This decision to avoid the new burdens or risks created by a treatment is not the same as directly intending to end life in order to avoid the burden of living in a disabled state.
(3) Sometimes a disabling condition may directly influence the benefits and burdens of a specific treatment for a particular patient. For example, a confused or demented patient may find medically assisted nutrition and hydration more frightening and burdensome than other patients do because he or she cannot understand what it is. The patient may even repeatedly pull out feeding tubes, requiring burdensome physical restraints if this form of feeding is to be continued. In such cases, ways of alleviating such special burdens should be explored before concluding that they justify withholding all food and fluids needed to sustain life.

These humane considerations are quite different from a "quality of life" ethic that would judge individuals with disabilities or limited potential as not worthy of care or respect. It is one thing to withhold a procedure because it would impose new disabilities on a patient, and quite another thing to say that patients who already have such disabilities should not have their lives preserved. A means considered ordinary or proportionate for other patients should not be considered extraordinary or disproportionate for severely impaired patients solely because of a judgment that their lives are not worth living.

In short, while considerations regarding a person's quality of life have some validity in weighing the burdens and benefits of medical treatment, at the present time in our society judgments about the quality of life are sometimes used to promote euthanasia. The church must emphasize the sanctity of life of each person as a fundamental principle in all moral decision-making.

6. DO PERSISTENTLY UNCONSCIOUS PATIENTS REPRESENT A SPECIAL CASE?

Even Catholics who accept the same basic moral principles may strongly disagree on how to apply them to patients who appear to be persistently unconscious—that is, those who are in a permanent coma or a "persistent vegetative state" (PVS). Some moral questions in this area have not been explicitly resolved by the church's teaching authority.

On some points there is wide agreement among Catholic theologians:

(1), An unconscious patient must be treated as a living human person with inherent dignity and value. Direct killing of such a patient is as morally reprehensible as the direct killing of anyone else. Even the medical terminology used to describe these patients as "vegetative" unfortunately tends to obscure this vitally important point, inviting speculation that a patient in this state is a "vegetable" or a subhuman animal.
(2) The area of legitimate controversy does not concern patients with conditions like mental retardation, senility, dementia or even temporary unconsciousness. Where serious disagreement begins is with the patient who has been diagnosed as completely and permanently unconscious after careful testing over a period of weeks or months.

Some moral theologians argue that a particular form of care or treatment is morally obligatory only when its benefits outweigh its burdens to a patient or the care providers. In weighing burdens, they say, the total burden of a procedure and the consequent requirements of care must be taken into account. If no benefit can be demonstrated, the procedure, whatever its burdens, cannot be obligatory. These moralists also hold that the chief criterion to determine the benefit of a procedure cannot be merely that it prolongs physical life, since physical life is not an absolute good but is relative to the spiritual good of the person. They assert that the spiritual good of the person is union with God, which can be advanced only by human acts, i.e., conscious, free acts. Since the best current medical opinion holds that persons in the persistent vegetative state (PVS) are incapable now or in the future of conscious, free human acts, these moralists conclude that, when careful diagnosis verifies this condition, it is not obligatory to prolong life by such interventions as a respirator, antibiotics or medically assisted hydration and nutrition. To decide to omit non-obligatory care, therefore, is not to intend the patient's death, but only to avoid the burden of the procedure. Hence, though foreseen, the patient's death is to be attributed to the patient's pathological condition and not to the omission of care. Therefore, these theologians conclude, while it is always wrong directly to intend or cause the death of such patients, the natural dying process which would have occurred without these interventions may be permitted to proceed.

While this rationale is convincing to some, it is not theologically conclusive and we are not persuaded by it. In fact, other theologians argue cogently that theological inquiry could lead one to a more carefully limited conclusion.

These moral theologians argue that while particular treatments can be judged useless or burdensome, it is morally questionable and would create a dangerous precedent to imply that any human life is not a positive good or "benefit." They emphasize that while life is not the highest good, it is always and everywhere a basic good of the human person and not merely a means to other goods. They further assert that if the "burden" one is trying to relieve by discontinuing medically assisted nutrition and hydration is the burden of remaining alive in the allegedly undignified condition of PVS, such a decision is unacceptable because one's intent is only achieved by deliberately ensuring the patient's death from malnutrition or dehydration. Finally, these moralists suggest that PVS is best seen as an extreme form of mental and physical disability—one whose causes, nature and prognosis are as yet imperfectly understood—and not as a terminal illness or fatal pathology from which patients should generally be allowed to die. Because the patient's life can often be sustained indefinitely by medically assisted nutrition and hydration that is not unreasonably risky or burdensome for that patient, they say, we are not dealing here with a case where "inevitable death is imminent in spite of the means used." Rather, because the patient will die in a few days if medically assisted nutrition and hydration are discontinued, but can often live a long time if they are provided, the inherent dignity and worth of the human person obligates us to provide this patient with care and support.

Further complicating this debate is a disagreement over what responsible Catholics should do in the absence of a final resolution of this question. Some point to our moral tradition of probabilism, which would allow individuals to follow the appropriate moral analysis that they find persuasive. Others point to the principle that in cases where one might risk unjustly depriving someone of life, we should take the safer course.

In the face of the uncertainties and unresolved medical and theological issues, it is important to defend and preserve important values. On the one hand, there is a concern that patients and families should not be subjected to unnecessary burdens, ineffective treatments and indignities when death is approaching. On the other hand, it is important to ensure that the inherent dignity of human persons, even those who are persistently unconscious, is respected and that no one is deprived of nutrition and hydration with the intent of bringing on his or her death.

It is not easy to arrive at a single answer to some of the real and personal dilemmas involved in this issue. In study, prayer and compassion we continue to reflect on this issue and hope to discover additional information that will lead to its ultimate resolution.

In the meantime, at a practical level we are concerned that withdrawal of all life support, including nutrition and hydration, not be viewed as appropriate or automatically indicated for the entire class of PVS patients simply because of a judgment that they are beyond the reach of medical treatment that would restore consciousness. We note the current absence of conclusive scientific data on the causes and implications of different degrees of brain damage, on the PVS patient's ability to experience pain and on the reliability of prognoses for many such patients. We do know that many of these patients have a good prognosis for long-term survival when given medically assisted nutrition and hydration, and a certain prognosis for death otherwise—and we know that many in our society view such an early death as a positive good for a patient in this condition. Therefore we are gravely concerned about current attitudes and policy trends in our society that would too easily dismiss patients without apparent mental faculties as non-persons or as undeserving of human care and concern. In this climate, even legitimate moral arguments intended to have a careful and limited application can easily be misinterpreted, broadened and abused by others to erode respect for the lives of some of our society's most helpless members. . . .

THE *WENDLAND* CASE AND THE TREACHEROUS ROAD TO NONPERSONHOOD

Wesley J. Smith

In 1993, Robert Wendland, then 42, suffered profound brain injuries in a truck accident. He spent the first sixteen months post-accident unconscious, a condition from which doctors did not expect him to emerge. Then, beginning in December 1994 or early January 1995, he began to stir.

It soon became apparent to all that Robert was conscious and he was given extensive therapy. Although the extent of his capabilities was disputed vigorously during the litigation that was to follow, it seems clear from medical records, court testimony, and the ruling of the California Supreme Court, that after he awakened, Robert improved to the point where he could:

- Maneuver a motorized wheelchair down a corridor;
- Respond to simple requests, such as "Hand me the ball," 80 to 100 percent of the time;
- Close his eyes upon command and open them when the therapist said the number "three";
- Support 110 pounds on one of his legs even though he was paralyzed on the other side;
- Write the letter "R" of his first name;
- Answer yes and no questions occasionally by pointing to the appropriate button (for example: "Is your name Michael?" No. "Is your name Robert?" Yes. "Do you have pain?" Yes. "Do your legs hurt?" No. Does your buttocks hurt?" No. "Do you want to die?" Silence, etc.);
- Exhibit emotional reactions such as crying and reaching out to kiss his mother's hand.[1]

Then in July 1995, Robert's wife, Rose Wendland, made a momentous decision: in consultation with Robert's doctors, she decided not to replace his feeding tube after it became detached from his body. The Lodi Memorial Hospital Ethics Committee ratified her decision unanimously—and anonymously. Disturbingly, the Committee apparently did not consult the nurses or other medical professionals who had continual interaction with Robert. Nor did they seek the perspective of Robert's mother, Florence Wendland, who had been visiting her son several times a week continually since his injury. (During the litigation, Florence's lawyer sought to cross-examine the committee members as to the bases for their decision. This effort was quashed by the trial court at the request of the Hospital.) Indeed, Florence and most of Robert's siblings were not informed that his dehydration was being planned. (One of his brothers was advised and supported Rose.)

The decision to make Robert die by dehydration did not sit well with many of the nurses and other hospital staffers who cared for him on a daily basis. "Wife requesting transfer [of Robert] to discontinue tube feeding for euthanasia," complained a nurse in the nursing notes that became a part of Robert's medical records. "The shock of this decision and committee approval! Is very difficult for obvious reason of his progression."[2]

Robert's life was saved when an anonymous nurse placed a telephone call to one of Robert's sisters revealing Rose's plan. Shocked, Florence and his sister Rebekah Vinson immediately sought a court injunction barring Rose from authorizing the termination of Robert's nutrition and hydration. That injunction set in motion a bitter six-year legal and public relations struggle that ended with Robert's death by pneumonia, followed a few weeks later by a landmark decision by the California Supreme Court in favor of Florence. For those who believe in the inherent equality of all human life, the high court's unanimous ruling provided significant and needed legal protections to the lives of conscious, cognitively disabled people—among society's most weak, vulnerable, and devalued patients.[3]

The litigation focused on the constitutionality of a rather oddly worded California statute, Probate Code 2355, that grants a conservator of the person the "exclusive authority to give consent" for medical treatment as he or she "in good faith based on medical advice determines to be necessary. . . ." Previous court cases had construed this statute as also covering the decision not to treat.

The essence of the legal argument made by those supporting Rose can be boiled down to this: when a petition is filed for a conservatorship of the person, the court's primary duty is to determine whether the patient is incompetent and, if so, to make a proper appointment.[4] Once an appointment has been made, the court is then powerless to overrule a conservator's decision to withhold or withdraw treatment—including tube-supplied food and fluids—so long as the conservator can demonstrate by a preponderance of the evidence (the lowest level of proof in civil court) that the decision was made in good faith in consultation with a doctor. This, Rose and her supporters argued vigorously, was in keeping with the fundamental right of all persons, including the cognitively disabled, to refuse unwanted medical treatment. Thus, those arguing for Robert's dehydration saw *Wendland* as a "right to die" case.

Florence's attorney and *amici* viewed the matter from a 180-degree different perspective, perceiving it instead as a crucial "right to live" case. They argued that a mere "good faith" standard would provide unconstitutionally inadequate protection to helpless patients since "putting the conservator on trial" and focusing on her motives, thought processes, and emotions would shift attention away from the best interests and previously expressed desires of the conservatee. Moreover, since the very life of the patient is literally at stake in the decision to remove food and fluids, the constitutional right to equal protection and the fundamental right to life must require proof supporting such a death decision by "clear and convincing" evidence—the most rigorous in civil law.[5]

The case proved to be a white-knuckle roller coaster ride. Florence won the first round when her attorney prevailed upon the trial judge to rule that those seeking Robert's dehydration had not presented clear and convincing evidence that he would have wanted to die under his circumstances or that dehydration would be in his best interests. That approach was reversed by the California Court of Appeal, which substantially upheld Rose's view, albeit requiring that she demonstrate her good faith by clear and convincing evidence. (Alarmingly, the Court of Appeal also ruled that "there should be no presumption for continued existence" in California law.[6]) The case reached its dramatic denouement when the California Supreme Court overruled the Court of Appeal and reinstated the trial judge's approach, noting, *inter alia,* that similarly fundamental decisions involving incompetent persons require very high standards of proof. For example, a California conservator must prove beyond a reasonable doubt that a decision to sterilize a developmentally disabled conservatee is in the conservatee's best interests. (As Florence's lawyer argued compellingly that to "provide greater legal protections against sterilization than death is to turn the overarching purposes of constitutional safeguards upside down."[7])

Responding to the concern expressed by the *amici* for Rose that a ruling supporting Florence would unduly inhibit family members from making end-of-life decisions, the Supreme Court limited the circumstances in which it applies. First, the ruling only controls those circumstances in which a court appointed conservator is making health decisions. Thus, families or other surrogates acting informally as medical decision makers for incompetent patients are not bound by the *Wendland* ruling. Next, the Court further limited the decision's scope by stating, "Only the decision to withdraw life-sustaining treatment because of its effect on a conscious conservatee's fundamental rights, justifies imposing that high [clear and convincing] standard of proof." Thus, other decisions by a conservator remain governed by the good faith standard established by Probate Code 2355. Finally, the Court stated that the decision "affects only a narrow class of persons: conscious conservatees who have not left formal directions for health care and those whose conservators propose to withhold life-sustaining treatment for the purpose of causing their conservatee's deaths."[8] In other words, a written advanced medical directive directing the withholding or removal of medically delivered hydration and nutrition will be honored.

Despite my strong view that the decision is too narrowly drawn—a matter I will discuss at the end of this essay—I do believe that in connection with other similar state high court decisions, *Wendland*'s giving the benefit of doubt to life erected a significant and important legal bulwark protecting the lives of many cognitively disabled people.[9] Moreover, given the national influence of California jurisprudence, the decision should serve as a model for other state courts facing similar legal controversies in the years to come. Given this likely national influence, it is thus not hyperbole to conclude that *Wendland* is one of the most important and beneficial court decisions in the field of bioethics since the United States Supreme Court ruled that there is no federal constitutional right to assisted suicide.[10]

DEHUMANIZING THE COGNITIVELY DISABLED

To fully understand the import of the decision, we must look beyond the ruling itself to the bioethical context in which the legal drama played itself out. It is an atmosphere in which people with profound cognitive disabilities are increasingly denigrated by many in bioethics as having less moral worth than people with normal cognitive capacities. Thus the crucial subtext of the litigation—at least from the perspective of the partisans who spent years striving to save Robert's life—was the issue of universal human equality.

One of the primary tenets of the modern bioethics movement is that there is such a thing as a born human being who is not a person.[11] Under this belief system (personhood theory), people who are not persons possess less moral worth—and thus should have fewer legal rights—than do persons. Thus, personhood theory seeks the creation of an explicit hierarchy of human life.

While the exact criteria for determining personhood are still being debated vigorously within bioethics, it is generally agreed that the decision about who is or is not a person should be based upon the cognitive capacity of the human being (or animal) being judged.[12] Indeed, it has been quite seriously suggested that determining which humans are and are not persons involves which "individuals have the highest moral value or importance."[13] Such a discriminatory "quality of life" approach for measuring the value of human life strips worth and dignity from people based on health and disability (particularly cognitive disability) just as surely as racism does based on skin pigment, hair texture, or facial characteristics.

In personhood theory, being denigrated as a non person removes the human in question from the moral community, leading to a loss of the right to life.[14] The label may also strip the human from the right to bodily integrity. Thus, Tom L. Beauchamp has written that "because many humans lack properties of personhood" they are "rendered equal or inferior in moral standing to some nonhumans." He further asserted:

> If this conclusion is defensible we will need to rethink our traditional view that these unlucky humans cannot be treated in the same way we treat relevantly similar nonhumans. For example, they might be aggressively used as human research subjects and sources of organs.[15]

The stripping of unconscious patients of their inherent human dignity has even gotten to the point where some of the most prominent voices in bioethics advocate "redefining" death to include a diagnosis of permanent unconsciousness for the purposes of organ procurement.[16] Such attitudes have seeped into the clinical setting. The *New York Times* published a troubling poll in 1996 finding that 54 percent of medical directors and 44 percent of neurologists believe that patients in persistent vegetative state should be "considered dead."[17] Thus, personhood theory not only threatens the lives of profoundly cognitively disabled people but poses the very real danger that they could, in the not too distant future, be dehumanized to the point that they are viewed as being akin to cattle herds or timber forests, mere natural resources available for the harvest and other forms of exploitation.

Along these lines, one of the most disturbing aspects of the *Wendland* case was the concerted effort to dehumanize and depersonalize Robert in order to make his dehydration easier for the courts to swallow. Thus, instead of celebrating Robert's progress as wonderful medical victories for someone who only months before had been unconscious, expert bioethicist witnesses denigrated his interactivity as mere "trained responses," rather than truly human behavior.[18] One went so far as to contend that Robert "is unable to think at all in the manner we conceive humans do."[19] Similarly, Robert's own court appointed appellate attorney argued that Robert "can respond to stimuli somewhat in the manner that an animal might."[20] Most disturbingly, illustrating how such dehumanizing and denigrating values can become embedded into law, the three-judge panel of the California Court of Appeals actively embraced his dehumanization in their discussion explaining why they wished to reverse the trial judge's ruling.

Thankfully, with the Supreme Court's contrary decision, the legal and moral equality of conscious, profoundly cognitively disabled people like Robert was forcefully reinforced and embedded into the jurisprudence of the State of California. Indeed, the Court's strong assertion of constitutional equality for conscious cognitively disabled people may be its most important contribution to the ongoing cultural debate over life, its meaning, and its value.

CREATING A DISPOSABLE CASTE

While there is certainly much to be celebrated about the *Wendland* decision, there is also a dark side to the ruling. Rather than protecting all cognitively disabled people equally, *Wendland* actually furthers the ongoing depersonalization of patients diagnosed as permanently unconscious.

Previous California Court of Appeals cases, most particularly *Conservatorship of Drabic*, gave virtually unfettered discretion to families or conservators who wish to remove tube-supplied nutrition and hydration from patients diagnosed as permanently unconscious.[21] The Supreme Court's reasoning in *Wendland* could have altered that legal/bioethical consensus. But instead of providing a single standard of protection for all Californians, whether conscious or unconscious, the justices instead ventured beyond *Drabic*—which had merely construed statutory law—by explicitly stripping crucial constitutional protections from unconscious Californians.[22] Not only does this approach discriminate against those diagnosed (or misdiagnosed) as being permanently unconscious, but it explicitly weaves the odious concept of the born, human nonperson into the fabric of California constitutional law.

To fully understand the nature of the problem, let's turn briefly to the wisdom of the late Paul Ramsey, who argued that only the "objective medical condition of the patient" should be considered when determining whether to cut off treatment "not the subjective, capricious, and often selfish evaluations of the quality of future life that are often to the detriment of the most vulnerable and voiceless."[23] Ramsey's point was that decisions to terminate life support should not be based on subjective value judgments of the worth of the patient's life or whether it was worth living, but exclusively upon determinations about what would be in the best medical interests of the patient.

Judge Bobby McNatt, the *Wendland* trial judge, took a properly "Ramseyan" approach to deciding the case. Thus, even though McNatt wholeheartedly believed in Rose's virtue, he ruled that good faith alone would provide insufficient protection for patients in Robert's condition:

> In our society, the rules under which Rose must make surrogate decisions are the same ones that someone less compassionate, less ethical would also operate. . . . To allow termination of Robert's life over the objections of other family members and on the legal basis of the evidence presented would allow the opening of a door that other families with less noble motives might follow through. . . . To allow it would be to start down a treacherous road.[24]

If that is true—and I strongly assert that it is—are not those diagnosed as permanently unconscious faced with an even greater danger since they are viewed widely as having even lesser value than are people like Robert? Unfortunately, not to the

California Supreme Court, which moved the state further down McNatt's "treacherous road" when it concluded that unconscious patients do not enjoy the same legal protections as do people who are conscious simply because unconscious patients cannot feel the discomfort of dehydration.[25] In other words, the court ruled that the fundamental constitutional right to life depends upon being able to perceive.

This is a dangerously slender reed upon which to support a constitutional guarantee as fundamental as the right to life! Not only does it create a two-tiered system of constitutional protections, but any patient—even the cognitively able—could be rendered "permanently unconscious" through the systematic application of consciousness-deadening drugs. Indeed, the neurologist Dr. Ronald Cranford, an expert witness and medical consultant for Rose, testified that he might return Robert to a comatose state to ensure that he felt no discomfort from having his nutrition and hydration removed.[26] Moreover, permanent unconsciousness is a notoriously difficult diagnosis to accurately make. (For example, it was reported in the June 1991 *Archives of Neurology* that 58 percent of patients with a firm diagnosis of PVS awakened within three years.) Besides, PVS patients sometimes unexpectedly awaken—just as Robert Wendland did.

CONCLUSION

By limiting constitutional rights to those with the ability to perceive pain and discomfort when it should have applied the same constitutional standards to all incompetent patients, the Supreme Court blundered badly. Consider this: before his accident, Robert Wendland enjoyed full constitutional rights. Then, during his 16-month period of unconsciousness, he lost them. But when he reawakened, his rights resurrected. In other words, his rights depended not upon his humanity but upon his medical condition. Such an on-again, off-again, on-again standard of legal protection is not only surreal but furthers personhood theory's attempt to craft an explicit hierarchy of human life.

Thus, as valuable as the *Wendland* ruling is—and it is very valuable indeed—in the end, it merely erected a speed bump that slows our pace but does not significantly alter our overall direction toward the embodiment of personhood theory into the bedrock of law. In this sense, *Wendland* may just be a rest stop on the path to a public policy that will eventually give official sanction to the odious concept of the human life deemed unworthy of life.

NOTES

1. Medical records of Robert Wendland. Testimony, affidavits, and other evidence from various court proceedings, *In re the Conservatorship of Robert Wendland,* Superior Court of California, County of Joaquin, Case No. 65669. The yes and no interaction between Robert and his doctor is cited by the California Supreme Court in *Conservatorship of the Person of Robert Wendland,* 26 Cal. 4th 519, 528 (2001).
2. Medical records of Robert Wendland, nurse's notes, July 25, 1995.
3. *Conservatorship of the Person of Robert Wendland,* 26 Cal. 4th 519, 524 (2001).
4. Among the *amici* who filed briefs supporting Rose were the American Civil Liberties Union, the California Medical Association, California Health Care Association, and 43 individual bioethicists.
5. The *amici* for Florence were the Coalition of Concerned Medical Professionals, a group that advocates for the poor (represented by this author), ADAPT, NOT DEAD YET, and other disability rights groups, the Nursing Home Action Group, and the National Legal Center for the Medically Dependent and Disabled, Inc.
6. *In re Conservatorship of Wendland,* 78 Cal. App. 4th 517.
7. *Conservatorship of Robert Wendland,* "Respondent's Opening Brief on the Merits," In the Supreme Court of California, Case No. S 087265, p. 29.
8. *Conservatorship of Wendland,* Supreme Court, Supra.
9. See *In Re Edna M.F.* 270 Wis.2d558 (1997, WI), in which the Wisconsin Supreme Court ruled that conscious cognitively disabled people may not have their feeding tubes removed; *In re Michael Martin,* 538 N.W. 2d 399 (1995, MI). *Martin v. Martin,* The Michigan Supreme Court ruled in a case strikingly similar to Wendland, that a conservator must demonstrate by clear and convincing evidence that standard in the case of *Martin v. Martin.*
10. *Washington v. Glucksburg,* 117 S. Ct. 2258 (1997), *Vacco v. Quill,* 117 S. Ct. 2293 (1997).
11. See, for example, John Harris, "The Concept of the Person and the Value of Life," *Kennedy Institute of Ethics Journal,* Vol. 9, No. 4 (December 1999), pp. 291–308.

12. Early in the bioethics movement, Joseph Fletcher crafted a "Criteria for Humanhood," that was first published in the *Hastings Center Report*, including "minimal intelligence," a "sense of futurity," the ability to communicate, and "neocortical function." (As republished in Joseph Fletcher, *Humanhood: Essays in Biomedical Ethics*, 1979, Prometheus Books, Buffalo, NY, pp. 16–17.) This approach evolved into alleged distinction between persons and nonpersons. For example, Princeton University's Peter Singer claims that there are two crucial characteristics of personhood, rationality, and self-consciousness. (*Practical Ethics*, 2d. ed., 1993, Cambridge University Press, Cambridge, England, p. 87.) Other prominent bioethicists have suggested other criteria while accepting the premise of the human being nonperson.
13. Harris, supra, p. 294.
14. Harris, supra, p. 294.
15. Tom L. Beauchamp, "The Failure of Theories of Personhood," *Kennedy Institute of Ethics Journal*, supra, pp. 310–324 at 320.
16. See for example, R. Hoffenbert, et al., "Should Organs from Patients in Permanent Vegetative State Be Used for Transplantation?" *The Lancet* 350 (Nov. 1, 1997).
17. Linda Carroll, "Debating the Definition of Death," Medical Tribune News Service, as published in the *New York Times*, July 29, 1996.
18. Trial testimony of Dr. Ronald Cranford.
19. Trial testimony of Dr. Ernest Bryant.
20. *In re the Conservatorship of Robert Wendland*, Court of Appeals, Third Appellate District, Case no Civil C-029439, "Appellant Robert Wendland's Opening Brief," p. 30.
21. *Conservatorship of Drabic*, 200 Cal. App. 3d 185 (1988).
22. Because of the peculiar facts of the case and with Robert's case literally hanging in the balance, the *amicus* brief authored by this writer supporting Florence did not argue for the overruling of *Drabic*—which I would have preferred—but rather, that the case had no applicability to the facts at bench. Indeed, in my opinion it was Robert Wendland's capabilities that made Florence's case "winnable" since Robert's undisputed conscious condition made his humanity easier for the court to grasp, appreciate, and protect. I believe that those arguing on Rose's behalf viewed the matter similarly and thus continually sought to convince the court that his condition was morally equivalent to unconsciousness, for example, through the repeated use of the term "minimally conscious state."
23. As quoted by Albert R. Jonsen, *The Birth of Bioethics* (1998, Oxford University Press, New York, NY), p. 259.
24. *Wendland*, Superior Court, Supra, "Bifurcated Decision: Findings of Fact and Conclusions of Law."
25. *Wendland*, Supreme Court, Supra, p. 537.
26. *Wendland*, Superior Court, Supra, Testimony of Ronald Cranford, M.D.

THE *WENDLAND* CASE

Lawrence Nelson

The significance of the dispute between Robert Wendland's wife and court appointed conservator, Rose, and his estranged mother over the legal and ethical propriety of Rose's decision to end his medically provided nutrition and hydration certainly does not lie in the result for Robert himself of the California Supreme Court's unanimously ruling against Rose. By stroke of ironic fate or divine grace, just a few weeks prior to the Court releasing its opinion, Robert developed a serious infection and died. After initial treatment failed, Rose had refused any further treatment and directed that he be kept comfortable and dignified as he was dying. In light of the Supreme Court's ruling, it is ironic that the superior court order at issue barred her only from discontinuing his gastrostomy tube feeding and left her free to refuse any other form of life-sustaining medical treatment. Had he survived, the Court's decision would have prevented Rose from refusing any life-sustaining treatment for Robert unless and until he became permanently unconscious or terminally ill—or unless she was willing to add to the 6 years of litigation she and her children had already suffered through by again attempting to prove in court that his wishes or best interest permitted treatment to be stopped.

The true significance of the case of Robert Wendland lies in other places. First, it is worth noting who (and how many of them) joined the parties as advocates in their respective legal efforts. Support for Rose and the validity of the law that authorized her to refuse medically provided nutrition and hydration came from organized medicine (e.g., the California Medical Association), a joint medical-legal group (Los Angeles Cty Medical Assoc./Bar Association Joint Committee on Biomedical Ethics), the statewide organization of hospitals (California Healthcare Association), three Catholic health care systems (e.g., Alliance of Catholic Health Care), the American Civil Liberties Union, the Los Angeles County Bar Association Bioethics Committee, and 43 individual bioethicists.

On the other side, support for the estranged mother's opposition to ending Robert's tube feedings as well as her efforts to have Probate Code §2355 struck down as unconstitutional came from a variety of disability rights and pro-life organizations: the Coalition of Concerned Medical Professionals (represented by Wesley Smith), the Ethics and Advocacy Task Force of the Nursing Home Action Group, the National Legal Center for the Medically Dependent & Disabled, Not Dead Yet, Adapt, Self-Advocates Becoming Empowered, the Association for Retarded Citizens, Brain Injury Association, Inc., Center for Self-Determination, the Center on Human Policy at Syracuse University, the Disability Rights Center, the National Council on Independent Living, the National Spinal Cord Injury Association, and The Association for the Severely Handicapped.

This particular arrayal of individuals and organizations is unique in the jurisprudence of bioethics. It seems to pit clinicians, hospitals, traditional civil libertarians, and professional bioethicists against advocacy groups for the disabled and symbolizes profound disagreement over surrogate medical decision making for the incompetent and the role of quality of life considerations in treatment choices that lead to the death of a conscious individual. The clash here also reflects a new depth of disagreement over the importance of the individual in question having *some*, however minimal, degree of consciousness and function (and *not* being in a permanently unconscious state). Rose argued that little or nothing turned either legally or morally on Robert having a minimal degree of consciousness, while the mother asserted that this meant a great deal and warned of the dire consequences for millions of disabled but conscious persons whose lives would be put in jeopardy without stringent limits being put on their surrogates and medical caretakers. The Court plainly endorsed the mother's point of view. These disagreements and what can now be called a judicial trend[1] toward imposing the clear and convincing evidentiary standard on decisions to forgo life-sustaining of conscious, incompetent, and disabled individuals are very likely to fuel more litigation in this area. The groups involved as friends of the court in the *Wendland* case will surely tangle again.

Second, *Wendland* is an important decision because it refused to apply as written an existing California statute that specified standards for the conservator's decision making commonly advanced by bioethicists and quite clearly made preponderance the applicable evidentiary standard.[2] In fact, the California legislature had expressly established uniform standards for all surrogate medical decision making in its Health Care Decisions Law, of which §2355 was a portion. Yet the Court found these standards constitutionally inadequate, but only as they applied to conservators and non-terminally ill, conscious conservatees. In other prominent cases involving incompetents such as *Conroy, Cruzan, Matter of Edna* and *In re Martin* the democratically elected legislature had been silent on surrogate decision making procedure when these courts made their rulings. But in *Wendland* the legislature had spoken clearly and directly about this subject, and yet the Court did not uphold the legislature's policy choice or adhere to its own rule that "courts 'must follow the language used [in the statute] and give to it its plain meaning, whatever may be thought of the wisdom, expediency, or policy of the act, even if it appears probable that a different object was in the mind of the legislature.'"[3]

Fortunately, *Conservatorship of Wendland* casts no doubt on the legal authority of surrogates or agents appointed by a competent adult to make any medical decision as authorized. The Court made a sharp distinction between a surrogate or agent appointed by the individual and one appointed by a court.

Consequently, these surrogates or agents do not have to show clear and convincing evidence of their principals' wishes relating to specific treatments, disease, or types of injuries; they can make medical decisions and refuse life-sustaining treatment as long as this is within their delegated authority.

In contrast, the underlying rationale of *Wendland*'s imposition of the clear and convincing evidentiary standard on conservators could have a tremendous impact on other cases involving the incompetent, depending on how this rationale is identified and interpreted. At one point, the Court finds "a serious constitutional problem" with stopping tube feedings because Robert "may consciously perceive the effects of dehydration and starvation." (26 Cal.4th 537, 543) Therefore, the constitutional problem in the case that the Court felt compelled to address was the expectation that Robert would suffer if treatment were stopped. But this amorphous "constitutional problem" exists when treatment is forgone for *any* conscious patient and assumes, both flippantly and in contravention of established ethics and clinical practice, that the patient would be denied medication to prevent him suffering.

At other points in the opinion, the Court seems to rest its conclusion on Robert's constitutional right to privacy and to life: "[A conservator's decision to withdraw tube feeding] with which the conservatee disagrees and which subjects [him] to starvation, dehydration and death . . . would represent the gravest possible affront to a conservatee's state constitutional right to privacy, in the sense of freedom from unwanted bodily intrusions, and to life." (26 Cal.4th 547) This reasoning is noteworthy for three reasons. One, it begs the question of the incompetent's choice regarding tube feeding and assumes stopping it would harm him. No evidence was in the record that Robert ever stated he wanted to be tube fed, and a great deal of testimony by his wife, brother, and children strongly he indicated he wouldn't. Yet, as mentioned above, the Court oddly assumes that he would want the tube feeding because he'd want to avoid the (completely unnecessary) attendant suffering.

Two, the conceptual essence of "privacy" is the maintenance of control by an individual over his or her own person and intimate, personal decisions and the authority to exclude other individuals—and most certainly the State—from these determinations. The *Wendland* Court turns privacy inside out by making it the individual's interest in keeping the bodily intrusion *in* him. Three, if it is Robert's constitutional right to (biological) life of any quality (though we don't know this is what the Court means because it never described this right or related it to any judicial precedent) that would have been violated by Rose's decision to end the tube feedings, then this same violation would occur if tube feedings were stopped on any incompetent patient—including a child or a permanently unconscious patient. Yet the Court explicitly stated that its holding did not apply to the unconscious. This position is inconsistent: the constitutional right to life as (poorly) articulated by this Court must apply to all persons equally, or the unconscious are being denied the equal protection of the laws.

In any event, the *Wendland* opinion's reasoning invites hard questions to be raised both about the nature and scope of the legal authority of parents to reject life-sustaining treatment for their conscious children and the authority of surrogates or close family to decide for never competent adults. As already mentioned, the Court drew a sharp distinction between choices made by competent adults or their personally appointed surrogates to refuse treatment and such choices made *for* an incompetent person (whether adult or minor) by someone else. Citing the U.S. Supreme Court's decision in *Cruzan*, the Court observed that the difference between these two kinds of choices is "so obvious" that "the State is warranted in establishing rigorous procedures for the latter class of cases which do not apply to the former." (26 Cal.4th 536) The Court's strong emphasis on the "[incompetent's] right to life [and] the state's interest in preserving life," (26 Cal.4th 537) factors equally applicable to a child, could also contribute to doubt being cast upon open-ended parental decision making authority and give a legislature grounds for imposing more "rigorous procedures" on parental refusals of life-sustaining treatment for their children.[4]

More important, *Wendland* is surely going to have a huge and unsettling impact on decisions to forgo life-sustaining treatment of conscious developmentally disabled persons who have reached majority age and are conserved, but who never were and will never be competent to make their own choices about accepting or refusing medical treatment. As these individuals have no autonomy they can delegate to another, a conservator could refuse life-sustaining treatment only by producing clear and convincing evidence that such a decision was in the patient's best interest.

Some of the most glaring deficiencies of the *Wendland* opinion can be seen when applied to this group of individuals. First, it provides no guidance whatsoever on how the patient's "best interest" is to be legally determined; it doesn't even allude to any factors that should be considered, despite their long-standing existence in California case law.[5] Second, as the *Wendland* opinion itself does not expressly require judicial review of a conservator's refusal of life-sustaining treatment, the identity of the one who is to ensure that the standard has been met is left unspecified: if not a judge, is it the attending physician? An institutional ethics committee? Finally, this very muddled state of the law gives close family members of a developmentally disabled individual a strong (albeit perverse in light of the opinion's own reasoning) incentive *not* to seek conservatorship authority over medical decisions. As *Wendland* expressly limits itself to decisions made by conservators and California law contains no requirement that conservatorship be sought, family members could actually have more latitude in making decisions to forgo treatment by invoking their common law authority recognized in *Barber v. Superior Court*.[6]

REFERENCES

1. *In re Martin*, 538 NW.2d 399 (Mich. 1995); *Matter of Edna M.F.*, 563 N.W.2d 485 (Wis. 1997), and now *Wendland*. Other courts have imposed the clear and convincing evidence standard on any decision to forgo life-sustaining treatment of any incompetent adult, e.g., *In re Westchester Medical Center* (O'Connor), 531 N.E.2d 607 (NY 1988) and *Cruzan v. Harmon*, 760 S:W.2d 408 (Mo. 1988).
2. The statute, Probate Code §2355, stated that: (a) the "conservator has the exclusive authority to make health care decisions for the conservatee that the conservator in good faith based on medical advice determines to be necessary"; (b) the conservator was required to make medical decisions "in accordance with the conservatee's individual health care instructions, if any, and other wishes to the extent known to the conservator"; and (c) if the conservatee's instructions or wishes were unknown, the conservator was mandated to make the decision "in accordance with the conservator's determination of the conservatee's best interest. In determining the conservatee's best interest, the conservator shall consider the conservatee's personal values to the extent known to the conservator." The California Law Revision Commission, a governmental body that studies the law and recommends legislation to make needed reforms, issued an Official Comment on §2355 that pointed out that the law "does not specify any specific evidentiary standard for the determination of the conservatee's wishes or best interest. Consequently, the general rule applies: the standard is by the preponderance of the evidence. Proof is not required by clear and convincing evidence." Curiously, the *Wendland* opinion itself calls the Commission's comments "persuasive evidence of the intent of the Legislature."
3. *People v. Weidert*, 39 Cal.3d 836, 843 (1985).
4. The U.S. Supreme Court has acknowledged that "state law vests decisional responsibility in the parents, in the first instance, subject to review in exceptional cases by the State acting as *parens patriae*" and noted there is a "presumption, strong but rebuttable, that parents are the appropriate decisionmakers for their infants." *Bowen v. American Hospital Association*, 476 U.S. 610, 627, 628 fn. 13 (1986). But this characterization of the scope of parental authority could be altered by either legislation or constitutional requirements.
5. "If it is not possible to ascertain the choice the patient would have made, the surrogate ought to be guided in his decision by the patient's best interests. Under this standard, such factors as the relief of suffering, the preservation or restoration of functioning and the quality as well as the extent of life sustained may be considered. Finally, since most people are concerned about the well-being of their loved ones, the surrogate may take into account the impact of the decision on those people closest to the patient. (President's Commission, ch. 4, pp. 134–135.) *Barber v. Superior Court* (1983) 147 Cal.App.3d 1006, 1022.
6. See 147 Cal.App.3d at 1021–22.

QUALITY OF LIFE AND NON-TREATMENT DECISIONS FOR INCOMPETENT PATIENTS: A CRITIQUE OF THE ORTHODOX APPROACH

Rebecca S. Dresser and John A. Robertson

Since the Quinlan decision in 1976, courts and legislatures have made substantial progress in defining rules to govern non-treatment of dying and debilitated patients. For example, the right of the competent patient to refuse necessary care is now widely established, and the legality of withdrawing respirators and even nutrition and hydration from permanently unconscious patients is increasingly recognized.

More difficult questions arise, however, when the patient is neither competent nor permanently unconscious, but instead is in a conscious, severely demented and debilitated state, with experiences that appear quite limited. Thousands of patients in this condition are cared for in private homes, hospitals, and nursing homes, the victims of stroke, senility, Alzheimer's disease, and other illnesses. Even though they usually require only low-tech, minimally supportive care, such patients can impose great stress on their families and high financial costs on the health care system.

As the population of frail elderly and demented patients grows, determining the limits of family and societal obligations to sustain them has become a major ethical, legal, and policy issue. Its resolution requires balancing the importance of life in such compromised conditions against the social and familial burdens that prolonging such lives entails. A conflict between a patient-centered and other-directed approach inevitably arises, testing the scope of society's respect for vulnerable and debilitated persons.

Unfortunately, the orthodox judicial approach to non-treatment decisions is not an adequate guide to resolution of these issues. Judicial analysis is too focused on the model of a competent person refusing treatment, even when the case involves a person who is incompetent and unable to choose. Although many of the decided cases have produced defensible results, the courts' efforts to fit incompetent patients to the model of a competent decision-maker are seriously flawed and ultimately threaten harm to many incompetent patients.

Courts, legislators, and physicians would do better to focus directly on the interests of the incompetent patient before them. Competing interests, such as family distress and financial costs, may then be directly evaluated and their role in such decisions properly assigned. Such an approach has the best chance of respecting incompetent persons, while giving due regard to the interests of families and society.

THE ORTHODOX APPROACH: ADVANCE DIRECTIVES AND SUBSTITUTED JUDGMENT

Starting with *In re Quinlan*, and continuing with such cases as *Superintendent of Belchertown* v. *Saikewicz*, *Eichner* v. *Dillon*, *Barber* v. *Superior Court*, *In re Conroy*, *Brophy* v. *New England Sinai Hospital, Inc.*, and *In re Jobes*, the courts have found that life-sustaining treatment may be withheld or withdrawn from incompetent patients in certain circumstances.

The cases adopt the same general pattern of reasoning. Adopting a patient-centered approach, they require that patient choices concerning their medical care be respected. The basic legal premise, derived from common law and constitutional rights to

Rebecca S. Dresser and John A. Robertson, "Quality of Life and Non-Treatment Decisions for Incompetent Patients," *Law, Medicine & Health Care* 17, no. 3 (Fall 1989):234–244. Reprinted by permission of Professors Dresser and Robertson and the American Society of Law, Medicine & Ethics.

Editors' note: Notes have been omitted. Readers wishing to follow up on sources should consult the original article.

self-determination and privacy, is that competent patients have a right to refuse necessary medical care when they face intrusive treatment or life in a compromised state. Countervailing state interests in preserving life, preventing suicide, and upholding the integrity of the medical profession are then found insufficient to override the patient's objection to treatment.

What, however, if the patient is incompetent and cannot make a choice about treatment? Here the courts in most jurisdictions make a conceptual move that determines the structure of subsequent analysis. They assume that respect for incompetent patients requires according such patients the same right to refuse treatment accorded competent patients. This assumption requires that the incompetent patient be viewed as a choosing individual and leads the courts to find or construct a competent person as decision-maker to determine the incompetent patient's choice.

Determining what the fictional competent person in the incompetent patient's situation would choose entails further moves. An incompetent patient's prior oral or written directive concerning treatment when incompetent is given great weight in determining that hypothetical choice. If no directive exists, courts typically adopt the substituted judgment doctrine and allow the family or other proxy to choose as they think the patients would have chosen when or if competent.

This approach to decision-making for incompetent patients was first enunciated in the landmark New Jersey Supreme Court case, *In re Quinlan*, when the court stated that the patient's guardian and family should determine whether she would herself choose non-treatment in her present circumstances: ". . . the only practical way to prevent destruction of the right [of privacy] is to permit the guardian and family of Karen to render their best judgment . . . as to whether she would exercise it in these circumstances."

This approach has shaped the reasoning and analysis in every subsequent non-treatment case involving incompetent patients. Indeed, eleven years later the New Jersey Supreme Court forcefully reiterated the accepted view in *Jobes*:

> . . . the patient's right to self-determination is the guiding principle in determining whether to continue or withdraw life-sustaining treatment; . . . therefore the goal of a surrogate decision-maker for an incompetent patient must be to determine and effectuate what that patient, if competent, would want.

The strategy of relying on prior expressed wishes or proxy inferred competent treatment preferences to determine treatment choices for incompetent patients has wide currency in ethical and policy analysis involving incompetent patients. Authoritative bodies such as the President's Commission for the Study of Ethical Problems in Medicine and the Hastings Center have also endorsed it. Living-will and durable-power-of-attorney legislation embodies a further acceptance of the theme. Health professionals and ethicists hail it as the best solution to the difficult problem of deciding when treatment should be withheld from incompetent patients. It has also been extended to govern medical treatment for patients who never were competent, psychiatric treatment for civilly committed persons, sterilization of retarded persons, and organ donation by incompetent persons.

THE ALLURE OF THE ORTHODOX APPROACH

The orthodox judicial approach of relying on the patient's prior directive or choice inferred by a proxy's substituted judgment has a strong allure for several reasons. One is the appearance of consistency with widely shared values of personal autonomy. When we look to what incompetent patients formerly wanted, or what we infer they would desire, if known, the patient as competent appears to be deciding. This position purportedly extends the freedom and autonomy of competent persons to situations of incompetency.

A second attraction is that the orthodox approach has generally operated to protect incompetent patients from overzealous medical interventions. Until recently, applications of the test in most jurisdictions have found that patients would have refused treatment if they were competent, and have thus permitted intrusive, expensive treatments to be forgone. Also, by ostensibly treating incompetent patients as choice-makers who control whether treatment occurs, the orthodox approach denies others the power, at least explicitly, to override the incompetent patient's interests for the sake of others.

The orthodox approach also attracts because it recognizes a central role for family discretion in treatment decisions for incompetent patients. Since families are so directly involved in the illness of loved ones, an approach that reposes authority in the family seems to respect present social mores. Although this discretion is couched in terms of ascertaining what the patient would choose if competent, or what the patient in fact once said, the family is usually the source of this information and hence is in a position to control it. Close scrutiny of the family's assessment of these questions is frequently omitted, thus giving them ultimate discretion to decide the matter.

Finally, the orthodox approach is attractive because it is comfortable. It enables decision-makers to finesse the dilemmas or tragic choices that make decisions for incompetent patients so difficult. By shifting the inquiry to what the patient when competent had or would have decided, it absolves decision-makers of the need to confront directly the value of debilitated life versus the burdens such life places on families, physicians, and society. It enables the courts to say, as they do in *Saikewicz* and *Brophy*, that they are not making quality of life choices or privileging other-directed interests but simply honoring what the patient has or would have chosen.

With these advantages, it is no surprise that the orthodox approach of treating the incompetent patient as a competent decision-maker so dominates legal and ethical thinking in this area. But its conceptual flaws and contradictions emerge when it is applied to the conscious, demented, and debilitated patients who now claim judicial and policy attention. When extended to this diverse group of individuals, the orthodox approach risks giving excessive and unexamined power to family and cost considerations in the guise of respecting patient autonomy.

THE ERRORS OF THE ORTHODOX APPROACH

Despite its allure and wide acceptance, the orthodox approach to non-treatment decisions for incompetent patients is conceptually confused and threatens to harm conscious incompetent patients. The problems arise from its concept of the incompetent patient, which excludes the patient's current needs, and from its implementation method, which allows family and other interests to take control. To demonstrate these points, we examine three erroneous assumptions of the orthodox approach.

1. Incompetent Persons Must Be Treated as Autonomous Choice-Makers.

A major error in the orthodox approach is the assumption that equal respect for incompetent patients requires that they be treated as competent patients—that is, as choice-making actors. Equal respect for incompetent patients requires that their interests be protected and that they not be abused simply because they are incompetent. However, it does not follow that they must be treated as if they were exercising autonomy.

Choice is irrelevant if one lacks the capacity to choose, and incompetent persons are by definition incapable of exercising choice or self-determination. Rather than engage in the fiction of asking what they would choose, we should determine what interests, if any, they currently have in receiving life-sustaining treatment. As we will show, the interests of incompetent patients are not respected by an approach that analyzes their situations as if they were competent individuals exercising choice about treatment and continued life.

2. Expressed or Inferred Prior Choices Are an Accurate Indicator of Incompetent Persons' Current Interests.

A second conceptual error implicit in the orthodox approach is the assumption that the incompetent patient's own treatment choice, if known, would incorporate the preferences the patient had as a competent person. It is wrong to assume that the incompetent patient's prior competent preferences are the best indicator of the patient's current interests. If we could determine the choice that these patients would make if suddenly able to speak—if they could tell us what their interests in their compromised states are—such choices would reflect their current and future interests as incompetent individuals, not their past preferences.

Linking incompetent patients' past competent treatment preferences to their existing welfare is highly problematic. The desires competent persons have concerning their future medical care reflect the activities and goals that make life worthwhile for them as competent, choosing individuals. To most competent persons, work, family, friendships, exercise, hobbies, and related pursuits seem integral to a life worth living. Self-determination, bodily integrity, and personal privacy are also matters of deep concern. Many competent persons would refuse life-sustaining treatment that severely compromised those interests.

When people become incompetent and seriously ill, however, their interests may radically change. With their reduced mental and physical capacities, what was once of extreme importance to them no longer matters, while things that were previously of little moment assume much greater significance. An existence that seems demeaning and unacceptable to the competent person may still be of value to the incompetent patient, whose abilities, desires, and interests have so greatly narrowed.

It is difficult, if not impossible, for competent individuals to predict their interests in future treatment situations when they are incompetent because their needs and interests will have so radically changed. As a result, the directives they issue for future situations of incompetency, though they reflect their current needs and interests, may have little relevance to their needs and interests once they become incompetent. Indeed, their advance directives may even be detrimental to their interests once in that state.

Philosophical concepts of personal identity are relevant to this analysis. One contemporary theory, which is articulated most clearly by the British philosopher Derek Parfit, holds that a person's life can be a series of successive selves, with a new self emerging as the individual undergoes significant changes in beliefs, desires, memories, and intentions. According to this theory, advance directives for non-treatment could be issued by a different person than the subsequently incompetent individual. In such a situation, the former self's preferences would have no particular authority to govern the incompetent patient's treatment.

Yet our analysis does not depend on acceptance of Parfit's theory of personal identity, which could have radical implications for contract, criminal, and other rules of law. According to an alternate widely held view of personal identity, an essential core of the individual persists over time. Persons retain a unitary identity during their entire lives, even though a person's interests may change dramatically as new personal situations arise. The position that a person's interests may change drastically once incompetency develops is consistent with this theory of a more unitary personal identity, and argues against taking the prior directive as an indication of the patient's current interests.

3. Personal Autonomy Includes the Right to Control the Future by Advance Directives.

Some persons might argue that the orthodox approach, especially in its reliance on advance directives, follows from the generally recognized right of autonomous persons to order their future in various ways. The advance directive against medical treatment is simply another way to exert control over one's fate, by minimizing the risk that one will be kept alive unnecessarily. If persons control their future by contract, will, and other self-binding arrangements, should they not also have the right to control their medical future by advance directives against life-prolonging treatment?

At the outset it should be noted that the argument from autonomy only partially supports the orthodox approach to non-treatment decisions regarding incompetent patients. Even if accepted, it would apply only to situations in which the person had issued an explicit directive concerning future conditions that have come to exist. This argument gives no support to the substituted judgment approach to decision-making for incompetent patients, for the proxy decision-maker is not then relying on an explicit directive issued by a person trying to exercise autonomy over her future. Instead, the proxy infers from general statements and behavior what the incompetent patient would have chosen if she had made a decision when competent or could now express a competent preference.

Even with this proviso, it is not clear why a person's directions concerning situations that arise when incompetent should be followed. Such directives are very different from ordering the future by contract or will. For example, unlike contracts, advance treatment directives are not promises on which other parties rely, in return for their own promise of performance or other consideration.

Other persons may have their own interests in enforcement of an advance directive, but they have no contractual right to enforcement, since they have not promised performance in return. Thus, an obligation to honor advance directives does not follow from the obligation to enforce contracts.

The advance directive is also dissimilar to a devise by will. At the time that a will takes effect the testator is dead and no longer has interests that can be harmed by a decision to honor the prior instructions. By contrast, honoring the advance directive occurs at a time when the maker is still alive and can very much be harmed by adherence to its provisions. Failing to honor a "living will" is, therefore, not inconsistent with honoring a "property will."

The argument from autonomy in effect represents a normative judgment that it is more important to give persons the advance certainty that they will not be overtreated than to prevent mistakes of undertreatment which their directives may cause. The security gained in empowering persons to control their medical future in this way is not cost-free. The cost—too often overlooked—is that adherence to the directive will lead to the death of incompetent patients who retain significant interests in continued life. Because interests change over time and the person executing the directive may not be assessing the situation from the perspective of the future incompetent patient, the interests of the competent person contemplating a hypothetical future and the interests of the incompetent person once that future occurs, may diverge. A policy favoring advance directives is not justified unless it recognizes and chooses to run this risk.

A recent New York case, *Evans* v. *Bellevue Hospital*, shows that this concern is more than theoretical. In *Evans*, an incompetent patient diagnosed with AIDS-related complex had when competent executed a document stating that life-sustaining treatment should be forgone if he suffered from "illness, disease or injury or experienced extreme mental deterioration, such that there is no reasonable expectation of recovering or regaining a meaningful quality of life." He also had executed a power of attorney authorizing another individual to make all medical decisions on his behalf.

The court case arose after physicians observed that the patient had multiple brain lesions, which they attributed to toxoplasmosis, a type of infection. The patient's proxy decision-maker asked physicians to withhold antibiotic treatment for the infection. They refused, arguing that the treatment was expected to produce recovery from toxoplasmosis and restore the patient's ability to communicate. The court authorized the treatment, on grounds that the document's reference to "meaningful quality of life" was too ambiguous to sanction non-treatment in this case. The judge noted, however, that if the document had specified conditions that clearly applied to the patient's situation, the proxy would have been permitted to decline the treatment.

Evans sheds light on several major problems with the advance treatment directive. First is the document's imprecision. Living wills and other non-treatment directives tend to consist of broad statements that may supply little guidance on specific treatment questions. In fact they may have no binding effect at all simply because they are too vague or general to be construed to authorize non-treatment in a variety of circumstances never explicitly contemplated by the maker.

A second problem is the strong possibility that individuals who execute directives are unaware that they may be authorizing actions or omissions that conflict with their subsequent well-being. The argument for enforcing a prior directive even when it conflicts with the incompetent patient's interests is hardly compelling if the person, when competent, had not been made aware that his future interests may radically change, and thus be in conflict with what he judged—through the eyes of his previously competent self—to be in his interest.

The *Evans* decision also raises the more serious policy issue of whether to honor advance directives that appear clearly to conflict with the incompetent patient's existing interests. (Of course, many competent patients' advance directives will represent the patients' current interests as well, but in those cases there is no real need for an advance directive to justify forgoing treatment.) Although there is insufficient information to determine if a conflict between past wishes and present interests existed in the *Evans* case, the scenario illustrates the need for courts and legislatures to address this issue.

Avoiding unnecessary, nonbeneficial treatment is clearly a valid individual, family, and policy concern. Patients should not be treated unnecessarily whether or not they have issued a prior directive against such treatment. Withholding treatment in those cases is thus not dependent on issuing an advance directive. As we discuss below, the need to treat should be assessed independently in each case regardless of a directive. Since the directive is unnecessary to this end and may in other situations threaten the welfare of incompetent patients, the policy judgment in its favor is open to serious question. Respect for autonomy thus does not automatically include an obligation to adopt the orthodox approach on prior directives.

THE DANGERS OF THE ORTHODOX APPROACH: UNDERTREATMENT AND INAPPROPRIATE ATTENTION TO COSTS AND FAMILY DISTRESS

The orthodox approach threatens incompetent patients with undertreatment, because it overlooks the interests they may have in continued life in their diminished state. Prior directives made when patients were competent, as well as choices proxy decision-makers infer patients would make under substituted judgment, may conflict with patients' current interests, thus leading to non-treatment decisions that harm incompetent patients.

The potential for conflict with patient interests is heightened under the substituted judgment doctrine. This standard will affect many more people than the advance directive approach, given that few people issue explicit treatment directives. In most applications of substituted judgment, there is no express evidence speaking to the situation at hand. Instead, the family is asked what the formerly competent person would have wanted, if confronted with a choice about this situation. The patient's relatives are seen as having an "intimate understanding of the patient's medical attitudes and general world view." But in answering the treatment question, strong pressures may also move the family to focus on considerations other than the needs of the patient before them.

First, the question itself shifts attention to the patient at another time—to the preferences and needs the patient had as a competent person. As we noted previously, these can differ from the incompetent patient's existing interests. Second, families often have their own interests in being relieved of the distress of seeing their loved ones in a chronic debilitated state. Although not conscious or directly influential, such distress may push the family to determine that the patient "would certainly have wanted treatment forgone." After all, they themselves would not want to be treated in those circumstances. Is it not reasonable to assume that the patient as a competent person would have wanted the same?

When the treatment decision is made, however, the patient is no longer competent, and thus, in most cases, lacks interests in privacy, dignity, and other values that presuppose some conscious appreciation of those concerns. Assigning these factors weight when they are no longer relevant to the patient actually gives priority to family interests and to generally held values of competent persons. Indeed, the real offense in maintaining debilitated patients is to competent observers, whose own concepts of what constitutes dignified and respectful medical treatment for seriously compromised human beings have been violated. Perhaps, as Justice Handler argued in his *Conroy* and *Jobes* opinions, these interests should be influential in the treatment setting. The orthodox approach, however, formally proclaims that they have no role while simultaneously permitting them *sub silentio* to shape non-treatment decisions that may conflict with the patient's current welfare.

The possibility of conflict between patients' interests and the outcomes permitted under the substituted judgment standard is not merely theoretical. Although the proxy's assumptions about the incompetent patient's choices "if competent" may coincide with the incompetent patient's current interests, they may also diverge in crucial ways. A key difference between the approaches emerges when the patient's current interests would seem to require treatment, contrary to the patient's inferred competent wishes.

This difficulty is evident in *Spring* and *Hier*, two Massachusetts cases that permitted life-sustaining care to be withheld from conscious incompetent patients. These cases illustrate how courts applying the substituted judgment approach have failed to examine and protect the actual interests of the individual incompetent patients before them. Both these opinions gave the patients' interests as incompetent individuals short shrift, focusing instead on their alleged interests in privacy and dignity, interests they appeared incapable of possessing at the time due to their incapacity. Moreover, the decisions are vulnerable to charges that family distress and cost considerations influenced the substituted judgment inquiry.

In re Spring concerned a 78-year-old senile but fully conscious nursing-home resident whose end-stage renal disease was being treated with dialysis. He sometimes resisted the procedure and required sedation during its administration. His family asked the court to authorize cessation of the dialysis. The court applied the substituted judgment test and, relying on the family's claim that if Spring were competent he would have refused treatment, held that the dialysis could be discontinued.

The judgment that Spring's competent decision would be to refuse dialysis ignored the possibility that in his incompetent state he obtained sufficient countervailing pleasure and satisfaction to make the benefits of continued life outweigh the discomforts of the dialysis necessary to preserve that life. Nor was there any examination of whether the burdens of dialysis could be reduced by less drastic means, such as behavior modification techniques. The court accepted with little scrutiny the family's view that the patient would have wanted treatment withheld because he had previously been an active outdoorsman.

While Spring's family might have been sincere in their assessment, they were really focusing on what some (certainly not all) competent persons in Spring's situation might choose, and not on what would serve the interests of a person who no longer was competent. The court also failed to consider the possibility that the family's own distress and expense in such a situation influenced their assessment of what the patient would have wanted. The opinion dispenses with any need to assess these possibilities by simply assuming that they would not influence the wishes of a family faced with chronic nursing-home care of a senile husband and father.

Similar conceptual weaknesses characterize the opinion in *In re Hier*, a case involving a 92-year-old nonterminally ill incompetent patient who required feeding by gastrostomy tube. When she pulled out the tube and resisted its reinsertion, the hospital sought judicial guidance. The Court refused to order the minor surgery necessary to replace the tube, stressing the procedure's risk and interpreting Hier's behavior as a "plea for privacy and personal dignity for a 92-year-old person who is seriously ill and for whom life has little left to offer."

The determination that Hier's resistance to feeding manifested a desire for privacy and personal dignity attributed the concerns of a competent individual to an incompetent patient who was probably expressing a simple response, such as irritation with the feeding apparatus or a demand for attention. As in *Spring*, the major deficiencies in this opinion are its omission of a systematic analysis of the patient's current capacities and experiences, and its failure to weigh and balance these elements in determining whether the patient had significant contemporaneous interests in continued life.

Particularly troubling is the *Hier* court's neglect of the pain and distress a conscious patient could experience if she were denied nourishment, as well as its omission of any inquiry into the possibility that she obtained pleasure and enjoyment from her restricted life. There also was evidence that one physician who testified against performing the surgery did so because Hier had already consumed "enough" health care resources. (After the appellate court decision, Hier's legal representative returned to the trial court, presented additional medical testimony, and convinced the lower court to order the surgery.)

These cases illustrate how the court's application of the substituted judgment standard opens the door to non-treatment of nursing-home residents and other severely debilitated persons based on what competent persons believe they would want in those situations, or on what meets the needs of their families and others, rather than on what serves the needs of the incompetent patients themselves. The more recent *Brophy* case reinforces this possibility. Although *Brophy* involved a patient who was irreversibly comatose, the court formulated the substituted judgment doctrine in broad terms that could affect all incompetent patients. The result is that respirators, antibiotics, nutrition, or any other treatment could be withheld from conscious incompetent patients whenever the family asserts that the incompetent patients would have found their current lives "degrading and without human dignity" when they were competent. Since many competent persons might so view such a diminished existence, *Brophy* opens the door legally to withdrawing treatment from any conscious, incompetent nursing-home resident.

THE ORTHODOX APPROACH AND THE RISKS OF OVERTREATMENT

Although the orthodox approach has been generally favorable to family requests for non-treatment, sometimes granting such requests even when unjustified, it could as easily be interpreted to deny proxy requests for non-treatment that should be granted. *In re O'Connor*, decided last year by New York's highest court, exemplifies this problem. Ms. O'Connor was an elderly woman who had suffered a series of strokes that left her paralyzed and bedridden. The court described her as "severely demented" and "profoundly incapacitated," able to respond to some simple commands, but with severe, irreparable neurological damage. Yet the court ruled against removal of a nasogastric tube because the evidence of her past preferences was insufficient to establish that she would have opted against such treatment if she were competent. Similarly, in *Cruzan* v. *Harmon*, the Missouri Supreme Court recently prohibited cessation of tube feeding for a permanently unconscious patient, emphasizing the lack of evidence that she had expressed desires to avoid such treatment.

As in *Spring* and *Hier*, these courts failed to inquire systematically into the patients' current interests in continued life. Instead, they sought to apply the orthodox approach, but took a stricter approach to what counted as sufficient evidence of the patients' competent wishes. Since it is difficult to know what an incompetent patient "if competent" would have wanted, the standard of proof applied to answering that question will control the outcome. Unlike the *Spring* and *Hier* judges, the courts in *O'Connor* and *Cruzan* applied a higher standard of proof to answering that question, finding insufficient evidence that they would have chosen non-treatment.

These cases illustrate the ultimate indeterminacy of the fiction of treating the incompetent patient as a self-determining individual. While the predominant danger of the orthodox approach is undertreatment, it also poses a risk that unjustified overtreatment will occur whenever the courts impose a strict standard for inferring the patient's choice if competent. In that case, medical zeal and rigid concern with right to life values may override patient and other interests. In either case, by focusing on the wrong question—the wishes of a past or hypothetical competent person—the interests of the incompetent patient as they now exist are ignored.

TOWARD A NEW LEGAL STANDARD: THE INCOMPETENT PATIENT'S CURRENT INTERESTS

The orthodox approach to non-treatment decisions for incompetent patients is seriously flawed and should be scrapped. It mistakenly assumes that incompetent patients should be regarded as choice-makers when they are incapable of decision, and then constructs a hypothetical competent decision-maker that confuses past or inferred preferences of patients with their current interests. By overlooking the conflict between past directives and current interests, it allows concerns with family stress and costs to override the real needs of incompetent patients, without an adequate evaluation of each. Alternatively, the test can be manipulated to require such a high standard of proof for inferring competent choice, that treatment can seldom be withheld, no matter how justified in terms of the patient's current interests.

An alternative approach that is more likely to protect conscious incompetent patients and to give factors external to patient welfare their proper role is to ask whether treatment actually serves the incompetent patient's existing interests. If treatment cannot succeed in supplying patients with an acceptable quality of life, then external considerations should be permitted to affect the decision. If treatment would serve patient interests but would impose heavy burdens on family or society, the conflict can be faced openly. Society's commitment to a patient-centered position can be reaffirmed or modified on the merits, not in the guise of determining what the incompetent patient would have chosen if competent.

To develop defensible standards governing the care of incompetent patients, legal decision-makers must directly assess the value to patients of their diminished or marginalized lives. The most appropriate method is to adopt a variation of the "best interests" standard and to ask whether treatment will advance the current and future welfare of the patient. This approach requires a systematic evaluation of the incompetent patient's personal contemporaneous interests, rather than the interests competent persons might have in those situations. Assessing these interests requires observers to evaluate, from the incompetent patient's perspective, indications of the patient's subjective state, and ultimately, to judge whether this state of existence is a sufficient good to justify further treatment of the patient. The question is not how a competent person would feel in such states, but whether these experiences are of value to a person in the incompetent person's situation. The important question is whether patients who cannot experience the richness of normal life still have experiences that make continued existence from their own perspective better than no life at all.

Such an approach has several advantages that recommend its adoption for all decision-making regarding incompetent patients. First, it is respectful of the individual whose treatment is at issue. The ethical commitment to a patient-centered approach requires a focus on the patient as she now is, and not on the desires that she previously had when her interests were quite different. This approach will better protect a debilitated patient's existing interests in continued life.

Second, it will permit non-treatment to occur when justified, e.g., when the patient cannot reasonably be said to have any continued interest in living because her level of awareness is so minimal that the patient is unable to appreciate being alive. For life to be of value to an individual, some capacity to interact with the environment must be present. Thus, incompetent patients with minimal "relational capacity," such as Nancy Cruzan, Claire Conroy, or Mary O'Connor, lack significant interests in having their lives maintained, and might have further treatment withheld under this test.

Third, the current-interests approach acknowledges the role of costs, family stress, and similar concerns, thus preventing them from influencing non-treatment decisions in an uncontrolled or unprincipled way. By focusing on the incompetent patient's current interests, room is given for these competing concerns when no significant patient interests are affected. Thus, for example, in cases involving permanently unconscious and barely conscious individuals, the family's burdens and financial costs may be taken into account because no interests of the patient are directly affected.

Fourth, a focus on current interests of the incompetent patient sharpens the conflict between a patient-centered and other-directed approach, thus requiring explicit consideration of the normative judgments supporting either approach. The desire to relieve family stress and reduce costs may operate at some level in treatment decisions affecting many severely debilitated patients. Unless these factors are candidly confronted, they risk influencing treatment decisions in an unprincipled fashion, potentially overriding the significant interests some incompetent patients have in obtaining life-sustaining treatment. While such directness may be discomforting, facing the question openly will keep other-directed concerns from operating subterraneously and hold them in check.

Finally, a current-interests approach still permits the family to be the initial or primary decision-maker—an important ingredient of any public policy. The family or other proxy will, in effect, be asked to determine whether the patient's life is so diminished that the patient has no further interests in living, not whether continued living is what the patient would have chosen. Doctors, courts, and others reviewing family decisions, however, will then explicitly apply a current-interests test to the proxy's choice. Ultimately a societal judgment about what states of diminished life are worth protecting will be brought to bear on those decisions.

Such an approach is not as radical a departure as it might initially sound, and is inevitable once the inability of the orthodox approach to handle more difficult cases becomes clear. Indeed, variations on this approach have already appeared. In *Saikewicz*, for example, the court purportedly applied the substituted judgment standard, couching its decision in terms of the patient's privacy and self-determination rights. In reality it performed a best interests analysis and concluded that in light of the patient's capacity to understand the pain that would be imposed to gain a few extra months of living, a decision against treatment would best serve his interests. Similarly, although its decision to require treatment might be questioned, the New York Court of Appeals in *Storar* based its decision on an individualized assessment of the burdens and benefits of continued treatment for the patient. Unfortunately it chose not to follow that lead in *O'Connor*, where a judgment that further treatment was not in the patient's interests could reasonably have been reached.

The New Jersey Supreme Court in *Conroy* partially accepted this approach when no explicit treatment directive or other clear evidence of a patient's past preferences was available. According to the court, if "the net burdens of the patient's life with the treatment . . . clearly and markedly outweigh the benefits that the patient derives from life" and "the recurring, unavoidable, and severe pain of the patient's life [are] such that the effect of administering life-sustaining treatment would be inhumane," life-sustaining treatment may be forgone.

In our view, however, *Conroy* articulates the benefit-burden analysis too narrowly to protect incompetent patients adequately, for it fails to include such factors as lack of awareness and relational capacity. Thus, it does not authorize nontreatment of permanently unconscious or barely conscious patients who obtain negligible benefits from life, but experience no pain and suffering. Moreover, *Conroy, Saikewicz,* and *Storar* limit the benefit-burden analysis to cases in which reliable evidence of the patients' competent treatment preferences is lacking, thus overlooking the possibility of conflict between such evidence and current interests. Nevertheless, the courts' partial recognition of the need to examine the incompetent patient's contemporaneous interests is encouraging, and may facilitate expanded acceptance of the current-interests standard.

DIFFICULTIES OF A CURRENT-INTERESTS APPROACH

The major difficulty in applying a current-interests approach lies in obtaining reliable information about a patient's subjective experiences and in evaluating their significance. The danger is that arbitrary assessments of patient interests will occur, to the detriment of patients and society's respect for life.

However, the difficulty in obtaining and evaluating data about the patient and thus determining her interests is surmountable in many cases. Even though these patients typically can furnish us with little or no verbal data on how they experience their lives, the observer can gain this information from assessing their behavior and physical condition. Evidence bearing on patients' perception of pain and other physical sensations, ability to interact with other persons and the environment, and ability to engage in cognitive activity are all relevant to the examination of what these patients' lives are like for them.

More daunting is the next step: to determine whether these experiences provide "a life worth living" to the patient and a corresponding obligation by family or society to preserve it, despite the burdens that doing so entails. Yet here too it is possible to make considerable progress before facing the toughest questions about quality of life and tradeoffs with other interests.

For example, a wide consensus already exists that certain states of being are not in a patient's interest, and therefore need not be provided if the family requests non-treatment. One such situation exists when the patient can experience only unremitting pain, without any countervailing pleasure and enjoyment. With modern techniques of pain relief, however, few patients may be in this category.

Permanently unconscious patients comprise a larger agreed-upon category of individuals lacking significant interests in prolonged life. All available medical evidence indicates that these individuals have no mental awareness. Although they suffer no pain or distress, they cannot experience any benefit from continued life. For them, there is only the remote possibility of restoration in the event of a mistaken diagnosis or an as yet undiscovered cure that supplies a reason for maintenance. With the exception of the *Cruzan* case in Missouri, every state court that has faced the question has permitted nontreatment of these individuals under the orthodox approach. It is likely that these decisions were influenced by the view that continued life fails to confer a significant benefit on such patients, although the opinions fail explicitly to incorporate this analysis.

Assessment of current interests of other groups of patients may also reasonably occur. "Barely conscious" individuals who cannot initiate purposeful activity, whose experiences are limited to physical sensations, and whose medical prognosis holds no reasonable chance of improvement, have clear interests in avoiding pain and discomfort. Their interests in continued life seem small, however, because they lack the cognitive capacity to interact with others and to appreciate being alive. Although some will argue that any minimally conscious human being has a significant stake in being maintained, it is difficult to see how life without greater awareness of self and others can confer a genuine benefit on these patients. Families who take this position and request non-treatment would not therefore be violating the right to life of such patients.

In contrast, conscious incompetent patients who can experience enjoyment and pleasure, and whose conditions and necessary treatment interventions impose on them small or moderate burdens, have more significant interests in obtaining life-sustaining care. The "pleasantly senile" and other debilitated individuals who appear to receive benefits from their restricted lives fall into this category. Even though their activities may seem unduly limited to some observers, these individuals appear to retain sufficient mental capacity for continued life to hold material value for them. If society is committed to a patient-centered approach, it should be willing to provide the resources necessary to protect these patients' lives. It should also find that these patients' former competent preferences against treatment and family distress are inadequate to override the patients' interests in receiving continued care.

The hardest cases will fall between those who are barely conscious and the pleasantly senile. For those patients it may be difficult to ascertain or meaningfully discuss their interests in living from their own limited perspective. "Objective" quality of life assessments are inevitably crude and subject to dispute. Disagreement and controversy may be unavoidable. In some cases, it will be impossible to reach a clear decision on what outcome would best serve the patient's existing interests. Moreover, extensive debate may be required to determine what level of awareness and benefit is sufficient to give incompetent patients a significant interest in continued life, notwithstanding the patients' former competent preferences against treatment and the burdens imposed on family and society.

But these problems are no greater than the problems under the orthodox approach of determining what the patient would choose if competent when that approach is scrupulously applied. The comparative advantage of the current-interests standard is that quality of life assessments and the conflicts they pose with other interests are faced openly, rather than in the guise of family or proxy decision of what the patient would choose if competent. In our view this openness constitutes a great advantage.

THE INEVITABILITY OF QUALITY OF LIFE ASSESSMENTS

Applying the current-interests test necessarily involves assessing the value of a particular existence to the incompetent patient in question, and its value relative to the burdens that providing it poses for family and society. Ultimately, the current-interests test brings us to the controversial task of making quality of life judgments—of deciding whether the duty to sustain life in marginalized states is obligatory, notwithstanding the burdens on others of doing so.

Although balancing patient quality of life against other interests has long been a taboo subject, we believe that an honest, direct approach to these issues is both warranted and manageable. Since quality of life judgments must inevitably be made, it is preferable to make them openly so that arbitrary or unjustified assessments can be identified. The alternative is a conceptually flawed approach that allows those judgments to be made covertly, thus risking even greater likelihood of damage to incompetent patients, their families, and society.

How do these considerations apply to actual decision-making for incompetent patients? Families will still retain primary decision-making authority, deciding whether the patient has further interests in living. In the great majority of instances their choices will reflect general societal judgments about the value to patients of greatly diminished states of existence. In cases that are less clear, the family or proxy's choice should be reviewed in light of the current-interests standard. If an objective viewer finds that the patient has significant interests in continued existence, then treatment providing that existence should continue unless the community at large reevaluates its overriding commitment to a patient-centered approach to these questions.

CONCLUSION

As the non-treatment debate moves to hard questions concerning conscious incompetent patients, it is essential that the issues be clearly posed and carefully analyzed. The orthodox judicial approach, which substitutes the fiction of a competent decision-maker for the reality of an incompetent person, is inadequate to this task and should be abandoned. That fiction confuses the issue, misleads families, doctors, and others struggling with treatment decisions, and harms the patients and families most directly affected.

An approach that focuses on the current interests of the incompetent patient—on her quality of life—is far preferable. Open assessment of quality of life will give incompetent patients their due, while at the same time acknowledging a proper role for family and cost concerns. While difficult questions will remain, the central normative questions will be directly faced. What quality of diminished life should be protected? At what cost? These are the questions that must be faced in decision-making at the margins of life.

THE LIMITS OF LEGAL OBJECTIVITY

Nancy K. Rhoden

PRIOR DIRECTIVES AND THE OBJECTIVE ENTERPRISE

The objective standard as articulated in *Conroy* was, of course, intended only for those situations in which the patient's prior beliefs were not determinative. If taken to its logical extension, however, the quest for a person-neutral standard may come to clash with the widespread acceptance of clear-cut prior directives as controlling. This conflict arises because if we focus solely on the incompetent's present interests, we so radically distinguish her from the author of the prior directive that it's hard to see why the prior choice should govern.

To illustrate how a completely present-oriented test can undermine the justification for honoring living wills, imagine for a moment that after the court evaluated Ms. Conroy objectively, her nephew discovered a valid and clearly applicable living will rejecting all medical treatment if "barely conscious." Given its preference for a subjective test, the *Conroy* court almost certainly would want to reconsider and let the document control. But this hypothetical discovery creates a "past-present" conflict, in which Ms. Conroy's present interests support treatment, while her prior choice is to forgo it. Although the court could simply hold that an applicable living will trumps current interests, this decision procedure seems rather arbitrary in light of the just-completed assessment of current interests. Why, one might ask, should a prior directive control if it thwarts a patient's present interests?

North Carolina Review 68, no. 5, June 1990: 845–865.

Editors' note: Professor Rhoden's article has been substantially edited and most of the footnotes have been omitted. Readers wishing to follow up on sources should consult the original article. Deleted sections noted the problems with the "subjective" tests articulated in the Conroy case (reprinted in this section) and challenged the adequacy of the "objective" tests on the grounds that they (1) set a standard that can almost never be met, and (2) focus narrowly on pain to the exclusion of other important subjective values. In the sections reprinted here, Rhoden argues that the objective approach advocated in the preceding article by Professors Dresser and Robertson also threatens the validity of prior directives.

One answer to this is that it should not. Dresser, as the most logical and consistent advocate of a present best interests test, essentially rejects living wills, except to the extent they provide useful reassurance in cases in which the objective choice would be to terminate treatment, so that the wills are largely redundant.[1] Hence my first task is to analyze her arguments and rebut them by setting forth a rights-based justification for honoring prior directives. . . .

The Impairment of the Incompetent's Interests

. . . [Dresser argues] that honoring a living will can compromise unacceptably the interests of an incompetent person. One cannot be sure that what the person chose then is what he would choose now, because views about what constitutes an acceptable level of functioning may change radically as function declines. Active, healthy persons often say they would never want to live if wheelchair-bound, on dialysis, or whatever, and then later embrace life despite their disabilities. Likewise, once capacity for complex intellectual pleasures is gone, simpler things take on greater importance. As Dresser and Robertson put it:

> If we truly could determine the choice that these patients would make if suddenly able to speak—if they could tell us what their interests in their compromised states are—such choices would be most likely to reflect their current and future interests as incompetent individuals, not their past preferences.[2]

Thus prior directives reflect competent persons' former interests, but the better, more caring way to make choices for incompetents is to focus on their current interests. The law should not allow someone to make a binding future choice for death, because to do so gives an unacceptable degree of primacy to the interests of competent persons over incompetent ones.

The strength of this argument is reinforced by a very troubling sort of example. Suppose a highly intellectual person makes a prior directive stating that if he becomes even somewhat mentally impaired, he wants no medical treatment. He then suffers a mild stroke and is in a nursing home. While he cannot comprehend his prior directive, and hence can neither affirm nor rescind it, he appears to enjoy his simple existence, watching television and sharing meals with other patients. Then he gets pneumonia. His directive clearly rejects antibiotics. If it is controlling, the staff must simply watch him die. But, Dresser quite reasonably argues, he has substantial present interests in life, and they must prevail. This sort of case may well incline us toward a Parfit-type view*—that this happy incompetent person *is* someone different from the intellectual who made the document—or, at least, should make us question the wisdom of necessarily subordinating present interests to prior choices, no matter how explicit and strongly held.

All this makes a strong case against prior directives. It suggests that the reason living wills have been so widely accepted is not that we have an abiding faith in future-oriented choices, but that the substantive choice in most living wills is an objectively reasonable one (to avoid prolongation of the dying process, or treatment when persistently vegetative). Hence a prior directive may well help bolster a decision to stop treatment for a patient who lacks present interests in living, but it should not justify termination when the patient has such interests. I will later deal with the case in which the incompetent patient has clear-cut and substantial interests in living and will suggest that the right to make binding future choices should be less absolute than the right to make present ones. But first I must resurrect prior directives in general as reflecting a moral preference for individual choice rather than merely reinforcing objective decisions. To do so, I will show that rejecting future-oriented choices threatens present ones.

The Continuum with Contemporaneous Choices

Assume that George is a Christian Scientist who rejects all surgical interventions. He makes a prior directive refusing surgery at any time for any condition. He subsequently develops a brain tumor which impairs his cognitive processes so that he is incapable of either affirming or rejecting his prior

---

Editors' note: See Dresser/Robertson article, this section.

directive. He is happily watching television, and the brain tumor could be removed, extending his life (though not restoring his competency). Dresser undoubtedly would say that decision makers should authorize surgery, on the grounds that the prior religious faith is no longer relevant and that his present interests in his happy, albeit limited, life should control.

George's case seems very similar to the intellectual's, except of course that his prior beliefs are religious rather than "merely" secular. A truly "hard-core" believer in prior directives may feel that in even these cases, the directive should prevail. Some proponents of precedent autonomy may feel otherwise, because the incompetent patients: (1) have such clear-cut interests in life; and (2) are so unlikely to retain beliefs in the primacy of the intellect or the tenets of the Christian Science faith. Hence some supporters of prior directives may wish to disavow them in one or both of these cases. To show, however, that this should not lead to a wholesale rejection of precedent autonomy, we merely need alter one of two variables. The first is the time frame; the second is the patient's mental status at the time of initial diagnosis and decision making.

First, the time frame. Assume our intellectual is also psychic—or at least aware that his blood pressure is 210 over 190. He anticipates his stroke and one day before it makes his prior directive. Although the stroke affects only his brain, one week later he contracts pneumonia. Despite his recent choice, made in anticipation of disability, a proponent of current interests undoubtedly still would protect the incompetent's present interests. After all, interests can change gradually over twenty years, or in one fell swoop when one's neocortex is damaged.

If this feels somewhat less comfortable to the proponent of patient autonomy, it is because the rapidity of the developments has blurred the distinction between present- and future-oriented choice. We can blur this distinction even further if, returning to George, the brain tumor is diagnosed while he is still competent. As a Christian Scientist, he refuses surgery. Because he knows incompetency may soon ensue, he makes a prior directive. One week later, he is incompetent. Rethinking his choice now seems to me like a wrong to George—the George who competently chose, based on considered religious beliefs, to reject treatment. Yet from the present-oriented perspective, I cannot see why this is any different from the other cases. *Now* George is an incompetent whose life could be prolonged by medical intervention. And *now* he lacks the mental structure to hold his former beliefs. Under a present-oriented view, we would respect choice as long as the person was competent, but then, once his powers dimmed, we would rethink it if treatment was still potentially efficacious. In other words, a competent choice will lose its force once the person is incapable of realizing it has been made, because now—whether this occurs gradually or suddenly—the incompetent is the only player in town.

If we accept this present focus, then the competent patient's "right" to refuse treatment will be upheld only for the few months, weeks, days, or hours she remains competent. After that, the treatment decision will be made on the basis of the objectively assessed present interests of the incompetent. Taken to an extreme, this could mean that a Jehovah's Witness could refuse a blood transfusion until he "bled out" and became incompetent, after which he could be transfused.

However an objective test would decide cases of intermittent incompetency, such as the typical Jehovah's Witness scenario, it seems to commit us to a wholesale reassessment of contemporaneous treatment refusals upon subsequent incompetency. Not all refusals will impair the interests of the now-incompetent: if he is terminally ill, he may be better-off dying more quickly. But many treatment refusals will, especially those based upon minority views about religion or modern medicine. Minority beliefs are usually considered to be precisely those for which protection of autonomy is most crucial. Once we recognize that present autonomy and precedent autonomy are simply two ends of a continuum, along which are choices initially made when competent, reaffirmed repeatedly, but subject to reexamination after the person becomes incompetent, we see that rejecting precedent autonomy threatens a fairly broad spectrum of present, prior, and mixed present/prior choices.

Viewing the Incompetent

This returns us to the dilemma of how to view incompetent patients. They can, of course, be viewed just in the present, with only their current, highly truncated interests taken into account. As so viewed, the prior directive clearly impairs the incompetent's interests. Back when the directive was made, however, the person was acting as a moral agent, and it is harder to take a completely present-oriented view toward moral agents and their interests. As Christine Korsgaard, who criticizes Parfit for viewing persons in a peculiarly passive sense as essentially the experiencers of various sensations, puts it:

> Perhaps it is natural to think of the present self as necessarily concerned with present satisfaction. But it is mistaken. In order to make deliberative choices, your present self must identify with something from which you will derive your reasons, but not necessarily with something present. The sort of thing you identify yourself with may carry you automatically into the future; and I have been suggesting that this will very likely be the case. Indeed, the choice of any action, no matter how trivial, takes you some way into the future. And to the extent that you regulate your choices by identifying yourself as the one who is implementing something like a particular plan of life, you need to identify with your future in order to be *what you are even now*. When the person is viewed as an agent, no clear content can be given to the idea of a merely present self.[3]

Dresser criticizes prior directives as giving moral and legal primacy to competent persons over incompetent ones. While incompetent persons of course warrant respect, I think it is nonetheless perfectly appropriate to give primacy to competent persons—at least if the incompetent person inhabits the formerly competent person's body. The competent person's primacy derives from his status as moral agent. Moral agency is inherently future-directed, and the future may, unfortunately, encompass one's incompetency. Prior directives are the tools for projecting one's moral and spiritual values into the future. These values seem to me worthy of respect even when they conflict with the subsequent, purely physical, interests of an incompetent. (I must admit here, though, that there may be an irreconcilable clash of instincts about whether the incompetent should be viewed as the moral agent he was or the more passive experiencer of physical sensations he is now.)

Another problem with the purely present perspective is that prior directives reflect concern for others. Many people make living wills because they do not want their family's resources to be consumed in sustaining a barely sentient existence. Consider another example of other-directed values. Suppose a pregnant woman is stricken with cancer. Her prognosis is better if she aborts, but she refuses, because having this baby is the most important thing to her. She makes out a document specifying this, and then lapses into incompetency. An abortion still could be performed. Someone who rejects prior directives would, it seems, have to reopen the issue of the abortion and endorse it if it promoted the now-incompetent woman's physical interests. Yet just as it is difficult to view moral agents only in the present, it is difficult to view them in total isolation. Surely it is misleading to view *this* woman in complete isolation. Her most cherished goal—to leave the legacy of a child—is attainable only via a prior directive that harms the incompetent. It reflects the values of the competent person she was, and these values warrant a degree of moral primacy.

All this suggests that while it may be true that the incompetent person, if suddenly able to speak, would choose based on her current interests, this should not be determinative, because her former values, though no longer consciously held, have not lost their moral force. Among other reasons, such values are still important because the formerly competent person made a choice—an exercise of her autonomy. Her living will should not be seen simply as evidence of what she (as an incompetent) might now want. Seen as mere evidence, a prior directive inevitably will fail, because even the most devastatingly impaired patient could now, at least hypothetically, want something else. Viewed as an actual choice, a living will can function fairly well. It of course has limitations, as do other prior choices such as testamentary wills. Much as one cannot know one's precise medical plight in advance, one cannot anticipate the changes in conduct, lifestyle, or fortune of one's heirs. A regular will clearly is not evidence of most recent desires, but is an actual choice, and a change in circumstances is simply the risk one runs in making future choices. The alternative is not to make such choices (or to designate a proxy rather than make a substantive choice). But if we believe in the right to make future choices, we should not complain about their inherent and inescapable limitations.

The analogy with testamentary wills, however, returns us to the troubling example of the intellectual's idiosyncratic directive, because a living will, unlike a testamentary will, can severely compromise a person's present interests. Are there no limits to the harmful future choices a person can make? It does not seem inconsistent with accepting precedent autonomy to place some limits on it. In a few cases, competent contemporaneous choices are overruled, because, for example, they place medical professionals in such an untenable position. This was the impetus for denying Elizabeth Bouvia the relief sought in her first lawsuit—the right to refuse food and water by mouth while receiving hygienic care in the psychiatric ward of a hospital. The court held, essentially, that individual autonomy could not transform medical professionals into attendants at a suicide parlor. Prior directives are made with far less knowledge of the medical situation and the patient's future interests than are current choices. Hence some restrictions could be placed on them (as the law currently does), so that the former intellectual could not demand that nursing home staff let a happy, otherwise healthy, but "pleasantly senile" person die. We can thus concede that such an unusual prior directive need not control—because other concerns can override our prima facie duty to honor it—without rejecting the basic principle of prior control. After all, challenging as this philosophical puzzle is, no one (at least at present) makes such directives. People make prior directives to avoid being tethered to medical technology when unconscious or in a state such as Claire Conroy's. When they start saying, "If I can't do higher mathematics, kill me," we will have to worry in earnest about the limits of precedent autonomy.

Finally, I do not deny that we can, when pressed, make quality-of-life assessments from a present-oriented perspective. Decision makers must do this for infants and for the never-competent. Something is wrong, however, when we treat formerly competent patients as if they were never competent. Someone who makes a prior directive sees herself as the unified subject of a human life. She sees her concern for her body, her goals, or her family as transcending her incapacity. It is at least one, if not an overriding, component of treating persons with respect, that we view them as they view themselves. If we are to do this, we must not ignore their prior choices and values.

Actual prior choices are an exercise of autonomy and hence deserve far more weight than informally expressed preferences. This is not only because of evidentiary concerns, but because a person who makes a living will has exercised her right to decide—a right that imposes upon others a prima facie duty to honor her choice. We have, however, no similar right that informally expressed preferences be honored. Yet many of the same reasons that make prior directives morally relevant also make prior preferences relevant. Primary among them is the sense that most persons, when competent, see their preferences, goals, and values as relevant to future choices about them, because they see themselves as unified subjects of their lives. Were we all Parfitians, this conclusion would change. But, I hazard to say, we are not. Hence, when making moral choices for formerly competent persons who left no explicit directives we should still consider their probable desires, although we should avoid succumbing to the illusion that such desires will necessarily be unambiguous or determinative.

THE ANALOGY TO WILLS AND THE PROBLEM OF THE SUBJECT

Someone might object that all this boils down to the claim that because many people feel that if they become incompetent they would want others to think of them as they were in their prime, the law should accept and reinforce this delusion. In other words, if there is no competent person there who will notice the dishonoring of his prior wishes, then thinking we must honor them is just as silly as thinking of the dead as they were when alive and imagining we have duties to them. The "problem of the subject"—the question of just who is harmed by posthumous betrayals—has received substantial philosophical consideration. I cannot treat it adequately here, but can offer some suggestions that relate back to the unconscious or barely conscious. One solution that is easy—perhaps too easy—is just to emphasize that competent people care about their future, and if word gets out that choices will be reassessed upon incompetency, everyone will be anxious and uneasy. This rule-utilitarian approach does yield a duty to honor prior directives, albeit one that does not run to anyone in particular. It clearly would be acceptable to someone whose general moral theory is a rule-utilitarian one. It is less satisfactory to a rights-based theorist, because it means that while failure to honor a present choice wrongs the chooser, failure to honor a prior choice is, in Joel Feinberg's words, merely a "diffuse public harm."

Because Feinberg believes that the dead can be wronged (and, indeed, harmed), he tackles this problem of who is harmed by a posthumous betrayal. Feinberg distinguishes two ways of conceptualizing the dead: as dead bodies ("postmortem persons") and as the persons they were when alive ("antemortem persons"). Postmortem persons cannot be harmed; they are mere corpses. But, Feinberg argues, antemortem persons can be harmed, because they can have "surviving interests" that can be invaded. Hence posthumous betrayals can count as harms to antemortem persons. Holding that the subject of the harm is the antemortem person is an attempt, and probably a successful one, to solve the problem of the subject.

Joan Callahan argues that although in postulating antemortem persons, Feinberg has devised a proper subject of harm, he faces another problem—that of "backward causation," or the implication that an event after a person's death can harm him prior to his death.[4] Feinberg seeks to avoid this implication by holding that the antemortem subject of posthumous harm was harmed all along, or at least at the point when he acquired the interest that would subsequently be defeated. It is just that until the harmful event actually occurs, no one could know of his harmed condition. As Feinberg puts it:

> [T]he financial collapse of the life-insurance company through which I have protected my loved dependents, occurring, let us imagine, five minutes after my death, several years in the future, makes it true that my present interest in my children's security is harmed, and therefore, that *I* am harmed too, though I know it not. When that time comes, my friends might feel sorry not only for my children but for me too, though I am dead.[5]

According to Feinberg, believing that the antemortem person is harmed before the event is no different from believing that a father whose son has just been killed is immediately harmed, even though he has not yet received the bad news.

Several closely related and, it seems, telling criticisms have been made of this notion that a person whose interests will be defeated after his death is in a harmed state from the time he acquires such interests. W. J. Waluchow notes that we do not think this way about future harms to existing persons; we do not consider ourselves already harmed by events that will happen in the future.[6] It seems he is correct that future harms should have the same logical structure whether the victim will be dead or alive when the harmful event occurs. As Callahan points out, Feinberg's theory implies that a person who will later perform a harmful action is, long before doing so, responsible for placing the victim in a harmed (though as-of-yet unrecognizably so) position. Sympathetic as I find Feinberg's overall approach, this particular aspect does seem to smack of predestination. If before a decedent's demise his future betrayer had not even formed his evil intent, it seems very strange to maintain that the decedent while alive was in a harmed state. Despite Feinberg's attempt to equate this with a father's lack of awareness of his son's recent death, there does seem to be a crucial asymmetry between being unaware of an event that has occurred, and being unaware of a future event that, unless we are fatalists, may not happen after all.

Even if Feinberg's attempted solution to the problem of backward causation fails, I believe that the basic moral intuition that we wrong the promisee when we breach a promise, even posthumously, remains firm, as Callahan's discussion itself illustrates. Callahan first tries to defend this duty by claiming that testamentary bequests generally merit respect in their own right; that we feel obligated to honor them because they usually coincide with other values we hold important, such as the good of individual heirs. To support this, she notes that we would feel less obligation to carry out an iniquitous or wasteful request (that all the paintings of a great artist be burned). But surely we don't feel that giving an estate to the decedent's spoiled, self-indulgent son (to whom it was bequeathed) is objectively preferable to giving it to his hard-working, saintly (but disinherited) daughter. If honoring his will is morally obligatory, this is because we believe the deceased had a right to distribute his estate as he saw fit, even if we abhor the end result. If truly heinous requests are not binding upon us, it is simply because other moral principles can sometimes override prima facie rights.

Callahan does admit that the independent moral value of bequests cannot fully account for what she recognizes as the genuine moral conviction that persons have a right to dispose of their property as they see fit. However, she claims that right yields a duty not to the decedent, but only to his heirs. That sounds initially plausible, but how would it apply to other promises made to a decedent? Suppose I leave my friend ten thousand dollars in my will in return for his promise to care for my cat. If, as soon as I die, he has my cat euthanized, it is hard not to think that he has breached a duty to me, rather than to my cat. It becomes even harder if the promise was to nurture my stamp collection. Moreover, when we turn to living wills, holding that the duty runs to the relatives is clearly unworkable, because surely the absence of family would not negate the duty to respect the prior directive. (And suggesting that duties run to persistently vegetative patients, viewed just in the present, is no more plausible than saying they run to corpses.) Thus Callahan is left recognizing the moral force of the duty to honor wills, but failing either to ground or direct such a duty.

The perplexities about harm predating the harmful event, and the opposite problem of being unable to justify the belief that there are duties to the dead, can each be avoided if we simply extrapolate from the observation that a right-holder need not have either the capacity or potential to discover a breach of duty. Clearly, if a person who has contracted for a statue to be erected in her honor moves to Australia, failure of the promisor to erect the statue is a breach of duty to the person in Australia, even if she never finds out. Why should the analysis change if the promisor procrastinates and breaches the contract after the emigrant has died? It is still a breach of duty, and of a duty that ran to the person who, while alive, held the right to performance. In other words, rights and duties, although correlative, need not be temporally coextensive.

This analysis relates back to the various ways persons can view themselves. Someone seeking a future-oriented promise sees herself as caring how her body, or property, or heirs, are treated. The promisor in turn incurs a duty of performance that entails an obligation to see the promisee as she envisioned herself. Thus the promisor cannot legitimately focus only upon the consequences of a breach (reasoning "she's a corpse now, she cannot care"), but instead must think of the promisee as she was in the past, and as she projected her goals and interests into the future. This duty in some sense runs backward: the object of its fulfillment or breach is most appropriately viewed as the person as she was when alive (Feinberg's "antemortem person"). But recognizing duties to antemortem persons does not mean we have to agree that dead persons can be harmed or that future victims of harms are harmed from the moment they acquire interests that will be defeated. All we need affirm is that living persons can have rights of future performance, and that breaches of duties to perform after death count as wrongs to the right-holder, thought of as she was when alive.

Although duties to persons who previously held the correlative right but who no longer exist are admittedly an unusual case, we might think of this as similar to other future-oriented promises made in anticipation of incapacity. Suppose Joe, a manic-depressive given to extravagant and disastrous business deals in his manic phase, makes a contract (during a lucid period) with a friend whereby the friend promises not to let him make any business deals while manic. Then Joe becomes manic. In adhering to the contract, the friend is upholding his duty to view Joe (and Joe's interests) as Joe saw things when lucid. This case differs from wills or living wills, because Joe himself will benefit in the future from having his present desires thwarted. But the cases are not so completely different, because each involves a duty to act upon wishes of a person that are no longer held and indeed to view the person, for moral purposes, as he viewed himself at a previous time, and as he projected the values held then into the future. The solution of saying a duty exists *now,* and breach of it is a breach of duty, and thus a wrong, to the person as he was *then,* is not unproblematic. If one accepts a rights-based justification for present and precedent autonomy, however, the backward-looking solution seems preferable to holding that upon death or incapacity, a formerly grounded duty suddenly runs in no direction at all.

CONCLUSION

Thus we must reject the premise of the present-oriented objective test—that if a subjective analysis does not yield a definitive answer, a fully objective approach must be used. Viewing the patient only in the present divides her from her history, her values, and her relationships—from all those things that made her a moral agent. It likewise undermines living wills. Living wills are not as unproblematic as often assumed: they are subject to the criticism that they subjugate the interests of incompetent persons to the values of competent ones. But as we have seen, many or most autonomous choices take the chooser some way into the future. Denying the right of future choice thus threatens the right of present choice. Hence the mirror image of the asserted problem with living wills is giving so much primacy to incompetents that one acts as if they never were competent. If a person has stated, "Treat me, when incompetent, as if my competent values still hold," respect for persons demands that we do so. This does give primacy to the competent person, but it is, after all, competent persons who have the considered moral values, life plans, and treatment preferences that underlie our respect. Finally, this analysis can apply, albeit less strongly, to formerly competent patients who did not make prior directives, because they, too, most likely held relevant views. If we believe that a competent person is, more likely than not, to see her values as still being relevant during incapacity, then respect for persons suggests that we consider those values in making treatment decisions, even while recognizing that they may be more difficult to assess, and hence far less determinative, than actual prior choices.

NOTES

1. R. Dresser, "Life, Death, and Incompetent Patients: Conceptual Infirmities and Hidden Values in the Law," 373 *Ariz v. Rev.* at 379–82, 394–95; Dresser, "Relitigating Life and Death," 51 *Ohio St. L. J.* 425 (1990), at 433.
2. "Quality of Life and Non-Treatment Decisions for Incompetent Patients: A Critique of the Orthodox Approach," 17 *Law, Med. & Health Care* 234, 236–37 (1989) [*supra* this section].
3. Korsgaard, "Personal Identity and the Unity of Agency: A Kantian Response to Parfit," 18 *Phil. & Pub. Aff.* 101, 113–14 (1989) (footnotes omitted).
4. *See* Callahan, "On Harming the Dead," 97 *Ethics* 341, 345 (1987).
5. J. Feinberg, *Harm to Others.* 91 (1984).
6. Waluchow, "Feinberg's Theory of 'Preposthumous' Harm," 25 *Dialogue* 727, 732–33 (1986).

EUTHANASIA AND PHYSICIAN-ASSISTED SUICIDE

DEATH AND DIGNITY: A CASE OF INDIVIDUALIZED DECISION MAKING

Timothy E. Quill

Diane was feeling tired and had a rash. A common scenario, though there was something subliminally worrisome that prompted me to check her blood count. Her hematocrit was 22, and the white-cell count was 4.3 with some metamyelocytes and unusual white cells. I wanted it to be viral, trying to deny what was staring me in the face. Perhaps in a repeated count it would disappear. I called Diane and told her it might be more serious than I had initially thought—that the test needed to be repeated and that if she felt worse, we might have to move quickly. When she pressed for the possibilities, I reluctantly opened the door to leukemia. Hearing the word seemed to make it exist. "Oh, shit!" she said. "Don't tell me that." Oh, shit! I thought, I wish I didn't have to.

Diane was no ordinary person (although no one I have ever come to know has been really ordinary). She was raised in an alcoholic family and had felt alone for much of her life. She had vaginal cancer as a young woman. Through much of her adult life, she had struggled with depression and her own alcoholism. I had come to know, respect, and admire her over the previous eight years as she confronted these problems and gradually overcame them. She was an incredibly clear, at times brutally honest, thinker and communicator. As she took control of her life, she developed a strong sense of independence and confidence. In the previous three-and-one-half years, her hard work had paid off. She was completely abstinent from alcohol, she had established much deeper connections with her husband, college-age son, and several friends, and her business and her artistic work were blossoming. She felt she was really living fully for the first time.

Not surprisingly, the repeated blood count was abnormal, and detailed examination of the

---

New England Journal of Medicine 324, No. 10, March 7, 1991: 691–694.

peripheral blood smear showed myelocytes. I advised her to come into the hospital, explaining that we needed to do a bone marrow biopsy and make some decisions relatively rapidly. She came to the hospital knowing what we would find. She was terrified, angry, and sad. Although we knew the odds, we both clung to the thread of possibility that it might be something else.

The bone marrow confirmed the worst: acute myelomonocytic leukemia. In the face of this tragedy, we looked for signs of hope. This is an area of medicine in which technological intervention has been successful, with cures 25 percent of the time—long-term cures. As I probed the costs of these cures, I heard about induction chemotherapy (three weeks in the hospital, prolonged neutropenia, probable infectious complications, and hair loss; 75 percent of patients respond, 25 percent do not). For the survivors, this is followed by consolidation chemotherapy (with similar side effects; another 25 percent die, for a net survival of 50 percent). Those still alive, to have a reasonable chance of long-term survival, then need bone marrow transplantation (hospitalization for two months and whole-body irradiation, with complete killing of the bone marrow, infectious complications, and the possibility for graft-versus-host disease—with a survival of approximately 50 percent, or 25 percent of the original group). Though hematologists may argue over the exact percentages, they don't argue about the outcome of no treatment—certain death in days, weeks, or at most a few months.

Believing that delay was dangerous, our oncologist broke the news to Diane and began making plans to insert a Hickman catheter and begin induction chemotherapy that afternoon. When I saw her shortly thereafter, she was enraged at his presumption that she would want treatment, and devastated by the finality of the diagnosis. All she wanted to do was go home and be with her family. She had no further questions about treatment and in fact had decided that she wanted none. Together we lamented her tragedy and the unfairness of life. Before she left, I felt the need to be sure that she and her husband understood that there was some risk in delay, that the problem was not going to go away, and that we needed to keep considering the options over the next several days. We agreed to meet in two days.

She returned in two days with her husband and son. They had talked extensively about the problem and the options. She remained very clear about her wish not to undergo chemotherapy and to live whatever time she had left outside the hospital. As we explored her thinking further, it became clear that she was convinced she would die during the period of treatment and would suffer unspeakably in the process (from hospitalization, from lack of control over her body, from the side effects of chemotherapy, and from pain and anguish). Although I could offer support and my best effort to minimize her suffering if she chose treatment, there was no way I could say any of this would not occur. In fact, the last four patients with acute leukemia at our hospital had died very painful deaths in the hospital during various stages of treatment (a fact I did not share with her). Her family wished she would choose treatment but sadly accepted her decision. She articulated very clearly that it was she who would be experiencing all the side effects of treatment and that odds of 25 percent were not good enough for her to undergo so toxic a course of therapy, given her expectations of chemotherapy and hospitalization and the absence of a closely matched bone marrow donor. I had her repeat her understanding of the treatment, the odds, and what to expect if there were no treatment. I clarified a few misunderstandings, but she had a remarkable grasp of the options and implications.

I have been a longtime advocate of active, informed patient choice of treatment or nontreatment, and of a patient's right to die with as much control and dignity as possible. Yet there was something about her giving up a 25 percent chance of long-term survival in favor of almost certain death that disturbed me. I had seen Diane fight and use her considerable inner resources to overcome alcoholism and depression, and I half expected her to change her mind over the next week. Since the window of time in which effective treatment can be initiated is rather narrow, we met several times that week. We obtained a second hematology consultation and talked at length about the meaning and implications of treatment and nontreatment. She talked to a psychologist she had seen in the past. I gradually understood the decision from her perspective and became convinced that it was the right decision for her. We arranged for home hospice care (although at that time Diane felt reasonably well, was active, and looked healthy), left the door open for her to change her mind, and tried to anticipate how to keep her comfortable in the time she had left.

Just as I was adjusting to her decision, she opened up another area that would stretch me profoundly. It was extraordinarily important to Diane to maintain control of herself and her own dignity during the time remaining to her. When this was no longer possible, she clearly wanted to die. As a former director of a hospice program, I know how to use pain medicines to keep patients comfortable and lessen suffering. I explained the philosophy of comfort care, which I strongly believe in. Although Diane understood and appreciated this, she had known of people lingering in what was called relative comfort, and she wanted no part of it. When the time came, she wanted to take her life in the least painful way possible. Knowing of her desire for independence and her decision to stay in control, I thought this request made perfect sense. I acknowledged and explored this wish but also thought that it was out of the realm of currently accepted medical practice and that it was more than I could offer or promise. In our discussion, it became clear that preoccupation with her fear of a lingering death would interfere with Diane's getting the most out of the time she had left until she found a safe way to ensure her death. I feared the effects of a violent death on her family, the consequences of an ineffective suicide that would leave her lingering in precisely the state she dreaded so much, and the possibility that a family member would be forced to assist her, with all the legal and personal repercussions that would follow. She discussed this at length with her family. They believed that they should respect her choice. With this in mind, I told Diane that information was available from the Hemlock Society that might be helpful to her.

A week later she phoned me with a request for barbiturates for sleep. Since I knew that this was an essential ingredient in a Hemlock Society suicide, I asked her to come to the office to talk things over. She was more than willing to protect me by participating in a superficial conversation about her insomnia, but it was important to me to know how she planned to use the drugs and to be sure that she was not in despair or overwhelmed in a way that might color her judgment. In our discussion, it was apparent that she was having trouble sleeping, but it was also evident that the security of having enough barbiturates available to commit suicide when and if the time came would leave her secure enough to live fully and concentrate on the present. It was clear that she was not despondent and that in fact she was making deep, personal connections with her family and close friends. I made sure that she knew how to use the barbiturates for sleep, and also that she knew the amount needed to commit suicide. We agreed to meet regularly, and she promised to meet with me before taking her life, to ensure that all other avenues had been exhausted. I wrote the prescription with an uneasy feeling about the boundaries I was exploring—spiritual, legal, professional, and personal. Yet I also felt strongly that I was setting her free to get the most out of the time she had left, and to maintain dignity and control on her own terms until her death.

The next several months were very intense and important for Diane. Her son stayed home from college, and they were able to be with one another and say much that had not been said earlier. Her husband did his work at home so that he and Diane could spend more time together. She spent time with her closest friends. I had her come into the hospital for a conference with our residents, at which she illustrated in a most profound and personal way the importance of informed decision making, the right to refuse treatment, and the extraordinarily personal effects of illness and interaction with the medical system. There were emotional and physical hardships as well. She had periods of intense sadness and anger. Several times she became very weak, but she received transfusions as an outpatient and responded with marked improvement of symptoms. She had two serious infections that responded surprisingly well to empirical courses of oral antibiotics. After three tumultuous months, there were two weeks of relative calm and well-being, and fantasies of a miracle began to surface.

Unfortunately, we had no miracle. Bone pain, weakness, fatigue, and fevers began to dominate her life. Although the hospice workers, family members, and I tried our best to minimize the suffering and promote comfort, it was clear that the end was approaching. Diane's immediate future held what she feared the most—increasing discomfort, dependence, and hard choices between pain and sedation. She called up her closest friends and asked them to come over to say goodbye, telling them that she would be leaving soon. As we had agreed, she let me know as well. When we met, it was clear that she knew what she was doing, that she was sad and frightened to be leaving, but that she would be even more terrified to stay and suffer. In our tearful goodbye, she promised a reunion in the future at her favorite spot on the edge of Lake Geneva, with dragons swimming in the sunset.

Two days later her husband called to say that Diane had died. She had said her final goodbyes to her husband and son that morning, and asked them to leave her alone for an hour. After an hour, which must have seemed an eternity, they found her on the couch, lying very still and covered by her favorite shawl. There was no sign of struggle. She seemed to be at peace. They called me for advice about how to proceed. When I arrived at their house, Diane indeed seemed peaceful. Her husband and son were quiet. We talked about what a remarkable person she had been. They seemed to have no doubts about the course she had chosen or about their cooperation, although the unfairness of her illness and the finality of her death were overwhelming to us all.

I called the medical examiner to inform him that a hospice patient had died. When asked about the cause of death, I said, "acute leukemia." He said that was fine and that we should call a funeral director. Although acute leukemia was the truth, it was not the whole story. Yet any mention of suicide would have given rise to a police investigation and probably brought the arrival of an ambulance crew for resuscitation. Diane would have become a "coroner's case," and the decision to perform an autopsy would have been made at the discretion of the medical examiner. The family or I could have been subject to criminal prosecution, and I to professional review, for our roles in support of Diane's choices. Although I truly believe that the family and I gave her the best care possible, allowing her to define her limits and directions as much as possible, I am not sure the law, society, or the medical profession would agree. So I said "acute leukemia" to protect all of us, to protect Diane from an invasion into her past and her body, and to continue to shield society from the knowledge of the degree of suffering that people often undergo in the process of dying. Suffering can be lessened to some extent, but in no way eliminated or made benign, by the careful intervention of a competent, caring physician, given current social constraints.

Diane taught me about the range of help I can provide if I know people well and if I allow them to say what they really want. She taught me about life, death, and honesty and about taking charge and facing tragedy squarely when it strikes. She taught me that I can take small risks for people that I really know and care about. Although I did not assist in her suicide directly, I helped indirectly to make it possible, successful, and relatively painless. Although I know we have measures to help control pain and lessen suffering, to think that people do not suffer in the process of dying is an illusion. Prolonged dying can occasionally be peaceful, but more often the role of the physician and family is limited to lessening but not eliminating severe suffering.

I wonder how many families and physicians secretly help patients over the edge into death in the face of such severe suffering. I wonder how many severely ill or dying patients secretly take their lives, dying alone in despair. I wonder whether the image of Diane's final aloneness will persist in the minds of her family, or if they will remember more the intense, meaningful months they had together before she died. I wonder whether Diane struggled in that last hour, and whether the Hemlock Society's way of death by suicide is the most benign. I wonder why Diane, who gave so much to so many of us, had to be alone for the last hour of her life. I wonder whether I will see Diane again, on the shore of Lake Geneva at sunset, with dragons swimming on the horizon.

PATIENT REQUEST FORM FOR OREGON'S DEATH WITH DIGNITY ACT

REQUEST FOR MEDICATION TO END MY LIFE IN A HUMANE AND DIGNIFIED MANNER

Authorized by ORS 127.800-127.897

I, ____ am an adult of sound mind.

I am suffering from ____
which my attending physician has determined is a terminal disease and which has been medically confirmed by a consulting physician.

I have been fully informed of my diagnosis, prognosis, the nature of medication to be prescribed and potential associated risks, the expected result, and the feasible alternatives, including comfort care, hospice care and pain control.

I request that my attending physician prescribe medication that will end my life in a humane and dignified manner.

INITIAL ONE:

[ ] I have informed my family of my decision and taken their opinions into consideration.

[ ] I have decided not to inform my family of my decision.

[ ] I have no family to inform of my decision.

I understand that I have the right to rescind this request at any time.

I understand the full import of this request and I expect to die when I take the medication to be prescribed.

I make this request voluntarily and without reservation, and I accept full moral responsibility for my actions.

I further understand that although most deaths occur within three hours, my death may take longer and my physician has counseled me about this possibility.

Signature:	Date:

DECLARATION OF WITNESSES

We declare that the person signing this request:

(a) Is personally known to us or has provided proof of identity;
(b) Signed this request in our presence;
(c) Appears to be of sound mind and not under duress, fraud or undue influence;
(d) Is not a patient for whom either of us is attending physician.

Signature:	Date:
Name (PRINTED)	
Signature:	Date:
Name (PRINTED)	

NOTE: One witness shall not be a relative (by blood, marriage or adoption) of the person signing this request, shall not be entitled to any portion of the person's estate upon death and shall not own, operate or be employed at a health care facility where the person is a patient or resident. If the patient is an inpatient at a health care facility, one of the witnesses shall be an individual designated by the facility.

REV 06/01

ASSISTED SUICIDE: THE PHILOSOPHERS' BRIEF

Ronald Dworkin

INTRODUCTION

The laws of all but one American state now forbid doctors to prescribe lethal pills for patients who want to kill themselves.* These cases[1] began when groups of dying patients and their doctors in Washington State and New York each sued asking that these prohibitions be declared unconstitutional so that the patients could be given, when and if they asked for it, medicine to hasten their death. The pleadings described the agony in which the patient plaintiffs were dying, and two federal Circuit Courts of Appeal—the Ninth Circuit in the Washington case and the Second Circuit in the New York case—agreed with the plaintiffs that the Constitution forbids the government from flatly prohibiting doctors to help end such desperate and pointless suffering.[2]

Washington State and New York appealed these decisions to the Supreme Court, and a total of sixty amicus briefs were filed, including briefs on behalf of the American Medical Association and the United States Catholic Conference urging the Court to reverse the circuit court decisions, and on behalf of the American Medical Students Association and the Gay Men's Health Crisis urging it to affirm them. The justices' comments during oral argument persuaded many observers that the Court would reverse the decisions, probably by a lopsided majority. The justices repeatedly cited two versions—one theoretical, the other practical—of the "slippery slope" argument: that it would be impossible to limit a right to assisted suicide in an acceptable way, once that right was recognized.

The theoretical version of the argument denies that any principled line can be drawn between cases in which proponents say a right of assisted suicide is appropriate and those in which they concede that it is not. The circuit courts recognized only a right for competent patients already dying in great physical pain to have pills prescribed that they could take themselves. Several justices asked on what grounds the right once granted could be so severely limited. Why should it be denied to dying patients who are so feeble or paralyzed that they cannot take pills themselves and who beg a doctor to inject a lethal drug into them? Or to patients who are not dying but face years of intolerable physical or emotional pain, or crippling paralysis or dependence? But if the right were extended that far, on what ground could it be denied to anyone who had formed a desire to die—to a sixteen-year-old suffering from a severe case of unrequited love, for example?

The philosophers' brief answers these questions in two steps. First, it defines a very general moral and constitutional principle—that every competent person has the right to make momentous personal decisions which invoke fundamental religious or philosophical convictions about life's value for himself. Second, it recognizes that people may make such momentous decisions impulsively or out of emotional depression, when their act does not reflect their enduring convictions; and it therefore allows that in some circumstances a state has the constitutional power to override that right in order to protect citizens from mistaken but irrevocable acts of self-destruction. States may be allowed to prevent assisted suicide by people who—it is plausible to think—would later be grateful if they were prevented from dying.

Introduction to "Assisted Suicide: The Philosophers' Brief" by Ronald Dworkin, *The New York Review of Books,* Vol. XLIV, No. 5, March 27, 1997, 41–47. Reprinted with permission from The New York Review of Books.

Editors' note: In June 1997 the Supreme Court decided two cases (*State of Washington* v. *Glucksberg* and *Vacco* v. *Quill*) posing the question whether dying patients have a right to physician-assisted suicide. We present here the amicus curiae brief of six moral philosophers, with an introduction by Ronald Dworkin.

*In November 1997, Oregon voters rejected Measure 51, which would have reversed Measure 16 (approved by the voters in 1994), thereby legalizing physician-assisted suicide in that state.

That two-step argument would justify a state's protecting a disappointed adolescent from himself. It would equally plainly not justify forcing a competent dying patient to live in agony a few weeks longer. People will of course disagree about the cases in between these extremes, and if the Court adopted this argument, the federal courts would no doubt be faced with a succession of cases in years to come testing whether, for example, it is plausible to assume that a desperately crippled patient in constant pain but with years to live, who has formed a settled and repeatedly stated wish to die, would one day be glad he was forced to stay alive. But though two justices dwelled, during the oral argument, on the unappealing prospect of a series of such cases coming before the courts, it seems better that the courts do assume that burden, which they could perhaps mitigate through careful rulings, than that they be relieved of it at the cost of such terrible suffering. The practical version of the slippery slope argument is more complex. If assisted suicide were permitted in principle, every state would presumably adopt regulations to insure that a patient's decision for suicide is informed, competent, and free. But many people fear that such regulations could not be adequately enforced, and that particularly vulnerable patients—poor patients dying in overcrowded hospitals that had scarce resources, for example—might be pressured or hustled into a decision for death they would not otherwise make. The evidence suggests, however, that such patients might be better rather than less well protected if assisted suicide were legalized with appropriate safeguards.

More of them could then benefit from relief that is already available—illegally—to more fortunate people who have established relationships with doctors willing to run the risks of helping them to die. The current two-tier system—a chosen death and an end of pain outside the law for those with connections and stony refusals for most other people—is one of the greatest scandals of contemporary medical practice. The sense many middle-class people have that if necessary their own doctor "will know what to do" helps to explain why the political pressure is not stronger for a fairer and more open system in which the law acknowledges for everyone what influential people now expect for themselves.

For example, in a recent study in the State of Washington, which guaranteed respondents anonymity, 26 percent of doctors surveyed said they had received explicit requests for help in dying, and had provided, overall, lethal prescriptions to 24 percent of patients requesting them.[3] In other studies, 40 percent of Michigan oncologists surveyed reported that patients had initiated requests for death, 18 percent said they had participated in assisted suicide, and 4 percent in "active euthanasia"—injecting lethal drugs themselves. In San Francisco, 53 percent of the 1,995 responding physicians said they had granted an AIDS patient's request for suicide assistance at least once.[4] These statistics approach the rates at which doctors help patients die in Holland, where assisted suicide is in effect legal.

The most important benefit of legalized assisted suicide for poor patients however, might be better care while they live. For though the medical experts cited in various briefs disagreed sharply about the percentage of terminal cases in which pain can be made tolerable through advanced and expensive palliative techniques, they did not disagree that a great many patients do not receive the relief they could have. The Solicitor General who urged the Court to reverse the lower court judgments conceded in the oral argument that 25 percent of terminally ill patients actually do die in pain. That appalling figure is the result of several factors, including medical ignorance and fear of liability, inadequate hospital funding, and (as the Solicitor General suggested) the failure of insurers and health care programs to cover the cost of special hospice care. Better training in palliative medicine, and legislation requiring such coverage, would obviously improve the situation, but it seems perverse to argue that the patients who would be helped were better pain management available must die horribly because it is not; and, as Justice Breyer pointed out, the number of patients in that situation might well increase as medical costs continue to escalate.

According to several briefs, moreover, patients whose pain is either uncontrollable or uncontrolled are often "terminally sedated"—intravenous drugs (usually barbiturates or benzodiazepenes) are injected to induce a pharmacologic coma during which the patient is given neither water nor nutrition and dies sooner than he otherwise would.[5]

Terminal sedation is widely accepted as legal, though it advances death.[6] But it is not subject to regulations nearly as stringent as those that a state forced to allow assisted suicide would enact, because such regulations would presumably include a requirement that hospitals, before accepting any request for assistance in suicide, must demonstrate that effective medical care including state-of-the art pain management had been offered. The guidelines recently published by a network of ethics committees in the Bay Area of California, for example, among other stringent safeguards, provide that a primary care physician who receives a request for suicide must make an initial referral to a hospice program or to a physician experienced in palliative care, and certify in a formal report filed in a state registry, signed by an independent second physician with expertise in such care, that the best available pain relief has been offered to the patient.[7]

Doctors and hospitals anxious to avoid expense would have very little incentive to begin a process that would focus attention on their palliative care practices. They would be more likely to continue the widespread practice of relatively inexpensive terminal care which is supplemented, perhaps, with terminal sedation. It is at least possible, however, that patients' knowledge of the possibility of assisted suicide would make it more difficult for such doctors to continue as before. That is the view of the Coalition of Hospice Professionals, who said, in their own amicus brief, "Indeed, removing legal bans on suicide assistance will enhance the opportunity for advanced hospice care for all patients because regulation of physician-assisted suicide would mandate that all palliative measures be exhausted as a condition precedent to assisted suicide."

So neither version of the slippery slope argument seems very strong. It is nevertheless understandable that Supreme Court justices are reluctant, particularly given how little experience we have so far with legalized assisted suicide, to declare that all but one of the states must change their laws to allow a practice many citizens think abominable and sacrilegious. But as the philosophers' brief that follows emphasizes, the Court is in an unusually difficult position. If it closes the door to a constitutional right to assisted suicide it will do substantial damage to constitutional practice and precedent, as well as to thousands of people in great suffering. It would face a dilemma in justifying any such decision, because it would be forced to choose between the two unappealing strategies that the brief describes.

The first strategy—declaring that terminally ill patients in great pain do not have a constitutional right to control their own deaths, even in principle —seems alien to our constitutional system, as the Solicitor General himself insisted in the oral argument. It would also undermine a variety of the Court's own past decisions, including the carefully constructed position on abortion set out in its 1993 decision in Casey. Indeed some amicus briefs took the occasion of the assisted suicide cases to criticize the abortion decisions—a brief filed on behalf of Senator Orrin Hatch of Utah and Representatives Henry Hyde of Illinois and Charles Canady of Florida, for example, declared that the abortion decisions were "of questionable legitimacy and even more questionable prudence." Protecting the abortion rulings was presumably one of the aims of the Clinton administration in arguing, through the Solicitor General, for the second strategy instead.

The first strategy would create an even more evident inconsistency within the practice of terminal medicine itself. Since the Cruzan decision discussed in the brief, lawyers have generally assumed that the Court would protect the right of any competent patient to have life sustaining equipment removed from his body even though he would then die. In the oral argument, several justices suggested a "common-sense" distinction between the moral significance of acts, on the one hand, and omissions, on the other. This distinction, they suggested, would justify a constitutional distinction between prescribing lethal pills and removing life support; for, in their view, removing support is only a matter of "letting nature take its course," while prescribing pills is an active intervention that brings death sooner than natural processes would.

The discussion of this issue in the philosophers' brief is therefore particularly significant. The brief insists that such suggestions wholly misunderstand the "common-sense" distinction, which is not between acts and omissions, but between acts or omissions that are designed to cause death and those that are not. One justice suggested that a patient who insists that life support be disconnected is not committing suicide. That is wrong: he is committing suicide if he aims at death, as most such patients do, just as someone whose wrist is cut in an accident is committing suicide if he refuses to try to stop the bleeding. The distinction between acts that aim at death and those that do not cannot justify a constitutional distinction between assisting in suicide and terminating life support. Some doctors, who stop life support only because the patient so demands, do not aim at death. But neither do doctors who prescribe lethal pills only for the same reason, and hope that the patient does not take them. And many doctors who terminate life support obviously do aim at death, including those who deny nutrition during terminal sedation, because denying nutrition is designed to hasten death, not to relieve pain.

There are equally serious objections, however, to the second strategy the philosophers' brief discusses. This strategy concedes a general right to assisted suicide but holds that states have the power to judge that the risks of allowing any exercise of that right are too great. It is obviously dangerous for the Court to allow a state to deny a constitutional right on the ground that the state lacks the will or resource to enforce safeguards if it is exercised, particularly when the case for the practical version of the "slippery slope" objection seems so weak and has been little examined.

NOTES

1. *State of Washington et al.* v. *Glucksberg et al.* and *Vacco et al.* v. *Quill et al.*, argued January 8, 1997.
2. I described the circuit court decisions in an earlier article, "Sex and Death in the Courts," *The New York Review*, August 8, 1996.
3. Anthony L. Back et al., "Physician-Assisted Suicide and Euthanasia in Washington State," *Journal of the American Medical Association*, Volume 275, No. 2, pp. 919, 920, 922 (1996).
4. See David I. Doukas et al., "Attitudes and Behaviors on Physician Assisted Death: A Study of Michigan Oncologists," *Clinical Oncology*, Volume 13, p. 1055 (1995); and L. Slome et al., "Attitudes Toward Assisted Suicide in AIDS: A Five Year Comparison Study," conference abstract now available on the World Wide Web (1996). The amicus brief of the Association of Law School Professors offers other statistics to the same effect taken from other states and from nurses.
5. According to one respondent's brief, "Despite some imprecision in the empirical evidence, it has been estimated that between 5 percent and 52 percent of dying patients entering home palliative care units have been terminally sedated." The brief cites Paul Rousseau, "Terminal Sedation in the Care of Dying Patients," *Archives of Internal Medicine*, Volume 156, p. 1785 (1996).
6. The amicus brief of the Coalition of Hospice Professionals raised a frightening question about terminal sedation. "Unfortunately, while a terminally sedated patient exhibits an outwardly peaceful appearance, medical science cannot verify that the individual ceases to experience pain and suffering. To the contrary, studies of individuals who have been anaesthetized (with the same kinds of drugs used in terminal sedation) for surgery (and who are in a deeper comatose state than terminally sedated patients since their breathing must be sustained by a respirator) have demonstrated that painful stimuli applied to the patient will cause a significant increase in brain activity, even though there is no external physical response." See, e.g., Orlando R. Hung et al., "Thiopental Pharmacodynamics: Quantitation of Clinical and Electroencephalographic Depth of Anesthesia," *Anesthesiology*, Volume 77, p. 237 (1992).
7. *BANEC-Generated Guidelines for Comprehensive Care of the Terminally Ill.* Bay Area Network of Ethics Committees, September, 1996.

THE PHILOSOPHERS' BRIEF

Ronald Dworkin, Thomas Nagel, Robert Nozick, John Rawls, Thomas Scanlon, and Judith Jarvis Thomson

Amici are six moral and political philosophers who differ on many issues of public morality and policy. They are united, however, in their conviction that respect for fundamental principles of liberty and justice, as well as for the American constitutional tradition, requires that the decisions of the Courts of Appeals be affirmed.

INTRODUCTION AND SUMMARY OF ARGUMENT

These cases do not invite or require the Court to make moral, ethical, or religious judgments about how people should approach or confront their death or about when it is ethically appropriate to hasten one's own death or to ask others for help in doing so. On the contrary, they ask the Court to recognize that individuals have a constitutionally protected interest in making those grave judgments for themselves, free from the imposition of any religious or philosophical orthodoxy by court or legislature. States have a constitutionally legitimate interest in protecting individuals from irrational, ill-informed, pressured, or unstable decisions to hasten their own death. To that end, states may regulate and limit the assistance that doctors may give individuals who express a wish to die. But states may not deny people in the position of the patient-plaintiffs in these cases the opportunity to demonstrate, through whatever reasonable procedures the state might institute—even procedures that err on the side of caution—that their decision to die is indeed informed, stable, and fully free. Denying that opportunity to terminally ill patients who are in agonizing pain or otherwise doomed to an existence they regard as intolerable could only be justified on the basis of a religious or ethical conviction about the value or meaning of life itself. Our Constitution forbids government to impose such convictions on its citizens.

Petitioners [i.e., the state authorities of Washington and New York] and the amici who support them offer two contradictory arguments. Some deny that the patient-plaintiffs have any constitutionally protected liberty interest in hastening their own deaths. But that liberty interest flows directly from this Court's previous decisions. It flows from the right of people to make their own decisions about matters "involving the most intimate and personal choices a person may make in a lifetime, choices central to personal dignity and autonomy." *Planned Parenthood* v. *Casey,* 505 U.S. 833, 851(1992).

The Solicitor General, urging reversal in support of Petitioners, recognizes that the patient-plaintiffs do have a constitutional liberty interest at stake in these cases. *See* Brief for the United States as Amicus Curiae Supporting Petitioners at 12, *Washington* v. *Vacco* (hereinafter Brief for the United States) ("The term 'liberty' in the Due Process Clause . . . is broad enough to encompass an interest on the part of terminally ill, mentally competent adults in obtaining relief from the kind of suffering experienced by the plaintiffs in this case, which includes not only severe physical pain, but also the despair and distress that comes from physical deterioration and the inability to control basic bodily functions."); *see also id.* at 13 ("*Cruzan* . . . supports the conclusion that a liberty interest is at stake in this case.").

The Solicitor General nevertheless argues that Washington and New York properly ignored this profound interest when they required the patient-plaintiffs to live on in circumstances they found intolerable. He argues that a state may simply declare that it is unable to devise a regulatory scheme that would adequately protect patients whose desire to die might be ill informed or unstable or foolish or not fully free, and that a state may therefore fall back on a blanket prohibition. This Court has never accepted that patently dangerous rationale for denying protection altogether to a conceded fundamental constitutional interest. It would be a serious mistake to do so now. If that rationale were accepted, an interest acknowledged to be constitutionally protected would be rendered empty.

ARGUMENT

I. THE LIBERTY INTEREST ASSERTED HERE IS PROTECTED BY THE DUE PROCESS CLAUSE

The Due Process Clause of the Fourteenth Amendment protects the liberty interest asserted by the patient-plaintiffs here.

Certain decisions are momentous in their impact on the character of a person's life decisions about religious faith, political and moral allegiance, marriage, procreation, and death, for example. Such deeply personal decisions pose controversial questions about how and why human life has value. In a free society, individuals must be allowed to make those decisions for themselves, out of their own faith, conscience, and convictions. This Court has insisted, in a variety of contexts and circumstances, that this great freedom is among those protected by the Due Process Clause as essential to a community of "ordered liberty." *Palko* v. *Connecticut,* 302 U.S. 319, 325 (1937). In its recent decision in *Planned Parenthood* v. *Casey,* 505 U.S. 833, 851 (1992), the Court offered a paradigmatic statement of that principle:

> matters [] involving the most intimate and personal choices a person may make in a lifetime, choices central to a person's dignity and autonomy, are central to the liberty protected by the Fourteenth Amendment.

That declaration reflects an idea underlying many of our basic constitutional protections. As the Court explained in *West Virginia State Board of Education* v. *Barnette,* 319 U.S. 624, 642 (1943):

> If there is any fixed star in our constitutional constellation, it is that no official . . . can prescribe what shall be orthodox in politics, nationalism, religion, or other matters of opinion or force citizens to confess by word or act their faith therein.

A person's interest in following his own convictions at the end of life is so central a part of the more general right to make "intimate and personal choices" for himself that a failure to protect that particular interest would undermine the general right altogether. Death is, for each of us, among the most significant events of life. As the Chief Justice said in *Cruzan* v. *Missouri,* 497 U.S. 261, 281 (1990), "[t]he choice between life and death is a deeply personal decision of obvious and overwhelming finality." Most of us see death—whatever we think will follow it—as the final act of life's drama, and we want that last act to reflect our own convictions, those we have tried to live by, not the convictions of others forced on us in our most vulnerable moment.

Different people, of different religious and ethical beliefs, embrace very different convictions about which way of dying confirms and which contradicts the value of their lives. Some fight against death with every weapon their doctors can devise. Others will do nothing to hasten death even if they pray it will come soon. Still others, including the patient-plaintiffs in these cases, want to end their lives when they think that living on, in the only way they can, would disfigure rather than enhance the lives they had created. Some people make the latter choice not just to escape pain. Even if it were possible to eliminate all pain for a dying patient—and frequently that is not possible—that would not end or even much alleviate the anguish some would feel at remaining alive, but intubated, helpless, and often sedated near oblivion.

None of these dramatically different attitudes about the meaning of death can be dismissed as irrational. None should be imposed, either by the pressure of doctors or relatives or by the fiat of government, on people who reject it. Just as it would be intolerable for government to dictate that doctors never be permitted to try to keep someone alive as long as possible, when that is what the patient wishes, so it is intolerable for government to dictate that doctors may never, under any circumstances, help someone to die who believes that further life means only degradation. The Constitution insists that people must be free to make these deeply personal decisions for themselves and must not be forced to end their lives in a way that appalls them, just because that is what some majority thinks proper.

II. THIS COURT'S DECISIONS IN *CASEY* AND *CRUZAN* COMPEL RECOGNITION OF A LIBERTY INTEREST HERE

A. Casey *Supports the Liberty Interest Asserted Here.* In *Casey,* this Court, in holding that a state cannot constitutionally proscribe abortion in all cases, reiterated that the Constitution protects a sphere of autonomy in which individuals must be permitted to make certain decisions for themselves. The Court began its analysis by pointing out that "[a]t the heart of liberty is the right to define one's own concept of existence, of meaning, of the universe, and of the mystery of human life." 505 U.S. at 851. Choices flowing out of these conceptions, on matters "involving the most intimate and personal choices a person may make in a lifetime, choices central to personal dignity and autonomy, are central to the liberty protected by the Fourteenth Amendment." *Id.* "Beliefs about these matters," the Court continued, "could not define the attributes of personhood were they formed under compulsion of the State." *Id.*

In language pertinent to the liberty interest asserted here, the Court explained why decisions about abortion fall within this category of "personal and intimate" decisions. A decision whether or not to have an abortion, "originat[ing] within the zone of conscience and belief," involves conduct in which "the liberty of the woman is at stake in a sense unique to the human condition and so unique to the law." *Id.* at 852. As such, the decision necessarily involves the very "destiny of the woman" and is inevitably "shaped to a large extent on her own conception of her spiritual imperatives and her place in society." *Id.* Precisely because of these characteristics of the decision, "the State is [not] entitled to proscribe [abortion] in all instances." *Id.* Rather, to allow a total prohibition on abortion would be to permit a state to impose one conception of the meaning and value of human existence on all individuals. This the Constitution forbids.

The Solicitor General nevertheless argues that the right to abortion could be supported on grounds other than this autonomy principle, grounds that would not apply here. He argues, for example, that the abortion right might flow from the great burden an unwanted child imposes on its mother's life. Brief for the United States at 14–15. But whether or not abortion rights could be defended on such grounds, they were not the grounds on which this Court in fact relied. To the contrary, the Court explained at length that the right flows from the constitutional protection accorded all individuals to "define one's own concept of existence, of meaning, of the universe, and of the mystery of human life." *Casey,* 505 U.S. at 851.

The analysis in *Casey* compels the conclusion that the patient-plaintiffs have a liberty interest in this case that a state cannot burden with a blanket prohibition. Like a woman's decision whether to have an abortion, a decision to die involves one's very "destiny" and inevitably will be "shaped to a large extent on [one's] own conception of [one's] spiritual imperatives and [one's] place in society." *Id.* at 852. Just as a blanket prohibition on abortion would involve the improper imposition of one conception of the meaning and value of human existence on all individuals, so too would a blanket prohibition on assisted suicide. The liberty interest asserted here cannot be rejected without undermining the rationale of *Casey.* Indeed, the lower court opinions in the Washington case expressly recognized the parallel between the liberty interest in *Casey* and the interest asserted here. *See Compassion in Dying* v. *Washington,* 79 F.3d 790, 801(9th Cir. 1996) (en banc) ("In deciding right-to-die cases, we are guided by the Court's approach to the abortion cases. *Casey* in particular provides a powerful precedent, for in that case the Court had the opportunity to evaluate its past decisions and to determine whether to adhere to its original judgment."), *aff'g.* 850 F. Supp. 1454,1459 (W. D. Wash. 1994) ("[T]he reasoning in *Casey* [is] highly instructive and almost prescriptive . . ."). This Court should do the same.

B. Cruzan *Supports the Liberty Interest Asserted Here.* We agree with the Solicitor General that this Court's decision in "*Cruzan* . . . supports the conclusion that a liberty interest is at stake in this case." Brief for the United States at 8. Petitioners, however, insist that the present cases can be distinguished because the right at issue in *Cruzan* was limited to a right to reject an unwanted invasion of one's body.[1] But this Court repeatedly has held that in appropriate circumstances a state may require individuals to accept unwanted invasions of the body. *See, e.g., Schmerber* v. *California,* 384 U.S. 757 (1966) (extraction of blood sample from individual suspected of driving while intoxicated, notwithstanding defendant's objection, does not violate privilege against self-incrimination or other constitutional rights); *Jacobson* v. *Massachusetts,* 197 U.S. 11 (1905) (upholding compulsory vaccination for smallpox as reasonable regulation for protection of public health).

The liberty interest at stake in *Cruzan* was a more profound one. If a competent patient has a constitutional right to refuse life-sustaining treatment, then, the Court implied, the state could not override that right. The regulations upheld in *Cruzan* were designed only to ensure that the individual's wishes were ascertained correctly. Thus, if *Cruzan* implies a right of competent patients to refuse life-sustaining treatment, that implication must be understood as resting not simply on a right to refuse bodily invasions but on the more profound right to refuse medical intervention when what is at stake is a momentous personal decision, such as the timing and manner of one's death. In her concurrence, Justice O'Connor expressly recognized that the right at issue involved a "deeply personal decision" that is "inextricably intertwined" with our notion of "self-determination." 497 U.S. at 287–89.

Cruzan also supports the proposition that a state may not burden a terminally ill patient's liberty interest in determining the time and manner of his death by prohibiting doctors from terminating life support. Seeking to distinguish *Cruzan,* Petitioners insist that a state may nevertheless burden that right in a different way by forbidding doctors to assist in the suicide of patients who are not on life-support machinery. They argue that doctors who remove life support are only allowing a natural process to end in death whereas doctors who prescribe lethal drugs are intervening to cause death. So, according to this argument, a state has an independent justification for forbidding doctors to assist in suicide that it does not have for forbidding them to remove life support. In the former case though not the latter, it is said, the state forbids an act of killing that is morally much more problematic than merely letting a patient die.

This argument is based on a misunderstanding of the pertinent moral principles. It is certainly true that when a patient does not wish to die, different acts, each of which foreseeably results in his death, nevertheless have very different moral status. When several patients need organ transplants and organs are scarce, for example, it is morally permissible for a doctor to deny an organ to one patient, even though he will die without it, in order to give it to another. But it is certainly not permissible for a doctor to kill one patient in order to use his organs to save another. The morally significant difference between those two acts is not, however, that killing is a positive act and not providing an organ is a mere omission, or that killing someone is worse than merely allowing a "natural" process to result in death. It would be equally impermissible for a doctor to let an injured patient bleed to death, or to refuse antibiotics to a patient with pneumonia—in each case the doctor would have allowed death to result from a "natural" process—in order to make his organs available for transplant to others. A doctor violates his patient's rights whether the doctor acts or refrains from acting, against the patient's wishes, in a way that is designed to cause death.

When a competent patient does want to die, the moral situation is obviously different, because then it makes no sense to appeal to the patient's right not to be killed as a reason why an act designed to cause his death is impermissible. From the patient's point of view, there is no morally pertinent difference between a doctor's terminating treatment that keeps him alive, if that is what he wishes, and a doctor's helping him to end his own life by providing lethal pills he may take himself, when ready, if that is what he wishes—except that the latter may be quicker and more humane. Nor is that a pertinent difference from the doctor's point of view. If and when it is permissible for him to act with death in view, it does not matter which of those two means he and his patient choose. If it is permissible for a doctor deliberately to withdraw medical treatment in order to allow death to result from a natural process, then it is equally permissible for him to help his patient hasten his own death more actively, if that is the patient's express wish.

It is true that some doctors asked to terminate life support are reluctant and do so only in deference to a patient's right to compel them to remove unwanted invasions of his body. But other doctors, who believe that their most fundamental professional duty is to act in the patient's interests and that, in certain circumstances, it is in their patient's best interests to die, participate willingly in such decisions: they terminate life support to cause death because they know that is what their patient wants. *Cruzan* implied that a state may not absolutely prohibit a doctor from deliberately causing death, at the patient's request, in that way and for that reason. If so, then a state may not prohibit doctors from deliberately using more direct and often more humane means to the same end when that is what a patient prefers. The fact that failing to provide life-sustaining treatment may be regarded as "only letting nature take its course" is no more morally significant in this context, when the patient wishes to die, than in the other, when he wishes to live. Whether a doctor turns off a respirator in accordance with the patient's request or prescribes pills that a patient may take when he is ready to kill himself, the doctor acts with the same intention: to help the patient die.

The two situations do differ in one important respect. Since patients have a right not to have life-support machinery attached to their bodies, they have, in principle, a right to compel its removal. But that is not true in the case of assisted suicide: patients in certain circumstances have a right that the state not forbid doctors to assist in their deaths, but they have no right to compel a doctor to assist them. The right in question, that is, is only a right to the help of a willing doctor.

III. STATE INTERESTS DO NOT JUSTIFY A CATEGORICAL PROHIBITION ON ALL ASSISTED SUICIDE

The Solicitor General concedes that "a competent, terminally ill adult has a constitutionally cognizable liberty interest in avoiding the kind of suffering experienced by the plaintiffs in this case." Brief for the United States at 8. He agrees that this interest extends not only to avoiding pain, but to avoiding an existence the patient believes to be one of intolerable indignity or incapacity as well. *Id.* at 12. The Solicitor General argues, however, that states nevertheless have the right to "override" this liberty interest altogether, because a state could reasonably conclude that allowing doctors to assist in suicide, even under the most stringent regulations and procedures that could be devised, would unreasonably endanger the lives of a number of patients who might ask for death in circumstances when it is plainly not in their interests to die or when their consent has been improperly obtained.

This argument is unpersuasive, however, for at least three reasons. *First*, in *Cruzan*, this Court noted that its various decisions supported the recognition of a general liberty interest in refusing medical treatment, even when such refusal could result in death. 497 U.S. at 278–79. The various risks described by the Solicitor General apply equally to those situations. For instance, a patient kept alive only by an elaborate and disabling life-support system might well become depressed, and doctors might be equally uncertain whether the depression is curable: such a patient might decide for death only because he has been advised that he will die soon anyway or that he will never live free of the burdensome apparatus, and either diagnosis might conceivably be mistaken. Relatives or doctors might subtly or crudely influence that decision, and state provision for the decision may (to the same degree in this case as if it allowed assisted suicide) be thought to encourage it.

Yet there has been no suggestion that states are incapable of addressing such dangers through regulation. In fact, quite the opposite is true. In *McKay v. Bergstedt*, 106 Nev. 808, 801 P.2d 617 (1990), for example, the Nevada Supreme Court held that "competent adult patients desiring to refuse or discontinue medical treatment" must be examined by two nonattending physicians to determine whether the patient is mentally competent, understands his prognosis and treatment options, and appears free of coercion or pressure in making his decision. *Id.* at 827–28, 801 P.2d at 630. See also: *id.* (in the case of terminally ill patients with natural life expectancy of less than six months, [a] patient's right of self-determination shall be deemed to prevail over state interests, whereas [a] non-terminal patient's decision to terminate life-support systems must first be weighed against relevant state interests by trial judge); [and] *In re Farrell*, 108 N.J. 335, 354, 529 A.2d 404, 413 (1987) ([which held that a] terminally-ill patient requesting termination of life-support must be determined to be competent and properly informed about [his] prognosis, available treatment options and risks, and to have made decision voluntarily and without coercion). Those protocols served to guard against precisely the dangers that the Solicitor General raises. The case law contains no suggestion that such protocols are inevitably insufficient to prevent deaths that should have been prevented.

Indeed, the risks of mistake are overall greater in the case of terminating life support. *Cruzan* implied that a state must allow individuals to make such decisions through an advance directive stipulating either that life support be terminated (or not initiated) in described circumstances when the individual was no longer competent to make such a decision himself, or that a designated proxy be allowed to make that decision. All the risks just described are present when the decision is made through or pursuant to such an advance directive, and a grave further risk is added: that the directive, though still in force, no longer represents the wishes of the patient. The patient might have changed his mind before he became incompetent, though he did not change the directive, or his proxy may make a decision that the patient would not have made himself if still competent. In *Cruzan,* this Court held that a state may limit these risks through reasonable regulation. It did not hold—or even suggest—that a state may avoid them through a blanket prohibition that, in effect, denies the liberty interest altogether.

Second, nothing in the record supports the [Solicitor General's] conclusion that no system of rules and regulations could adequately reduce the risk of mistake. As discussed above, the experience of states in adjudicating requests to have life-sustaining treatment removed indicates the opposite. The Solicitor General has provided no persuasive reason why the same sort of procedures could not be applied effectively in the case of a competent individual's request for physician-assisted suicide.

Indeed, several very detailed schemes for regulating physician-assisted suicide have been submitted to the voters of some states and one has been enacted. In addition, concerned groups, including a group of distinguished professors of law and other professionals, have drafted and defended such schemes. *See, e.g.,* Charles H. Baron, *et al., A Model State Act to Authorize and Regulate Physician-Assisted Suicide,* 33 Harv. J. Legis. 1 (1996). Such draft statutes propose a variety of protections and review procedures designed to insure against mistakes, and neither Washington nor New York attempted to show that such schemes would be porous or ineffective. Nor does the Solicitor General's brief: it relies instead mainly on flat and conclusory statements. It cites a New York Task Force report, written before the proposals just described were drafted, whose findings have been widely disputed and were implicitly rejected in the opinion of the Second Circuit below. *See generally Quill* v. *Vacco,* 80 F.3d 716 (2d Cir. 1996). The weakness of the Solicitor General's argument is signaled by his strong reliance on the experience in the Netherlands which, in effect, allows assisted suicide pursuant to published guidelines. Brief for the United States at 23–24. The Dutch guidelines are more permissive than the proposed and model American statutes, however. The Solicitor General deems the Dutch practice of ending the lives of people like neonates who cannot consent particularly noteworthy, for example, but that practice could easily and effectively be made illegal by any state regulatory scheme without violating the Constitution.

The Solicitor General's argument would perhaps have more force if the question before the Court were simply whether a state has any rational basis for an absolute prohibition; if that were the question, then it might be enough to call attention to risks a state might well deem not worth running. But as the Solicitor General concedes, the question here is a very different one: whether a state has interests sufficiently compelling to allow it to take the extraordinary step of altogether refusing the exercise of a liberty interest of constitutional dimension. In those circumstances, the burden is plainly on the state to demonstrate that the risk of mistakes is very high, and that no alternative to complete prohibition would adequately and effectively reduce those risks. Neither of the Petitioners has made such a showing.

Nor could they. The burden of proof on any state attempting to show this would be very high. Consider, for example, the burden a state would have to meet to show that it was entitled altogether to ban public speeches in favor of unpopular causes because it could not guarantee, either by regulations short of an outright ban or by increased police protection, that such speeches would not provoke a riot that would result in serious injury or death to an innocent party. Or that it was entitled to deny those accused of crime the procedural rights that the Constitution guarantees, such as the right to a jury trial, because the security risk those rights would impose on the community would be too great. One can posit extreme circumstances in which some such argument would succeed. *See, e.g., Korematsu* v. *United States,* 323 U.S., 214 (1944) (permitting United States to detain individuals of Japanese ancestry during wartime). But these circumstances would be extreme indeed, and the *Korematsu* ruling has been widely and severely criticized.

Third, it is doubtful whether the risks the Solicitor General cites are even of the right character to serve as justification for an absolute prohibition on the exercise of an important liberty interest. The risks fall into two groups. The first is the risk of medical mistake, including a misdiagnosis of competence or terminal illness. To be sure, no scheme of regulation, no matter how rigorous, can altogether guarantee that medical mistakes will not be made. But the Constitution does not allow a state to deny patients a great variety of important choices, for which informed consent is properly deemed necessary, just because the information on which the consent is given may, in spite of the most strenuous efforts to avoid mistake, be wrong. Again, these identical risks are present in decisions to terminate life support, yet they do not justify an absolute prohibition on the exercise of the right.

The second group consists of risks that a patient will be unduly influenced by considerations that the state might deem it not in his best interests to be swayed by, for example, the feelings and views of close family members. Brief for the United States at 20. But what a patient regards as proper grounds for such a decision normally reflects exactly the judgments of personal ethics—of why his life is important and what affects its value—that patients have a crucial liberty interest in deciding for themselves. Even people who are dying have a right to hear and, if they wish, act on what others might wish to tell or suggest or even hint to them, and it would be dangerous to suppose that a state may prevent this on the ground that it knows better than its citizens when they should be moved by or yield to particular advice or suggestion in the exercise of their right to make fateful personal decisions for themselves. It is not a good reply that some people may not decide as they really wish—as they would decide, for example, if free from the "pressure" of others. That possibility could hardly justify the most serious pressure of all—the criminal law which tells them that they may not decide for death if they need the help of a doctor in dying, no matter how firmly they wish it.

There is a fundamental infirmity in the Solicitor General's argument. He asserts that a state may reasonably judge that the risk of "mistake" to some persons justifies a prohibition that not only risks but insures and even aims at what would undoubtedly be a vastly greater number of "mistakes" of the opposite kind—preventing many thousands of competent people who think that it disfigures their lives to continue living, in the only way left to them, from escaping that—to them—terrible injury. A state grievously and irreversibly harms such people when it prohibits that escape. The Solicitor General's argument may seem plausible to those who do not agree that individuals are harmed by being forced to live on in pain and what they regard as indignity. But many other people plainly do think that such individuals are harmed, and a state may not take one side in that essentially ethical or religious controversy as its justification for denying a crucial liberty.

Of course, a state has important interests that justify regulating physician-assisted suicide. It may be legitimate for a state to deny an opportunity for assisted suicide when it acts in what it reasonably judges to be the best interests of the potential suicide, and when its judgment on that issue does not rest on contested judgments about "matters involving the most intimate and personal choices a person may make in a lifetime, choices central to personal dignity and autonomy." *Casey*, 505 U.S. at 851. A state might assert, for example, that people who are not terminally ill, but who have formed a desire to die, are, as a group, very likely later to be grateful if they are prevented from taking their own lives. It might then claim that it is legitimate, out of concern for such people, to deny any of them a doctor's assistance [in taking their own lives].

This Court need not decide now the extent to which such paternalistic interests might override an individual's liberty interest. No one can plausibly claim, however—and it is noteworthy that neither Petitioners nor the Solicitor General does claim—that any such prohibition could serve the interests of any significant number of terminally ill patients. On the contrary, any paternalistic justification for an absolute prohibition of assistance to such patients would of necessity appeal to a widely contested religious or ethical conviction many of them, including the patient-plaintiffs, reject. Allowing *that* justification to prevail would vitiate the liberty interest.

Even in the case of terminally ill patients, a state has a right to take all reasonable measures to insure that a patient requesting such assistance has made an informed, competent, stable and uncoerced decision. It is plainly legitimate for a state to establish procedures through which professional and administrative judgments can be made about these matters, and to forbid doctors to assist in suicide when its reasonable procedures have not been satisfied. States may be permitted considerable leeway in designing such procedures. They may be permitted, within reason, to err on what they take to be the side of caution. But they may not use the bare possibility of error as justification for refusing to establish any procedures at all and relying instead on a flat prohibition.

CONCLUSION

Each individual has a right to make the "most intimate and personal choices central to personal dignity and autonomy." That right encompasses the right to exercise some control over the time and manner of one's death.

The patient-plaintiffs in these cases were all mentally competent individuals in the final phase of terminal illness and died within months of filing their claims.

Jane Doe described how her advanced cancer made even the most basic bodily functions such as swallowing, coughing, and yawning extremely painful and that it was "not possible for [her] to reduce [her] pain to an acceptable level of comfort and to retain an alert state." Faced with such circumstances, she sought to be able to "discuss freely with [her] treating physician [her] intention of hastening [her] death through the consumption of drugs prescribed for that purpose." *Quill* v. *Vacco,* 80 F.2d 716, 720 (2d Cir. 1996) (quoting declaration of Jane Doe).

George A. Kingsley, in advanced stages of AIDS which included, among other hardships, the attachment of a tube to an artery in his chest which made even routine functions burdensome and the development of lesions on his brain, sought advice from his doctors regarding prescriptions which could hasten his impending death. *Id.*

Jane Roe, suffering from cancer since 1988, had been almost completely bedridden since 1993 and experienced constant pain which could not be alleviated by medication. After undergoing counseling for herself and her family, she desired to hasten her death by taking prescription drugs. *Compassion in Dying* v. *Washington,* 850 F. Supp. 1454, 1456 (1994).

John Doe, who had experienced numerous AIDS-related ailments since 1991, was "especially cognizant of the suffering imposed by a lingering terminal illness because he was the primary caregiver for his long-term companion who died of AIDS" and sought prescription drugs from his physician to hasten his own death after entering the terminal phase of AIDS. *Id.* at 1456–57.

James Poe suffered from emphysema which caused him "a constant sensation of suffocating" as well as a cardiac condition which caused severe leg pain. Connected to an oxygen tank at all times but unable to calm the panic reaction associated with his feeling of suffocation even with regular doses of morphine, Mr. Poe sought physician-assisted suicide. *Id.* at 1457.

A state may not deny the liberty claimed by the patient-plaintiffs in these cases without providing them an opportunity to demonstrate, in whatever way the state might reasonably think wise and necessary, that the conviction they expressed for an early death is competent, rational, informed, stable, and uncoerced.

Affirming the decisions by the Courts of Appeals would establish nothing more than that there is such a constitutionally protected right in principle. It would establish only that some individuals, whose decisions for suicide plainly cannot be dismissed as irrational or foolish or premature, must be accorded a reasonable opportunity to show that their decision for death is informed and free. It is not necessary to decide precisely which patients are entitled to that opportunity. If, on the other hand, this Court reverses the decisions below, its decision could only be justified by the momentous proposition—a proposition flatly in conflict with the spirit and letter of the Court's past decisions—that an American citizen does not, after all, have the right, even in principle, to live and die in the light of his own religious and ethical beliefs, his own convictions about why his life is valuable and where its value lies.

NOTE

1. In that case, the parents of Nancy Cruzan, a woman who was in a persistent vegetative state following an automobile accident, asked the Missouri courts to authorize doctors to end life support and therefore her

life. The Supreme Court held that Missouri was entitled to demand explicit evidence that Ms. Cruzan had made a decision that she would not wish to be kept alive in those circumstances, and to reject the evidence the family had offered as inadequate. But a majority of justices assumed, for the sake of the argument, that a competent patient has a right to reject life-preserving treatment, and it is now widely assumed that the Court would so rule in an appropriate case.

PHYSICIAN-ASSISTED SUICIDE: A TRAGIC VIEW

John D. Arras

INTRODUCTION

For many decades now, the call for physician-assisted suicide (PAS) and euthanasia have been perennial lost causes in American society. Each generation has thrown up an assortment of earnest reformers and cranks who, after attracting their fifteen minutes of fame, inevitably have been defeated by the combined weight of traditional law and morality. Incredibly, two recent federal appellate court decisions suddenly changed the legal landscape in this area, making the various states within their respective jurisdictions the first governments in world history, excepting perhaps the Nazi regime in Germany, to officially sanction PAS. Within the space of a month, both an eight to three majority of the United States Court of Appeals for the Ninth Circuit[1] on the West Coast, and a three-judge panel in the United States Court of Appeals for the Second Circuit,[2] in the Northeast, struck down long-standing state laws forbidding physicians to aid or abet their patients in acts of suicide. Within a virtual blink of an eye, the unthinkable had come to pass: PAS and euthanasia had emerged from their exile beyond the pale of law to occupy center stage in a dramatic public debate that eventually culminated in the United States Supreme Court's unanimous reversal of both lower court decisions in June 1997. . . .[3]

As a firm believer in patient autonomy, I find myself to be deeply sympathetic to the central values motivating the case for PAS and euthanasia; I have concluded, however, that these practices pose too great a threat to the rights and welfare of too many people to be legalized in this country at the present time. Central to my argument in this paper will be the claim that the recently overturned decisions of the circuit courts employ a form of case-based reasoning that is ill-suited to the development of sound social policy in this area. I shall argue that in order to do justice to the very real threats posed by the widespread social practices of PAS and euthanasia, we need to adopt precisely the kind of policy perspective that the circuit courts rejected on principle. Thus, this essay presents the case for a forward-looking, legislative approach to PAS and euthanasia, as opposed to an essentially backward-looking, judicial or constitutional approach.[4] Although I suggest below that the soundest legislative policy at the present time would be to extend the legal prohibition of PAS into the near future, I remain open to the possibility that a given legislature, presented with sufficient evidence of the reliability of various safeguards, might come to a different conclusion.

ARGUMENTS AND MOTIVATIONS IN FAVOR OF PAS/EUTHANASIA

Let us begin, then, with the philosophical case for PAS and euthanasia, which consists of two distinct

From *Journal of Contemporary Health Law and Policy* 13: 361–389 (1997). Reprinted by permission.

Editors' note: This article has been heavily edited. Many footnotes have been deleted and the remainder have been renumbered. Readers wishing to follow up on sources should consult the original article.

prongs, both of which speak simply, directly, and powerfully to our commonsensical intuitions. First, there is the claim of autonomy, that all of us possess a right to self-determination in matters profoundly touching on such religious themes as life, death, and the meaning of suffering. . . . Second, PAS and/or euthanasia are merciful acts that deliver terminally ill patients from painful and protracted death. . . . For patients suffering from the final ravages of end-stage AIDS or cancer, a doctor's lethal prescription or injection can be, and often is, welcomed as a blessed relief. Accordingly, we should treat human beings at least as well as we treat grievously ill or injured animals by putting them, at their own request, out of their misery.

These philosophical reflections can be supplemented with a more clinical perspective addressed to the motivational factors lying behind many requests to die. Many people advocate legalization because they fear a loss of control at the end of life. They fear falling victim to the technological imperative; they fear dying in chronic and uncontrolled pain; they fear the psychological suffering attendant upon the relentless disintegration of the self; they fear, in short, a bad death. All of these fears, it so happens, are eminently justified. Physicians routinely ignore the documented wishes of patients and all-too-often allow patients to die with uncontrolled pain.[5] Studies of cancer patients have shown that over fifty percent suffer from unrelieved pain,[6] and many researchers have found that uncontrolled pain, particularly when accompanied by feelings of hopelessness and untreated depression, is a significant contributing factor for suicide and suicidal ideation.

Clinical depression is another major factor influencing patients' choice of suicide. Depression, accompanied by feelings of hopelessness, is the strongest predictor of suicide for both individuals who are terminally ill and those who are not. Yet most doctors are not trained to notice depression, especially in complex cases such as the elderly suffering from terminal illnesses. Even when doctors succeed in diagnosing depression, they often do not successfully treat it with readily available medications in sufficient amounts.

Significantly, the New York Task Force found that the vast majority of patients who request PAS or euthanasia can be treated successfully both for their depression and their pain, and that when they receive adequate psychiatric and palliative care, their requests to die usually are withdrawn.[7] In other words, patients given the requisite control over their lives and relief from depression and pain usually lose interest in PAS and euthanasia.

With all due respect for the power of modern methods of pain control, it must be acknowledged that a small percentage of patients suffer from conditions, both physical and psychological, that currently lie beyond the reach of the best medical and humane care. Some pain cannot be alleviated short of inducing a permanent state of unconsciousness in the patient, and some depression is unconquerable. For such unfortunate patients, the present law on PAS/euthanasia can represent an insuperable barrier to a dignified and decent death.[8]

OBJECTIONS TO PAS/EUTHANASIA

Opponents of PAS and euthanasia can be grouped into three main factions. One strongly condemns both practices as inherently immoral, as violations of the moral rule against killing the innocent. Most members of this group tend to harbor distinctly religious objections to suicide and euthanasia, viewing them as violations of God's dominion over human life. They argue that killing is simply wrong in itself, whether or not it is done out of respect for the patient's autonomy or out of concern for her suffering. Whether or not this position ultimately is justifiable from a theological point of view, its imposition on believers and non-believers alike is incompatible with the basic premises of a secular, pluralistic political order.

A second faction primarily objects to the fact that physicians are being called upon to do the killing. While conceding that killing the terminally ill or assisting in their suicides might not always be morally wrong for others to do, this group maintains that the participation of physicians in such practices undermines their role as healers and fatally compromises the physician-patient relationship.

Finally, a third faction readily grants that neither PAS nor active euthanasia, practiced by ordinary citizens or by physicians, are always morally wrong. On the contrary, this faction believes that in certain rare instances early release from a painful or intolerably degrading existence might constitute both a positive good and an important exercise of personal autonomy for the individual. Indeed, many members of this faction concede that should such a terrible fate befall them, they would hope to find a thoughtful, compassionate, and courageous physician to release them from their misery. But in spite of these important concessions, the members of this faction shrink from endorsing or regulating PAS and active euthanasia due to fears bearing on the social consequences of liberalization. This view is based on two distinct kinds of so-called "slippery slope" arguments: one bears on the inability to cabin PAS/euthanasia within the confines envisioned by its proponents; the other focuses on the likelihood of abuse, neglect, and mistake.

An Option Without Limits

The first version of the slippery slope argument contends that a socially sanctioned practice of PAS would in all likelihood prove difficult, if not impossible, to cabin within its originally anticipated boundaries. Proponents of legalization usually begin with a wholesomely modest policy agenda, limiting their suggested reforms to a narrow and highly specified range of potential candidates and practices. "Give us PAS," they ask, "not the more controversial practice of active euthanasia, for presently competent patients who are terminally ill and suffering unbearable pain." But the logic of the case for PAS, based as it is upon the twin pillars of patient autonomy and mercy, makes it highly unlikely that society could stop with this modest proposal once it had ventured out on the slope. As numerous other critics have pointed out, if autonomy is the prime consideration, then additional constraints based upon terminal illness or unbearable pain, or both, would appear hard to justify. Indeed, if autonomy is crucial, the requirement of unbearable suffering would appear to be entirely subjective. Who is to say, other than the patient herself, how much suffering is too much? Likewise, the requirement of terminal illness seems an arbitrary standard against which to judge patients' own subjective evaluation of their quality of life. If my life is no longer worth living, why should a terminally ill cancer patient be granted PAS but not me, merely because my suffering is due to my "non-terminal" amyotrophic lateral sclerosis (ALS) or intractable psychiatric disorder?

Alternatively, if pain and suffering are deemed crucial to the justification of legalization, it is hard to see how the proposed barrier of contemporaneous consent of competent patients could withstand serious erosion. If the logic of PAS is at all similar to that of forgoing life-sustaining treatments, and we have every reason to think it so, then it would seem almost inevitable that a case soon would be made to permit PAS for incompetent patients who had left advance directives. That would then be followed by a "substituted judgment" test for patients who "would have wanted" PAS, and finally an "objective" test would be developed for patients (including newborns) whose best interests would be served by PAS or active euthanasia even in the absence of any subjective intent (see Part 3, Section 4 above).

In the same way, the joint justifications of autonomy and mercy combine to undermine the plausibility of a line drawn between PAS and active euthanasia. As the authors of one highly publicized proposal have come to see, the logic of justification for active euthanasia is identical to that of PAS.[9] Legalizing PAS, while continuing to ban active euthanasia, would serve only to discriminate unfairly against patients who are suffering and wish to end their lives, but cannot do so because of some physical impairment. Surely these patients, it will be said, are "the worst-off group," and therefore they are the most in need of the assistance of others who will do for them what they can no longer accomplish on their own.

None of these initial slippery slope considerations amount to knock-down objections to further liberalization of our laws and practices. After all, it is not obvious that each of the highly predictable shifts (e.g., from terminal to "merely" incurable, from contemporaneous consent to best interests, and from PAS to active euthanasia), are patently immoral and unjustifiable. Still, in pointing out this likely slippage, the consequentialist opponents of PAS/euthanasia are calling on society to think about the likely consequences of taking the first tentative step onto the slope. If all of the extended practices predicted above pose substantially greater risks for vulnerable patients than the more highly circumscribed initial liberalization proposals, then we need to factor in these additional risks even as we ponder the more modest proposals.[10]

The Likelihood of Abuse

The second prong of the slippery slope argument argues that whatever criteria for justifiable PAS and active euthanasia ultimately are chosen, abuse of the system is highly likely to follow. In other words, patients who fall outside the ambit of our justifiable criteria will soon be candidates for death. This prong resembles what I have elsewhere called an "empirical slope" argument, as it is based not on the close logical resemblance of concepts or justifications, but rather on an empirical prediction of what is likely to happen when we insert a particular social practice into our existing social system.

In order to reassure skeptics, the proponents of PAS/euthanasia concur that any potentially justifiable social policy in this area must meet at least the following three requirements. The policy would have to insist first, that all requests for death be truly voluntary; second, that all reasonable alternatives to PAS and active euthanasia must be explored before acceding to a patient's wishes; and, third, that a reliable system of reporting all cases must be established in order to effectively monitor these practices and respond to abuses. As a social pessimist on these matters, I believe, given social reality as we know it, that all three assumptions are problematic.

With regard to the voluntariness requirement, we pessimists contend that many requests would not be sufficiently voluntary. In addition to the subtly coercive influences of physicians and family members, perhaps the most slippery aspect of this slope is the highly predictable failure of most physicians to diagnose reliably and treat reversible clinical depression, particularly in the elderly population. As one geriatric psychiatrist testified before the New York Task Force, we now live in the "golden age" of treating depression, but the "lead age" of diagnosing it. We have the tools, but physicians are not adequately trained and motivated to use them. Unless dramatic changes are effected in the practice of medicine, we can predict with confidence that many instances of PAS and active euthanasia will fail the test of voluntariness.

Second, there is the lingering fear that any legislative proposal or judicial mandate would have to be implemented within the present social system marked by deep and pervasive discrimination against the poor and members of minority groups. We have every reason to expect that a policy that worked tolerably well in an affluent community like Scarsdale or Beverly Hills, might not work so well in a community like Bedford-Stuyvesant or Watts, where your average citizen has little or no access to basic primary care, let alone sophisticated care for chronic pain at home or in the hospital. There is also reason to worry about any policy of PAS initiated within our growing system of managed care, capitation, and physician incentives for delivering less care. Expert palliative care no doubt is an expensive and time-consuming proposition, requiring more, rather than less, time spent just talking with patients and providing them with humane comfort. It is highly doubtful that the context of physician-patient conversation within this new dispensation of "turnstile medicine" will be at all conducive to humane decisions untainted by subtle economic coercion.

In addition, given the abysmal and shameful track record of physicians in responding adequately to pain and suffering,[11] we also can confidently predict that in many cases all reasonable alternatives will not have been exhausted. Instead of vigorously addressing the pharmacological and psychosocial needs of such patients, physicians no doubt will continue to ignore, undertreat or treat many of their patients in an impersonal manner. The result is likely to be more depression, desperation, and requests for physician-assisted death from patients who could have been successfully treated. The root causes of this predictable failure are manifold, but high on the list is the inaccessibility of decent primary care to over thirty-seven million Americans. Other notable causes include an appalling lack of training in palliative care among primary care physicians and cancer specialists alike; discrimination in the delivery of pain control and other medical treatments on the basis of race and economic status; various myths shared by both physicians and patients about the supposed ill effects of pain medications; and restrictive state laws on access to opioids.

Finally, with regard to the third requirement, pessimists doubt that any reporting system would adequately monitor these practices. A great deal depends here on the extent to which patients and practitioners will regard these practices as essentially private matters to be discussed and acted upon within the privacy of the doctor-patient relationship. As the Dutch experience has conclusively demonstrated, physicians will be extremely loath to report instances of PAS and active euthanasia to public authorities, largely for fear of bringing the harsh glare of publicity upon the patients' families at a time when privacy is most needed. The likely result of this predictable lack of oversight will be society's inability to respond appropriately to disturbing incidents and long-term trends. In other words, the practice most likely will not be as amenable to regulation as the proponents contend.

The moral of this story is that deeply seated inadequacies in physicians' training, combined with structural flaws in our health care system, can be reliably predicted to secure the premature deaths of many people who would in theory be excluded by the criteria of most leading proposals to legalize PAS. If this characterization of the status quo is at all accurate, then the problem will not be solved by well meaning assurances that abuses will not be tolerated, or that patients will, of course, be offered the full range of palliative care options before any decision for PAS is ratified.[12] While such regulatory solutions are possible in theory, and may well justly prevail in the future, we should be wary of legally sanctioning any negative right to be let alone by the state when the just and humane exercise of that right will depend upon the provision of currently nonexistent services. The operative analogy here, I fear, is our failed and shameful policy of "deinstitutionalization," which left thousands of vulnerable and defenseless former residents of state psychiatric hospitals to fend for themselves on the streets, literally "rotting with their rights on." It is now generally agreed that the crucial flaw in this well-intended but catastrophic policy was our society's willingness to honor such patients' negative right to be free of institutional fetters without having first made available reliable local alternatives to institutionalization. The operative lesson for us here is that judges and courts are much better at enunciating negative rights than they are at providing the services required for their successful implementation. . . .

TOWARDS A POLICY OF PRUDENT (LEGAL) RESTRAINT AND AGGRESSIVE (MEDICAL) INTERVENTION

In contrast to the judicial approach, which totally vindicates the value of patient autonomy at the expense of protecting the vulnerable, my own preferred approach to a social policy of PAS and euthanasia conceives of this debate as posing an essentially "tragic choice."[13] It frankly acknowledges that whatever choice we make, whether we opt for a reaffirmation of the current legal restraints or for a policy of legitimization and regulation, there are bound to be "victims." The victims of the current policy are easy to identify: They are on the news, the talk shows, the documentaries, and often on Dr. Kevorkian's roster of so-called "patients." The victims of legalization, by contrast, will be largely hidden from view; they will include the clinically depressed eighty-year-old man who could have lived for another year of good quality if only he had been adequately treated, and the fifty-year-old woman who asks for death because doctors in her financially stretched HMO cannot, or will not, effectively treat her unrelenting, but mysterious, pelvic pain. Perhaps eventually, if we slide far enough down the slope, the uncommunicative stroke victim, whose distant children deem an earlier death to be a better death, will fall victim. There will be others besides these, many coming from the ranks of the uninsured and the poor. To the extent that minorities and the poor already suffer from the effects of discrimination in our health care system, it is reasonable to expect that any system of PAS and euthanasia will exhibit similar effects, such as failure to access adequate primary care, pain management, and psychiatric diagnosis and treatment. Unlike Dr. Kevorkian's "patients," these victims will not get their pictures in the papers, but they all will have faces and they will all be cheated of good months or perhaps even years.

This "tragic choice" approach to social policy on PAS/euthanasia takes the form of the following argument formulated at the legislative level. First, the number of "genuine cases" justifying PAS, active euthanasia, or both, will be relatively small. Patients who receive good personal care, good pain relief, treatment for depression, and adequate psychosocial supports tend not to persist in their desire to die.

Second, the social risks of legalization are serious and highly predictable. They include the expansion of these practices to nonvoluntary cases, the advent of active euthanasia, and the widespread failure to pursue readily available alternatives to suicide motivated by pain, depression, hopelessness, and lack of access to good primary medical care.

Third, rather than propose a momentous and dangerous policy shift for a relatively small number of "genuine cases"—a shift that would surely involve a great deal of persistent social division and strife analogous to that involved in the abortion controversy—we should instead attempt to redirect the public debate toward a goal on which we can and should all agree, namely the manifest and urgent need to reform the way we die in America. Instead of pursuing a highly divisive and dangerous campaign for PAS, we should attack the problem at its root with an ambitious program of reform in the areas of access to primary care and the education of physicians in palliative care. At least as far as the "slippery slope" opponents of PAS are concerned, we should thus first see to it that the vast majority of people in this country have access to adequate, affordable, and nondiscriminatory primary and palliative care. At the end of this long and arduous process, when we finally have an equitable, effective, and compassionate health care system in place, one that might be compared favorably with that in the Netherlands, then we might well want to reopen the discussion of PAS and active euthanasia.

Finally, there are those few unfortunate patients who truly are beyond the pale of good palliative, hospice, and psychiatric care. The opponents of legalization must face up to this suffering remnant and attempt to offer creative and humane solutions. One possibility is for such patients to be rendered permanently unconscious by drugs until such time, presumably not a long time, as death finally claims them. Although some will find such an option to be aesthetically unappealing, many would find it a welcome relief. Other patients beyond the reach of the best palliative and hospice care could take their own lives, either by well-known traditional means, or with the help of a physician who could sedate them while they refused further food and (life extending) fluids. Finally, those who find this latter option to be unacceptable might still be able to find a compassionate physician who, like Dr. Timothy Quill, will ultimately be willing, albeit in fear and trembling, to "take small risks for people they really know and care about." Such actions will continue to take place within the privacy of the patient-physician relationship, however, and thus will not threaten vulnerable patients and the social fabric to the same extent as would result from full legalization and regulation.

As the partisans of legalized PAS correctly point out, the covert practice of PAS will not be subject to regulatory oversight, and is thus capable of generating its own abuses and slippery slope. Still, I believe that the ever-present threat of possible criminal sanctions and revocation of licensure will continue to serve, for the vast majority of physicians, as powerful disincentives to abuse the system. Moreover, as suggested earlier, it is highly unlikely that the proposals for legalization would result in truly effective oversight.

CONCLUSION

Instead of conceiving this momentous debate as a choice between, on the one hand, legalization and regulation with all of their attendant risks, and on the other hand, the callous abandonment of patients to their pain and suffering, enlightened opponents must recommend a positive program of clinical and social reforms. On the clinical level, physicians must learn how to really listen to their patients, to unflinchingly engage them in sensitive discussions of their needs and the meaning of their requests for assisted death, to deliver appropriate palliative care, to distinguish fact from fiction in the ethics and law of pain relief; to diagnose and treat clinical depression, and finally, to ascertain and respect their patients' wishes for control regarding the forgoing of life-sustaining treatments. On the social level, opponents of PAS must aggressively promote major initiatives in medical and public education regarding pain control, in the sensitization of insurance companies and licensing agencies to issues of the quality of dying, and in the reform of state laws that currently hinder access to pain-relieving medications.

In the absence of an ambitious effort in the direction of aggressive medical and social reform, I fear that the medical and nursing professions will have lost whatever moral warrant and credibility they might still have in continuing to oppose physician-assisted suicide and active euthanasia. As soon as these reforms are in place, however, we might then wish to proceed slowly and cautiously with experiments in various states to test the overall benefits of a policy of legalization. Until that time, however, we are not well served as a society by court decisions allowing for legalization of PAS. The Supreme Court has thus reached a sound decision in ruling out a constitutional right to PAS. As the Justices acknowledged, however, this momentous decision will not end the moral debate over PAS and euthanasia. Indeed, it should and hopefully will intensify it.

NOTES

1. *Compassion in Dying* v. *Washington,* 79 F.3d 790, 838 (9th Cir. 1996).
2. *Quill* v. *Vacco,* 80 F.3d 716, 731(2nd Cir. 1996).
3. *Vacco, Attorney General of New York. et al.* v. *Quill et al.* certiorari to the United States Court of Appeals for the Second Circuit, No. 95-1858. Argued January 8, 1997—Decided June 26, 1997. *Washington et al.* v. *Glucksberg et al.,* certiorari to the United States Court of Appeals for the Ninth Circuit, No. 96-110. Argued January 8, 1997—Decided June 26, 1997.
4. My stance on these issues has been profoundly influenced by my recent work with the New York State Task Force on Life and the Law (hereinafter "Task Force") to come to grips with this issue.
5. "A Controlled Trial to Improve Care for Seriously Ill Hospitalized Patients: The Study to Understand Prognoses and Preferences for Outcomes and Risks of Treatments" (SUPPORT), *Journal of the American Medical Association* 274 (Nov. 22, 1995): 1591–92.
6. Task Force, *When Death Is Sought,* x–xi.
7. Task Force, *When Death Is Sought,* xiv.
8. The preceding section thus signals two important points of agreement with the so-called "Philosophers' Brief" submitted to the Supreme Court in *Compassion in Dying* and *Vacco* by Ronald Dworkin, Thomas Nagel, Robert Nozick, John Rawls, Thomas Scanlon, and Judith Jarvis Thomson [in this volume, pp. 386–94]. I agree that individuals in the throes of a painful or degrading terminal illness may well have a very strong moral and even legal interest in securing PAS. I also agree that the pain and suffering of a small percentage of dying patients cannot be adequately controlled by currently available medical interventions. As we shall see, however, I disagree with the philosophers' conclusion that this interest is sufficiently strong in the face of current medical and social inadequacies as to justify a legal right that would void the reasonably cautious prohibitions of PAS and euthanasia in effect in every state.
9. Cassel et al., "Care of the Hopelessly Ill," 1380–84. See also Franklin G. Miller et al., "Regulating Physician-Assisted Death," *New England Journal of Medicine* 331(1994): 199–23 (conceding by the untenability of the previous distinction).
10. Professors Dworkin, et al. consistently fail to mention the possibility, let alone the high likelihood, of this first sort of slippage; I take this to be a serious omission both in their joint brief and in Dworkin's individually authored articles on this subject. These authors simply assume (with the plaintiffs and circuit court majority opinions) that this right will be restricted by means of procedural safeguards to presently competent, incurably ill individuals manifesting great pain and suffering due to physical illness. (For evidence of Dworkin's continuing failure to acknowledge this problem, see his assessment of the Supreme Court opinions in "Assisted Suicide: What the Court Really Said," *New York Review of Books* 44, no. 14 (Sept. 25, 1997): 40–44. Failure to notice this sort of dynamic might be due either to the philosophers' lack of familiarity with the recent history of bioethics or to their belief that the social risks of PAS are equivalent to the risks inherent in the widely accepted practice of forgoing life-sustaining treatments, and thus that such slippage would not present any additional risk. The latter assumption is, of course, vigorously contested by the opponents of PAS and euthanasia.
11. Task Force, *When Death Is Sought,* 43–47. "Despite dramatic advances in pain management, the delivery of pain relief is grossly inadequate in clinical practice . . . Studies have shown that only 2 to 60 percent of cancer pain is treated adequately." *Ibid.,* 43.
12. See, e.g., Ronald Dworkin, "Introduction to the Philosophers' Brief," *New York Review of Books,* 41–42 [in this volume, 382–85]; and Dworkin, "Assisted Suicide: What the Court Really Said," 44.
13. For an explication of the notion of a "tragic choice" in the sense that I employ here, see Guido Calabresi and Philip Bobbit, *Tragic Choices* (New York: W.W. Norton, 1978).

EUTHANASIA: THE WAY WE DO IT, THE WAY THEY DO IT

End-of-Life Practices in the Developed World

Margaret P. Battin

Because we tend to be rather myopic in our discussions of death and dying, especially about the issues of active euthanasia and assisted suicide, it is valuable to place the question of how we go about dying in an international context. We do not always see that our own cultural norms may be quite different from those of other nations and that our background assumptions and actual practices differ dramatically—even when the countries in question are all developed industrial nations with similar cultural ancestries, religious traditions, and economic circumstances. I want to explore the three rather different approaches to end-of-life dilemmas prevalent in the United States, the Netherlands, and Germany—developments mirrored in Australia, Belgium, Switzerland, and elsewhere in the developed world—and consider how a society might think about which model of approach to dying is most appropriate for it.

THREE BASIC MODELS OF DYING

The Netherlands, Germany, and the United States are all advanced industrial democracies. They all have sophisticated medical establishments and life expectancies over 75 years of age; their populations are all characterized by an increasing proportion of older persons. They are all in what has been called the fourth stage of the epidemiologic transition[1]—that stage of societal development in which it is no longer the case that the majority of the population dies of acute parasitic or infectious diseases, often with rapid, unpredictable onsets and sharp fatality curves (as was true in earlier and less developed societies); rather, in modern industrial societies, the majority of a population—as much as perhaps 70–80%—dies of degenerative diseases, especially delayed-degenerative diseases that are characterized by late, slow onset and extended decline. This is the case throughout the developed world. Accidents and suicide claim some, as do infectious diseases like AIDS, pneumonia, and influenza, but most people in highly industrialized countries die from heart disease (by no means always suddenly fatal); cancer; atherosclerosis; chronic obstructive pulmonary disease; diabetes; liver, kidney, or other organ disease; or degenerative neurological disorders. In the developed world, we die not so much from attack by outside diseases but from gradual disintegration. Thus, all three of these modern industrial countries—the United States, the Netherlands, and Germany—are alike in facing a common problem: how to deal with the characteristic new ways in which we die.

Dealing with Dying in the United States

In the United States, we have come to recognize that the maximal extension of life-prolonging treatment in these late-life degenerative conditions is often inappropriate. Although we could keep the machines and tubes—the respirators, intravenous lines, feeding tubes—hooked up for extended periods, we recognize that this is inhumane, pointless, and financially impossible. Instead, as a society we have developed a number of mechanisms for dealing with these hopeless situations, all of which involve withholding or withdrawing various forms of treatment.

Some mechanisms for withholding or withdrawing treatments are exercised by the patient who is confronted by such a situation or who anticipates it. These include refusal of treatment, the patient-executed Do Not Resuscitate (DNR) order, the Living Will, and the Durable Power of Attorney. Others are mechanisms for decision by second parties

Originally appeared in the *Journal of Pain and Symptom Management*, vol. 6, no. 5, 1991, pp. 298–305. Revised and updated multiple times by the author, most recently December 2001.

about a patient who is no longer competent or never was competent, reflected in a long series of court cases from *Quinlan; Saikewicz; Spring; Eichner; Barber; Bartling; Conroy; Brophy;* the trio *Farrell, Peter,* and *Jobes,* to *Cruzan.* These cases delineate the precise circumstances under which it is appropriate to withhold or withdraw various forms of therapy, including respiratory support, chemotherapy, dialysis, antibiotics in intercurrent infections, and artificial nutrition and hydration. Thus, during the past quarter-century, roughly since *Quinlan* (1976), the U.S. has developed an impressive body of case law and state statutes that protects, permits, and facilitates the characteristic American strategy of dealing with end-of-life situations. These cases provide a framework for withholding or withdrawing treatment when physicians and family members believe there is no medical or moral point in going on. This has sometimes been termed *passive euthanasia;* more often, it is simply called *allowing to die.*

Indeed, "allowing to die" has become ubiquitous in the United States. For example, a 1988 study found that of the 85% of deaths in the United States that occurred in health care institutions, including hospitals, nursing homes, and other facilities, about 70% involved electively withholding some form of life-sustaining treatment.[2] A 1989 study found that 85–90% of critical care professionals said they were withholding or withdrawing life-sustaining treatments from patients who were "deemed to have irreversible disease and are terminally ill."[3] A 1997 study of limits to life-sustaining care found that between 1987–88 and 1992–93, recommendations to withhold or withdraw life support prior to death increased from 51% to 90% in the intensive-care units studied.[4] Rates of withholding therapy such as ventilator support, surgery, and dialysis were found in yet another study to be substantial, and to increase with age.[5] A 1994/95 study of 167 intensive-care units—all the ICUs associated with U.S. training programs in critical care medicine or pulmonary and critical care medicine—found that in 75% of deaths, some form of care was withheld or withdrawn.[6] It has been estimated that 1.3 million American deaths a year follow decisions to withhold life support;[7] this is a majority of the just over 2 million American deaths per year.

In recent years, the legitimate use of withholding and withdrawing treatment has increasingly been understood to include practices likely or certain to result in death. The administration of escalating doses of morphine in a dying patient, which, it has been claimed, will depress respiration and so hasten death, is acceptable under the (Catholic) principle of double effect provided the medication is intended to relieve pain and merely foreseen but not intended to result in death; this practice is not considered killing or active hastening of death. The use of "terminal sedation," in which a patient dying in pain is sedated into unconsciousness while artificial nutrition and hydration are withheld, is also recognized as medically and legally acceptable; it too is understood as a form of "allowing to die," not active killing. With the single exception of Oregon, where physician-assisted suicide became legal in 1997,[8] withholding and withdrawing treatment and related forms of allowing to die are the only legally recognized ways we in the United States go about dealing with dying. A number of recent studies have shown that many physicians—in all states studied—do receive requests for assistance in suicide or active euthanasia and that a substantial number of these physicians have complied with one or more such requests; however, this more direct assistance in dying takes place entirely out of sight of the law. Except in Oregon, *allowing to die,* but not *causing to die,* has been the only legally protected alternative to maximal treatment legally recognized in the United States; it remains America's—and American medicine's—official posture in the face of death.

Dealing with Dying in the Netherlands

In the Netherlands, although the practice of withholding and withdrawing treatment is similar to that in the United States, voluntary active euthanasia and physician assistance in suicide are also available responses to end-of-life situations.[9] Active euthanasia is the more frequent form of assistance in dying and most discussion in the Netherlands has concerned it rather than assistance in suicide, though the conceptual difference is not regarded as great: many cases of what the Dutch term *voluntary active euthanasia* involve initial self-administration of the lethal dose by the patient but procurement of death by the physician, and many cases of what is termed *physician-assisted suicide* involve completion of the lethal process by the physician if a self-administered drug does not prove fully effective. Although until 2001 they were still technically illegal under statutory law, and even with legalization remain an "exception" to those provisions of the Dutch Penal Code which prohibit killing on request and intentional assistance in suicide, active euthanasia and assistance in suicide have long been widely regarded as legal, or rather *gedoogd,* legally "tolerated," and have in fact been deemed justified (not only nonpunishable) by the courts when performed by a physician if certain conditions were met. Voluntary active euthanasia (in the law, called "life-ending on request") and physician-assisted suicide are now fully legal by statute under these guidelines. Dutch law protects the physician who performs euthanasia or provides assistance in suicide from prosecution for homicide if these guidelines, known as the conditions of "due care," are met.

Over the years, the guidelines have been stated in various ways. They contain six central provisions:

1. that the patient's request be voluntary and well-considered;
2. that the patient be undergoing or about to undergo intolerable suffering, that is, suffering which is lasting and unbearable;
3. that all alternatives acceptable to the patient for relieving the suffering have been tried, and that the patient believes there is no other reasonable solution;
4. that the patient have full information about his situation and prospects;
5. that the physician consult with a second physician who has examined the patient and whose judgment can be expected to be independent;
6. that in performing euthanasia or assisting in suicide, the physician act with due care.

Of these criteria, it is the first that is held to be central: euthanasia may be performed only at the *voluntary* request of the patient. This criterion is also understood to require that the patient's request be a stable, enduring, reflective one—not the product of a transitory impulse. Every attempt is to be made to rule out depression, psychopathology, pressures from family members, unrealistic fears, and other factors compromising voluntariness, though depression is not in itself understood to preclude such choice. Euthanasia may be performed *only* by a physician, not by a nurse, family member, or other party.

In 1990, a comprehensive, nationwide study requested by the Dutch government, popularly known as the Remmelink Commission report, provided the first objective data about the incidence of euthanasia.[10] This study also provided information about other medical decisions at the end of life: withholding or withdrawal of treatment; the use of life-shortening doses of opioids for the control of pain; and direct termination, including not only voluntary active euthanasia and physician-assisted suicide but life-ending procedures not termed euthanasia. The Remmelink study was supplemented by a second empirical examination, focusing particularly carefully on the characteristics of patients and the nature of their euthanasia requests.[11] Five years later, the researchers from these two studies jointly conducted a major new nationwide study replicating much of the previous Remmelink inquiry, providing empirical data both about current practice in the Netherlands and change over a five-year period.[12] A third such study is to be published in fall 2003.

About 135,000 people die in the Netherlands every year, and of these deaths, about 30% are acute and unexpected, while about 70% are predictable and foreseen, usually the result of degenerative illness comparatively late in life. Of the total deaths in the Netherlands, about 20% involve decisions to withhold or withdraw treatment in situations where continuing treatment would probably have prolonged life; another 20% involve the "double effect" use of opioids to relieve pain but in dosages probably sufficient to shorten life.[13]

The 1990 study revealed that about 2,300 people, 1.8% of the total deaths in the Netherlands at that time, died by euthanasia—understood as the termination of the life of the patient at the patient's explicit and persistent request; close to another 400 people, 0.3% of the total, chose physician-assisted suicide. However, the study also revealed that another 0.8% of patients who died did so as the result of life-terminating procedures not technically called euthanasia, without explicit, current request. These cases, known as "the 1000 cases," unleashed highly exaggerated claims that patients were being killed against their wills. In fact, in about half of these cases, euthanasia had been previously discussed with the patient or the patient had expressed in a previous phase of the disease a wish for euthanasia if his or her suffering became unbearable ("Doctor, please don't let me suffer too long"); and in the other half, the patient was no longer competent and was near death, clearly suffering grievously although verbal contact had become impossible.[14] In 91% of these cases without explicit, current request, life was shortened by less than a week, and in 33% by less than a day.

By 1995, although the proportion of cases of assisted suicide had remained about the same, the proportion of cases of euthanasia had risen to about 2.4% (associated, the authors conjectured, with the aging of the population and an increase in the proportion of deaths due to cancer, that condition in which euthanasia is most frequent). However, the proportion of cases of life termination without current explicit request had declined slightly to 0.7%. In 1990, a total of 2.9% of all deaths had involved euthanasia and related practices; by 1995 this total was 3.3%. Not all cases are reported as required, though there has been a dramatic gain since the physician has no longer been required to report them directly to the police or the Ministry of Justice. However, there are no major differences between reported and unreported cases in terms of the patient's characteristics, clinical conditions, or reasons for the action.[15] Euthanasia is performed in about 1:25 of deaths that occur at home, about 1:75 of hospital deaths, and about 1:800 of nursing home deaths.

Although euthanasia is thus not frequent, a small fraction of the total annual mortality, it is nevertheless a conspicuous option in terminal illness, well-known to both physicians and the general public. There has been very widespread public discussion of the issues that arise with respect to euthanasia during the last quarter-century, and surveys of public opinion show that public support for a liberal euthanasia policy has been growing: from 40% in 1966 to 81% in 1988,[16] then to about 90% by 2000. Doctors, too, support the practice, and although there has been a vocal opposition group, it has remained in the clear minority. Some 53% of Dutch physicians say that they have performed euthanasia or provided assistance in suicide, including 63% of general practitioners. An additional 35% of all physicians said that although they had not actually done so, they could conceive of situations in which they would be prepared to do so. Nine percent say they would never perform it, and just 3% say they not only would not do so themselves but would not refer a patient who requested it to a physician who would. Thus, although many physicians who had practiced euthanasia mentioned that they would be most reluctant to do so again and that "only in the face of unbearable suffering and with no alternatives would they be prepared to take such action,"[17] both the 1990 and 1995 studies showed that the majority of Dutch physicians accept the practice in some cases. Surveying the changes over the 5-year period between 1990–1995, the study authors also commented that the data do not support claims of a slippery slope.[18]

In general, pain alone is not the basis for deciding upon euthanasia, since pain can, in most cases, be effectively treated. Rather, the "intolerable suffering" mentioned in the second criterion is understood to mean suffering that is intolerable in the patient's (rather than the physician's) view and can include a fear of or unwillingness to endure *entluistering,* that gradual effacement and loss of personal identity that characterizes the end stages of many terminal illnesses. In very exceptional circumstances, the Supreme Court ruled in the Chabot case of 1994, physician-assisted suicide may be justified for a patient with non-somatic, psychiatric illness like intractable depression, but such cases are extremely rare. Of patients who do receive euthanasia or physician-assisted suicide, about 80% have cancer, while just 3% have cardiovascular disease and 4% neurological disease.

In a year, almost 35,000 patients seek reassurance from their physicians that they will be granted euthanasia if their suffering becomes severe; there are about 9,700 explicit requests, and about two-thirds of these are turned down, usually on the grounds that there is some other way of treating the patient's suffering. In 14% of cases in 1990, the denial was based on the presence of depression or psychiatric illness.

In the Netherlands, many hospitals now have protocols for the performance of euthanasia; these serve to ensure that the legal guidelines have been met. However, euthanasia is often practiced in the patient's home, typically by the general practitioner who is the patient's long-term family physician. Euthanasia is usually performed after aggressive hospital treatment has failed to arrest the patient's terminal illness; the patient has come home to die, and the family physician is prepared to ease this passing. Whether practiced at home or in the hospital, it is believed that euthanasia usually takes place in the presence of the family members, perhaps the visiting nurse, and often the patient's pastor or priest. Many doctors say that performing euthanasia is never easy but that it is something they believe a doctor ought to do for his or her patient when the patient genuinely wants it and nothing else can help.

Thus, in the Netherlands a patient who is facing the end of life has an option not openly practiced in the United States: to ask the physician to bring his or her life to an end. Although not everyone does so—indeed, almost 97% of people who die in a given year do not do so—it is a choice legally recognized and widely understood.

Facing Death in Germany

In part because of its very painful history of Nazism, Germany medical culture has insisted that doctors should have no role in directly causing death. As in the other countries with advanced medical systems, withholding and withdrawing of care is widely used to avoid the unwanted or inappropriate prolongation of life when the patient is already dying, but there has been vigorous and nearly universal opposition in German public discourse to the notion of active euthanasia, at least in the horrific, politically-motivated sense associated with Nazism. In the last ten years, some Germans have begun to approve of euthanasia in the Dutch sense, based on the Greek root *eu-thanatos,* or "good death," a voluntary choice by the patient for an easier death, but many Germans still associate euthanasia with the politically-motivated exterminations by the Nazis, and view the Dutch as stepping out on a dangerously slippery slope.

However, although under German law killing on request (including voluntary euthanasia) is illegal, German law has not prohibited assistance in suicide since the time of Frederick the Great (1742), provided the person is *tatherrschaftsfähig,* capable of exercising control over his or her actions, and also acting out of *freiverantwortliche Wille,* freely responsible choice. Doctors are prohibited from assistance in suicide not by law but by the policies and code of ethics of the *Bundesärtzekammer,* the German medical association. Furthermore, any person, physician or otherwise, has a duty to rescue a person who is unconscious. Thus, assistance in suicide is limited, but it is possible for a family member or friend to assist in a person's suicide, for instance by providing a lethal drug, as long as the person is competent and acting freely and the assister does not remain with the person after unconsciousness sets in.

Taking advantage of this situation, there has developed a private organization, the *Deutsche Gesellschaft für Humanes Sterben* (DGHS), or German Society for Dying with Dignity, which provides support to its very extensive membership in many end-of-life matters, including choosing suicide as an alternative to terminal illness. Of course, not all Germans are members of this organization and many are not sympathetic with its aims, yet the notion of self-directed ending of one's own life in terminal illness is widely understood as an option. Although the DGHS does not itself supply such information, it tells its members how to obtain a booklet published in Scotland with information about ending life, if they request it, provided they have not received medical or psychotherapeutic treatment for depression or other psychiatric illness during the last two years. The information includes a list of prescription drugs, together with the specific dosages necessary for producing a certain, painless death. The DGHS does not itself sell or supply lethal drugs;[19] rather, it recommends that the member approach a physician for a prescription for the drug desired, asking, for example, for a barbiturate to help with sleep. If necessary, the DGHS has been willing to arrange for someone to obtain drugs from neighboring countries, including France, Italy, Spain, Portugal, and Greece, where they may be available without prescription. It also makes available the so-called Exit Bag, a plastic bag used with specific techniques for death by asphyxiation. The DGHS provides and trains family members in what it calls *Sterbebegleitung* (accompaniment in dying), which may take the form of simple presence with a person who is dying, but may also involve direct assistance to a person who is committing suicide, up until unconsciousness sets in. The *Sterbebegleiter* is typically a layperson, not someone medically trained, and physicians play no role in assisting in these cases of suicide. Direct active *Sterbehilfe*—active euthanasia—is illegal under German law. But active indirect *Sterbehilfe,* understood as assistance in suicide, is not illegal, and the DGHS provides counseling in how a "death with dignity" may be achieved in this way.

To preclude suspicion by providing evidence of the person's intentions, the DGHS also provides a form—printed on a single sheet of distinctive purple paper—to be signed once when joining the organization, documenting that the person has reflected thoroughly on the possibility of "free death" *(Freitod)* or suicide in terminal illness as a way of releasing oneself from severe suffering, and expressing the intention to determine the time and character of one's own death. The person then signs this form again at the time of the suicide, leaving it beside the body as evidence that the act is not impetuous or coerced. The form also requests that, if the person is discovered before the suicide is complete, no rescue measures be undertaken. Because assisting suicide is not illegal in Germany (provided the person is competent and in control of his or her own will, and thus not already unconscious), there is no legal risk for family members, the *Sterbebegleiter,* or others in reporting information about the methods and effectiveness of suicide attempts, and at least in the past the DGHS has encouraged its network of regional bureaus, located in major cities throughout the country, to facilitate feedback. On this basis, it has regularly updated and revised the drug information provided.

Open, legal assistance in suicide is supported by a feature of the German language that makes it possible to conceptualize it in a comparatively benign way. While English, French, Spanish, and many other languages have just a single primary word for suicide, German has four: *Selbstmord, Selbsttötung, Suizid,* and *Freitod,* of which the latter has comparatively positive, even somewhat heroic connotations.[20] Thus German-speakers can think about the deliberate termination of their lives in a linguistic way not easily available to speakers of other languages. The negatively-rooted term *Selbstmord* ("self-murder") can be avoided; the comparatively neutral terms *Selbsttötung* ("self-killing") and *Suizid* ("suicide") can be used, and the positively-rooted term *Freitod* ("free death") can be reinforced. The DGHS has frequently used *Freitod* rather than German's other, more negative terms to describe the practice with which it provides assistance. No reliable figures are available about the number of suicides with which this organization has assisted, and, as in the Netherlands, the actual frequency of directly assisted death is probably small. Yet it is fair to say, both because of the legal differences and the different conceptual horizons of German-speakers, that the option of self-produced death outside the medical system is more clearly open in Germany than it has been in the Netherlands or the United States.

In recent years, the DGHS has decreased its emphasis on suicide, now thinking of it as a "last resort" when pain control is inadequate—and turned much of its attention to the development of other measures for protecting the rights of the terminally ill, measures already available in many other countries. It distributes newly legalized advance directives, including living wills and durable powers of attorney, as well as organ-donation documents. It provides information about pain control, palliative care, and Hospice. It offers information about suicide prevention. Yet it remains steadfast in defense of the terminally ill patient's right to self-determination, including the right to suicide, and continues to be supportive of patients who make this choice.

To be sure, assisted suicide is not the only option open to terminally ill patients in Germany, and the choice may be infrequent. Reported suicide rates in Germany are only moderately higher than in the Netherlands or the United States,[21] though there is reason to think that terminal-illness suicides in all countries are often reported as deaths from the underlying disease. Although there is political pressure from right-to-die organizations to change the law to permit voluntary active euthanasia in the way understood in the Netherlands, Germany is also seeing increasing emphasis on help in dying, like that offered by Hospice, that does not involve direct termination. Whatever the pressures, the DGHS is a conspicuous, widely known organization, and many Germans appear to be aware that assisted suicide is available and not illegal even if they do not use its services.

OBJECTIONS TO THE THREE MODELS OF DYING

In response to the dilemmas raised by the new circumstances of death, in which the majority of people in the advanced industrial nations die after an extended period of terminal deterioration, different countries develop different practices. The United States, with the sole exception of Oregon, legally permits only withholding and withdrawal of treatment conceived of as "allowing to die," understood to include "double effect" uses of high doses of opiates and terminal sedation. The Netherlands permits these, but also permits voluntary active euthanasia and physician-assisted suicide. Germany rejects physician-performed euthanasia, but it permits assisted suicide not assisted by a physician. These three serve as the principal types or models of response to end-of-life dilemmas in the developed world. To be sure, all of these practices are currently undergoing evolution, and in some ways they are becoming more alike: Germany is paying new attention to the rights of patients to execute advance directives and thus to have treatment withheld or withdrawn, and public surveys reveal considerable support for euthanasia in the Dutch sense, voluntary active aid-in-dying under careful controls. In the Netherlands, a 1995 policy statement of the Royal Dutch Medical Association expressed a careful preference for physician-assisted suicide in preference to euthanasia, urging that physicians encourage patients who request euthanasia to administer the lethal dose themselves as a further protective of voluntary choice. And, in the United States, the Supreme Court's 1997 ruling there is no constitutional right to physician-assisted suicide has been understood to countenance the emergence of a "laboratory of the states" in which individual states, following the example of Oregon, may in the future move to legalize physician-assisted suicide, though following an attempt in 2001 by the U.S. Attorney General to undercut Oregon's law by prohibiting the use of scheduled drugs for the purpose of causing death, it appears that the issue will return to the U.S. Supreme Court. Nevertheless, among these three countries that serve as the principal models of approaches to dying, there remain substantial differences, and while there are ethical and practical advantages to each approach, each approach also raises serious moral objections.

Objections to the German Practice

German law does not prohibit assisting suicide, but postwar German culture and the Germany physicians' code of ethics discourages physicians from taking an active role in causing death. This gives rise to distinctive moral problems. For one thing, if the physician is not permitted to assist in his or her patient's suicide, there may be little professional help or review provided for the patient's choice about suicide. If patients make such choices essentially outside the medical establishment, medical professionals may not be in a position to detect or treat impaired judgment on the part of the patient, especially judgment impaired by depression. Similarly, if the patient must commit suicide assisted only by persons outside the medical profession, there are risks that the patient's diagnosis and prognosis will be inadequately confirmed, that the means chosen for suicide will be unreliable or inappropriately used, that the means used for suicide will fall into the hands of other persons, and that the patient will fail to recognize or be able to resist intrafamilial pressures and manipulation. While it now makes efforts to counter most of these objections, even the DGHS itself has been accused in the past of promoting rather than simply supporting choices of suicide. Finally, as the DGHS now emphasizes, assistance in suicide can be a freely chosen option only in a legal context that also protects the many other choices a patient may make—declining treatment, executing advance directives, seeking Hospice care—about how his or her life shall end.

Objections to the Dutch Practice

The Dutch practice of physician-performed active voluntary euthanasia and physician-assisted suicide also raises a number of ethical issues, many of which have been discussed vigorously both in the

Dutch press and in commentary on the Dutch practices from abroad. For one thing, it is sometimes said that the availability of physician-assisted dying creates a disincentive for providing good terminal care. There is no evidence that this is the case; on the contrary, Peter Admiraal, the anesthesiologist who has been perhaps the Netherlands' most vocal defender of voluntary active euthanasia, insists that pain should rarely or never be the occasion for euthanasia, as pain (in contrast to suffering) is comparatively easily treated.[22] In fact, pain is the primary reason for the request in only about 5% of cases. Instead, it is a refusal to endure the final stages of deterioration, both mental and physical, that primarily motivates the majority of requests.

It is also sometimes said that active euthanasia violates the Hippocratic Oath. The original Greek version of the Oath does prohibit the physician from giving a deadly drug, even when asked for it; but the original version also prohibits the physician from performing surgery and from taking fees for teaching medicine, neither of which prohibitions has survived into contemporary medical practice. At issue is whether deliberately causing the death of one's patient—killing one's patient, some claim—can ever be part of the physician's role. "Doctors must not kill," insist opponents,[23] but Dutch physicians often say that they see performing euthanasia—where it is genuinely requested by the patient and nothing else can be done to relieve the patient's condition—as part of their duty to the patient, not as a violation of it. As the 1995 Remmelink report commented, "a large majority of Dutch physicians consider euthanasia an exceptional but accepted part of medical practice."[24] The Dutch do worry, however, that too many requests for euthanasia or assistance in suicide are refused—only about ⅓ of explicit requests are actually honored. One well-known Dutch commentator points to another, seemingly contrary concern: that some requests are made too early in a terminal course, even shortly after diagnosis, when with good palliative care the patient could live a substantial amount of time longer.[25] However, these are concerns about how euthanasia and physician-assisted suicide are practiced, not whether they should be legal at all.

The Dutch are also often said to be at risk of starting down the slippery slope, that is, that the practice of voluntary active euthanasia for patients who meet the criteria will erode into practicing less-than-voluntary euthanasia on patients whose problems are not irremediable and perhaps by gradual degrees will develop into terminating the lives of people who are elderly, chronically ill, handicapped, mentally retarded, or otherwise regarded as undesirable. This risk is often expressed in vivid claims of widespread fear and wholesale slaughter—claims based on misinterpretation of the 1,000 cases of life-ending treatment without explicit, current request, claims that are often repeated in the right-to-life press in both the Netherlands and the U.S. although they are simply not true. However, it is true that the Dutch have begun to agonize over the problems of the incompetent patient, the mentally ill patient, the newborn with serious deficits, and other patients who cannot make voluntary choices, though these are largely understood as issues about withholding or withdrawing treatment, not about direct termination.[26]

What is not often understood is that this new and acutely painful area of reflection for the Dutch—withholding and withdrawing treatment from incompetent patients—has already led in the United States to the emergence of a vast, highly developed body of law: namely, that long series of cases beginning with *Quinlan* and culminating in *Cruzan*. Americans have been discussing these issues for a long time and have developed a broad set of practices that are regarded as routine in withholding and withdrawing treatment from persons who are no longer or never were competent. The Dutch see Americans as much further out on the slippery slope than they are because Americans have already become accustomed to second-party choices that result in death for other people. Issues involving second-party choices are painful to the Dutch in a way they are not to Americans precisely because *voluntariness* is so central in the Dutch understanding of choices about dying. Concomitantly, the Dutch see the Americans' squeamishness about first-party choices—voluntary euthanasia, assisted suicide—as evidence that we are not genuinely committed to recognizing voluntary choice after all. For this reason, many Dutch commentators believe that the Americans are at a much greater risk of sliding down the slippery slope into involuntary killing than they are.

Objections to the American Practice

The German, Dutch, and American practices all occur within similar conditions—in industrialized nations with highly developed medical systems where a majority of the population die of illnesses exhibiting characteristically extended downhill courses—but the issues raised by the American response to this situation—relying on withholding and withdrawal of treatment—may be even more disturbing than those of the Dutch or the Germans. We Americans often assume that our approach is "safer" because, except in Oregon, it involves only letting someone die, not killing them; but it, too, raises very troubling questions.

The first of these issues is a function of the fact that withdrawing and especially withholding treatment are typically less conspicuous, less pronounced, less evident kinds of actions than direct killing, even though they can equally well lead to death. Decisions about nontreatment have an invisibility that decisions about directly causing death do not have, even though they may have the same result, and hence there is a much wider range of occasions in which such decisions can be made. One can decline to treat a patient in many different ways, at many different times—by not providing oxygen, by not instituting dialysis, by not correcting electrolyte imbalances, and so on—all of which will cause the patient's death. Open medical killing also brings about death, but is much more overt and conspicuous. Consequently, letting die invites many fewer protections. In contrast to the standard slippery-slope argument, which sees killing as riskier than letting die, the more realistic slippery-slope argument warns that because our culture relies primarily on decisions about nontreatment and practices like terminal sedation construed as "allowing to die," grave decisions about living or dying are not as open to scrutiny as they are under more direct life-terminating practices, and hence are more open to abuse. Indeed, in the view of one well-known commentator, the Supreme Court's 1997 decision in effect legalized active euthanasia, voluntary and nonvoluntary, in the form of terminal sedation, even as it rejected physician-assisted suicide.[27]

Second, reliance on withholding and withdrawal of treatment invites rationing in an extremely strong way, in part because of the comparative invisibility of these decisions. When a health care provider does not offer a specific sort of care, it is not always possible to discern the motivation; the line between believing that it would not provide benefit to the patient and that it would not provide benefit worth the investment of resources in the patient can be very thin. This is a particular problem where health care financing is decentralized, profit-oriented, and nonuniversal, as in the United States, and where rationing decisions without benefit of principle are not always available for easy review.

Third, relying on withholding and withdrawal of treatment can often be cruel. Even with hospice or with skilled palliative care, it requires that the patient who is dying from one of the diseases that exhibits a characteristic extended, downhill course (as the majority of patients in the developed world all do) must, in effect, wait to die until the absence of a certain treatment will cause death. For instance, the cancer patient who forgoes chemotherapy or surgery does not simply die from this choice; he or she continues to endure the downhill course of the cancer until the tumor finally destroys some crucial bodily function or organ. The patient with amyotrophic lateral sclerosis who decides in advance to decline respiratory support does not die at the time this choice is made but continues to endure increasing paralysis until breathing is impaired and suffocation occurs. Of course, attempts are made to try to ameliorate these situations by administering pain medication or symptom control at the time treatment is withheld—for instance, by using opiates and paralytics as a respirator is withdrawn—but these are all ways of disguising the fact that we are letting the disease kill the patient rather than directly bringing about death. But the ways diseases kill people can be far more cruel than the ways physicians kill patients when performing euthanasia or assisting in suicide.

END-OF-LIFE PRACTICES IN OTHER COUNTRIES

In most of the developed world dying looks much the same. As in the United States, the Netherlands, and Germany, the other industrialized nations also have sophisticated medical establishments, enjoy extended life expectancies, and find themselves in the fourth stage of the epidemiological transition, in which the majority of their populations die of diseases with extended downhill courses. Dying takes place in much the same way in all these countries, though the exact frequency of withholding and withdrawing treatment, of double-effect use of opiates, and euthanasia and physician-assisted suicide varies among them. Indeed, new data is rapidly coming to light.

In Australia, a replication of the Remmelink Commission study originally performed in the Netherlands found that of deaths in Australia that involved a medical end-of-life decision, 28.6% involved withholding or withdrawing treatment; 30.9% involved the use of opiates under the principle of double effect, and 1.8% involved voluntary active euthanasia (including 0.1% physician-assisted suicide), though neither are legal.[28] But the study also found—this is the figure that produced considerable surprise—that some 3.5% of deaths involved termination of the patient's life without the patient's concurrent explicit request. This figure is five times as high as that in the Netherlands. In slightly more than a third of these cases (38%), there was some discussion with the patient, though not an explicit request for death to be hastened, and in virtually all of the rest, the doctor did not consider the patient competent or capable of making such a decision. In 0.5% of all deaths involving medical end-of-life decisions, doctors did not discuss the choice of hastening of death with the patient because they thought it was "clearly the best one for the patient" or that "discussion would have done more harm than good."[29]

Replication of the same study in Flanders, Belgium, revealed a similar picture. Withholding and/or withdrawing treatment was involved in 16.4% of deaths; the double-effect use of opiates in 18.5%, euthanasia and physician-assisted suicide in 1.3%, and—a figure just slightly lower than that of Australia, but substantially higher than that of the Netherlands, termination of life without current, explicit consent from the patient in 3.2%.[30] While data is not yet available for actual end-of-life decision-making and practices for the full range of developed countries, a thorough study of end-of-life decisions in five European countries will be published in 2003.

End-of-life practices in other developed countries tend to follow one of the three models explored here. For example, Canada's practices are much like those of the United States, in that it relies on withholding and withdrawing treatment and other forms of allowing to die, but, in the 1993 case *Rodriquez* v. *British Columbia*, the Canadian Supreme Court narrowly rejected physician-assisted suicide. Australia's Northern Territory briefly legalized assisted dying in 1997, but the law was overturned after just four cases. The United Kingdom, the birthplace of the Hospice movement, stresses palliative care but also rejects physician-assisted suicide and active euthanasia. Late in 2001, Belgium's parliament voted to legalize voluntary active euthanasia and physician-assisted suicide; Belgium's law is patterned fairly closely after the Dutch law. Switzerland's law, like that of Germany, does not criminalize assisted suicide, but does not impose a duty to rescue that makes assistance in suicide difficult. The Swiss organization Exit, the analogue of Germany's DGHS, follows the same general model as the German organization in providing information, counseling, and other support to terminally ill patients who choose suicide, *Freitod,* but the Swiss group also provides such a patient an accompaniment team which consults with the patient to make sure that the choice of suicide is voluntary, secures a prescription from a sympathetic physician, and delivers the lethal medication to the person at a pre-appointed time. It encourages family members to be present when the patient takes the drug, if he or she still wants to use it, and operates at least one "safe house" for patients traveling from abroad for this purpose. In general, the Swiss organization provides extensive help to the patient who chooses this way of dying, though in keeping with Swiss law, it insists that the patient take the drug him- or herself: assisted suicide is legal, but euthanasia is not.

In contrast, practices in less developed countries look very, very different. In these countries, especially the least developed, background circumstances are different: lifespans are significantly shorter, health care systems are only primitively equipped and grossly underfunded, and many societies have not passed through to the fourth stage of the epidemiologic transition: in these countries, people die earlier, they are more likely to die of infectious and parasitic disease, and degenerative disease is more likely to be interrupted early by death from pneumonia, sepsis, malnutrition, and other factors in what would otherwise have been a long downhill course. Dying in the poorer countries remains different from dying in the richer countries, and the underlying ethical problem in the richer countries—what practices concerning the end of life to adopt when the majority of a population dies of late-life degenerative diseases with long downhill courses—is far less applicable in the less developed parts of the world.

THE PROBLEM: A CHOICE OF CULTURES

In the developed world, we see three sorts of models in the three countries we've examined in detail. While much of medical practice in them is similar, they do offer three quite different basic options in approaching death. All three of these options generate moral problems; none of them, nor any others we might devise, is free of moral difficulty. The question, then, is this: for a given society, which practices about dying are, morally and practically speaking, best?

It is not possible to answer this question in a less-than-ideal world without attention to the specific characteristics and deficiencies of the society in question. In asking which of these practices is best, we must ask which is best *for us.* That we currently employ one set of these options rather than others does not prove that it is best for us; the question is, would practices developed in other cultures or those not yet widespread in any culture be better for our own culture than that which has so far developed here? Thus, it is necessary to consider the differences between our own society and these other societies in the developed world that have real bearing on which model of approach to dying we ought to adopt. This question can be asked by residents of any country or culture: which model of dying is best *for us?* I have been addressing this question from the point of view of an American, but the question could be asked by any member of any culture, anywhere.

First, notice that different cultures exhibit different degrees of closeness between physicians and patients—different patterns of contact and involvement. The German physician is sometimes said to be more distant and more authoritarian than the American physician; on the other hand, the Dutch physician is often said to be closer to his or her patients than either the American or the German is. In the Netherlands, basic primary care is provided by the *huisarts,* the general practitioner or family physician, who typically lives in the neighborhood, makes house calls frequently, and maintains an office in his or her own home. This physician usually also provides care for the other members of the patient's family and will remain the family's physician throughout his or her practice. Thus, the patient for whom euthanasia becomes an issue—say, the terminal cancer patient who has been hospitalized in the past but who has returned home to die—will be cared for by the trusted family physician on a regular basis. Indeed, for a patient in severe distress, the physician, supported by the visiting nurse, may make house calls as often as once a day, twice a day, or even more frequently (after all, the physician's office is right in the neighborhood) and is in continuous contact with the family. In contrast, the traditional American institution of the family doctor who makes house calls has largely become a thing of the past, and although some patients who die at home have access to hospice services and receive house calls from their long-term physician, many have no such long-term care and receive most of it from staff at a clinic or from house staff rotating through the services of a hospital. Most Americans die in institutions, including hospitals and nursing homes; in the Netherlands, in contrast, the majority of people die at home. The degree of continuing contact that the patient can have with a familiar, trusted physician and the degree of institutionalization clearly influence the nature of his or her dying and also play a role in whether physician-performed active euthanasia, assisted suicide, and/or withholding and withdrawing treatment is appropriate.

Second, the United States has a much more volatile legal climate than either the Netherlands or Germany; its medical system is highly litigious, much more so than that of any other country in the world. Fears of malpractice actions or criminal prosecution color much of what physicians do in managing the dying of their patients. Americans also tend to develop public policy through court decisions and to assume that the existence of a policy puts an end to any moral issue. A delicate legal and moral balance over the issue of euthanasia, as has been the case in the Netherlands throughout the time it was understood as *gedoogd*, tolerated but not fully legal, would hardly be possible here.

Third, we in the United States have a very different financial climate in which to do our dying. Both the Netherlands and Germany, as well as virtually every other industrialized nation, have systems of national health insurance or national health care. Thus the patient is not directly responsible for the costs of treatment, and consequently the patient's choices about terminal care and/or euthanasia need not take personal financial considerations into account. Even for the patient who does have health insurance in the United States, many kinds of services are not covered, whereas the national health care or health insurance programs of many other countries provide multiple relevant services, including at-home physician care, home-nursing care, home respite care, care in a nursing home or other long-term facility, dietitian care, rehabilitation care, physical therapy, psychological counseling, and so on. The patient in the United States needs to attend to the financial aspects of dying in a way that patients in many other countries do not, and in this country both the patient's choices and the recommendations of the physician are very often shaped by financial considerations.

There are many other differences between the United States, on the one hand, and the Netherlands and Germany, with their different options for dying, on the other hand, including differences in degrees of paternalism in the medical establishment, in racism, sexism, and ageism in the general culture, and in awareness of a problematic historical past, especially Nazism. All of these cultural, institutional, social, and legal differences influence the appropriateness or inappropriateness of practices such as active euthanasia and assisted suicide. For instance, the Netherlands' tradition of close physician-patient contact, its absence of malpractice-motivated medicine, and its provision of comprehensive health insurance, together with its comparative lack of racism and ageism and its experience in resistance to Nazism, suggest that this culture is able to permit the practice of voluntary active euthanasia, performed by physicians, as well as physician-assisted suicide, without risking abuse. On the other hand, it is sometimes said that Germany still does not trust its physicians, remembering the example of Nazi experimentation, and given a comparatively authoritarian medical climate in which the contact between physician and patient is quite distanced, the population could not be comfortable with the practice of physician-performed active euthanasia or physician-assisted suicide. There, only a wholly patient-controlled response to terminal situations, as in non-physician-assisted suicide, is a reasonable and prudent practice.

But what about the United States? This is a country where (1) sustained contact with a personal physician has been decreasing, (2) the risk of malpractice action is perceived as substantial, (3) much medical care is not insured, (4) many medical decisions are financial decisions as well, (5) racism has been on the rise, and (6) the public has not experienced direct contact with Nazism or similar totalitarian movements. Thus, the United States is in many respects an untrustworthy candidate for practicing active euthanasia. Given the pressures on individuals in an often atomized society, encouraging solo suicide, assisted if at all only by nonprofessionals, might well be open to considerable abuse too.

However, there are several additional differences between the United States and both the Netherlands and Germany that may seem peculiarly relevant here. First, American culture is more confrontational than many others, including Dutch culture. While the Netherlands prides itself rightly on a long tradition of rational discussion of public issues and on toleration of others' views and practices, the United States (and to some degree also Germany) tends to develop highly partisan, moralizing oppositional groups, especially over social issues like abortion. In general, this is a disadvantage, but in the case of euthanasia it may serve to alert the public to issues and possibilities it might not otherwise consider, especially the risks of abuse. Here the role of religious groups may be particularly strong, since in discouraging or prohibiting suicide and euthanasia (as many, though by no means all, religious groups do), they may invite their members to reinspect the reasons for such choices and encourage families, physicians, and health care institutions to provide adequate, humane alternatives.

Second, though this may at first seem to be not only a peculiar but a trivial difference, it is Americans who are particularly given to self-analysis.

This tendency not only is evident in the United States' high rate of utilization of counseling services, including religious counseling, psychological counseling, and psychiatry, but also is more clearly evident in its popular culture: its diet of soap operas, situation comedies, and pop psychology books. It is here that the ordinary American absorbs models for analyzing his or her personal relationships and individual psychological characteristics. While, of course, things are changing rapidly and America's cultural tastes are widely exported, the fact remains that the ordinary American's cultural diet contains more in the way of professional and do-it-your-self amateur psychology and self-analysis than anyone else's. This long tradition of self-analysis may put Americans in a better position for certain kinds of end-of-life practices than many other cultures. Despite whatever other deficiencies U.S. society has, we live in a culture that encourages us to inspect our own motives, anticipate the impact of our actions on others, and scrutinize our own relationships with others, including our physicians. This disposition is of importance in euthanasia and assisted-suicide contexts because these are the kinds of fundamental choices about which one may have somewhat mixed motives, be subject to various interpersonal and situational pressures, and so on. If the voluntary character of choices about one's own dying is to be protected, it may be a good thing to inhabit a culture in which self-inspection of one's own mental habits and motives, not to mention those of one's family, physician, and others who might affect one's choices, is culturally encouraged. Counseling specifically addressed to end-of-life choices is not yet easily or openly available, especially if physician-assisted suicide is at issue—though some groups like Seattle-based Compassion in Dying now provide it—but I believe it will become more frequent in the future as people facing terminal illnesses characterized by long downhill, deteriorative courses consider how they want to die.

Finally, the United States population, varied as it is, is characterized by a kind of do-it-yourself ethic, an ethic that devalues reliance on others and encourages individual initiative and responsibility. (To be sure, this ethic is little in evidence in the series of court cases from *Quinlan* to *Cruzan,* but these were all cases about patients who had become or always were incapable of decisionmaking.) This ethic seems to be coupled with a sort of resistance to authority that perhaps also is basic to the American temperament, even in all its diversity. If this is really the case, Americans might be especially well-served by end-of-life practices that emphasize self-reliance and resistance to authority.

These, of course, are mere conjectures about features of American culture relevant to the practice of euthanasia or assisted suicide. These are the features that one would want to reinforce should these practices become general, in part to minimize the effects of the negative influences. But, of course, these positive features will differ from one country and culture to another, just as the negative features do. In each country, a different architecture of antecedent assumptions and cultural features develops around end-of-life issues, and in each country the practices of euthanasia and assisted or physician-assisted suicide, if they are to be free from abuse, must be adapted to the culture in which they take place.

What, then, is appropriate for the United States' own cultural situation? Physician-performed euthanasia, even if not in itself morally wrong, is morally jeopardized where legal, time-related, and especially financial pressures on both patients and physicians are severe; thus, it is morally problematic in our culture in a way that it is not in the Netherlands. Solo suicide outside the institution of medicine (as in Germany) may be problematic in a country (like the United States) that has an increasingly alienated population, offers deteriorating and uneven social services, is increasingly racist and classist, and in other ways imposes unusual pressures on individuals, despite opportunities for self-analysis. Reliance only on withholding and withdrawing treatment and allowing to die (as in the United States) can be cruel, and its comparative invisibility invites erosion under cost-containment and other pressures. These are the three principal alternatives we have considered, but none of them seems wholly suited to our actual situation for dealing with the new fact that most of us die of extended-decline, deteriorative diseases.

Perhaps, however, there is one that would best suit the United States, certainly better than its current reliance on allowing to die, and better than the Netherlands' more direct physician involvement or Germany's practices entirely outside medicine. The "arm's-length" model of physician-assisted suicide—permitting physicians to supply their terminally ill patients who request it with the means for ending their own lives (as has become legal in Oregon) still grants physicians some control over the circumstances in which this can happen—only, for example, when the prognosis is genuinely grim and the alternatives for symptom control are poor—but leaves the fundamental decision about whether to use these means to the patient alone. It is up to the patient then—the independent, confrontational, self-analyzing, do-it-yourself, authority-resisting patient—and his or her advisors, including family members, clergy, the physician, and other health care providers, to be clear about whether he or she really wants to use these means or not. Thus, the physician is involved but not directly, and it is the patient's decision, although the patient is not making it alone. Thus also it is the patient who performs the action of bringing his or her own life to a close, though where the patient is physically incapable of doing so or where the process goes awry the physician must be allowed to intercede. We live in an imperfect world, but of the alternatives for facing death—which we all eventually must—I think that the practice of permitting this somewhat distanced though still medically supported form of physician-assisted suicide is the one most nearly suited to the current state of our own flawed society. This is a model not yet central in any of the three countries examined here—the Netherlands, Germany, or (except in Oregon) the United States, or any of the other industrialized nations with related practices—but it is the one, I think, that suits us best.

NOTES

1. S. J. Olshansky and A. B. Ault, "The Fourth Stage of the Epidemiological Transition: The Age of Delayed Degenerative Diseases," *Milbank Memorial Fund Quarterly Health and Society* 64 (1986): 355–91.
2. S. Miles and C. Gomez, *Protocols for Elective Use of Life-Sustaining Treatment* (New York: Springer-Verlag, 1988).
3. C. L. Sprung, "Changing Attitudes and Practices in Forgoing Life-Sustaining Treatments," *JAMA* 262 (1990):2213.
4. T. J. Prendergast and J. M. Luce, "Increasing Incidence of Withholding and Withdrawal of Life Support from the Critically Ill," *American Journal of Respiratory and Critical Care Medicine* 155 (1):1–2 (January 1997).
5. M. B. Hamel et al. (SUPPORT Investigators), "Patient age and decisions to withhold life-sustaining treatments from seriously ill, hospitalized adults," *Annals of Internal Medicine* 130(2):116–125 (Jan. 19, 1999).
6. John M. Luce, "Withholding and Withdrawal of Life Support: Ethical, Legal, and Clinical Aspects," *New Horizons* 5(1):30–37 (Feb. 1997).
7. *New York Times,* 23 July 1990. A13.
8. Accounts of the use of Measure 16 in Oregon are to be found in A. E. Chin, K. Hedberg, G. K. Higginson, D. W. Fleming, "Legalized Physician-Assisted Suicide in Oregon—the first year's experience," *New England Journal of Medicine* 340:577–83 (1999); A. D. Sullivan, K. Hedberg, D. W. Fleming, "Legalized Physician-Assisted Suicide in Oregon—the second year," *New England Journal of Medicine* 342:598–604 (2000); and A. D. Sullivan, K. Hedberg, D. Hopkins, "Legalized Physician-Assisted Suicide in Oregon, 1998–2000," *New England Journal of Medicine* 344:605 (2001). The 70 cases of legal physician-assisted suicide that have taken place in the first three years since it became legal in Oregon—a three-year period during which a total of about 6 million deaths occurred in the U.S.—represent at most about 0.00116% of the total annual mortality. As of this writing new legal challenges have been directed against this law; the outcome remains in question.
9. For a fuller account, see my remarks "A Dozen Caveats Concerning the Discussion of Euthanasia in the Netherlands," in Margaret P. Battin, *The Least Worst Death: Essays in Bioethics on the End of Life* (New York and London: Oxford University Press, 1994): 130–44.
10. P. J. van der Maas, J. J. M. van Delden, L. Pijnenborg, "Euthanasia and Other Medical Decisions Concerning the End of Life," published in full in English as a special issue of *Health Policy,* 22, nos. 1–2 (1992) and, with C. W. N. Looman, in summary in *The Lancet* 338 (1991):669–674.
11. G. van der Wal et al., "Euthanasie en hulp bij zelfdoding door artsen in de thuissituatie," parts 1 and 2, *Nederlands Tijdschrift voor Geneesekunde* 135 (1991): 1593–98, 1600–03.
12. P. J. van der Maas, G. van der Wal, et al., "Euthanasia, Physician-Assisted Suicide, and Other Medical Practices Involving the End of Life in the Netherlands, 1990–1995," *New England Journal of Medicine* 335:22 (1996): 1699–1705.
13. The precise figures are 17.9% (1990) and 20.2% (1995) deaths involving decisions to forgo treatment; 18.8% (1990) and 19.1% (1995) deaths involving opioids in large doses; 1.7% (1990) and 2.4% (1995) euthanasia;

0.2% (1990) and 0.2 (1995) physician-assisted suicide; and 0.8% (1990) and 0.7% (1995), life-ending without patient's explicit request. Source: van der Maas et al., Table 1, p. 1701.
14. L. Pijnenborg, P. J. van der Maas, J. J. M. van Delden, C. W. N. Looman, "Life Terminating Acts without Explicit Request of Patient, *The Lancet* 341 (1993):1196–99.
15. G. van der Wal et al., "Evaluation of the Notification Procedure for Physician-Assisted Death in the Netherlands," *New England Journal of Medicine* 335:22 (1996): 1706–1711.
16. E. Borst-Eilers, "Euthanasia in the Netherlands: Brief Historical Review and Present Situation," in Robert I. Misbin, ed., *Euthanasia: The Good of the Patient, the Good of Society* (Frederick, Md.: University Publishing Group, 1992): 59.
17. van der Maas et al., "Euthanasia and other Medical Decisions Concerning the End of Life," 673.
18. van der Maas et al., "Euthanasia, Physician-Assisted Suicide, and Other Medical Practices Involving the End of Life in the Netherlands, 1990–1995," p. 1705.
19. That is, it no longer sells or supplies such drugs. A scandal in 1992–93 engulfed the original founder and president of the DGHS, Hans Hennig Atrott, who had been secretly providing some members cyanide in exchange for substantial contributions; he was convicted of violating the drug laws and tax evasion, though not charged with or convicted of assisting suicides.
20. See my "Assisted Suicide: Can We Learn from Germany?" in Margaret P. Battin, *The Least Worst Death: Essays in Bioethics on the End of Life* (New York and London: Oxford University Press, 1994): 254–70.
21. The World Health Organization provides the following data concerning suicide rates, provided here for the years indicated for the various countries discussed in this paper:
Australia (1997) 14.3 (per 100,000 population)
Austria (1999) 19.2
Belgium (1995) 21.3
Canada (1997) 12.3
Germany (1998) 14.2
Netherlands (1997) 10.1
Switzerland (1996) 20.2
USA (1998) 11.3
Courtesy of John L. McIntosh, American Association of Suicidology.
22. P. Admiraal, "Euthanasia in a General Hospital," paper read at the Eighth World Congress of the International Federation of Right-to-Die Societies, Maastricht, the Netherlands, June 8, 1990.
23. See the editorial "Doctors Must Not Kill," *Journal of the American Medical Association* 259:2139–40 (1988), signed by Willard Gaylin, M.D., Leon R. Kass, M.D., Edmund D. Pellegrino, M.D., and Mark Siegler, M.D.
24. van der Maas et al., "Euthanasia, Physician-Assisted Suicide, and Other Medical Practices," 1705.
25. Govert den Hartogh, personal communication.
26. H. ten Have, "Coma: Controversy and Consensus," *Newsletter of the European Society for Philosophy of Medicine and Health Care* (May 1990): 19–20.
27. David Orentlicher, "The Supreme Court and Terminal Sedation: Rejecting Assisted Suicide, Embracing Euthanasia," *Hastings Constitutional Law Quarterly* 24(4):947–968 (1997); see also *The New England Journal of Medicine* 337(17):1236–39 (1997).
28. Physician-assisted suicide was briefly legal in the Northern Territory of Australia in 1997 and four cases were performed before the law was overturned, but these cases did not occur during the study period.
29. Helga Kuhse, Peter Singer, Peter Baume, Malcolm Clark, and Maurice Rickard, "End-of-life Decisions in Australian Medical Practice," *The Medical Journal of Australia* 166:191–196 (1997).
30. Luc Deliens, Freddy Mortier, Johan Bilsen, Marc Cosyns, Robert Vander Stichele, Johan Vanoverloop, Koen Ingels, "End-of-life Decisions in Medical Practice in Flanders, Belgium: a nationwide survey," *The Lancet* 356:1806–11 (2000).

IS THERE A DUTY TO DIE?

John Hardwig

Many people were outraged when Richard Lamm claimed that old people had a duty to die. Modern medicine and an individualistic culture have seduced many to feel that they have a right to health care and a right to live, despite the burdens and costs to our families and society. But in fact there are circumstances when we have a duty to die. As modern medicine continues to save more of us from acute illness, it also delivers more of us over to chronic illnesses, allowing us to survive far longer than we can take care of ourselves. It may be that our technological sophistication coupled with a commitment to our loved ones generates a fairly widespread duty to die.

When Richard Lamm made the statement that old people have a duty to die, it was generally shouted down or ridiculed. The whole idea is just too preposterous to entertain. Or too threatening. In fact, a fairly common argument against legalizing physician-assisted suicide is that if it were legal, some people might somehow get the idea that they have a duty to die. These people could only be the victims of twisted moral reasoning or vicious social pressure. It goes without saying that there is no duty to die.

But for me the question is real and very important. I feel strongly that I may very well some day have a duty to die. I do not believe that I am idiosyncratic, mentally ill, or morally perverse in thinking this. I think many of us will eventually face precisely this duty. But I am first of all concerned with my own duty. I write partly to clarify my own convictions and to prepare myself. Ending my life might be a very difficult thing for me to do.

This notion of a duty to die raises all sorts of interesting theoretical and metaethical questions. I intend to try to avoid most of them because I hope my argument will be persuasive to those holding a wide variety of ethical views. Also, although the claim that there is a duty to die would ultimately require theoretical underpinning, the discussion needs to begin on the normative level. As is appropriate to my attempt to steer clear of theoretical commitments, I will use "duty" "obligation," and "responsibility" interchangeably, in a pretheoretical or preanalytic sense.[1]

CIRCUMSTANCES AND A DUTY TO DIE

Do many of us really believe that no one ever has a duty to die? I suspect not. I think most of us probably believe that there is such a duty, but it is very uncommon. Consider Captain Oates, a member of Admiral Scott's expedition to the South Pole. Oates became too ill to continue. If the rest of the team stayed with him, they would all perish. After this had become clear, Oates left his tent one night, walked out into a raging blizzard, and was never seen again.[2] That may have been a heroic thing to do, but we might be able to agree that it was also no more than his duty. It would have been wrong for him to urge—or even to allow—the rest to stay and care for him.

This is a very unusual circumstance—a "lifeboat case"—and lifeboat cases make for bad ethics. But I expect that most of us would also agree that there have been cultures in which what we would call a duty to die has been fairly common. These are relatively poor, technologically simple, and especially nomadic cultures. In such societies, everyone knows that if you manage to live long enough, you will eventually become old and debilitated. Then you will need to take steps to end your life. The old people in these societies regularly did precisely that. Their cultures prepared and supported them in doing so.

Those cultures could be dismissed as irrelevant to contemporary bioethics; their circumstances are so different from ours. But if that is our response, it is instructive. It suggests that we assume a duty to die is irrelevant to us because our wealth and technological sophistication have purchased exemption

Hastings Center Report, Vol. 27, No. 2, 1997, 34–42.

for us . . . except under very unusual circumstances like Captain Oates's.

But have wealth and technology really exempted us? Or are they, on the contrary, about to make a duty to die common again? We like to think of modern medicine as all triumph with no dark side. Our medicine saves many lives and enables most of us to live longer. That is wonderful, indeed. We are all glad to have access to this medicine. But our medicine also delivers most of us over to chronic illnesses and it enables many of us to survive longer than we can take care of ourselves, longer than we know what to do with ourselves, longer than we even are ourselves.

The costs—and these are not merely monetary—of prolonging our lives when we are no longer able to care for ourselves are often staggering. If further medical advances wipe out many of today's "killer diseases"—cancers, heart attacks, strokes,—ALS, AIDS, and the rest—then one day most of us will survive long enough to become demented or debilitated. These developments could generate a fairly widespread duty to die. A fairly common duty to die might turn out to be only the dark side of our life-prolonging medicine and the uses we choose to make of it.

Let me be clear. I certainly believe that there is a duty to refuse life-prolonging medical treatment and also a duty to complete advance directives refusing life-prolonging treatment. But a duty to die can go well beyond that. There can be a duty to die before one's illnesses would cause death, even if treated only with palliative measures. In fact, there may be a fairly common responsibility to end one's life in the absence of any terminal illness at all. Finally, there can be a duty to die when one would prefer to live. Granted, many of the conditions that can generate a duty to die also seriously undermine the quality of life. Some prefer not to live under such conditions. But even those who want to live can face a duty to die. These will clearly be the most controversial and troubling cases; I will, accordingly, focus my reflections on them.

THE INDIVIDUALISTIC FANTASY

Because a duty to die seems such a real possibility to me, I wonder why contemporary bioethics has dismissed it without serious consideration. I believe that most bioethics still shares in one of our deeply embedded American dreams: the individualistic fantasy. This fantasy leads us to imagine that lives are separate and unconnected, or that they could be so if we chose. If lives were unconnected, things that happened in my life would not or need not affect others. And if others were not (much) affected by my life, I would have no duty to consider the impact of my decisions on others. I would then be free morally to live my life however I please, choosing whatever life and death I prefer for myself. The way I live would be nobody's business but my own. I certainly would have no duty to die if I preferred to live.

Within a health care context, the individualistic fantasy leads us to assume that the patient is the only one affected by decisions about her medical treatment. If only the patient were affected, the relevant questions when making treatment decisions would be precisely those we ask: What will benefit the patient? Who can best decide that? The pivotal issue would always be simply whether the patient wants to live like this and whether she would consider herself better off dead.[3] "Whose life is it, anyway?" we ask rhetorically.

But this is morally obtuse. We are not a race of hermits. Illness and death do not come only to those who are all alone. Nor is it much better to think in terms of the bald dichotomy between "the interests of the patient" and "the interests of society" (or a third-party payer), as if we were isolated individuals connected only to "society" in the abstract or to the other, faceless members of our health maintenance organization.

Most of us are affiliated with particular others and most deeply, with family and loved ones. Families and loved ones are bound together by ties of care and affection, by legal relations and obligations, by inhabiting shared spaces and living units, by interlocking finances and economic prospects, by common projects and also commitments to support the different life projects of other family members, by shared histories, by ties of loyalty. This life together of family and loved ones is what defines and sustains us; it is what gives meaning to most of our lives. We would not have it any other way. We would not want to be all alone, especially when we are seriously ill, as we age, and when we are dying.

But the fact of deeply interwoven lives debars us from making exclusively self-regarding decisions, as the decisions of one member of a family may dramatically affect the lives of all the rest. The impact of my decisions upon my family and loved ones is the source of many of my strongest obligations and also the most plausible and likeliest basis of a duty to die. "Society," after all, is only very marginally affected by how I live, or by whether I live or die.

A BURDEN TO MY LOVED ONES

Many older people report that their one remaining goal in life is not to be a burden to their loved ones. Young people feel this, too: when I ask my undergraduate students to think about whether their death could come too late, one of their very first responses always is, "Yes, when I become a burden to my family or loved ones." Tragically, there are situations in which my loved ones would be much better off—all things considered, the loss of a loved one notwithstanding—if I were dead.

The lives of our loved ones can be seriously compromised by caring for us. The burdens of providing care or even just supervision twenty-four hours a day, seven days a week are often overwhelming.[4] When this kind of caregiving goes on for years, it leaves the caregiver exhausted, with no time for herself or life of her own. Ultimately, even her health is often destroyed. But it can also be emotionally devastating simply to live with a spouse who is increasingly distant, uncommunicative, unresponsive, foreign, and unreachable. Other family members' needs often go unmet as the caring capacity of the family is exceeded. Social life and friendships evaporate, as there is no opportunity to go out to see friends and the home is no longer a place suitable for having friends in.

We must also acknowledge that the lives of our loved ones can be devastated just by having to pay for health care for us. One part of the recent SUPPORT study documented the financial aspects of caring for a dying member of a family. Only those who had illnesses severe enough to give them less than a 50 percent chance to live six more months were included in this study. When these patients survived their initial hospitalization and were discharged about one-third required considerable caregiving from their families; in 20 percent of cases a family member had to quit work or make some other major lifestyle change; almost one-third of these families lost all of their savings; and just under 30 percent lost a major source of income.[5]

If talking about money sounds venal or trivial, remember that much more than money is normally at stake here. When someone has to quit work, she may well lose her career. Savings decimated late in life cannot be recouped in the few remaining years of employability, so the loss compromises the quality of the rest of the caregiver's life. For a young person, the chance to go to college may be lost to the attempt to pay debts due to an illness in the family, and this decisively shapes an entire life.

A serious illness in a family is a misfortune. It is usually nobody's fault; no one is responsible for it. But we face choices about how we will respond to this misfortune. That's where the responsibility comes in and fault can arise. Those of us with families and loved ones always have a duty not to make selfish or self-centered decisions about our lives. We have a responsibility to try to protect the lives of loved ones from serious threats or greatly impoverished quality, certainly an obligation not to make choices that will jeopardize or seriously compromise their futures. Often, it would be wrong to do just what we want or just what is best for ourselves; we should choose in light of what is best for all concerned. That is our duty in sickness as well as in health. It is out of these responsibilities that a duty to die can develop.

I am not advocating a crass, quasi-economic conception of burdens and benefits, nor a shallow, hedonistic view of life. Given a suitably rich understanding of benefits, family members sometimes do benefit from suffering through the long illness of a loved one. Caring for the sick or aged can foster growth, even as it makes daily life immeasurably harder and the prospects for the future much bleaker. Chronic illness or a drawn-out death can also pull a family together, making the care for each other stronger and more evident. If my loved ones are truly benefiting from coping with my illness or debility, I have no duty to die based on burdens to them.

But it would be irresponsible to blithely assume that this always happens, that it will happen in my family, or that it will be the fault of my family if they cannot manage to turn my illness into a positive experience. Perhaps the opposite is more common: a hospital chaplain once told me that he could not think of a single case in which a family was strengthened or brought together by what happened at the hospital.

Our families and loved ones also have obligations, of course—they have the responsibility to stand by us and to support us through debilitating illness and death. They must be prepared to make significant sacrifices to respond to an illness in the family. I am far from denying that. Most of us are aware of this responsibility and most families meet it rather well. In fact, families deliver more than 80 percent of the long-term care in this country, almost always at great personal cost. Most of us who are a part of a family can expect to be sustained in our time of need by family members and those who love us.

But most discussions of an illness in the family sound as if responsibility were a one-way street. It is not, of course. When we become seriously ill or debilitated, we too may have to make sacrifices. To think that my loved ones must bear whatever burdens my illness, debility, or dying process might impose upon them is to reduce them to means to my well-being. And that would be immoral. Family solidarity, altruism, bearing the burden of a loved one's misfortune, and loyalty are all important virtues of families, as well. But they are all also two-way streets.

OBJECTIONS TO A DUTY TO DIE

To my mind, the most serious objections to the idea of a duty to die lie in the effects on my loved ones of ending my life. But to most others, the important objections have little or nothing to do with family and loved ones. Perhaps the most common objections are: (1) there is a higher duty that always takes precedence over a duty to die; (2) a duty to end one's own life would be incompatible with a recognition of human dignity or the intrinsic value of a person; and (3) seriously ill, debilitated, or dying people are already bearing the harshest burdens and so it would be wrong to ask them to bear the additional burden of ending their own lives.

These are all important objections; all deserve a thorough discussion. Here I will only be able to suggest some moral counterweights—ideas that might provide the basis for an argument that these objections do not always preclude a duty to die.

An example of the first line of argument would be the claim that a duty to God, the giver of life, forbids that anyone take her own life. It could be argued that this duty always supersedes whatever obligations we might have to our families. But what convinces us that we always have such a religious duty in the first place? And what guarantees that it always supersedes our obligations to try to protect our loved ones?

Certainly, the view that death is the ultimate evil cannot be squared with Christian theology. It does not reflect the actions of Jesus or those of his early followers. Nor is it clear that the belief that life is sacred requires that we never take it. There are other theological possibilities.[6] In any case, most of us—bioethicists, physicians, and patients alike—do not subscribe to the view that we have an obligation to preserve human life as long as possible. But if not, surely we ought to agree that I may legitimately end my life for other-regarding reasons, not just for self-regarding reasons.

Secondly, religious considerations aside, the claim could be made that an obligation to end one's own life would be incompatible with human dignity or would embody a failure to recognize the intrinsic value of a person. But I do not see that in thinking I had a duty to die I would necessarily be failing to respect myself or to appreciate my dignity or worth. Nor would I necessarily be failing to respect you in thinking that you had a similar duty. There is surely also a sense in which we fail to respect ourselves if in the face of illness or death, we stoop to choosing just what is best for ourselves. Indeed, Kant held that the very core of human dignity is the ability to act on a self-imposed moral law, regardless of whether it is in our interest to do so.[7] We shall return to the notion of human dignity.

A third objection appeals to the relative weight of burdens and thus, ultimately, to considerations of fairness or justice. The burdens that an illness creates for the family could not possibly be great enough to justify an obligation to end one's life—the sacrifice of life itself would be a far greater burden than any involved in caring for a chronically ill family member.

But is this true? Consider the following case:

> An 87-year-old woman was dying of congestive heart failure. Her APACHE score predicted that she had less than a 50 percent chance to live for another six months.

> She was lucid, assertive, and terrified of death. She very much wanted to live and kept opting for rehospitalization and the most aggressive life-prolonging treatment possible. That treatment successfully prolonged her life (though with increasing debility) for nearly two years. Her 55-year-old daughter was her only remaining family, her caregiver, and the main source of her financial support. The daughter duly cared for her mother. But before her mother died, her illness had cost the daughter all of her savings, her home, her job, and her career.

This is by no means an uncommon sort of case. Thousands of similar cases occur each year. Now, ask yourself which is the greater burden:

(a) To lose a 50 percent chance of six more months of life at age 87?

(b) To lose all your savings, your home, and your career at age 55?

Which burden would you prefer to bear? Do we really believe the former is the greater burden? Would even the dying mother say that (a) is the greater burden? Or has she been encouraged to believe that the burdens of (b) are somehow morally irrelevant to her choices?

I think most of us would quickly agree that (b) is a greater burden. That is the evil we would more hope to avoid in our lives. If we are tempted to say that the mother's disease and impending death are the greater evil, I believe it is because we are taking a "slice of time" perspective rather than a "lifetime perspective."[8] But surely the lifetime perspective is the appropriate perspective when weighing burdens. If (b) is the greater burden, then we must admit that we have been promulgating an ethics that advocates imposing greater burdens on some people in order to provide smaller benefits for others just because they are ill and thus gain our professional attention and advocacy.

A whole range of cases like this one could easily be generated. In some, the answer about which burden is greater will not be clear. But in many it is. Death—or ending your own life—is simply not the greatest evil or the greatest burden.

This point does not depend on a utilitarian calculus. Even if death were the greatest burden (thus disposing of any simple utilitarian argument), serious questions would remain about the moral justifiability of choosing to impose crushing burdens on loved ones in order to avoid having to bear this burden oneself. The fact that I suffer greater burdens than others in my family does not license me simply to choose what I want for myself, nor does it necessarily release me from a responsibility to try to protect the quality of their lives.

I can readily imagine that, through cowardice, rationalization, or failure of resolve, I will fail in this obligation to protect my loved ones. If so, I think I would need to be excused or forgiven for what I did. But I cannot imagine it would be morally permissible for me to ruin the rest of my partner's life to sustain mine or to cut off my sons' careers, impoverish them, or compromise the quality of their children's lives simply because I wish to live a little longer. This is what leads me to believe in a duty to die.

WHO HAS A DUTY TO DIE?

Suppose, then, that there can be a duty to die. Who has a duty to die? And when? To my mind, these are the right questions, the questions we should be asking. Many of us may one day badly need answers to just these questions.

But I cannot supply answers here, for two reasons. In the first place, answers will have to be very particular and contextual. Our concrete duties are often situated, defined in part by the myriad details of our circumstances, histories, and relationships. Though there may be principles that apply to a wide range of cases and some cases that yield pretty straightforward answers, there will also be many situations in which it is very difficult to discern whether one has a duty to die. If nothing else, it will often be very difficult to predict how one's family will bear up under the weight of the burdens that a protracted illness would impose on them. Momentous decisions will often have to be made under conditions of great uncertainty.

Second and perhaps even more importantly, I believe that those of us with family and loved ones should not define our duties unilaterally, especially not a decision about a duty to die. It would be isolating and distancing for me to decide without consulting them what is too much of a burden for my loved ones to bear. That way of deciding about my moral duties is not only atomistic, it also treats my family and loved ones paternalistically. They must be allowed to speak for themselves about the burdens my life imposes on them and how they feel about bearing those burdens.

Some may object that it would be wrong to put a loved one in a position of having to say, in effect, "You should end your life because caring for you is too hard on me and the rest of the family." Not only will it be almost impossible to say something like that to someone you love, it will carry with it a heavy load of guilt. On this view, you should decide by yourself whether you have a duty to die and approach your loved ones only after you have made up your mind to say good-bye to them. Your family could then try to change your mind, but the tremendous weight of moral decision would be lifted from their shoulders.

Perhaps so. But I believe in family decisions. Important decisions for those whose lives are interwoven should be made together, in a family discussion. Granted, a conversation about whether I have a duty to die would be a tremendously difficult conversation. The temptations to be dishonest could be enormous. Nevertheless, if I am contemplating a duty to die, my family and I should, if possible, have just such an agonizing discussion. It will act as a check on the information, perceptions, and reasoning of all of us. But even more importantly, it affirms our connectedness at a critical juncture in our lives and our life together. Honest talk about difficult matters almost always strengthens relationships.

However, many families seem unable to talk about death at all, much less a duty to die. Certainly most families could not have this discussion all at once, in one sitting. It might well take a number of discussions to be able to approach this topic. But even if talking about death is impossible, there are always behavioral clues—about your caregiver's tiredness, physical condition, health, prevailing mood, anxiety, financial concerns, outlook, overall well-being, and so on. And families unable to talk about death can often talk about how the caregiver is feeling, about finances, about tensions within the family resulting from the illness, about concerns for the future. Deciding whether you have a duty to die based on these behavioral clues and conversation about them honors your relationships better than deciding on your own about how burdensome you and your care must be.

I cannot say when someone has a duty to die. Still, I can suggest a few features of one's illness, history, and circumstances that make it more likely that one has a duty to die. I present them here without much elaboration or explanation.

(1) A duty to die is more likely when continuing to live will impose significant burdens—emotional burdens, extensive caregiving, destruction of life plans, and, yes, financial hardship—on your family and loved ones. This is the fundamental insight underlying a duty to die.
(2) A duty to die becomes greater as you grow older. As we age, we will be giving up less by giving up our lives, if only because we will sacrifice fewer remaining years of life and a smaller portion of our life plans. After all, it's not as if we would be immortal and live forever if we could just manage to avoid a duty to die. To have reached the age of, say, seventy-five or eighty years without being ready to die is itself a moral failing, the sign of a life out of touch with life's basic realities.[9]
(3) A duty to die is more likely when you have already lived a full and rich life. You have already had a full share of the good things life offers.
(4) There is greater duty to die if your loved ones' lives have already been difficult or impoverished, if they have had only a small share of the good things that life has to offer (especially if through no fault of their own).
(5) A duty to die is more likely when your loved ones have already made great contributions—perhaps even sacrifices—to make your life a good one. Especially if you have not made similar sacrifices for their well-being or for the well-being of other members of your family.
(6) To the extent that you can make a good adjustment to your illness or handicapping condition, there is less likely to be a duty to die. A good adjustment means that smaller sacrifices will be required of loved ones and there is more compensating interaction for them. Still, we must also recognize that some diseases—Alzheimer [*sic*] or Huntington [*sic*] chorea—will eventually take their toll on

your loved ones no matter how courageously, resolutely, even cheerfully you manage to face that illness.

(7) There is less likely to be a duty to die if you can still make significant contributions to the lives of others, especially your family. The burdens to family members are not only or even primarily financial, neither are the contributions to them. However, the old and those who have terminal illnesses must also bear in mind that the loss their family members will feel when they die cannot be avoided, only postponed.

(8) A duty to die is more likely when the part of you that is loved will soon be gone or seriously compromised. Or when you soon will no longer be capable of giving love. Part of the horror of dementing disease is that it destroys the capacity to nurture and sustain relationships, taking away a person's agency and the emotions that bind her to others.

(9) There is a greater duty to die to the extent that you have lived a relatively lavish lifestyle instead of saving for illness or old age. Like most upper middle-class Americans, I could easily have saved more. It is a greater wrong to come to your family for assistance if your need is the result of having chosen leisure or a spendthrift lifestyle. I may eventually have to face the moral consequences of decisions I am now making.

These, then, are some of the considerations that give shape and definition to the duty to die. If we can agree that these considerations are all relevant, we can see that the correct course of action will often be difficult to discern. A decision about when I should end my life will sometimes prove to be every bit as difficult as the decision about whether I want treatment for myself.

CAN THE INCOMPETENT HAVE A DUTY TO DIE?

Severe mental deterioration springs readily to mind as one of the situations in which I believe I could have a duty to die. But can incompetent people have duties at all? We can have moral duties we do not recognize or acknowledge, including duties that we never recognized. But can we have duties we are unable to recognize? Duties when we are unable to understand the concept of morality at all? If so, do others have a moral obligation to help us carry out this duty? These are extremely difficult theoretical questions. The reach of moral agency is severely strained by mental incompetence.

I am tempted to simply bypass the entire question by saying that I am talking only about competent persons. But the idea of a duty to die clearly raises the specter of one person claiming that another—who cannot speak for herself—has such a duty. So I need to say that I can make no sense of the claim that someone has a duty to die if the person has never been able to understand moral obligation at all. To my mind, only those who were formerly capable of making moral decisions could have such a duty.

But the case of formerly competent persons is almost as troubling. Perhaps we should simply stipulate that no incompetent person can have a duty to die, not even if she affirmed belief in such a duty in an advance directive. If we take the view that formerly competent people may have such a duty, we should surely exercise extreme caution when claiming a formerly competent person would have acknowledged a duty to die or that any formerly competent person has an unacknowledged duty to die. Moral dangers loom regardless of which way we decide to resolve such issues.

But for me personally, very urgent practical matters turn on their resolution. If a formerly competent person can no longer have a duty to die (or if other people are not likely to help her carry out this duty), I believe that my obligation may be to die while I am still competent, before I become unable to make and carry out that decision for myself. Surely it would be irresponsible to evade my moral duties by temporizing until I escape into incompetence. And so I must die sooner than I otherwise would have to. On the other hand, if I could count on others to end my life after I become incompetent, I might be able to fulfill my responsibilities while also living out all my competent or semicompetent days. Given our society's reluctance to permit physicians, let alone family members, to perform aid-in-dying, I believe I may well have a duty to end my life when I can see mental incapacity on the horizon.

There is also the very real problem of sudden incompetence—due to a serious stroke or automobile accident, for example. For me, that is the real nightmare. If I suddenly become incompetent, I will fall into the hands of a medical-legal system that will conscientiously disregard my moral beliefs and do what is best for me, regardless of the consequences for my loved ones. And that is not at all what I would have wanted!

SOCIAL POLICIES AND A DUTY TO DIE

The claim that there is a duty to die will seem to some a misplaced response to social negligence. If our society were providing for the debilitated, the chronically ill, and the elderly as it should be, there would be only very rare cases of a duty to die. On this view, I am asking the sick and debilitated to step in and accept responsibility because society is derelict in its responsibility to provide for the incapacitated.

This much is surely true: there are a number of social policies we could pursue that would dramatically reduce the incidence of such a duty. Most obviously, we could decide to pay for facilities that provided excellent long-term care (not just health care!) for all chronically ill, debilitated, mentally ill, or demented people in this country. We probably could still afford to do this. If we did, sick, debilitated, and dying people might still be morally required to make sacrifices for their families. I might, for example, have a duty to forgo personal care by a family member who knows me and really does care for me. But these sacrifices would only rarely include the sacrifice of life itself. The duty to die would then be virtually eliminated.

I cannot claim to know whether in some abstract sense a society like ours should provide care for all who are chronically ill or debilitated. But the fact is that we Americans seem to be unwilling to pay for this kind of long-term care, except for ourselves and our own. In fact, we are moving in precisely the opposite direction—we are trying to shift the burdens of caring for the seriously and chronically ill onto families in order to save costs for our health care system. As we shift the burdens of care onto families, we also dramatically increase the number of Americans who will have a duty to die.

I must not, then, live my life and make my plans on the assumption that social institutions will protect my family from my infirmity and debility. To do so would be irresponsible. More likely, it will be up to me to protect my loved ones.

A DUTY TO DIE AND THE MEANING OF LIFE

A duty to die seems very harsh, and often it would be. It is one of the tragedies of our lives that someone who wants very much to live can nevertheless have a duty to die. It is both tragic and ironic that it is precisely the very real good of family and loved ones that gives rise to this duty. Indeed, the genuine love, closeness, and supportiveness of family members is a major source of this duty: we could not be such a burden if they did not care for us. Finally, there is deep irony in the fact that the very successes of our life-prolonging medicine help to create a widespread duty to die. We do not live in such a happy world that we can avoid such tragedies and ironies. We ought not to close our eyes to this reality or pretend that it just doesn't exist. We ought not to minimize the tragedy in any way.

And yet, a duty to die will not always be as harsh as we might assume. If I love my family, I will want to protect them and their lives. I will want not to make choices that compromise their futures. Indeed, I can easily imagine that I might want to avoid compromising their lives more than I would want anything else. I must also admit that I am not necessarily giving up so much in giving up my life: the conditions that give rise to a duty to die would usually already have compromised the quality of the life I am required to end. In any case, I personally must confess that at age fifty-six, I have already lived a very good life, albeit not yet nearly as long a life as I would like to have.

We fear death too much. Our fear of death has led to a massive assault on it. We still crave after virtually any life-prolonging technology that we might conceivably be able to produce. We still too often feel morally impelled to prolong life—virtually any form of life—as long as possible. As if the best death is the one that can be put off longest.

We do not even ask about meaning in death, so busy are we with trying to postpone it. But we will not conquer death by one day developing a technology so magnificent that no one will have to die. Nor can we conquer death by postponing it ever longer. We can conquer death only by finding meaning in it.

Although the existence of a duty to die does not hinge on this, recognizing such a duty would go some way toward recovering meaning in death. Paradoxically, it would restore dignity to those who are seriously ill or dying. It would also reaffirm the connections required to give life (and death) meaning. I close now with a few words about both of these points.

First, recognizing a duty to die affirms my agency and also my moral agency. I can still do things that make an important difference in the lives of my loved ones. Moreover, the fact that I still have responsibilities keeps me within the community of moral agents. My illness or debility has not reduced me to a mere moral patient (to use the language of the philosophers). Though it may not be the whole story, surely Kant was onto something important when he claimed that human dignity rests on the capacity for moral agency within a community of those who respect the demands of morality.

By contrast, surely there is something deeply insulting in a medicine and an ethic that would ask only what I want (or would have wanted) when I become ill. To treat me as if I had no moral responsibilities when I am ill or debilitated implies that my condition has rendered me morally incompetent. Only small children, the demented or insane, and those totally lacking in the capacity to act are free from moral duties. There is dignity, then, and a kind of meaning in moral agency, even as it forces extremely difficult decisions upon us.

Second, recovering meaning in death requires an affirmation of connections. If I end my life to spare the futures of my loved ones, I testify in my death that I am connected to them. It is because I love and care for precisely these people (and I know they care for me) that I wish not to be such a burden to them. By contrast, a life in which I am free to choose whatever I want for myself is a life unconnected to others. A bioethics that would treat me as if I had no serious moral responsibilities does what it can to marginalize, weaken, or even destroy my connections with others.

But life without connection is meaningless. The individualistic fantasy, though occasionally liberating, is deeply destructive. When life is good and vitality seems unending, life itself and life lived for yourself may seem quite sufficient. But if not life, certainly death without connection is meaningless. If you are only for yourself, all you have to care about as your life draws to a close is yourself and your life. Everything you care about will then perish in your death. And that—the end of everything you care about—is precisely the total collapse of meaning. We can, then, find meaning in death only through a sense of connection with something that will survive our death.

This need not be connections with other people. Some people are deeply tied to land (for example, the family farm), to nature, or to a transcendent reality. But for most of us, the connections that sustain us are to other people. In the full bloom of life, we are connected to others in many ways—through work, profession, neighborhood, country, shared faith and worship, common leisure pursuits, friendship. Even the guru meditating in isolation on his mountain top is connected to a long tradition of people united by the same religious quest.

But as we age or when we become chronically ill, connections with other people usually become much more restricted. Often, only ties with family and close friends remain and remain important to us. Moreover, for many of us, other connections just don't go deep enough. As Paul Tsongas has reminded us, "When it comes time to die, no one says, 'I wish I had spent more time at the office.'"

If I am correct, death is so difficult for us partly because our sense of community is so weak. Death seems to wipe out everything when we can't fit it into the lives of those who live on. A death motivated by the desire to spare the futures of my loved ones might well be a better death for me than the one I would get as a result of opting to continue my life as long as there is any pleasure in it for me. Pleasure is nice, but it is meaning that matters.

. . .

I don't know about others, but these reflections have helped me. I am now more at peace about facing a duty to die. Ending my life if my duty required might still be difficult. But for me, a far greater horror would be dying all alone or stealing the futures of my loved ones in order to buy a little more time for myself. I hope that if the time comes when I have a duty to die, I will recognize it, encourage my loved ones to recognize it too, and carry it out bravely.

ACKNOWLEDGMENTS

I wish to thank Mary English, Hilde Nelson, Jim Bennett, Tom Townsend, the members of the Philosophy Department at East Tennessee State University, and anonymous reviewers of the *Report* for many helpful comments on earlier versions of this paper. In this paper, I draw on material in John Hardwig, "Dying at the Right Time; Reflections on (Un)Assisted Suicide" in *Practical Ethics,* ed. H. LaFollette (London: Blackwell, 1996), with permission.

NOTES

1. Given the importance of relationships in my thinking, "responsibility"—rooted as it is in "respond"—would perhaps be the most appropriate word. Nevertheless, I often use "duty" despite its legalistic overtones, because Lamm's famous statement has given the expression "duty to die" a certain familiarity. But I intend no implication that there is a law that grounds this duty, nor that someone has a right corresponding to it.
2. For a discussion of the Oates case, see Tom L. Beauchamp, "What Is Suicide?" in *Ethical Issues in Death and Dying,* ed. Tom L. Beauchamp and Seymour Perlin (Englewood Cliffs, N.J.: Prentice-Hall, 1978).
3. Most bioethicists advocate a "patient-centered ethics"—an ethics which claims only the patient's interests should be considered in making medical treatment decisions. Most health care professionals have been trained to accept this ethic and to see themselves as patient advocates. For arguments that a patient-centered ethics should be replaced by a family-centered ethics see John Hardwig, "What About the Family?" *Hastings Center Report* 20, no. 2 (1990): 5–10; Hilde L. Nelson and James L. Nelson, *The Patient in the Family* (New York: Routledge, 1995).
4. A good account of the burdens of caregiving can be found in Elaine Brody, *Women in the Middle: Their Parent-Care Years* (New York: Springer Publishing Co., 1990). Perhaps the best article-length account of these burdens is Daniel Callahan, "Families as Caregivers; the Limits of Morality" in *Aging and Ethics: Philosophical Problems in Gerontology,* ed. Nancy Jecker (Totowa N.J.: Humana Press, 1991).
5. Kenneth E. Covinsky et al., "The Impact of Serious Illness on Patients' Families," *JAMA* 272 (1994): 1839–44.
6. Larry Churchill, for example, believes that Christian ethics takes us far beyond my present position: "Christian doctrines of stewardship prohibit the extension of one's own life at a great cost to the neighbor . . . And such a gesture should not appear to us a sacrifice, but as the ordinary virtue entailed by a just, social conscience." Larry Churchill, *Rationing Health Care in America* (South Bend, Ind.: Notre Dame University Press, 1988), p. 112.
7. Kant, as is well known, was opposed to suicide. But he was arguing against taking your life out of self-interested motives. It is not clear that Kant would or we should consider taking your life out of a sense of duty to be wrong. See Hilde L. Nelson, "Death with Kantian Dignity," *Journal of Clinical Ethics* 7 (1996): 215–21.
8. Obviously, I owe this distinction to Norman Daniels. Norman Daniels, *Am I My Parents' Keeper? An Essay on Justice Between the Young and the Old* (New York: Oxford University Press, 1988). Just as obviously, Daniels is not committed to my use of it here.
9. Daniel Callahan, *The Troubled Dream of Life* (New York: Simon & Schuster, 1993).

"FOR NOW HAVE I MY DEATH"[1]: THE "DUTY TO DIE" VERSUS THE DUTY TO HELP THE ILL STAY ALIVE

Felicia Ackerman

For the last three days he screamed incessantly. It was unendurable. I cannot understand how I bore it; you could hear him three rooms off. Oh, what I have suffered![2]

I

Suppose you are a sixty-year-old who has worked hard and made sacrifices for your family. Now you are ill and the care necessary to keep you alive is taking up a lot of time and money, including almost all your spouse's free time and much of the money you previously set aside for your child's college education. You and your family still love one another, but you all have strong self-interested desires as well. You want to stay alive as long as possible. Your spouse, a dedicated amateur athlete who used to spend much time playing tennis, is tired of being your caregiver. Your child wants to go to college. Who has a duty to do what? Here are four possible answers.

1. You have a duty to die (possibly including a duty to commit suicide) in order to avoid burdening your family.
2. Your spouse has a duty to accept the loss of leisure time and take care of you (that is why "in sickness and in health" is in the marriage vows) and your child has a duty to accept the loss of your financial contribution to his education, in order to avoid burdening you with the premature loss of your life.
3. Either course of action can be justified; it is not a matter of duty.
4. It depends.

John Hardwig has recently argued in favor of (1), at least in some circumstances. This paper will criticize his views and argue for alternatives.

One way Hardwig seeks to support his view is by pointing out that

> [m]any older people report that their one remaining goal in life is not to be a burden to their loved ones. Young people feel this, too: when I ask my undergraduate students to think about whether their death could come too late, one of their very first responses always is, "Yes, when I become a burden to my family or loved ones."[3]

Hardwig thinks this reflects "moral wisdom." He does not consider the possibility that it reflects our society's bias against and systematic devaluation of the old and ill, a devaluation some old people accept uncritically, just as many women used to accept the idea that women should be subordinate to men. After all, it would hardly be surprising to discover that fifty years ago, most married women reported that they did not want careers that would burden their families. But people (or at least liberals) nowadays would have second thoughts about calling this moral wisdom, let alone using it to support an argument that married women had a duty to avoid careers that would burden their families. We now recognize two factors. First, fifty years ago there was so much social pressure on married women, if they worked outside the home at all, not to let their work inconvenience their families that any woman who dissented from this outlook risked being instantly condemned as selfish (which is not to deny that some women genuinely felt this way). Second, there was bias involved in seeing women's careers, but not men's, as a burden to their families. Many people recognize these things nowadays. But how many recognize that the same factors apply to Hardwig's uncritical report of present-day expressions of attitudes toward old age and illness? To illustrate the first factor, imagine the social reaction

Reprinted with permission of the author and publisher from *Midwest Studies in Philosophy*, XXIV (2000).

Editor's note: Some footnotes have been deleted. Students who want to follow up on sources should consult the original article.

to a sick old person who said, "I'm sorry if it burdens my family, but my life comes first." The fact that sick old people do make "burdensome" choices often enough to give the question of a duty to die practical as well as theoretical interest suggests that many of the old and ill are less self-sacrificing than the sentiments they pay lip service to may suggest. To illustrate the second factor, consider the (deliberate) oddness of my formulation of (2), above. Sick old people are routinely called burdens to their families, but college-bound teenagers are not. It is surprising that someone who believes "life without connection is meaningless" would think it shows moral wisdom for people to talk as though they did not realize that accepting the burdens of taking care of one another is part of what a family is all about. If Hardwig really holds, as much of his writing claims, the more moderate position that there are *limits* to the burdens families can be expected to assume (although I will argue that his limits are unacceptably stringent), then why does he think it shows moral wisdom to speak as though any burden, no matter how small, would be unacceptable?

Similar concerns apply to Hardwig's use of such loaded words as 'individualistic' and 'selfish.' I doubt that anyone actually believes what he condemns as "the individualistic fantasy . . . that the patient is the only one affected by decisions about her medical treatment." And few would find fault, except on grounds of triteness, with his claim that "[t]hose of us with families and loved ones always have a duty not to make selfish . . . decisions about our lives." We normally use the pejorative term 'selfish' only for things we want to condemn. But in order to see what sorts of decisions Hardwig condemns as selfish or unduly individualistic, we must look at the family burdens he thinks can give rise to a duty to die. He says:

> The lives of our loved ones can be seriously compromised by caring for us. The burdens of providing care or even just supervision twenty-four hours a day, seven days a week are often overwhelming. When this kind of caregiving goes on for years, it leaves the caregiver exhausted, with no time for herself or life of her own. Ultimately, even her health is often destroyed. But it can also be emotionally devastating simply to live with a spouse who is increasingly distant, uncommunicative, unresponsive, foreign, and unreachable. Other family members' needs often go unmet as the caring capacity of the family is exceeded. Social life and friendships evaporate, as there is no opportunity to go out to see friends and the home is no longer a place suitable for having friends in.
>
> We must also acknowledge that the lives of our loved ones can be devastated just by having to pay for health care for us. One part of [a] recent . . . study documented the financial aspects of caring for a dying member of a family. Only those who had illnesses severe enough to give them less than a 50 percent chance to live six more months were included in this study. When these patients survived their initial hospitalization and were discharged about one-third required considerable caregiving from their families; in 20 percent of cases a family member had to quit work or make some other major lifestyle change; almost one-third of these families lost all of their savings; and just under 30 percent lost a major source of income.
>
> If talking about money sounds venal or trivial, remember that much more than money is normally at stake here. When someone has to quit work, she may well lose her career. Savings decimated late in life cannot be recouped in the few remaining years of employability, so the loss compromises the quality of the rest of the caregiver's life. For a young person, the chance to go to college may be lost to the attempt to pay debts due to an illness in the family, and this decisively shapes an entire life.

These remarks cry out for critical examination. For one thing, Hardwig's conception of what can constitute an unacceptable family burden seems astonishingly weak. Several questions immediately arise. Should being "distant, uncommunicative, unresponsive, foreign, and unreachable" really be a capital offense anywhere, let alone in a "loving" family? Does a loving family really welcome a beloved member's suicide in order to keep a young person from having to work and/or borrow his way through college? Does the view that you have a duty to spend your hard-earned money to put your able-bodied child through college rather than to prolong your own life reflect a devaluation of the old and the ill that will someday be as offensive to liberals as 1950s attitudes toward women are today?

Hardwig's bias is also reflected in his failure to extend his criticism of selfishness and individualism to a teenager's decision to accept the college tuition money that could be used to extend his father's life or to a husband's self-interested encouragement of the suicide of his ailing wife. Such failure illustrates how terms like 'selfish' and 'individualistic' can serve in a worldview promoting not altruism, but the favoring of the interests of some *individuals* over those of others. Hardwig says, "We fear death too much." But to the extent that his views are widespread, I think that what we fear too much is having our lives and plans disrupted by the medical needs of our loved ones. This fear may cause us to magnify such disruptions out of proportion, to the point where having to work and borrow one's way through college or live with a distant and uncommunicative spouse seems so terrible that the sick person's death seems preferable and perhaps even obligatory.

There are other elements of bias in the quoted passage. The burden of providing "care or even just supervision twenty-four hours a day, seven days a week," far from being unbearable or unique to caretakers of the ill, is routine for many stay-at-home single mothers of babies and toddlers (and for stay-at-home married mothers whose husbands do no child care). . . . It is likewise common for "a family member [to have] to quit work or make some other major lifestyle change" or for a family to lose "a major source of income" when a baby is born. (Of course, people are aware of such needs when they choose to have children, but people who choose to marry are likewise aware of the strong possibility that their spouse will someday be ill and need care. I will discuss this matter more in the next section.) And Hardwig's claim that "[s]ocial life and friendships evaporate, as there is no opportunity to go out to see friends and the home is no longer a place suitable for having friends in" raises three questions. First, hasn't Hardwig ever heard of the telephone or e-mail? Why is he so ready to see the hardships of taking care of a sick person as reasons why that sick person has a duty to die, rather than as practical problems open to practical remedies? Second, precisely why is a home with a seriously ill person "no longer a place suitable for having friends in"? Suppose that person is unpredictable and incontinent. Is a home with a rambunctious toddler who is not yet toilet trained no longer a suitable place for having friends in? Third, does a loving spouse really welcome the suicide of a beloved partner in order to preserve the spouse's social life? What sort of values and what sort of love would this priority indicate?

The foregoing may make Hardwig look like a bigot with respect to age and health. So it is important to consider other aspects of his arguments, including the following case:

> An 87-year-old woman was dying of congestive heart failure. [The prognosis was] that she had less than a 50 percent chance to live for another six months. She was lucid, assertive, and terrified of death. She very much wanted to live and kept opting for rehospitalization and the most aggressive life-prolonging treatment possible. That treatment successfully prolonged her life (though with increasing debility) for nearly two years. Her 55-year-old daughter was her only remaining family, her caregiver, and the main source of her financial support. The daughter duly cared for her mother. But before her mother died, her illness had cost the daughter all of her savings, her home, her job, and her career.

I will return to this case after looking at some general features of Hardwig's views.

II

Hardwig's approach has one great strength: he acknowledges the existence of genuine conflicts of interest between patients and their families. This contrasts favorably with the sentimentality of the hospice approach, on which "[p]atients, their families and loved ones are the unit of care."[4] In contrast, Hardwig points out that "[t]he conflicts of interests, beliefs, and values among family members are often too real and too deep to treat all members as 'the patient.'"[5] He also refuses to hide behind the claim that many of the conditions he thinks can generate a duty to die can also impair patients' lives to the point where they have self-interested reasons for wanting to die. He recognizes that the most problematic cases are those where the burdensome patient wants to live. I follow him in focusing on such cases. In fact, unless otherwise specified, I assume as a background condition that the patient *greatly* wants to stay alive, and that the family's competing wants are equally strong.

Elsewhere, however, Hardwig is not so clear-headed. He uses the phrase 'duty to die' indiscriminately to apply to a duty to eschew aggressive life-prolonging medical care and a duty to commit suicide. He holds that "[t]here can be a duty to die before one's illness would cause death, even if treated only with palliative measures," and that "there may be a fairly common responsibility to end one's life in the absence of any terminal illness at all," and he offers a detailed discussion of whether a person with a duty to die should carry out his own suicide or solicit suicide assistance from his loving family or from doctors.

Hardwig's use of the phrase 'duty to die' to cover both a duty to commit suicide and a duty to eschew aggressive life-prolonging medical treatment leads him to exaggerate the originality and daringness of his position. The view that sick people can have a duty to commit suicide may indeed strike people as "just too preposterous to entertain. Or too threatening." But this is hardly true of the view that the old and/or terminally ill have a duty not to burden their families and society by insisting on the most aggressive life-prolonging treatment possible, regardless of financial and other costs. This latter view is popular nowadays to the point of cliché. It occurs with varying degrees of explicitness in numerous newspaper and magazine pieces, as well as in highly praised, widely read, and widely influential books by Daniel Callahan[6] and Sherwin B. Nuland,[7] the latter a *New York Times* bestseller and National Book Award winner. The *denial* of this latter view is what strikes people as "just too preposterous to entertain. Or too threatening." (When did you last hear anyone, bioethicist or otherwise, say that terminally ill old people are entitled to extend their lives as long as possible and by the most aggressive care possible, regardless of the cost to their families and society?) Hardwig is conventional, not original, when he says that "we must now face the fact: deaths that come too late are only the other side of our miraculous, life-prolonging modern medicine."[8] What is amazing is his claim (in 1996!) that "[w]e have so far avoided looking at this dark side of our medical triumphs."[9]

Unsurprisingly, Daniel Callahan, who is hostile to aggressive life-extending care for the old and ill but to whom suicide is anathema, has criticized Hardwig's moral equation of suicide and the refusal of aggressive life-prolonging medical care. Since I accept neither Callahan's views about suicide nor his views about aggressive life-prolonging medical care, I will not defend this sort of criticism. Instead, I find Callahan and Hardwig similar in the low value they place on the lives of the old and the ill. Callahan's objection to Hardwig that

> it trivializes the relationship of family members to each other to act as if their mutual obligations to each other are to be judged by some benefit-burden calculus. Hardwig seems to be saying in effect: "for better or worse, in sickness and in health—well, sort of, it all depends"[10]

should be read in light of things he says elsewhere. For example:

> It is not improper for people to worry about being a burden on their families. . . . A family member should reject [a technologically extended death] for the sake of the family's welfare after he or she is gone.[11]

Callahan even says that "the *primary* aspiration of the old [should be] to serve the young."[12] He also says, "We do not need a . . . set of moral values that will impose upon families the drain of extended illness and death."[13] (Note the bias in Callahan's use of "we" here. Who are the "we" who do not need such a set of moral values? Families eager to free themselves of burdensome sick "loved ones" do not need such a set of moral values, but the sick people themselves may, if they want to stay alive. What "we" (i.e., such actual and potential sick people) do not need is a set of moral values that impose on us the drain of being pressured to forgo high-tech life-extending care and die sooner than necessary, in order to avoid burdening our families—a description of the situation that is no more biased than Callahan's own. "We" old people also do not need a set of moral values that tell us our primary aspiration should be to serve the young.) Callahan's real objection thus seems to be to suicide, rather than to a benefit-burden calculation. In contrast, I have only a practical reason for finding Hardwig's views about the duty to commit suicide more objectionable than Callahan's views about the duty to refuse aggressive life-prolonging medical care: the former duty casts a much wider net. This paper will not distinguish further between these two possible duties, but will follow Hardwig's practice of using 'duty to die' to apply indiscriminately to both.

Hardwig's second conflation is also interesting. He makes no distinction between the duty to die in order to avoid burdening your children and the duty to die in order to avoid burdening your spouse. (Interestingly, none of his examples mentions young adults with a duty to die in order to avoid burdening their caregiving parents.) But there are obvious differences between parental and "adult child" cases, on the one hand, and spousal cases on the other. Parents have often made great sacrifices for their children, including an approximation of the hyperbolically described "twenty-four hours a day, seven days a week" care that Hardwig considers so onerous in the case of the old and the ill. There is a large literature on what, if anything, grown children owe their parents, but, to my mind, nothing that refutes Joel Feinberg's "My benefactor once freely offered me his services when I needed them. . . . But now circumstances have arisen in which he needs help, and I am in a position to help him. Surely I *owe* my services now, and he would be entitled to resent my failure to come through."[14] He would also be entitled to resent my hypocrisy if I claimed to love him. (What if I have significant obligations elsewhere? This issue will be touched upon later.)

Marriages differ from parent-child relationships in two ways that are relevant here. First, they do not normally begin with a long period of one-sided caregiving, let alone one-sided caregiving by the party most likely to need care later on. Second, marriages are freely entered into by both parties. This gives couples the opportunity for prenuptial discussions and agreements that will generate their own agreed-upon caregiving duties. Of course, such an approach has its own problems. The first, which also applies to living wills, is that it may be virtually impossible for many healthy young people to enter imaginatively into hypothetical situations in which they would be seriously ill and debilitated. As Ellen Goodman puts it, "No one . . . wants to live to be senile. But once senile, he may well want to live."[15] The second problem, which also applies to prenuptial financial agreements, is that such an arrangement may seem cold-blooded and destructive to the loving spirit of the marriage. Hardwig also advocates discussions in families. He even advocates having them once a person is ill, which avoids the first problem and enables people to consider the "particular and contextual" details of their actual situation. But it enormously intensifies the second problem. Hardwig's sentimental claim that "[h]onest talk about difficult matters almost always strengthens relationships" raises the question of just how it would strengthen a relationship to say to your father, even in response to his query, "Well, Dad, you're not pleasant to have around anymore, and if you don't die soon, your care will use up all the money you saved for my college education, so I'd really appreciate it if you killed yourself now or at least stopped getting treatment." This may be a crude formulation, but what could be a better one of such a crude thought? The plain fact is that letting your father know you value his life less than your college tuition is unlikely to strengthen your relationship. It is surprising that someone hard-headed enough to see that the slogan "the patient is the family" glosses over genuine conflicts of interest (see the material leading up to note [5]) would slip into the sentimentality of supposing that honest discussion of such conflicts will almost always strengthen relationships. Prenuptial agreements may seem cold-blooded, but at least they do not involve the cruelty of telling a sick and vulnerable person that you would welcome his death. Prenuptial discussions also give a couple the option of calling off the wedding if they find that their values are too far apart.

III

Hardwig realizes that a duty to die may seem harsh. "And yet," he says, "a duty to die will not always be as harsh as we might assume. If I love my family, I will want to protect them and their lives. I will not want to make choices that compromise their futures." But if he loves his ill wife, will he want to protect her and her life? Will he want to avoid compromising her future by encouraging her to commit suicide so he will be free of the burden of caregiving? Hardwig says that "there is something deeply insulting in . . . an ethic that . . . [treats] me as if I had no moral responsibilities when I am ill or debilitated." Will he also be insulted if his ill wife commits suicide because she thinks he is the sort of person who would rather have her dead than take care of her? I would be enormously insulted if a loved one had such a view of me. Hardwig tells us that his "own grandfather committed suicide after his heart attack as a final gift to his wife—he had plenty of life insurance but not nearly enough health insurance, and he feared that she would be left homeless and destitute if he lingered on in an incapacitated state."[16] Hardwig does not tell us whether his grandmother appreciated this "gift." What sort of person would she be if she did? If she welcomed this sacrifice, how could she be worth it? What sort of love could she have felt for her husband? What sort of love could he have thought she felt for him? And was there no one else in this loving family who could help his grandmother so she would not have to be left "homeless and destitute" if her husband lingered on?

This brings me to a discussion of what I have elsewhere called "the paradox of the selfless invalid." In its most extreme form, the paradox goes as follows. Either the patient's loved ones want him to die quickly in order to save money or otherwise make their lives easier, or they do not. If they do not, the patient does not respect them by dying for their sake. If they do, then why is the patient sacrificing what would otherwise be left of his life for people who love him so little that they value his life less than money and/or freedom from encumbrance? Wouldn't a truly loving family find such a sacrifice appalling? Of course, families can have mixed feelings, which include both the desire to have the patient stay alive and the self-interested desire to get it all over with and to keep expenses down. But the basic point remains. Decent and loving families, as part of their decency and lovingness, will recognize the latter desire as ignoble and, on balance, will not want patients to pander to it.

This extreme view is itself open to objections. Just as it is inhumane to suppose a sick person has a duty to forgo an extra year of life in order to conserve money for a child's college tuition, it is unreasonable to suppose there are no limits to what a loving family can be expected to do for a sick member, even to the point of selling literally everything they own in order to give him a minute of extra life. The devil is in the details, or, as Hardwig puts it, "the really serious moral questions are . . . how far family and friends can be asked to support and sustain the patient."[17] I have argued that some of Hardwig's answers are ludicrous. Where should we draw the line? I hardly have an exact answer, nor does Hardwig. But here are his general guidelines.

(1) A duty to die is more likely when continuing to live will impose significant burdens—emotional burdens, extensive caregiving, destruction of life plans, and yes, financial hardship—on your family and loved ones. This is the fundamental insight underlying a duty to die.

(2) A duty to die becomes greater as you grow older. As we age, we will be giving up less by giving up our lives, if only because we will sacrifice fewer remaining years of life and a smaller portion of our life plans. After all, it's not as if we would be immortal and live forever if we could just manage to avoid a duty to die. To have reached the age of, say, seventy-five or eighty years without being ready to die is itself a moral failing, the sign of a life out of touch with life's basic realities.

(3) A duty to die is more likely when you have already lived a full and rich life. You have already had a full share of the good things life offers.

(4) There is a greater duty to die if your loved ones' lives have already been difficult or impoverished, if they have had only a small share of the good things that life has to offer (especially if through no fault of their own).

(5) A duty to die is more likely when your loved ones have already made great contributions—perhaps even sacrifices—to make your life a good one. Especially if you have not made similar sacrifices for their well-being or for the well-being of other members of your family.

(6) To the extent that you can make a good adjustment to your illness or handicapping condition, there is less likely to be a duty to die. A good adjustment means that smaller sacrifices will be required of loved ones and there is more compensating interaction for them. Still, we must also recognize that some diseases—Alzheimer [*sic*] or Huntington [*sic*] chorea—will eventually take their toll on your loved ones no matter how courageously, resolutely, even cheerfully you manage to face that illness.

(7) There is less likely to be a duty to die if you can still make significant contributions to the lives of others, especially your family. The burdens to family members are not only or

even primarily financial, neither are the contributions to them. However, the old and those who have terminal illnesses must also bear in mind that the loss their family members will feel when they die cannot be avoided, only postponed.

(8) A duty to die is more likely when the part of you that is loved will soon be gone or seriously compromised. Or when you soon will no longer be capable of giving love. Part of the horror of dementing disease is that it destroys the capacity to nurture and sustain relationships, taking away a person's agency and the emotions that bind her to others.

(9) There is a greater duty to die to the extent that you have lived a relatively lavish lifestyle instead of saving for illness or old age. . . . It is a greater wrong to come to your family for assistance if your need is the result of having chosen leisure or a spendthrift lifestyle.

I suggest we reconceptualize the problem by asking how these and related conditions might affect the duty to make sacrifices in order to extend the life of a burdensomely ill loved one. I will call this "a duty to aid." Here are nine conditions parallel to Hardwig's.

1. A duty to aid is more likely when failing to do so will impose significant burdens, when the ill loved one wants very much to go on living and needs your help. This is the fundamental insight underlying a duty to aid.
2. Perhaps a duty to aid becomes greater as you grow older, because you will be sacrificing a smaller portion of your life plans. Alternatively, a duty to aid may be greater when you are young, because you have more stamina as well as more life ahead of you, with more opportunity to recoup your losses. At any rate, to have reached adulthood without being ready to undertake major financial burdens and changes in "lifestyle" in order to aid a seriously ill loved one is itself a moral failing, a sign of a life out of touch with life's basic realities.
3. A duty to aid is more likely when you have already lived a full and rich life. You have already had a full share of the good things life offers.
4. There is a greater duty to aid if your ill loved one's life has already been difficult or impoverished, if he has had only a small share of the good things that life has to offer (especially if through no fault of his own).
5. A duty to aid is more likely when your loved one has already made great contributions—perhaps even sacrifices—to make your life a good one. Especially if you have not made similar sacrifices for his well-being. This imbalance frequently exists between grown children and the parents who raised them.
6. To the extent that there are others able to share the burden of aiding, there is less you have a duty to do. To the extent that you cannot make a good adjustment to the duty of aiding, there is less of a duty to aid. Still, we must also recognize that unwillingness to make a good adjustment does not constitute inability to do so, nor does making a good adjustment mean you must enjoy aiding.
7. There is less of a duty to aid if you have significant obligations elsewhere. However, you must also bear in mind that your obligations to your children do not automatically outweigh your obligations to your parents. The popular slogan "The best thing you can do for your parents is to take good care of their grandchildren" is obviously false if your father needs and wants a heart transplant, which he cannot afford without your help, and your son "needs" and wants four years at Yale.
8. A duty to aid is more likely when your loved one is painfully aware that the part of him that was loved will soon be gone or seriously compromised and is terrified that his loved ones will abandon him. And if you genuinely love your "loved one," then to the extent that the part that is loved is *not* compromised, you will have a strong self-interested reason for wanting to help him stay alive; you would hate never seeing him again.
9. There is a greater duty to provide physical care to the extent that you have lived a relatively lavish "lifestyle" that has prevented you from saving enough to provide financial help.

These guidelines are not formally incompatible with Hardwig's. He grants that families "must be prepared to make significant sacrifices to respond to an illness in the family, although his examples I quoted earlier of what can constitute an intolerable family burden raise the question of just what sort of "significant sacrifices" he has in mind. His statement "I cannot imagine that it would be morally permissible for me to . . . compromise the quality of [my grandchildren's] lives simply because I wish to live a little longer" illustrates the importance of this question. What deprivation could *not* be said to compromise the quality of one's grandchildren's lives? Going without private schooling? Going without summer camp? Going without tennis lessons? At any rate, my guidelines and Hardwig's reflect (although they do not entail) different orientations. Hardwig believes we can find meaning in death by recognizing our duty to die, thus engaging in an "affirmation of connections." I am less inclined to find meaning in death at all. I find Malory's "Let me lie down and wail with you"[18] a much more humane response to adversity than today's relentless tendency to insist we turn adversity into an opportunity for "growth," a tendency Hardwig at any rate follows very selectively. His selectivity reflects his characteristic bias. After all, if we are going to urge people to regard death and dying as opportunities for growth and "affirmation of connections," why not urge families to seize the opportunity to grow and "affirm connections" by making loving sacrifices to prolong the life of a seriously ill loved one? Hardwig says, "Caring for the sick or aged can foster growth. . . . But it would be irresponsible to blithely assume that this always happens, that it will happen in my family, or that it will be the fault of my family if they cannot manage to turn my illness into a positive experience." He does not criticize such unsuccessful families for having a "sense of community [that] is so weak." He reserves this harsh judgment for old and/or ill people who are unwilling to unburden their families by dying (although he does grant that "[a] man who can leave his wife the day after she learns she has cancer, on the grounds that he has his own life to live, is to be deplored").[19]

Hardwig's guidelines, as well as his whole approach, raise another question. Why does he fail to consider cases where the sacrificial suicide of someone who is healthy and far from old could benefit his (not overly) loving family? Suppose you are a forty-year-old mid-level executive who has been downsized. The only job you can get pays the minimum wage, not enough to support your family, even with the added income of your wife, who now has to work fifty hours a week as a home health aide, doing the caregiving Hardwig finds so onerous when done for a family member. Your family is about to lose their home; you will all have to move to a rat-infested apartment in an unsafe inner-city, neighborhood. "For [your children], the chance to go to college [will] be lost" (if we assume, as Hardwig inexplicably does in cases involving illness, that young people's working and/or borrowing their way through college is not an option). There is, however, a solution. Like Hardwig's grandfather, you have excellent life insurance. (If your life insurance has the common two-year "suicide clause" denying payment if the insured person commits suicide within two years of purchasing the policy, that clause has long since expired.) In accord with Hardwig's guidelines, we can build in that your life so far has been rich and full, your wife has had a difficult, impoverished childhood, and your family has made sacrifices for your career (your wife sacrificed her own career and also spent much time in the tedious pseudosocializing necessary to further your ambitions, and your children endured the dislocation of frequent moves). We can even say that you lost your job not through downsizing but through your own fault and that you have little in the way of savings because you lived a "relatively lavish lifestyle instead of saving." Would Hardwig then say you could have a duty to commit suicide instead of burdening your family by depriving them of your life insurance money? If not, why not?

Like Hardwig, I cannot lay down a series of precise rules saying who owes whom what when a sick family member needs care. In Hardwig's case of the eighty-seven-year-old woman, for example, I think much hinges on her prior relationship with her daughter. How much did that mother sacrifice for her daughter? Did the mother pay, and make sacrifices to pay, for the education that enabled the daughter to have the career Hardwig is so distressed about her losing? What was their relationship like once the daughter grew up? Did the mother, like many parents nowadays, give her daughter some of the money that enabled the daughter to buy the home Hardwig is so distressed about her losing? What happened after the mother died? Did the daughter ever find another job? Hardwig does not tell us any of these things. But I think it is clear that in my own example with which I opened this paper, alternative (2) is the right answer. A teenager should work and borrow his way through college in order to free up money to prolong the life of a beloved parent who raised him and sacrificed for him. A spouse should forgo tennis (even if it is not a trivial recreation but an important part of his life) in order to take care of the beloved partner "that he promised his faith unto."[20] "Sometimes, it's simply the only loving thing to do."[21]

NOTES

1. Sir Thomas Malory, *Le Morte D'Arthur* (London: Penguin, 1969), v.2, 515.
2. Leo Tolstoy, *The Death of Ivan Ilych* (New York: New American Library of World Literature, 1960), 10. Tolstoy, of course, intended this remark (by a cancer patient's widow) to show monumental selfishness and callousness.
3. John Hardwig, "Is There a Duty to Die?" *Hastings Center Report* 27, no. 2 (1997), 36.
4. See B. Manard and C. Perrone, *Hospice Care: An Introduction and Review of the Evidence* (Arlington, VA: National Hospice Organization, 1994), 4.
5. John Hardwig, "What about the Family?" *Hastings Center Report* (March/April 1990), 5.
6. See Daniel Callahan, *Setting Limits* (Washington, DC: Georgetown University Press, 1987), *What Kind of Life?* (Washington, DC: Georgetown University Press, 1990), and *The Troubled Dream of Life* (New York: Simon and Schuster, 1993).
7. Sherwin B. Nuland, *How We Die* (New York: Knopf, 1994).
8. Hardwig, "Dying at the Right Time," 63.
9. Ibid.
10. Callahan, letter to the editor, *Hastings Center Report* (November/December 1997), 4.
11. Callahan, *The Troubled Dream of Life*, 218–19.
12. Callahan, *Setting Limits*, 43 (italics in original).
13. Callahan, *The Troubled Dream of Life*, 218–9.
14. Joel Feinberg, "Duties, Rights, and Claims," *American Philosophical Quarterly* 3, no. 2 (1966), 139 (italics in original).
15. Ellen Goodman, "Who Lives? Who Dies? Who Decides?" in E. Goodman, *At Large* (New York: Simon and Schuster, 1981), 161. (The first part of Goodman's statement is false. I want to live to be senile. I would rather be mentally intact than senile, of course, but I would rather be senile than dead.)
16. Hardwig, "What about the Family?" 6.
17. Hardwig, "What about the Family?" 6.
18. Malory, *Le Morte D'Arthur*, v.2, 172.
19. Hardwig, "What about the Family?" 7.
20. Malory, *Le Morte D'Arthur*, v. 2, 426.
21. This is a claim Hardwig makes about killing yourself in order to avoid burdening your loved ones: "Dying at the Right Time," 57.

RECOMMENDED SUPPLEMENTARY READING

GENERAL WORKS

Annas, George J. *Standard of Care: The Law of American Bioethics.* Oxford: Oxford University Press, 1993.

Beauchamp, Tom L., and Veatch, Robert M., eds. *Ethical Issues in Death and Dying.* 2nd ed. Upper Saddle River, NJ: Prentice-Hall, 1996.

Brock, Dan. *Life and Death: Philosophical Essays in Biomedical Ethics.* New York: Cambridge University Press, 1993.

Brody, Baruch. *Life and Death Decision Making.* New York: Oxford University Press, 1988.

Buchanan, Allen, and Brock, Dan. *Deciding for Others: The Ethics of Surrogate Decision Making.* Cambridge: Cambridge University Press, 1989.

Byock, Ira. *Dying Well: The Prospect for Growth at the End of Life.* New York: Riverhead Books, 1997.

Cantor, Norman L. *Legal Frontiers of Death and Dying.* Bloomington: Indiana University Press, 1987.

———. "Twenty-Five Years after *Quinlan:* A Review of the Jurisprudence of Death and Dying." *Journal of Law, Medicine, & Ethics* 29 (2001): 182–196.

Englehardt, H. Tristram, Jr. *The Foundations of Bioethics.* New York: Oxford University Press, 1986.

Gorovitz, Samuel. *Drawing the Line: Life, Death, and Ethical Choice in an American Hospital.* Oxford: Oxford University Press, 1991.

Kamm, F. M. *Morality, Mortality.* 2 vols. New York: Oxford University Press, 1993–1996.

Lynn, Joanne. "Serving Patients Who May Die Soon and Their Families: The Role of Hospice and Other Services." *JAMA* 285 (February 21, 2001): 925–932.

McMahan, Jeff. *The Ethics of Killing: Killing at the Margins of Life.* New York: Oxford University Press, 2001.

Meisel, Alan. *The Right to Die.* New York: John Wiley and Sons, 1989.

Moller, David Wendell. *Confronting Death.* New York: Oxford University Press, 1996.

President's Commission for the Study of Ethical Problems in Medicine and Biomedical and Behavioral Research. *Deciding to Forego Life-Sustaining Treatment.* Washington, DC: U.S. Government Printing Office, 1983.

Ramsey, Paul. *Ethics at the Edges of Life, Part Two.* New Haven, CT: Yale University Press, 1978.

Thomasma, David C., and Kushner, Thomasine, eds. *Birth to Death: Science and Bioethics.* New York: Cambridge University Press, 1996.

Veatch, Robert. *Death, Dying, and the Biological Revolution.* 2nd ed. New Haven, CT: Yale University Press, 1989.

Weir, Robert F. *Abating Treatment with Critically Ill Patients.* New York: Oxford University Press, 1989.

———, ed. *Ethical Issues in Death and Dying.* 2nd ed. New York: Columbia University Press, 1986.

THE DEFINITION OF DEATH

Agich, George, and Jones, Royce P. "Personal Identity and Brain Death: A Critical Response." *Philosophy and Public Affairs* 15 (Summer 1986): 267–274.

Bernat, James L. "Refinements in the Definition and Criterion of Death." In *The Definition of Death: Contemporary Controversies* edited by Stuart J. Youngner, Robert M. Arnold, and Renie Schapiro. Baltimore: The Johns Hopkins University Press, 1999.

Brody, Baruch. "Special Ethical Issues in the Management of PVS Patients." *Law, Medicine & Health Care* 20 (1992): 104–115.

Capron, Alexander M. "Anencephalic Donors: Separate the Dead from the Dying." *Hastings Center Report* 17, no. 1 (1987): 5–9.

———. "Brain Death—Well Settled Yet Still Unresolved." *New England Journal of Medicine* 344 (2001): 1244–1246.

Cole, David. "Statutory Definitions of Death and the Management of Terminally Ill Patients Who May Become Organ Donors after Death." *Kennedy Institute of Ethics Journal* 3, no. 2 (1993): 145–155.

Cranford, Ronald E. "The Persistent Vegetative State: The Medical Reality (Getting the Facts Straight)." *Hastings Center Report* 18, no. 1 (1988): 27–32.

Emanuel, Linda L. "Reexamining Death: The Asymptomatic Model and a Bounded Zone

Definition." *Hastings Center Report* (July–August 1995): 27–35.

Gervais, Karen Grandstrand. *Redefining Death.* New Haven, CT: Yale University Press, 1986.

———. "Advancing the Definition of Death: A Philosophical Essay," *Medical Humanities Review* 3, no. 2 (1989): 7–19.

Green, Michael, and Wikler, Daniel. "Brain Death and Personal Identity." *Philosophy and Public Affairs* 9, no. 2 (Winter 1980): 105–133.

Greenberg, Gary. "As Good as Dead." *The New Yorker* (August 13, 2001): 36–41.

Harvard Medical School Committee to Examine the Definition of Brain Death. "A Definition of Irreversible Coma." *JAMA* 205, no. 6 (August 5, 1968): 337–340.

McMahan, Jeff. "The Metaphysics of Brain Death." *Bioethics* 9, no. 2 (April 1995): 91–126.

Pernick, Martin S. "Brain Death in a Cultural Context: The Reconstruction of Death, 1967–1981." In *The Definition of Death: Contemporary Controversies,* edited by Stuart J. Youngner, Robert M. Arnold, and Renie Schapiro. Baltimore: The Johns Hopkins University Press, 1999.

Potts, Michael; Byrne, Paul A.; and Nilges, Richard G.; eds. *Beyond Brain Death: The Case against Brain Based Criteria for Human Death.* Dordrecht, The Netherlands: Kluwer Academic Publishers, 2000.

Shewmon, D. A.; Capron, A. M.; Peacock, W. J.; and Shulman, B. L. "The Use of Anencephalic Infants as Organ Sources: A Critique. *JAMA* 261, no. 12 (March 24–31, 1989): 1773–1781.

Shinnar, Shlomo, and Arras, John. "Ethical Issues in the Use of Anencephalic Infants as Organ Donors." *Neurologic Clinics* 7, no. 4 (November 1989): 729–743.

Steinbock, Bonnie. "Recovery from Persistent Vegetative State? The Case of Carrie Coons." *Hastings Center Report* 19, no. 4 (1989): 14–15.

Tomlinson, Tom. "The Irreversibility of Death: Reply to Cole." *Kennedy Institute of Ethics Journal* 3, no. 2 (1993): 157–165.

Truog, Robert D. "Is It Time to Abandon Brain Death?" *Hastings Center Report* 27 (1997): 29–37.

Wijdicks, Eelco F. M. "The Diagnosis of Brain Death." *New England Journal of Medicine* 344, (2001): 1215–1221.

Wikler, Daniel. "Not Dead, Not Dying? Ethical Categories and Persistent Vegetative State." *Hastings Center Report* 18, no. 1 (1988): 41–47.

———. "Brain Death: A Durable Consensus?" *Bioethics* 7, nos. 2–3 (1993): 239–246.

Youngner, Stuart, et al. "'Brain Death' and Organ Retrieval: A Cross-Sectional Survey of Knowledge and Concepts among Health Professionals." *JAMA* 261 (1989): 2205–2210.

Youngner, Stuart J.; Arnold, Robert M., and Schapiro, Renie, eds. *The Definition of Death: Contemporary Controversies.* Baltimore: The Johns Hopkins University Press, 1999.

Zaner, Richard M., ed. *Death: Beyond Whole-Brain Criteria.* Dordrecht, Holland: Kluwer Academic Press, 1988.

DECISIONAL CAPACITY AND THE RIGHT TO REFUSE TREATMENT

Brink, Susan. "Taking Charge," *U.S. News & World Report* (July 28, 1997): 17–21 (An update on the Dax Cowart Story).

Brock, Dan W. "Decision-Making Competence and Risk." *Bioethics* 5, no. 2 (1991): 105–112.

Callahan, Daniel. "Terminating Life-Sustaining Treatment of the Demented." *Hastings Center Report* (November–December 1995): 25–31.

Connors, Russell B., Jr., and Smith, Martin L. "Religious Insistence on Medical Treatment: Christian Theology and Imagination." *Hastings Center Report* (July–August 1996): 23–30.

Freedman, Benjamin. "Competence, Marginal and Otherwise: Concepts and Ethics." *International Journal of Law and Psychiatry* 4 (1981): 53–72.

Kliever, Lonnie D., ed. *Dax's Case: Essays in Medical Ethics and Human Meaning.* Dallas, TX: Southern Methodist University Press, 1989.

Kopehnan, Loretta M. "On the Evaluative Nature of Competency and Capacity Judgments." *International Journal of Law and Psychiatry* (1990): 309–329.

Macklin, Ruth. "Consent, Coercion and Conflicts of Rights." *Perspectives in Biology and Medicine* 20, no. 3 (1977): 360–371.

May, Larry. "Challenging Medical Authority: The Refusal of Treatment by Christian Scientists." *Hastings Center Report* (January–February 1995): 15–21.

Meisel, Alan. "Legal Myths about Terminating Life Support." *Archives of Internal Medicine* 109 (1991):1497–1502.

Powell, Tia, and Lowenstein, Bruce. "Refusing Life-Sustaining Treatment after Catastrophic Injury: Ethical Implications." *Journal of Law, Medicine and Ethics* 24, no. 1 (Spring 1996): 54–61.

Roth, Loren H.; Meisel, Alan; and Lidz, Charles. "Tests of Competency to Consent to Treatment." *American Journal of Psychiatry* 134, no. 3 (March 1977): 279–284.

Sheldon, Mark. "Ethical Issues in the Forced Transfusion of Jehovah's Witness Children," *The Journal of Emergency Medicine* 14, no. 2 (1996): 251–257.

Skene, Loane. "Risk-Related Standard Inevitable in Assessing Competence." *Bioethics* 5, no. 2 (1991): 113–122.

Wicclair, Mark R. "Patient Decision-Making Capacity and Risk." *Bioethics* 5, no. 2 (1991): 91–104.

ADVANCE DIRECTIVES

"Advance Directives: Expectations, Experience, and Future Practice." *Journal of Clinical Ethics* 4, no. 1 (1993): 1–104.

Brett, Allan S. "Advance Directives and the Personal Identity Problem." *Philosophy and Public Affairs* 17 (Fall 1988): 277–302.

———. "Limitations of Listing Specific Medical Interventions in Advance Directives," *JAMA* 266, no. 6 (August 14, 1991): 825–828.

Cantor, Norman. *Advance Directives and the Pursuit of Death with Dignity.* Bloomington: Indiana University Press, 1993.

———. "Making Advance Directives Meaningful." *Psychology, Public Policy, and Law* 4 (1998): 629–652.

Dresser, Rebecca. "Confronting the Near Irrelevance of Advance Directives." *Journal of Clinical Ethics* 5 (1994): 55–56.

Hackler, C. R.; Moseley, R.; and Vawter, D. E., eds. *Advance Directives in Medicine.* New York: Praeger Publishers, 1989.

"Patient Self-Determination Act." *Cambridge Quarterly of Healthcare Ethics* 2, no. 2 (special section, 1992): 97–126.

Robertson, John. "Second Thoughts on Living Wills." *Hastings Center Report* 21, no. 6 (1991): 6–9.

Teno, Joan, et al. "Do Formal Advance Directives Affect Resuscitation Decisions and the Use of Resources for Seriously Ill Patients?" *Journal of Clinical Ethics* 5, no. 1 (Spring 1994): 23–30.

CHOOSING FOR OTHERS

Arras, John. "Beyond Cruzan: Individual Rights, Family Autonomy and the Persistent Vegetative State." *Journal of the American Geriatrics Society* 39 (1991): 1018–1024.

Blustein, Jeffrey. "The Family in Medical Decision-making." *Hastings Center Report* 23, no. 3 (May–June 1993): 6–13.

Cantor, Norman. "Discarding Substituted Judgment and Best Interests: Toward a Constructive Preference Standard for Dying, Previously Competent Patients without Advance Instructions." *Rutgers Law Review* 48 (1996): 1193–1272.

Capron, Alexander M., ed. "Medical Decision-Making and the 'Right to Die' after Cruzan." *Law, Medicine & Health Care* 19, nos. 1–2 (Spring/Summer 1991): 5–104.

"Children and Bioethics: Uses and Abuses of the Best Interests Standard." *Journal of Medicine and Philosophy* 22, no. 3 (Symposium; June 1997).

Dresser, Rebecca. "Missing Persons: Legal Perceptions of Incompetent Patients." *Rutgers Law Review* 46, no. 2 (Winter 1994): 609–719.

———. "Dworkin on Dementia: Elegant Theory, Questionable Policy." *Hastings Center Report* (November–December 1995): 32–38.

Emanuel, Ezekiel J. *The Ends of Human Life: Medical Ethics in a Liberal Polity.* Cambridge, MA: Harvard University Press, 1991.

Emanuel, Ezekiel J., and Emanuel, Linda L. "Decisions at the End of Life: Guided by Communities of Patients." *Hastings Center Report* 23, no. 5 (1993): 6–14.

Freedman, Benjamin. "Respectful Service and Reverent Obedience: A Jewish View on Making Decisions for Incompetent Parents." *Hastings Center Report* (July–August 1996): 31–37.

Kadish, Sanford H. "Letting Patients Die: Legal and Moral Reflections." *California Law Review* 80, no. 4 (1992): 857–888.

Lynn, Joanne, ed. *By No Extraordinary Means: The Choice to Forego Life-Sustaining Food and Water.* Bloomington: Indiana University Press, 1986.

May, William E., et al. "Feeding and Hydrating the Permanently Unconscious and Other Vulnerable Persons." *Issues in Law and Medicine* 3, no. 3 (1987): 203–211.

Meisel, Alan. "The Legal Consensus about Forgoing Life-Sustaining Treatment: Its Status and

Prospects." *Kennedy Institute of Ethics Journal* 2, no. 4 (December 1992): 309–342.

Nelson, James Lindermann. "Taking Families Seriously." *Hastings Center Report* 22, no. 4 (1992): 6–12.

———. "Critical Interests and Sources of Familial Decision-Making Authority for Incapacitated Patients." *Journal of Law, Medicine and Ethics* 23, no. 2 (Summer 1995): 143–148.

New York State Task Force on Life and the Law. *Life-Sustaining Treatment: Making Decisions and Appointing a Health Care Agent.* 1987.

———. *When Others Must Choose: Deciding for Patients without Capacity.* 1992.

"Pediatric Decision Making." *Journal of Law, Medicine and Ethics* 23, no. 1 (Symposium; Spring 1995).

Rhoden, Nancy K. "Litigating Life and Death." *Harvard Law Review* 102, no. 2 (December 1988): 375–446.

Solomon, Mildred Z., et al. "Decisions Near the End of Life: Professional Views on Life-Sustaining Treatments." *American Journal of Public Health* 83, no. 1 (January 1993): 14–23.

Veatch, Robert M. "Forgoing Life-Sustaining Treatment Limits to the Consensus." *Kennedy Institute of Ethics Journal* 3, no. 1 (March 1993): 1–19.

White, Patricia D., ed. "Essays in the Aftermath of Cruzan." *Journal of Medicine and Philosophy* 17, no. 6 (December 1992): 563ff.

EUTHANASIA AND PHYSICIAN-ASSISTED SUICIDE

"Aid in Dying: The Supreme Court and the Public Response." *Hastings Center Report* (September–October, 1997).

Arras, John D. "The Right to Die on the Slippery Slope." *Social Theory and Practice* 8, no. 3 (Fall 1982): 285–328.

Battin, Margaret P. *The Least-Worst Death: Essays in Bioethics on the End of Life.* New York: Oxford University Press, 1994.

———. "A Dozen Caveats Concerning the Discussion of Euthanasia in the Netherlands." In *Arguing Euthanasia: The Controversy over Mercy Killing, Assisted Suicide and the "Right to Die,"* edited by Jonathan Moreno. New York: Simon & Schuster, 1995.

———. *The Death Debate: Ethical Issues in Suicide.* Englewood Cliffs, NJ: Prentice Hall, 1996.

Battin, Margaret P.; Rhodes, Rosamond; and Silvers, Anita; eds. *Physician-Assisted Suicide: Expanding the Debate.* New York and London: Routledge, 1998.

Beauchamp, Tom L., ed. *Intending Death: The Ethics of Assisted Suicide and Euthanasia.* Upper Saddle River, NJ: Prentice-Hall, 1996.

Brock, Dan W. "Voluntary Active Euthanasia." *Hastings Center Report* (March–April 1992).

Brody, Baruch. *Suicide and Euthanasia.* Dordrecht, Holland: Kluwer Academic Press, 1989.

Brody, Howard. "Assisted Death: A Compassionate Response to Medical Failure." *New England Journal of Medicine* 327, no. 19 (November 5, 1992): 1384–1388.

Callahan, Daniel. *The Troubled Dream of Life: Living with Mortality.* New York: Simon & Schuster, 1993.

Cohen, Cynthia B. "Christian Perspectives on Assisted Suicide and Euthanasia: The Anglican Tradition." *Journal of Law, Medicine and Ethics* 24, no. 4 (Winter 1996): 369–379.

Downing, A. B.; and Smoker, Barbara; eds. *Voluntary Euthanasia: Experts Debate the Right to Die.* London: Peter Owen Publishers, 1986.

Dworkin, Gerald; Frey, R. G.; and Bok, Sissela. *Euthanasia and Physician-Assisted Suicide: For and Against.* Cambridge: Cambridge University Press, 1998.

Dworkin, Ronald. *Life's Dominion: An Argument about Abortion, Euthanasia, and Individual Freedom.* New York: Alfred A. Knopf, 1993.

"Dying Well? A Colloquy on Euthanasia and Assisted Suicide." *Hastings Center Report* 22, no. 2 (special issue; 1992): 6–55.

"Euthanasia and Physician-Assisted Suicide: Murder or Mercy." *Cambridge Quarterly of Healthcare Ethics* 2, no. I (special section; 1993): 9–88.

Feinberg, Joel. "Voluntary Euthanasia and the Inalienable Right to Life." *Philosophy and Public Affairs* 7, no. 2 (Winter 1978): 93–123.

Foot, Philippa. "Euthanasia." *Philosophy and Public Affairs* 6, no. 2 (Winter 1977): 85–112.

Gaylin, Willard, et al. "Doctors Must Not Kill." *JAMA* 259, no. 14 (April 8, 1988): 2139–2140.

Glover, Jonathan. *Causing Death and Saving Lives.* New York: Penguin Books, 1977.

Jennings, Bruce. "Active Euthanasia and Forgoing Life-Sustaining Treatment: Can We Hold the Line?" *Journal of Pain and Symptom Management* 6, no. 5 (July 1991): 312–316.

Kamisar, Yale. "Some Non-Religious Views against Proposed 'Mercy-Killing' Legislation." *Minnesota Law Review* 42 (1958): 969–1042.

———. "Are Laws against Assisted Suicide Unconstitutional?" *Hastings Center Report* 23, no. 3 (1993): 32–41.

Kass, Leon. "Is There a Right to Die?" *Hastings Center Report* 23, no. 1 (1993): 34–43.

Kevorkian, Jack. *Prescription Medicine: The Goodness of Planned Death.* Buffalo, NY: Prometheus Books, 1991.

Kuhse, Helga. "Voluntary Euthanasia and Other Medical End-of-Life Decisions: Doctors Should Be Permitted to Give Death a Helping Hand." In *Birth to Death: Science and Bioethics,* edited by David C. Thomasma and Thomasine Kushner. Cambridge: Cambridge University Press, 1996.

Mappes, Thomas A., and Zembaty, Jane S. "Patient Choices, Family Interests, and Physician Obligations." *Kennedy Institute of Ethics Journal* 4 (1994): 27–46.

Momeyer, Richard. "Does Physician-Assisted Suicide Violate the Integrity of Medicine?" *Journal of Medicine and Philosophy* 20, no. 1 (February 1995): 13–24.

Moreno, Jonathan D. *Arguing Euthanasia: The Controversy over Mercy Killing, Assisted Suicide, and the "Right to Die."* New York: Simon & Schuster, 1995.

New York State Task Force on Life and the Law. *When Death Is Sought: Assisted Suicide and Euthanasia in the Medical Context.* 1994.

———. *When Death Is Sought: Assisted Suicide and Euthanasia in the Medical Context, Supplement to Report.* April 1997.

Orentlicher, David. "The Legalization of Physician-Assisted Suicide: A Very Modest Revolution." *Boston College Law Review* 38, no. 3 (1997): 443–475.

"Physician-Assisted Suicide in Context: Constitutional, Regulatory, and Professional Challenges." *Journal of Law, Medicine & Ethics* 24, no. 3 (Symposium; Fall 1996): 181–242.

Pratt, David A. "Too Many Physicians: Physician-Assisted Suicide after Glucksberg/Quill." *Albany Journal of Law, Science & Technology* 9 (1999): 161–234.

Pratt, David A., and Steinbock, Bonnie. "Death with Dignity or Unlawful Killing: The Ethical and Legal Debate Over Physician-Assisted Death." *Criminal Law Bulletin* (May–June 1997): 226–261.

Quill, Timothy E. *Death and Dignity: Making Choices and Taking Charge.* New York: Oxford University Press, 1986.

———. "The Ambiguity of Clinical Intentions." *New England Journal of Medicine* 329 (1992): 1039–1040.

———. *A Midwife through the Dying Process: Stories of Healing and Hard Choices at the End of Life.* Baltimore: Johns Hopkins University Press, 1996.

Quill, Timothy E.; Cassel, Christine K.; and Meier, Diane E. "Care of the Hopelessly Ill: Proposed Clinical Criteria for Physician-Assisted Suicide." *New England Journal of Medicine* 327, no. 19 (November 5, 1992): 1380–1384.

Rachels, James. *The End of Life: Euthanasia and Morality.* New York: Oxford University Press, 1986.

Steinbock, Bonnie, and Norcross, Alastair, eds. *Killing and Letting Die.* 2nd ed. New York: Fordham University Press, 1994.

Symposium on Assisted Suicide. *Hastings Center Report* (May–June 1995).

Thomasma, David C.; Kimbrough-Kushner, Thomasine; Kimsma, Gerrit K.; and Cisesielski-Carlucci, Chris. *Asking to Die: Inside the Dutch Debate about Euthanasia.* Dordrecht, The Netherlands: Kluwer Academic Publishers, 1998.

Velleman, J. David. "Against the Right to Die." *Journal of Medicine and Philosophy* 17, no. 6 (December 1992): 664–681.

Weir, R. F. "The Morality of Physician-Assisted Suicide." *Law, Medicine & Health Care* 20 (1992): 116–126.

PART FOUR

REPROGENETICS

The term "reprogenetics" was coined by Princeton biologist Lee Silver in his 1997 book, *Remaking Eden*, to characterize the merging of assisted reproductive technology (ART) with genetic interventions. For example, a couple at risk of passing on a genetic disorder can use in vitro fertilization (IVF) to create embryos, and then test the embryos for genetic defects using preimplantation genetic diagnosis (PGD). Embryos that have the genetic disorder will be discarded and only unaffected embryos will be replaced in the woman's uterus. Recently PGD has been used not only to prevent the births of children with genetic diseases but also to create children whose genome makes them possible donors for existing siblings with fatal genetic diseases, as in the case study of Molly and Adam Nash. Someday it may be possible to do more than discard affected embryos. It may be possible to genetically modify embryos or gametes to prevent disease in offspring. However, genetic interventions need not be limited to gene therapy, that is, the treatment or prevention of disease. Genetic enhancement, the manipulation of genes to produce desired physical and psychological traits, such as greater intelligence, improved athletic ability, or an outgoing personality, may one day be possible. The union of genetics and reproduction has opened an era in which parents may have an unprecedented ability to select the attributes of their offspring, with profound implications for the entire species.

All of these technologies, as well as cloning and stem cell research, involve creating, manipulating, and discarding embryos. Deciding whether this is morally acceptable means addressing an issue familiar from the abortion debate: the moral status of the human embryo. Part 4 begins with the topic of abortion, in part because abortion remains a morally controversial topic in its own right, in part because of the implications for reprogenetics.

THE MORALITY OF ABORTION

Law and Policy

Nearly thirty years have passed since the Supreme Court struck down restrictive abortion statutes in the landmark decision of *Roe* v. *Wade* (1973), yet the moral battle over abortion continues to rage. On the one side are those who defend the unborn child's right to life; on the other, those who insist that women must be able to make their own decisions about whether to bear a child.

In recent years, the battle over abortion has focused on late-term abortions, which many Americans, even the majority who generally support abortion rights, find morally troubling. In a procedure described by its opponents as "partial-birth abortion" (known medically as intact dilation and extraction), the fetus is partly delivered and its brain suctioned out in order to collapse the skull so that it can pass through the cervix. Congress twice attempted to ban partial-birth abortions, and twice the legislation was vetoed by President Clinton. A number of states passed laws banning partial-birth abortions, laws which were challenged in court. On June 29, 2000, the Supreme Court, in a 5 to 4 decision *(Stenberg* v. *Carhart),* invalidated a Nebraska law banning partial-birth abortions, a decision which rendered similar laws in thirty other states unconstitutional as well. The Court ruled that because the procedure may be the most medically appropriate way of terminating some pregnancies, it cannot constitutionally be banned.

At present, then, the law on abortion is clear. As the Supreme Court has consistently ruled, the constitutional right of privacy protects a woman's decision to terminate her pregnancy up until viability, and even thereafter when necessary to protect her life or health. The morality of abortion, however, remains hotly debated.

Moral Perspectives

The five selections in Section 1 offer philosophical discussions that illuminate the basic moral structure behind the issue of abortion. The abortion controversy poses two fundamental and extraordinarily difficult ethical questions. The first question relates to the moral status of the fetus, and is usually framed as asking whether the fetus is a "human being" or a "person" with a right to life. The second question relates to the moral obligation of a pregnant woman to continue gestating the fetus. It has often been assumed that the answer to the first question determines the answer to the second. That is, it is assumed that if the fetus is a person with a right to life, then abortion is morally wrong. As we will see, things are not that simple. Nevertheless, if the fetus is a full-fledged person, with a right to life, the usual reasons for supporting abortion—that the world is already overpopulated, that children are better-off if they are wanted, that bearing and raising unwanted children imposes serious burdens on women—would appear to be inadequate. We do not think it is right to kill people to prevent overpopulation, nor that parents can kill their unwanted newborns. As for the burdens imposed on women by unwanted pregnancies, it may be objected that the situation is not unique. For example, women are the primary caretakers of elderly parents, but no one thinks that old and senile people may be killed to relieve the burden on their daughters. If abortion is different, it must be because of a difference in moral status between born human beings and fetuses. At the core of the abortion debate is the question of the moral status of the fetus.

This issue is addressed in the first three selections of Section 1. The traditional conservative position is represented in the first selection which comes from the *Evangelium Vitae* by Pope John Paul II. Abortion, according to the Pope, is an "unspeakable crime" because it is "the deliberate and direct killing of a human being." The Pope acknowledges that the decision to have an abortion is often made not for selfish reasons or out of convenience, but to protect important values such as the woman's own health, or to procure a decent standard of living for her family. Nevertheless, he maintains that such reasons "can never justify the deliberate killing of an innocent human being." As for the claim that a fertilized egg is not yet a human being, the Pope responds, "It would never be made human if it were not human already." Nor does this claim rest on religious views such as the occurrence of ensoulment. Rather, "modern genetic science" demonstrates that at fertilization there is a new, individual human being. This human being is to be respected and treated as a person, with a right to life, from the moment of conception.

The classic article by Mary Anne Warren, "On the Moral and Legal Status of Abortion," has set the stage for contemporary debates on abortion, and requires a summary here. Warren argues that the conservative on abortion fails to notice that the term "human being" has two different meanings. The genetic or biological meaning ascribes species membership to an entity. Human embryos and fetuses clearly are human beings in this sense; they are not members of any other species. However, there is another sense of "human being," the moral sense. To ascribe moral humanity to a being is to say that it has full membership in the moral community and is the possessor of certain rights (human rights). Warren thinks that the conservative confuses these two meanings, and that this confusion is responsible for the view that all genetic humans, even human embryos, are moral humans.

In the second selection, "Why Abortion Is Immoral," Don Marquis agrees that it is hard to see why it is reasonable to base moral status on something as arbitrary as the number of chromosomes in one's cells. At the same time, the "person view," which holds that moral status is based on such abilities as self-consciousness, rationality, and language use, has its own difficulties. Proponents of the person view have to explain why their principle, which justifies abortion, does not justify the killing of newborn infants, or the elderly senile, or the severely mentally impaired as well.

Whatever else might be said for the person view, it certainly does not seem to square with or explain our repugnance to infanticide. For this reason, a number of theorists (Sumner 1981, Steinbock 1992) have suggested a weaker criterion of moral status, namely, sentience—the ability to experience pain and pleasure. Sentience theorists maintain that sentience is a necessary condition for having interests and a welfare, and that only beings that have interests and a welfare have moral status. In the third selection, "Why Most Abortions Are Not Wrong," Steinbock outlines this conception of moral status, calling it "the interest view." The implications of the interest view for abortion depend on the factual question: when do fetuses become sentient? Undoubtedly the onset of sentience is gradual, but it probably occurs during the second trimester. Prior to the onset of sentience, abortion is not seriously wrong. Any reason why a woman does not want to become a mother suffices to justify abortion: After the fetus becomes sentient, its interests must be balanced against those of the pregnant woman. This accords with a moderate view on abortion in which the reasons for having an abortion must be proportionately more compelling as the fetus develops and acquires more of the characteristics of born human beings.

One difficulty for sentience theorists is the status of nonhuman animals. Just as the challenge for person theorists is to explain why it would be wrong to kill human infants, the challenge for sentience theorists is to explain why it is not seriously wrong to kill (most) animals. Some theorists in both camps are willing to "bite the bullet" and accept the counterintuitive implications of their views. Michael Tooley, a person theorist, thinks infanticide is not generally wrong (Tooley 1983), and Peter Singer, a sentience theorist, thinks the killing of animals is usually wrong (Singer 1975). Sentience theorists who want to ascribe a greater moral status to sentient human beings than to animals must explain why this is rational. One possibility is to differentiate among sentient beings, giving greater moral status to sentient beings who are also persons or potentially persons, because of the centrality of personhood to moral agency and responsibility (Steinbock 1992).

Marquis maintains that the sentience view is no improvement over the person view, and both are as flawed as the genetic humanity criterion for moral status. The solution, Marquis suggests, is to stop looking for what gives an entity human moral status. Instead, we should develop a general account of the wrongness of killing people, and then see if abortion is included in this account. What makes killing wrong is the loss of the victim's future—in particular, a future like ours (or FLO, as it has come to be called). This principle differs from the traditional pro-life position in two ways. First, it is not based on the special value of human life; it is not "speciesist." If there are nonhuman aliens or animals with a future like ours, however that is interpreted, they too have a right to life. Second, Marquis notes that his principle does not rule out practices opposed by most pro-lifers. For example, on Marquis's view, it might not be wrong to kill someone in a persistent vegetative state (PVS), who will never regain consciousness, because such a person no longer has a valuable future. A fetus, however, usually does have a valuable future and therefore abortion is almost always immoral. It is immoral for the same reason that it would be wrong to kill you or me: to do so would deprive us of our valuable futures.

Marquis thinks that the FLO account is superior to the interest view because the FLO account can explain what is wrong with killing people who are temporarily unconscious, while the interest view, he says, cannot. Bonnie Steinbock responds to this objection by saying that someone who is temporarily unconscious has had desires and preferences in the past, which form the basis for saying he would not want to be killed now. However, even if the FLO account is the correct account of the wrongness of killing, it is not clear it has the implications for abortion that Marquis claims. Steinbock argues that this depends on the theory of personal identity one accepts. On a psychological theory of identity, it is not clear that the adult is "the same person" as the preconscious fetus, as it lacks any thoughts, memories, or experiences that could connect them. There is continuous physical development between the fetus and the adult, and this could justify the claim that they are "the same individual," given a physical continuity view of identity. However, there is also physical continuity between the fetus and the embryo, and between the embryo and the gametes that combined to produce it. Why, then, is it only fetuses that have FLO; why not gametes? But if gametes have FLO, then Marquis, it seems, is committed to regarding contraception as being as morally wrong as abortion—a consequence that Marquis strenuously wishes to avoid.

So far, we have been looking only at arguments that focus on the status of the fetus. This leaves out entirely the pregnant woman whose body sustains the fetus. Judith Jarvis Thomson's novel contribution to the abortion debate is to point out that settling the moral status of the fetus does not necessarily determine the morality of abortion. In "A Defense of Abortion," Thomson argues that the anti-abortion argument based on the fetus's right-to-life argument is logically flawed. The conclusion—that abortion is wrong—does not follow from the premise that the fetus is a person, with a right to life. For the argument does not show that killing the fetus *violates* its right to life. This may sound paradoxical: if the fetus has a right to life, and abortion kills it, surely its right to life is violated? But this is precisely what Thomson wishes to deny. The core of her argument is that a right to life does not carry with it the right to whatever one may need to stay alive. Much of Thomson's article discusses whether the woman's (partial) responsibility for the fetus's existence in her body does give the fetus-person a right to use her body. If her responsibility for the fetus does give it a right to use her body, then her refusal to let it remain in her body could be seen as depriving the fetus of what it has a right to, and this would make abortion unjust killing. Somewhat ironically, although Thomson's article is intended as a defense of abortion, her argument has great appeal for people who think that abortion is generally wrong, but wish to make an exception in the case of rape. If the woman was clearly not responsible for her pregnancy, as in the case of rape, then she cannot be said to have given the fetus a right to use her body. Thus, abortion in the case of rape is not unjust killing, and does not violate the fetus's right to life.

Thomson tries to show that nonresponsibility extends beyond the rape scenario; that, for example, a woman who has a contraceptive failure also has not given the fetus a right to use her body. She then goes on to consider whether a woman *ought*—out of common decency—to allow the fetus-person to use her body, even if it has no right to do so. Thomson rejects this suggestion, however, saying that the sacrifice on the part of the pregnant woman is too great. No one is morally required to make large sacrifices in order to keep another person alive. This part of Thomson's article inspired an "equal protection" argument against restrictive abortion laws, on the grounds that requiring women, but not men, to be "Good Samaritans" violates equal protection (Regan 1979). Despite its title, Thomson's article is best read not as a general defense of abortion, but rather as a focused critique of the conservative argument against abortion, in particular, the claim that abortion is immoral because the fetus has a right to life. However, even if Thomson is correct about the limitations of rights in general, and the right to life in particular, it could still be possible to argue that abortion is wrong. If the fetus is a person, then it is a special person, namely, the pregnant woman's child. Parents have special obligations, that strangers do not, to nurture and protect their children.

Margaret Olivia Little takes up this issue in the last selection. She maintains that even if abortion is not a "wrongful interference," as Thomson has argued, it might still be morally wrong. "If fetuses are persons, the question we really need to decide is what positive responsibilities, if any, do pregnant women have to continue gestational assistance? This is a question that takes us into far richer, and far more interesting, territory than that occupied by discussions of murder." In part, this is a question of what we owe others as a matter of general beneficence. It is much more than that, however, due to the unique nature of gestation. This has been virtually ignored in mainstream philosophical discussions of abortion, and this "has ended up deeply underselling the moral complexity of abortion."

Just as pro-lifers oversimplify the situation by assuming that the wrongness of abortion follows from the personhood of the fetus, so too pro-choicers oversimplify matters by assuming that it follows from the nonpersonhood of the fetus that abortion is morally neutral. Even if fetuses are not persons, and not owed the respect due to persons, they still might be, as Little put it, *"respect-worthy."* Exactly what this means and entails is an issue revisited in Section 5.

Most women have abortions because they do not want to have a child. A subset of abortions are undertaken by women who want to have a child, but wish to avoid having a child who will have a serious genetic disease. Section 2 addresses the moral and policy implications of genetic testing for reproductive decisions.

CARRIER SCREENING, PRENATAL TESTING, AND REPRODUCTIVE DECISIONS

Approximately 3 percent of all children are born with a severe disorder that is presumed to be genetic in origin, and several thousand definite or suspected "single-gene" diseases have been described. Among the better known are cystic fibrosis (CF), Tay-Sachs disease, and Huntington's disease (HD). Most genetic diseases manifest early in life, though some inherited diseases—and many others that have a genetic component—have their onset later in life: for example, HD and hemochromatosis. There are many disorders in which both genetic and environmental factors play major roles, including coronary heart disease, obesity, and hypertension. The more we learn about genetics, the more we learn about the genetic causes of disease. "It has become increasingly evident that virtually all human afflictions, from cancer to psychiatric disorders, and susceptibility to infection, are rooted in our genes" (Merz, 2001).

Since 1990, much of our understanding of "the new genetics" has been propelled by the Human Genome Project (HGP). An international project, involving hundreds of scientists worldwide, the HGP has facilitated the discovery of thousands of gene markers, and new tests are being developed every day. Its goal is to find the location of all human genes and to sequence the chemical bases in human DNA, all 3 billion bits of information, by the year 2005. At one point, scientists estimated the number of human genes at around 100,000, though this estimation was reduced in the rough draft of the HGP, which put the number at around 30,000–35,000. Nevertheless, some scientists believe that the number of human genes will ultimately be shown to be much higher. The HGP will help scientists find the source of nearly 4,000 known genetic disorders, as well as diseases that are produced in part by genetic malfunctions and various normal human traits.

A distinction is often drawn between genetic screening and genetic testing. Genetic screening usually refers to a public health program performed on a whole population, or some subset, such as an ethnic group at high risk for a particular disease. Screening could be done to discover which people have or are likely to develop a disease, although they are as yet asymptomatic, or it could be done to identify carriers, that is, those who will not develop the disease but who could pass it to offspring. By contrast, genetic testing, or clinical genetic testing, as it is sometimes called, refers to a procedure performed on an individual because of that individual's risk factors. Many geneticists think that the distinction is very important because the purposes are different. Screening is done to decide where best to target public health programs aimed at reducing the incidence of disease in the group as a whole, whereas genetic testing is done to help individuals make personal medical (and other) decisions, including reproductive decisions. However, Norman Fost says that he does not find the distinction a particularly useful one in considering the ethical issues.

> All screening programs involve performing a test on individuals. If the program is voluntary, then at least minimal standards for consent are implied and the issues overlap substantially with what is called testing. Conversely, some forms of testing are so widespread as to constitute a standard of practice and have become de facto screening programs. The central question is what ethical principles and policies should guide proposals to perform a test on an asymptomatic individual or population of individuals. (Fost 1992, p. 2813)

An example that illustrates the fine line between testing and screening is prenatal genetic testing. In the United States, it is recommended that pregnant women over the age of 35 be offered prenatal testing for Down syndrome. Should this be regarded as clinical genetic testing based on the individual's risk factor (age)? Perhaps, but today many pregnant women under 35 undergo prenatal testing for Down syndrome. It has become so routine that it might be viewed as a screening program, rather than genetic testing based on individual risk factors. Moreover, prenatal testing for Down syndrome can be used both to help individuals make reproductive decisions and to reduce the incidence of Down syndrome in the population.

The number of genetic tests developed and employed is rapidly expanding. The tests assist in medical diagnosis, including diagnosis where it was previously impossible (e.g., presymptomatic diagnosis or identification of unaffected carriers of a gene), or where swift diagnosis can be helpful (e.g., prenatal diagnosis and newborn screening). Better understanding of the complex interactions among environment, behavior, and genes enables public health officials to identify appropriate populations to target for public health interventions (Gostin, Hodge, and Calvo 2001). Genetic screening can help to promote the public's health, but also raises both pragmatic questions about the efficacy and cost-effectiveness of screening programs, as well as ethical questions relating to informed consent, confidentiality, privacy, and discrimination. One question for public policy is whom to test for which genetic disease, since it would be prohibitively expensive to test everyone for everything. Since many genetic diseases are associated with ethnic, racial, or geographic heritage, targeting tests to members of specific groups is a possibility. However, such targeting can be problematic. For one thing, race and ethnicity are not biological, but cultural constructions. Some people who consider themselves "white" may have the same number of African ancestors as others who are considered "black." A person's racial identity is at best a guide to his or her genetic inheritance. For this reason, *all* newborns in New York State are screened for sickle-cell anemia, not just those who appear to be African-Americans. Another problem with genetic testing based on ethnic or racial grouping is that this may lead to stigmatization (Fost 1992).

Using the example of cystic fibrosis (CF), Wilfond and Fost provide several reasons in the section's first article for being cautious about instituting screening programs, especially mass screening programs. About 30,000 Americans have cystic fibrosis (CF), the most common fatal hereditary disorder affecting white people in the United States. CF is an autosomal recessive disorder. This means that in order to get the disease, a child must receive one mutant allele from each parent. The parents usually do not have the disease, but rather are carriers. If two carriers reproduce, they have a 25 percent chance with every pregnancy of having a child with CF. The chance that the child will be a carrier is 50 percent, and the chance that the child will be entirely unaffected is 25 percent. The prevalence of CF is related to ethnic background. The chance of being a carrier for CF is about 1 in 30 (3 percent) for those of European descent, 1 in 46 for Hispanic Americans, 1 in 65 for African Americans, and 1 in 90 for Asian Americans. Severity of the disease varies greatly. While in general people with CF have a shortened life span, some die in childhood, and others live into their 40s or even longer. There is no cure for CF, although research on more effective treatments is under way. Despite breathing and digestive problems, many people with CF attend school, have careers, and have fulfilling lives.

In 1989, when scientists isolated the gene that causes CF, many of them believed that screening for the gene would provide the prototype for national screening programs to combat other dread diseases, in addition to providing widespread prenatal diagnosis for couples who are found to carry the mutated CF gene. However, the issue has proven to be more complex than originally thought. Nearly 1000 mutations that can cause CF have been identified. The current test picks out the most common mutation, the Delta F508 mutation, which accounts for about 70 percent of cases. However, there are some mutations in the CF gene that the current test cannot find. For this reason, a negative test is not a guarantee that a couple will not have a baby with CF, though the likelihood of this happening is very small.

In addition to carrier testing, prenatal testing can be performed on fetuses. One of the problems with such testing in the past is that a positive result did not invariably signify that the child, if born, would develop full-blown cystic fibrosis. Their symptoms might be much less serious disorders, including infertility, asthma, or chronic bronchitis. Many couples who would abort a pregnancy if the fetus were affected with the severe lung and digestive problems characteristic of CF would not abort for these less-serious disorders, complicating decisions about being tested and how to respond to test results. In recent years, testing has become more sophisticated and more precise. The different clinical forms of CF can be tied to specific mutations in the CF gene, which means that a more precise prognosis can be given to prospective parents on the basis of DNA testing.

Some geneticists think that since the current test can pick up approximately 90 percent of carriers, it is appropriate to offer it, and they argue that it should be up to patients to decide whether they want to be tested. Others say that it is pointless, even harmful, to offer testing to individuals who do not have a family history of the disease, since it would offer uncertainty rather than reassurance or guidance to most of them. In 1997, a panel of experts from the National Institutes of Health recommended that genetic testing for CF should be offered to all couples currently planning a pregnancy and to couples seeking prenatal testing, whether or not they have a family history of CF. A similar recommendation was recently made by the American College of Medical Genetics (ACMG) and the American College of Gynecologists and Obstetricians (ACGO), endorsing carrier screening for *all* reproductive couples for 25 specified mutations (the most common ones) of CF. It is not clear who would offer genetic testing for CF to couples *planning* a pregnancy, since couples without a family history of CF are unlikely to consult a genetics counselor or physician before starting a family. ACGO also recommends offering pregnant women carrier testing for CF on a voluntary basis, noting that it is a very personal decision which belongs to the pregnant woman and the father of her baby.

Prenatal testing for genetic disease can be seen from a public health perspective, which has the reduction of genetic disease as a principal goal, or from the perspective of individuals and couples making reproductive decisions. At the present time, genetic defects can be detected, but most cannot be corrected. Thus, testing can be used by the prospective parents to prepare for the birth of an affected child or, more commonly, as the basis for selective abortion. Thus, the prospective parents' views on the morality of abortion are relevant to their attitudes toward prenatal testing. Other relevant factors include their attitudes toward disability, and which traits they consider serious enough to test for. In the second selection in Section 2, "Ethical Issues Related to Prenatal Genetic Testing," the American Medical Association's Council on Ethical and Judicial Affairs says that a misuse of prenatal genetic testing would be "to ensure that children possess certain characteristics that should be irrelevant in an egalitarian society" and gives sex selection as a prime example. The council acknowledges the potential for discrimination, even when prenatal testing is used only to avoid genetic disease, because this might increase negative attitudes toward the disabled. Nevertheless, the council maintains that the use of genetic technology to avoid the birth of a child with a genetic disorder is in accordance with the physician's therapeutic role, although abortion or discard based on nondisease traits would be inappropriate. In the next selection, Adrienne Asch rejects the disease/nondisease distinction characteristic of the medical model. She argues that the medical paradigm contains a profound misunderstanding of disability. Most people with disabilities are healthy, not sick, and the problems they face stem not from the disability itself, but from discriminatory social arrangements. A public health approach, according to Asch, should not be focused on testing to prevent the births of children who will have disabilities, but rather on changing social arrangements so that all children, whatever their abilities, can reach their full potential.

Preimplantation genetic diagnosis (PGD) may seem morally less problematic than prenatal testing and abortion, because affected embryos are discarded at a very early stage in their development and before a pregnancy has been instantiated. However, as Jeffrey R. Botkin points out in the fourth selection, for those who view the fertilized human egg to be of equal moral status with the late-gestation fetus (and indeed any born human being), PGD is worse than abortion, since it involves a greater loss of human life. PGD also has the disadvantage of requiring the creation of embryos through IVF, with all the attendant risk and expense of that procedure. Furthermore, most clinicians recommend that PGD be followed up with prenatal diagnosis, which means that the abortion decision may still have to be faced. All of these considerations make PGD less attractive as a method of prenatal diagnosis than it might at first appear. Botkin also considers the disability critique, acknowledging that "If prenatal diagnosis and PGD specifically were to have a significantly negative effect on the millions of disabled individuals in society, this would be a powerful argument for limiting or discouraging its use, at least for less than serious medical conditions." However, he does not think that it would have this effect. Despite the use of prenatal diagnosis for several decades, individuals with disabilities have never had more social support than they have today. Of greater concern, from Botkin's perspective, is the use of PGD to select against minor conditions or for desirable characteristics.

Bonnie Steinbock presents a case study in which PGD was used not simply to avoid having a child with a lethal genetic disease, but also to provide a tissue match for an existing child. Does this treat the child who is created as "spare parts," and thus violate the Kantian dictum against treating others merely as means to our ends? Steinbock argues that this depends on whether the child will be loved and cherished for his own sake, regardless of the reasons for creating him in the first place. Nevertheless, the potential for misuse of PGD that was of concern to Botkin is raised by the Nash case study. Will screening embryos for tissue type lead to screening for other characteristics, such as gender, height, or even intelligence? Is this the kind of choice prospective parents should have? And if not, are the dangers of the misuse of PGD sufficient to deny people in the Nashes' situation from using PGD to save an existing child?

So far, we have been discussing whether it is morally permissible for prospective parents to use prenatal testing to avoid the birth of a child with a genetic disease. In the last selection in Section 2 Allen Buchanan, Dan W. Brock, Norman Daniels, and Daniel Wikler raise the question of whether parents might have a moral obligation to use genetic testing to avoid the birth of a child with a severe genetic impairment. When, if ever, is it wrong to have a child who might have a serious disability? This question raises both practical and conceptual questions. The practical question is, what are prospective parents morally required to do to avoid the birth of a severely disabled child? Everyone would agree that prospective parents should take reasonable steps to prevent the "not-yet-born child" from developing a disability (Steinbock 1992). For example, pregnant women should not smoke (and prospective fathers should not smoke around their wives) or drink or use unprescribed drugs. They should take prenatal vitamins, including folic acid, to prevent the fetus from developing spina bifida, a neural tube disorder. But should prospective parents use genetic testing to learn if they are at risk of having a child with a genetic disease, and if so, either avoid conception or terminate a pregnancy to avoid that outcome? Some, like Asch, would argue that there is no moral obligation to prevent the births of people with genetic diseases. Indeed, while she stops short of claiming that there is a moral obligation *not* to engage in selective abortion or embryo discard, she implies that those who wish to do so are either ignorant of disability or lacking in virtues ideally possessed by parents. By contrast, Buchanan et al. argue that there is a moral obligation to prevent the births of people with serious genetic diseases. The deeply philosophical issue is the explanation of that obligation.

In the Introduction of *From Chance to Choice*, the book from which the last selection is taken, the authors say, ". . . we argue that the most straightforward and compelling case for developing and using genetic interventions is to fulfill one of the most basic moral obligations human beings have: the obligation to prevent harm" (Buchanan et al. 2000, p. 18). However, in many cases, the only way to prevent the genetic harm is to prevent the child's birth. That is, the choice facing a couple at risk of transmitting a genetic disease to their offspring is *not* between having this child in an impaired condition and having this child "healthy and whole." The choice is rather between having this child in an impaired condition and not having this child. This raises the troubling questions: Can one protect a child by preventing it from being born? Can birth in an impaired condition be unfair to the child?

This problem has been much discussed in the philosophical literature, notably by Derek Parfit, so that it is often referred to as "the Parfit problem." It is also the basis of a novel tort, the tort of "wrongful life." The tort is very controversial, for reasons that are legal, philosophical, and political, and it is recognized as a cause of action in only three states (New Jersey, California, and Washington). From a philosophical perspective, the wrong to the child is based on the idea that when life is filled with suffering and bereft of compensating pleasures, life is not a benefit but a harm (Steinbock 1986, Feinberg 1987). The child has been wronged by being given a life that is not a good to the child, from his or her own perspective. Some would argue that life is *always* worth living, no matter how great the suffering, no matter how limited the child's existence. But this seems to be more a matter of faith (or perhaps a failure of imagination) than a defensible position. Nevertheless, as Asch points out, and Buchanan et al. agree, most people with disabilities, even severe disabilities, find their lives worth living. Buchanan et al. term such cases "wrongful disabilities" to distinguish them from "wrongful life" cases. The challenge is to say what the "wrong" is in "wrongful disability" cases. Why is it wrong to have children who will have lives that are, on balance, worth living?

John Robertson has forcefully argued that, as long as the child can be expected to have a life worth living, procreation is not a wrong to the child (Robertson 1994). He concludes that protecting offspring is never, or hardly ever, a rationale for restricting procreative choice. This may sound startling. Surely, it may be asked, we should think about the welfare of children when assessing new reproductive technologies? (This is an explicit requirement of the Human Fertilization and Embryology Authority, which licenses fertility clinics in the United Kingdom.) For example, if a reproductive technique was found to be associated with a higher incidence of disability in offspring, that would presumably be a reason to ban it. Suppose we discovered that intracytoplasmic sperm injection (ICSI), in which a single sperm is injected directly into the egg, increased the risk of having a child with cystic fibrosis. One theory is that some men are infertile because they have a mild case of CF. They do not have any of the lung or digestive problems associated with CF, but only infertility. Enabling them to reproduce via ICSI, when ordinarily they would not be able to reproduce, means that some of them will transmit the mutated allele to their child, and (if the mother is also a carrier) might result in the birth of a child with CF. Robertson does not think that this would justify banning ICSI. The decision to use ICSI, or any other reproductive technology, should be up to the infertile couple. They may, of course, wish to avoid having a child with CF, and they should be told of the risk so that they can make an informed decision. However, it does not make sense to ban the technique in order to protect *the child*, for banning the technique would also prevent the child, who has no other way of getting born, from existing. As Robertson puts it, "But for the technique in question, the child never would have been born. Whatever psychological or social problems arise, they hardly rise to the level of severe handicap or disability that would make the child's very existence a net burden, and hence a wrongful life" (Robertson 1994, p. 122).

In other words, Robertson is willing to acknowledge that birth can be seen as a harm and a wrong to the child if, but only if, the child's life is likely to be so awful that it constitutes "wrongful life" (a life that, from the child's own perspective, is not worth living). Buchanan et al. agree. Such cases are likely to be rare, but in these few cases, they conclude that "it would be clearly and seriously morally wrong for individuals to risk conceiving and having . . . a child." They hasten to add that they do not support forced abortion, which would be "so deeply invasive of [the woman's] reproductive freedom, bodily integrity, and right to decide about her own health care as to be virtually never morally justified."

What about wrongful disability cases? Again, Buchanan et al. agree with Robertson: the child in a wrongful disability case has not been harmed in the ordinary sense of harm. However, they disagree that no serious moral wrong has been done. The wrong is allowing the birth of a child in a harmful condition, when this could have been prevented. This is brought out in their example, P1, in which a woman can avoid having a child with moderate mental retardation by taking medication and delaying pregnancy for one month. However, delaying pregnancy means that a different child will be born, one conceived from a different egg (and sperm). Thus, delaying pregnancy changes the identity of the child, making this a "nonidentity" problem. If the woman decides not to wait, she cannot be said to have harmed the child who gets born, for that child could not have been born any other way, and moderate mental retardation is not a plausible candidate for wrongful life. Nevertheless, the harm is "avoidable by substitution" (Peters 1989). That is, the woman could have a mentally normal child simply by taking the medication and delaying pregnancy for one month. Since this imposes virtually no hardship on her, and prevents the birth of a moderately retarded child, waiting is the right thing to do. This suggests that we need to revise or extend our conception of harm to fit wrongful disability cases by including in our moral theory some non-person-affecting principles.

There has been considerable experience with newborn screening, prenatal diagnosis, and carrier testing in high-risk populations. New genetic tests are being developed for diseases with a significant genetic component that manifest in middle and late life, diseases like coronary heart disease and diabetes. Whereas the older genetic tests are used to discover relatively rare genetic conditions, the new tests will identify susceptibility to fairly common disorders. This could have a significant benefit for the public's health, but also poses potential risks of discrimination and stigmatization. Another new development made possible by advances in genetics is genomic medicine, in which drugs are tailored to the individual's genetic make-up. In November 2001, researchers reported in *JAMA* that giving women who have the BRCA2 mutation the drug tamoxifen while they are still healthy can prevent them from developing breast cancer, while women with the BRCA1 mutation got little or no benefit from the drug ("Genetic Testing of Women Aids in Cancer Fight," *New York Times*, November 14, 2001, p. A16). On the horizon is the possibility of genetic interventions to prevent or cure disease: gene therapy. These issues are taken up in Section 3.

MAPPING THE HUMAN GENOME: IMPLICATIONS FOR GENETIC TESTING, GENETIC COUNSELING, AND GENETIC INTERVENTIONS

Science is moving closer to understanding the genetics of adult disorders such as Alzheimer's disease, various cancers, heart disease, and arthritis, to name a few. We do not yet understand why some people with a certain gene develop a disease and others do not. The complexities involved in determining susceptibility, sorting out environmental influences, and devising strategies for genetic counseling and treatment will pose tremendous challenges in the future.

Predictive or presymptomatic testing and screening can help determine which adults are at higher risk for genetic disease. For monogenic disorders of late onset, such as Huntington's disease, the test is usually highly predictive. Anyone who inherits the mutant allele for HD will almost certainly develop the disease. Many common diseases, including coronary artery disease, cancer, high blood pressure, rheumatoid arthritis, and some psychiatric diseases have multifactorial causation, including both multiple genetic and environmental factors. Because the etiology of these diseases is so complex, the prediction that a particular individual will develop a disease at some point in his or her life is much less certain. In the first selection in Section 3, Francis S. Collins, Lowell Weiss, and Kathy Hudson give a short and trenchant introduction to the complexity of genetic influence and the importance of avoiding the fallacies of genetic determinism and reductionism.

Genetic testing of presymptomatic individuals enables them to benefit from early intervention (if it is available). It may enable them to protect their health by making the right decisions about diet, workplace, and lifestyle. However, the potential benefits of presymptomatic interventions must be weighed against the potential anxiety they may induce, stigmatization, and other possible harms to individuals who are informed that they are at increased risk of developing future disease. An example of anxiety induced by predictive testing is the reaction that some women have had upon learning that they have the genetic mutations for breast cancer. They have had their breasts prophylactically removed, although radical mastectomy is not always necessary even after breast cancer is diagnosed. Some see a significant danger of discrimination from genetic testing. "Several studies in scientific journals suggest that many people have been asked questions about genetic diseases on job applications, and some workers report that they have been denied jobs or dismissed from jobs because of genetic conditions in the family" (Robert Pear, "Clinton Bans Use of Genetic Makeup in Federal Employment," *New York Times*, February 9, 2000, p. A16). Others maintain that most of the studies merely collect anecdotal claims by people who think they have been discriminated against. With no way to check out their stories, these self-reported claims are not evidence of existing genetic discrimination. Nevertheless, there is a concern that, unless legislative barriers are put in place, employers might not hire people at high risk for genetic disease, or those genetically susceptible to environmental contaminants in the workplace. Insurers might use genetic information as a basis for denying people health or life insurance.

Thomas H. Murray argues that this would be discriminatory and unfair. In a relatively early (1992) article on the topic of genetic discrimination in health insurance, "Genetics and the Moral Mission of Health Insurance," Murray questions whether the concept of "actuarial fairness" (charging people premiums based on their expected risk) is an adequate criterion of fairness in health insurance. As Norman Daniels, using a Rawlsian analysis, has argued, justice requires that we protect fair equality of opportunity for individuals. Reasonable access to health care is a necessary condition of fair equality of opportunity. Murray writes, "The social purpose of health insurance, understood in this way, is to provide access to the health care that people need to have a fair opportunity in life." A similar view was adopted by a committee created by the Institute of Medicine (IOM) of the National Academy of Sciences. In its 1994 report, *Assessing Genetic Risks,* the committee recommended that legislation be adopted to prevent medical risks, including genetic risks, from being taken into account in decisions whether to issue or how to price health insurance. "Because health insurance differs significantly from other types of insurance in that it regulates access to health care—an important social good—risk-based health insurance should be eliminated" (Andrews et al. 1994, p. 24). Access to health care, the report maintained, should be available to every American without regard to an individual's present health status or condition.

The federal government has developed genetic law and policy within all three branches in response to the proliferation of genetic information. The most important examples of federal legislation include the Americans with Disabilities Act of 1990 (ADA), which forbids employers, government agencies, and public accommodations from discriminating against persons with disabilities, where these disabilities are unrelated to job performance, and the Health Insurance Portability and Accountability Act of 1996 (HIPAA). This law prevents the disclosure of health information for purposes unrelated to health care (e.g., employment, insurance, or mortgage eligibility) without explicit patient authorization and also prohibits discrimination in access to health insurance based on an individual's health status or health status–related factors. While this law offers considerable protection in theory, many commentators are pessimistic about its ability to protect the privacy and confidentiality of medical records, if only because these records are available to so many people. In addition, while the law prohibits insurance companies from considering genetic susceptibility to disease in providing coverage or setting prices, it may be difficult to prove that a company has violated the law. Beyond the ADA and HIPAA, Congress has also proposed multiple genetic-specific privacy and anti-discrimination bills. "Some proposed laws would restrict group health plans and issuers of health insurance coverage in connection to a group health plan from evaluation eligibility based on requests for genetic services, requesting genetic tests and information, and disclosing predictive genetic testing information to certain parties" (Gostin, Hodge, and Calvo 2001).

Another controversial area is genetic counseling. There is a strong tradition of nondirectiveness in medical genetics, particularly in reproductive decision making. Roughly, the term "nondirectiveness" means that patients should make their own decisions about genetic testing, based on their own values, without being pressured or unduly influenced by the values of the counselor. However, this tradition of nondirectiveness contrasts sharply with other areas of medicine. Most physicians recognize an obligation to provide appropriate medical *advice,* not simply information (see Part 1, "Foundations of the Health Professional Patient-Relationship.") Why, then, it may be asked, should there be such strong support for the principle of nondirective counseling for *reproductive* decisions? One important reason is the history of eugenics during the late nineteenth and early twentieth centuries in the United States (Reilly 1991) and Europe. Forcible sterilizations of the "feeble-minded" were carried out as late as the 1970s. Some of those who were sterilized on eugenic grounds were not, in fact, mentally retarded. Many were poor or members of minority groups, or institutionalized for other reasons, such as becoming pregnant out of wedlock. Sterilization programs were often instituted not to protect children from incompetent parents who might neglect or abuse them, but out of the belief that some individuals or "races" are inferior and ought not to reproduce. In light of this sordid chapter in our history, it is no surprise that genetics counselors have been reluctant to impose their own values regarding the births of children with disabling conditions on prospective parents.

In addition, some writers on genetic counseling are pessimistic that such counseling can ever be genuinely nondirective (Bernhardt 1997). These issues are addressed in "Patient Autonomy and Value-Neutrality in Nondirective Genetic Counseling" by Robert Wachbroit and David Wasserman. Part of the problem is that the term "nondirective" is used to cover two distinct concerns: value-neutrality and patient autonomy. Value-neutrality is probably impossible, but they argue that genetics counselors do not need to be value-neutral in order to promote patient autonomy. This does not imply, however, that respecting the patient's autonomy is an easy or obvious task, for a range of psychological and philosophical reasons. They end with a discussion of the role of genetic counselors regarding individual reproductive decisions that may, in the aggregate, have harmful social consequences. Sex selection is an obvious example, but this is only the tip of the iceberg. For example, should genetics counselors inform patients about prenatal tests for conditions that are not life-threatening but impairing or socially undesirable, such as obesity or homosexuality, as these become available? Does respect for autonomy entail giving people all the procreative choices they may wish to make? This question brings us back to the issue raised in Part 1: the nature and scope of autonomy.

With the advent of molecular biology in the 1960s and of the recombinant deoxyribonucleic acid (DNA) era in the early 1970s came the possibility for a new kind of treatment: gene therapy. Gene therapy attempts to treat diseases that result from errors in the structure or function of genes by adding new genes to cells or by substituting new genes for original malfunctioning genes. Sickle cell anemia, cystic fibrosis, rheumatoid arthritis, familial hypercholesterolemia, coronary artery disease, cancer, and AIDS are among the diseases that might someday be successfully treated with gene therapy.

A thorough overview of the ethical issues in human gene transfer research—the research that may one day produce genuine gene therapies—is provided by Eric Juengst and LeRoy Walters in the fourth selection in Section 3. One issue concerns the distinction between somatic cell gene therapy and germ-line gene therapy. Somatic cell gene therapy is directed toward somatic cells, that is, all the cells of the body except for gametes. By contrast, germ-line genetic interventions would aim to correct genetic defects in gametes (sperm and ova) and embryos. All of the usual ethical issues in experimental treatment (safety, efficacy, informed consent) apply to both kinds of gene therapy, but germ-line gene therapy is thought to pose special ethical issues because changes in the germ-line can be passed on to the patient's offspring. This means that any mistakes could affect generations to come, making questions of safety even more pressing than in other types of experimental therapies. In addition, changing the germ-line offers an unprecedented, and some would say frightening, potential for deliberately changing the human species.

So far, all of this is in the future. Although gene therapy has grown enormously from its beginnings in 1990, when a 4-year-old girl became the first patient to be treated with genes, it remains experimental. Prior to 2000, despite hundreds of studies involving thousands of patients suffering from a variety of diseases, the field had yet to document its first cure. A 1996 report from the National Institutes of Health (NIH) Recombinant DNA Advisory Committee (RAC) stated, "It is clearly too early . . . to assess the therapeutic efficacy of gene therapy or even to predict its promise. Numerous studies have reported the ability to express recombinant DNA in vivo, but few have reported clinical efficacy. . . . The few 'dramatic' successes claimed are not dissimilar to those that were reported with a variety of other therapeutic techniques for which enthusiasm ultimately dampened over time" (Ross 1996, p. 1789). Reviewing the history of gene therapy, LeRoy Walter writes, "In retrospect, one can discern a clear, though gradual downward trajectory in human gene transfer research in the U.S. from the end of 1995 through late 1999" (Walters 2000, p. 340).

Gene transfer research received an enormous blow on September 17, 1999 when Jesse Gelsinger, an 18-year-old young man who had ornithine transcarbamylase (OTC) deficiency, died as a direct result of having received gene transfer with an adenoviral vector. "The tragedy was compounded by the fact that Mr. Gelsinger's disease had been relatively well controlled through all of 1999 by a combination of drugs and diet" (Walters 2000, p. 340). In January 2000, the federal government halted all gene therapy studies at the University of Pennsylvania's Institute for Human Gene Therapy, saying that the school's program was in serious disarray. Penn could not provide investigators with proof that any of the volunteers in the fatal study had been eligible to participate or had been adequately warned of the risks of the research. At a Senate hearing in February 2000, Mr. Gelsinger's father asserted that he and his son had not been told that monkeys in preclinical trials of earlier generations of adenoviral vectors had died. Mr. Gelsinger also reported that he and his son had been led to believe that the son's participation in the gene transfer study was likely to be clinically beneficial, even though the study was a Phase I trial. Phase I trials are done simply to test for safety and are not intended or expected to have any clinical benefit to participants. Nevertheless, it is not uncommon for patients who enroll in Phase I trials to think that they will benefit from the trial, and researchers who want them to enroll may fail to disabuse them of this notion with sufficient vigor. Walters comments, "The future success of gene transfer in the treatment of disease cannot be guaranteed. What can definitively be achieved, however, is the creation of a transparent, accountable oversight system that assures that the human subjects who make this research possible will be dealt with honestly and with the highest measure of respect" (Walters 2000, p. 341). (See Part 5 for further discussion of research with human subjects.)

Gene therapy had its first real success in April 2000. Researchers in Paris announced that they had successfully treated three babies with gene therapy for severe combined immune deficiency, or SCID. The only other treatment for SCID is a bone marrow transplant, which works just 60 percent of the time. Otherwise, patients with SCID must live in germ-free bubbles. "The success proves that gene therapy can work, researchers said, but the patients had a disease that is especially suited for the treatment. The researchers cautioned that the method might not be immediately applicable to other diseases" (Gina Kolata, "Scientists Report the First Success of Gene Therapy," *New York Times,* April 28, 2000, p. Al). Some researchers, acknowledging the premature celebration of gene therapy in the mid-90s, point to recent successes as the real beginning of the new revolution in medicine. Others remain skeptical.

If somatic cell gene therapy is just beginning to be successful, germ-line gene therapy is even further in the future. As Juengst and Walters point out, "For gene-therapy techniques to be effective, the genes must be stably integrated, expressed correctly and only in the appropriate tissues, and reliably targeted to the correct location on a chromosome. . . . Critics maintain that, given the complexity of gene regulation and expression during human development germ-line gene-transfer experiments will always involve too many unpredictable long-term iatrogenic risks to the transformed subjects and their offspring to be justifiable." However, proponents argue that this justifies not a permanent ban, but only a postponement of human trials. Recent successes in animal research raises the possibility that we will eventually have the technical capacity to modify genes that are transmitted to future generations. The question then is whether we ought to develop these techniques, and the answer to that question depends on the potential benefits and harms. Germ-line gene therapy would, in theory, have several advantages over somatic cell gene therapy. If successful, it could prevent the inheritance of some genetically based diseases within families without having to repeat somatic therapy generation after generation. Because germ-line intervention would influence the earliest stage of human development, it might prevent irreversible damage caused by defective genes before it occurs. Over time, germ-line gene therapy might decrease the incidence of certain inherited diseases in the human gene pool.

Those opposed to germ-line modifications argue that it is unlikely that their use would be confined to the treatment of disease, but would also be aimed at enhancement, to make some children (and their future offspring through the ages) taller, stronger, healthier, smarter. Though such inequalities already exist in our society, some worry that the ability to buy genetic interventions will widen the gap between haves and have-nots. Another concern is that such technologies will encourage parents to think of their children as "products" that can be ordered to specification, thus commodifying reproduction and fostering attempts to have "perfect" children

(Frankel and Chapman 2000). After reviewing the arguments for and against germ-line gene therapy, LeRoy Walters and Julie Gage Palmer conclude that it is ethically acceptable in principle. By contrast, David Danks maintains that it has no place in the treatment of genetic disease. For one thing, the number of cases in which germ line interventions might be used is very small. For another, germ-line gene therapy would require the creation of embryos using IVF, as in PGD. But in virtually all genetic diseases, the risk of transmission is not 100 percent, which means that both affected and unaffected embryos will be created. The question, then, is why would it make sense to attempt to correct an embryo with a genetic defect? "Surely one should discard the affected and reimplant one of the unaffected." Thus, the method for accomplishing germ-line gene therapy would make its use superfluous. Nor is Danks optimistic about the possibility of doing germ-line gene therapy on gametes prior to fertilization, due to the difficulty of getting the inserted DNA into exactly the right place in the chromosome that carries the mutant gene. Even if this could be done, it is very unlikely that the corrective effect of the inserted gene would survive genetic recombination, and thus persist for more than one generation. The alleged advantage of germ-line interventions—their heritability—is unlikely to be achieved. Danks thinks that genetic interventions might be done to alter normal characteristics, but says, "It requires an extraordinary combination of arrogance and ignorance to propose that we will soon understand these matters well enough to indulge in genetic manipulation to 'improve the human race.' "

ASSISTED REPRODUCTIVE TECHNOLOGIES

We have already seen how assisted reproductive technologies (ART) such as IVF can be used for the purpose of genetic testing and might be used for genetic modifications. Section 4 presents some of the arguments for and against ART when used for reproductive purposes. Assisted reproductive technologies run the gamut from the low-tech (though not without risk) administration of fertility drugs to more high-tech procedures, such as IVF and cryopreservation of embryos. In addition to IVF, gamete intrafallopian transfer (GIFT), zygote intrafallopian transfer (ZIFT), and a slew of other acronyms identify each new procedure. Many new techniques are improvements of earlier techniques, although many fertility experts in the United States complain that restrictions on federal funding for embryo research hamper progress in fertility treatments.

All of these procedures are expensive and are not always covered by insurance. A single attempt at IVF costs anywhere from $5,000 to $12,000, and most couples attempt more than one cycle in the pursuit of parenthood. GIFT and ZIFT may be even more expensive. All of these techniques have discouragingly low "take-home baby" rates. Even the best clinics treating the least-impaired couples report success rates only in the mid-30 percent range. Physical and emotional risks are always involved, raising medical, legal, and ethical questions.

John Robertson is perhaps the most prominent defender of the rights of infertile couples to have biologically related offspring. The first selection in Section 4, "The Presumptive Primacy of Procreative Liberty," comes from his book, *Children of Choice*. Robertson supports allowing individuals to make their own reproductive decisions, including decisions about fertility treatments and collaborative reproduction. He believes that attempts to ban or restrict reproductive rights violate the constitutional rights of infertile people, in the absence of demonstrable proof that such techniques would cause tangible harm to existing people. By contrast, the Catholic Church opposes virtually every assisted reproductive technique, including artificial insemination by husband (AIH), at least where AIH is a substitute for, as opposed to a facilitator of, the conjugal act, or sexual intercourse within marriage. The usual objections to ART, such as commercialization of reproduction and the introduction of a "third party" into the marital relationship are not present in AIH. Nevertheless, the church objects to AIH for the same reason it objects to contraception: Both are seen as severing the connection between procreation and the conjugal act. The one ART technique the Vatican appears willing to accept is a variation on the IVF protocol that begins with the infertile couple undergoing intercourse while the husband wears a special condom in which small holes have been cut, so as not to violate the

Church's edict against contraception. After intercourse, sperm are retrieved from the condom and placed in a laboratory dish next to eggs that have been retrieved from the wife's ovary. Then the whole mixture is quickly inserted back into the wife's fallopian tube so that fertilization can take place inside her body. "This protocol has been given the acronym GIFT, not only to distinguish it from the morally suspect IVF technology, but also to provide the image of a "gift of life" that comes directly from God" (Silver, 1997, p. 76).

ART allows for "collaborative reproduction" or using the reproductive parts and abilities of several people in the production of one child. Such arrangements as surrogate motherhood and gamete donation make it possible for a child to have as many as five potential parents: a rearing mother and father, a biological father, a genetic mother, who donates the egg, and a gestational mother, who provides the womb. Indeed, with a technique known as "ooplasmic transfer," two women can provide one egg, one providing the nucleus containing most of the DNA and one providing the cytoplasm. Nor is the multiplication of parents merely a theoretical possibility. It actually happened in a 1998 California case, *in re Buzzanca,* in which the couple, both of whom had fertility problems, used sperm donation, egg donation, and a surrogate. Before the child, Jaycee, was born, the couple divorced and the husband, John Buzzanca, refused to pay child support, arguing that the resulting child was not a child of the marriage. The trial court agreed. Indeed, it held that Jaycee Buzzanca, *had* no legal parents. Since Luanne Buzzanca, who had cared for the child from birth, had neither contributed an egg nor gestated Jaycee, she was not Jaycee's mother and would have to adopt her to become her legal mother. The appeals court disagreed. It overturned the decision, holding that the intent to parent made John and Luanne the lawful parents of Jaycee. Luanne Buzzanca was given legal custody of Jaycee, while the matter of child support was remanded. The court issued a plea to the Legislature "to sort out the parent rights and responsibilities of those involved in artificial reproduction," saying:

> No matter what one thinks of artificial insemination, traditional and gestational surrogacy (in all its permutations), and—as now appears in the not-too-distant future, cloning and even gene splicing—courts are still going to be faced with the problem of determining legal parentage. A child cannot be ignored. Even if all means of artificial reproduction were outlawed with draconian criminal penalties visited on the doctors and parties involved, courts will still be called upon to decide who the lawful parents really are and who—other than the taxpayers—is obligated to provide maintenance and support for the child. These cases will not go away. (In re Marriage of John A. and Luanne H. Buzzanca, 61 Cal App. 4th 1410)

It is not only questions about custody and child support that are raised by the multiplication of parents. In addition, concern has been expressed about lineage, kinship, and identity when children have more (or less) than one mother and one father (Kass 1997). One of the biggest concerns arising from collaborative reproduction stems from its commercial aspect. In the third selection in Section 4, Ruth Mackin considers the claim that commercial egg donation is objectionable because it "commodifies" reproduction. Macklin asks whether paying women to provide eggs is ethically different from paying models or athletes for their bodily attributes. She concludes that while there is something "unsavory" about commercial egg donation, it is not immoral (does not violate anyone's rights) and should not be prohibited. Sara Ann Ketchum argues that "contracted motherhood" (CM) is wrong on several grounds. First, there is the Kantian argument that selling people treats them as means instead of ends, as objects instead of persons. Second, CM is baby selling and "any selling of a human being should be prohibited because it devalues human life and human individuals." It is wrong for the same reason that slavery is wrong. Third, CM sells women's bodies. Ketchum suggests that selling one's reproductive capacity is akin to selling one's body for sex—it is a form of prostitution. This raises the question whether, and why, prostitution is wrong. It is possible that the wrongness of prostitution stems from the actual history of the practice, rather than the intrinsic wrongness of selling one's body or sexual favors. If, indeed, it is the degradation and exploitation of women by men that is immoral, perhaps this could be prevented by regulating, rather than banning, contracted motherhood and commercial egg donation.

HUMAN CLONING AND STEM CELL RESEARCH

The last section of Part 4 takes up two relatively new reprogenetic techniques: cloning, or more precisely, somatic cell nuclear transfer cloning, and embryonic stem (ES) cell research. In July 1997, Dr. Ian Wilmut announced that he had successfully cloned a lamb, Dolly, using SCNT cloning. Wilmut's team took the DNA from a somatic cell (in this case, a mammary cell) of an adult ewe and placed it in an egg cell from another ewe, from which the nucleus had been removed. The resulting embryo was carried to term by yet a third sheep, creating Dolly who was a (nearly) identical genetic copy, or "delayed" genetic twin, of the sheep whose mammary cell was used. (She was not totally identical to the sheep from whom she was cloned because a small amount of mitchondrial DNA remained in the enucleated egg cell.)

President Clinton immediately imposed a temporary ban on federal funding of human cloning research. He directed the National Bioethics Advisory Commission (NBAC) to undertake a thorough review of the legal and ethical issues and to report back to him within ninety days with recommendations on possible federal actions to prevent the abuse of this new technology. To no one's surprise, the NBAC report recommended that the President's moratorium be continued. It held, almost exclusively on the basis of safety considerations, that it was morally unacceptable at this time for anyone, privately or publicly funded, to engage in SCNT cloning research aimed at creating a child. The report stressed the medical and scientific potential of cloning technology for such uses as the creation of tissue for burn victims or bone marrow for transplantation, and it emphasized the need to make a distinction between "human cloning" (now usually called "therapeutic cloning") and "cloning a human being" ("reproductive cloning") so as not to hinder important areas of scientific research. As for the use of SCNT cloning to create human beings, the report recommended further dialogue on the nonsafety objections (ethical, religious, and policy) and suggested that the issue be revisited in three to five years.

However, in August 2001, the U.S. House of Representatives passed legislation outlawing both therapeutic and reproductive cloning. Soon afterwards, two fertility specialists, Severino Antinori and Panayiotis Zavos, along with Brigitte Boisselier, a scientist for the Raelian cult (which believes the human race was created by advanced extraterrestrials) announced at a meeting of the National Academy of Sciences that they plan to begin cloning babies this year. Most experts agree that cloning humans would not be safe yet. The chief problem in cloning mammals so far is its inefficiency. It takes a lot of failed embryos to produce one healthy cloned animal. "Right now, only 2 percent to 4 percent of mammalian clones are long-term survivors, and even most of them are not healthy" (Ronald Bailey, "There'll Never Be Another You," *Wall Street Journal,* August 10, 2001). The reason for such a low survival rate may be that the genes from the nuclei of mature cells may have lost their proper imprinting. When these mature nuclei are inserted into enucleated eggs to produce embryos, their imprinting is wrong. Either paternal or maternal genes affecting fetal growth may end up being dominant, creating the severe developmental imbalances seen in cloned animals. Moreover, there is currently no test available to check whether genes are properly imprinted or not. This means that the testing of clones for abnormalities, promised by Drs. Antinori and Boisselier, will be prenatal testing followed either by selective abortion or the birth of abnormal offspring, neither of which are desirable outcomes. As one commentator suggests, "A good benchmark for deciding to proceed with human reproductive cloning would be when researchers are reasonably sure that clones would suffer no more likelihood of birth defects (about 2 percent) than do children produced by sexual reproduction. It's too early now" (Bailey 2001). However, one's view on this depends on the stance one takes on the nonidentity problem: since cloned children would have no other way of getting born, would their suffering from birth defects be a justification for preventing their births? On the other side, many people think that cloning human beings will never be ethically acceptable. In August 2001, France and Germany requested the United Nations to approve a worldwide ban on reproductive cloning, calling it an "offense to human dignity." Some experts think that, regardless of any bans, reproductive cloning will occur, and indeed may have already occurred. Some predict that when the first healthy baby produced by cloning is born, the ethical debate will be over, just as the debate over "test-tube babies" ended with the birth of Louise Brown on July 25, 1978.

In the first selection in Section 5, Dan W. Brock examines the main moral arguments for and against cloning human beings. Brock argues that the moral right to reproductive freedom creates a presumption that individuals should be free to choose the means of reproduction that best serves their interests and desires. SCNT cloning might be used by a couple whose inability to reproduce results from male-factor infertility. Rather than resort to donor insemination, which brings a third party into their reproductive project, the couple might prefer to take DNA from a somatic cell of the husband, put it into an enucleated egg cell of the wife, and implant the resulting embryo into her uterus. Both parents would have a biological connection with the resulting child, although the child would be (nearly) genetically identical to the husband. The motivation in this case would be the same as that of other infertile couples: to have a child of their own. Would cloning in these circumstances be morally objectionable? After examining possible objections, Brock concludes that the ethical pros and cons are "sufficiently balanced and uncertain that there is not an ethically decisive case either for or against" cloning human beings. He urges careful public oversight of research and wider public debate before the technique is used on human beings.

A diametrically opposed view is presented by Leon Kass, who views cloning human beings as another step toward "Brave New World." Although Kass is primarily opposed to "clonal baby-making," he has come to believe that we need "an all-out ban on human cloning, including the creation of embryonic clones" for purposes of research. The reason is that he thinks it will be impossible to enforce a ban on reproductive cloning once research cloning is permitted. If labs and clinics can produce cloned embryos, it will be virtually impossible to monitor what becomes of them. And if a cloned embryo ends up in a woman's womb, what public authority is going to force her to have an abortion or prosecute her for bringing the baby to term (at least if it is healthy and normal)? Kass calls for a global legal ban if possible, and a unilateral national ban at a minimum. In sharp disagreement, Mark Eibert argues that such a ban would be unconstitutional. While there is not a great deal of case law on procreative liberty, such law as exists suggests that infertile couples have a constitutional right to use IVF and other high-tech assistance to help them have children. Eibert thinks that the safety considerations against cloning have been greatly exaggerated and that, in any event, prospective parents and their doctors, not the government, should make the risk-benefit calculation. We end the discussion of cloning with a moving essay by Tom Murray specifically about the use of cloning to replace a dead or dying child.

One nonreproductive use of cloning technology is to create embryos to extract their stem cells. The most extraordinary stem cells are found in the early stage embryo. These *embryonic stem (ES) cells,* unlike the more differentiated adult stem cells, retain the special ability to develop into nearly any cell type. ES cells might be used to treat injuries or diseases, such as Alzheimer's disease, Parkinson's disease, heart disease, diabetes, and kidney failure. In addition, scientists regard these cells as an important means for understanding the earliest stages of human development and as an important tool in the development of life-saving drugs and cell-replacement therapies to treat disorders caused by early cell death (NBAC 1999). However, the source of ES cells—aborted fetuses or preimplantation embryos—makes such research morally and politically controversial.

Long before human ES cells were isolated and cultured in 1998, the question of rules for research on embryos had been considered. In the late 1970s, Congress created an Ethics Advisory Board (EAB) to recommend and apply guidelines for federally funded research into improving IVF. In May 1979, the EAB issued a report recommending support for embryo research, including the creation of embryos for research purposes. The EAB report stirred enormous controversy, and when its charter expired in 1979, its membership was not renewed and no funding was provided. Since U.S. law required that all research in this area funded by the federal government be reviewed by the EAB, the result was a de facto moratorium on federal support for embryo research in the United States.

In June 1993, Congress passed a law that nullified the requirement of EAB approval of federal funding for infertility and embryo research projects. For the first time in fifteen years, NIH was free to respond to research proposals in this area, of which more than forty were already in the pipeline. Wanting guidelines to instruct members of IRBs when they considered the proposals, the NIH created the Human Embryo Research Panel (HERP) in late 1993. In September 1994, HERP issued a report, recommending that the federal government fund important research that used embryos, provided that the research could not be done on animals. It also recommended limiting research on embryos to the fourteenth day of development, at the formation of the primitive streak, the precursor of the nervous system. HERP's recommendations were largely ignored (Green 2001). President Clinton said that he did not believe that federal funds should be used to support the creation of embryos for research purposes and he directed NIH not to allocate any resources for such research. This appears to conflict with his later views about creating embryos for research purposes using somatic cell nuclear transfer (SCNT). In February 1998, the administration announced that it could support a bill to prohibit using SCNT to produce children only if it met four conditions, the second of which was that the bill should "permit [SCNT] using human cells for the purpose of developing stem-cell . . . technology to prevent and treat serious and life-threatening diseases" (Parens 2000, pp. 1-3).

Federal law forbids the use of federal funds for the creation of a human embryo for research purposes or for research in which human embryos are destroyed, discarded, or knowingly subjected to the risk of injury or death. What are the implications for stem cell research? The answer depends on how the law is interpreted. In January of 1999, the director of NIH, Harold Varmus, asked for a legal opinion on whether federal funds may be used for research conducted with ES cells. General Counsel Harriet Rabb opined that the statutory prohibition on the use of funds for human embryo research would not apply to research using ES cells, because such cells are not embryos: They are not capable of developing into a new individual as an embryo is. Under Raab's ruling, federal research funding could be provided for research with ES cells as long as the actions involved in removing the ES cells were not federally funded. Critics called this interpretation of the law sophistical. The ban on embryo research, they argue, applies to the initial collection of cells from the embryo, even if the stem cells themselves are not and could not become embryos. As Douglas Johnson, legislative director for the National Right to Life Committee, told the *Los Angeles Times*, the NIH "may think it can protect itself by requiring that the embryos actually be killed by someone not receiving federal funds, or by requiring the federally funded researcher to clock out when he kills the embryos, but these would be subterfuges and do violence to the clear intent of the law."

ES cells could be derived from "surplus" embryos, embryos left over from fertility treatment, which will either be discarded or perpetually frozen. (Just how many surplus embryos would be available is not known. Tens of thousands of embryos are in storage worldwide, but whether their progenitors would agree to their being used in research, as opposed to being kept for reproductive purposes, is a matter of speculation.) Many people have been perplexed at the idea that it would be wrong to derive stem cells from embryos that are going to be discarded anyway. If embryos are not going to be used for reproduction, is it not better that some good come from their creation? President Bush considered this point in his speech to the nation on August 9, 2001, but ultimately he rejected it. He decided that only stem cell lines that had been derived before 9 p.m. on August 9 could be used in federally funded research. This was clearly intended as a compromise between those who want the research to go forward and those who would ban it (or at least not fund it) altogether. By limiting the funding to existing stem cell lines (estimated at over sixty), the President would not be encouraging any further destruction of embryos.

There are three main ethical issues raised by ES cell research. One is the issue of complicity. If it is wrong to destroy embryos, as Bush's policy suggests, is it morally acceptable to use the results of the wrongful act? Or would that make one morally complicit and therefore also guilty of wrongdoing? This was an issue addressed by the Human Tissue Fetal Transplant Research Panel in 1988, when it considered whether it was acceptable public policy to support transplant research with fetal tissue from aborted fetuses. A majority of the panel (18–3) found that it was, either because the source of the tissue posed no moral problem, or because "the immorality of its source could be ethically isolated from the morality of its use in research." The ethical isolation claim is based on an analogy with using organs from transplant from murder victims. If organs from murder victims can be used without complicity in murder, then fetal remains can be used without complicity in the abortion. On this view, there is complicity only if one's action is causally related to the wrongful act, that is, if the wrongful act would not have been done but for the later act. If the wrongful act would have been done anyway, there's no complicity on the causative theory.

Others might argue that one is complicit in evil not only if one's action is causally related to it, but also if one benefits from it. To benefit from a wrongful act, it might be argued, *legitimizes* it: this is basically the moral argument against using data derived from Nazi experiments on concentration camp inmates. The question, then, is whether those who are anti-abortion should regard using fetal tissue as more like using the organs of murder victims (which is permissible) or more like using Nazi data (which is impermissible). However, some argue that using Nazi data is not necessarily wrong. Even though the Nazi experiments were wrong and should never have been done, to use their results to save lives salvages good from evil. It shows more respect for the victims of the Nazis, it has been argued, to use the data and save lives, than to ignore them. (This assumes that Nazi data have scientific validity, which may be dubious.)

A second ethical issue concerns the source of stem cells. Should stem cells be derived only from embryos left over from fertility treatment, or is it morally permissible to create embryos as a source of stem cells? Embryos could be created by IVF, using gametes donated for that purpose, or they could be created using somatic cell nuclear transfer. NBAC recommended that an exception should be made to the present ban on federal funding of embryo research to permit funding of research using spare embryos, but it also recommended that federal agencies should not fund research involving the derivation of human ES cells from embryos made solely for research purposes. NBAC said:

> The primary objection to creating embryos specifically for research is that there is a morally relevant difference between generating an embryo for the sole purpose of creating a child and producing an embryo with no such goal. Those who object to creating embryos for research often appeal to arguments about respecting human dignity by avoiding instrumental use of human embryos (i.e., using embryos merely as a means to some other goal does not treat them with appropriate respect or concern as a form of human life). (NBAC 1999, Vol. 1, p. v)

The question is why research that uses embryos that were created for reproductive purposes, but are no longer needed for that purpose, treats them with appropriate respect and concern as a form of human life, while research that uses embryos created specifically for that purpose does not. NBAC's answer brings us to the third, and most central, ethical issue in stem cell research: the moral status of preimplantation embryos. According to NBAC, only surplus embryos may be used in research because:

> Embryos that are discarded following the completion of IVF treatment were presumably created by individuals who had the primary intention of implanting them for reproductive purposes. . . . By contrast, research embryos are created for use in research and, in the case of stem cell research, their destruction in the process of research. Hence, one motivation that encourages serious consideration of the "discarded-created" distinction is a concern about instrumentalization—treating the embryo as a mere object—a practice that may increasingly lead us to think of embryos generally as means to our ends rather than as ends in themselves. (NBAC, 1999, Vol. 1, p. 56)

The assumption here is that embryos are the kinds of things that can be ends in themselves. In "Respect for Human Embryos," Bonnie Steinbock denies this. Whatever "respect for embryos" might mean, it differs from the respect that is due to persons. Respect for *persons,* as Kant instructs us, means never treating persons as mere means to our ends, but always treating them as ends in themselves. This means that we must take seriously other people's ends—their projects and goals—and not just our own. This kind of respect, then, is of necessity limited to beings who can have projects and goals, and thus is not appropriate to preimplantation embryos, beings which do not even yet have a nervous system, much less any form of sentience. Nevertheless, embryos are a "potent symbol of human life" and for that reason, are worthy of respectful treatment. This rules out frivolous or trivial uses of human embryos, such as using embryos in high school science classes, to test the safety of cosmetics or to create jewelry. These are situations in which there is no pressing need to use human embryos and their use displays contempt rather than respect for human life.

Maura Ryan gives a respectful account of the "interest view" that lies beyond Steinbock' s analysis, calling her argument "very persuasive." However, she does not think that the only relevant moral question is whether embryos have interests. The question is "what it means to display respect for embryos not as persons but as potent symbols of human life." Ryan remains unconvinced that the human interests to be served by stem cell research "are compelling enough to override widespread moral and religious anxieties about the production of research embryos." Moreover, if the embryo is a powerful symbol of human life, and not just a commodity or convenient tool for research, is this not because it has "a transcendent value, a moral standing that, even if not equivalent to full personhood, distinguishes it from things and non-human forms of life?" Finally, Ryan suggests that there is something intrinsically wrong with severing the initiating of human life from intentions and commitments to care for and sustain it. She acknowledges that her argument "rests on a particular account of the intrinsic relationship between sexuality, procreation, and parenthood, an account with which many in this society may disagree and one with important theological influences," and asks the important question, what weight should such religiously based arguments have in public and policy-oriented debates? The debate over stem cell research, it turns out, is fascinating not only for the ethical questions it raises, but also for the political question of how to create public policy in a pluralistic and deeply divided democratic society (Charo 1995).

THE MORALITY OF ABORTION

THE UNSPEAKABLE CRIME OF ABORTION

Pope John Paul II

Among all the crimes which can be committed against life, procured abortion has characteristics making it particularly serious and deplorable. The Second Vatican Council defines abortion, together with infanticide, as an "unspeakable crime."[1]

But today, in many people's consciences, the perception of its gravity has become progressively obscured. The acceptance of abortion in the popular mind, in behaviour and even in law itself, is a telling sign of an extremely dangerous crisis of the moral sense, which is becoming more and more incapable of distinguishing between good and evil, even when the fundamental right to life is at stake. Given such a grave situation, we need now more than ever to have the courage to look the truth in the eye and *to call things by their proper name*, without yielding to convenient compromises or to the temptation of self-deception. In this regard the reproach of the Prophet is extremely straightforward: "Woe to those who call evil good and good evil, who put darkness for light and light for darkness" (*Is* 5:20). Especially in the case of abortion there is a widespread use of ambiguous terminology, such as "interruption of pregnancy," which tends to hide abortion's true nature and to attenuate its seriousness in public opinion. Perhaps this linguistic phenomenon is itself a symptom of an uneasiness of conscience. But no word has the power to change the reality of things: procured abortion is *the deliberate and direct killing, by whatever means it is carried out, of a human being in the initial phase of his or her existence, extending from conception to birth.*

The moral gravity of procured abortion is apparent in all its truth if we recognize that we are dealing with murder and, in particular, when we consider the specific elements involved. The one eliminated is a human being at the very beginning of life. No one more absolutely *innocent* could be imagined. In no way could this human being ever be considered an aggressor, much less an unjust

From John Paul II. *Evangelium Vitae,* Encyclical Letter, August 16, 1993.

aggressor! He or she is *weak*, defenseless, even to the point of lacking that minimal form of defence consisting in the poignant power of a newborn baby's cries and tears. The unborn child is *totally entrusted* to the protection and care of the woman carrying him or her in the womb. And yet sometimes it is precisely the mother herself who makes the decision and asks for the child to be eliminated, and who then goes about having it done.

It is true that the decision to have an abortion is often tragic and painful for the mother, insofar as the decision to rid herself of the fruit of conception is not made for purely selfish reasons or out of convenience, but out of a desire to protect certain important values such as her own health or a decent standard of living for the other members of the family. Sometimes it is feared that the child to be born would live in such conditions that it would be better if the birth did not take place. Nevertheless, these reasons and others like them, however serious and tragic, can never justify the deliberate killing of an innocent human being.

As well as the mother, there are often other people too who decide upon the death of the child in the womb. In the first place, the father of the child may be to blame, not only when he directly pressures the woman to have an abortion, but also when he indirectly encourages such a decision on her part by leaving her alone to face the problems of pregnancy:[2] in this way the family is thus mortally wounded and profaned in its nature as a community of love and in its vocation to be the "sanctuary of life." Nor can one overlook the pressures which sometimes come from the wider family circle and from friends. Sometimes the woman is subjected to such strong pressure that she feels psychologically forced to have an abortion: certainly in this case moral responsibility lies particularly with those who have directly or indirectly obliged her to have an abortion. Doctors and nurses are also responsible, when they place at the service of death skills which were acquired for promoting life.

But responsibility likewise falls on the legislators who have promoted and approved abortion laws, and, to the extent that they have a say in the matter, on the administrators of the health-care centres where abortions are performed. A general and no less serious responsibility lies with those who have encouraged the spread of an attitude of sexual permissiveness and a lack of esteem for motherhood, and with those who should have ensured—but did not—effective family and social policies in support of families, especially larger families and those with particular financial and educational needs. Finally, one cannot overlook the network of complicity which reaches out to include international institutions, foundations and associations which systematically campaign for the legalization and spread of abortion in the world. In this sense abortion goes beyond the responsibility of individuals and beyond the harm done to them, and takes on a distinctly social dimension. It is a most serious *wound* inflicted on society and its culture by the very people who ought to be society's promoters and defenders. As I wrote in my *Letter to Families*, "we are facing an immense threat to life: not only to the life of individuals but also to that of civilization itself."[3] We are facing what can be called a *"structure of sin" which opposes human life not yet born.*

Some people try to justify abortion by claiming that the result of conception, at least up to a certain number of days, cannot yet be considered a personal human life. But in fact, "from the time that the ovum is fertilized, a life is begun which is neither that of the father nor the mother; it is rather the life of a new human being with his own growth. It would never be made human if it were not human already. This has always been clear, and . . . modern genetic science offers clear confirmation. It has demonstrated that from the first instant there is established the programme of what this living being will be: a person, this individual person with his characteristic aspects already well determined. Right from fertilization the adventure of a human life begins, and each of its capacities requires time—a rather lengthy time—to find its place and to be in a position to act."[4] Even if the presence of a spiritual soul cannot be ascertained by empirical data, the results themselves of scientific research on the human embryo provide "a valuable indication for discerning by the use of reason a personal presence at the moment of the first appearance of a human life: how could a human individual not be a human person?"[5]

Furthermore, what is at stake is so important that, from the standpoint of moral obligation, the mere probability that a human person is involved would suffice to justify an absolutely clear prohibition of any intervention aimed at killing a human embryo. Precisely for this reason, over and above all scientific debates and those philosophical affirmations to which the Magisterium has not expressly committed itself, the Church has always taught and continues to teach that the result of human procreation, from the first moment of its existence, must be guaranteed that unconditional respect which is morally due to the human being in his or her totality and unity as body and spirit: "*The human being is to be respected and treated as a person from the moment of conception;* and therefore from that same moment his rights as a person must be recognized, among which in the first place is the inviolable right of every innocent human being to life."[6] . . .

NOTES

1. Pastoral Constitution on the Church in the Modern World *Gaudium et Spes*. 51: "Abortius necnon infanticidium nefanda sunt crimina."
2. Cf. John Paul II. Apostolic Letter *Muliens Dignitatem* (15 August 1988), 14:*AAS* 80 (1988), 1686.
3. No. 21:*AAS* 86 (1994), 920.
4. Congregation for the Doctrine of the Faith, *Declaration on Procured Abortion* (18 November 1974), Nos. 12–13: *AAS* 66 (1974), 738.
5. Congregation for the Doctrine of the Faith, Instruction on Respect for Human Life in Its Origin and on the Dignity of Procreation *Donum vitae* (22 February 1987), I, No. 1:*AAS* 80 (1988), 78–79.
6. *Ibid., loc. cit:.*, 79.

WHY ABORTION IS IMMORAL

Don Marquis

I

. . . Consider the way a typical anti-abortionist argues. She will argue or assert that life is present from the moment of conception or that fetuses look like babies or that fetuses possess a characteristic such as a genetic code that is both necessary and sufficient for being human. Anti-abortionists seem to believe that (1) the truth of all of these claims is quite obvious, and (2) establishing any of these claims is sufficient to show that abortion is morally akin to murder.

A standard pro-choice strategy exhibits similarities. The pro-choicer will argue or assert that fetuses are not persons or that fetuses are not rational agents or that fetuses are not social beings. Pro-choicers seem to believe that (1) the truth of any of these claims is quite obvious, and (2) establishing any of these claims is sufficient to show that an abortion is not a wrongful killing.

In fact, both the pro-choice and the anti-abortion claims do seem to be true, although the "it looks like a baby" claim is more difficult to establish the earlier the pregnancy. We seem to have a standoff. How can it be resolved? . . .

Note what each partisan will say. The anti-abortionist will claim that her position is supported by such generally accepted moral principles as "It is always prima facie seriously wrong to take a human life" or "It is always prima facie seriously wrong to end the life of a baby." Since these are generally accepted moral principles, her position is certainly not obviously wrong. The pro-choicer will claim that her position is supported by such plausible moral principles as, "Being a person is what gives an individual intrinsic moral worth," or, "It is only seriously prima facie wrong to take the life of a member of the human community." Since these are generally accepted moral principles, the pro-choice

Journal of Philosophy LXXXVI, No. 4, April 1989, 183–202. Reprinted by permission.

position is certainly not obviously wrong. Unfortunately, we have again arrived at a standoff.

Now, how might one deal with this standoff? The standard approach is to try to show how the moral principles of one's opponent lose their plausibility under analysis. It is easy to see how this is possible. On the one hand, the anti-abortionist will defend a moral principle concerning the wrongness of killing which tends to be broad in scope in order that even fetuses at an early stage of pregnancy will fall under it. The problem with broad principles is that they often embrace too much. In this particular instance, the principle, "It is always prima facie wrong to take a human life," seems to entail that it is wrong to end the existence of a living human cancer-cell culture, on the grounds that the culture is both living and human. Therefore, it seems that the anti-abortionist's favored principle is too broad.

On the other hand, the pro-choicer wants to find a moral principle concerning the wrongness of killing which tends to be narrow in scope in order that fetuses will *not* fall under it. The problem with narrow principles is that they often do not embrace enough. Hence, the needed principles such as, "It is prima facie seriously wrong to kill only persons," or, "It is prima facie wrong to kill only rational agents," do not explain why it is wrong to kill infants or young children or the severely retarded or even perhaps the severely mentally ill. Therefore, we seem again to have a standoff. The anti-abortionist charges, not unreasonably, that pro-choice principles concerning killing are too narrow to be acceptable; the pro-choicer charges, not unreasonably, that anti-abortionist principles concerning killing are too broad to be acceptable.

Attempts by both sides to patch up the difficulties in their positions run into further difficulties. The anti-abortionist will try to remove the problem in her position by reformulating her principle concerning killing in terms of human beings. Now we end up with: "It is always prima facie seriously wrong to end the life of a human being." This principle has the advantage of avoiding the problem of the human cancer-cell culture counterexample. But this advantage is purchased at a high price. For although it is clear that a fetus is both human and alive, it is not at all clear that a fetus is a human *being*. There is at least something to be said for the view that something becomes a human being only after a process of development, and that, therefore, first trimester fetuses, and perhaps all fetuses, are not yet human beings. Hence, the anti-abortionist, by this move, has merely exchanged one problem for another.

The pro-choicer fares no better. She may attempt to find reasons why killing infants, young children, and the severely retarded is wrong which are independent of her major principle that is supposed to explain the wrongness of taking human life, but which will not also make abortion immoral. This is no easy task. Appeals to social utility will seem satisfactory only to those who resolve not to think of the enormous difficulties with a utilitarian account of the wrongness of killing and the significant social costs of preserving the lives of the unproductive. A pro-choice strategy that extends the definition of 'person' to infants or even to young children seems just as arbitrary as an anti-abortion strategy that extends the definition of 'human being' to fetuses. Again, we find symmetries in the two positions and we arrive at a standoff.

There are even further problems that reflect symmetries in the two positions. In addition to counterexample problems, or the arbitrary application problems that can be exchanged for them, the standard anti-abortionist principle, "It is prima facie seriously wrong to kill a human being," or one of its variants, can be objected to on the grounds of ambiguity. If 'human being' is taken to be a *biological* category, then the anti-abortionist is left with the problem of explaining why a merely biological category should make a moral difference. Why, it is asked, is it any more reasonable to base a moral conclusion on the number of chromosomes in one's cells than on the color of one's skin? If 'human being', on the other hand, is taken to be a *moral* category, then the claim that a fetus is a human being cannot be taken to be a premise in the anti-abortion argument, for it is precisely what needs to be established. Hence, either the anti-abortionist's main category is a morally irrelevant, merely biological category, or it is of no use to the anti-abortionist in establishing (noncircularly, of course) that abortion is wrong.

Although this problem with the anti-abortionist position is often noticed, it is less often noticed that the pro-choice position suffers from an analogous problem. The principle, "Only persons have the right to life" also suffers from an ambiguity. The term 'person' is typically defined in terms of psychological characteristics, although there will certainly be disagreement concerning which characteristics are most important. Supposing that this matter can be settled, the pro-choicer is left with the problem of explaining why *psychological* characteristics should make a *moral* difference. If the pro-choicer should attempt to deal with this problem by claiming that an explanation is not necessary, that in fact we do treat such a cluster of psychological properties as having moral significance, the sharp-witted anti-abortionist should have a ready response. We do treat being both living and human as having moral significance. If it is legitimate for the pro-choicer to demand that the anti-abortionist provide an explanation of the connection between the biological character of being a human being and the wrongness of being killed (even though people accept this connection), then it is legitimate for the anti-abortionist to demand that the pro-choicer provide an explanation of the connection between psychological criteria for being a person and the wrongness of being killed (even though that connection is accepted).

[Joel] Feinberg has attempted to meet this objection (he calls psychological personhood "commonsense personhood"):

> The characteristics that confer commonsense personhood are not arbitrary bases for rights and duties, such as race, sex or species membership; rather they are traits that make sense out of rights and duties and without which those moral attributes would have no point or function. It is because people are conscious; have a sense of their personal identities; have plans, goals, and projects; experience emotions; are liable to pains, anxieties, and frustrations; can reason and bargain, and so on—it is because of these attributes that people have values and interests, desires and expectations of their own, including a stake in their own futures, and a personal well-being of a sort we cannot ascribe to unconscious or nonrational beings. Because of their developed capacities they can assume duties and responsibilities and can have and make claims on one another. Only because of their sense of self, their life plans, their value hierarchies, and their stakes in their own futures can they be ascribed fundamental rights. There is nothing arbitrary about these linkages. [Feinberg 1986]

The plausible aspects of this attempt should not be taken to obscure its implausible features. There is a great deal to be said for the view that being a psychological person under some description is a necessary condition for having duties. One cannot have a duty unless one is capable of behaving morally, and a being's capability of behaving morally will require having a certain psychology. It is far from obvious, however, that having rights entails consciousness or rationality, as Feinberg suggests. We speak of the rights of the severely retarded or the severely mentally ill, yet some of these persons are not rational. We speak of the rights of the temporarily unconscious. The New Jersey Supreme Court based their decision in the Quinlan case on Karen Ann Quinlan's right to privacy, and she was known to be permanently unconscious at that time. Hence, Feinberg's claim that having rights entails being conscious is, on its face, obviously false. . . .

There is a way out of this apparent dialectical quandary. . . .

II

. . . We can start from the following unproblematic assumption concerning our own case: it is wrong to kill us. Why is it wrong? Some answers can be easily eliminated. It might be said that what makes killing us wrong is that a killing brutalizes the one who kills. But the brutalization consists of being inured to the performance of an act that is hideously immoral; hence, the brutalization does not explain the immorality. It might be said that what makes killing us wrong is the great loss others would experience due to our absence. Although such hubris is understandable, such an explanation does not account for the wrongness of killing hermits, or those whose lives are relatively independent and whose friends find it easy to make new friends.

A more obvious answer is better. What primarily makes killing wrong is neither its effect on the murderer nor its effect on the victim's friends and relatives, but its effect on the victim. The loss of one's life is one of the greatest losses one can suffer. The loss of one's life deprives one of all the experiences, activities, projects, and enjoyments that would otherwise have constituted one's future. Therefore, killing someone is wrong, primarily because the killing inflicts (one of) the greatest possible losses on the victim. . . . When I am killed, I am deprived both of what I now value which would have been part of my future personal life, but also what I would come to value. Therefore, when I die, I am deprived of all of the value of my future. Inflicting this loss on me is ultimately what makes killing me wrong. This being the case, it would seem that what makes killing *any* adult human being prima facie seriously wrong is the loss of his or her future. . . .

The claim that what makes killing wrong is the loss of the victim's future is directly supported by two considerations. In the first place, this theory explains why we regard killing as one of the worst of crimes. Killing is especially wrong, because it deprives the victim of more than perhaps any other crime. In the second place, people with AIDS or cancer who know they are dying believe, of course, that dying is a very bad thing for them. They believe that the loss of a future to them that they would otherwise have experienced is what makes their premature death a very bad thing for them. A better theory of the wrongness of killing would require a different natural property associated with killing which better fits with the attitudes of the dying. What could it be?

The view that what makes killing wrong is the loss to the victim of the value of the victim's future gains additional support when some of its implications are examined. In the first place, it is incompatible with the view that it is wrong to kill only beings who are biologically human. It is possible that there exists a different species from another planet whose members have a future like ours. Since having a future like that is what makes killing someone wrong, this theory entails that it would be wrong to kill members of such a species. Hence, this theory is opposed to the claim that only life that is biologically human has great moral worth, a claim which many anti-abortionists have seemed to adopt. This opposition, which this theory has in common with personhood theories, seems to be a merit of the theory.

In the second place, the claim that the loss of one's future is the wrong-making feature of one's being killed entails the possibility that the futures of some actual nonhuman mammals on our own planet are sufficiently like ours that it is seriously wrong to kill them also. Whether some animals do have the same right to life as human beings depends on adding to the account of the wrongness of killing some additional account of just what it is about my future or the futures of other adult human beings which makes it wrong to kill us. No such additional account will be offered in this essay. Undoubtedly, the provision of such an account would be a very difficult matter. Undoubtedly, any such account would be quite controversial. Hence, it surely should not reflect badly on this sketch of an elementary theory of the wrongness of killing that it is indeterminate with respect to some very difficult issues regarding animal rights.

In the third place, the claim that the loss of one's future is the wrong-making feature of one's being killed does not entail, as sanctity-of-human-life theories do, that active euthanasia is wrong. Persons who are severely and incurably ill, who face a future of pain and despair, and who wish to die will not have suffered a loss if they are killed. It is, strictly speaking, the value of a human's future which makes killing wrong in this theory. This being so, killing does not necessarily wrong some persons who are sick and dying. Of course, there may be other reasons for a prohibition of active euthanasia, but that is another matter. Sanctity-of-human-life theories seem to hold that active euthanasia is seriously wrong even in an individual case where there seems to be good reason for it independently of public policy considerations. This consequence is most implausible, and it is a plus for the claim that the loss of a future of value is what makes killing wrong that it does not share this consequence.

In the fourth place, the account of the wrongness of killing defended in this essay does straightforwardly entail that it is prima facie seriously wrong to kill children and infants, for we do presume that they have futures of value. Since we do believe that it is wrong to kill defenseless little babies, it is important that a theory of the wrongness of killing easily account for this. Personhood theories of the wrongness of killing, on the other hand, cannot straightforwardly account for the wrongness of killing infants and young children. Hence, such theories must add special ad hoc accounts of the wrongness of killing the young. The plausibility of such ad hoc theories seems to be a function of how desperately one wants such theories to work. The claim that the primary wrong-making feature of a killing is the loss to the victim of the value of its future accounts for the wrongness of killing young children and infants directly; it makes the wrongness of such acts as obvious as we actually think it is. This is a further merit of this theory. Accordingly, it seems that this value of a future-like-ours theory of the wrongness of killing shares strengths of both sanctity-of-life and personhood accounts while avoiding weaknesses of both. In addition, it meshes with a central intuition concerning what makes killing wrong.

The claim that the primary wrong-making feature of a killing is the loss to the victim of the value of its future has obvious consequences for the ethics of abortion. The future of a standard fetus includes a set of experiences, projects, activities, and such which are identical with the futures of adult human beings and are identical with the futures of young children. Since the reason that is sufficient to explain why it is wrong to kill human beings after the time of birth is a reason that also applies to fetuses, it follows that abortion is prima facie seriously morally wrong.

This argument does not rely on the invalid inference that, since it is wrong to kill persons, it is wrong to kill potential persons also. The category that is morally central to this analysis is the category of having a valuable future like ours; it is not the category of personhood. The argument that abortion is prima facie seriously morally wrong proceeded independently of the notion of person or potential person or any equivalent. Someone may wish to start with this analysis in terms of the value of a human future, conclude that abortion is, except perhaps in rare circumstances, seriously morally wrong, infer that fetuses have the right to life, and then call fetuses "persons" as a result of their having the right to life. Clearly, in this case, the category of person is being used to state the *conclusion* of the analysis rather than to generate the *argument* of the analysis. . . .

III

How complete an account of the wrongness of killing does the value of a future-like-ours account have to be in order that the wrongness of abortion is a consequence? This account does not have to be an account of the necessary conditions for the wrongness of killing. Some persons in nursing homes may lack valuable human futures, yet it may be wrong to kill them for other reasons. Furthermore, this account does not obviously have to be the sole reason killing is wrong where the victim did have a valuable future. This analysis claims only that, for any killing where the victim did have a valuable future like ours, having that future by itself is sufficient to create the strong presumption that the killing is seriously wrong.

One way to overturn the value of a future-like-ours argument would be to find some account of the wrongness of killing which is at least as intelligible and which has different implications for the ethics of abortion. Two rival accounts possess at least some degree of plausibility. One account is based on the obvious fact that people value the experience of living and wish for that valuable experience to continue. Therefore, it might be said, what makes killing wrong is the discontinuation of that experience for the victim. Let us call this the *discontinuation account*. Another rival account is based upon the obvious fact that people strongly desire to continue to live. This suggests that what makes killing us so wrong is that it interferes with the fulfillment of a strong and fundamental desire, the fulfillment of which is necessary for the fulfillment of any other desires we might have. Let us call this the *desire account*. . . .

One problem with the desire account is that we do regard it as seriously wrong to kill persons who have little desire to live or who have no desire to live or, indeed, have a desire not to live. We believe it is seriously wrong to kill the unconscious, the sleeping, those who are tired of life, and those who are suicidal. The value-of-a-human-future account renders standard morality intelligible in these cases; these cases appear to be incompatible with the desire account.

The desire account is subject to a deeper difficulty. We desire life, because we value the goods of this life. The goodness of life is not secondary to our desire for it. If this were not so, the pain of one's own premature death could be done away with merely by an appropriate alteration in the configuration of one's desires. This is absurd. Hence, it would seem that it is the loss of the goods of one's future, not the interference with the fulfillment of a strong desire to live, which accounts ultimately for the wrongness of killing.

It is worth noting that, if the desire account is modified so that it does not provide a necessary, but only a sufficient, condition for the wrongness of killing, the desire account is compatible with the value of a future-like-ours account. The combined accounts will yield an anti-abortion ethic. This suggests that one can retain what is intuitively plausible about the desire account without a challenge to the basic argument of this paper.

It is also worth noting that, if future desires have moral force in a modified desire account of the wrongness of killing, one can find support for an anti-abortion ethic even in the absence of a value of a future-like-ours account. If one decides that a morally relevant property, the possession of which is sufficient to make it wrong to kill some individual, is the desire at some future time to live—one might decide to justify one's refusal to kill suicidal teenagers on these grounds, for example—then, since typical fetuses will have the desire in the future to live, it is wrong to kill typical fetuses. Accordingly, it does not seem that a desire account of the wrongness of killing can provide a justification of a pro-choice ethic of abortion which is nearly as adequate as the value of a human-future justification on an anti-abortion ethic.

The discontinuation account looks more promising as an account of the wrongness of killing. It seems just as intelligible as the value of a future-like-ours account, but it does not justify an anti-abortion position. Obviously, if it is the continuation of one's activities, experiences, and projects, the loss of which makes killing wrong, then it is not wrong to kill fetuses for that reason, for fetuses do not have experiences, activities, and projects to be continued or discontinued. Accordingly, the discontinuation account does not have the anti-abortion consequences that the value of a future-like-ours account has. Yet, it seems as intelligible as the value of a future-like-ours account, for when we think of what would be wrong with our being killed, it does seem as if it is the discontinuation of what makes our lives worthwhile which makes killing us wrong.

Is the discontinuation account just as good an account as the value of a future-like-ours account? The discontinuation account will not be adequate at all, if it does not refer to the *value* of the experience that may be discontinued. One does not want the discontinuation account to make it wrong to kill a patient who begs for death and who is in severe pain that cannot be relieved short of killing. (I leave open the question of whether it is wrong for other reasons.) Accordingly, the discontinuation account must be more than a bare discontinuation account. It must make some reference to the positive value of the patient's experiences. But, by the same token, the value of a future-like-ours account cannot be a bare future account either. Just having a future surely does not itself rule out killing the above patient. This account must make some reference to the value of the patient's future experiences and projects also. Hence, both accounts involve the value of experiences, projects, and activities. So far we still have symmetry between accounts.

The symmetry fades, however, when we focus on the time period of the value of the experiences, etc., which has moral consequences. Although both accounts leave open the possibility that the patient in our example may be killed, this possibility is left open only in virtue of the utterly bleak future for the patient. It makes no difference whether the patient's immediate past contains intolerable pain, or consists in being in a coma (which we can imagine is a situation of indifference), or consists in a life of value. If the patient's future is a future of value, we want our account to make it wrong to kill the patient. If the patient's future is intolerable, whatever his or her immediate past, we want our account to allow killing the patient. Obviously, then, it is the value of that patient's future which is doing the work in rendering the morality of killing the patient intelligible.

This being the case, it seems clear that whether one has immediate past experiences or not does no work in the explanation of what makes killing wrong. The addition the discontinuation account makes to the value of a human future account is otiose. Its addition to the value-of-a-future account plays no role at all in rendering intelligible the wrongness of killing. Therefore, it can be discarded with the discontinuation account of which it is a part.

IV

The analysis of the previous section suggests that alternative general accounts of the wrongness of killing are either inadequate or unsuccessful in getting around the anti-abortion consequences of the value of a future-like-ours argument. A different strategy for avoiding these anti-abortion consequences involves limiting the scope of the value of a future argument. More precisely, the strategy involves arguing that fetuses lack a property that is essential for the value-of-a-future argument (or for any anti-abortion argument) to apply to them.

One move of this sort is based upon the claim that a necessary condition of one's future being valuable is that one values it. Value implies a valuer. Given this one might argue that, since fetuses cannot value their futures, their futures are not valuable to them. Hence, it does not seriously wrong them deliberately to end their lives.

This move fails, however, because of some ambiguities. Let us assume that something cannot be of value unless it is valued by someone. This does not entail that my life is of no value unless it is valued by me. I may think, in a period of despair, that my future is of no worth whatsoever, but I may be wrong because others rightly see value—even great value—in it. Furthermore, my future can be valuable to me even if I do not value it. This is the case when a young person attempts suicide, but is rescued and goes on to significant human achievements. Such young people's futures are ultimately valuable to them, even though such futures do not seem to be valuable to them at the moment of attempted suicide. A fetus's future can be valuable to it in the same way. Accordingly, this attempt to limit the anti-abortion argument fails.

Another similar attempt to reject the anti-abortion position is based on [Michael] Tooley's claim that an entity cannot possess the right to life unless it has the capacity to desire its continued existence. It follows that, since fetuses lack the conceptual capacity to desire to continue to live, they lack the right to life. Accordingly, Tooley concludes that abortion cannot be seriously prima facie wrong. . . .

What could be the evidence for Tooley's basic claim? Tooley once argued that individuals have a prima facie right to what they desire and that the lack of the capacity to desire something undercuts the basis of one's right to it. . . . This argument plainly will not succeed in the context of the analysis of this essay, however, since the point here is to establish the fetus's right to life on other grounds. Tooley's argument assumes that the right to life cannot be established in general on some basis other than the desire for life. This position was considered and rejected in the preceding section of this paper.

One might attempt to defend Tooley's basic claim on the grounds that, because a fetus cannot apprehend continued life as a benefit, its continued life cannot be a benefit, or cannot be something it has a right to, or cannot be something that is in its interest. This might be defended in terms of the general proposition that, if an individual is literally incapable of caring about or taking an interest in some X, then one does not have a right to X, or X is not a benefit, or X is not something that is in one's interest.

Each member of this family of claims seems to be open to objections. As John C. Stevens has pointed out, one may have a right to be treated with a certain medical procedure (because of a health insurance policy one has purchased), even though one cannot conceive of the nature of the procedure. And, as Tooley himself has pointed out, persons who have been indoctrinated, or drugged, or rendered temporarily unconscious may be literally incapable of caring about or taking an interest in something that is in their interest, or is something to which they have a right, or is something that benefits them. Hence, the Tooley claim that would restrict the scope of the value of a future-like-ours argument is undermined by counterexamples.

Finally, Paul Bassen has argued that, even though the prospects of an embryo might seem to be a basis for the wrongness of abortion, an embryo cannot be a victim and therefore cannot be wronged [Bassen 1982, 332–326]. An embryo cannot be a victim, he says, because it lacks sentience. His central argument for this seems to be that, even though plants and the permanently unconscious are alive, they clearly cannot be victims. What is the explanation of this? Bassen claims that the explanation is that their lives consist of mere metabolism and mere metabolism is not enough to ground victimizability. Mentation is required.

The problem with this attempt to establish the absence of victimizability is that both plants and the permanently unconscious clearly lack what Bassen calls "prospects" or what I have called "a future life like ours." Hence, it is surely open to one to argue that the real reason we believe plants and the permanently unconscious cannot be victims is that killing them cannot deprive them of a future life like ours; the real reason is not their absence of present mentation.

Bassen recognizes that his view is subject to this difficulty, and he recognizes that the case of children seems to support this difficulty, for "much of what we do for children is based on prospects." He argues, however, that, in the case of children and in other such cases, "potentiality comes into play only where victimizability has been secured on other grounds" [Bassen 1982, 333]. . . .

Bassen's defense of his view is patently question-begging, since what is adequate to secure victimizability is exactly what is at issue. His examples do not support his own view against the thesis of this essay. Of course, embryos can be victims: when their lives are deliberately terminated, they are deprived of their futures of value, their prospects. This makes them victims, for it directly wrongs them.

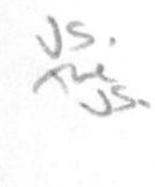

The seeming plausibility of Bassen's view stems from the fact that paradigmatic cases of imagining someone as a victim involve empathy, and empathy requires mentation of the victim. The victims of flood, famine, rape, or child abuse are all persons with whom we can empathize. That empathy seems to be part of seeing them as victims.

In spite of the strength of these examples, the attractive intuition that a situation in which there is victimization requires the possibility of empathy is subject to counterexamples. Consider a case that Bassen himself offers: "Posthumous obliteration of an author's work constitutes a misfortune for him only if he had wished his work to endure" [Bassen 1982, 318]. . . . The conditions Bassen wishes to impose upon the possibility of being victimized here seem far too strong. Perhaps this author, due to his unrealistic standards of excellence and his low self-esteem, regarded his work as unworthy of survival, even though it possessed genuine literary merit. Destruction of such work would surely victimize its author. In such a case, empathy with the victim concerning the loss is clearly impossible.

Of course, Bassen does not make the possibility of empathy a necessary condition of victimizability; he requires only mentation. Hence, on Bassen's actual view, this author, as I have described him, can be a victim. The problem is that the basic intuition that renders Bassen's view plausible is missing in the author's case. In order to attempt to avoid counterexamples, Bassen has made his thesis too weak to be supported by the intuitions that suggested it.

Even so, the mentation requirement on victimizability is still subject to counterexamples. Suppose a severe accident renders me totally unconscious for a month, after which I recover. Surely killing me while I am unconscious victimizes me, even though I am incapable of mentation during that time. It thus follows that Bassen's thesis fails. Apparently, attempts to restrict the value of a future-like-ours argument so that fetuses do not fall within its scope do not succeed.

V

In this essay, it has been argued that the correct ethic of the wrongness of killing can be extended to fetal life and used to show that there is a strong presumption that any abortion is morally impermissible. If the ethic of killing adopted here entails, however, that contraception is also seriously immoral, then there would appear to be a difficulty with the analysis of this essay.

But this analysis does not entail that contraception is wrong. Of course, contraception prevents the actualization of a possible future of value. Hence, it follows from the claim that futures of value should be maximized that contraception is prima facie immoral. This obligation to maximize does not exist, however; furthermore, nothing in the ethics of killing in this paper entails that it does. The ethics of killing in this essay would entail that contraception is wrong only if something were denied a human future of value by contraception. Nothing at all is denied such a future by contraception, however.

Candidates for a subject of harm by contraception fall into four categories: (1) some sperm or other, (2) some ovum or other, (3) a sperm and an ovum separately, and (4) a sperm and an ovum together. Assigning the harm to some sperm is utterly arbitrary, for no reason can be given for making a sperm the subject of harm rather than an ovum. Assigning the harm to some ovum is utterly arbitrary, for no reason can be given for making an ovum the subject of harm rather than a sperm. One might attempt to avoid these problems by insisting that contraception deprives both the sperm and the ovum separately of a valuable future like ours. On this alternative, too many futures are lost. Contraception was supposed to be wrong, because it deprived us of one future of value, not two. One might attempt to avoid this problem by holding that contraception deprives the combination of sperm and ovum of a valuable future like ours. But here the definite article misleads. At the time of contraception, there are hundreds of millions of sperm, one (released) ovum and millions of possible combinations of all of these. There is no actual combination at all. Is the subject of the loss to be a merely possible combination? Which one? This alternative does not yield an actual subject of harm either. Accordingly, the immorality of contraception is not entailed by the loss of a future-like-ours argument simply because there is no nonarbitrarily identifiable subject of the loss in the case of contraception.

VI

The purpose of this essay has been to set out an argument for the serious presumptive wrongness of abortion subject to the assumption that the moral permissibility of abortion stands or falls on the moral status of the fetus. Since a fetus possesses a property, the possession of which in adult human beings is sufficient to make killing an adult human being wrong, abortion is wrong. This way of dealing with the problem of abortion seems superior to other approaches to the ethics of abortion, because it rests on an ethics of killing which is close to self-evident, because the crucial morally relevant property clearly applies to fetuses, and because the argument avoids the usual equivocations on 'human life', 'human being', or 'person'. The argument rests neither on religious claims nor on papal dogma. It is not subject to the objection of "speciesism." Its soundness is compatible with the moral permissibility of euthanasia and contraception. It deals with our intuitions concerning young children.

Finally, this analysis can be viewed as resolving a standard problem—indeed, *the* standard problem—concerning the ethics of abortion. Clearly, it is wrong to kill adult human beings. Clearly, it is not wrong to end the life of some arbitrarily chosen single human cell. Fetuses seem to be like arbitrarily chosen human cells in some respects and like adult humans in other respects. The problem of the ethics of abortion is the problem of determining the fetal property that settles this moral controversy. The thesis of this essay is that the problem of the ethics of abortion, so understood, is solvable.

WHY MOST ABORTIONS ARE NOT WRONG

Bonnie Steinbock

I. INTRODUCTION

The focus of this chapter is the morality of abortion, not whether it should be legal. Some people who believe that many or even most abortions are morally wrong take a prochoice stance as regards the law. They think that the decision to abort properly belongs to the woman herself because the state ought not to be involved in so personal and intimate a decision as whether to bear a child. Such people maintain that women should think long and hard about whether their circumstances justify abortion, but they want the choice to remain the woman's, as it is she who will bear the burden of an unwanted pregnancy. Other arguments for keeping abortion safe and legal are based on the horrendous health consequences of illegal abortion or the inequalities that result when women, especially poor and minority women, are unable to control their fertility (Graber, 1996). Someone can cite these reasons for keeping abortion legal without believing, as I do, that abortion is almost always a morally permissible option. My belief that abortion is not wrong is based on two considerations: the moral status of the embryo and fetus and the burdens

---

Advances in Bioethics. Volume 5, pages 245–267. ISBN: 0-7623-0559-2

Editor's note: Most footnotes have been deleted. Students who want to follow up on sources should consult the original article.

imposed by pregnancy and childbirth on women. I begin by presenting briefly the view of moral status that I take to be correct, that is, the interest view. The interest view limits moral status to beings who have interests and restricts the possession of interests to conscious, sentient beings. The implication for abortion is that it is not seriously wrong to kill a nonconscious, nonsentient fetus where there is an adequate reason for doing so, such as not wanting to be pregnant. Next I discuss Don Marquis' challenge to the interest view (Marquis, 1989). According to Marquis, killing is prima facie wrong when it deprives a being of a valuable future like ours. If a being has a valuable future, the fact that it is now nonconscious and nonsentient is irrelevant. Marquis' account of the wrongness of killing implies that abortion is almost always wrong. I try to show that his view has serious problems, in particular, that it applies to gametes as well as fetuses, and it makes contraception as well as abortion seriously wrong.

I then discuss whether abortion can be a serious moral issue at all, given the interest view, and conclude by addressing some problematic abortions that many people, prochoice as well as prolife, have considered to be morally wrong.

II. THE MORAL STATUS OF THE FETUS

I use the term "fetus" to refer to the unborn at all stages of pregnancy, even though this is not, strictly speaking, correct. Between conception and 8 weeks, the correct term is "embryo"; the term "fetus" is correctly used between 8 weeks gestation age and birth. I will use the term "fetus" throughout, both in order to avoid the inconvenience of the phrase "embryo or fetus" and because using the term "embryo" which refers to the earliest weeks of pregnancy, might convey an unfair advantage to my argument. Everything I have to say about abortion in this essay applies as much to a 12-week-old fetus as it does to a newly fertilized egg.

I will not discuss the morality of abortion beyond the first trimester of pregnancy (approximately 12 weeks long) since the vast majority of abortions (approximately 90 percent) take place by then. I am quite willing to accept that late abortions, especially those that occur after 24 weeks, are morally problematic; but since these are quite rare (about one percent of all abortions) and almost always done for very serious moral reasons such as to preserve the life or health of the mother or to prevent the birth of an infant with a serious disability, I will not discuss these abortions. Instead, I will focus on so-called elective abortions, those chosen to avoid the burdens of pregnancy, childbearing, and childrearing.

Most opponents of abortion say that abortion is wrong because it is the killing of an innocent human being. They see no morally relevant difference between an early gestation fetus and a newborn baby. If it would be wrong to kill a newborn because it is unwanted (something on which there is virtually unanimous agreement), then, according to this thinking, it is equally wrong to perform an abortion, which deliberately kills the fetus.

The question, then, is whether an early gestation fetus (or simply "fetus" as I will say from now on) is morally equivalent to a newborn baby. This seems to me completely implausible. A newborn can feel, react, and perceive. It cries when it is hungry or stuck with needles. Very soon after birth it cries from boredom or loneliness as well and can be soothed by being rocked and held. By contrast, the first-trimester fetus cannot think, feel, or perceive anything. It is certainly alive and human, but it feels and is aware of nothing; it is more like a gamete (a sperm or an ovum), which is also alive and human, than a baby. While early abortion is not the psychological equivalent of contraception, it is morally closer to contraception than to homicide.

My thesis is that killing fetuses is morally different from killing babies because fetuses are not, and babies are, sentient. By sentience, I mean the ability to experience pain and pleasure. But what is the moral significance of sentience? I have argued (Steinbock, 1992) that sentience is important because nonsentient beings, whether mere things (e.g., cars and rocks and works of art) or living things without nervous systems (e.g., plants), lack interests of their own. Therefore, nonsentient beings are not among those beings whose interests we are required to consider. To put it another way, nonsentient beings lack moral status. I refer to this view of moral status as "the interest view."

Critics of the interest view ask why a being has to feel or experience anything to have interests. Leaving a bicycle out in the rain will cause it to rust, affecting adversely both its appearance and its performance. Why can we not say that this is contrary to its interests? Stripping the bark off a tree will cause it to die. Why can't we say that this is against the tree's interest? Limiting interests to sentient beings (namely, animals—human and otherwise) seems to limit unduly the arena of our concern. What about rivers and forests and mountains? What about the environment?

However, this objection misconceives the interest view. The claim is not that we should be concerned to protect and preserve only sentient beings, but rather that only sentient beings can have an interest or a stake in their own existence. It is only sentient beings to whom anything matters, which is quite different from saying that only sentient beings matter. The interest view can acknowledge the value of many nonsentient beings, from works of art to wilderness areas. It recognizes that we have all kinds of reasons—economic, aesthetic, symbolic, even moral reasons—to protect or preserve nonsentient beings. The difference between sentient and nonsentient beings is not that sentient beings have value and nonsentient ones lack value. Rather, it is that since nonsentient beings cannot be hurt or made to suffer, it does not matter *to them* what is done to them. In deciding what we should do, we cannot consider *their* interests since they do not have any. It might be wrong to deface a work of art or to burn a flag, but it is not a wrong *to* the painting or the flag. Put another way "golden rule"–type reasons do not apply to nonsentient beings. That is, no one would explain opposition to burning the flag of the United States of America by saying, "How would you like it if you were a flag and someone burned you?" Instead, such opposition would have to be based on the symbolic importance of the flag and the message that is conveyed when it is burned in a political demonstration. (I am not saying that flag-burning *is* wrong, only contrasting an intelligible reason for opposing flag-burning, based on the symbolic value of the flag, with an absurd reason.)

The interest view is a general theory about moral status, but it has implications for the morality of abortion. During early gestation, fetuses are nonsentient beings and, as such, they do not have interests. Scientists do not agree on precisely when fetuses become sentient, but most agree that first-trimester fetuses are not sentient. The reason is that, in the first trimester, the fetal nervous system is not sufficiently developed to transmit pain messages to the brain. Since the brain cannot receive pain messages, the first-trimester fetus is not sentient; it cannot feel anything. The synaptic connections necessary for pain perception are established in the fetal brain between 20 and 24 weeks of gestation (Anand and Hickey, 1987). This means not only that premature infants *are* capable of experiencing pain—something that doctors rejected until very recently—but also that, throughout the first and most of the second trimester, fetuses do not experience pain or any other sensation. Despite the claims of propaganda films like *The Silent Scream,* first-trimester fetuses do not suffer when they are aborted.

Prolifers may think that I have missed the point of their opposition to abortion. They need not claim that abortion *hurts* the fetus, or causes it to experience pain, but rather that abortion deprives the fetus of its *life*. I quite agree that this is the important issue, but I maintain that a nonsentient being is not deprived of anything by being killed. In an important sense, it does not have a life to lose.

Now this claim may strike some people as odd. If the fetus is alive, then surely it has a life to lose? But this is just what I am denying. It seems to me that unless there is conscious awareness of some kind, a being does not have a life to lose. Consider all the living cells in our bodies which die or are killed. Surely it would be absurd to speak of all of them as losing their lives or being deprived of their lives. Or consider those in a state of permanent unconsciousness, with no hope of regaining consciousness. I would say that such persons have already lost their lives in any sense that matters, even though they are still biologically alive. It is not biological life that matters, but rather conscious existence. Killing the fetus before it becomes conscious and aware deprives it of nothing. To put it another way, the first-trimester fetus has a biological life, but its biographical life has not yet begun (Rachels, 1986). The interest view suggests that it is *prima facie* wrong to deprive beings of their biographical lives, but not wrong to end merely biological lives, at least where there are good reasons for doing so, such as not wanting to bear a child.

III. THE ARGUMENT FROM POTENTIAL

Of course, there is one difference between a human fetus and any other living, nonsentient being, namely, that if the fetus is not killed, but allowed to develop and grow, it will become a person, just like you or me. Some opponents of abortion cite the potential of the fetus to become a sentient being, with interests and a welfare of its own, as the reason for ascribing to it the moral status belonging to sentient beings. Equally, on this view, the potential of the fetus to become a person gives it the same rights as other persons, including the right to life.

The potentiality principle has been criticized on several grounds. Firstly, it does not follow from the fact that something is a potential *x* that it should be treated as an actual *x*. This is often called "the logical problem with potentiality." As John Harris (1985) puts it, we're all potentially dead, but that's no reason to treat living people as if they were corpses. Secondly, it is not clear why potential personhood attaches only to the fertilized egg. Why aren't unfertilized eggs and sperm also potential people? If certain things happen to them (like meeting a gamete) and certain other things do not (like meeting a contraceptive), they too will develop into people. Admittedly, the chance of any particular sperm becoming a person is absurdly low, but why should that negate its potential? Isn't every player a potential winner in a state lottery, even though the chances of winning are infinitesmal? We should not confuse potentialities with probabilities. So if abortion is wrong because it kills a potential person, then using a spermicide as a contraceptive is equally wrong because it also kills a potential person. Few opponents of abortion are willing to accept this conclusion, which means either giving up the argument from potential or finding a way to differentiate morally between gametes and embryos.

IV. MARQUIS' ARGUMENT

Don Marquis (1989) argues that traditional arguments on abortion, both those of opponents of abortion and those of proponents of a woman's right to choose, are seriously flawed. His argument against abortion derives from a general principle about the wrongness of killing. Killing adult human beings is *prima facie* wrong because it deprives them of their worthwhile future. Marquis writes:

> The loss of one's life is one of the greatest losses one can suffer. The loss of one's life deprives one of all the experiences, activities, projects, and enjoyments that would otherwise have constituted one's future. Therefore, killing someone is wrong, primarily because the killing inflicts (one of) the greatest possible losses on the victim. . . . When I am killed, I am deprived both of what I now value which would have been part of my future personal life, but also what I would come to value. Therefore, when I die, I am deprived of all of the value of my future. Inflicting this loss on me is ultimately what makes killing me wrong. This being the case, it would seem that what makes killing *any* adult human being *prima facie* seriously wrong is the loss of his or her future (Marquis, 1989, p. 592; in this volume, pp. 463–71).

This argument for the wrongness of killing applies only to those who in fact have a future with experiences, activities, projects, and enjoyments. In Marquis' view, it might not be wrong to kill someone in a persistent vegetative state (PVS), for example, who will never regain consciousness, because such a person no longer has a valuable future. (There might be other reasons against killing PVS patients, but these would not refer to the loss inflicted on the patient.) Similarly, persons who are severely and incurably ill and who face a future of pain and despair and who wish to die may not be wronged if they are killed, because the future of which they are deprived is not considered by them to be a valuable one. However, most fetuses (leaving aside those with serious anomalies) do have valuable futures. If they are not aborted, they will come to have lives they will value and enjoy, just as you and I value and enjoy our lives. Therefore, abortion is seriously wrong for the same reason that killing an innocent adult human being is seriously wrong: it deprives the victim of his or her valuable future.

Marquis' argument against abortion is similar to arguments based on the principle of potentiality in that the wrongness of killing is derived from the loss of the valuable future the fetus will have, if allowed to grow and develop, rather than being based on any characteristic, such as genetic humanity, the fetus now has. However, Marquis' view differs from traditional potentiality arguments in two ways. Firstly, most arguments from potential maintain that it is wrong not only to kill persons, but also to kill potential persons. Though a human fetus is not now a person, it will develop into one if allowed to grow and develop. By contrast, Marquis' argument says nothing about the wrongness of killing persons and therefore nothing about the wrongness of killing potential persons. Marquis is explicit about his argument not necessarily being limited to persons but applying to any beings who have valuable futures like ours. Some nonpersons (e.g., some animals) also might have such futures, and so it might be wrong to kill them in Marquis' account. Admittedly, the concept of a person is not coextensive with the capacity to have a valuable future, and there are heated debates about what it is to be a person. However, if we use the term "person" simply to mean an individual with a valuable future like ours and hence one it would be seriously wrong to kill, we can reword Marquis' account in terms of the wrongness of killing persons.

Another way in which Marquis differs from potentiality theorists is that his argument is not based on the potential of the fetus to become something different from what it is now. Rather, it is wrong to kill a fetus because killing it deprives it of its valuable future—the very same reason why it is wrong to kill you or me. Thus, although Marquis focuses on a certain kind of potential, namely, the fetus's potential to have experiences in the future, this potential is no different from the potential that any born human being has to have future experiences. Thus, he cannot be accused of basing the wrongness of killing born human beings on a feature that we actually possess, while basing the wrongness of abortion on a (merely) potential feature of the fetus.

Marquis thinks that his view is superior to other accounts of moral status in that it is able to explain what is wrong with killing people who are temporarily unconscious, something the interest view seems incapable of doing. If it is morally permissible to kill nonsentient beings, why is it wrong to kill someone in a reversible coma? Such a person is not now conscious or sentient. And if we appeal to his future conscious states, the same argument seems to apply to the fetus, who will become conscious and sentient if we just leave it alone.

Two responses can be made to this objection to the interest view. The first is to note an important difference between a temporarily unconscious person and a fetus. The difference is that the person who is now unconscious has had experiences, plans, beliefs, desires, etc. in the past. These past experiences are relevant because they form the basis for saying that the comatose person wants not to be killed while unconscious. "He valued his life," we might say. "Of course he would not want to be killed." This desire or preference is the basis for saying that the temporarily unconscious person has an interest in not being killed. But the same cannot be said of a nonsentient fetus. A nonsentient fetus cannot be said to want anything, and so cannot be said to want not to be killed. By contrast, if I am killed while sleeping or temporarily comatose, I am deprived of something I want very much, namely, to go on living. This is not an *occurrent* desire; that is, it is rarely if ever a desire of which I am consciously aware, but it is certainly one of my desires. We have all sorts of desires of which we are not at any particular moment consciously aware, and it would be absurd to limit our desires to what we are actually thinking about. Nor do our desires, plans, and goals, or the interests composing them, vanish when we fall into dreamless sleep.

However, our interests are not limited to what we take an interest in, as Tom Regan (1976) has correctly noted. Our interests also include what is *in* our interest, whether or not we are interested in it. For example, getting enough sleep, eating moderately, and forgoing tobacco might be in the interest of a person who has no interest in following such a regime. Now even if the nonconscious fetus is not interested in continuing to live, could we not say that continued existence is *in* its interest? If the fetus will go on to have a valuable future, is not that future in its interest?

The issue raised here is whether the future the fetus will go on to have is in an important sense *its* future. Marquis considers the existence of past experiences to be entirely irrelevant to the question of whether an entity can be deprived of its future. But this is not at all clear. Killing embryos or early gestation fetuses differs from killing adult human beings because adult human beings have a life that they (ordinarily) value and which they would prefer not to lose: a biographical as opposed to merely biological life. How might the idea of having a biographical life be connected with the possibility of having a personal future, a future of one's own? In an unpublished manuscript, "The Future-Like-Ours Argument Against Abortion and The Problem of Personal Identity," David Boonin uses a plausible theory of personal identity—the psychological continuity account—to argue that nonsentient fetuses do not have a personal future.[1] According to the psychological continuity account of personal identity, having a certain set of past experiences is what makes me the person I am, and the experiences that I have, *my* experiences. What makes experiences at two different times experiences of the same person is that they are appropriately related by a chain of memories, desires, intentions, and the like. So an individual's past experiences are not, as Marquis claims, otiose to an account of the value of his future; indeed, they are precisely what makes his future *his*.

On this account of personal identity, then, there is an important difference between someone who is temporarily unconscious and a fetus. The difference is this: when the unconscious person regains consciousness, "there will be a relationship of continuity involving memories, intentions, character traits, and so on between his subsequent experiences and those which he had before he lapsed into the coma" (Boonin, 1996, p. 11).

This is what makes his future experiences (those he will have if he is not killed) *his*. The situation of the preconscious fetus is quite different.

> When he gains (rather than regains) consciousness, there will be no relationship of continuity involving memories, intentions, character traits, and so on between his subsequent experiences and those which he had before he gained consciousness precisely because he *had* no experiences before he gained consciousness. This is what permits us to say of the preconscious fetus that it is not he who will have these later experiences if he is not killed. And this, in turn, is what permits us to deny that *he* will be harmed if we prevent those experiences from occurring (Boonin, 1996, p. 12).

If we accept the psychological continuity account of personal identity, then past experiences do matter because without past experiences there is no one with a personal future. This is not to say that this provides us with a reason to kill the presentient fetus but rather that we lack the strong reason for not killing it that we have in the case of people like you and me. The justificatory reason for killing the fetus stems from the woman's rights to bodily autonomy and self-determination, to which I will return in the next section.

However, perhaps the psychological continuity account is wrong. Perhaps personal identity is better based on physical continuity. In that case, even if the born human being has no memories connecting her to the fetal stage, we can still say that she is the same individual because there is physical continuity between the born human and the fetal human.

There are certain advantages to a physical continuity account of personal identity. It allows us to say of someone who develops total amnesia that he has a history of which he has absolutely no memory, and this seems to be a plain statement of fact. Similarly, most people have very few memories about anything that occurred before the ages of four or five; yet most of us are convinced that we are the same individuals we were when very young. Of course, there could be psychological connections of which we have no memory. For example, providing an infant with secure, loving experiences as opposed to terrifying or traumatic ones is likely to affect the psychological development of the eventual adult, whether or not she remembers what happened. So it may be that a more sophisticated psychological account, one that is not entirely dependent on memory, is the better account of identity, but I will not pursue that issue.

Boonin argues that the trouble with basing identity on physical continuity is that this implies that contraception is as wrong as abortion, something most people, including Marquis, want to reject. Thus, the claim that contraception prevents a gamete from enjoying a future like ours takes the form of a *reductio ad absurdum:* the argument (allegedly) commits one to an absurd (or at least unacceptable) conclusion. A physical continuity account of personal identity is vulnerable to the objection that it makes contraception as wrong as abortion because there seems to be no reason why embryos have and gametes do not have valuable futures. For the embryo does not appear *ex nihilo.* Its physical history goes back to the conjoining of the sperm and ovum. Thus, if you prevent the sperm and ovum from conjoining, you deprive each of them of the future they would have had if fertilization had taken place.

Marquis says that his view does not apply to contraception because, prior to fertilization, there is no entity that has a future. It is only after fertilization, when there is a being with a specific genetic code, that there is an individual with a future who can be deprived of that future by being killed. But why should this be so? Admittedly, neither gamete can have a future all by itself, but that is also true of the embryo, which cannot develop all by itself. It needs a uterus and adequate nutrients to develop into a fetus and a baby. Admittedly, the future the sperm will have is not its future alone; it shares its future with the ovum it fertilizes. This makes the situation of gametes unusual, perhaps unique, but does not seem to provide a reason why gametes cannot have futures if the criterion of identity is physical continuity.

Sometimes it is said that a sperm is not a unique individual in the way that a fetus is. For who the sperm turns out to be depends on which ovum it unites with. Why, however, should this lack of uniqueness deprive the sperm of being a potential person, or to use Marquis' language, why should its lack of uniqueness prevent it from having "a future like ours"? Although we cannot specify which future existence the sperm will have, if it is allowed to fertilize an egg, it will become *somebody* and that somebody will have a valuable future.

I think the reason we do not usually think of sperm as having futures is that, in the ordinary reproductive context, literally millions of sperm are released, and only one can fertilize the egg. The rest are doomed. So it seems implausible to say that by killing sperm, we are depriving them of a future. Still, *one* of them might fertilize the egg, even though we cannot say which one it will be, and that one sperm will not get to develop into an embryo and eventual person if it is killed before conception occurs.

Moreover, assisted reproductive technology (ART) facilitates the tracing of an embryo back to its constituent gametes in a way never before possible. In the context of *in vitro* fertilization (IVF), where an egg and sperm are placed in a petri dish for fertilization to occur, we *can* identify the particular gametes who might unite. If dumping out the contents of the petri dish after fertilization has occurred would be immoral because doing that deprives the fertilized egg of "a future like ours," why is it not equally wrong to dump out the contents of the petri dish seconds before fertilization occurs? The ability to identify which gametes make up the embryo is even greater in the micromanipulation technique known as intracytoplasmic sperm injection (ICSI). The ICSI technique enables patients with male factor infertility, where not enough motile sperm can be recovered for ordinary *in vitro* fertilization (IVF), to be considered for assisted reproductive intervention. In ICSI, a single sperm is injected directly into the egg. The isolation of a single sperm makes it possible for us to identify with certainty which sperm conjoined with the egg in the resultant embryo. Thus, the individual who comes to be after fertilization is physically continuous with the sperm in the pipette and the egg in the petri dish. Killing the gametes before fertilization deprives both of them of the future they would have had.

Marquis might respond to the ART examples by maintaining, in his account, that embryos *in vitro* do not have valuable futures like ours. It is only after implantation, when twinning is no longer possible, that we have an individual who can be said to have a personal future. Thus, Marquis need not be backed into claiming a moral difference between dumping out a petri dish just before or just after conception. Equally, his view is compatible with allowing contraceptives and abortifacients that kill the embryo before implantation occurs. These are seen as importantly morally different from terminating a clinical pregnancy, that is, after implantation occurs. Certainly most of us do regard abortion, even in the first trimester, as morally different from contraception or even a morning-after pill. It seems to me, however, that the reason is not that the status of the embryo radically changes with implantation. Rather, it is that most people have very different feelings toward the termination of a pregnancy than they have toward the prevention of pregnancy. I will return to this point later.

In any event, I do not think Marquis has adequately explained why embryos have valuable futures and gametes do not. For this reason, I consider his account of why abortion is immoral to be vulnerable to the usual objection to potentiality arguments, namely, that they make contraception seriously wrong. The interest view avoids this difficulty. As for its alleged difficulty with explaining why it is wrong to kill sleeping and temporarily comatose people, I maintain that this can be explained in terms of the interests of the nonconscious person, interests that a fetus does not yet have. For these reasons, the interest view seems to me a better account of moral status than the future-like-ours account.

V. THE ARGUMENT FROM BODILY SELF-DETERMINATION

Suppose I am right about the first trimester fetus's lack of moral status. This does not mean, as I said earlier, that this gives us a reason for killing the fetus. Wantonly killing living things, even if they lack moral status, may well be wrong. To show that most abortions are not wrong, I have to do more than show that fetuses lack moral status. I have to explain why there are good reasons for killing them. These reasons stem from the fact that sustaining the life of a fetus requires the pregnant woman to serve as its life-support system. Thus, the morality of abortion depends not only on whether the fetus is the kind of being it is seriously wrong to kill, but also on whether women have serious moral obligations to sustain the lives of presentient fetuses by not terminating their pregnancies.

The first person to make this point about abortion was Judith Thomson (1971). Thomson argues that even if the fetus is a person with a right to life, it does not follow that abortion is wrong. For the right to life does not give its possessor an unlimited right to whatever it needs to stay alive. In particular, the right to life does not give anyone a right to use another person's body without permission. In at least some cases of pregnancy (e.g., rape and possibly also unintended pregnancy due to contraceptive failure), the fetus was not given even tacit permission to use the woman's body, and therefore it has no right to use it. Having an abortion does not violate the fetus's right to life, even though it kills it.

Thomson's main concern is with the anti-abortion argument based on the fetus's right to life. Therefore, she is primarily interested in whether abortion violates the fetus's right to life. However, she acknowledges that even if no right of the fetus is violated, abortion might still be wrong if the woman has a moral obligation to let the fetus stay in her body until it can survive in the world. After all, we can and do have obligations to help others that do not stem from their rights. Whether the pregnant woman is morally obligated to allow the fetus to stay inside her body depends, according to Thomson, on the degree of burden and sacrifice this imposes on her. For no one is morally obligated, Thomson says, to make large sacrifices to keep another person alive; and pregnancy—unwanted pregnancy—does impose very great sacrifices.

Firstly, there are the physical complaints of pregnancy: weight gain, soreness in the breasts, tiredness, nausea, heartburn, leg cramps, the need to urinate frequently, the difficulty of sleeping in the last trimester, and so forth. Then there is labor and delivery, which can be protracted and painful. These are not insignificant burdens even in a normal pregnancy where there is no serious risk of harm to the pregnant woman. In "problem pregnancies," the woman may experience much more serious difficulties, including death. Don Regan (1979) argues that outside the abortion context there is no situation in which anyone is required to undergo significant risks and burdens to preserve another person's life. Restrictive abortion laws thus impose burdens on pregnant women that are not imposed on others in comparable situations and so violate the principle of "equal protection."

Although this argument may be successful in showing that abortion should remain legal, its moral force is less clear. Consider the moral obligations of parents to their children, and the sacrifices we think parents should be willing to make for their sakes. In the context of parenthood, it seems false to maintain that no one is morally obligated to make large sacrifices to keep another person alive. Would we think that a parent was under no obligation to take a dying child to the doctor if this were very inconvenient? Suppose the child needed a bone marrow or even a kidney transplant and the parent was a match. Would it be morally permissible for the parent to refuse because of the pain, inconvenience, or bodily invasion? We might not want a society in which judges could force parents to be donors, but surely there *is* a moral obligation to undergo even large sacrifices involving bodily invasion for the sake of one's children. If the fetus is a person, then it presumably has the same status as any other child, and the same claim on its parents that any born children have, including the obligation to make significant sacrifices on its behalf. Of course the burden falls primarily on the woman, since only women can be pregnant (so far), but that biological fact is not intrinsically unfair.

However, if the fetus is importantly different from a born child, as I argued in the last section, then it is hard to see why a woman is morally required to undertake significant risks and burdens to keep the fetus alive. These burdens are not all physical. If abortion is morally wrong, then either the woman will have to raise a child when she does not want to do so, or she will have to endure the pregnancy, labor, and delivery and give the baby up for adoption. Some prolifers talk as if this should be easy enough; after all, she was ready to kill her baby. Why should giving it away upset her? But this cruel attitude ignores the realities. Terminating a pregnancy—especially in the first trimester—is nothing like giving a child up for adoption, in terms of the grief the mother is likely to feel. I can imagine few sacrifices more difficult. One might be morally obligated to make a sacrifice of this magnitude for one's *child,* but no one has a moral obligation to make this huge sacrifice for a merely potential person.

VI. IS ABORTION A SERIOUS MORAL ISSUE?

Some people think not merely that a woman has the right to decide whether to have an abortion, but that no decision she makes can be criticized on moral grounds. For example, Mary Anne Warren (1973) once claimed that abortion is a "morally neutral" issue, comparable to the decision to have one's hair cut. Most people, regardless of their position on abortion, find this extremely implausible, even outrageous. Are we forced to view abortion this way, if we deny that the fetus has moral status? Surely not. In the first place, terminating a pregnancy is typically connected with powerful emotions in a way that deciding to get one's hair cut is not. The pregnant woman may feel ashamed, embarrassed, or guilty about her pregnancy; and all of these feelings may influence how she feels about an abortion. Her feelings about her partner and their relationship, her attitudes toward sexuality and motherhood are all likely to play a part in her decision; and these topics are fraught with emotional significance in a way that a decision to cut one's hair generally is not. She may be ambivalent about the pregnancy, wishing she could keep the baby, although recognizing that she would make a better mother if she waits until she is older or married or more established in a career. Even a woman who is certain she does not want a child (now) may experience some sadness (as well as relief) at ending a pregnancy—sadness at not being able to welcome and enjoy what is ideally a joyous occasion and something to be celebrated. All of these factors help to explain why so many people do not have the same emotional attitudes toward abortion that they have toward contraception. For most people, even most American Catholics, contraception is likely to be regarded as morally neutral, a sensible preventive health habit, like flossing your teeth. It has none of the sadness or sense of loss that may accompany abortions.

These are all reasons why abortion feels different from contraception; but does this emotional difference support a moral difference if fetuses lack moral status? The answer depends on one's conception of morality. In one conception of morality, actions are wrong only if they harm others. On a different conception of morality, virtue ethics, the morality of actions is not limited to the harm they are likely to cause, but includes our assessment of the character traits or attitudes of the agent. It is possible that some people have abortions too casually or for unimportant reasons, and this may affect our moral appraisal of what they do. For example, I once heard a 15-year-old girl announce that she was about to have her third abortion. Surprised that so young a girl had had so many unwanted pregnancies when birth control was readily available, I asked her why she kept getting pregnant. "Oh," she said, "I can never remember to put in a diaphragm, and the pill makes me fat." Such an offhand attitude toward sex and pregnancy seems immature, callow, and superficial. Young people should not become sexually active until they are prepared to take precautions to prevent pregnancy. In addition, this girl's insouciant attitude toward having abortions, which would not be necessary if she were more responsible about contraception, indicates a cavalier, indeed, wanton attitude toward potential human life.

Nevertheless, though I deplore the attitudes revealed by the girl's easy acceptance of abortion, I do not think that her decision to have an abortion was wrong. In fact, the very opposite is true. We hear today that quite a lot of young teenagers of 15 or 16 decide to keep their babies because they want the status and prestige that comes with being a mother, or they want the unconditional love they think a baby will provide, or they hope that this will induce a straying boyfriend to stick around. All of these are, in my opinion, terrible reasons for having a child. Before committing oneself to the responsibilities of parenthood, one should have reasonable grounds for thinking that one will be able to be a good—or good enough—parent. Although some 15-year-olds may be capable of being good mothers, most lack the maturity this requires: the patience, experience, knowledge, and ability to put the interests of someone else first. In my view, a 15-year-old who knows that she cannot be a "good enough" parent and has an abortion partly for this reason acts more responsibly, more morally, than the girl who has a baby without thinking about her responsibilities to her future child.

VII. WHICH ABORTIONS ARE IMMORAL?

As the title of my essay suggests, I believe that most abortions are not wrong. Most abortions occur because the woman does not want to have a child, and I think that this is a very good reason to terminate a pregnancy. However, some abortions may be immoral for a variety of reasons.

A. Trivial Reasons

Consider the following story. A man learns that his girlfriend is pregnant. He is ecstatic and would like to marry her and raise the child together. However, she tells him that she does not want to continue the pregnancy because she does not want to be pregnant in the summer when she would be unable to wear a bikini. This is certainly a very trivial reason for having an abortion. Would the triviality of the reason make the abortion morally wrong? Certainly her willingness to abort for so slight a reason reflects very badly on her character, but perhaps we should be glad that someone so ditzy is not planning on motherhood, just as we are glad when the immature girl in the previous section decides to abort. There is one difference between this case and the one discussed above, namely, that in this case the girl's partner is willing to take on the childrearing responsibilities by himself if necessary. Assuming that he will be a good parent, bringing the child into the world would not be unfair to the child. If it were really the case that she has no other reason for wanting to avoid pregnancy (such as the usual risks and burdens) and is only worried about not being able to wear a bikini, we might reasonably judge her abortion to be immoral. So trivial a reason does not seem to justify killing a fetus or depriving a man of his desperately wanted child. However, it is scarcely plausible that this could ever be a woman's sole reason for wishing to avoid pregnancy.

B. Sex Selection

A more realistic example is abortion for sex selection. In some cultures, the desire for a male child is so strong that women will request prenatal diagnosis for the sole purpose of learning the sex of the fetus in order to abort if it is a girl. Most people in our culture consider the destruction of a healthy fetus just because of its sex to be immoral, either because of the sexist attitude it expresses or because such abortions reflect insufficient respect for potential human life, or both. However, it is not clear that abortion for sex selection is always or necessarily wrong. Imagine a woman in her late 40s who has already borne five sons and finds to her amazement that she is again pregnant. If she were to decide to abort, few people would regard her decision as unjustified or her reason—that she has completed her family and is through with childbearing and rearing—as trivial. Now suppose that the woman has always wanted a girl. She could face a sixth child, she thinks, if it were the longed-for daughter. If it is morally permissible for her to terminate the pregnancy, I do not see why it would be wrong for her to terminate if the fetus would be another son. Wanting a daughter after five boys is not an unreasonable or sexist preference. It seems to me that it is up to the woman to decide if another pregnancy would be too burdensome, and that the decision that it would not be if the child were a girl does not demonstrate insufficient respect for prenatal life.

In some countries, the desire for a son is so strong that women undergo numerous pregnancies in order to have a male child. We may regard such a preference as sexist and unenlightened, but it exists and has large implications for the lives of women living in these cultures. Repeated pregnancies take a serious toll on their health and force them to bear more children than they can adequately feed and clothe. The lives of the girls who are born in the attempt to get a son are often substandard as they typically receive less food and medical attention than their brothers. Preventing the births of girls by abortion seems a morally preferable option to requiring that they be born, then neglected, or allowed to starve to death. So while we may regard abortion for sex selection to be generally wrong, at least in our country, the automatic and absolute rejection of sex selection fails to take into consideration the social realities in which it may occur.

C. Fetal Reduction

Most fetal reductions are done when there are more fetuses than can be safely expected to be carried to term. Typically, this is due to the woman's having taken fertility drugs, which greatly increases the chance of having multiple fetuses. Fertility drugs were responsible for the first surviving set of septuplets born in Iowa in November 1997 to Bobbi and Kenny McCaughey. Doctors usually advise women pregnant with more than three fetuses to undergo selective reduction. The reasoning behind fetal reduction is that if some of the fetuses are not killed, the chances that any of them will survive, especially without disability, are greatly reduced. If a reduction is not performed, the couple may lose the entire pregnancy. The mother's health is also put at risk in a multiple pregnancy.

Fetal reduction of a much-wanted pregnancy is likely to be a heartrending choice, even though this improves the chances of survival of the remaining fetuses. For some, like the McCaugheys, selective reduction may be completely unacceptable. Some people criticized the McCaugheys for their decision not to reduce, arguing that while Bobbi McCaughey was entitled to risk her own life and health by carrying seven fetuses, she had no right to subject her future children to the substantial risks of mental retardation, cerebral palsy, and blindness. These critics say that the fact that "the gamble paid off," and all the babies appear to be healthy so far (although it may be some time before any damage is evident), does not make the risk-taking more justifiable. Indeed, some doctors who have had very bad outcomes with multiple births are no longer willing to prescribe fertility drugs for women who would not consider selective reduction. Others think that the choice must remain that of the individual patient.

The choice to reduce a multiple pregnancy to twins is invariably regarded as permissible by those who think that abortion can ever be justified, since the aim is to preserve the life and health of the mother and remaining fetuses. What if the pregnant woman wants a fetal reduction from twins to a singleton, not because of the objective risk of a multiple birth, but because she would prefer to have just one baby? In August 1996, Dr. Phillip Bennett of Queen Charlotte's Hospital in London told *The Sunday Express* that he had recommended abortion of one fetus as a solution when the woman told him she could not continue her 16-week-old pregnancy if it meant having twins. He felt that it would be better to do the reduction and leave one alive than to lose two babies.

The first reports of the story maintained that the woman was a 28-year-old single mother with one child, who was too poor to raise twins. The public reacted with shock, anger, and dismay. Life, a British national charity, said it was deluged with calls and was able immediately to offer the woman upward of $16,000 to give birth to both twins and give one up for adoption. Many commentators were appalled by the doctor's willingness to perform a selective reduction in this situation. One called it selective murder, saying, "I mean, we know they have aborted healthy babies before, but to leave one and kill the other is abhorrent" (Ibrahim, 1996).

As it later turned out, the woman was a middle-class professional who was not motivated by lack of funds. Apparently, she simply did not want to cope with twins. This does not seem unduly callous or selfish. Even carrying twins puts considerable extra burdens on the pregnant woman, and caring for twins is a great deal more work than caring for one child. The justification for abortion in this case is very similar to the standard case: it is based on the amount of sacrifice and burden the pregnancy will impose. In this case, as in all the rest, only the woman herself can judge if the burdens are too great for her to bear. If aborting both twins is both legally and morally permissible (and indeed would have passed unnoticed), it is hard to see why aborting one of the twins would be morally wrong. If the woman had felt she had no choice but to abort one fetus because of poverty, that would indeed have been tragic—though no more tragic than the decision to abort a single fetus due to poverty. Yet such cases, which surely occur, do not get written up in the newspapers; and no one offers these poor women money so they will be able to keep their babies.

D. Vengeful Abortion

Abortion could also be immoral if done for morally bad, as opposed to trivial, reasons. For example, imagine a woman who has an abortion to take revenge on her husband when she learns that he was unfaithful to her earlier in the marriage. She does not want to end the marriage, or even not to have his child, but only to make him suffer as she has suffered. Once she feels that he has adequately made amends, she intends to get pregnant again. Let us further imagine that she already has two children to whom she has been an excellent mother. This variation of the *Medea* story, with its jealousy, vengefulness, spite, and cruelty, is a pretty clear example of an immoral abortion. My qualification is due to the fact that the woman seems psychotic and thus possibly not morally responsible.

VIII. CONCLUSION

Of course, most women do not have abortions for the bizarre reasons given above. A very common reason for abortion, perhaps the most common, is birth control failure. Women get pregnant using diaphragms, IUDs, even on the pill. The possibility of birth control failure makes abortion a necessity if women are to have genuine choice about when and whether they reproduce. Even if the pregnancy is someone's "fault," that is, due to a failure to use birth control, that bears no relation to the morality of abortion. Given that fetuses are not the sorts of entities whom it is seriously wrong to kill, women have the moral right to decide for themselves if they are willing to endure the burdens of pregnancy and childbirth. In most cases, their reasons for wishing to terminate their pregnancies are sensible ones. In fact, in light of the number of abused and neglected children in the world, it might make more sense to ask that people justify their decisions to have children, instead of their decisions to terminate pregnancies.

NOTES

1. For a statement of Boonin's more recent critique of Marquis's argument, see his book, *A Defense of Abortion* (Cambridge University Press, forthcoming, section 2.8).

REFERENCES

Anand, K.J.S. & Hickey, P.R. (1987). Pain and its effects in the human neonate and fetus. N. Engl. J. Med. 317, 1322.

Boonin, D. (1996). The future-like-ours argument against abortion and the problem of personal identity. (Unpublished.)

Graber, M.A. (1996). Rethinking Abortion: Equal Choice, the Constitution, and Reproductive Politics. Princeton University Press, Princeton, NJ.

Harris, J. (1985). The Value of Life: An Introduction to Medical Ethics. Routledge & Kegan Paul, London.

Ibrahim, Y.M. (1996). Planned abortion of one twin stirs furor in Britain. The New York Times, August 6, p. A3.

Marquis, D. (1989). Why abortion is immoral. J. of Phil. 76, 183-202.

McCormick, J. and Kantrowitz, B. (1997). The magnificent seven. Newsweek, December 1, pp. 58-62.

Rachels, J. (1986). The End of Life: Euthanasia and Morality. Oxford University Press, New York.

Regan, D. (1979). Rewriting *Roe* v. *Wade*. Mich. L. Rev. 77.

Regan, T. (1976). Feinberg on what sorts of beings can have rights. Southern J. of Phil. 14, 485-498.

Robertson, J.A. (1994). Children of Choice: Freedom and the New Reproductive Technologies. Princeton University Press, Princeton, NJ.

Steinbock, B. (1992). Life Before Birth: The Moral and Legal Status of Embryos and Fetuses. Oxford University Press, New York.

Thomson, J. (1971). A defense of abortion. Phil. & Pub. Affairs 1, 47-66.

Warren, M.A. (1973). On the moral and legal status of abortion. Monist 57, 43-61.

A DEFENSE OF ABORTION[1]

Judith Jarvis Thomson

Most opposition to abortion relies on the premise that the fetus is a human being, a person, from the moment of conception. The premise is argued for, but, as I think, not well. Take, for example, the most common argument. We are asked to notice that the development of a human being from conception through birth into childhood is continuous; then it is said that to draw a line, to choose a point in this development and say "before this point the thing is not a person, after this point it is a person" is to make an arbitrary choice, a choice for which in the nature of things no good reason can be given. It is concluded that the fetus is, or anyway that we had better say it is, a person from the moment of conception. But this conclusion does not follow. Similar things might be said about the development of an acorn into an oak tree, and it does not follow that acorns are oak trees, or that we had better say they are. Arguments of this form are sometimes called "slippery slope arguments"—the phrase is perhaps self-explanatory—and it is dismaying that opponents of abortion rely on them so heavily and uncritically.

I am inclined to agree, however, that the prospects for "drawing a line" in the development of the fetus look dim. I am inclined to think also that we shall probably have to agree that the fetus has already become a human person well before birth. Indeed, it comes as a surprise when one first learns how early in its life it begins to acquire human characteristics. By the tenth week, for example, it already has a face, arms and legs, fingers and toes; it has internal organs, and brain activity is detectable.[2] On the other hand, I think that the premise is false, that the fetus is not a person from the moment of conception. A newly fertilized ovum, a newly implanted clump of cells, is no more a person than an acorn is an oak tree. But I shall not discuss any of this. For it seems to me to be of great interest to ask what happens if, for the sake of argument, we allow the premise. How, precisely, are we supposed to get from there to the conclusion that abortion is morally impermissible? Opponents of abortion commonly spend most of their time establishing that the fetus is a person, and hardly any time explaining the step from there to the impermissibility of abortion. Perhaps they think the step too simple and obvious to require much comment. Or perhaps instead they are simply being economical in argument. Many of those who defend abortion rely on the premise that the fetus is not a person, but only a bit of tissue that will become a person at birth; and why pay out more arguments than you have to? Whatever the explanation, I suggest that the step they take is neither easy nor obvious, that it calls for closer examination than it is commonly given, and that when we do give it this closer examination we shall feel inclined to reject it.

I propose, then, that we grant that the fetus is a person from the moment of conception. How does the argument go from here? Something like this, I take it. Every person has a right to life. So the fetus has a right to life. No doubt the mother has a right to decide what shall happen in and to her body; everyone would grant that. But surely a person's right to life is stronger and more stringent than the mother's right to decide what happens in and to her body, and so outweighs it. So the fetus may not be killed; an abortion may not be performed.

It sounds plausible. But now let me ask you to imagine this. You wake up in the morning and find yourself back to back in bed with an unconscious violinist. A famous unconscious violinist. He has been found to have a fatal kidney ailment, and the Society of Music Lovers has canvassed all the available medical records and found that you alone have the right blood type to help. They have therefore kidnapped you, and last night the violinist's circulatory system was plugged into yours, so that your kidneys can be used to extract poisons from his

From *Philosophy and Public Affairs*, Vol. 1, No. 1, 47–66.

blood as well as your own. The director of the hospital now tells you, "Look, we're sorry the Society of Music Lovers did this to you—we would never have permitted it if we had known. But still, they did it, and the violinist now is plugged into you. To unplug you would be to kill him. But never mind, it's only for nine months. By then he will have recovered from his ailment, and can safely be unplugged from you." Is it morally incumbent on you to accede to this situation? No doubt it would be very nice of you if you did, a great kindness. But do you *have* to accede to it? What if it were not nine months, but nine years? Or longer still? What if the director of the hospital says, "Tough luck, I agree, but you've now got to stay in bed, with the violinist plugged into you, for the rest of your life. Because remember this. All persons have a right to life, and violinists are persons. Granted you have a right to decide what happens in and to your body, but a person's right to life outweighs your right to decide what happens in and to your body. So you cannot ever be unplugged from him." I imagine you would regard this as outrageous, which suggests that something really is wrong with that plausible-sounding argument I mentioned a moment ago.

In this case, of course, you were kidnapped; you didn't volunteer for the operation that plugged the violinist into your kidneys. Can those who oppose abortion on the ground I mentioned make any exception for a pregnancy due to rape? Certainly. They can say that persons have a right to life only if they didn't come into existence because of rape; or they can say that all persons have a right to life, but that some have less of a right to life than others, in particular, that those who came into existence because of rape have less. But these statements have a rather unpleasant sound. Surely the question of whether you have a right to life at all, or how much of it you have, shouldn't turn on the question of whether or not you are the product of a rape. And in fact the people who oppose abortion on the ground I mentioned do not make this distinction, and hence do not make an exception in case of rape.

Nor do they make an exception for a case in which the mother has to spend the nine months of her pregnancy in bed. They would agree that would be a great pity, and hard on the mother; but all the same, all persons have a right to life, the fetus is a person, and so on. I suspect, in fact, that they would not make an exception for a case in which, miraculously enough, the pregnancy went on for nine years, or even the rest of the mother's life.

Some won't even make an exception for a case in which continuation of the pregnancy is likely to shorten the mother's life; they regard abortion as impermissible even to save the mother's life. Such cases are nowadays very rare, and many opponents of abortion do not accept this extreme view. All the same, it is a good place to begin: a number of points of interest come out in respect to it.

1. Let us call the view that abortion is impermissible even to save the mother's life "the extreme view." I want to suggest first that it does not issue from the argument I mentioned earlier without the addition of some fairly powerful premises. Suppose a woman has become pregnant, and now learns that she has a cardiac condition such that she will die if she carries the baby to term. What may be done for her? The fetus, being a person, has a right to life, but as the mother is a person too, so has she a right to life. Presumably they have an equal right to life. How is it supposed to come out that an abortion may not be performed? If mother and child have an equal right to life, shouldn't we perhaps flip a coin? Or should we add to the mother's right to life her right to decide what happens in and to her body, which everybody seems to be ready to grant—the sum of her rights now outweighing the fetus's right to life?

The most familiar argument here is the following. We are told that performing the abortion would be directly killing[3] the child, whereas doing nothing would not be killing the mother, but only letting her die. Moreover, in killing the child, one would be killing an innocent person, for the child has committed no crime, and is not aiming at his mother's death. And then there are a variety of ways in which this might be continued. (1) But as directly killing an innocent person is always and absolutely impermissible, an abortion may not be performed. Or, (2) as directly killing an innocent person is murder, and murder is always and absolutely impermissible, an abortion may not be performed.[4] Or, (3) as one's duty to refrain from directly killing an innocent person is more stringent than one's duty to keep a person from dying, an abortion may not be performed. Or, (4) if one's only options are directly killing an innocent person or letting a person die, one must prefer letting the person die, and thus an abortion may not be performed.[5]

Some people seem to have thought that these are not further premises which must be added if the conclusion is to be reached, but that they follow from the very fact that an innocent person has a right to life.[6] But this seems to me to be a mistake, and perhaps the simplest way to show this is to bring out that while we must certainly grant that innocent persons have a right to life, the theses in (1) through (4) are all false. Take (2), for example. If directly killing an innocent person is murder, and thus is impermissible, then the mother's directly killing the innocent person inside her is murder, and thus is impermissible. But it cannot seriously be thought to be murder if the mother performs an abortion on herself to save her life. It cannot seriously be said that she *must* refrain, that she *must* sit passively by and wait for her death. Let us look again at the case of you and the violinist. There you are, in bed with the violinist, and the director of the hospital says to you "It's all most distressing, and I deeply sympathize, but you see this is putting an additional strain on your kidneys, and you'll be dead within the month. But you *have* to stay where you are all the same. Because unplugging you would be directly killing an innocent violinist, and that's murder, and that's impermissible." If anything in the world is true, it is that you do not commit murder, you do not do what is impermissible, if you reach around to your back and unplug yourself from that violinist to save your life. . . .

2. The extreme view could of course be weakened to say that while abortion is permissible to save the mother's life, it may not be performed by a third party, but only by the mother herself. But this cannot be right either. For what we have to keep in mind is that the mother and the unborn child are not like two tenants in a small house which has, by an unfortunate mistake, been rented to both: the mother *owns* the house. The fact that she does adds to the offensiveness of deducing that the mother can do nothing from the supposition that third parties can do nothing. But it does more than this: it casts a bright light on the supposition that third parties can do nothing. Certainly it lets us see that a third party who says "I cannot choose between you" is fooling himself if he thinks this is impartiality. If Jones has found and fastened on a certain coat, which he needs to keep him from freezing, but which Smith also needs to keep him from freezing, then it is not impartiality that says "I cannot choose between you" when Smith owns the coat. Women have said again and again "This body is *my* body!" and they have reason to feel angry, reason to feel that it has been like shouting into the wind. Smith, after all, is hardly likely to bless us if we say to him, "Of course it's your coat, anybody would grant that it is. But no one may choose between you and Jones who is to have it."

We should really ask what it is that says "no one may choose" in the face of the fact that the body that houses the child is the mother's body. It may be simply a failure to appreciate this fact. But it may be something more interesting, namely the sense that one has a right to refuse to lay hands on Jones, a right to refuse to do physical violence to people, even where it would be just and fair to do so, even where justice seems to require that somebody do so. Thus justice might call for somebody to get Smith's coat back from Jones, and yet you have a right to refuse to be the one to lay hands on Jones, a right to refuse to do physical violence to him. This, I think, must be granted. But then what should be said is not "no one may choose" but only "*I* cannot choose," and indeed not even this, but "*I* will not *act*," leaving it open that somebody else can or should, and in particular that anyone in a position of authority, with the job of securing people's rights, both can and should. So this is no difficulty. I have not been arguing that any given third party must accede to the mother's request that he perform an abortion to save her life, but only that he may.

I suppose that in some views of human life the mother's body is only on loan to her, the loan not being one which gives her any prior claim to it. One who held this view might well think it impartiality to say "I cannot choose." But I shall simply ignore this possibility. My own view is that if a human being has any just, prior claim to anything at all, he has a just, prior claim to his own body. And perhaps this needn't be argued for here anyway, since, as I mentioned, the arguments against abortion we are looking at do grant that the woman has a right to decide what happens in and to her body.

But although they do grant it, I have tried to show that they do not take seriously what is done in granting it. I suggest the same thing will reappear even more clearly when we turn away from cases in which the mother's life is at stake, and attend, as I propose we now do, to the vastly more common cases in which a woman wants an abortion for some less weighty reason than preserving her own life.

3. Where the mother's life is not at stake, the argument I mentioned at the outset seems to have a much stronger pull. "Everyone has a right to life, so the unborn person has a right to life." And isn't the child's right to life weightier than anything other than the mother's own right to life, which she might put forward as ground for an abortion?

This argument treats the right to life as if it were unproblematic. It is not, and this seems to me to be precisely the source of the mistake.

For we should now, at long last, ask what it comes to, to have a right to life. In some views having a right to life includes having a right to be given at least the bare minimum one needs for continued life. But suppose that what in fact *is* the bare minimum a man needs for continued life is something he has no right at all to be given? If I am sick unto death, and the only thing that will save my life is the touch of Henry Fonda's cool hand on my fevered brow, then all the same, I have no right to be given the touch of Henry Fonda's cool hand on my fevered brow. It would be frightfully nice of him to fly in from the West Coast to provide it. It would be less nice, though no doubt well meant, if my friends flew out to the West Coast and carried Henry Fonda back with them. But I have no right at all against anybody that he should do this for me. Or again, to return to the story I told earlier, the fact that for continued life that violinist needs the continued use of your kidneys does not establish that he has a right to be given the continued use of your kidneys. He certainly has no right against you that *you* should give him continued use of your kidneys. For nobody has any right to use your kidneys unless you give him such a right; and nobody has the right against you that you shall give him this right—if you do allow him to go on using your kidneys, this is a kindness on your part, and not something he can claim from you as his due. Nor has he any right against anybody else that *they* should give him continued use of your kidneys. Certainly he had no right against the Society of Music Lovers that they should plug him into you in the first place. And if you now start to unplug yourself, having learned that you will otherwise have to spend nine years in bed with him, there is nobody in the world who must try to prevent you, in order to see to it that he is given something he has a right to be given.

Some people are rather stricter about the right to life. In their view, it does not include the right to be given anything, but amounts to, and only to, the right not to be killed by anybody. But here a related difficulty arises. If everybody is to refrain from killing that violinist, then everybody must refrain from doing a great many different sorts of things. Everybody must refrain from slitting his throat, everybody must refrain from shooting him—and everybody must refrain from unplugging you from him. But does he have a right against everybody that they shall refrain from unplugging you from him? To refrain from doing this is to allow him to continue to use your kidneys. It could be argued that he has a right against us that *we* should allow him to continue to use your kidneys. That is, while he has no right against us that we should give him the use of your kidneys, it might be argued that he anyway has a right against us that we shall not now intervene and deprive him of the use of your kidneys. I shall come back to third-party interventions later. But certainly the violinist has no right against you that *you* shall allow him to continue to use your kidneys. As I said, if you do allow him to use them, it is a kindness on your part, and not something you owe him.

The difficulty I point to here is not peculiar to the right to life. It reappears in connection with all the other natural rights; and it is something which an adequate account of rights must deal with. For present purposes it is enough just to draw attention to it. But I would stress that I am not arguing that people do not have a right to life—quite to the contrary, it seems to me that the primary control we must place on the acceptability of an account of rights is that it should turn out in that account to be a truth that all persons have a right to life. I am arguing only that having a right to life does not guarantee having either a right to be given the use of or a right to be allowed continued use of another person's body—even if one needs it for life itself. So the right to life will not serve the opponents of abortion in the very simple and clear way in which they seem to have thought it would.

4. There is another way to bring out the difficulty. In the most ordinary sort of case, to deprive someone of what he has a right to is to treat him unjustly. Suppose a boy and his small brother are jointly given a box of chocolates for Christmas. If the older boy takes the box and refuses to give his brother any of the chocolates, he is unjust to him, for the brother has been given a right to half of them. But suppose that, having learned that otherwise it means nine years in bed with that violinist, you unplug yourself from him. You surely are not being unjust to him, for you gave him no right to use your kidneys, and no one else can have given him any such right. But we have to notice that in unplugging yourself, you are killing him; and violinists, like everybody else, have a right to life, and thus in the view we were considering just now, the right not to be killed. So here you do what he supposedly has a right you shall not do, but you do not act unjustly to him in doing it.

The emendation which may be made at this point is this: the right to life consists not in the right not to be killed, but rather in the right not to be killed unjustly. This runs a risk of circularity, but never mind: it would enable us to square the fact that the violinist has a right to life with the fact that you do not act unjustly toward him in unplugging yourself, thereby killing him. For if you do not kill him unjustly, you do not violate his right to life, and so it is no wonder you do him no injustice.

But if this emendation is accepted, the gap in the argument against abortion stares us plainly in the face: it is by no means enough to show that the fetus is a person, and to remind us that all persons have a right to life—we need to be shown also that killing the fetus violates its right to life, i.e., that abortion is unjust killing. And is it?

I suppose we may take it as a datum that in a case of pregnancy due to rape the mother has not given the unborn person a right to the use of her body for food and shelter. Indeed, in what pregnancy could it be supposed that the mother has given the unborn person such a right? It is not as if there were unborn persons drifting about the world, to whom a woman who wants a child says "I invite you in."

But it might be argued that there are other ways one can have acquired a right to the use of another person's body than by having been invited to use it by that person. Suppose a woman voluntarily indulges in intercourse, knowing of the chance it will issue in pregnancy, and then she does become pregnant; is she not in part responsible for the presence, in fact the very existence, of the unborn person inside her? No doubt she did not invite it in. But doesn't her partial responsibility for its being there itself give it a right to the use of her body?[7] If so, then her aborting it would be more like the boy's taking away the chocolates, and less like your unplugging yourself from the violinist—doing so would be depriving it of what it does have a right to, and thus would be doing it an injustice.

And then, too, it might be asked whether or not she can kill it even to save her own life: If she voluntarily called it into existence, how can she now kill it, even in self-defense?

The first thing to be said about this is that it is something new. Opponents of abortion have been so concerned to make out the independence of the fetus, in order to establish that it has a right to life, just as its mother does, that they have tended to overlook the possible support they might gain from making out that the fetus is *dependent* on the mother, in order to establish that she has a special kind of responsibility for it, a responsibility that gives it rights against her which are not possessed by any independent person—such as an ailing violinist who is a stranger to her.

On the other hand, this argument would give the unborn person a right to its mother's body only if her pregnancy resulted from a voluntary act, undertaken in full knowledge of the chance a pregnancy might result from it. It would leave out entirely the unborn person whose existence is due to rape. Pending the availability of some further argument, then, we would be left with the conclusion that unborn persons whose existence is due to rape have no right to the use of their mothers' bodies, and thus that aborting them is not depriving them of anything they have a right to and hence is not unjust killing.

And we should also notice that it is not at all plain that this argument really does go even as far as it purports to. For there are cases and cases, and the details make a difference. If the room is stuffy, and I therefore open a window to air it, and a burglar climbs in, it would be absurd to say, "Ah, now he can stay, she's given him a right to the use of her house—for she is partially responsible for his presence there, having voluntarily done what enabled him to get in, in full knowledge that there are such things as burglars, and that burglars burgle." It would be still more absurd to say this if I had had bars installed outside my windows, precisely to prevent burglars from getting in, and a burglar got in only because of a defect in the bars. It remains equally absurd if we imagine it is not a burglar who climbs in, but an innocent person who blunders or falls in. Again, suppose it were like this: people-seeds drift about in the air like pollen, and if you open your windows, one may drift in and take root in your carpets or upholstery. You don't want children, so you fix up your windows with fine mesh screens, the very best you can buy. As can happen, however, and on very, very rare occasions does happen, one of the screens is defective; and a seed drifts in and takes root. Does the person-plant who now develops have a right to the use of your house? Surely not—despite the fact that you voluntarily opened your windows, you knowingly kept carpets and upholstered furniture, and you knew that screens were sometimes defective. Someone may argue that you are responsible for its rooting, that it does have a right to your house, because after all you *could* have lived out your life with bare floors and furniture, or with sealed windows and doors. But this won't do—for by the same token anyone can avoid a pregnancy due to rape by having a hysterectomy, or anyway by never leaving home without a (reliable!) army.

It seems to me that the argument we are looking at can establish at most that there are *some* cases in which the unborn person has a right to the use of its mother's body, and therefore *some* cases in which abortion is unjust killing. There is room for much discussion and argument as to precisely which, if any. But I think we should sidestep this issue and leave it open, for at any rate the argument certainly does not establish that all abortion is unjust killing.

5. There is room for yet another argument here, however. We surely must all grant that there may be cases in which it would be morally indecent to detach a person from your body at the cost of his life. Suppose you learn that what the violinist needs is not nine years of your life, but only one hour: all you need do to save his life is to spend one hour in that bed with him. Suppose also that letting him use your kidneys for that one hour would not affect your health in the slightest. Admittedly you were kidnapped. Admittedly you did not give anyone permission to plug him into you. Nevertheless it seems to me plain you *ought* to allow him to use your kidneys for that hour—it would be indecent to refuse.

Again, suppose pregnancy lasted only an hour, and constituted no threat to life or health. And suppose that a woman becomes pregnant as a result of rape. Admittedly she did not voluntarily do anything to bring about the existence of a child. Admittedly she did nothing at all which would give the unborn person a right to the use of her body. All the same it might well be said, as in the newly emended violinist story, that she *ought* to allow it to remain for that hour—that it would be indecent of her to refuse.

Now some people are inclined to use the term "right" in such a way that it follows from the fact that you ought to allow a person to use your body for the hour he needs, that he has a right to use your body for the hour he needs, even though he has not been given that right by any person or act. They may say that it follows also that if you refuse, you act unjustly toward him. This use of the term is perhaps so common that it cannot be called wrong; nevertheless it seems to me to be an unfortunate loosening of what we would do better to keep a tight rein on. Suppose that box of chocolates I mentioned earlier had not been given to both boys jointly, but was given only to the older boy. There he sits, stolidly eating his way through the box, his small brother watching enviously. Here we are likely to say "You ought not to be so mean. You ought to give your brother some of those chocolates." My own view is that it just does not follow from the truth of this that the brother has any right to any of the chocolates. If the boy refuses to give his brother any, he is greedy, stingy, callous—but not unjust. I suppose that the people I have in mind will say it does follow that the brother has a right to some of the chocolates, and thus that the boy does act unjustly if he refuses to give his brother any. But the effect of saying this is to obscure what we should keep distinct, namely the difference between the boy's refusal in this case and the boy's refusal in the earlier case, in which the box was given to both boys jointly, and in which the small brother thus had what was from any point of view clear title to half.

A further objection to so using the term "right" that from the fact that A ought to do a thing for B, it follows that B has a right against A that A do it for him, is that it is going to make the question of whether or not a man has a right to a thing turn on how easy it is to provide him with it; and this seems not merely unfortunate, but morally unacceptable. Take the case of Henry Fonda again. I said earlier that I had no right to the touch of his cool hand on my fevered brow even though I needed it to save my life. I said it would be frightfully nice of him to fly in from the West Coast to provide me with it, but that I had no right against him that he should do so. But suppose he isn't on the West Coast. Suppose he has only to walk across the room, place a hand briefly on my brow—and lo, my life is saved. Then surely he ought to do it; it would be indecent to refuse. Is it to be said, "Ah, well, it follows that in this case she has a right to the touch of his hand on her brow, and so it would be an injustice for him to refuse"? So that I have a right to it when it is easy for him to provide it, though no right when it's hard? It's rather a shocking idea that anyone's rights should fade away and disappear as it gets harder and harder to accord them to him.

So my own view is that even though you ought to let the violinist use your kidneys for the one hour he needs, we should not conclude that he has a right to do so—we should say that if you refuse, you are, like the boy who owns all the chocolates and will give none away, self-centered and callous, indecent in fact, but not unjust. And similarly, that even supposing a case in which a woman pregnant due to rape ought to allow the unborn person to use her body for the hour he needs, we should not conclude that he has a right to do so; we should conclude that she is self-centered, callous, indecent, but not unjust, if she refuses. The complaints are no less grave; they are just different. However, there is no need to insist on this point. If anyone does wish to deduce "he has a right" from "you ought," then all the same he must surely grant that there are cases in which it is not morally required of you that you allow that violinist to use your kidneys, and in which he does not have a right to use them, and in which you do not do him an injustice if you refuse. And so also for mother and unborn child. Except in such cases as the unborn person has a right to demand it—and we were leaving open the possibility that there may be such cases—nobody is morally *required* to make large sacrifices, of health, of all other interests and concerns, of all other duties and commitments, for nine years, or even for nine months, in order to keep another person alive.

6. We have in fact to distinguish between two kinds of Samaritan: the Good Samaritan and what we might call the Minimally Decent Samaritan. The story of the Good Samaritan, you will remember, goes like this:

> A certain man went down from Jerusalem to Jericho, and fell among thieves, which stripped him of his raiment, and wounded him, and departed, leaving him half dead.
>
> And by chance there came down a certain priest that way; and when he saw him, he passed by on the other side.
>
> And likewise a Levite, when he was at the place, came and looked on him, and passed by on the other side.
>
> But a certain Samaritan, as he journeyed, came where he was; and when he saw him he had compassion on him.
>
> And went to him, and bound up his wounds, pouring in oil and wine, and set him on his own beast, and brought him to an inn, and took care of him.
>
> And on the morrow, when he departed, he took out two pence, and gave them to the host, and said unto him, "Take care of him; and whatsoever thou spendest more, when I come again, I will repay thee."
>
> (Luke 10:30–35)

The Good Samaritan went out of his way, at some cost to himself, to help one in need of it. We are not told what the options were, that is, whether or not the priest and the Levite could have helped by doing less than the Good Samaritan did, but assuming they could have, then the fact they did nothing at all shows they were not even Minimally Decent Samaritans, not because they were not Samaritans, but because they were not even minimally decent.

These things are a matter of degree, of course, but there is a difference, and it comes out perhaps most clearly in the story of Kitty Genovese, who, as you will remember, was murdered while thirty-eight people watched or listened, and did nothing at all to help her. A Good Samaritan would have rushed out to give direct assistance against the murderer. Or perhaps we had better allow that it would have been a Splendid Samaritan who did this, on the ground that it would have involved a risk of death for himself. But the thirty-eight not only did not do this, they did not even trouble to pick up a phone to call the police. Minimally Decent Samaritanism would call for doing at least that, and their not having done it was monstrous.

After telling the story of the Good Samaritan, Jesus said, "Go, and do thou likewise." Perhaps he meant that we are morally required to act as the Good Samaritan did. Perhaps he was urging people to do more than is morally required of them. At all events it seems plain that it was not morally required of any of the thirty-eight that he rush out to give direct assistance at the risk of his own life, and that it is not morally required of anyone that he give long stretches of his life—nine years or nine months—to sustaining the life of a person who has no special right (we were leaving open the possibility of this) to demand it.

Indeed, with one rather striking class of exceptions, no one in any country in the world is *legally* required to do anywhere near as much as this for anyone else. The class of exceptions is obvious. My main concern here is not the state of the law in respect to abortion, but it is worth drawing attention to the fact that in no state in this country is any man compelled by law to be even a Minimally Decent Samaritan to any person; there is no law under which charges could be brought against the thirty-eight who stood by while Kitty Genovese died. By contrast, in most states in this country women are compelled by law to be not merely Minimally Decent Samaritans, but Good Samaritans to unborn persons inside them. This doesn't by itself settle anything one way or the other, because it may well be argued that there should be laws in this country—as there are in many European countries—compelling at least Minimally Decent Samaritanism.[8] But it does show that there is a gross injustice in the existing state of the law. And it shows also that the groups currently working against liberalization of abortion laws, in fact working toward having it declared unconstitutional for a state to permit abortion, had better start working for the adoption of Good Samaritan laws generally, or earn the charge that they are acting in bad faith.

I should think, myself, that Minimally Decent Samaritan laws would be one thing, Good Samaritan laws quite another, and in fact highly improper. But we are not here concerned with the law. What we should ask is not whether anybody should be compelled by law to be a Good Samaritan, but whether we must accede to a situation in which somebody is being compelled—by nature, perhaps—to be a Good Samaritan. We have, in other words, to look now at third-party interventions. I have been arguing that no person is morally required to make large sacrifices to sustain the life of another who has no right to demand them, and this even where the sacrifices do not include life itself; we are not morally required to be Good Samaritans or anyway Very Good Samaritans to one another. But what if a man cannot extricate himself from such a situation? What if he appeals to us to extricate him? It seems to me plain that there are cases in which we can, cases in which a Good Samaritan would extricate him. There you are, you were kidnapped, and nine years in bed with that violinist lie ahead of you. You have your own life to lead. You are sorry, but you simply cannot see giving up so much of your life to the sustaining of his. You cannot extricate yourself, and ask us to do so. I should have thought that—in light of his having no right to the use of your body—it was obvious that we do not have to accede to your being forced to give up so much. We can do what you ask. There is no injustice to the violinist in our doing so.

7. Following the lead of the opponents of abortion, I have throughout been speaking of the fetus merely as a person, and what I have been asking is whether or not the argument we began with, which proceeds only from the fetus's being a person, really does establish its conclusion. I have argued that it does not.

But of course there are arguments and arguments, and it may be said that I have simply fastened on the wrong one. It may be said that what is important is not merely the fact that the fetus is a person, but that it is a person for whom the woman has a special kind of responsibility issuing from the fact that she is its mother. And it might be argued that all my analogies are therefore irrelevant—for you do not have that special kind of responsibility for that violinist, Henry Fonda does not have that special kind of responsibility for me. And our attention might be drawn to the fact that men and women both *are* compelled by law to provide support for their children.

I have in effect dealt (briefly) with this argument in section 4 above; but a (still briefer) recapitulation now may be in order. Surely we do not have any such "special responsibility" for a person unless we have assumed it, explicitly or implicitly. If a set of parents do not try to prevent pregnancy, do not obtain an abortion, and then at the time of birth of the child do not put it out for adoption, but rather take it home with them, then they have assumed responsibility for it, they have given it rights, and they cannot *now* withdraw support from it at the cost of its life because they now find it difficult to go on providing for it. But if they have taken all reasonable precautions against having a child, they do not simply by virtue of their biological relationship to the child who comes into existence have a special responsibility for it. They may wish to assume responsibility for it, or they may not wish to. And I am suggesting that if assuming responsibility for it would require large sacrifices, then these parents may refuse. A Good Samaritan would not refuse—or anyway, a Splendid Samaritan, if the sacrifices that had to be made were enormous. But then so would a Good Samaritan assume responsibility for that violinist; so would Henry Fonda, if he is a Good Samaritan, fly in from the West Coast and assume responsibility for me.

8. My argument will be found unsatisfactory on two counts by many of those who want to regard abortion as morally permissible. First, while I do argue that abortion is not impermissible, I do not argue that it is always permissible. There may well be cases in which carrying the child to term requires only Minimally Decent Samaritanism of the mother, and this is a standard we must not fall below. I am inclined to think it a merit of my account precisely that it does *not* give a general yes or a general no. It allows for and supports our sense that, for example, a sick and desperately frightened fourteen-year-old schoolgirl, pregnant due to rape, may *of course* choose abortion, and that any law which rules this out is an insane law. And it also allows for and supports our sense that in other cases resort to abortion is even positively indecent. It would be indecent in the woman to request an abortion, and indecent in a doctor to perform it, if she is in her seventh month, and wants the abortion just to avoid the nuisance of postponing a trip abroad. The very fact that the arguments I have been drawing attention to treat all cases of abortion, or even all cases of abortion in which the mother's life is not at stake, as morally on a par ought to have made them suspect at the outset.

Secondly, while I am arguing for the permissibility of abortion in some cases, I am not arguing for the right to secure the death of the unborn child. It is easy to confuse these two things in that up to a certain point in the life of the fetus it is not able to survive outside the mother's body; hence removing it from her body guarantees its death. But they are importantly different. I have argued that you are not morally required to spend nine months in bed, sustaining the life of that violinist; but to say this is by no means to say that if, when you unplug yourself, there is a miracle and he survives, you then have a right to turn round and slit his throat. You may detach yourself even if this costs him his life; you have no right to be guaranteed his death, by some other means, if unplugging yourself does not kill him. There are some people who will feel dissatisfied by this feature of my argument. A woman may be utterly devastated by the thought of a child, a bit of herself, put out for adoption and never seen or heard of again. She may therefore want not merely that the child be detached from her, but more, that it die. Some opponents of abortion are inclined to regard this as beneath contempt—thereby showing insensitivity to what is surely a powerful source of despair. All the same, I agree that the desire for the child's death is not one which anybody may gratify, should it turn out to be possible to detach the child alive.

At this place, however, it should be remembered that we have only been pretending throughout that the fetus is a human being from the moment of conception. A very early abortion is surely not the killing of a person, and so is not dealt with by anything I have said here.

NOTES

1. I am very much indebted to James Thomson for discussion, criticism, and many helpful suggestions.
2. Daniel Callahan, *Abortion: Law, Choice and Morality* (New York, 1970), p. 373. This book gives a fascinating

survey of the available information on abortion. The Jewish tradition is surveyed in David M. Feldman, *Birth Control in Jewish Law* (New York, 1968), Part 5, the Catholic tradition in John T. Noonan, Jr., "An Almost Absolute Value in History," in *The Morality of Abortion*, ed. John T. Noonan, Jr. (Cambridge, Mass., 1970).

3. The term "direct" in the arguments I refer to is a technical one. Roughly, what is meant by "direct killing" is either killing as an end in itself, or killing as a means to some end; for example, the end of saving someone else's life. See note 5 below, for an example of its use.
4. Cf. *Encyclical Letter of Pope Pius XI on Christian Marriage*, St. Paul Editions (Boston, n.d.), p. 32: "however much we may pity the mother whose health and even life is gravely imperiled in the performance of the duty allotted to her by nature, nevertheless what could ever be a sufficient reason for excusing in any way the direct murder of the innocent? This is precisely what we are dealing with here." Noonan (*The Morality of Abortion*, p. 43) reads this as follows: "What cause can ever avail to excuse in any way the direct killing of the innocent? For it is a question of that."
5. The thesis in (4) is in an interesting way weaker than those in (1), (2), and (3): they rule out abortion even in cases in which both mother *and* child will die if the abortion is not performed. By contrast, one who held the view expressed in (4) could consistently say that one needn't prefer letting two persons die to killing one.
6. Cf. the following passage from Pius XII, *Address to the Italian Catholic Society of Midwives:* "The baby in the maternal breast has the right to life immediately from God.—Hence there is no man, no human authority, no science, no medical, eugenic, social, economic or moral 'indication' which can establish or grant a valid juridical ground for a direct deliberate disposition of an innocent human life, that is a disposition which looks to its destruction either as an end or as a means to another end perhaps in itself not illicit.—The baby, still not born, is a man in the same degree and for the same reason as the mother" (quoted in Noonan, *The Morality of Abortion*, p. 45).
7. The need for a discussion of this argument was brought home to me by members of the Society for Ethical and Legal Philosophy, to whom this paper was originally presented.
8. For a discussion of the difficulties involved, and a survey of the European experience with such laws, see *The Good Samaritan and the Law*, ed. James M. Ratcliffe (New York, 1966).

THE MORALITY OF ABORTION

Margaret Olivia Little

INTRODUCTION

It is often noted that the public discussion of abortion's moral status is disappointingly crude. The positions staked out and the reasoning proffered seem to reflect little of the subtlety and nuance—not to mention ambivalence—that mark more private reflections on the subject. Despite attempts by various parties to find middle ground, the debate remains largely polarized—at its most dramatic, with extreme conservatives claiming abortion the moral equivalent of murder even as extreme liberals think it devoid of moral import.

To some extent, this polarization is due to the legal battle that continues to shadow moral discussions: admission of ethical nuance, it is feared, will play as concession on the deeply contested question of whether abortion should be a legally protected option for women. But to some extent, blame for the continued crudeness can be laid at the doorstep of moral theory itself.

For one thing, the ethical literature on abortion has focused its attention almost exclusively on the thinnest moral assessment—on whether and when abortion is "morally permissible." That question is, of course, a crucial one, its answer often desperately sought. But many of our deepest struggles with the morality of abortion concern much more textured questions about its placement on the scales of *decency, respectfulness,* and *responsibility.* It is one thing to decide that an abortion was permissible, quite another to decide that it was *honorable;* one thing to decide that an abortion was impermissible, quite another to decide that it was *monstrous*. It is these latter categories that determine what we might call the thick moral interpretation of the act—and, with it, the meaning the woman must live with, and the reactive attitudes such as disgust, forbearance, or admiration that she and others think the act deserves. A moral theory that moves too quickly or focuses too exclusively on moral permissibility won't address these crucial issues.

Moreover, the tools that mainstream moral theory has used for analyzing abortion fit only awkwardly to this subject-matter. Many treatments analyze abortion in the same terms used for assessing when war is justified, or the extent of our obligations to needy strangers, or the protection owed Da Vinci paintings. While there is some overlap of issues, such treatments end up leaving to the side many of the most important themes relevant to the ethics of gestation: what it means to play a role in *creating* a person, how to assess responsibilities that involve *sharing*, not just risking, one's body and life, what follows from the fact that the entity in question is or would be *one's child*. Nor are such lacunae incidental glitches. As theorists such as Catharine MacKinnon (1991) and Robin West (1993) have pointed out, our moral and political theories have been forged, by and large, to deal with interactions between independently situated and relatively equal strangers. However well this might work for soldierly heroism and barroom brawls (a question worth pressing in its own right), such a theory might not be expected to do well with moral questions dealing with the sort of intertwinement at issue in pregnancy.

If this is right, it means it is especially important not to focus all our energies, as many treatments are wont to do, arbitrating the question of fetal personhood. The question certainly matters: the moral contours of abortion, as we shall see, are importantly different depending on the answer we give it. The question is, moreover, a genuinely complex one, pressing, in essence, on the extent to which moral status is a function of the sort of being something already is, as judged by its occurrent properties, and the sort of creature it would become if it developed. (My own view, which I won't defend here, is that full moral status is in part anticipatory and in part something achieved; the fetus's status becomes progressively more weighty as pregnancy continues.) Complex as the issue of personhood is, though, the temptation to think our work done if only we could settle it—as though the moral status of abortion follows lockstep from the moral status of the fetus—has led theorists to ignore the rich ethical issues that are raised by the, shall we say, rather distinctive situation in which the fetus is located.

To make progress on abortion's moral status, it thus turns out, requires us not just to arbitrate already familiar controversies in metaphysics and ethics, but to attend to the distinctive aspects of pregnancy that often stand at their margins. In the following, I want to argue that if we acknowledge gestation as an *intimacy*, motherhood as a *relationship*, and creation as a *process*, we will be in a far better position to appreciate the moral textures of abortion. I explore these textures, in the first half on stipulation that the fetus is a person, in the second half under supposition that early human life has an important value worthy of respect.

FETAL PERSONHOOD: FROM WRONGFUL INTERFERENCE TO POSITIVE RESPONSIBILITIES

If fetuses are persons, then abortion is surely an enormously serious matter: What is at stake is nothing less than the life of a creature with full moral standing. To say that the stakes are high, though, is not to say that moral analysis is obvious (which is why elsewhere in moral theory, conversation usually starts, not stops, once we realize people's lives are at issue). I think the most widely held objection to abortion is badly misguided; more importantly, it obscures the deeper ethical question at issue.

On the usual view, it is perfectly obvious what to say about abortion on supposition of fetal personhood: if fetuses are persons, then abortion is murder. Persons, after all, have a fundamental right to life, and abortion, it would seem, counts as its gross violation. On this view, we can assess the status of abortion quite cleanly. In particular, we needn't delve too deeply into the burdens that continued gestation might present for women—not because their lives don't matter or because we don't sympathize with their plight, but because we don't take hardship as justification for murder.

In fact, though, abortion's assimilation to murder will seem clear-cut only if we have already ignored key features of gestation. While certain metaphors depict gestation as passive carriage—as though the fetus were simply occupying a room until it is born—the truth is of course far different. One who is gestating is providing the fetus with sustenance—donating nourishment, creating blood, delivering oxygen, providing hormonal triggers for development—without which it could not live. For a fetus, to live *is* to be receiving aid. And whether the assistance is delivered by way of intentional activity (as when the woman eats or takes her prenatal vitamins) or by way of biological mechanism, assistance it plainly is. But this has crucial implications for abortion's alleged status as murder. To put it simply, the right to life, as Judith Thomson famously put it, does not include the right to have all assistance needed to maintain that life (Thomson, 1971). Ending gestation will, at early stages at least, certainly lead to the fetus's demise, but that does not mean that doing so would constitute murder.

Now Thomson herself illustrated the point with an (in)famous thought experiment in which one person is kidnapped and used as life support for another: staying connected to the Famous Violinist, she points out, may be the kind thing to do, but disconnecting oneself does not violate the Violinist's rights. The details of this rather esoteric example have led to widespread charges that Thomson's point ignores the distinction between killing and letting die, and would apply at any rate only to cases in which the woman was not responsible for procreation occurring. In fact, though, I think the central insight here is broader than the example, or Thomson's own analysis, indicates.

As Frances Kamm's work points out (Kamm, 1992), in the usual case of a killing—if you stab a person on the street, for instance—you interfere with the trajectory the person had independently of you. She faced a happy enough future, we'll say; your action changed that, taking away from her something she would have had but for your action. In ending gestation, though, what you are taking away from this person is something she wouldn't have had to begin with without your aid. She comes to you with a downward trajectory, as it were: but for you she would already be dead. In removing that assistance, you are not violating the person's right to life, judged in the traditional terms of a right against interference. While all killings are tragedies, then, not all are alike: some killings, as Kamm puts it, share the crucial "formal" feature of letting die, which is that they leave the person no worse off than before she encountered you.

The argument is not some crude utilitarian one, according to which you get to kill the person because you saved her life (as though, having given you a nice lamp for your birthday, I may therefore later steal it with impunity). The point, rather, is that where I am still in the process of saving—or sustaining or enabling—your life, and that life cannot be thusly saved or sustained by anyone else, ending that assistance, even by active means, does not violate your right to life.

Now some, of course, will argue that matters change when the woman is causally responsible for procreation. In such cases, it will be said, she is responsible for introducing the person's need. She isn't like someone happening by an accident on the highway who knows CPR; she's like the person who *caused* the accident. Her actions introduced a set of vulnerabilities or needs, and we have a special duty to lessen vulnerabilities and repair harms we have inflicted on others.

But there is a deep disanalogy between causing the accident and procreating. The fact of causing a crash itself introduces a harm to surrounding drivers: they are in a worse position for having encountered that driver. But the simple act of procreating does not worsen the fetus's position: without procreation, the fetus wouldn't exist at all; and the mere fact of being brought into existence is not a bad thing. To be sure, creating a human is creating someone who comes with needs. But this, crucially, is not the same as inflicting a need *onto* someone (see Silverstein, 1987). It isn't as though the fetus already existed with one level of needs and the woman added a new one (as does happen, for instance, if a woman takes a drug after conception that increases the fetus's vulnerability to, say, certain cancers). The woman is (partially) responsible for creating a life, and it's a life that necessarily includes needs, but that is not the same as being responsible for the person being needy rather than not. The pregnant woman has not made the fetus more vulnerable than it would otherwise have been: absent her procreative actions, it wouldn't have existed at all.

Even if the fetus is a person, then, abortion would not be murder. More broadly put, abortion, whatever its rights and wrongs, isn't a species of *wrongful interference*.

None of this, though, is to say that abortion under such supposition is therefore unproblematic. It is to argue, instead, that the crucial moral issue needs to be re-located. Wrongful interference is a central concern in morality, but it isn't the only one. We are also concerned with notions of *neglect*, *abandonment* and *disregard*. These are issues that involve abrogations of positive responsibilities to help others, not injunctions against interfering with them. If fetuses are persons, the question we really need to decide is what positive responsibilities, if any, do pregnant women have to continue gestational assistance? This is a question that takes us into far richer, and far more interesting, territory than that occupied by discussions of murder.

One issue it raises is: what do pregnant women owe to the fetuses they carry as a matter of *general beneficence?* Philosophers, of course, familiarly divide over the ambitions of beneficence, generically construed; but abortion raises distinct difficulties of its own. On the one hand, the beneficence called for here is of a particularly urgent kind: the stakes are life and death, and the pregnant woman is the *only* one who can render the assistance needed. It's a rare (and, many of us will think, dreadful) moral theory that will think she faces no responsibilities to assist here: passing a drowning person for mere convenience when no one else is within shouting distance is a very good example of moral indecency. On the other hand, gestation is not just any activity. It involves sharing one's very body. It brings with it an emotional intertwinement that can reshape one's entire life. It brings another person into one's family. Being asked to gestate another person, that is, isn't like being asked to write a check to support an impoverished child; it's like being asked to adopt the child. Doing so is a caring, compassionate act; it is also an enormous undertaking that has reverberations for an entire lifetime. Deciding whether, and if so when, such action is obligatory rather than admirable is no light matter.

I don't think moral theory has begun to address the rich questions at issue here. When are intimate actions owed to generic others? How do we weigh the sacrifice morality requires of us when it is measured, not in terms of risk, but of intertwinement? What should we think of such obligations if the required acts would be performed under conditions of profound self-alienation? The *type* of issue paradigmatically represented by gestation—an assistance that combines life and death stakes with deep intimacy— is virtually nowhere discussed in ethical theory. (We aren't called upon in the usual course of events to save people's lives by, say, having sexual intercourse with them.) By ignoring these issues, mainstream moral theory has ended up deeply underselling the moral complexity of abortion.

Difficult as these questions are, though, it is actually a second issue, I suspect, that is responsible for much of the passion that surrounds abortion on supposition of fetal personhood. On reflection, many will say, the issues confronting the pregnant woman aren't about generic beneficence at all. The considerations she faces are not just those that would face someone uniquely well placed to serve as Good Samaritan to some stranger—as when one passes the drowning person: for the pregnant woman and fetus, crucially, aren't strangers. If the fetus is a person, many will say, it is *her child;* and for this reason she has special responsibilities to meet its needs. In the end, I believe, much of the animating concern with abortion is not about what we owe to generic others; it's about what parents owe their children.

But if it's parenthood that is carrying normative weight, then we need an ethics of parenthood—a theory of what makes someone a parent in this thickly normative sense and what the contours of its responsibilities really are. This should raise something of a warning flag. Philosophers, it must be said, have by and large done a rather poor job when it comes to parenthood—variously avoiding it, romanticizing it, or assimilating it to categories, like contractual relations, to which it stands in paradigmatic contrast. This general shortcoming is evident in discussions of abortion, where two remarkably unhelpful models dominate.

One position, advocated by Judith Thomson and some of the most recent treatments of abortion, is a classically liberal one. It agrees that special responsibilities attach to parenthood but argues that parenthood is thereby a status that is entered into only by consent. That consent is usually tacit, to be sure—taking the baby home from the hospital qualifies; nonetheless, special responsibilities to a child accrue only when one voluntarily assumes them.

Such a model is surely an odd one. The model yields the plausible view that the rape victim does not face the very same set of duties as many other pregnant women, but it does so by implying that a man who fathers a child during a one-night stand has no special responsibilities toward that child unless he decides he does. Perhaps most strikingly, such a view has no resources for acknowledging that there may be moral reasons why one *should* consent to the status. Those who sustain a biological connection may have a tendency to enter the role of parent, but on this scheme it's a mere psychological proclivity that rides atop nothing normative.

Another position is classically conservative. According to this view, the special responsibilities of parenthood are grounded in biological progenitorship. It is blood ties, to use the old-fashioned vernacular—"passing on one's genes," in more current translation—that makes one a parent and grounds heightened responsibilities. This view has its own blind spot. It has the resources for agreeing that a man who fathers a child from a one-night stand faces special responsibilities for the child whether he likes it or not, but none for distinguishing between the responsibilities of someone who has served as the special steward for a child—who has engaged for years in the *activity* of parenting—and the responsibilities of someone who bears literally no connection beyond a genetic or causal contribution to existence. On this view, a sperm donor faces all the responsibilities of a social father.

What both positions have in common is the supposition that parenthood is an all or nothing affair. Applied to pregnancy, the gestating woman either owes everything we imagine we owe to the children we love and rear or she owes nothing beyond general beneficence unless she decides she does. But parenthood—like all familial relations—is surely a more complicated moral notion than this. Parenthood, and its attendant responsibilities, admit of *layers*. It has a crucial existence as a social *role*—something with institutionally defined entrances, exits, and expectations that can attach to us quite independently of what our self-conceptions might say. It also has a crucial existence as a *relationship*—an emotional connection, a shared history, an intertwinement of lives. It is because of that intertwinement that parents' motivation to sacrifice is so often immediate. But it is also because of that relationship that even especially ambitious sacrifices are legitimately expected, and why failure to undertake them would be so problematic: absent unusual circumstances, it becomes a betrayal of the relationship itself. In short, parenthood is not monolithic: some of the responsibilities we paradigmatically associate as parental attach, not to the role, but to the relationship that so often accompanies it.

These layers matter especially when we get to gestation, for the pregnant woman stands precisely at their intersection. If a fetus is a person, then there is surely an important sense in which she is its mother: to regard her as just a passing stranger uniquely able to help it would grossly distort the situation. But she is not yet a mother most thickly described—a mother in standing relationship with a child, with the responsibilities born of shared history and the enterprise of caretaking.

These demarcations are integral, I think, to understanding the distinctive sorts of conflicts that pregnancy can represent—including, most notably, the conflicts it can bring *within* the mantle of motherhood. Women sometimes decide to abort even though they regard the fetus they carry as their child, because they realize, grimly, that bringing this child into the world will leave too little room to care adequately for the children they are already raising. This is a conflict we cannot even name, much less arbitrate, on standard views—if the fetus is her child, how could she possibly choose to sacrifice its life unless the stakes are literally equivalent for the others? But this is to ignore the layers of parenthood. She occupies the *role* of mother to the fetus, but with the other children, she is, by dint of time, interaction, and intertwinement, in a *relationship* of motherhood. The fetus is her baby, then,—not just some passing stranger she alone can help—which is why this conflict brings the kind of agony it does. But if it is her child in the role sense only, she does not yet owe all that she owes to her other children. Depending on the circumstances, other family members with whom she is already in relationship may, tragically, come first.

None of this is to make light of the responsibilities pregnant women face on supposition of fetal personhood. If fetuses are persons, such responsibilities are surely profound. It is, rather, to insist that they admit of layer and degree, and that these distinctions, while delicate, are crucial to capturing the *types* of tragedy—and the types of moral compromise—abortion can here represent.

THE SANCTITY OF LIFE: RESPECT REVISITED

Just as we cannot assume that abortion is monstrous if fetuses are persons, so too we cannot assume that abortion is empty of moral import if they are not. Given all the ink that has been spilt on arbitrating the question of fetal personhood, one might be forgiven for having thought so: on some accounts, decisions about whether to continue or end a pregnancy really are, from a moral point of view, just like decisions about whether to cut one's hair.

But as Ronald Dworkin has urged (Dworkin, 1993), to think abortion morally weighty does not require supposition that the fetus is a person, or even a creature with interests in continued life. Destruction of a Da Vinci painting, he points out, is not bad *for the painting*—the painting has no interests. Instead, it is regrettable because of the deep value it has. So, too, one of the reasons we might regard abortion as morally weighty does not have to do with its being bad for *the fetus*—a setback to its interests, for it may not satisfy the criteria of having interests. Abortion may be weighty, instead, because there is something precious and significant about germinating human life that deserves our deep respect. This, as Dworkin puts it, locates issues of abortion in a different neighborhood of our moral commitments: namely, the accommodation we owe to things of value. That an organism is a potential person may not make it a claims-bearer, but it does mean it has a kind of stature that is worthy of respect.

This intuition, dismissed by some as mere sentimentality, is, I think, both important and broadly held. Very few people regard abortion as the moral equivalent of contraception. Most think a society better morally—not just by public health measures—if it regards abortion as a backup to failed contraception rather than as routine birth control. Reasons adequate for contracepting do not translate transparently as reasons adequate for aborting. Indeed, there is a telling shift in presumption: for most people, it takes no reason at all to justify contracepting; it takes *some* reason to justify ending a pregnancy. That a human life has now begun matters morally.

Burgeoning human life, we might put it, is *respect-worthy*. This is why we care not just whether, but how, abortion is done—while crass jokes are made or with solemnity, and why we care how the fetal remains are treated. It is why the thought of someone aborting for genuinely trivial reasons—to fit into a favorite party dress, say—makes us morally queasy. Perhaps most basically, it is why the thought of someone aborting with casual indifference fills us with misgiving. Abortion involves loss. Not just loss of the hope that various parties might have invested, but loss of something valuable in its own right. To respect something is to appreciate fully the value it has and the claims it presents to us; someone who aborts but never gives it a second thought hasn't exhibited genuine appreciation of the value and moral status of that which is now gone.

But if many share the intuition that early human life has a value deserving of respect, there is considerable disagreement about what that respect looks like. There is considerable conflict, that is, over what accommodation we owe to burgeoning human life. In part, of course, this is due to disagreement over the *degree* of value such life should be accorded: those for whom it is thoroughly modest will have very different views on issues, from abortion to stem cell research, than those for whom it is transcendent. But this is only part of the story. Obscured by analogies to Da Vinci paintings, some of the most important sources of conflict, especially for the vast middle rank of moderates, ride atop rough agreement on fetal value. If we listen to women's own struggles about when it is morally decent to end pregnancy, what we hear are themes about *motherhood* and *respect for creation*. These themes are enormously complex, I want to argue; for they enter stories on both sides of the ledger—for some women, as reasons to continue, and for some, as reasons to end, pregnancy. Let me start with motherhood.

For many women who contemplate abortion, the desire to end pregnancy is not, or not centrally, a desire to avoid the nine months of pregnancy; it is to avoid what lies on the far side of those months—namely, motherhood. If gestation were simply a matter of rendering, say, somewhat risky assistance to help a burgeoning human life they've come across—if they could somehow render that assistance without thereby adding a member to their family—the decision faced would be a far different one. But gestation doesn't just allow cells to become a person; it turns one into a mother.

One of the most common reasons women give for wanting to abort is that they do not want to become a mother—now, ever, again, with this partner, or no reliable partner, with these few resources, or these many that are now, after so many years of mothering, slated finally to another cause. Nor does adoption represent a universal solution. To give up a child would be for some a life-long trauma; others occupy fortunate circumstances that would, by their own lights, make it unjustified to give over a child for others to rear. Or again—and most frequently—she doesn't want to raise a child just now but knows that if she *does* carry the pregnancy to term, she won't *want* to give up the child for adoption. Gestation, she knows, is likely to reshape her heart and soul, transforming her into a mother emotionally, not just officially; and it is precisely that transformation she does not want to undergo. It is because continuing pregnancy brings with it this new identity and, likely, relationship, then, that many feel it legitimate to decline.

But pregnancy's connection to motherhood also enters the phenomenology of abortion in just the opposite direction. For some women, that it would be her child is precisely why she feels she must continue the pregnancy—even if motherhood is not what she desired. To be pregnant is to have one's potential child knocking at one's door; to abort is to turn one's back on it, a decision, many women say, that would haunt them forever. On this view, the desire to avoid motherhood, so compelling as a reason to contracept, is uneasy grounds to abort: for once an embryo is on the scene, it isn't about rejecting motherhood, it's about rejecting one's *child*. Not literally, of course, since there is no child yet extant to stand as the object of rejection. But the stance one should take to pregnancy, sought or not, is one of *acceptance:* when a potential family member is knocking at the door, one should move over, make room, and welcome her in.

These two intuitive stances represent just profoundly different ways of gestalting the situation of ending pregnancy. On the first view, abortion is closer to contraception—hardly equivalent, because it means the demise of something of value. But the desire to avoid the enterprise and identity of motherhood is an understandable and honorable basis for deciding to end a pregnancy. Given that there is no child yet on the scene, one does not owe special openness to the relationship that stands at the end of pregnancy's trajectory. On the second view, abortion is closer to exiting a parental relationship—hardly equivalent, for one of the key relata is not yet fully present. But one's decision about whether to continue the pregnancy already feels specially constrained: that one would be related to the resulting person exerts now some moral force. It would take especially grave reasons to refuse assistance here, for the norms of parenthood already have a toehold. Assessing the moral status of abortion, it turns out, then, is not just about assessing the contours of generic respect owed to burgeoning human life, it's about assessing the salience of *impending relationship.* And this is an issue that functions in different ways for different women—and, sometimes, in one and the same woman.

In my own view, until the fetus is a person, we should recognize a moral prerogative to decline parenthood and end the pregnancy. Not because motherhood is necessarily a burden (though it can be); but because it so thoroughly changes what we might call one's fundamental practical identity. The enterprise of mothering restructures the self—changing the shape of one's heart, the primary commitments by which one lives one's life, the terms by which one judges one's life a success or a failure. If the enterprise is eschewed and one decides to give the child over to another, the identity of mother still changes the normative facts that are true of one, as there is now someone by whom one does well or poorly. And either way—whether one rears the child or lets it go—to continue a pregnancy means that a piece of one's heart, as the saying goes, will forever walk outside one's body. As profound as the respect we should have for burgeoning human life, we should acknowledge moral prerogatives over identity-constituting commitments and enterprises as profound as motherhood.

But I also don't think this is the whole of the moral story. If women find themselves with different ways of gestalting the prospective relationship involved in pregnancy, it is in part because they have different identities, commitments, and ideals that such a prospect intersects with—commitments which, while permissibly idiosyncratic, are morally authoritative for *them*. If a woman feels already duty-bound by the norms of parenthood to nurture this creature, it may be for the very good reason that, in an important personal sense, she already *is* its mother. She finds herself—perhaps to her surprise, happy or otherwise—with a maternal commitment to this creature. As philosophers forget but women and men have long known, something can be your child even if it is not yet a person. But taking on the identity of mother towards something just *is* to take on certain imperatives about its well-being as categorical. Her job is thus clear—it's to help this creature reach its fullest potential. For other women, the identity is still something that can be assessed—tried on, perhaps accepted, but perhaps declined: in which case respect is owed, but is saved, or confirmed, for others—other relationships, other projects, other passions.

And again, if a woman feels she owes a stance of welcome to burgeoning human life that comes her way, it may be, not because she thinks such a stance authoritative for all, but because of the virtues around which her practical identity is now oriented: receptivity to life's agenda, for instance, or responsiveness to that which is most vulnerable. For another woman, the executive virtues to be exercised tug in just the other direction: loyalty to treasured life plans, a commitment that it be she, not the chances of biology, that should determine her life's course, bolstering self-direction after a life too long ruled by serendipity and fate.

Deciding when it is morally decent to end a pregnancy, it turns out, is an admixture of settling impersonally or universally authoritative moral requirements, and of discovering and arbitrating—sometimes after agonizing deliberation, sometimes in a decision no less deep for its immediacy—one's own commitments, identity, and defining virtues.

A similarly complex story appears when we turn to the second theme. Another thread that appears in many women's stories in the face of unsought pregnancy is respect for the weighty responsibility involved in creating human life. Once again, it is a theme that pulls and tugs in different directions.

In its most familiar direction, it shows up in many stories of why an unsought pregnancy is continued. Many people believe that one's responsibility to nurture new life is importantly amplified if one is responsible for bringing about its existence in the first place. Just what it takes to count as responsible here is a point on which individuals diverge (whether voluntary but contracepted intercourse is different from intercourse without use of birth control, and again from intentionally deciding to become pregnant at the IVF clinic). But triggering the relevant standard of responsibility for creation, it is felt, brings with it a heightened responsibility to nurture: it is disrespectful to create human life only to allow it to wither. Put more rigorously, one who is responsible for bringing about a creature that has intrinsic value in virtue of its potential to become a person has a special responsibility to enable it to reach that end state.

But the idea of respect for creation is also, if less frequently acknowledged, sometimes the reason why women are moved to *end* pregnancies. As Barbara Katz Rothman (1985) puts it, decisions to abort often represent, not a decision to destroy, but a refusal to create. Many people have deeply felt convictions about the circumstances under which they feel it right for them to bring a child into the world—can it be brought into a decent world, an intact family, a society that can minimally respect its agency? These considerations may persist even after conception has taken place; for while the *embryo* has already been created, a person has not. Some women decide to abort, that is, not because they do not *want* the resulting child—indeed, they may yearn for nothing more, and desperately wish that their circumstances were otherwise—but because they do not think bringing a child into the world the right thing for them to do.

These are abortions marked by moral language. A woman wants to abort because she knows she couldn't give up a child for adoption but feels she couldn't give the child the sort of life, or be the sort of parent, she thinks a child *deserves;* a woman who would have to give up the child thinks it would be *unfair* to bring a child into existence already burdened by rejection, however well grounded its reasons; a woman living in a country marked by poverty and gender apartheid wants to abort because she decides it would be *wrong* for her to bear a daughter whose life, like hers, would be filled with so much injustice and hardship.

Some have thought that such decisions betray a simple fallacy: unless the child's life were literally going to be worse than non-existence, how can one abort out of concern for the future child? But the worry here isn't that one would be imposing a *harm* on the child by bringing it into existence (as though children who are in the situations mentioned have lives that aren't worth living). The claim is that bringing about a person's life in these circumstances would do violence to her ideals of creating and parenthood. She does not want to bring into existence a daughter she cannot love and care for, she does not want to bring into existence a person whose life will be marked by disrespect or rejection.

Nor does the claim imply judgment on women who *do* continue pregnancies in similar circumstances—as though there were here an obligation to abort. For the norms in question, once again, need not be impersonally authoritative moral chums. Like ideals of good parenting, they mark out considerations all should be sensitive to, perhaps, but equally reasonable people may adhere to different variations and weightings. Still, they are normative for those who do have them; far from expressing mere matters of taste, the ideals one does accept carry an important kind of categoricity, issuing imperatives whose authority is not reducible to mere desire. These are, at root, issues about *integrity*, and the importance of maintaining integrity over one's participation in this enterprise precisely because it is so normatively weighty.

What is usually emphasized in the morality of abortion is the ethics of destruction; but there is a balancing ethics of creation. And for many people, conflict about abortion is a conflict *within* that ethics. On the one hand, we now have on hand an entity that has a measure of sanctity: that it has begun is reason to help it continue—perhaps especially if one had a role in its procreation—which is why even early abortion is not normatively equivalent to contraception. On the other hand, not to end a pregnancy *is* to do something else, namely, to continue creating a person, and for some women, pregnancy strikes in circumstances in which they cannot countenance that enterprise. For some, the sanctity of developing human life will be strong enough to tip the balance towards continuing the pregnancy; for others, their norms of respectful creation will hold sway. For those who believe that the norms governing creation of a person are mild relative to the normative telos of embryonic life, being a responsible creator means continuing to gestate, and doing the best one can to bring about the conditions under which that creation will be more respectful. For others, though, the normativity of fetal telos is mild and their standards of respectful creation high, and the lesson goes in just the other direction: it is a sign of respect not to continue creating when certain background conditions, such as a loving family or adequate resources, are not in place.

However one thinks these issues settle out, they will not be resolved by austere contemplation of the value of human life. They require wrestling with the rich meanings of creation, responsibility, and kinship. And these issues, I have suggested, are just as much issues about one's integrity as they are about what is impersonally obligatory. On many treatments of abortion, considerations about whether or not to continue a pregnancy are exhausted by preferences, on the one hand, and universally authoritative moral demands, on the other; but some of the most important terrain lies in between.

REFERENCES

Dworkin, R. (1993) *Life's dominion: an argument about abortion, euthanasia, and individual freedom.* New York: Alfred A. Knopf.

Kamm, F. M. (1992). *Creation and abortion: a study in moral and legal philosophy.* New York: Oxford University Press.

MacKinnon, C. A. Reflections on sex equality under law. *The Yale Law Journal,* 100:5 (March 1991), 1281–1328, p. 1314.

Rothman, B. K. (1989). *Recreating motherhood: ideology and technology in a patriarchal society.* New York: Norton.

Silverstein, H. S. (1987). On a woman's 'responsibility' for the fetus. *Social Theory and Practice,* 13, 103–19.

Thomson, J. J. (1971) A defense of abortion. *Philosophy and Public Affairs,* 1, 47–66.

West, R. (1993). Jurisprudence and gender. In D. Kelly Weisberg (Ed.). *Feminist legal theory: foundations* (pp. 75–98). Philadelphia: Temple University Press.

CARRIER SCREENING, PRENATAL TESTING, AND REPRODUCTIVE DECISIONS

THE INTRODUCTION OF CYSTIC FIBROSIS CARRIER SCREENING INTO CLINICAL PRACTICE: POLICY CONSIDERATIONS

Benjamin S. Wilfond and Norman Fost

Since the identification of the gene associated with cystic fibrosis (CF), interest in general population CF carrier screening has been growing. Screening has the potential to allow individuals to make more informed reproductive decisions and to increase the choices available to them for avoiding the birth of a child with CF while offering society the potential public health benefit of a reduced incidence of individuals with CF. With the anticipated expansion of genetic knowledge resulting from the Human Genome Initiative, the experience of providing CF screening to the general population may become a model for developing new genetic tests and subsequently integrating them into clinical medical practice. More important, the potential magnitude of CF carrier testing in the reproductive-aged population gives this issue immediate relevance.

Soon after the CF gene mutation sequence was published, several biotechnology companies offered this service to physicians. However, enthusiasm for screening has been tempered by two policy statements, one issued by the American Society of Human Genetics (ASHG) in November 1989, and the other by the National Institutes of Health (NIH) during a workshop on population screening for the CF gene held in March 1990, both recommending a moratorium on routine screening. The statements concur on several key points:

1. Routine screening should be delayed until pilot studies are completed, as "there is little experience in the delivery of such complex information to large populations." The complexity of the information derives from the ambiguity of

Milbank Quarterly, Vol. 70, No. 4, 1992, 629–659. Used with permission.

Editors' note: References have been omitted; those wishing to follow up on sources should consult the original article.

negative test results and the variable prognosis for CF, complicating the education and counseling process, which would be formidable for a large population even with a simpler test.

2. If the test had a greater detection rate, then it might be appropriate to consider mass population screening. The NIH workshop report recommends that "screening could be offered to all persons of reproductive age if a 95 [percent] level of carrier detection were achieved," but only if additional conditions were met.
3. "Carrier testing should be offered couples in which either partner has a close relative affected with CF."
4. The "optimal setting for carrier testing is through primary health care providers."

Although these recommendations have dampened the initial drive for screening while articulating the current consensus on practice recommendations, they have not been analyzed in detail. Our purpose in this article is to review critically the ASHG and the NIH workshop recommendations, to evaluate some of the legal and ethical issues that will influence physicians' screening practices for cystic fibrosis, and to propose guidelines for their screening practices to primary care physicians and genetics services providers.

CLINICAL BACKGROUND

Cystic fibrosis is one of the most common significant autosomal recessive diseases affecting the white population. The median life expectancy of about 28 years has been steadily rising for more than two decades. The median survival of patients born in 1990 has been estimated to be 40 years, based on an observed decline in infant mortality of CF patients. Current investigational therapies, such as DNase, offer the potential for even longer survival. Patients are variably affected, dying in infancy from meconium ileus, a neonatal intestinal obstruction, some severely disabled with chronic obstructive pulmonary disease (COPD) as children, whereas others are rarely hospitalized, play competitive sports, and may not even develop symptoms until adulthood. However, most people with CF develop moderate lung disease by adolescence or early adulthood.

The CF incidence in whites ranges from 1 in 1,700 to 1 in 6,500 in various populations, but is generally estimated to be 1 in 2,500 live births. Assuming this incidence, approximately 1 in 25 white individuals (4 percent) are heterozygotes—asymptomatic carriers with a 1 in 4 chance of having a child with CF if their partners are also carriers. Recent newborn screening data from Colorado and Wisconsin suggest that the incidence of CF in whites may be the range of from 1 in 3,000 to 1 in 3,500. The Cystic Fibrosis Patient Registry estimates the incidence to be 1 in 3,400 in whites and 1 in 15,000 in blacks, with a corresponding carrier frequency of 1 in 30 for whites and 1 in 62 for blacks. Risk calculations in this article will be based on the most current data.

Cystic fibrosis results from mutations in a gene mapped to a chromosome that codes for a protein, the cystic fibrosis transmembrane conductance regulator (CFTR), which facilitates chloride transport. In the United States, the most common CFTR mutation, ΔF508, a three-base pair deletion, has been found on approximately 75 percent of chromosomes from CF patients. Over 175 additional mutations have been identified, most of them rare, but analysis of from four to seven of the most common mutations, using polymerase chain reaction (PCR) amplification and gel electrophoresis, could increase the carrier detection rate in the U.S. population to about 85 percent. With this detection rate, 72 percent (85 x 85) of at-risk couples will be identifiable. For varying ethnic and geographic groups, different mutations occur more commonly, which may require individualizing the testing protocol. Although the charge for the test is currently between $150 and $200, if screening is done on a mass scale, and with improved technology, the charge may be reduced to a range of from $30 to $50.

DEFERMENT OF POPULATION SCREENING UNTIL PILOT STUDIES DEMONSTRATE ITS SAFETY AND EFFECTIVENESS

The ASHG and the NIH workshop statements advocate that mass CF carrier-screening programs should only be implemented after pilot studies are completed. Pilot studies prior to mass genetic testing have been recommended by reports from the

Hastings Center, the National Academy of Sciences, and the President's Commission for the Study of Ethical Problems in Medicine and Biomedical and Behavioral Research. The rationale for pilot testing is that previous experiences with genetic testing have demonstrated serious problems such as confusion, stigmatization, and discrimination when no comprehensive infrastructure was in place to provide education, informed consent, and counseling. The primary purpose of pilot studies is to establish effective educational methods, to determine interest in testing, to evaluate the influence of test results on reproductive behavior, and to document the occurrence of adverse psychological and social effects.

Support for pilot studies of CF carrier screening has been articulated in the medical literature by ethicists, geneticists, obstetricians, pediatricians, and pulmonologists. Recently, the American Medical Association adopted a report affirming the same position, as did the American College of Obstetrics and Gynecology. As a result of the professional consensus for pilot studies, the NIH Ethical, Legal, and Social Implications Program of the National Center for Human Genome Research funded seven pilot programs for CF screening in October 1991.

However, many individuals with a commercial interest suggest that mass screening should be instituted without prior pilot studies. In 1989, Keith Brown, president of Gene Screen, a biotechnology company that markets the test, suggested that pilot studies were not reasonable and that mass screening was inevitable: "to [expect us to] wait until we get 99 percent of the mutations and a national program is defined in 2½ years, that's kind of dreaming. The genetics community is thinking about how to make it happen ideally. Forget it, that game is already lost." Others believe the potential benefits of testing sufficiently outweigh the possible risks and suggest that empirical verification of benefit is not necessary. For example, Schulman et al., writing for the Genetics and IVF [In Vitro Fertilization] Institute, a private laboratory and clinic in Virginia, argue that it is "neither necessary nor desirable to delay access to a test now capable of detecting the large majority of CF carriers and families [and that the] benefits to the general public must take priority over possible perturbations within the healthcare delivery system (expanded education and counseling efforts) if CF screenings were implemented without delay."

The central ethical dilemma is how to balance the benefit to persons who may wish to avoid the birth of a child with CF against the potential harm that would result from the confusion, stigmatization, and discrimination associated with testing. Although the rationale for pilot studies prior to population testing is based on the duty to avoid harm, it does not mean that interventions must carry no risks because this requirement would preclude most medical care. Rather, risks are expected to have at least the potential of compensating benefits: in this case, that patients have sufficient information to allow an informed choice. The problem with Schulman's argument is that weighing the potential benefits and harms of mass screening cannot be performed without the empirical evidence from pilot studies.

Brock, who runs a pilot screening program in Scotland, puts forth a different argument in favor of screening, focusing on the autonomy of the patient. He asks "whether we have the right to withhold, largely because of our own unresolved worries about the capacity to provide adequate counseling, screening from those who request it." He implies that patients' requests for testing should outweigh paternalistic actions to withhold testing. However, such paternalism is consistent with long-standing policies that limit the use of experimental drugs and devices unless there has been institutional review and patient consent after being informed about the experimental nature of the medical intervention. There is no clear obligation to provide experimental interventions to persons who request them. However, what is actually experimental in CF carrier testing is not the test itself, but the mechanism to provide the test to large groups of people.

The mechanism to provide education, consent, and counseling should be evaluated because these activities will determine the balance between benefits and harms. Before deciding whether the benefits of screening are worth the risks, potential screenees must be educated so they can make a preliminary judgment about their reproductive options. In CF carrier testing, the major benefit is the opportunity to avoid the birth of an affected child, but this benefit disappears if test results would not affect a couple's reproductive plans. Unless the person identified another potential benefit, there would be no reason to conduct the tests. Other benefits of testing would include reassurance that a fetus does not have CF or emotional preparation for the birth of an affected child. The knowledge of an affected fetus may offer families the following practical benefits:

1. arranging for adequate medical insurance
2. providing for perinatal assessment
3. moving closer to a CF center that provides medical care
4. moving closer to family or other support networks
5. changing employment for the purpose of providing home care

Whether such potential benefits will be sufficient motivators to obtain testing is unknown.

In deciding whether to be tested, an individual would also need accurate, balanced information about the medical aspects of cystic fibrosis and, in order to comprehend their reproductive options, about the potential risks of being identified as a carrier and the implications of a negative test. Using current standards, such informed consent may require one to two hours of a genetic counselor's time. The use of alternative delivery systems, including pamphlets, videos, computers, or group sessions, will reduce personnel time, but these, too, need to be studied. The results of the NIH-funded pilot studies, which may not be available for at least two years, may not answer these questions sufficiently. Further studies may be required before population testing can be adequately assessed.

THE LIMITED RELEVANCE OF THE DETECTION RATE

Both documents cite the limited sensitivity of the tests as a major impediment to mass screening. Several biotechnology companies also acknowledge this factor, but their opinions vary as to what degree of sensitivity would justify mass screening. One commercial brochure states: "We would like the test to detect at least 90 [percent] of CF carriers before advising routine screening." Others claim that, at 75 percent, the necessary threshold had been reached. In fact, as early as February 1990, the Genetics and IVF Institute began offering prenatal ΔF508 screening of fetuses to all white couples undergoing amniocentesis or chorionic villus sampling (CVS) (Bick et al. 1990)

The NIH workshop noted the 95 percent threshold because of a concern for couples in which one partner is a carrier while the other has a negative test (table 1). Approximately 5 percent (1 in 18) of

TABLE 1

Cystic Fibrosis Carrier Testing—Changes after Mutation Analysis[a]

Percent of cystic fibrosis mutations detectable	Chance of being a carrier risk for person after a negative test	Chance of cystic fibrosis in offspring		
		One partner tested	Both partners tested	
		Negative	Both negative	One positive/ one negative
0	1 in 30	1 in 3,400	1 in 3,400	1 in 3,400
55	1 in 66	1 in 7,900	1 in 17,400	1 in 264
75	1 in 118	1 in 14,200	1 in 55,700	1 in 472
85	1 in 196	1 in 23,500	1 in 154,000	1 in 784
90	1 in 294	1 in 35,300	1 in 346,000	1 in 1,180
95	1 in 587	1 in 70,400	1 in 1,380,000	1 in 2,350
96	1 in 838	1 in 101,000	1 in 2,810,000	1 in 3,350

[a]Calculations described in Lemna et al. (1990). The chance of being a carrier (assuming an incidence of 1 in 3,400) after a negative test (assuming a detection rate [d]) is obtained by calculating the joint probability that a person is a carrier and has a negative test ($.033 \times [1 - d]$) divided by the sum of the joint probabilities that a person is a carrier and has a negative test plus that of a person being a noncarrier and having a negative test ($.097 \times 1$).

the couples in the general population would fall into this category (table 2). These couples cannot be reassured that they are not at risk. The complexities associated with an imperfect CF test will be difficult to convey and understand, as evidenced by this confusing excerpt from the consent form of one commercial company:

> Due to the present inability to detect all CYSTIC FIBROSIS CARRIERS, if I am a carrier of the cystic fibrosis gene, and if the other parent of any child I may have is also a carrier of the cystic fibrosis gene, and if either of us are [*sic*] not detected to be carriers of the CYSTIC FIBROSIS GENE using the test presently available, then a child born to us may be affected with CYSTIC FIBROSIS.

The challenge for education and consent posed by these complexities has been a deterrent to mass screening. Ten-Kate has argued that once the detection rate is greater than 95 percent, the major barrier to mass population screening will have been removed because the risk to couples with only one detected carrier of having a child with CF will be no greater than the a priori risk in the general population (table 1). Although an improved detection rate is necessary, it is not sufficient, as indicated in the NIH workshop statement:

> These difficulties would be substantially reduced if testing could detect at least 90 to 95 percent of carriers. There is a consensus that population-based screening for carriers could be offered to all persons of reproductive age if a 95 percent level of carrier detection were achieved. The offering of population-based screening would still require that substantial educational and counseling guidelines be satisfied.

However, the NIH workshop statement has been misrepresented by at least one commercial company, whose brochure implies that a 90 percent detection rate would be sufficient:

> The members of that workshop also suggested that testing of individuals with no family history of the disease should not begin until, among other things, the test could detect "at least 90–95 [percent] of carriers." *This new CF carrier test satisfies that requirement* for Caucasians of northern European ancestry.
>
> For those individuals who are found not to carry any of these ten mutations, the negative results will, in effect, reduce their chance of being a CF carrier to only about 1 in 250. Thus, this new test may be of interest to ANYONE who has not yet completed their reproductive plans. (emphasis in original)

The brochure creates the impression that the NIH workshop would endorse screening for "anyone" because 90 percent of carriers are detectable. However, the consensus was 95 percent, not 90 percent. More important, the counseling and educational guidelines for population testing have not been sufficiently developed because the necessary research is still in progress.

Concern About Persistent Uncertainty

Although a higher detection rate will simplify the information, a detection rate of 93 percent is not sufficient justification for mass screening. It is still possible that families with one positive and one negative test will be left with uncertainty and a sense of increased risk. Basic concepts of probability and risk are not easily understood. A study of

TABLE 2
Genetic Counseling Hours for 3 Million Couples

Carrier status	Frequency (%)[a]	Total couples	Minutes per couple	Hours
No carriers	94.47	2,834,100	10	472,400
One carrier	5.45	163,500	60	163,500
Two carriers	.08	2,400	60	2,400
Total	—	—	—	638,300

[a]Calculated given a carrier frequency $q = .033$ and detection rate $d = .85$; $(1 - dq)^2 + 2\,dq(1 - dq) + (dq)^2 = 1$.

middle-class, pregnant women found that 25 percent interpreted a 1 in 1,000 chance to mean 10 percent or greater. People also tend to translate uncertainty into a binary form that focuses on the numerator of one, projecting from it that the event either will occur or not. Even though the majority of couples is not at risk of having a child with CF, some might alter their reproductive plans (including the abortion of healthy fetuses) because they are confused about the impression of risk created by testing results.

Even with a 95 percent rate, as a result of the testing process, a couple with one positive test may falsely *perceive* their risk for having an affected child to be higher than before testing. Without testing, the couple may have given little thought to CF, unaware of the baseline risk. The process of carrier testing may heighten a couple's concern about CF, causing anxiety or irrational changes in reproductive plans, particularly if genetic counseling is inadequate. For example, although few couples' reproductive plans are influenced by the theoretical 2 percent risk of serious congenital problems, a couple that was informed about a "test" result showing a 2 percent chance of their child having a major birth defect may become anxious or change their reproductive plans. An effective, research-based counseling program for avoiding these problems and the practical ability to provide such a system are necessary criteria for population testing.

The Need for an Effective Infrastructure

Even with 100 percent sensitivity, an effective program to provide education, consent, and counseling is still necessary. This lesson was demonstrated by the experience of the sickle cell screening programs of the early 1970s. Even though the sickle cell tests had a specificity and sensitivity of virtually 100 percent, the early programs generally did not adequately provide for education. Misunderstanding about the difference between being a sickle cell carrier and having the disease, sickle cell anemia, led to persons being stigmatized and experiencing discrimination in their access to employment and ability to obtain life insurance.

In contrast, Kaback and Zeiger established an effective pretesting education program for the voluntary Tay–Sachs screening program piloted in the Baltimore and Washington Jewish community in the early 1970s. In addition to informed consent, Kaback emphasized community support and multimedia educational information; more than one year was devoted to educating the community before the first person was tested. The program was well received by the community and there was an effective transfer of information with minimal adverse psychological effects. This program differed from the sickle cell program in that there were no racial issues involved in the screening, prenatal diagnosis was available, and the population was better educated.

Public education will be important in shaping attitudes toward genetic disorders and genetic testing to avoid stigmatization. Genetic counseling is necessary, but not sufficient, to prevent problems of stigmatization. A study of the long-term effects of a screening program for Tay–Sachs disease among high school students in Montreal revealed that, eight years later, 19 percent of carriers still attached some anxiety to being a carrier. A seven-year follow-up study of the sickle cell carrier screening program in Orchomenos, Greece revealed that 34 percent of couples perceived the trait as a mild disease. Twenty percent of these families felt that sickle cell trait meant a restriction of freedom and a risk of social stigmatization. Frequently, carrier status was concealed at the time of marriage arrangements, and engagements between carriers and unaffected individuals were broken once carrier status was disclosed. Furthermore, the study found no reduction in sickle cell births. However, experiences with heterozygote detection for other diseases have fared better than those with sickle cell anemia. For example, screening for β-thalassemia in Sardinia resulted in a decline in incidence from 1 in 250 to 1 in 1,200.

Genetic counseling for CF will require extensive explanation about CF and the potential risks associated with screening, particularly the possibility of insurance or employment discrimination (Billings et al. 1992). Medical insurers may attempt to coerce reproductive decisions. For example, a Los Angeles couple who already had a child with CF was informed that their health maintenance organization (HMO) would cover either prenatal diagnosis or the medical care of an affected child, but not both. The fetus was diagnosed with CF and the couple elected to continue the pregnancy. The HMO told the family that they would not cover the medical expenses of the child. When challenged, the HMO reversed its decision, but the case demonstrates the potential for coercion. Potential screenees will at least need to be aware of these risks before they consent to testing. Recently, Wisconsin enacted legislation to prevent medical insurers either from requiring individuals to reveal whether a genetic test has been obtained, and, if so, the results, or from requesting genetic tests as a condition of coverage or in order to set rates.[1] The impact of this legislation is unclear, as the subsequent regulations are still being developed.

Given the complexities of genetic counseling for CF carrier testing, the development of an effective mass population screening program will be challenging because of its potential to screen the entire childbearing population. Pilot studies will be needed to determine the amount of personnel time required and whether there are sufficient resources to provide effective counseling. Even if ten minutes of direct personnel time were devoted to prescreening consent and education, an annual screening program for three million couples (an estimate of the potential magnitude if screening was provided to 75 percent of the four million women who become pregnant annually) would require at least 638,000 hours (table 2). Counseling provided by the approximately 1,000 certified clinical geneticists and genetic counselors would require each provider to spend 16 weeks every year on CF testing. Therefore, a mass screening program would require a tremendous increase in trained personnel to achieve only a minimum standard of consent and counseling. The only current alternative is to assign this very complex counseling task to persons not trained in genetics or genetic counseling, and unlikely to be informed about the rapidly changing complexities of CF testing. Alternative mechanisms for counseling, including multimedia resources (such as interactive computers and video), community-based programs, and improved training of primary care providers, especially nurses, need to be developed and assessed.

Cost-Effectiveness Considerations

Even if a safe and effective delivery infrastructure were developed, policy makers will need to look carefully at the program costs per case of CF prevented. Commonly the public health goal of reducing disease as the raison d'être of genetic counseling is disavowed; the purpose instead is generally described as one of allowing more informed reproductive decisions by individuals. Policy makers must consider whether it would be a fair or prudent use of resources to spend money on this arguably discretionary program at a time when approximately 33 million Americans are without basic health insurance. It is not enough to point out that most of the money for screening would be spent in the private sector because this does not address the question of whether such services should be available to Medicaid recipients or persons with no third-party coverage. Moreover, dollars spent for CF screening are unavailable for other social needs. If costs incurred through population screening did not avert a single case of cystic fibrosis, it would be difficult to defend the expenditure for the sole benefit of providing more informed decisions. Evidence that testing does result in the reduction of disease, and at what cost, will be needed before funding of such a program could be justified from a public health perspective.

The impact of a screening program on the incidence of CF is uncertain, but preliminary evidence suggests that many people may not be interested in undergoing testing, prenatal diagnosis, or aborting a fetus with CF. CF differs from many other diseases for which there is interest in prenatal diagnosis because the severity of symptoms in a particular individual is unpredictable, there is the potential for survival into middle age, and normal intelligence is preserved. In a survey of parents of children with CF, Wertz et al. found that only 20 percent indicated a willingness to abort a fetus with CF, compared with 79 percent of this group who indicated a willingness to abort a pregnancy to save the mother's life, 75 percent for rape, and 58 percent for severe mental retardation. In another study, 214 pregnant women in the general population were surveyed after reading educational materials on CF. Although 98 percent believed carrier testing should be available, only 84 percent would have taken the test prior to pregnancy. If found to be at risk, 67 percent would be interested in prenatal diagnosis, whereas only 29 percent indicated a willingness to abort an affected fetus.

If these preliminary findings reflect actual practices, the direct costs to avoid one CF birth could be close to 2.4 million dollars and might involve

TABLE 3

Cost of General Population CF Carrier Testing to Avoid One CF Birth[a]

Number of families		Services	Costs ($)
Total couples approached	27,010	Education and consent @ $10	270,100
Couples tested (.8)	21,607	Testing and counseling @ $100	2,160,700
Couples at risk $(.033 \times .85)^2$	17	Counseling @ $100	1,700
Prenatal diagnosis (.7)	12	CVS and CF testing @ $1,200	14,400
Affected fetuses (.25)	3	Counseling @ $100	300
Abortions (.33)	1	Abortion @ $2,000	2,000
		Total	$2,449,200

[a]Based on estimates of utilization and direct costs. Abbreviation: CVS, chorionic villus sampling.

screening as many as 27,000 couples (table 3). An accurate cost-effective analysis will require further empiric assessment of behaviors. However, there may be less test-seeking behavior than these studies suggest because responses in questionnaires do not always translate to behavior. For example, although approximately 70 percent of at-risk people for Huntington's disease indicated an interest in being tested, when the test was offered fewer than 15 percent actually responded. In fact, in one of the few reports of CF testing, from a self-paying CF screening program, only 43 percent of CVS patients and 19 percent of amniocentesis patients agreed also to have their fetus tested for CF.

THE ROLE OF PRIMARY HEALTH CARE PROVIDERS

The NIH workshop statement concluded that the "optimal setting for carrier testing is through primary health care providers." Involvement of primary care providers is attractive for mass population genetic testing because of the apparent logistical advantage of using a large personnel reservoir. However, the primary care setting may not be ideal for population carrier screening. Primary health care providers may not have the time, information, training, experience, or interest to provide this service well.

Physicians may not be sufficiently informed about the genetic testing and reproductive counseling to provide the necessary information. For example, a study involving pediatricians found that 54 percent could not accurately state the risk of phenylketonuria (PKU) in a neonate with a moderately elevated test result. In another study, Holtzman found that only 22 percent of a sample of obstetricians could describe the recommended clinical course of action following an elevated maternal serum alpha fetoprotein (MSAFP). Some respondents may have recommended abortion instead of first repeating the test or obtaining sonography, as recommended by the American College of Obstetrics and Gynecology.

The NIH workshop statement on CF states: "Providers of screening services have an obligation to ensure [that] adequate education and counseling are included in the program." The National Academy of Sciences report recommended that a comprehensive program include an ongoing assessment of patients' comprehension of information. Such standards would be difficult for most primary care providers to fulfill. It is not clear whether primary care providers will be willing or able to spend the time for education, consent, test interpretation, counseling, and assessment that is necessary in a CF screening program. However, it may be feasible to train primary care nurses, perhaps under the supervision of genetic counselors, to provide at least such services as prescreening education and consent.

Some primary care settings may pose additional problems. For example, prenatal visits appear to be an efficient setting for population CF carrier testing. However, the NIH workshop concluded that, ideally, population screening should be done prior to conception so that patients could avail themselves of preconception alternatives such as adoption or artificial insemination, and decisions would not be complicated by the urgency and emotional burden of an existing pregnancy.

Carrier screening during pregnancy is also likely initially to involve testing only women, which is not desirable for several reasons. First, any adverse effects of carrier identification would fall disproportionately on women. Second, testing both partners together would reduce the anxiety associated with the time delay in obtaining the partner's results after the woman has a positive test. Finally, the test results of the partner would greatly alter the risk assessment. For example, at an 85 percent detection rate, a person with a negative test has an apparent risk of 1 in 23,500 of having a child with CF (table 1). If the partner was negative, the risk would be reduced to 1 in 154,000; if the partner was positive, the risk would be 1 in 784. Testing the partner is desirable because these results could alter the apparent risk by close to 200-fold.

RELEVANCE OF A FAMILY HISTORY OF CF

The ASHG and the NIH workshop statements acknowledged that people with a family history of CF should be offered testing. Testing of family members has been available since the late 1980s, using linkage analysis. Combining this with mutation analysis could allow carrier testing of blood relatives to be informative at close to 100 percent, provided that a proband's chromosomes were available. The chance of a relative of a CF patient being a carrier is 67 percent for a sibling, 50 percent in an aunt or uncle, 33 percent in a niece or nephew, and 25 percent in a first cousin. Relatives of identified carriers are also at increased risk.

Testing a population whose a priori chance of being a carrier is higher will result in proportionately fewer false positives for a given specificity, increasing the positive predictive value of the test. Although the specificity of mutation analysis is unknown, false positives should be uncommon. However, laboratory or clerical errors will still cause a low proportion of false positive results and even this will become a finite number if screening is done on a mass scale.

The potential benefits of testing individuals with a positive family history are greater than for the general population. Some may already be anxious about their uncertain carrier status. Couples may otherwise have chosen not to bear children. High-risk couples with negative results could be reassured; the knowledge may allow some to bear children without fear. A couple found to be at a one in four risk prior to conception would be able to apply that knowledge to a full range of reproductive options. These families should be easier to counsel than the general population, as they are more likely to be familiar with the clinical course of CF and the associated burden of care. However, because more than 85 percent of CF patients are born to families without a prior family history, testing this high-risk population is not likely to result in substantial reduction in CF incidence.

A screening program directed toward relatives of CF patients would limit the size and cost of the program. Cystic fibrosis centers could facilitate such a program by informing their patients that carrier testing is available for interested family members. Interested persons could be referred to genetic counseling programs, or counseled directly in centers that have genetic counselors or other clinicians competent in genetic counseling. Physicians and other health professionals in the CF centers would be able to play a substantial role in providing education and counseling. The CF Foundation could establish criteria for quality control of the test, as is currently done for the diagnostic test for CF known as the "sweat test." The resources for counseling and quality control of testing even within such a limited program remain to be organized, but an infrastructure using existing resources has a greater potential of being developed to meet these needs. . . .

GUIDELINES FOR PRIMARY CARE PHYSICIANS

Physicians could fulfill the potential legal and ethical duty to inform all patients about test availability without necessarily being prepared to provide testing. However, they must recognize the potential for this information to influence behavior, depending on what information is given and how it is framed and delivered. Although the goal of disclosure should be to provide nondirective information, how the information is presented may motivate people to be tested. For example, Goodman and Goodman have commented that some of the brochures used in Tay–Sachs screening programs successfully promoted screening because they generated anxiety. Private companies with financial interests in promoting screening are also likely to present information in a potentially misleading fashion. A brochure from the Genetics and IVF Institute states: "Could I have a child with CF? The answer is probably yes. Almost any couple is at risk for having children with CF". In fact, fewer than 1 in 900 couples are at risk, but information presented in this way may be a strong motivation for screening.

Decisions to be tested for CF may also be influenced by how information about the disease is presented. An illustration of the possible impact of an arguably biased presentation is provided by the following excerpt from a consent form used in a pilot study from Denmark:

> Cystic fibrosis is a serious disease that causes a marked tendency to pneumonia and a reduced function of the pancreas. Today, the disease is incurable and, if untreated, it leads to death in childhood as a result of increasing damage to the lung tissue. A very intensive life-long treatment of the lung disease now enables many patients to reach adulthood, but many still risk acquiring some degree of lung disablement at an early stage. At present, most patients are hospitalized every three months for two weeks of intensive treatment of infections; they also are treated daily for several hours in their homes.

Not surprisingly, more than 90 percent of clients who read this description accepted testing. Consider the difference in a client's reaction to the following alternative hypothetical version:

> CF is an inherited disease which used to be fatal, but now half of all patients will live into their fourth decade. CF does not affect intelligence; many people with CF go to college, enter professional occupations, get married, and have children. CF affects the respiratory and digestive systems, but symptoms can be controlled by taking enzyme capsules to help digestion, as well as antibiotics to fight off lung infections. Average life expectancy is steadily increasing, with rapidly advancing research producing the potential for better controls in the near future, and perhaps even a cure.

Both descriptions provide accurate, but limited, information. The second version, if read and understood, would almost certainly lead to a lower interest in testing than the Danish model. The point is not that either description is better, but only that the information sent by the counselor and the way it is sent, or more important, the way it is received by the client, will have a profound impact on what reproductive decisions are made.

Therefore, CF testing will need to be presented in a balanced fashion. If, once informed, patients then want to learn more about the test, they could be referred to a genetics counseling program. A proposal for a more balanced disclosure follows:

> There is now a blood test to identify carriers of the cystic fibrosis gene. Carriers are healthy but may be at risk for having a child with CF. CF occurs in about 1 in 3,400 births, but it is more likely to happen if there is a history of CF in your family. People with CF have chronic lung disease, but normal intelligence, and usually live into early adulthood. Testing is done in conjunction with genetic counseling, which may require one to two hours of your time before you would be in a position to know whether you would want to be tested. If you are interested in hearing more about this, please let your doctor know.

One argument for mentioning CF testing to all white patients, not just those with a family history, is because CF is a relatively common genetic disease in that population. However, what counts as common is arbitrary. Because the CF carrier frequency in blacks is close to half that of whites, some might suggest that blacks also be tested. Others might claim that CF is a relatively infrequent occurrence, even in whites. These potentially conflicting interpretations suggest that the frequency of the disease is not itself the central issue, but one of several that must be considered.

As physicians become more oriented to initiating discussions about reproductive health issues with their patients, information about CF testing, and genetic testing in general, should be discussed with patients along with such issues as family planning and contraception. However, there are over a hundred conditions for which carrier detection and prenatal diagnosis are potentially available and the Human Genome Initiative will increase this number. Primary care physicians are not likely to have the time to inquire about a family history, ethnic background, or interest in testing for each of these diseases. The patient's genuine interest in being informed of available tests could be supported by a checklist to be completed in the physician's waiting room and reviewed during the visit. The checklist might include a list of genetic diseases with brief descriptions, as well as a list of symptoms suggestive of genetic disease. If the patient is interested in further testing, the primary care practitioner could provide it if he or she is prepared also to provide genetics counseling; if not, the patient could be referred to a genetics counselor. This approach has been implemented in family planning clinics in New England.

GUIDELINES FOR GENETICISTS AND GENETIC COUNSELORS

Geneticists and genetic counselors are more likely to have the time and training to provide the education, consent, and counseling needed for CF screening. However, because providing CF testing to all genetics clients who are seen for other reasons would place a great strain on these counseling programs, an additional hour might be required for each visit. Like primary care physicians, clinicians could acknowledge the availability of the CF test during a visit by asking patients to review a checklist and arranging an additional appointment for those interested in further testing. A generic list of testable genetic disorders may be less likely to raise anxiety about CF than a brochure specifically about CF. Persons interested in CF testing should be informed that the test is not yet routine, and may not be covered by insurance. Finally, the patient should be aware that prescreening counseling, ideally for both partners, is necessary, and this may take up to an hour. Unless the interest in CF testing exceeds the resources of a particular genetics clinic, counseling and testing should be provided to anyone who requests it. It is possible that referrals from primary care physicians and interest among existing genetics counseling clients still could exceed the resources of a particular clinic, in which case the clinic might consider giving priority to patients who have a relative with a CF mutation.

The distinction between informing and providing draws attention to the ethical obligation to inform patients about the test. Although this distinction is valuable in determining the extent of a physician's obligation toward patients, it may be lost on other practicing clinicians whose manner of informing may motivate patients to be tested, but who do not provide adequate education, consent, and counseling. Geneticists' practice of informing patients about CF testing might result in other less qualified practitioners informing, offering, and providing testing to their patients. This might result in de facto mass testing with a great potential to cause harm. Thus a geneticist's decision of whether to inform patients about CF testing must not only include an evaluation of his or her obligation to promote the autonomy of the patient at hand, but must also account for the social consequences of this action on other patients, who may be harmed by an unevaluated mass testing program. Because providing specific information about CF is more likely than mentioning CF as one of many potentially available tests to result in the rapid diffusion of testing, we recommend that genetics providers meet their ethical obligation to inform patients by providing a generic checklist.

CONCLUSION

The ASHG and NIH workshop reports concluded that mass population CF screening should be deferred until pilot studies demonstrating effective mechanisms for delivery of these services are completed. The NIH statement emphasized the importance of a 95 percent detection rate in deciding whether population screening should be initiated. We have argued that a high detection rate is not the central issue. It is a necessary, but not sufficient, reason for population screening. Even with 100 percent detection of carriers, the personnel and logistical resources needed to meet education and counseling needs must be developed and evaluated. Furthermore, policy makers must determine whether the goals of a population program—prevention of CF or informed reproductive decision making—warrant public funding or private reimbursement preferentially over other urgent health care needs of the American public.

Primary care physicians may not be the ideal providers of mass population carrier screening programs. Alternative mechanisms of community-organized programs with trained providers and multimedia educational resources should be developed and evaluated. There is no clear legal duty for primary care physicians to provide patients who have no family history with direct access to the test. Primary care physicians who are concerned about liability may discharge their ethical and legal duty by *informing* patients that CF carrier testing is available. *Providing* testing requires adherence to strict standards of education and consent. This should include information about CF, reproductive options, the meaning of a negative test, and the risks of testing. Providers may be liable if information is not communicated accurately or clearly. Therefore, primary care physicians who are not equipped to provide such services should refer interested patients to qualified genetics counseling programs. Ideally, geneticists and genetics counselors should inform patients about the availability of CF carrier testing. However, because this might result in de facto mass testing, as the distinction between informing and providing is easily blurred, geneticists should exercise restraint in informing patients about CF testing except in the context of a general description of potentially available tests.

In response to the ASHG and NIH workshop statements, most physicians have not provided CF screening to patients. Biotechnology companies have backed off from initial marketing positions. The NIH has funded pilot studies. In one to two years, we will have more data from which to develop a rational screening policy for CF. The initial experience with CF carrier testing indicates that it is possible to learn from past mistakes. This is encouraging, in light of the anticipated mapping and sequencing of the human genome, which will continue to raise the question of whether or not to screen.

ACKNOWLEDGMENTS

Some of this work was part of a report prepared for the National Institutes of Health–Department of Energy Working Group on Ethical, Legal, and Social Implications (ELSI) of Human Genome Research. We thank John Robertson, JD, and Ellen Wright Clayton, JD, MD, for their criticism and suggestions on the report submitted to ELSI.

NOTES

1. Wis. Stat. § 631.89.

Authors' note: Between 1991 and 1994, there were eight studies of CF carrier testing in the United States funded by the Ethical, Legal, and Social Implications Program (ELSI) at the National Institutes of Health. Some studies, in the general population, found a minimal level of interest in the general population, from 4 to 20 percent. However, prenatal studies demonstrated a level of interest between 50 and 70 percent. There have been similar results in the United Kingdom, and one study in particular suggested that even in the general population, the level of interest in testing is influenced by active versus passive presentation of information, convenience of testing, and whether the information is presented by a health care professional. The results of these studies raise questions about how decisions regarding the structure of the screening program could influence the interest rate.

In 1997, a Consensus Development Conference sponsored by the NIH recommended that CF testing be offered to the prenatal population but not to the general population. The report seemed to assume that programs with higher interest rates should be supported more than those with lower interest rates. However, the report never explicitly considered the malleability of interest rates and did not seem to give much weight to the complexities of effectively educating people. Professional organizations have not adopted these recommendations, in part because the Consensus Development Conference did not adequately address these issues. Thus in 1998, CF carrier testing is not yet the standard of care.

ETHICAL ISSUES RELATED TO PRENATAL GENETIC TESTING

The Council on Ethical and Judicial Affairs, American Medical Association

This report examines ethical issues related to prenatal genetic testing, including the physician's role in promoting informed reproductive decisions and physician involvement in genetic selection and manipulation. In general, it would be ethically permissible to participate in genetic selection (abortion or embryo discard) or genetic manipulation to prevent, cure, or treat genetic disease. It would not be ethical to engage in selection on the basis of benign characteristics. Genetic manipulation of benign traits, though generally unacceptable, may be permissible under exceptional circumstances. At a minimum, three criteria would have to be satisfied: there would have to be a clear and meaningful benefit to the child, there could be no trade-off with other characteristics or traits, and all citizens would have to have equal access to the genetic technology, irrespective of income or other socioeconomic characteristics.

BACKGROUND

The Human Genome Project

The Human Genome Project, begun in October 1990, is part of an international effort to expand current genetic knowledge. The ultimate goal of the project is the construction of a detailed map of human chromosomes. The knowledge that is expected to be gained from the project could aid in the identification and cure of diseases at the genetic level and expand the understanding of genetic influences on human behavior.

Significantly, of the total funding for the project, a percentage has been designated for its ethical evaluation. Prominent among the ethical issues implied by the project is the appropriate use of new information about the genome and new procedures developed for genetic analysis and manipulation. The Council on Ethical and Judicial Affairs of the American Medical Association, Chicago, Ill, has already addressed several issues related to genetic testing, including genetic testing by employers and insurers and carrier screening for cystic fibrosis and other disorders.

In this report, the Council will consider ethical issues related to prenatal genetic testing, the examination of the genetic makeup of a fetus during gestation or of an embryo at the preimplantation stage of artificial reproductive techniques. Currently, prenatal genetic testing is performed through amniocentesis, chorionic villi sampling, or fetal blood sampling during fetal gestation or through in vitro analysis of a preimplantation embryo. Other prenatal tests, such as ultrasonography or embryoscopy, provide anatomical information about the fetus that may lead to the detection of a genetic defect. Maternal serum α-fetoprotein screening can also aid in the identification of women at an elevated risk of having a child with neural tube defects, Down syndrome, or other genetic disorders. If a genetic defect is discovered, it generally cannot be corrected, and the parents can avoid the defect only by aborting the fetus or discarding the preimplantation embryo. In the future, other methods for prenatal genetic testing may develop, and it may be possible to correct genetic defects through manipulation.

As much as possible, this report concentrates on the ethical dimensions of existing prenatal testing practices. However, genetic technologies are developing at a rapid rate and will, in all likelihood, develop even faster as the Human Genome Project progresses. Many commentators recognize the possibility that increased understanding of the genetic component of human characteristics may one day make it possible to alter human traits through manipulations at the genetic level. Thus, in addition to examining current practices, this report also explores some of the possible future uses of current and emerging genetic technologies, particularly those that relate to genetic manipulation.

Editor's note: All footnotes have been deleted. Students who want to follow up on sources should consult the original article.

Prenatal genetic testing is still, in many ways, an emerging science. The Council's recommendations on future practices in prenatal genetic testing must be seen as only preliminary. As genetic technologies advance in the coming years, further consideration of the ethical application of those technologies will inevitably be warranted.

Current Abilities to Select or Manipulate for Genetic Disorders and Traits

When couples suspect they are at high risk for having a child with a genetic disease, they may respond to the risk in one of four ways. They may choose to not reproduce at all, to accept the risk and reproduce anyway, to undergo prenatal diagnosis for detectable disorders and possibly abort an affected fetus, or to reproduce with the aid of artificial reproductive technologies.

When artificial reproductive technologies are used, an affected child can be avoided in a number of ways. A couple may use artificial insemination or surrogacy to have a child who is biologically related to one parent but who would not inherit the undesired gene from the other parent. Couples may undergo in vitro fertilization or make use of other reproductive technologies in which the gametes or zygotes may be examined in vitro. Couples may then discard the gametes or zygotes that would result in a child with a genetic disorder.

Generally, the ability to detect a genetic abnormality precedes the ability to correct the abnormality. Consequently, when a fetus or a preimplantation embryo is found to have a genetic abnormality, abortion or discard may be the only means of avoiding the birth of an affected child. Selective abortion or discard refers to the abortion of a fetus or the discard of a preimplantation embryo with a genetic abnormality. Though some view selective discard of a preimplantation embryo as equivalent to abortion, some distinction between the two can be drawn, as discussed later in this report.

Currently, selective abortion or discard is used to control a number of genetic diseases, including Down syndrome and Tay-Sachs disease. The possibility of selecting for benign (i.e., non-disease-related) genetic traits is less advanced and is currently limited essentially to sex selection. Both prenatal testing during gestation and in vitro analysis of preimplantation embryos identify the sex of the fetus in most cases, thus creating the possibility of aborting fetuses of the undesired sex. In some cases, sex selection is performed to be able to avoid the birth of a male infant with an X-linked disorder. However, the ability to select for sex also allows for the possibility of doing so for nontherapeutic reasons.

Genetic manipulation, the alteration of genetic material through gene therapy or other means, is in the early stages of investigation. Gene therapy is the replacement or repair of an undesired gene with a desired gene and may prove to be a promising treatment for genetic disorders that result from a single gene defect. Gene therapy has been attempted with encouraging results for a few disorders, such as cystic fibrosis, adenosine deaminase deficiency, and advanced melanoma, it is also theoretically possible in preimplantation embryos. In addition, although resources have been focused on the diagnosis and cure of genetic diseases, genetic manipulation could potentially be used to alter benign genetic traits.

Fundamental Ethical Issues

Because physicians will play a critical part in the future application of reproductive genetic technology, it is important for the medical profession to define its role in the overall process. It is also important for the profession to consider the potential social effects of genetic technology when defining its role because genetic technology will have a major impact on all of society. Several broad ethical issues present themselves.

The Role of Parental Choice One underlying ethical issue is how to balance the rights of individuals to make choices about the health and characteristics of their children against the social values and needs that may be in conflict with individual preferences. Traditionally, parents have been given great (but not unlimited) latitude in making decisions regarding their children. In some cases, individuals may make choices for their children that others may regard as wrong but that are not prohibited because of the larger interest in preserving choice in general. The dilemma posed by new genetic technologies is the question of how far parents' authority over their children should extend and, in particular, how completely parents should be able to control the genetic composition of their children.

Abortion to Avoid Genetic Disorders A second issue is the appropriate role of abortion to avoid the birth of a child with a genetic disorder. Several genetic disorders can be detected in utero but cannot be treated or cured satisfactorily. Presently, the detection and elimination of genetic disorders generally relies on a combination of prenatal diagnosis and the abortion of an affected fetus. Many individuals, regardless of their views regarding abortion, consider prenatal diagnosis plus abortion a less than optimal solution to the problem of genetic disease.

Modifying the Human Genome Even if abortion or discard of preimplantation embryos is not used to avoid disease, many ethical questions remain about the use of genetic technologies to modify the genes of a fetus or a preimplantation embryo. Genetic manipulation introduces larger questions about the potential effects of genetic technologies on human relationships, questions that also exist with the abortion or discard of preimplantation embryos.

Uncertain Future Developments A final issue is the difficulty inherent in providing ethical guidelines for the use of a technology that is still in its rudimentary stages. The depth of information that will come out of the Human Genome Project is uncertain, as well as the extent to which it can be applied to select for and manipulate human genes. There is little direct empirical evidence to predict how genetic technology will be used, which complicates attempts to formulate ethical guidelines for its use.

DEFENSES OF THE USE OF PRENATAL TESTING AND GENETIC REPRODUCTIVE TECHNOLOGIES FOR SELECTION AND MANIPULATION

Reproductive Choice

The increased ability to understand the genetic causes of diseases and traits may enhance reproductive choice. Previously, many couples at high risk for having a child with a genetic disorder might have foregone reproduction due to the risks. In addition, high-risk couples who did conceive a child might have aborted the fetus because it was highly probable, although not certain, that the fetus was affected. Now, because of the increasing ability to test accurately for fetal genetic disorders, these high-risk couples may be willing to have children. The availability of prenatal genetic testing not only enhances the reproductive choices for high-risk couples but may also reduce the number of abortions to avoid disease and may increase the number of wanted children.

Reproductive choice may also be enhanced for couples who are not at high risk. For many women or couples, regardless of whether they have an increased risk of having a child with a genetic disease, the results of prenatal genetic testing could provide reassurance about the status of their current pregnancy. Furthermore, increasing abilities to select or manipulate for specific diseases or traits may expand parents' potential control over the health, appearance, or talents of the child.

Elimination of Disease

A primary goal of prenatal genetic testing and genetic manipulation is to increase the capacity to diagnose, treat, and eliminate disorders that are genetically caused. Of the 4000 known genetic disorders, many already can be detected through prenatal testing, and others may be identified through the analysis of preimplantation embryos. Genetically detectable disorders include Tay-Sachs disease, cystic fibrosis, pseudohypertrophic muscular dystrophy, Lesch-Nyhan syndrome, Down syndrome, and sickle cell anemia.

Although genetic disorders vary widely in their severity, some of the more severe involve substantial functional abnormality and early death. The affected child may be both severely disabled and subject to great physical or emotional suffering. In addition, caring for children with severe disorders is often psychologically draining on parents. Being able to avoid or effectively treat genetic disorders, perhaps through fetal therapy, would, of course, be highly desirable.

Early Detection

Early detection of genetic disorders gives parents the time to prepare for the birth of an affected child.

Advance knowledge of a child's genetic defect allows more time for educating parents about the disorder before the baby is born. Early detection, education, and preparation may help reduce any psychological trauma experienced by the parents at the time of the birth, promote maternal-fetal bonding, and positively influence the future relationship between the parents and their child. In addition, early detection gives parents time to make any financial and medical arrangements necessary to care for their child.

Improvement of Individuals

It may be possible to enhance a person's intellectual or physical abilities through genetic manipulation. Although such a use of genetic technologies would be highly problematic, some view it as a natural extension of nongenetic efforts to improve personal capacities. Society considers it acceptable to improve individual abilities through behavioral modification, instruction in the schools, and other approaches; genetic manipulation might be a more effective way to accomplish the same goals. In addition, it is argued that if it is permissible to use genetic technologies to improve intelligence by avoiding mental retardation, then it should be permissible to improve intelligence to achieve wisdom.

OBJECTIONS TO THE USE OF GENETIC REPRODUCTIVE TECHNOLOGIES FOR SELECTION AND MANIPULATION

The benefits of prenatal genetic testing, including the enhancement of reproductive autonomy, the elimination of genetic disease, and the early detection of genetic disorders, are widely recognized and accepted. The objections to some uses of prenatal genetic testing and other reproductive technologies, however, continue to create controversy and debate. In the following section, the merits and flaws of some of the more common objections are considered in detail.

Judicious Use of Societal Resources to Improve Health

Most objections or warnings against using reproductive genetic technology to improve overall health anticipate the misuse of genetic technology. However, apart from the issue of misuse, expenditures on new genetic technologies may be an inefficient use of scarce societal resources.

Currently, the use of genetic technology is expensive and is unlikely to become easily affordable in the foreseeable future. Justice requires that benefits and burdens be distributed fairly. Under the current system of access to genetic technology, the benefits primarily accrue to a relatively small number of people. It may not be justifiable to concentrate resources on a technology that will benefit few, at the expense of other projects that would provide a more general benefit to health. Although concerns over cost and inequitable access are likely to remain important considerations for the foreseeable future, these concerns may be mollified if information gained from the Human Genome Project leads to the development of inexpensive testing techniques and more affordable prenatal genetic testing.

Concern over the expense of developing and implementing reproductive technology becomes more serious, however, in light of the uncertainty regarding the possibility of ultimately curing or eradicating genetic disease. The development of genetic technology is likely to be time-consuming and may not result in optimal or even significant reduction of disease. Some disorders are likely to remain extremely difficult to treat or cure. It may not be appropriate to devote resources to speculative improvements in overall health when other solutions are known but lack sufficient resources.

Potential for Exacerbation of Discriminatory Practices

The potential misuse of genetic technology for discriminatory purposes comes from several sources. One is the misinterpretation of data, particularly if the misinterpreted results are used as a reason to punish individuals or eliminate them from the gene pool. For example, early investigation of males with XYY chromosomes seemed to show that they were more prone to criminal behavior than XY males. For several years, the public and some physicians eagerly embraced the idea that some violent behavior could be avoided by identifying males with XYY chromosomes and trying to alter their behavior. Eventually, the connection between XYY chromosomes and behavior was found to be too tenuous to justify screening programs or reeducation efforts.

A second potential source of discrimination is the use of genetic reproductive technologies to ensure that children possess certain characteristics that should be irrelevant in an egalitarian society. Sex selection is the most evident example of the discriminatory potential of selection for benign genetic traits. Despite the increasing social equality of men and women, even recent studies show a marked preference for male children in general and especially for male firstborn children. Sex selection is problematic because it implicitly fosters the value of one sex over the other, it confirms that sex is a governing factor in human behavior, and it treats gender, a genetic trait, as a disease. Sex selection might result in a significant disruption of usual social relationships, and discrimination and violence against women might increase. It may be true that not every instance of nontherapeutic sex selection would be sexist. Some sex selection may be motivated by a desire to have children of both sexes, each valued equally. Still, sex selection must be considered a dangerous practice both because of the possible negative social impact on the status of women and because of arbitrary and ethically unacceptable motivations.

Even when genetic reproductive technologies are used only to avoid genetic disease, they may still have some adverse discriminatory consequences. Selection on the basis of genetic disease could increase negative attitudes toward the disabled in a manner similar to attitudes toward women under sex selection. The number of disabled individuals may decrease to levels at which the needs of those remaining are not given attention or sufficient priority in resource allocation. Some commentators have observed that the active elimination of all genetic disorders from populations sends a profoundly devaluing message to individuals who have the diseases that are being eliminated. It may be difficult to maintain a general social structure in which people are valued on an individual basis for their potential and achievements while some people have disorders that are being eradicated from the gene pool. Also, the range of general diversity of genetic characteristics may be limited to the critical point at which the appreciation of similarity overpowers the appreciation of differences and fuels further discrimination.

Eugenics

Many discussions about the future of genetic technologies include consideration of human eugenics, the improvement of hereditary qualities or traits through genetic selection and manipulation. The immediate concern for most is not that the advancement of genetic technology would necessarily lead to compulsory eugenic programs, although some fear that may be an ultimate result. Rather, most fear a subtle or passive eugenics brought about through a combination of social pressures. These social pressures could include disapproval of or blame for parents who have an affected child or who fail to maximize their child's genetic capacities. In addition, lack of social and economic support for the disabled might dissuade parents who would otherwise bear and raise an affected child from choosing to reproduce.

Despite common perceptions to the contrary, new reproductive technology may not enhance the voluntariness of reproductive choices. Even without formal coercion to participate in selection technology or to make particular choices, other influences and pressures can make some options more difficult to choose than others. For instance, in one study, a significant percentage of women (15%) said they felt an obligation to consent to prenatal testing; they did not feel they were undergoing testing completely voluntarily. In addition, the majority of women (75% to 97%) said it was difficult to turn down the option of prenatal testing once it was offered, leading the conductors of the study to hypothesize that the women's autonomy was limited despite formal voluntariness. Such findings raise important concerns about the voluntariness of decisions to undergo prenatal testing, despite the fact that women who do have testing usually judge it to be a positive experience overall.

Decisions based on the results of testing may also be affected by outside pressures. For instance, although a couple may not believe in genetic manipulation or abortion and therefore may prefer to raise a child with a genetic disability, societal, familial, and peer pressure may deter them from exercising their own preferences. The development and availability of genetic technology may increase a parent's feelings of guilt or responsibility for bearing an affected child. Some commentators have suggested that parents should not be allowed to attempt reproduction if there is a risk of genetic disease in their offspring and that the parents be held liable if they do produce a child with a genetic disorder.

With existing genetic reproductive technologies, it is already true that decisions about life and an individual's worth are made on the basis of genetic factors. This may constitute an extremely dilute but acceptable form of eugenic selection. However, even this limited selection, usually based on eliminating the most severe genetic diseases, makes many individuals uncomfortable. This discomfort probably reflects the belief that eugenics is inherently an unacceptable philosophy, even if pursued voluntarily. Some fear that genetic selection and manipulation may set us on a slippery slope in which genetic intervention, once begun, would eventually lead to the alteration of humanity itself through the maximization of select genetic traits. Given the lack of empirical evidence concerning how people would deal with advancing genetic technologies, it is difficult to evaluate such speculations. Still, the fact that present practices can be seen as precursors to more extreme scenarios indicates that the possibility of voluntary or passive eugenics should be included in evaluations of genetic reproductive technology.

There is also the prospect of a more limited eugenic tendency based on class or cultural factors. If access to genetic technologies is dependent on individual wealth, then the more well-off financially could also become the more healthy overall. Also, individuals from different cultural backgrounds, regardless of economic class, have different definitions of health, sickness, and treatment. Some cultural groups may not consider the genetic origins of disease to be important. Concern has been expressed that certain classes or groups may be excluded from the health benefits accruing to others, relegated to the fringes of society, and consequently made more vulnerable to elimination through eugenics.

Treating Children as Products: A Consumeristic View of Reproduction

In general, children are regarded and valued as autonomous beings, subject to the limitations of their particular developmental and cognitive capacities. Wide leeway is given to parents concerning child raising because it is believed that they are in the best position to assess and act on the needs and best interests of their child. However, parental control is subject to limitations. Children are legally subject to parental authority only until the age of majority, children must be given an education, and the state can intervene to protect children in a variety of situations. For instance, a parent cannot refuse a lifesaving cure or intervention for a child based on the parent's own religious beliefs (*Prince v Massachusetts,* 321 US 158 [1944]; *Hoener v Bertinato,* 171 A2d 140 [1961]).

New genetic technologies suggest the possibility that parents will one day be able to control many aspects of their child's genetic makeup. If parents use genetic technologies to affect benign traits, such as sex or height, it is not clear that they are acting in the best interests of their future child. Although it is reasonable to assume that children would prefer to be free of disease, persons' preferences concerning benign traits or characteristics will depend on their own particular values. Consequently, decisions about traits or characteristics may not always be best left to parents.

A further consequence of using genetic technologies to enhance benign traits is that it may dehumanize the reproductive process by treating fetuses as products rather than as potentially autonomous human beings. Subjecting a child's core physical appearance and potential talents to the whims of his or her parents impinges on the child's ability to develop an autonomous self. Allowing parents to manipulate a child's most basic characteristics fosters a consumeristic attitude toward a child's development and personality.

ROLE OF MEDICINE IN THE APPLICATION OF REPRODUCTIVE GENETIC TECHNOLOGIES

Although reproductive genetic technologies have many legitimate medical uses, participation in some aspects of genetic technologies for selection and manipulation is antithetical to the professional role of the physician as caregiver and provider of therapeutic benefit. In addition to undermining the physician's traditional role, participation in these inappropriate practices can also lead to social harm, primarily in the form of discrimination based on gender or other characteristics.

Definition of the Physician's Role

The provision of therapeutic benefit lies at the core of the physician's professional role. Although the physician typically may perform auxiliary functions during the course of the physician-patient relationship, these functions are secondary to the primary goal of preventing or treating disease. It is the presence of or potential for a disease state that generates this relationship. It is specifically in response to the illness that the physician reacts, striving to reduce harm and suffering while also trying to restore the patient to a state of both psychological and physiological health. Technology often serves as the physician's assistant in performing the central aspects of the professional role, providing medical benefit.

In recent years, there has been a broadening of the physician's professional role with greater recognition of the factors that can affect a person's sense of well-being. For example, physicians employ cosmetic surgery to improve a person's psychological health. As the physician's role extends beyond the traditional concepts of disease, great care must be taken to ensure that the practice of medicine is not misused.

Prenatal Testing and Selective Abortion or Discard

Given the therapeutic focus of the physician's role, it is inappropriate for physicians to participate in non-medical uses of the information gleaned from prenatal testing. The use of genetic technology to avoid the birth of a child with a genetic disorder is in accordance with the ethical principles associated with the physician's therapeutic role. However, abortion or discard based on non-disease-related traits would be inappropriate. Selective practices, such as sex selection, may result in lasting social harms, such as the exacerbation of discrimination, a tendency to view children as products, and eugenics. Recognizing the potential for social harms, the President's Commission for the Study of Ethical Problems in Medicine and Biomedical and Behavioral Research strongly discouraged the use of prenatal testing for sex selection, stressing the need to confine such testing to "seeking genetic information in order to correct or avoid unambiguous disabilities or to improve the well-being of the fetus.

Selection to avoid genetic disorders would not always be appropriate. Abortion because of genetic disease is most understandable when the disease would have serious manifestations, such as with Tay-Sachs disease or Huntington's chorea. Conversely, selection becomes more problematic as the effects of the disease become milder and as they become manifest later in life. For example, the justification for abortion would be weaker if the purpose is to avoid a disorder that does not prevent a full lifespan and for which medical therapy can achieve good control of the complications until late in life. It is not possible to indicate precisely when a disease would not be serious enough to justify the abortion of a fetus or discard of a preimplantation embryo. Any such situations are only hypothetical at this time, and other factors would affect the acceptability of selection. For instance, over the next several years, it may become possible to make prenatal genetic diagnoses earlier during gestation (*New York Times*. September 24, 1992:A1, B10).Just as the justification for abortion weakens as the disease to be avoided becomes milder, the objection to abortion becomes weaker the earlier during the pregnancy that it occurs. Discard at the preimplantation embryo stage of development is less problematic than abortion after viability. In deciding whether selection is acceptable, a number of factors need to be considered: the severity of the disease, the probability of its occurrence, the age at onset, and the time of gestation at which selection would occur.

The potential use of prenatal testing to select for benign traits or milder disorders urges caution to physicians practicing in that area. In counseling women or couples about prenatal testing, physicians should discuss the ethical issues involved and indicate when and for what purposes it is appropriate to employ prenatal testing. Physicians should make clear to patients their opposition to abortion or discard based on benign traits and discourage testing of fetuses when it is clear that inappropriate selection is the sole motive for the testing request.

There are limits to how far physicians' counseling efforts can go in discouraging inappropriate selection. Physicians cannot always be certain about parents' motives, and excessive second-guessing of parents' wishes could jeopardize the trust so crucial to the physician-patient relationship. Physicians' efforts alone cannot ensure that inappropriate selection will never take place. Rather, prevention of inappropriate selection ultimately depends on societal educative efforts that promote the appreciation of genetic diversity as an important component of egalitarian ideals.

Some observers believe that aside from misuse of prenatal diagnostic findings, overuse of prenatal genetic testing presents dangers of its own. Reasons include the possible risks to the fetus from invasive testing techniques, a reduction in women's reproductive freedom as a result of increased professional or societal management of pregnancies, and the imposition of unwarranted levels of stress and anxiety on pregnant women who do not have an elevated risk of passing on a genetic disorder. This stress can arise from the testing procedure itself, from the information revealed about the fetus, from a fear of false-negative results, and from other sources. Because of this anxiety and the risk to the fetus, prenatal testing may not be desirable in cases involving couples whose medical histories and family backgrounds do not indicate an elevated risk of fetal genetic disorders. The physician should inform such couples of their statistical probability of having an affected fetus and warn them of the chances of damage to the fetus or of miscarriage. Women or couples without an elevated risk of genetic disease can legitimately request prenatal testing, provided they understand and accept the risks involved.

If prenatal testing is performed, the principle of patient autonomy requires that all medically relevant information that is generated from fetal tests be passed along to the parent(s), with appropriate counseling, so that the parent(s) can make informed decisions about the pregnancy. Although the physician should generally discourage requests for information about benign genetic traits, the physician may not ethically refuse to pass along any requested information in his or her possession. Some may argue that prenatal diagnosis involves a duty to promote the welfare of the fetus as well as to provide choice-enhancing information to the parent(s). In light of this duty to the fetus, it is argued that information that is not relevant to the health of the fetus, such as its gender, may be withheld from the parent(s). The perception that the fetus must be protected from the parent(s) is prompted by a concern that the information divulged will be abused (e.g., parents will wish to know the gender of the fetus to engage in inappropriate sex selection). However, the solution to the problem of potential abuse is not to withhold information that parents may have good reasons for wanting to know. Rather, as noted earlier, strong educational efforts are needed to promote appreciation of genetic diversity and gender equality.

Furthermore, while the interests of both the parent(s) and the fetus are important, it is the parent(s) who actively seeks prenatal testing as part of prenatal care. It is the parent(s) who must weigh the risks and benefits not only of testing but also of any future interventions on behalf of the fetus. Therefore, the parent(s) must be considered the primary patient. Accordingly, the final decision as to what information is deemed appropriate for disclosure can only fall to the parent(s), informed by the facts and recommendations presented to their physician.

Genetic Manipulation

At the present time, selection through abortion or discard of preimplantation embryos is the only way to avoid the effects or an undesired gene that has been detected through prenatal testing. In the future, however, genetic manipulation may allow the correction of an undesired gene without the need for abortion or discard.

Treatment of Genetic Disease The use of genetic manipulation to avoid disease is consistent with ethical principles. The tools of medicine are designed to prevent functional abnormalities, such as occur in Tay-Sachs disease, Down syndrome, or cystic fibrosis, and the fact that genetics are used rather than surgery or antibiotics does not make the treatment unacceptable. Genetic manipulation in this instance would be a legitimate extension of the physician's preexisting and fundamental duty to combat disease.

Debate continues over whether only somatic-cell gene therapy should be used to combat disease or whether germline therapy could also be used. In somatic-cell therapy, genetic alterations affect only the fetus at hand; in germline therapy, alterations would be inherited by the fetus' future off-spring as well. At least two reasons initially suggest that genetic manipulation should be limited to somatic cells only. First, the profound impact of germline manipulations on future generations requires that we proceed with extreme caution. Until the effects of a genetic manipulation, both long- and short-term, are certain, germline manipulations should not be attempted. Second, germline manipulations give parents unprecedented control over the lives of multiple generations of descendants. Such far-reaching control could potentially curtail the autonomy of future generations. One view holds that there is a moral obligation to refrain from tampering with mankind's "collective genetic heritage, whose unique worth is above any individual interest" and that therefore germline interventions should be prohibited. At the very least, germline interventions would impose on future generations a previous generation's conception of health, which may not turn out to be the best conception in light of future conditions and adaptive requirements.

Limits on germline manipulations also follow from existing societal practices that limit parents' abilities to extend their authority beyond their own immediate offspring. In property law, for instance, individuals are prevented from dictating the fate of their estate in perpetuity. If society has an interest in protecting future generations' autonomy in property matters, it may very well have an even stronger interest in protecting that autonomy in matters of genetic control over offspring. Initially, then, it would seem appropriate to limit genetic intervention to somatic cells only, although further consideration of this issue may be advisable in the future.

There may be exceptional situations in which genetic manipulation would not be appropriate to treat or cure disease, such as when the manipulation might damage or interfere with other genes, with deleterious effects. At some point, the potential adverse effects would be so serious that it would no longer be appropriate to assume that the future child would prefer the intervention.

Manipulation of Benign Traits When genetic technology would be used to change characteristics that are not disease causing, the dangers of abuse discussed in this report require that extreme caution be exercised. In general, it would not be appropriate to use genetic technology to manipulate the traits or characteristics of a fetus or a preimplantation embryo. Such manipulation risks the severe adverse consequences discussed earlier: the exacerbation of discriminatory practices, the treatment of children as commodities, and the prospects of repugnant eugenic practices. These considerations counsel against genetic manipulation of benign characteristics.

Nevertheless, there may be some very exceptional circumstances in which generic manipulation would be reasonable. Society already employs a number of strategies to improve the abilities or characteristics of its citizens. For example, the education system generally aims at improving the lives of citizens by making them more intelligent and more socially responsible. Parental choices of schools and extracurricular activities are often designed to maximize the capacities and life chances of their children. Individual self-improvement of all kinds is generally viewed as both laudable and one of the distinguishing capacities of human beings. These considerations suggest that under certain circumstances, genetic manipulation could be justified as an extension of the continuing efforts of society, parents, and individuals to enhance the capacities and improve the lives of citizens.

Because they are still speculative, it is difficult to say whether genetic manipulations can be justified as extensions of current practices. Until more is known, a total ban on manipulation would be premature. However, because of the potentially grave dangers and drawbacks of manipulation, genetic interventions to enhance traits should be considered permissible only in severely restricted situations. The kinds of criteria that would have to be satisfied include the following.

First, there would have to be a clear and meaningful benefit to the fetus or the child who will be born. This criterion would ensure that parents do not impose their own idiosyncratic values on their children but only engage in genetic manipulation when there would be an important improvement for the child.

Second, there could be no trade-off with other characteristics or traits. A genetic manipulation would be permissible only if the benefit could be gained without a change in some other characteristic or trait. Whether a gain in one area is worth a loss in another area is a choice that depends on subjective values. Consequently, only the individual who would experience the consequences of the trade-off should be able to decide whether the trade-off should be made. There also would have to be clear evidence that no trade-off will occur. It would not be sufficient to show merely that no trade-off was known because adverse effects often are unanticipated. Instead, the mechanisms of genetic manipulation would have to be understood in enough detail to ensure certainty that trade-offs would not occur.

Third, there would have to be equal access to genetic technologies, irrespective of income or other socioeconomic characteristics. If access depended on wealth, social divisions would widen, and the promise of equal opportunity for all citizens would quickly become an illusion.

These potential criteria should be viewed as a minimal, not an exhaustive, test of the ethical propriety of non–disease-related genetic intervention. As genetic technology and knowledge of the human genome develop further, additional restrictions or guidelines may be required.

CONCLUSIONS

Currently, prenatal genetic testing is available for serious disorders like Tay-Sachs disease, Down syndrome, and cystic fibrosis. In the future, genetic testing may become available for milder genetic disorders. As the ability to test for genetic disorders increases, the possibility of genetic selection will also increase. It is not possible to give precise guidelines on when selection would be ethically acceptable. Many situations in which selection would be possible are only hypothetical at this time, and other factors would affect the acceptability of selection. Nevertheless, it is important to begin discussion of the issue now to ensure that appropriate ethical guidelines are in place when new applications become available.

Physicians should promote informed reproductive choices by counseling prospective parents on the availability and the role of prenatal genetic testing. Counseling should include discussion of the reasons for and against testing as well as discussion of the inappropriate uses of genetic testing. Prenatal genetic testing is most appropriate for women or couples whose medical histories or family backgrounds indicate an elevated risk of fetal genetic disorders. Physicians should inform women or couples without an elevated risk of the reasons why prenatal diagnosis may not be desirable in their case. Women or couples without an elevated risk of genetic disease can legitimately request prenatal diagnosis, provided they understand and accept the risks involved.

In general, it would be ethically permissible for physicians to participate in genetic selection to prevent, cure, or treat genetic disease. Selection to avoid genetic disease would not always be appropriate. In some cases, the disease would have such mild manifestations that prenatal selection would not be justified. In deciding whether genetic selection is acceptable, a number of factors need to be considered: the severity of the disease, the probability of its occurrence, the age at onset, and the time of gestation at which selection would occur. It would not be ethical to engage in selection on the basis of non–disease-causing characteristics or traits.

As genetic understanding and technology continue to develop, prenatal manipulation of genetic material may become possible. In general, it would be ethically acceptable for physicians to participate in the manipulation of genetic material to prevent, cure, or treat genetic disease. There might be exceptional situations in which genetic manipulation would not be appropriate to treat or cure disease, such as when manipulation would cause serious adverse side effects.

Manipulation of genetic material to alter benign characteristics or traits should be approached with extreme reservation. In general, such manipulation is inappropriate, and its use should be strongly discouraged. There may be exceptional circumstances in which genetic manipulation to alter traits or characteristics would be acceptable. At a minimum, three criteria would have to be satisfied: there would have to be a clear and meaningful benefit to the child; there could be no trade-off with other characteristics or traits; and all citizens would have to have equal access to the genetic technology, irrespective of income or other socioeconomic characteristics.

Currently, when prenatal genetic testing is performed for Down syndrome or other disorders, the sex of the fetus is an incidental finding. In the future, prenatal genetic testing may yield other, more varied, incidental findings. If that occurs, incidental findings relative to the health of the fetus should be given to the parents. Whether incidental findings related to genetic characteristics should be released is a more complicated issue and would depend on whether it would be acceptable to engage in genetic manipulation of the characteristics. If it would be permissible to manipulate the characteristics, the incidental findings should be released to allow the parents to decide whether to seek manipulation. No information should be withheld when requested, but it may be appropriate to discuss with parents their motivation for wanting to know the child's characteristics.

The ability to treat genetic diseases through prenatal genetic manipulation should not divert attention from efforts to find postnatal treatment or cures for those diseases.

PRENATAL DIAGNOSIS AND SELECTIVE ABORTION: A CHALLENGE TO PRACTICE AND POLICY

Adrienne Asch

Although sex selection might ameliorate the situation of some individuals, it lowers the status of women in general and only perpetuates the situation that gave rise to it. . . . If we believe that sexual equality is necessary for a just society, then we should oppose sex selection.

Wertz and Fletcher[1(pp242–243)]

The very motivation for seeking an "origin" of homosexuality reveals homophobia. Moreover, such research may lead to prenatal tests that claim to predict for homosexuality. For homosexual people who live in countries with no legal protections these dangers are particularly serious.

Schuklenk et al.[2(p6)]

The tenor of the preceding statements may spark relatively little comment in the world of health policy, the medical profession, or the readers of this journal, because many recognize the dangers of using the technology of prenatal testing followed by selective abortion for the characteristic of fetal sex. Similarly, the medical and psychiatric professions, and the world of public health, have aided in the civil rights struggle of gays and lesbians by insisting that homosexuality is not a disease. Consequently, many readers would concur with those who question the motives behind searching for the causes of homosexuality that might lead scientists to develop a prenatal test for that characteristic. Many in our society, however, have no such misgivings about prenatal testing for characteristics regarded as genetic or chromosomal diseases, abnormalities, or disabilities:

> Attitudes toward congenital disability per se have not changed markedly. Both premodern as well as contemporary societies have regarded disability as undesirable and to be avoided. Not only have parents recognized the birth of a disabled child as a potentially

---

Editor's note: Many footnotes have been deleted. Students who want to follow up on sources should consult the original article.

Reprinted with permission of the author and publisher from *American Journal of Public Health* 89, no. 11 (November 1999): 1649–1657.

> divisive, destructive force in the family unit, but the larger society has seen disability as unfortunate (p 89). . . . Our society still does not countenance the elimination of diseased/disabled people; but it does urge the termination of diseased/disabled fetuses. The urging is not explicit, but implicit (p 90).[3]

Writing in the *American Journal of Human Genetics* about screening programs for cystic fibrosis, A. L. Beaudet acknowledged the tension between the goals of enhancing reproductive choice and preventing the births of children who would have disabilities:

> Although some would argue that the success of the program should be judged solely by the effectiveness of the educational programs (i.e., whether screenees understood the information), it is clear that prevention of [cystic fibrosis] is also, at some level, a measure of a screening program, since few would advocate expanding the substantial resources involved if very few families wish to avoid the disease.[4(p603)]

Prenatal tests designed to detect the condition of the fetus include ultrasound, maternal serum α-fetoprotein screening, chorionic villus sampling, and amniocentesis. Some (ultrasound screenings) are routinely performed regardless of the mother's age and provide information that she may use to guide her care throughout pregnancy; others, such as chorionic villus sampling or amniocentesis, do not influence the woman's care during pregnancy but provide information intended to help her decide whether to continue the pregnancy if fetal impairment is detected. Amniocentesis, the test that detects the greatest variety of fetal impairments, is typically offered to women who will be 35 years or older at the time they are due to deliver, but recently commentators have urged that the age threshold be removed and that the test be available to women regardless of age. Such testing is increasingly considered a standard component of prenatal care for women whose insurance covers these procedures, including women using publicly financed clinics in some jurisdictions.

These tests, which are widely accepted in the field of bioethics and by clinicians, public health professionals, and the general public, have nonetheless occasioned some apprehension and concern among students of women's reproductive experiences, who find that women do not uniformly welcome the expectation that they will undergo prenatal testing or the prospect of making decisions depending on the test results. Less often discussed by clinicians is the view, expressed by a growing number of individuals, that the technology is itself based on erroneous assumptions about the adverse impact of disability on life. Argument from this perspective focuses on what is communicated about societal and familial acceptance of diversity in general and disability in particular. Like other women-centered critiques of prenatal testing, this article assumes a pro-choice perspective but suggests that unreflective uses of testing could diminish, rather than expand, women's choices. Like critiques stemming from concerns about the continued acceptance of human differences within the society and the family, this critique challenges the view of disability that lies behind social endorsement of such testing and the conviction that women will, or should, end their pregnancies if they discover that the fetus has a disabling trait.

If public health frowns on efforts to select for or against girls or boys and would oppose future efforts to select for or against those who would have a particular sexual orientation, but promotes people's efforts to avoid having children who would have disabilities, it is because medicine and public health view disability as extremely different from and worse than these other forms of human variation. At first blush this view may strike one as self-evident. To challenge it might even appear to be questioning our professional mission. Characteristics such as chronic illnesses and disabilities (discussed together throughout this article) do not resemble traits such as sex, sexual orientation, or race, because the latter are not in themselves perceived as inimical to a rewarding life. Disability is thought to be just that—to be incompatible with life satisfaction. When public health considers matters of sex, sexual orientation, or race, it examines how factors in social and economic life pose obstacles to health and to health care, and it champions actions to improve the well-being of those disadvantaged by the discrimination that attends minority status. By contrast, public health fights to eradicate disease and disability or to treat, ameliorate, or cure these when they occur. For medicine and public health, disease and disability is the problem to solve, and so it appears natural to use prenatal testing and abortion as one more means of minimizing the incidence of disability.

In the remainder of this article I argue, first, that most of the problems associated with having a disability stem from discriminatory social arrangements that are changeable, just as much of what has in the past made the lives of women or gays difficult has been the set of social arrangements they have faced (and which they have begun to dismantle). After discussing ways in which the characteristic of disability resembles and differs from other characteristics, I discuss why I believe the technology of prenatal testing followed by selective abortion is unique among means of preventing or ameliorating disability, and why it offends many people who are untroubled by other disease prevention and health promotion activities. I conclude by recommending ways in which health practitioners and policymakers could offer this technology so that it promotes genuine reproductive choice and helps families and society to flourish.

CONTRASTING MEDICAL AND SOCIAL PARADIGMS OF DISABILITY

The definitions of terms such as "health," "normality," and "disability" are not clear, objective, and universal across time and place. Individual physical characteristics are evaluated with reference to a standard of normality, health, and what some commentators term "species-typical functioning." These commentators point out that within a society at a particular time, there is a shared perception of what is typical physical functioning and role performance for a girl or boy, woman or man. Boorse's definition of an undesirable departure from species-typicality focuses on the functioning of the person rather than the cause of the problem: "[A] condition of a part or process in an organism is pathological when the ability of the part or process to perform one or more of its species-typical biological functions falls below some central range of the statistical distribution for that ability."[5(p370)] Daniels writes, "Impairments of normal species functioning reduce the range of opportunity open to the individual in which he may construct his plan of life or conception of the good."[6 (p27)]

Chronic illness, traumatic injury, and congenital disability may indeed occasion departures from "species-typical functioning," and thus these conditions do constitute differences from both a statistical average and a desired norm of well-being. Certainly society prizes some characteristics, such as intelligence, athleticism, and musical or artistic skill, and rewards people with more than the statistical norm of these attributes; I will return to this point later. Norms on many health-related attributes change over time; as the life span for people in the United States and Canada increases, conditions that often lead to death before 40 years of age (e.g., cystic fibrosis) may become even more dreaded than they are today. The expectation that males will be taller than females and that adults will stand more than 5 feet in height leads to a perception that departures from these norms are not only unusual but undesirable and unhealthy. Not surprisingly, professionals who have committed themselves to preventing illness and injury or to ameliorating and curing people of illnesses and injuries, are especially attuned to the problems and hardships that affect the lives of their patients. Such professionals, aware of the physical pain or weakness and the psychological and social disruption caused by acute illness or sudden injury, devote their lives to easing the problems that these events impose.

What many scholars, policymakers, and activists in the area of disability contend is that medically oriented understandings of the impact of disability on life contain 2 erroneous assumptions with serious adverse consequences: first, that the life of a person with a chronic illness or disability is forever disrupted, as one's life might be temporarily disrupted as a result of a back spasm, an episode of pneumonia, or a broken leg; second, that if a disabled person experiences isolation, powerlessness, unemployment, poverty, or low social status, these are inevitable consequences of biological limitation. Body, psyche, and social life do change immediately following an occurrence of disease, accident, or injury, and medicine, public health, and bioethics all correctly appreciate the psychological and physical vulnerability of patients and their families and friends during immediate medical crises. These professions fail people with disabilities, however, by concluding that because there may never be full physical recovery there is never a regrouping of physical, cognitive, and psychological resources with which to participate in a rewarding life.

Chronic illness and disability are not equivalent to acute illness or sudden injury, in which an active disease process or unexpected change in physical function disrupts life's routines. Most people with conditions such as spina bifida, achondroplasia, Down syndrome, and many other mobility and sensory impairments perceive themselves as healthy, not sick, and describe their conditions as givens of their lives—the equipment with which they meet the world. The same is true for people with chronic conditions such as cystic fibrosis, diabetes, hemophilia, and muscular dystrophy. These conditions include intermittent flare-ups requiring medical care and adjustments in daily living, but they do not render the person as unhealthy as most of the public—and members of the health profession—imagine. . . .

The second way in which medicine, bioethics, and public health typically err is in viewing all problems that occur to people with disabilities as attributable to the condition itself, rather than to external factors. When ethicists, public health professionals, and policymakers discuss the importance of health care, urge accident prevention, or promote healthy lifestyles, they do so because they perceive a certain level of health not only as intrinsically desirable but as a prerequisite for an acceptable life. One commentator describes such a consensual view of types of life in terms of a "normal opportunity range": "The normal opportunity range for a given society is the array of life plans reasonable persons in it are likely to construct for themselves.[6(p33)] Health care includes that which is intended to "maintain, restore, or provide functional equivalents where possible, to normal species functioning.[6(p32)]

The paradigm of medicine concludes that the gaps in education, employment, and income that persist between adults with disabilities and those without disabilities are inevitable because the impairment precludes study or limits work. The alternative paradigm, which views people with disabilities in social, minority-group terms, examines how societal arrangements—rules, laws, means of communication, characteristics of buildings and transit systems, the typical 8-hour workday—exclude some people from participating in school, work, civic, or social life. This newer paradigm is expressed by enactment of the Individuals with Disabilities Education Act and the Americans with Disabilities Act and is behind the drive to ensure that employed disabled people will keep their access to health care through Medicaid or Medicare. This paradigm—still more accepted by people outside medicine, public health, and bioethics than by those within these fields—questions whether there is an inevitable, unmodifiable gap between people with disabilities and people without disabilities. Learning that in 1999, nine years after the passage of laws to end employment discrimination, millions of people with disabilities are still out of the work force, despite their readiness to work[7]; the social paradigm asks what remaining institutional factors bar people from the goal of productive work. Ethical and policy questions arise in regard to the connection that does or should exist between health and the range of opportunities open to people in the population. . . .

The Americans with Disabilities Act, signed into law in 1990, is a ringing indictment of the nation's history with regard to people with disabilities:

> Congress finds that . . . (3) discrimination against individuals with disabilities persists in such critical areas as employment, . . . education, recreation, . . . health services, ... and access to public services; (7) individuals with disabilities are a discrete and insular minority who have been faced with restrictions and limitations, subjected to a history of purposeful unequal treatment, and relegated to a position of political powerlessness in our society, based on characteristics that are beyond the control of such individuals and resulting from stereotypic assumptions not truly indicative of the individual ability of such individuals to participate in, and contribute to, society.[8]

Eight years after the passage of the Americans with Disabilities Act, disabled people reported some improvements in access to public facilities and that things are getting better in some areas of life, but major gaps between the disabled and the nondisabled still exist in income, employment, and social participation. To dramatically underscore the prevalence of social stigma and discrimination: "fewer than half (45%) of adults with disabilities say that people generally treat them as an equal after they learn they have a disability."[7]

It is estimated that 54 million people in the United States have disabilities, of which impairments of mobility, hearing, vision, and learning; arthritis; cystic fibrosis; diabetes; heart conditions; and back problems are some of the most well-known.[7] Thus, in discussing discrimination, stigma, and unequal treatment for people with disabilities, we are considering a population that is larger than the known gay and lesbian population or the African American population. These numbers take on new significance when we assess the rationale behind prenatal diagnosis and selective abortion as a desirable strategy to deal with disability.

Prenatal Diagnosis for Disability Prevention

If some forms of disability prevention are legitimate medical and public health activities, and if people with disabilities use the health system to improve and maintain their own health, there is an acknowledgment that the characteristic of disability may not be desirable. Although many within the disability rights movement challenge prenatal diagnosis as a means of disability prevention, no one objects to public health efforts to clean up the environment, encourage seat-belt use, reduce tobacco and alcohol consumption, and provide prenatal care to all pregnant women. All these activities deal with the health of existing human beings (or fetuses expected to come to term) and seek to ensure their well-being. What differentiates prenatal testing followed by abortion from other forms of disability prevention and medical treatment is that prenatal testing followed by abortion is intended not to prevent the disability or illness of a born or future human being but to prevent the birth of a human being who will have one of these undesired characteristics. In reminding proponents of the Human Genome Project that gene therapy will not soon be able to cure disability, James Watson declared,

> [W]e place most of our hopes for genetics on the use of antenatal diagnostic procedures, which increasingly will let us know whether a fetus is carrying a mutant gene that will seriously proscribe its eventual development into a functional human being. By terminating such pregnancies, the threat of horrific disease genes contributing to blight many family's prospects for future success can be erased. [9(p19)]

But Watson errs in assuming that tragedy is inevitable for the child or for the family. When physicians, public health experts, and bioethicists promote prenatal diagnosis to prevent future disability, they let disability become the only relevant characteristic and suggest that it is such a problematic characteristic that people eagerly awaiting a new baby should terminate the pregnancy and "try again" for a healthy child. Professionals fail to recognize that along with whatever impairment may be diagnosed come all the characteristics of any other future child. The health professions suggest that once a prospective parent knows of the likely disability of a future child, there is nothing else to know or imagine about who the child might become: disability subverts parental dreams.

The focus of my concern here is not on the decision made by the pregnant woman or by the woman and her partner. I focus on the view of life with disability that is communicated by society's efforts to develop prenatal testing and urge it on every pregnant woman. If public health espouses goals of social justice and equality for people with disabilities, as it has worked to improve the status of women, gays and lesbians, and members of racial and ethnic minorities, it should reconsider whether it wishes to continue endorsing the technology of prenatal diagnosis. If there is an unshakable commitment to the technology in the name of reproductive choice, public health should work with practitioners to change the way in which information about impairments detected in the fetus is delivered.

Rationales for Prenatal Testing

The medical professions justify prenatal diagnosis and selective abortion on the grounds of the *costs* of childhood disability—the costs to the child, to the family, and to the society. Some proponents of the Human Genome Project from the fields of science and bioethics argue that in a world of limited resources, we can reduce disability-related expenditures if all diagnoses of fetal impairment are followed by abortion.

On both empirical and moral grounds, endorsing prenatal diagnosis for societal reasons is dangerous. Only a small fraction of total disability can now be detected prenatally, and even if future technology enables the detection of predisposition to diabetes, forms of depression, Alzheimer [*sic*] disease, heart disease, arthritis, or back problems—all more prevalent in the population than many of the currently detectable conditions—we will never manage to detect and prevent most disability. Rates of disability increase markedly with age, and the gains in life span guarantee that most people will deal with disability in themselves or someone close to them. Laws and services to support people with disabilities will still be necessary, unless society chooses a campaign of eliminating disabled people in addition to preventing the births of those who would be disabled. Thus, there is small cost-saving in money or in human resources to be achieved by even the vigorous determination to test every pregnant woman and abort every fetus found to exhibit disabling traits.

My moral opposition to prenatal testing and selective abortion flows from the conviction that life with disability is worthwhile and the belief that a just society must appreciate and nurture the lives of all people, whatever the endowments they receive in the natural lottery. I hold these beliefs because—as I show throughout this article—there is abundant evidence that people with disabilities can thrive even in this less than welcoming society. Moreover, people with disabilities do not merely take from others, they contribute as well—to families, to friends, to the economy. They contribute neither in spite of nor because of their disabilities, but because along with their disabilities come other characteristics of personality, talent, and humanity that render people with disabilities full members of the human and moral community.

IMPLICATIONS FOR PEOPLE WITH DISABILITIES

Implications for children and adults with disabilities, and for their families, warrant more consideration. Several prominent bioethicists claim that to knowingly bring into the world a child who will live with an impairment (whether it be a "withered arm," cystic fibrosis, deafness, or Down syndrome) is unfair to the child because it deprives the child of the "right to an open future" by limiting some options. Green's words represent a significant strand of professional thinking: "In the absence of adequate justifying reasons, a child is morally wronged when he/she is knowingly, deliberately, or negligently brought into being with a health status likely to result in significantly greater disability or suffering, or significantly reduced life options relative to the other children with whom he/she will grow up."[10(p10)] Green is not alone in his view that it is irresponsible to bring a child into the world with a disability.

The biology of disability can affect people's lives, and not every feature of life with a disability is socially determined or medicated. People with cystic fibrosis cannot now expect to live to age 70. People with type 1 diabetes can expect to have to use insulin and to have to think carefully and continuously about what and how much they eat and about their rest and exercise, perhaps more than typical sedentary people who are casual about the nutritional content of their food. People who use a wheelchair for mobility will not climb mountains; people with the intellectual disabilities of Down syndrome or fragile X chromosome are not likely to read this article and engage in debate about its merits and shortcomings. Yet, as disability scholars point out, such limitations do not preclude a whole class of experiences, but only certain instances in which these experiences might occur. People who move through the world in wheelchairs may not be able to climb mountains, but they can and do participate in other athletic activities that are challenging and exhilarating and call for stamina, alertness, and teamwork. Similarly, people who have Down syndrome or fragile X chromosome are able to have other experiences of thinking hard about important questions and making distinctions and decisions. Thus, they exercise capacities for reflection and judgment, even if not in the rarified world of abstract verbal argument (P. Ferguson, e-mail, March 5, 1999).

The child who will have a disability may have fewer options for the so-called open future that philosophers and parents dream of for children. Yet I suspect that disability precludes far fewer life possibilities than members of the bioethics community claim. That many people with disabilities find their lives satisfying has been documented. For example, more than half of people with spinal cord injury (paraplegia) reported feeling more positively about themselves since becoming disabled. Similarly, Canadian teenagers who had been extremely-low-birthweight infants were compared with nondisabled teens and found to resemble them in terms of their own subjective ratings of quality of life. "Adolescents who were [extremely-low-birthweight] infants suffer from a greater burden of morbidity, and rate their health-related quality of life as significantly lower than control teenagers. Nevertheless, the vast majority of the [extremely-low-birthweight] respondents view their health-related quality of life as quite satisfactory and are difficult to distinguish from controls."[11(p453)]

Interestingly, professionals faced with such information often dismiss it and insist that happy disabled people are the exceptions.[12] . . .

. . . The 1998 survey of disabled people in the United States conducted by Louis Harris Associates found gaps in education, employment, income, and social participation between people with disabilities and people without disabilities and noted that fewer disabled than nondisabled people were "extremely satisfied" with their lives. The reasons for dissatisfaction did not stem from anything inherent in the impairments; they stemmed from disparities in attainments and activities that are not inevitable in a society that takes into account the needs of one sixth of its members.[7] . . .

For children whose disabling conditions do not cause early degeneration, intractable pain, and early death, life offers a host of interactions with the physical and social world in which people can be involved to their and others' satisfaction. Autobiographical writings and family narratives testify eloquently to the rich lives and the even richer futures that are possible for people with disabilities today. . . .

Nonetheless, I do not deny that disability can entail physical pain, psychic anguish, and social isolation—even if much of the psychological and social pain can be attributed to human cruelty rather than to biological givens. In order to imagine bringing a child with a disability into the world when abortion is possible, prospective parents must be able to imagine saying to a child, "I wanted you enough and believed enough in who you could be that I felt you could have a life you would appreciate even with the difficulties your disability causes." If parents and siblings, family members and friends can genuinely love and enjoy the child for who he or she is and not lament what he or she is not; if child care centers, schools, and youth groups routinely include disabled children; if television programs, children's books, and toys take children with disabilities into account by including them naturally in programs and products, the child may not live with the anguish and isolation that have marred life for generations of disabled children.

IMPLICATIONS FOR FAMILY LIFE

Many who are willing to concede that people with disabilities could have lives they themselves would enjoy nonetheless argue that the cost to families of raising them justifies abortion. Women are seen to carry the greatest load for the least return in caring for such a child. Proponents of using the technology to avoid the births of children with disabilities insist that the disabled child epitomizes what women have fought to change about their lives as mothers: unending labor, the sacrifice of their work and other adult interests, loss of time and attention for the other children in the family as they juggle resources to give this disabled child the best available support, and uncertain recompense in terms of the mother's relationship with the child. . . .

Assuming for a moment that there are "extra burdens" associated with certain aspects of raising children with disabilities, consider the "extra burdens" associated with raising other children: those with extraordinary (above statistical norm) aptitude for athletics, art, music, or mathematics. In a book on gifted children, Ellen Winner writes,

> [A]ll the family's energy becomes focused on this child. . . . Families focus in two ways on the gifted child's development: either one or both parents spend a great deal of time stimulating and teaching the child themselves, or parents make sacrifices so that the child gets high-level training from the best available teachers. In both cases, family life is totally arranged around the child's needs. Parents channel their interests into their child's talent area and become enormously invested in their child's progress.[13(p187)]

Parents, professionals working with the family, and the larger society all value the gift of the violin prodigy, the talent of the future Olympic figure skater, the aptitude of a child who excels in science and who might one day discover the cure for cancer. They perceive that all the extra work and rearrangement associated with raising such children will provide what people seek in parenthood: the opportunity to give ourselves to a new being who starts out with the best we can give, who will enrich us, gladden others, contribute to the world, and make us proud.

If professionals and parents believed that children with disabilities could indeed provide their parents many of the same satisfactions as any other child in terms of stimulation, love, companionship, pride, and pleasure in influencing the growth and development of another, they might reexamine their belief that in psychological, material, and social terms, the burdens of raising disabled children outweigh the benefits. A vast array of literature, both parental narrative and social science quantitative and qualitative research, powerfully testifies to the rewards—typical and atypical—of raising children with many of the conditions for which prenatal testing is considered de rigeur and abortion is expected (Down syndrome, hemophilia, cystic fibrosis, to name only some). Yet bioethics, public health, and genetics remain woefully—scandalously—oblivious, ignorant, or dismissive of any information that challenges the conviction that disability dooms families. . . .

The literature on how disability affects family life is, to be sure, replete with discussions of stress; anger at unsupportive members of the helping professions; distress caused by hostility from extended family, neighbors, and strangers; and frustration that many disability-related expenses are not covered by health insurance. And it is a literature that increasingly tries to distinguish why—under what conditions—some families of disabled children founder and others thrive. Contrary to the beliefs still much abroad in medicine, bioethics, and public health, recent literature does not suggest that, on balance, families raising children who have disabilities experience more stress and disruption than any other family.

IMPLICATIONS FOR PROFESSIONAL PRACTICE

Reporting in 1997 on a 5-year study of how families affected by cystic fibrosis and sickle cell anemia viewed genetic testing technologies, Duster and Beeson learned to their surprise that the closer the relationship between the family member and the affected individual, the more uncomfortable the family member was with the technology.

> [The] closer people are to someone with genetic disease the more problematic and usually unacceptable genetic testing is as a strategy for dealing with the issues. The experience of emotional closeness to someone with a genetic disease reduces, rather than increases, the acceptability of selective abortion. A close relationship with an affected person appears to make it more difficult to evaluate the meaning or worth of that person's existence solely in terms of their genetic disease. Family members consistently affirm the value of the person's life in spite of the disorders, and see value for their family in their experiences with (and) of this member, and in meeting the challenges the disease poses.[14(p43)]

This finding is consistent with other reports that parents of children with disabilities generally reject the idea of prenatal testing and abortion of subsequent fetuses, even if those fetuses are found to carry the same disabling trait.

Professionals charged with developing technologies, offering tests, and interpreting results should assess their current assumptions and practice on the basis of the literature on disability and family life generally and data about how such families perceive selective abortion. Of the many implications of such data, the first is that familiarity with disability as one characteristic of a child one loves changes the meaning of disability for parents contemplating a subsequent birth. The disability, instead of being the child's sole, or most salient, characteristic, becomes only one of the child's characteristics, along with appearance, aptitudes, temperament, interests, and quirks. The typical woman or couple discussing prenatal testing and possible pregnancy termination knows very little about the conditions for which testing is available, much less what these conditions might mean for the daily life of the child and the family. People who do not already have a child with a disability and who are contemplating prenatal testing must learn considerably more than the names of some typical impairments and the odds of their child's having one.

To provide ethical and responsible clinical care for anyone concerned about reproduction, professionals themselves must know far more than they now do about life with disability; they must convey more information, and different information, than they now typically provide. Shown a film about the lives of families raising children with Down syndrome, nurses and genetic counselors—but not parents—described the film as unrealistic and too positive a portrayal of family life. Whether the clinician is a genetics professional or (as is increasingly the case) an obstetrician promoting prenatal diagnosis as routine care for pregnant women, the tone, timing, and content of the counseling process cry out for drastic overhaul. . . .

Until their own education is revamped, obstetricians, midwives, nurses, and genetics professionals cannot properly counsel prospective parents. With broader exposure themselves, they would be far more likely to engage in discussions with their patients that would avoid problems such as those noted by Lippmann and Wilfond in a survey of genetic counselors. These researchers found that counselors provided far more positive information about Down syndrome and cystic fibrosis to parents already raising children diagnosed with those conditions than they did to prospective parents deciding whether to continue pregnancies in which the fetus had been found to have the condition. . . .

. . . I call for change to ensure that everyone obtaining testing or seeking information about genetic or prenatally diagnosable disability receives sufficient information about predictable difficulties, supports, and life events associated with a disabling condition to enable them to consider how a child's disability would fit into their own hopes for parenthood. Such information for all prospective parents should include, at a minimum, a detailed description of the biological, cognitive, or psychological impairments associated with specific disabilities, and what those impairments imply for day-to-day functioning; a discussion of the laws governing education, entitlements to family support services, access to buildings and transportation, and financial assistance to disabled children and their families; and literature by family members of disabled children and by disabled people themselves.

If prenatal testing indicates a disabling condition in the fetus, the following disability-specific information should be given to the prospective parents: information about services to benefit children with specific disabilities in a particular area, and about which of these a child and family are likely to need immediately after birth; contact information for a parent-group representative; and contact information for a member of a disability rights group or independent living center. In addition, the parents should be offered a visit with both a child and family and an adult living with the diagnosed disability.

Although some prospective parents will reject some or all of this information and these contacts, responsible practice that is concerned with genuine informed decision making and true reproductive choice must include access to this information, timed so that prospective parents can assimilate general ideas about life with disability before testing and obtain particular disability-relevant information if they discover that their fetus carries a disabling trait. These ideas may appear unrealistic or unfeasible, but a growing number of diverse voices support similar versions of these reforms to encourage wise decision making. Statements by Little People of America, the National Down Syndrome Congress, the National Institutes of Health workshop, and the Hastings Center Project on Prenatal Testing for Genetic Disability all urge versions of these changes in the process of helping people make childbearing decisions.

These proposals may be startling in the context of counseling for genetically transmitted or prenatally diagnosable disability, but they resonate with the recent discussion about childbearing for women infected with the HIV virus:

> The primary task of the provider would be to engage the client in a meaningful discussion of the implications of having a child and of not having a child for herself, for the client's family and for the child who would be born. . . . Providers would assist clients in examining what childbearing means to them. . . . Providers also would assist clients in gaining an understanding of the factual information relevant to decisions about childbearing . . . however, the conversation would cover a range of topics that go far beyond what can be understood as the relevant *medical* facts, and the direction of the conversation would vary depending on each person's life circumstances and priorities [emphasis added].[15(pp453–454)]

. . . Along with others who have expressed growing concern about needed reforms in the conduct of prenatal testing and counseling, I urge a serious conversation between prospective parents and clinicians about what the parents seek in childrearing and how a disabling condition in general or a specific type of impairment would affect their hopes and expectations for the rewards of parenthood. For some people, any mobility, sensory, cognitive, or health impairment may indeed lead to disappointment of parental hopes; for others, it may be far easier to imagine incorporating disability into family life without believing that the rest of their lives will be blighted.

Ideally, such discussions will include mention of the fact that every child inevitably differs from parental dreams, and that successful parenting requires a mix of shaping and influencing children and ruefully appreciating the ways they pick and choose from what parents offer, sometimes rejecting tastes, activities, or values dear to the parents. If prospective parents cannot envision appreciating the child who will depart in particular, known ways from the parents' fantasy, are they truly ready to raise would-be athletes when they hate sports, classical violinists when they delight in the Grateful Dead? Testing and abortion guarantee little about the child and the life parents create and nurture, and all parents and children will be harmed by inflated notions of what parenting in an age of genetic knowledge can bring in terms of fulfilled expectations.

Public health professionals must do more than they have been doing to change the climate in which prenatal tests are offered. Think about what people would say if prenatal clinics contained pamphlets telling poor women or African American women that they should consider refraining from childbearing because their children could be similarly poor and could endure discrimination or because they could be less healthy and more likely to find themselves imprisoned than members of the middle class or than Whites. Public health is committed to ending such inequities, not to endorsing them, tolerating them, or asking prospective parents to live with them. Yet the current promotion of prenatal testing condones just such an approach to life with disability.

Practitioners and policymakers can increase women's and couples' reproductive choice through testing and counseling, and they can expend energy and resources on changing the society in which families consider raising disabled children. If families that include children with disabilities now spend more money and ingenuity on after-school care for those children because they are denied entrance into existing programs attended by their peers and siblings, public health can join with others to ensure that existing programs include *all* children. The principle of education for all, which is reforming public education for disabled children, must spread to incorporate those same children into the network of services and supports that parents count on for other children. Such programs, like other institutions, must change to fit the people who exist in the world, not claim that some people should not exist because society is not prepared for them. We can fight to reform insurance practices that deny reimbursement for diabetes test strips; special diets for people with disabilities; household modifications that give disabled children freedom to explore their environment; and modifications of equipment, games, and toys that enable disabled children to participate in activities comparable to those of their peers. Public health can fight to end the catch-22 that removes subsidies for life-sustaining personal assistance services once disabled people enter the workforce, a policy that acts as a powerful disincentive to productivity and needlessly perpetuates poverty and dependence. . . .

Despite the strides of the past few decades, our current society is far from the ideal . . . toward which the disability community strives. Medicine, bioethics, and public health can put their efforts toward promoting such a society; with such efforts, disability could become nearly as easy to incorporate into the familial and social landscape as the other differences these professions respect and affirm as ordinary parts of the human condition. Given that more than 50 million people in the US population have disabling traits and that prenatal tests may become increasingly available to detect more of them, we are confronting the fact that tests may soon be available for characteristics that we have until now considered inevitable facts of human life, such as heart disease.

In order to make testing and selecting for or against disability consonant with improving life for those who will inevitably be born with or acquire disabilities, our clinical and policy establishments must communicate that it is as acceptable to live with a disability as it is to live without one and that society will support and appreciate everyone with the inevitable variety of traits. We can assure prospective parents that they and their future child will be welcomed whether or not the child has a disability. If that professional message is conveyed, more prospective parents may envision that their lives can be rewarding, whatever the characteristics of the child they are raising. When our professions can envision such communication and the reality of incorporation and appreciation of people with disabilities, prenatal technology can help people to make decisions without implying that only one decision is right. If the child with a disability is not a problem for the world, and the world is not a problem for the child, perhaps we can diminish our desire for prenatal testing and selective abortion and can comfortably welcome and support children of all characteristics.

REFERENCES

1. Wertz DC, Fletcher JC. Sex selection through prenatal diagnosis. In: Holmes HB, Purdy LM, eds. *Feminist Perspectives in Medical Ethics.* Bloomington: Indiana University Press; 1992: 240–253.
2. Schuklenk U, Stein E, Kerin J, Byne W. The ethics of genetic research on sexual orientation. *Hastings Center Rep.* 1997;27(4):6–13.
3. Retsinas J. Impact of prenatal technology on attitudes toward disabled infants. In: Wertz D. *Research in the Sociology of Healthcare* Westport, Conn: JAI Press; 1991:75–102.
4. Beaudet AL. Carrier screening for cystic fibrosis. *Am J Hum Genet* 1990;47:603–605.
5. Boorse C. Concepts of health. In: Van de Veer D, Regan T, eds. *Health Care Ethics.* Philadelphia, Pa: Temple University Press; 1987:359–393.
6. Daniels NL. *Just Health Care: Studies in Philosophy and Health Policy.* Cambridge, England: Cambridge University Press; 1985.
7. National Organization on Disability's 1998 Harris Survey of Americans With Disabilities. Available at: http://www.nod.org/press.html #poll. Accessed August 29, 1999.
8. Americans with Disabilities Act (Pub L No. 101–336, 1990, § 2).
9. Watson JD. President's essay: genes and politics. *Annual Report Cold Springs Harbor*. 1996: 1–20.
10. Green R. Prenatal autonomy and the obligation not to harm one's child genetically. *J Law Med Ethics*. 1996; 25(1):5–16.
11. Saigal S, Feeny D, Rosenbaum P, Furlong W, Burrows E, Stoskopf B. Self-perceived health status and health-related quality of life of extremely low-birth-weight infants at adolescence. *JAMA.* 1996;276: 453–459.
12. Tyson JE, Broyles RS. Progress in assessing the long-term outcome of extremely low-birth-weight infants. *JAMA.* 1996;276:492–493.
13. Winner E. *Gifted children: Myths and Realities.* New York, NY: Basic Books; 1996.
14. Duster T, Beeson D. *Pathways and Barriers to Genetic Testing and Screening: Molecular Genetics Meets the "High-Risk" Family.* Final report. Washington, DC: US Dept of Energy; October 1997.
15. Faden RR, Kass NE, Acuff KL, et al. HIV infection and childbearing: a proposal for public policy and clinical practice. In: Faden R, Kass N, eds. *HIV, Aids and Childbearing: Public Policy. Private Lives.* New York NY: Oxford University Press; 1996:447–461.

ETHICAL ISSUES AND PRACTICAL PROBLEMS IN PREIMPLANTATION GENETIC DIAGNOSIS

Jeffrey R. Botkin

Preimplantation genetic diagnosis (PGD) is a new method of prenatal diagnosis that is developing from a union of in vitro fertilization (IVF) technology and molecular biology. Briefly stated, PGD involves the creation of several embryos in vitro from the eggs and sperm of an interested couple. The embryos are permitted to develop to a 6-to-10-cell stage, at which point one of the embryonic cells is removed from each embryo and the cellular DNA is analyzed for chromosomal abnormalities or genetic mutations. An embryo or several embryos found to be free of genetic abnormalities are subsequently transferred to the woman's uterus for gestation. Embryos found to carry a genetic abnormality are discarded or frozen. Extra normal embryos may be frozen for future transfer or donation to another couple.

The rationale for this approach to prenatal diagnosis is straight-forward: "Preimplantation diagnosis for some couples at risk of transmitting inherited disorders to their children is an alternative to prenatal diagnosis and recurrent abortion." But, as with other forms of prenatal diagnosis, the use of PGD need not be restricted to couples at high risk for inherited disorders. No doubt, continued developments in molecular biology will permit a detailed genetic analysis of a potential child for a wide range of conditions, susceptibilities and, perhaps, behavioral tendencies before gestation even begins.

As an alternative to an existing clinical practice, the ethics of PGD can be considered in reference to prenatal diagnosis using better established techniques such as amniocentesis and chorionic villus sampling (CVS)—hereafter termed "traditional" prenatal diagnosis. Because PGD does not involve abortion it has been offered as a less morally problematic alternative to prenatal diagnosis. I will argue that PGD does circumvent the problem of abortion, but it raises an interesting array of other practical and ethical issues. A primary conclusion is that PGD will not provide a solution to some of the most serious ethical concerns in prenatal diagnosis.

The emphasis of this discussion will be on the ethically relevant distinctions between PGD and traditional prenatal diagnostic techniques, and I will not develop in detail the many ethical issues involved with prenatal diagnosis in general. I also will not address the ethical issues raised by storage of embryos or the potential use of normal or abnormal embryos for research purposes—both of which are relevant to PGD.

IS THERE A DEMAND FOR PGD?

As a backdrop to the discussion of this technology, we should consider the extent to which PGD might be utilized as an alternative to traditional prenatal diagnosis. Utilization will depend as much, or more, on the complexity of the procedures as it will on its perceived ethical advantages. The basic notions of placing eggs and sperm in a dish, testing the resulting embryos and transferring the healthy ones to a receptive uterus are, in principle, quite simple and elegant. Yet the retrieval of multiple eggs, the growing of embryos, the complexities of their analysis, and the subsequent induction of an initially fragile pregnancy require remarkable dedication by a couple and collaboration of a small army of physicians, scientists, and technicians. Willy Lissens et al. describe PGD:

> Preimplantation diagnosis is . . . a procedure requiring the multidisciplinary collaboration of a clinical IVF unit, a laboratory IVF unit with micromanipulation facilities, a molecular biology and cytogenetics laboratory, and a clinical genetics unit. Most centres still

Reprinted with permission from *Journal of Law, Medicine & Ethics*, 26 (1998): 17–28.

Editor's note: All footnotes have been deleted. Students who want to follow up on sources should consult the original article.

> consider [PGD] an experimental method and request and advise follow-up prenatal diagnosis in cases of pregnancy.

But this orchestrated creation is not a one-shot deal for most couples—two or more cycles of egg retrieval, testing, and implantation usually are required to establish a successful pregnancy. For any individual couple, PGD involves months of time, multiple drugs, invasive procedures, a team of subspecialists at a center for reproductive medicine, and it requires the will to endure the failures of implantation or the loss of early pregnancies. Once a pregnancy is established, subsequent traditional prenatal diagnosis is still recommended to check the accuracy of the process.

Related to the complexity and physical burdens and risks of the procedures are their costs. PGD remains experimental, meaning there is no established set of services provided, and there is yet to emerge a literature on its associated costs. However, there is literature on the cost of IVF for infertile couples. In a 1994 article, Peter Neumann et al. estimate that the total direct and indirect cost of IVF per cycle of egg retrieval ranges from $67,000 for the first cycle to $114,000 for the sixth cycle. In a 1997 publication, Bradley Van Voorhis et al. calculate the cost per delivery of IVF in 71 couples to be $43,000 per delivery of an infant. Assuming PGD is on the same order of magnitude, it is an extraordinarily expensive intervention. It is likely that customers for PGD will have to pay for this service out-of-pocket because it is unlikely that insurance carriers or government funding agencies will cover these costs given the nonessential nature of this intervention, the cheaper alternatives, and the controversial nature of prenatal diagnosis in general. Currently, 85 percent of the costs of IVF are not covered by insurance in the United States. Many individuals using PGD to date have their costs covered by the experimental programs developing the technology.

The market demand for PGD will depend on several factors: (1) the number of people interested in prenatal diagnosis; (2) the proportion of those interested who would strongly desire to avoid abortion; and (3) the proportion of those reluctant to consider abortion who would be willing to meet the monetary and nonmonetary costs of PGD procedures. Remarkably, despite these apparent constraints on its appeal, Yuri Verlinski notes that most experimental PGD cycles at present are being done for maternal age–related chromosomal aneuploidy (trisomy 21, trisomy 18, and so forth). For many or most of these older couples, PGD probably is being used as an adjunct to IVF for infertility. PGD by older women outside the context of infertility is an unlikely market due to two considerations. First, the risk of bearing a child with a chromosomal aneuploidy for, say, a forty-year-old women, is approximately 2.5 percent. Second, the efficiency of IVF declines significantly with age. Richard Legro et al. summarize the literature, which indicates that the pregnancy rate per cycle is 5 percent or less in women over forty years of age. Assuming future costs will not be covered by experimental programs or insurance, it is unlikely that many older mothers will be willing to undergo multiple interventions at high cost to address a modest risk that can otherwise be addressed through CVS or amniocentesis (or, perhaps, through adoption). To be more specific, how many women would spend $40,000 for a procedure with a 5 percent success rate to ensure an outcome that would occur 97.5 percent of the time anyhow? Traditional prenatal diagnosis, counseling, and pregnancy termination would avoid the same outcome at a cost of under $3,000, and this full expense would occur only if a pregnancy is achieved and a fetus with an abnormality is detected.

Further, for a number of genetic conditions, there has been a marked ambivalence about the use of prenatal diagnosis in some populations—cystic fibrosis (CF) and sickle cell disease are notable examples because they are the most common genetic conditions in Caucasians and African Americans, respectively. In 1991, a prospective trial of population screening for sickle cell disease found that less than half of those couples identified as at risk pursued prenatal diagnosis. Further, for those couples who pursued prenatal diagnosis and learned of an affected fetus, a termination rate of 39 percent was documented in a 1987 survey of U.S. and Canadian centers performing prenatal diagnosis for sickle cell disease. If these attitudes remain prevalent in the African American community, utilization of PGD for sickle cell disease is likely to be unusual. The ability to do prenatal testing for CF in recent years is being met with limited interest in the United States on the part of at-risk families. The reluctance of many at-risk couples to use prenatal diagnosis and to terminate pregnancies for these conditions is due, in part, to a reluctance to abort a pregnancy—precisely the issue addressed by PGD. But this ambivalence about selective termination is more complex than this one issue of a reluctance to abort per se. Additional dimensions include cultural attitudes about the use of prenatal diagnosis in general, the presence of other options, such as having no more children, and concerns about what abortion may imply for the value of the life of an existing affected child.

These limitations suggest that PGD in the *commercial* market will be a boutique service for the foreseeable future, even if the efficiency rates increase considerably. It is questionable whether many couples will believe that the added benefits of PGD will justify its costs and other burdens. This raises the broader question of whether the development of this extraordinary technology is born more of consumer demand for an alternative to prenatal diagnosis, or more of a technical fascination with the manipulation of human life, albeit for justifiable reasons. The relevance of this question comes, in part, from wondering how we will respond if we build it and they do not come. There will be other uses for PGD, beyond that for serious genetic disabilities, that may emerge as attractive if this powerful technology has limited use for its currently designated purpose. Alternative [*sic*] uses, such as for genetic enhancement, will be discussed below.

THE PURPOSE OF PGD

Despite reasons to question the future demand for this technology, there is at least a clarity of purpose for PGD compared with more established prenatal diagnostic techniques. The literature on traditional prenatal diagnosis offers a variety of potential purposes for these interventions. One purpose is to reduce the risk of bearing a child with an unwanted genetic condition or congenital malformation. This purpose is the same for PGD, although this purpose must be clearly focused and understood by clients. With all prenatal diagnostic approaches, the reduction in risk applies only to the conditions being evaluated by the technology. PGD does not guarantee that the child will be free of genetic or congenital conditions (a "perfect" baby), only that the child will be free of conditions for which testing is done. Two points are relevant here. First, the current literature is reassuring that the use of PGD does not appear to cause an increase in the risk congenital malformation in the resulting child—a reasonable concern because the procedure removes a substantial portion of the mass of the developing embryo. Joe Simpson and Inge Liebaers reviewed the literature in 1996 and report that pregnancy outcome data suggest that the prevalence of congenital malformation in infants following IVF with or without micromanipulation is about 3 to 4 percent, that is, the same as that in the general population. So although PGD does not appear to increase the overall risk, it does not decrease it below the general population level. Of course, it is important to emphasize that reduction of risk to the population level may look quite good to couples at high risk of bearing a child with a specific genetic condition.

The point here is that couples undergoing PGD should have the clear understanding that the child retains the same base-line risk of a congenital abnormality as children in the general population. More specifically, PGD is not useful for predicting congenital malformations or diseases that do not have an identified genetic basis. For couples who will not consider abortion, PGD alone will not reduce the risk of bearing a child with conditions such as spina bifida, anencephaly, encephalocele, omphalocele, hypoplastic left heart, bladder extrophy, renal agenesis, or many other conditions, because these malformations often do not have their origins in single-gene defects or in detectable chromosomal aberrations. It is interesting to note that Asangla Ao et al. report that more than 50 percent of the couples who underwent PGD for CF in their series did not want additional prenatal diagnostic evaluations of the fetus beyond routine ultrasound. Such decisions may be quite reasonable, as long as the couples understand the limitations of PGD technology.

Another purpose often mentioned for prenatal diagnosis is simply to provide couples with information about the pregnancy. This is a more neutral goal for prenatal diagnostic services consistent with the nondirective tradition of genetic counseling. Because this goal appears less problematic than goals that entail abortion, it may be promoted in patient information materials or in physician-patient encounters. Nancy Press and Carol Browner's work demonstrates how issues surrounding pregnancy termination were not explicitly mentioned in materials and initial encounters in the alpha-fetoprotein screening program in California. Many women did not understand that the principal implication of a decision to be screened was a decision about abortion if an affected child was detected. At the public policy level, it remains a challenge to decide whether prenatal screening programs are a success when at-risk couples are identified and informed of the risk, or whether success requires a significant reduction in the number of affected children born to screened couples. In the prospective screening trial for hemoglobinopathies noted above, 18,907 women were screened to identify 810 carrier women, leading to one pregnancy termination (for hemoglobin H disease). The women generally were grateful for the information—a success. Nevertheless, the limited use of the information by the women indicates that the program was largely a failure in terms of reducing the incidence of serious hemoglobinopathies—at least for the pregnancies followed in the study.

These clinical and policy problems associated with trying to provide neutral information as a purpose for prenatal diagnosis are not relevant to PGD. It would make little sense to go through IVF procedures and genetic analyses only to be nondirective about which embryos to place in the uterus. The purpose of PGD is not simply to inform couples about the genetic nature of their embryos. The explicit purpose is also to transfer healthy embryos and to discard those destined to be affected. Once a couple has chosen PGD, nondirectiveness is no longer relevant.

Similarly, a third purpose often claimed for prenatal diagnosis is that it permits parents to prepare for the birth of an affected child. Several scholars question whether emotional preparation by parents can be effective prior to actually holding and experiencing the child. Nevertheless, the claim is plausible, particularly for conditions requiring immediate surgical interventions that would be facilitated by delivery at a tertiary center. In any case, this purpose for prenatal diagnosis is not relevant to PGD. Embryo diagnosis would not be necessary or appropriate as a mechanism to prepare for the birth of an affected child. . . .

ETHICAL ISSUES

An initial set of ethical issues to consider are ones that are shared by other forms of prenatal diagnosis and selective termination. These include the destruction of prenatal life, defining the appropriate uses of the technology, the broader social effects of prenatal diagnosis for those with disabilities, allocation of resource issues, and informed consent concerns. PGD presents some new and interesting ethical concerns in each of these familiar domains. Following this discussion, I turn briefly to two new issues that are raised by PGD alone: germ-line gene therapy and genetic enhancement.

Destruction of Prenatal Life

The advantage of PGD over traditional prenatal diagnosis hinges largely on the ethical distinction between discarding an affected embryo and aborting an affected fetus. The range of positions on the moral status of prenatal life will be familiar to most readers. The conservative position, consistent with the position taken by the Catholic church, is that all prenatal life post-fertilization is of full and equal moral status to that of all other persons. Under this conception, no distinction exists between discarding an embryo and aborting a fetus—both are morally unacceptable. The opposite position, characterized by the arguments of Michael Tooley, is the claim that moral status is conferred by cognitive traits that are probably lacking in newborns, and clearly absent in fetuses and embryos. Under this conception, fetuses and embryos are equal in their lack of significant moral standing. However, the majority of scholars and official bodies who have addressed the issue have adopted positions within a broad center ground. These positions are similar in that they maintain that all prenatal human life should be afforded a special moral status, but a moral status that is not equal to that of a full-fledged person. Further, these views typically hold that the relative moral status is influenced by the developmental status of the embryo or fetus. Some commentators argue that development is a seamless continuum, therefore, the moral status of the embryo and fetus increases incrementally with development. However, the predominant set of arguments confer moral status based on the achievement of certain milestones in the developmental process that have moral significance. Developmental milestones that have been promoted as conferring increased (although not necessarily full) moral status for the developing human include formation of the primitive streak at 14 days, "quickening" at about 18 weeks, development of "brain life" at about 20 to 22 weeks, a sapient or sentient state emerging at about 22 to 24 weeks, and viability at 23 to 24 weeks of gestation. As Carson Strong notes, this developmental conception of moral status is in agreement with widely held moral intuitions that intrauterine devices are morally acceptable even though they destroy the preimplantation embryo, that early abortion is better than late abortion, and that infanticide is wrong. The recent partial birth abortion debate also illustrates the heightened ethical concern over pregnancy termination as the fetus approaches term.

The National Institutes of Health's Human Embryo Research Panel in 1994, in its review of the moral status of the embryo, observed that only the conservative position attributed personhood and full moral status to the preimplantation embryo. Other philosophical positions, the panel concluded, accord the preembryo either limited or no moral status. The panel preferred not to adopt any single criterion as determinative of the moral status of the embryo but rather what it called a "pluralistic approach."

> As gestation continues, the further development of human form, the onset of a heartbeat, the development of the nervous system leading to brain activity and with this at least some of the physical basis for future sentience, relational presence to the mother, and capacity for independent existence all counsel toward according an increasing degree of protectability.

Broad recognition of this pluralistic approach in our society provides solid support for the claim that the fetus has greater moral standing than the preimplantation embryo does. A preference by individual couples for discarding embryos versus terminating a fetus is ethically justified through reference to this widely accepted social standard. Therefore, PGD is ethically acceptable on this basis as a method of prenatal diagnosis and selective termination. Conversely, however, given the debatable nature of the moral status of prenatal life and the burdens and expense of PGD, it obviously cannot be claimed that PGD is ethically *obligatory,* as a method of prenatal diagnosis in contrast to more traditional methods.

One further point on the moral status of the preimplantation embryo deserves emphasis. For those who hold the conservative position, PGD will be seen as *more* ethically problematic than traditional prenatal diagnosis. PGD requires the creation of numerous embryos for each live birth produced. In a recent report by Ao et al., twelve couples utilized PGD to screen for CF. The couples produced 137 embryos, of which 26 were transferred to a woman's uterus and 5 births resulted. The loss of prenatal life was substantially greater through PGD than would have resulted had the twelve at-risk couples pursued traditional prenatal diagnosis and selective termination. Clearly, PGD does not resolve the ethical concerns in prenatal diagnosis for many who have fundamental objections to abortion—indeed, it makes the situation considerably worse.

Setting Limits On the Use of PGD

In general, there is social support for prenatal diagnosis for so-called "serious" conditions, including conditions like Tay Sachs disease, spina bifida, CF, sickle cell disease, hemophilia, muscular dystrophy, and a number of others. There is also a general conviction that prenatal diagnosis and abortion for "trivial" or minor conditions is ethically troubling, although a number of professionals and commentators could permit such use of prenatal diagnosis based on a respect for parental autonomy in reproductive matters. Gender selection is often used as an extreme example of selective abortion for frivolous reasons. Nevertheless, the majority of U.S. geneticists surveyed by Dorothy Wertz and John Fletcher in 1985 would either perform prenatal diagnosis for a couple who did not want a fifth daughter or refer them to a colleague who would. Therefore, with traditional prenatal diagnosis, a conflict in social values arises between a reluctance to validate termination of a fetus for a less than a serious medical condition and a desire to respect parental autonomy in this most intimate of enterprises.

This fundamental problem with traditional prenatal diagnosis will be exacerbated by the rapid increase in genetic tests for a wide range of conditions, including late-onset conditions, conditions with a limited impact on health, and, possibly, behavioral or physical characteristics that fall within the normal range. This is not to suggest that genes play a predominant role in complex human behaviors and characteristics. Increasingly, it could be found that, for all but the simplest genetic conditions, dozens or hundreds of genes interact with each other and with thousands of biochemical and environmental agents over extended periods of time to produce the phenotype. Such complexity could frustrate any meaningful predictions based on genetic tests alone. Richard Strohman argues that much of the contemporary interest in genetic testing will collapse as our overly deterministic genetic paradigm progressively fails. Nevertheless, we only may need a popular *perception* of genetic determinism, fueled by creative marketing and weak regulation, to move poorly predictive tests from the lab into the clinic.

If indeed, an extensive battery of genetic tests become available for prenatal diagnosis, what tests should be offered to couples and what tests should professionals provide on request? Should we draw a line, indicating which tests should and should not be provided by an ethical practitioner? Several general positions on the "line-drawing" question are beginning to emerge. John Robertson concedes the morally problematic nature of prenatal diagnosis for "minor" conditions, but argues that our respect for procreative liberty should be paramount, at least until some definitive harm is demonstrated from unfettered use. Robertson places no limits on the parents' ability to obtain prenatal testing for any condition. Strong advocates use of prenatal diagnosis for all diseases or susceptibilities to diseases, but not for nondisease conditions. Strong's analysis places a heavy emphasis on the value of nondirectiveness in prenatal diagnostic services, suggesting that line drawing between disease categories undermines this important value. In contrast, Stephen Post, Peter Whitehouse, and I have argued that minor and late-onset conditions do not justify testing. Angus Clark supports prenatal diagnosis only for the most serious conditions. Adrienne Asch, although deeply troubled by the termination of embryos and fetuses for disabling conditions, believes that a policy of line drawing would be enormously detrimental to those in the disabled community who fall below the line. She, therefore, opposes line drawing, but would couple prenatal diagnosis with better education, emphasizing a fuller understanding of life's prospects with a disabled child. The Institute of Medicine has taken the position that "prenatal diagnosis not be used for minor conditions or characteristics." These positions illustrate a balancing of a number of considerations, including the moral status of the embryo and fetus, the limits of professional authority; the limits, if any, of our respect for parental autonomy, and the impact of individuals with disabilities on the family and society. Also to be considered in this dilemma is the impact of prenatal diagnosis on those who live with disabilities and the impact of broad choice on the parent-child relationship. Much more work needs to be done on this line-drawing question for prenatal diagnosis in general to achieve some resolution at a societal level.

PGD will serve to complicate this dilemma by reducing the concern over one significant element in the equation—abortion. The technology, by its very design, offers each couple a range of choices in offspring. Choice in offspring through PGD is not contingent on abortion. Whether to transfer an affected embryo is not a dilemma with PGD, because this is its explicit purpose; but other more subtle choices are made possible by the technology. Imagine a couple who has 8 embryos in vitro, 2 of which are homozygous for CF, 2 are heterozygous, and 4 are neither carriers nor affected (termed *homozygous normal*). At the request of the parents, the embryos are sexed and three of the four homozygous normal embryos are female and both of the heterozygous embryos are male. The couple desires a son, so the homozygous normal male embryo is split—one-half (now a viable embryo itself) is implanted and the other is cryopreserved along with the other unaffected embryos.

Is there a problem with this scenario? No embryos have been destroyed on the basis of gender and the couple fulfills its wishes. Does this form of gender selection strike us as less problematic than gender selection by abortion? After all, the couple has quite a few embryos from which to choose—a primary choice has been made to discard the affected embryos, but why not choose the specific one to be implanted on the basis of secondary characteristics? By producing a number of embryos with each cycle and by eliminating the moral hurdle of abortion in the selection of offspring, PGD facilitates a broad range of possibilities for selecting the biologic characteristics of children.

If we are entering an age of genetic testing for a wide range of conditions, the extensive analysis of potential children may be a popular application. One example of a particularly interesting development is the chip technology in which tens of thousands of DNA fragments are imbedded in a glass slide that is used to analyze a target DNA sample. It is anticipated that these chips will enable a DNA sample to be evaluated for tens of thousands or hundreds of thousands of mutations or alleles. Backed by a powerful computer, it may be possible to correlate the results of such a DNA analysis with complex physical or psychological traits in individuals. For example, assuming intelligence has some genetic components, correlating a DNA chip analysis of, say, 100,000 random coding sites in the genome with traditional IQ scores may reveal patterns of results that are associated with higher or lower IQ scores in healthy individuals. Note that such a "test" can function with no true knowledge about the genetic influences on IQ. The same kind of testing might be used for any physical or psychological characteristic for which there are objective measures and any meaningful genetic contributions. As noted, these tests need not be very predictive to be adopted by some couples who want the very best that their sperm, eggs, and money can provide.

If such genetic tests are perceived as useful for predicting the physical and psychological characteristics of future children, some couples may pursue PGD for no other reason than to select their ideal embryo. This could well be a growth industry in the coming century for couples who can afford it.

For those who are uneasy with this notion, the challenge is to articulate the ethical problem with this approach to child bearing when abortion is no longer a concern (and assuming one does not hold the conservative position with respect to the moral weight of embryo destruction). One consistent criticism of prenatal diagnosis is the message of rejection that it sends to people with disabilities. It is feared that prenatal diagnosis will lead to heightened intolerance of disability as forces are marshaled to eliminate those embryos and fetuses with disabilities rather than to develop a society in which the disabled can live as welcomed partners. If prenatal diagnosis and PGD specifically were to have a significantly negative effect on the millions of disabled individuals in society, this would be a powerful argument for limiting or discouraging its use, at least for less than serious medical conditions.

The speculative nature of this concern, both in terms of whether people will use PGD or traditional prenatal diagnosis for a broad range of conditions, and whether such use will produce additional discrimination for the disabled, makes this concern difficult to weigh as a moral issue. There is no evidence of this kind of effect to date on a broad scale, despite the use of prenatal diagnosis for several decades. In contrast, individuals with disabilities have never had *more* social support than they do today, as reflected in the sentiment and substance of the Americans with Disabilities Act. Certainly, more social support is still due, but a generally improved social stature for the disabled has occurred in recent decades in parallel with the development and use of prenatal diagnostic techniques. Changes in technology economics, and attitudes could adversely change the situation for the disabled in the future, but current experience indicates that society can simultaneously promote respect and opportunity for the disabled while enabling couples to prevent the birth of a disabled child through prenatal diagnosis.

However, distinctions may be made in the future between those disabled from genetic conditions that are detectable prenatally and the majority of the disabled who have limitations from a broad range of other causes (injury, stroke, infection, and so forth). Given the potential power of PGD to select the genetic characteristics of future children, it could promote societal expectations of "perfectibility" in children, thus fostering a more narrow intolerance of those disabled from genetic and congenital etiologies and, perhaps, of the parents who choose to have such a child. This is a serious concern that deserves scrutiny and persistent efforts to combat discriminatory attitudes toward the disabled.

It is likely, however, that broad changes in social attitudes concerning perfectibility and disability will be affected more by prenatal diagnostic techniques that may have much greater appeal than will PGD. For example, techniques that will enable the isolation of fetal cells from maternal blood samples early in pregnancy, in conjunction with medications to terminate early pregnancies privately and relatively painlessly, are more likely to have widespread utilization than PGD. There are even developments that may enable the determination of fetal sex through a maternal urine test. I suspect that any new approaches that make prenatal diagnosis accurate and selective termination substantially easier early in pregnancy would be widely adopted. For whatever benefits this technology may bring, widespread use could significantly reduce societal tolerance for "less than perfect" babies.

A second concern raised by the use of PGD to select against minor conditions (or for desirable characteristics) is the potential effect such control might have on the parent-child relationship. As noted, PGD facilitates the selection of children, as compared with traditional prenatal diagnosis, because it offers a range of choices with each set of embryos produced rather than the single choice of accepting or terminating an established pregnancy.

The most compelling argument from my perspective as a pediatrician is the adverse effect detailed selection may have on the parent-child relationship, whether by PGD or traditional prenatal diagnosis. Parents always have had hopes and expectations at the birth of a child, but these are layered on the knowledge that children will grow up and in directions over which they ultimately will have little control. We have all lived through our own parents' expectations and we all understand how supportive and damaging these can be. What would it mean for parents to have very specific expectations for a child based in prenatal testing and selection?

From the age of nine months onward when an infant begins to crawl, her project becomes increasingly one of independence. Her parents' project, in contrast, is one of control, indoctrination, and education to protect, to prepare, to bypass the mistakes made by others (often their own), and to fulfill their own conception of a life of value. This tension between the child's striving for independence and the parents' need for nurturing is fundamental to the parent-child relationship. Ultimately, we establish ourselves as independent—often to be quite different from what our parents had in mind. But remarkably, there need be no love lost in this clash of projects, although there sometimes is. For the most part, we continue to love our children (and our parents) as they are.

What influence could PGD technology have on this most important relationship? How might the knowledge that a child was deliberately selected for her biological characteristics affect how an individual regards her parents, how her parents regard her, and how she regards herself? Could the selection enhance the expectations of parents and alter the child's self-perception of strengths and weaknesses? Would children be strongly channeled in directions of the parents' choosing? To what extent would children resent such an intrusion on their own autonomy? Oscar Wilde observed: "Children begin by loving their parents. After a time they judge them. Rarely, if ever, do they forgive them." I suspect that the greater the power parents have over the biological nature of their children, the more this observation will hold true. This is not because the child would be directly harmed by the biological selection, but because the selection may well come with a stifling set of expectations. The question is whether the child's future autonomy—her right to an "open future"—will be sacrificed through a uncompromising respect for parental liberty in reproductive decisions.

My purpose here is to outline ethical concerns over the unfettered use of PGD that extend beyond the destruction of embryos alone. These concerns over the parent-child relationship are quite speculative and there is certainly no data as yet to support or refute these possibilities. Nevertheless, the fundamental importance of the parent-child relationship suggests that a burden of justification must rest with parents or professionals who would use PGD for the selection of offspring for characteristics other than significant health conditions. Parental desires to use technology in the fine-grained selection of children must be justified through claims of legitimate interest. Parents traditionally have had only a *prima facie* right to liberty in reproductive decisions—not an absolute right in the face of potential countervailing harms. . . .

Why would parents want to select the biological characteristics of their children, beyond a selection against conditions causing significant disability? Is there a convincing rationale for such an intervention? If the claim is that such selections ultimately will make the resulting children happier with their lives, then the credibility of this claim can be challenged. Each of us can point to a number of biological characteristics that have influenced our lives favorably and unfavorably, but this provides little evidence for what characteristics our children will find beneficial or harmful in their lives as they unfold in very different ways, times, and places. Do we know which biological characteristics promote a contented life? If we were to look in detail at a list of genetic characteristics of a set of infants, would we presume to predict which children would experience the most fulfilling lives, by whatever definition we choose? We probably do have a list of traits that would make our children more *competitive* in contemporary society, but success in competition and contentment are two very different things. There is less moral force to the claim that parents should be supported in their efforts to gain competitive advantage for their children, particularly when competitive advantage remains possible through traditional means such as education, wealth, and hard work. . . .

It is essential that the appropriate uses and misuses of this technology be debated and defined. This is perhaps the greatest ethical challenge raised by PGD. At present, concerns over the impact on those with disabilities and the impact on the parent-child relationship suggest a limited use of PGD (and other prenatal diagnostic approaches) for significant health concerns. (This conclusion does not necessitate legal prohibitions on some uses of the technology, only the development of standards for which tests should be offered and/or provided by the ethical practitioner.) PGD avoids the problem of abortion, but it heightens more subtle and longer-term concerns over the limits of parental control over the biological nature of their children. . . .

ISSUES UNIQUE TO PGD: GERM-LINE GENE THERAPY AND GENETIC ENHANCEMENT

PGD could be a component of two controversial interventions that are not relevant to traditional prenatal diagnosis: germ-line gene therapy and genetic enhancement. The ability to manipulate the in vitro embryo will greatly facilitate the insertion of genetic material, either to treat a medical condition or, potentially, to enhance its genetic characteristics. Such gene therapy is germ-line therapy because the genetic insertion into an individual embryonic cell (or zygote), which is then grown as a separate embryo, would result in the transformation of all of the cells in the resulting individual, including the gametes. PGD could be used prior to and after insertion of genetic material in order first to identify a suitable embryo and then to evaluate the success of the genetic transfer.

Germ-line gene therapy has been the subject of a growing volume of literature, even though gene therapy in general has proven to be much more difficult than originally hoped. Leroy Walters and Judy Palmer outline eight arguments from the literature against germ-line gene therapy. The most compelling, at least for this purpose, is that the emergence of PGD has virtually eliminated the *need* for germ-line therapy. For many medical conditions in which genetic mutations produce structural or developmental abnormalities from early in gestation, successful therapy and prevention will require that the genetic material be inserted into the gamete(s) of the parents or into the early embryo. In this circumstance, the gene therapy becomes germ-line as a by-product of the primary therapeutic intent. However, in the foreseeable future, the difficulty of reliably introducing a stable, functional genetic element into in vivo human eggs and sperm will be very difficult to surmount. In contrast, the possibility of introducing functional genes into an in vitro zygote or embryo seems quite reasonable in the foreseeable future.

The basic question is why a couple would bother to treat an affected embryo with gene therapy when they could simply discard any affected embryos and transfer the ones destined to be healthy. Because embryos have little moral stature, there is no mandate to rescue them with gene therapy. Further, the failure of the gene therapy protocol would result in miscarriage or a choice over abortion later in the pregnancy, both highly undesirable in comparison with discarding the affected embryo in the first place. The only rational reasons to undertake gene therapy in an embryo would be (1) if a couple were opposed to discarding or freezing embryos, in which case PGD technology is unlikely to be attractive at the outset, or (2) if a couple were both homozygous for a recessive condition, say, a couple both of whom had sickle cell disease. This latter possibility hardly seems a solid basis for the development of an experimental gene therapy intervention for human embryos, particularly if gene therapy were developed to where somatic gene therapy could treat the affected children.

The only plausible reason to insert genetic material into embryos would be for genetic enhancement. PGD to select the best embryo followed by insertion of advantageous genetic material would be the most logical method to produce genetic enhancement. The ethics of genetic enhancement is complex and beyond the scope of this paper. Suffice it to say that, in my view, some forms of genetic enhancement may be justifiable, in principle. An enhancement of the immune system to assist in fighting infectious diseases and/or to reduce the risk of cancer or autoimmune diseases may be an example of a justifiable intervention. Enhancement of other characteristics like intelligence or physical stature or coordination, assuming such things will ever be possible, are much more problematic. In any case, enhancement created through embryo manipulation (including PGD) rather than enhancement of fetuses or children brings no new concerns to the debate, other than those created by potential differences in risk or efficacy. Research in PGD could facilitate the development of genetic enhancement, so it is imperative that we clearly articulate the appropriate uses of the technology.

CONCLUSIONS

First, PGD is ethically permissible for its primary purpose, that is, to offer couples at high risk of bearing a child with a significant genetic condition the opportunity to have a healthy child without resorting to selective abortion.

Second, PGD currently is inefficient, burdensome, and expensive. When the costs are not being subsidized by research protocols, few couples are likely to find PGD attractive for its primary purpose.

Third, as with other forms of prenatal diagnosis, socially sanctioned uses need to be defined through broad social discourse. The option to avoid aborting a fetus through PGD does not justify the selection of embryos for less than serious genetic conditions. The definition of *serious* in this context needs much more work. . . .

And, [fourth], PGD provides a logical avenue for genetic enhancement, but ethical concerns over enhancement possibilities do not invalidate PGD for its contemporary use.

PGD provides a new opportunity for couples who desire prenatal diagnosis, but who want to avoid abortion of an affected fetus. Yet the potential power of this technology to manipulate human embryos raises a host of new concerns about the nature of the parent-child relationship and the limits of our biological control over succeeding generations. It remains to be determined whether this is a good trade of ethical concerns.

USING PREIMPLANTATION GENETIC DIAGNOSIS TO SAVE A SIBLING: THE STORY OF MOLLY AND ADAM NASH[1]

Bonnie Steinbock

Molly Nash was born on July 4, 1994 with multiple birth defects due to Fanconi anemia, a deadly genetic disease that causes bone marrow failure, eventually resulting in leukemia and other forms of cancer. Her best chance for survival was a bone marrow transplant from a perfectly matched sibling donor. Lisa and Jack Nash had considered having another child, not as a source of bone marrow but because they very much wanted another child. They had decided against it because there was a one-in-four chance that the infant would have the same illness as Molly, and aborting an affected fetus was not an option Mrs. Nash would consider. Then they learned about preimplantation genetic diagnosis (PGD), which would enable them to screen embryos for the disease, and implant only the healthy ones. Moreover, the embryos could also be tested to find which ones shared Molly's tissue type. The baby would be not only disease-free, but could also provide bone marrow to Molly. Moreover, because blood cells saved from the baby's umbilical cord and placenta could be used, there would be no need to extract the bone marrow from the baby's body, a procedure which is both painful and carries some risk.

The odds of producing an embryo that is disease-free, a perfect match, and capable of initiating a pregnancy are daunting. In January 1999, Lisa Nash produced 12 eggs, 2 of which were healthy matches. She became pregnant, but miscarried. In June she produced only four eggs, one of which was a match, but she did not become pregnant. In September, she produced eight eggs, only one of which was a healthy match, but again she did not become pregnant. Molly was getting sicker and her physician recommended proceeding with a transplant from a nonrelated donor, although the odds that such a transplant would work were virtually nil. The Nashes decided to try a different IVF clinic, one known for being more aggressive. Lisa's hormone regimen was changed and in December 1999, 24 eggs were retrieved. Only one was a match, but this time she became pregnant. She was confined to bed to prevent a miscarriage. On August 29, 2000, after 52 hours of labor (Lisa resisted a cesarean section because more cord blood could be collected during a vaginal birth), Adam Nash was delivered by C-section. In October 2000, doctors at Fairview-University Hospital in Minneapolis, which specializes in bone marrow transplants for children with Fanconi anemia, successfully transferred tissue from Adam's umbilical cord into Molly's body. Molly, by all accounts, is doing very well. She is back at school, or rather a visiting teacher, who must wear a mask during lessons, comes to her home. She takes ballet lessons. Her transplant did not cure her of Fanconi anemia, but merely prevented her developing leukemia. She is likely to suffer Fanconi's other complications, particularly cancers of the mouth and neck, but that is far off in the future.

Adam Nash was not unique in being conceived to save a sibling. Ten years earlier, another couple, Abe and Mary Ayala, decided to have Abe's vasectomy reversed, in the hopes that Mary would become pregnant with a child who could be a bone marrow donor for their daughter, Anissa, aged 17, who had been diagnosed with leukemia. Surprisingly, the reversal worked and Mary, aged 42, became pregnant. Moreover, the baby, Marissa Eve, born on April 3, 1990, turned out to be a compatible donor. At the time, the reaction from medical ethicists was generally negative. Philip Boyle, an associate at the Hastings Center, said, "It's troublesome, to say the least. It's outrageous that people would go to this length." Alexander Capron, professor of law and medicine at the University of Southern California, suggested that having a baby to save another child was ethically unacceptable because it violated the Kantian principle that persons are never to be used solely as a means to another person's ends. Others, however, challenged the view that Marissa was being used as a means only, or that she was not given the respect due to persons. The crucial thing, they argued, was that her parents and siblings intended to love the new addition to the family as much as her older brother and sister, whether or not she could donate bone marrow. The risk to Marissa was minimal; indeed, if Anissa already had a baby sister with compatible marrow, no one would have questioned using the infant as a donor. Why should the moral situation be different if the choice is to create a child in the hopes that she will be a donor?

Unlike the Ayalas, who thought they had completed their family, the Nashes wanted another child. When they were told that the same technique that could prevent the birth of a child with Fanconi might also identify a compatible donor for Molly, they jumped at the chance. As Mrs. Nash put it, "You could say it was an added perk to have Adam be the right bone marrow type, which would not hurt him in the least and would save Molly's life. We didn't have to think twice about it."[2]

Are there ethical objections to what the Nashes did? Some oppose PGD even for its ordinary use, to prevent the birth of a child with a serious disability.[3] Others do not oppose PGD in principle, but think that it should not be used to save the lives of existing children. One concern is that the parents of fatally ill children will be unable to refuse to go through IVF if it is presented as their only chance for saving their child. Furthermore, not every story of a Fanconi child has the happy ending afforded the Nash family. Some women go through cycle after cycle of IVF, only to fail to produce a compatible embryo, or to suffer repeated miscarriages.[4] It may be argued that this is not a choice that doctors should offer desperate parents, given that the odds of success are relatively low. At the same time, many women choose to undergo the rigors of IVF to have babies. If it is not unethical to give them this choice, is it unethical to give them the chance to save their child's life, if they are fully informed about the burdens and risks, and the odds of success?

Some ethicists object to the idea of having a baby for "spare parts." Clearly it would be wrong to create a baby for spare parts if that would be harmful to the child. One could not create a baby for his heart or lungs or even kidney. In what sense has Adam Nash been harmed? He owes his very existence to the fact that he was a perfect match for Molly. Of course, many embryos were discarded and this is considered immoral by those who view preimplantation embryos as tiny children. This, however, is not an objection to using PGD to create donors, but to PGD generally, and indeed to all of IVF.

Finally, many are profoundly disturbed by the possibility of "having babies to spec," of choosing who will be born based on their genetic characteristics. "If we can screen an embryo for tissue type, won't we one day screen for eye color or intelligence?"[5] Some ethicists fear that the use of PGD to get compatible donors today will lead to a world in which parents will be able to select their children's physical, mental, and emotional traits. From one perspective, PGD offers parents of desperately ill children the hope of a miracle. From another, it opens the door to "genetic engineering" and a new eugenics.

NOTES

1. Much of the factual material in this case study comes from Lisa Belkin, "The Made-to-Order Savior," *The New York Times Magazine*, July 1, 2001.
2. Denise Grady, "Son Conceived to Provide Blood Cells for Daughter," *The New York Times*, October 4, 2000, A24.
3. See Adrienne Asch, "Prenatal Diagnosis and Selective Abortion: A Challenge to Practice and Policy," *American Journal of Public Health*, Vol. 89, no. 11 (November 1999): 1649–1657. In this volume, pp. 523–533. Though Asch does not specifically discuss PGD, her objections to selective abortion extend to embryo selection and discard as well.
4. See Belkin, *op. cit.*
5. *Ibid.*

REPRODUCTIVE FREEDOM AND PREVENTION OF GENETICALLY TRANSMITTED HARMFUL CONDITIONS

Allen Buchanan, Dan W. Brock, Norman Daniels, and Daniel Wikler

Public Policy and Wrongful Life Issues It is perhaps fortunate that despite the great expansion of genetic information that will be available in the future both from pre-conception testing for genetic risks to potential offspring and from prenatal diagnosis of the genetic condition of a fetus, public policy may be able largely to avoid the most contentious and intractable wrongful life issues for at least two reasons. First, only a very small proportion of genetic abnormalities and diseases are both compatible with life and also so severe as to result in the affected child having a life not worth living. Second, courts and legislatures are likely to continue to be reluctant to permit wrongful life legal suits, both because damages covering the child's medical and extra care expenses can usually be obtained by a suit brought in the name of the parents instead of a wrongful life suit in the name of the child, and because uncertainty exists about how to assess damages for wrongful life. But regardless of what occurs in the courts, moral choice about whether conceiving a child or carrying a pregnancy to term would constitute an action of wrongful life will be increasingly faced in the future by parents or would-be parents.

A complicating factor is that the woman or couple making the choice will often face only a risk, not a certainty, that the child will not have a life worth living and that risk can vary from very low to approaching certainty. Whether it is morally wrong to conceive in the face of such risks' will depend in part on the woman's willingness and intention to do appropriate prenatal genetic testing and to abort her fetus if it is found to have a disease or condition incompatible with a worthwhile life.

As noted before, pursuing the moral complexities of abortion would take us too far afield here. Nevertheless, suppose, as the authors of this book believe, that the fetus at least through the first two trimesters is not a person and so aborting it then is morally permissible. Aborting a fetus found during the first two trimesters to have a disease that would make life a burden to the child prevents the creation of a person with a life not worth living; no wrongful life then occurs, so there is no question of moral wrong-doing. Even conceiving when there is a relatively high risk of genetic transmission of a disease incompatible with a life worth living could be morally acceptable so long as the woman firmly intends to test the fetus for the disease and to abort it if the disease is present.

On the other hand, a woman may intend not to test her fetus and abort it if such a disease is present, either because she considers abortion morally wrong or for other reasons. In that case, the higher the risk that the child will have a genetic disease or condition incompatible with a life worth living, the stronger the moral case that she does a serious moral wrong to that child in conceiving it and carrying it to term.

If a mother or anyone else knowingly and responsibly caused harm to an already born child so serious as to make its life no longer worth living, that would constitute extremely serious child abuse and be an extremely serious moral and legal wrong. In that case, however, the child would have had a worthwhile life that was taken away by whomever was guilty of the child abuse; the wrong to the child then is depriving it of a worthwhile life that it otherwise would have had. That is a different and arguably more serious wrong than wrongful life, where the alternative to the life not worth living is never having a life at all, and so not having a worthwhile life taken away. The wrong in nearly all cases of wrongful life is bringing into existence a child who will have a short life dominated by severe and

Reprinted with permission of the authors and publisher from their book, *From Chance to Choice* (Cambridge, UK: Cambridge University Press, 2000).

unremitting suffering—that is, being caused to undergo that suffering without compensating benefits.

How high must the risk be of a child having a genetic disease incompatible with a worthwhile life be for it to be morally wrong for the parents to conceive it and allow it to be born? There is, of course, no precise probability at which the risk of the harm makes it morally wrong to conceive or not to abort; different cases fall along a spectrum in the degree to which undertaking the risk is morally justified. How seriously wrong, if a wrong at all, it is to risk the conception and birth of a child with such a life will depend on several factors. How bad is the child's life, and in particular how severe and unremitting is its suffering? How high is the probability of the child having a genetic disease incompatible with a worthwhile life? How weighty are its parents' interests in having the child? For example, is this likely its parents' only opportunity to become parents, or are they already parents seeking to have additional children? How significant is the possibility of the parents having an unaffected child if this pregnancy is terminated and another conception pursued? How willing and able are the parents to support and care for the child while it lives?

These factors, and no doubt others unique to specific cases, will determine how strong the moral case is against individuals risking having a child who will not have a life worth living. It is worth underlining that any case for the wrongness of parents conceiving and bringing to term such a child depends on their having reasonable access to genetic testing, contraception, and abortion services, and this can require public provision and funding of these services for those who otherwise cannot afford them.

We hope that our analysis so far makes it clear why we believe that there are some cases, albeit very few, in which it would be clearly and seriously morally wrong for individuals to risk conceiving and having such a child. However, use of government power to force an abortion on an unwilling woman would be so deeply invasive of her reproductive freedom, bodily integrity, and right to decide about her own health care as to be virtually never morally justified. Allowing the child to be born and then withholding life support even over its parents' objections would probably be morally preferable. The government's doing this forcibly and over the parents' objections would be extraordinarily controversial, both morally and legally, but in true cases of wrongful life, the wrong done is sufficiently serious as to possibly justify doing so in an individual case. However, at the present time as a practical matter, the common and strong bias in favor of life, even in the face of serious suffering, makes it nearly inconceivable that public policy might authorize the government forcibly to take an infant from its parents, not for the purpose of securing beneficial treatment for it, but instead to allow it to die because it could not have a worthwhile life. Moreover, the risk of abuse of such a governmental power to intervene forcibly in reproductive choices to prevent a wrongful life is too great to warrant granting that power.

There is a stronger moral case for the use of government coercive power to prevent conception in some wrongful life cases. Similar power is now exercised by government over severely mentally disabled people who are sterilized to prevent them from conceiving. In such cases, the individual sterilized is typically deemed incompetent to make a responsible decision about conception, as well as unable to raise a child. Forced sterilization of a competent individual is more serious morally, but the harm to be prevented of wrongful life is more serious than the harm prevented in typical involuntary sterilization cases where the child would have a worthwhile life if raised by others. Nevertheless, the historical abuses of "eugenic sterilizations" . . . are enough to warrant not giving government the coercive power to prevent wrongful life conceptions unless their occurrence was very common and widespread. Wrongful life conceptions are sufficiently uncommon, and practical and moral difficulties in using the coercive power of government to prevent them sufficiently great, to rule out policies that prevent people from conceiving wrongful lives. Coercive government intrusion into reproductive freedom to prevent wrongful life would be wrong.

PRE-CONCEPTION INTERVENTIONS TO PREVENT CONDITIONS COMPATIBLE WITH A WORTHWHILE LIFE

The Human Genome Project and related research will produce information permitting genetic screening for an increasing number of genetically transmitted diseases, or susceptibilities to diseases and other harmful conditions. In the foreseeable future, our capacities for conception and prenatal screening for these diseases and conditions will almost certainly far outstrip our capacities for genetic or other therapy to correct for the harmful genes and their effects. The vast majority of decisions faced by prospective parents, consequently, will not be whether to pursue genetic or other therapy for their fetus or child, but instead whether to test for particular genetic risks and/or conditions and, when they are found to be present, whether to avoid conception or to terminate a pregnancy. Moreover, the vast majority of genetic risks that will be subject to testing will not be for conditions incompatible with a life worth living—the wrongful life cases—but rather for less severe conditions compatible with having a life well worth living.

These genetically transmitted conditions and diseases will take different forms. Sometimes their disabling features will be manifest during much of the individual's life, but still will permit a worthwhile life, as with most cases of Down syndrome, which is caused by a chromosomal abnormality. Sometimes the disease or condition will result in significant disability and a significantly shorter than normal life span, but not so disabling or short as to make the life not worth living, as with cystic fibrosis. Sometimes the disease or condition; although devastating in its effects on the afflicted individual's quality of life, will only manifest symptoms after a substantial period of normal life and unction, as with Huntington's chorea and Alzheimer's dementia.

When the genetically transmitted conditions could and should have been prevented, they will constitute what we have called cases of wrongful disability. But in which cases will the failure to prevent a genetically transmitted disability be morally wrong? Again, different cases fall along a spectrum in the degree of moral justification for undertaking or not undertaking to prevent the disability.

Whether failure to prevent a disability is wrong in specific cases will typically depend on many features of that case. For example, what is the relative seriousness of the disability for the child's well-being and opportunities? What measures are available to the child's parents to prevent the condition—such as abortion, artificial insemination by donor, or oocyte donation—how acceptable are these means to the prospective parents? Is it possible, and if so how likely, that they can conceive another child without the disabling condition, or will any child they conceive have or be highly likely to have the condition? If the disability can only be prevented by not conceiving at all, do the couple have alternative means, such as adoption, of becoming parents? When the condition can be prevented or its adverse impact compensated for, what means are necessary to do so?

These and other considerations can all bear on the threshold question: Is the severity of a genetically transmitted disability great enough that particular parents are morally obligated to prevent it, given the means necessary for them to do so; or is it sufficiently limited and minor that it need not be prevented, but is instead a condition that the child can reasonably be expected to live with?

Different prospective parents will answer this threshold question differently because they differ about such matters as the burdensomeness and undesirability of particular alternative methods of reproduction that may be necessary to prevent the disability, the seriousness of the impact of the particular disability on a person's well-being and opportunity, aspects of reproductive freedom such as the importance of having children and of having biologically related as opposed to adopted or only partially biologically related children, the extent of society's obligation and efforts to make special accommodations to eliminate or ameliorate the disability, and their willingness to assume the burdens of raising a child with the disability in question.

Because there are these multiple sources of reasonable disagreement bearing on the threshold question, and because the aspects of reproductive freedom at stake will usually be of substantial importance, public policy should usually permit prospective parents to make and act on their own judgments about whether they morally ought to prevent particular genetically transmitted disabilities for the sake of their child. But there is a systematic objection to all preconception wrongful disability cases that must be met in order to clear the way for individual judgments about specific cases.

To fix attention on the general problem in question, which is restricted to cases of genetically transmitted disease, let us imagine, a case, call it P1, in which a woman is told by her physician that she should not attempt to become pregnant now because she has a condition that is highly likely to result in moderate mental retardation in her child. Her condition is easily and fully treatable by taking a safe medication for one month. If she takes the medication and delays becoming pregnant for a month, the risk to her child will be eliminated and there is every reason to expect that she will have a normal child. Because the delay would interfere with her vacation travel plans, however, she does not take the medication, gets pregnant now, and gives birth to a child who is moderately retarded.

According to commonsense moral views, this woman acts wrongly, and in particular, wrongs her child by not preventing its disability for such a morally trivial reason, even if for pragmatic reasons people would oppose government intrusion into her decision. According to commonsense morality, her action is no different morally if she failed to take the medicine in a case, P2, in which the condition is discovered, and so the medicine must be taken, after conception when she is already pregnant. Nor is it different morally than if she failed to provide a similar medication to her born child, in a case, P3, if doing so is again necessary to prevent moderate mental retardation in her child. It is worth noting that in most states in this country, her action in P3 would probably constitute medical neglect, and governmental child protection agencies could use coercive measures, if necessary, to ensure the child's treatment.

This suggests that it might only be because her reproductive freedom and her right to decide about her own health care are also involved in P1 that we are reluctant to coerce her decision, if necessary, there as well. On what Derek Parfit has called the "no difference" view, the view of commonsense morality, her failure to use the medication to prevent her child's mental retardation would be equally seriously wrong, and for the same reason, in each of the three cases (Parfit 1984). But her action in P1, which is analogous in relevant respects to preconception genetic screening to prevent disabilities, has a special feature that makes it not so easily shown to be wrong as commonsense morality might suppose.

What is the philosophical problem at the heart of wrongful disability cases like P1? As with wrongful life cases, in which the necessary comparison of life with nonexistence is thought to create both philosophical and policy problems, so also in wrongful disability cases do the philosophical and policy problems arise from having to compare a disabled existence with not having existed at all. But the nature of the philosophical problems in wrongful life and wrongful disability cases are in fact quite different. The philosophical objections we considered wrongful life cases centered on whether it is coherent to compare an individual's quality of life with never having existed at all—that is, with nonexistence—and whether merely possible persons can have moral rights or be owed moral obligations. In wrongful disability cases, a person's disability uncontroversially leaves him or her with a worthwhile life. The philosophical problem, as noted earlier, is how this is compatible with the commonsense view that it would be wrong to prevent the disability.

The special difficulty in wrongful disability cases, which Derek Parfit has called the "nonidentity problem," is that it would not be better for the person with the disability to have had it prevented, since that could only be done by preventing him or her from ever having existed at all. Preventing the disability would deny the disabled individual a worthwhile, although disabled life. That is because the disability could only have been prevented either by conceiving at a different time and/or under different circumstances (in which case a different child would have been conceived) or by terminating the pregnancy (in which case this child also never would have been born, although a different child may or may not have been conceived instead). None of these possible means of preventing the disability would be better for the child with the disability—all would deny him or her a worthwhile life.

But if the mother's failure to prevent the disability did not make her child worse off than he or she would have been without the intervention, then her failure to prevent it seems not to harm her child. And if she did not harm her child by not preventing its disability, then why does she wrong her child morally by failing to do so? How could making her child better off, or at least not worse off, by giving it a life worth living, albeit a life with a significant disability, wrong it? A wrong action must be bad for someone, but her choice to create her child with its disability is bad for no one, so she does no wrong. Of course, there is a sense in which it is bad for her child to have the disability, in comparison with being without it, but there is nothing the mother could have done to enable that child to be born without the disability, and so nothing she does or omits doing is bad for her child.

So actions whose harmful effects would constitute seriously wrongful child abuse if done to an existing child are no harm, and so not wrong, if their harmful effects on a child are inextricable from the act of bringing that child into existence with a worthwhile life! This argument threatens to undermine common and firmly held moral judgments, as well as public policy measures, concerning prevention of such disabilities for children.

Actual versus Possible Persons David Heyd has accepted the implications of this argument and concludes that in all of what he calls "genesis" choices—that is, choices that inextricably involve whether a particular individual will be brought into existence—only the interest of actual persons, not those of possible persons such as the disabled child in case P1, are relevant to the choice (Heyd 1992). So in case P1, the effects on the parents and the broader society, such as the greater childrearing costs and burdens of having the moderately retarded child instead of taking the medication and having a normal child a month later are relevant to the decision. But the effects on and interests of the child who would be moderately retarded are not relevant. In cases P2 and P3, on the other hand, Heyd presumably would share the commonsense moral view that the fundamental reason the woman's action would be wrong is the easily preventable harm that she allows her child to suffer. In these situations, the preventable harm to her child is the basis of the moral wrong she does her child.

In Parfit's "no difference" view, the woman's action in P1 is equally wrong, and for the same reason, as her action in P2 and P3. We share with Parfit, in opposition to Heyd, the position that the woman's action in P1 is wrong because of the easily preventable effect on her child. But we do not accept the "no difference" thesis. We will suggest a reason why her action in P1 may not be as seriously wrong as in P2 or P3, and also suggest that the reason her action is wrong in P1 is similar to but nevertheless importantly different from the reason it is wrong in P2 and P3.

As Parfit notes, the difficulty is identifying and formulating a moral principle that implies that the woman's action in P1 is seriously wrong, but does not have unacceptable implications for other cases. Before proceeding further, we must emphasize that we cannot explore this difficulty fully here. The issues are extraordinarily complex and involve testing the implications of such a principle in a wide variety of cases outside of the genetic context that is our concern here (e.g., in population policy contexts and, in particular, avoiding what Parfit calls the "Repugnant Conclusion" and explaining what he calls the Asymmetry"). Its relationship to other principles and features of a moral theory must also be explained, including that to the principle applicable to P2 and P3 (Parfit 1984).

The apparent failure to account for common and firmly held moral views in the genetics cases of wrongful disabilities like P1 constitutes one of the most important practical limitations (problems of population policy are another) of traditional ethical theories and of their principles of beneficence—doing good—and nonmaleficence—not causing or preventing harm. Where the commonsense moral judgment about cases like P1 is that the woman is morally wrong to go ahead and have the disabled child instead of waiting and having a normal child, the principles of traditional ethical theories apparently fail to support that judgment. New or revised moral principles appear to be needed. What alternatives and resources, either within or beyond traditional moral principles or theories, could account for and explain the wrong done in wrongful disability cases?

Person-Affecting Moral Principles Perhaps the most natural way to account for the moral wrongful disability cases like P1 is to abandon the specific feature of typical moral principles about obligations to prevent or not cause harm which generates difficulty when we move from standard cases of prevention of harm to existing persons, as in P3, to harm prevention in genesis cases like P1. That feature is what philosophers have called the "person-affecting" property of principles of beneficence and nonmaleficence. Recall that earlier we appealed to principle M: Those individuals responsible for a child's, or other dependent person's, welfare are morally required not to let her suffer a serious harm or disability or a serious loss of happiness or good that they could have prevented without imposing substantial burdens or costs or loss of benefits on themselves or others.

The person-affecting feature of M is that the persons who will suffer the harm if it is not prevented and not suffer it if it is prevented must be one and the same distinct individual. If M is violated, a distinct child or dependent person is harmed without good reason, and so the moral wrong is done to that person. Since harms to persons must always be harms to some person, it may seem that there is no alternative to principles that are person-affecting, but that is not so. The alternative is clearest if we follow Derek Parfit by distinguishing "same person" from "same number" choices.

In same person choices, the same persons exist in each of the different alternative courses of action from which an agent chooses. Cases P2 and P3 above were same person choices (assuming in P2 that the fetus is or will become a person, though that is not essential to the point)—the harm of moderate retardation prevented is to the woman's fetus or born child. In same number choices, the same number of persons exist in each of the alternative courses of action from which an agent chooses, but the identities of some of the persons—that is, who exists in those alternatives—is affected by the choice. P1 is a same number but not a same person choice—the woman's choice affects which child will exist. If the woman does not take the medication and wait to conceive, she gives birth to a moderately retarded child, whereas if she takes the medication and waits to conceive, she gives birth to a different child who is not moderately retarded.

The concept of "harm," arguably, is necessarily comparative, so the concept of "harm prevention" may seem necessarily person-affecting; this is why harm prevention principles seem not to apply to same number, different person choices like P1. But it would be a mistake to think that non-person-affecting principles, even harm prevention principles, are not coherent. Suppose for simplicity that the harm in question in P1 from the moderate retardation is suffering and limited opportunity. Then in P1, if the woman chooses to have the moderately retarded child, she causes suffering and limited opportunity to exist that would be prevented and not exist if she chooses to take the medication and wait to conceive a different normal child. An example of a non-person-affecting principle that applies to P1 is:

> N: Individuals are morally required not to let any child or other dependent person for whose welfare they are responsible experience serious suffering or limited opportunity or serious loss of happiness or good, if they can act so that, without affecting the number of persons who will exist and without imposing substantial burdens or costs or loss of benefits on themselves or others, no child or other dependent person for whose welfare they are responsible will experience serious suffering or limited opportunity or serious loss of happiness or good.

Any suffering and limited opportunity must, of course, be experienced by some person—they cannot exist in disembodied form—and so in that sense N remains person-affecting. But N does not require that the same individuals who experience suffering and limited opportunity in one alternative exist without the suffering and limited opportunity in the other alternative; it is a same number, not a same person, principle. N allows the child who does not experience the suffering and limited opportunity to be a different person from the child who does; that is why the woman's action in P1 is morally wrong according to N, but not according to M. If the woman in P1 does take the medication and wait to conceive a normal child, she acts so as to make the suffering and limited opportunity "avoidable by substitution," as Philip G. Peters, Jr. has put it (Peters 1989).

A different way of making the same point is to say that this principle for the prevention of suffering applies not to distinct individuals, so that the prevention of suffering must make a distinct individual better off than if he or she would have been, as M requires, but to the classes of individuals who will exist if the suffering is or is not prevented, as N does (Peters 1989; Bayles 1976). Assessing the prevention of suffering by the effect on classes of persons, as opposed to distinct individuals, also allows for avoidability by substitution—an individual who does not suffer if one choice is made is substituted for a different person who does suffer if the other choice is made. A principle applied to the classes of all persons who will exist in each of two or more alternative courses of action will be a non–person-affecting principle.

The preceding discussion referred only to the prevention of harm or loss of opportunity because that is the focus of this chapter. However, it should be noted that N allows, for the same reasons as does M, the weighing of securing happiness or good against preventing suffering and loss of opportunity. If it did not, but required only preventing serious suffering, then N would require not creating a child who would experience serious suffering, but also great happiness and good, in favor of creating a child who would suffer less, but experience no compensating happiness or good, even though the latter child on balance would have a substantially worse life. We note as well that we have not defined "serious" as it functions in either M or N; it is difficult to do so in a sufficiently general yet precise way to make the application of the principle simple and straightforward for a wide range of cases. Judgment must be used in applying N. The seriousness of suffering and loss of opportunity, or loss of happiness and good, that could be prevented must be assessed principally in light of their potential impact on the child's life, the probability of that impact, and the possibility and probability of compensatory measures to mitigate that impact. Applying N requires judgment as well regarding what are "substantial burdens or costs, or loss of benefits, on themselves or others." For example, how serious are possible moral objections by the parents to the use of abortion, and how great are the financial costs or medical risks of having an alternative child using assisted reproduction technologies, and so forth?

We do not claim that all moral principles concerning obligations to prevent harm, or of beneficence and nonmaleficence more generally, are non–person-affecting, and so we do not reject principle M. In typical cases of harm where a distinct individual is made worse off, the moral principles most straightforwardly applicable to them are person-affecting. Our claim is only that an adequate moral theory should include as well non–person-affecting principles like N. How these principles are related, as well as what principles apply to different number cases in a comprehensive moral theory, involves deep difficulties in moral theory that we cannot pursue here. In this respect, we do not propose a full solution to the nonidentity problem. . . .

REFERENCES

Bayles, M. 1976. "Harm to the Unconceived." *Philosophy and Public Affairs* 5(3): 292–304.

Heyd, D. 1992. *Genetics: Moral Issues in the Creation of People.* Berkeley, CA: University of California Press.

Parfit, D. 1984. *Reasons and Persons.* Oxford: Clarendon Press.

Peters, P.G. 1989. "Protecting the Unconceived: Nonexistence, Avoidability, and Reproductive Technology." *Arizona Law Review* 31(3): 487–548.

MAPPING THE HUMAN GENOME

Implications for Genetic Testing, Genetic Counseling, and Genetic Interventions

HEREDITY AND HUMANITY

Have No Fear. Genes Aren't Everything.

Francis S. Collins, Lowell Weiss, and Kathy Hudson

Forty-eight years ago, James Watson and Francis Crick introduced DNA's elegant double helix to the world in the pages of *Nature*. With extravagant understatement, they began their report by noting that DNA's "structure has novel features which are of considerable biological interest." Four months ago, with the publication of the sequence and the analysis of the human genome, scientists offered further evidence of just how considerable. Researchers gained a wealth of fresh insights into the miracle of life, and uncovered new mysteries that will occupy biomedical researchers for years to come.

Unfortunately the new focus on the genome has left some people with the impression that DNA's power is perhaps *too* considerable—that is, that genes are too great a factor in defining who we are. This fear is understandable. It seems that every morning we awake to a news story presenting yet another way in which our genes appear to be controlling us, like the proverbial tail that wags the dog: "Scientists Zero in on 'Genius Gene'"; "Kennedy Tragedies Linked to 'Risk-Taking Gene'"; "Diabetes Gene Poses Risk for Latinos"; "Scientists Say a Study of Brothers Proves Existence of a 'Gay Gene.'"

With a torrent of headlines such as these, reasonable people have come to fear that the more we learn about the human genome, the more we will see that every aspect of the human condition—from illness to intelligence to fear itself—is just the inevitable product of an unyielding, unfeeling genetic code. For this reason, they worry that our new genomic knowledge represents not a giant leap for humankind but rather a giant demotion. Perhaps we are just marionettes being tugged along by the strands of our DNA. Perhaps our lives are nothing more than a formulaic drama, with a plot line that was finalized before our birth.

Reprinted with permission from *The New Republic*, June 25, 2001.

Fortunately, ten years of intensive study of the human genome have provided ample evidence that these fears of genetic determinism are unwarranted. It has shown us definitively that we human beings are far more than the sum of our genetic parts. Needless to say, our genes play a major, formative role in human development—and in many of the processes of human disease; but high-tech molecular studies as well as low-tech (but still eminently useful) studies of identical and fraternal twins make it perfectly evident that our genes are not all-determining factors in the human experience.

To put it starkly, we have seen nothing in recent studies to suggest that nature's role in development is larger, or nurture's role smaller, than we previously thought. This is certainly an exciting time in genetic research; but if nature were to take advantage of this klieg-lights moment and boldly declare that it is in charge, history would remember it the same way we remember Alexander Haig.

In large measure, the fear of genetic determinism stems from misconceptions of how genetics works. As high school students, our first exposure to genetics came through the story of Gregor Mendel's experiments with his garden peas. First, we learned that each parent pea plant contributed one copy of each of its genes to its offspring. Second, we learned that certain genes were "dominant" and others "recessive. (The gene for white flowers [*W*] is dominant, while the gene for purple flowers [*w*] is recessive.) And third, we learned that a plant would need to inherit two copies of a recessive gene to manifest a recessive trait, but only one copy of a dominant gene to manifest a dominant trait. Offspring—to use the example of flower color—would grow white flowers if they inherited any of the following gene patterns: *Ww, wW,* or *WW.* Purple flowers, in contrast result only from one combination: *ww.*

All of the above is correct—for flowers and for pea plants. But when it comes to the study of complex human beings, we must take Mendel's peas with a giant shake of salt. Despite what your high school biology teacher told you, Mendelian rules do not apply even to eye color or hair color. Truth be told, they do not apply to most characteristics of peas or other plants, either. As Robin Marantz Henig documented in her wonderful book *The Monk in the Garden,* Mendel himself came to question the validity of his work on peas when he turned to the study of the hawkweed and got much more complex and confusing results.

This is not to say that deterministic Mendelian rules never apply to human traits and disorders. One classic case in which they certainly apply is sickle-cell anemia, a painful and often life-threatening disease that is caused by the presence of an abnormal form of hemoglobin (hemoglobin S); and that disproportionately afflicts families of African descent. Like purple flowers in pea plants, sickle-cell anemia is a recessive trait; it manifests itself in those who inherit two copies of the hemoglobin S gene.

And yet even in this case, human genetics proves far more complicated, and far less deterministic, than Mendel's pea flowers. It turns out that every case of sickle-cell anemia is not created equal. Even when patients have the same two copies of the hemoglobin S gene, the disease may manifest itself in different ways. This is in part because a separate set of genes in the genome—genes that code for fetal hemoglobin—can counteract some of the ill effects of the adult hemoglobin S genes. In most people, fetal hemoglobin genes turn off a few months after birth and the adult hemoglobin genes take over; but sometimes the fetal hemoglobin genes are "leaky," and they continue to produce fetal hemoglobin even into adulthood. When people with two copies of the hemoglobin S gene also inherit leaky fetal hemoglobin genes, their sickle-cell symptoms are usually much less severe. So sickle-cell anemia, widely considered to be the classic single-gene Mendelian disease, is not so clear-cut after all.

Phenylketonuria (PKU), a rare disorder that can cause severe mental retardation, is an even better example of how the most deterministic of genes may not determine much in real life. Like sickle-cell anemia, PKU is a recessive trait. If a child inherits two copies of the PKU gene, then he will get the disease. And yet, thanks to the newborn screening program now in place in all fifty states, the child will never experience mental retardation or the other devastating effects of PKU. Since the illness results from an inability to metabolize the amino acid phenylalanine, if you simply remove foods with phenylalanine from the child's diet, he or she will live a normal and healthy life. PKU is one hundred percent hard-wired in the genes. Yet it can be effectively cured with a one hundred percent environmental intervention.

Keep in mind also that sickle-cell anemia and PKU are about the closest people come to following Mendel's rules. When we look at other human diseases, the picture is far more complicated, with many more genes involved and an even greater involvement of environmental factors. Consider the case of juvenile (or type I) diabetes. Despite what researchers and reporters may have projected to the public over the past two years, there is no single "gene for diabetes." Instead, there are fifteen or more genes that may team up in an array of combinations to produce diabetes. In one person, having variants in five of these genes might be enough to cause symptoms, while in another it might take nine variants.

These gene-gene interactions represent just one layer of complexity. Gene-environment interactions represent an entirely different story. We now believe that type I cases require not only a series of gene variants but also an external environmental trigger—probably a childhood viral infection. If that is the case, it is entirely possible that in the near future researchers will identify the viral offender, produce a childhood vaccine against it for those who are genetically at risk, and ease the fears of parents all over the world.

It follows from all this that the common use of the shorthand term "the gene for illness X" by scientists and journalists is deeply misleading. If illness X is not one of the rare single-gene Mendelian diseases, then the so-called "gene for illness X" is more correctly described as "a gene variant that may, in combination with other genetic and environmental factors, increase the risk of developing illness X." Just think of how many times in recent years we have heard the inherently deterministic label "the gene for breast cancer" in reference to the gene BRCA1 and BRCA2. For starters, BRCA1 and BRCA2 are actually *anti*-cancer genes. It is when someone inherits an abnormality in these genes that she can develop breast cancer or ovarian cancer.

But the larger point that not everyone who has abnormalities in the BRCA1 or BRCA2 genes develops breast cancer, and not everyone who develops breast cancer has BRCA1 or BRCA2 abnormalities. Calling them "the genes for breast cancer" hopelessly confuses a correlation with a cause. And recall also the case of PKU: despite the fact that it is a single-gene Mendelian disease, nurture (in the form of a change of diet) still can trump nature. So yes, gene variants can and do increase our risk of developing diseases. But only extremely rarely do they determine our fate.

Why, then, all the fuss about the genomic revolution in medicine? If disease susceptibility is not deterministic, will it be all that revealing to discover the glitches that all of us have within our DNA? It most certainly will. First, identifying our individual predispositions to future illness will allow individualized programs of preventive medicine, in which we modify lifestyle, diet, and medical surveillance to reduce the risk of illness. In most cases, the resulting treatments will not be the all-or-nothing scenario of PKU; they will have much more in common with the steps that many of us are already taking to reduce our serum cholesterol (for which the set point has strong genetic roots) in an effort to lower our risk of heart disease.

More importantly, perhaps, every disease-susceptibility gene that scientists identify will shine a bright light on the molecular pathway by which that illness comes about. The proper understanding of those pathways offers us the best opportunity ever to develop targeted therapies that work. Even if someone's case of heart disease or cancer has only weak genetic roots, the knowledge of the pathway involved, discerned by the study of genetics, can form the basis of a treatment that may cure his or her disease.

But what about non-disease-related traits, such as intelligence and violent behavior? When it comes to behavioral traits like these, after all, a little genetic determinism can go a long way. The discovery of a prevalent gene variant strongly correlated with violence could have a profound effect upon our millennia-old understanding of free will, and weigh down the scales of justice in two equally dangerous ways. If someone who commits a violent crime has the gene variant, his lawyer could use a DNA defense ("If it's in the gene, the man is clean!"), and the defendant could well be seen by a judge and jury as not responsible for his actions. Yet it is also possible to imagine a scenario in which someone who has never even contemplated a violent act is found to have the gene variant and then subjected to the presumption of guilt (or even sent away to a postmodern-day leper colony) for the rest of his life.

If genes truly controlled behavior, our justice system and its guiding principle of equal protection would not be the only casualties. How would our concept of equal opportunity survive? What about the idea of merit? Just think of the frightening "genetocracy" depicted in the movie *Gattaca* (and note the letters that make up its name), a world in which children are assigned to castes at birth, based on an assessment of their intellectual capacity and professional potential as inscribed in their DNA.

These fears, too, are unwarranted. To be sure, scientists will find many behavioral factors in the genes. Researchers have long known that there is one extremely common genetic factor that confers at least a tenfold increase in the propensity to exhibit criminally violent behavior. It is called the Y chromosome. No one has suggested that all those who possess this genetic marker—that is, all males—ought to be seen as lacking free will or inherently possessing criminal intent. More to the point, the case of the Y chromosome is an almost absurd extreme. In the vast majority of cases, genetic factors exert a much smaller influence on patterns of behavior and capability.

In 1998, for example, a researcher reported the discovery of the first gene correlated with general cognitive ability. Reports in the press lauded it as the "genius gene." Given humankind's history of eugenics (the hard diabolical Hitler kind and the soft insidious *Bell Curve* kind), the discovery of a gene linked to intelligence was genuinely explosive stuff. In reality, however, the so-called "genius gene" was found to give a boost of exactly two points on IQ tests. That's right: two points. Valuable science, yes. Society-altering discovery, no.

New findings that flow from the completion of the human genome draft are likely to follow the same complicated and undeterministic pattern. According to the combined wisdom of twin studies and molecular studies, human behaviors appear to be like the most complex diseases: if a particular behavior has a heritable component at all, it involves the interaction of numerous genes and numerous environmental influences. Surely this should come as no surprise. After all, behavior is a product of the brain, which is by far our most complex organ, and one that continues to develop throughout a lifetime of living and learning.

To build on a metaphor offered by the biologist Johnjoe McFadden, looking for genes that encode our unique behaviors and the other products of our minds is like analyzing the strings of a violin or the keys of a piano in the hope of finding the *Emperor* Concerto. Indeed, the human genome can be thought of as the grandest of orchestras, with each of our approximately thirty thousand genes representing a unique instrument playing in the wondrous and massive concert that is molecular biology. Each instrument is essential, and each must be in tune to produce the proper (and highly sophisticated) musical sound. Likewise, genes are essential to the development of the brain, and must be "in tune" to produce functioning neurons and neurotransmitters. But this emphatically does not imply that genes make minds any more than a viola or a piccolo makes a sonata.

For many of us, there is still another powerful reason, wholly apart from the mechanics of science, to reject the notion that DNA is the core substance of our humanity. It is the belief that a higher power must also play some role in who we are and what we become. Of course, some scientists and writers dismiss this spiritual notion as pure superstition. Thus Richard Dawkins has observed that "we are machines built by DNA whose purpose is to make copies of the same DNA. . . . It is every living object's sole reason for living." Really? Is there nothing about being human that is different from being a bacterium or a slug?

Can the study of genetics and molecular biology really account for the universal intrinsic knowledge of right and wrong common to all human cultures in all eras (though all of us have trouble acting on this knowledge)? Can it account for the unselfish form of love that the Greeks called *agape?* Can it account for the experience of feeling called to sacrifice for others even when our own DNA may be placed at risk? While evolutionary biologists proffer various explanations for human behaviors that undermine the efficient propagation of our genes, there is something about those claims that rings hollow to us.

The notion that science alone holds all the secrets of our existence has become a religion of its own. The faith of Dawkins and others in biology seems even greater than the faith of the simple believer in God. Science is the proper way to understand the natural, of course; but science gives us no reason to deny that there are aspects of human identity that fall outside the sphere of nature, and hence outside the sphere of science. For most believers, God has no meaning unless God is more than nature. If God is more than nature, then studying the natural may never reveal the true mystery.

In the end, we must acknowledge that we human beings have only scratched the surface of self-understanding. The structure of DNA does hold considerable interest for this line of inquiry; but it would be the purest form of hubris to take our rudimentary knowledge of our genetic code, craft theories about it with our puny minds, and declare that nature has once and for all trumped nurture and toppled God. This is the kind of arrogance that humans alone seem to possess, and that genes alone could never explain.

GENETICS AND THE MORAL MISSION OF HEALTH INSURANCE

Thomas H. Murray

All men are created equal. So reads one of the United States of America's founding political documents. This stirring affirmation of equality was not meant as a claim that all people are equivalent in all respects. Surely the drafters of the Declaration of Independence and the Constitution were as aware then as we are now of the wondrous variety of humankind. People differ in their appearance, their talents, and their character, among other things, and those differences matter enormously.

The commitment to equality embodied in our political tradition is not a claim that people, in fact, are indistinguishable from one another. Rather it is an assertion that before this government, this system of laws and courts, all persons are to be given equal standing, and all persons must be treated with equal regard.

Human genetics, in contrast, is a *science of inequality*—a study of human particularity and difference. One of the most difficult challenges facing us in the coming flood tide of genetic information is how to assimilate these evidences of human differences without undermining our commitment to political, legal, and moral equality.

The information about human differences pouring forth from the science of human genetics provides us with a multitude of opportunities to treat people differently according to some aspect of their genetic makeup. Deciding which uses of this information are just and which are unjust will require us to reexamine the ethical significance of a wide variety of human differences and the larger social purposes of a variety of institutions, among them health, life, and other forms of insurance.

Health insurance in the United States has moved from a system based mostly on community rating where, in a given community, all people pay comparable rates, to a system where the cost to the purchasers of insurance is based on the expected claims—a risk- or experience-based system. This movement has significant ethical as well as economic overtones. Community rating was a system that reflected a notion of community responsibility for providing health care for its members, where the qualifying principle was community membership. Other differences, such as preexisting risks, did not count as morally relevant distinctions. Risk- and experience-based systems presume that it is fair to charge different prices, or to refuse to insure people entirely, if they will need expensive health care.

Reprinted with permission from Thomas H. Murray, "Genetics and the Moral Mission of Health Insurance," *Hastings Center Report* 22, no. 6 (1992): 12–17.

Editor's note: Most footnotes have been deleted. Students who want to follow up on sources should consult the original article.

Such systems treat predicted need for care as a morally relevant difference among persons that justifies differential access to health insurance, and through it, to health care. But this presumes precisely what is in question: what are good moral reasons for treating people differently with respect to access to health insurance and health care?

Risk- and experience-rated systems are now dominant in private health insurance in the United States, having largely replaced community rating. This trend, coupled with the rapid growth in the cost of health insurance for employers, creates a situation in which risk-oriented genetic testing could become an important, complicating feature.

We may create a catch-22 so that only people who are unlikely to need health insurance can afford it. Genetic testing may permit a much more complete and refined classification of people into risk categories, and so move us further away from sharing the financial burdens of illness and further in the direction of individualized premiums based on individual risk factors. Genetic risk testing is important because it exposes the logic of a system that provides access to health insurance to those least likely to need it.

GENETICS AND DISTRIBUTIVE JUSTICE

Distributive justice, as the term implies, concerns the distribution of social goods or ills: in its simplest formulation it holds that like cases are to be treated alike and unlike cases are to be treated differently. All depends, obviously, on how we fill in the material conditions of this purely formal statement of comparative justice. When we are asking about a particular occasion of just or unjust treatment, the question commonly takes the form, What makes these cases like or unlike in a morally relevant way? Failure to state a morally relevant reason for treating people differently opens one to the charge that one's action was arbitrary, capricious, and unjust.

Human genetics provides a large and rapidly growing set of differences among persons that may be used to try to justify unequal treatment. For many genetic differences and many distributions of social goods, the moral relevance of the difference seems transparently obvious. Height, for example, is largely determined by genetics. Does it make any sense to say that it was unfair to allow Kareem Abdul Jabaar to play center in the National Basketball Association for many years, but not me, just because he is taller than I am, and our differences in height are genetic, rather than anything we can claim credit for accomplishing? Most people would judge that to be absurd. In this instance a genetic difference—height—constitutes a morally relevant difference that justifies treating people differently. That same difference, however, would not justify treating us differently if, for example, we were accused of a crime, or being judged on our literary accomplishments, or in need of health care.

A judgment that something is or is not a morally relevant reason does not take place in a social vacuum. As in the case of height, a particular attribute or trait can count as a relevant difference under some circumstances but be utterly irrelevant in others. Whether some particular difference is relevant depends upon what conception of distributive justice applies to the specific case. Michael Walzer describes three concepts that are often taken as primary: free exchange, desert, and need.[1] Free exchange is exemplified by the market where people exchange goods, services, and money. Desert appears to be the operative principle where prizes or championships are being distributed. It is also important in, for example, determining which individuals will be given positions requiring certain skills. Need seems to be an appropriate criterion for allocating certain goods, for example food in a time of scarcity. Most would judge the hoarding of or gorging on food by people whose neighbors are starving as indecent and unjust. This would be true even if the hungry neighbors had nothing to exchange that the person with food wanted; and it would be true even if the starving people had done nothing to "deserve" food—indeed the notion of having to "deserve" a good here seems grossly out of place.

No one of these three criteria for distribution can cover all cases. Variants of one or the other, or sometimes combinations of more than one, can typically be found underlying our considered social judgments about what constitutes a fair distribution of a particular social good. The question that must be addressed here is whether and in what ways genetic (or other health-related) differences among individuals count as morally relevant reasons for treating people differently with respect to insurance, especially health insurance. That, in turn, requires asking what kind of good health care is, and what principle or principles should guide its distribution.

WHAT KIND OF GOOD IS HEALTH CARE?

Citizens of the United States do not speak with one voice on the question. We do not all agree as to what kind of good health care is, on what principle or principles it should be allocated, or on what count as morally relevant differences among persons in such allocation. In fact, voices can be found that call for health care to be distributed in whole or in part through the free exchange of the market, desert, or need. Nevertheless, we can examine our public policies and public debates for evidences of what we consider just in the allocation of health care. We have two massive public programs, Medicare and Medicaid, to provide health care to groups of people who would otherwise find it difficult or impossible to obtain—the old and the poor. The concerns manifested by these two programs cannot be explained by principles of free exchange or desert; rather they appear to reflect an underlying notion of health care as a response to need.

Health insurance, whether public or private, figures in to the extent that it affects access to health care. If one's access to health care were perfectly correlated with whether one had health insurance—that is, one could get health care if and only if one had health insurance—then whatever we concluded about justice and health care would apply equally to health insurance as the instrument by which people gain access to care. In practice, the correlation is far from perfect. People with health insurance may not get the care they need for a variety of reasons, such as other obstacles to access—for example, geography. Also, lack of health *insurance* does not automatically mean lack of health *care;* people with acute health care needs can usually find an individual or institution to treat them. Such "uncompensated care" does not solve the problem of lack of access to care via public programs or private insurance, as the timing of care is often far from optimal and the struggle to get it humiliating. But it does provide a further clue that we regard health care as a response to a need, rather than something that can be left entirely to the market or treated as a matter of desert.

Imagine someone entering an electronics store and pleading to be given a VCR. They cannot pay for it (free exchange). They might try to claim they deserve it (perhaps because they actually can operate the timed-record function), but that is unlikely to persuade the store owner. They could say that they need a VCR. But in the absence of some highly unusual circumstances tying possession of a VCR into some genuine need, their request will be dismissed. People do not *need* VCRs, certainly not in the way they sometimes need health care. In contrast, imagine someone going to a hospital emergency room bleeding badly. We know that such a person should be treated immediately and the problem of how to pay for that treatment sorted out afterwards.

Having health insurance is a way to pay for such treatment—the cost of treating a serious illness can easily exceed an average family's ability to pay for it. Health insurance is, for most people, the means to the end of health care. It is not the good of health care itself. But to the extent that it determines who does and who does not have access to care, and who has the peace of mind that comes with knowing that if care is needed it will be available, access to health insurance is a matter of justice.

GENETIC TESTING: THE CHALLENGE FOR HEALTH INSURANCE

Research in human genetics, such as the Genome Project, is likely to increase dramatically our ability to predict whether individuals are at risk for particular diseases. There are tests currently offered for diseases such as Huntington's, where the presence of the gene assures that the individual will develop the disease if he or she lives long enough. There are tests for carrier status such as cystic fibrosis where two copies of the defective gene—one from each parent—must be inherited in order for symptomatic disease to occur. And there will be tests for diseases of complex etiology such as heart disease, cancer, stroke, lung disease, and the like. For certain relatively rare genes there will be a strong connection between having the gene and having the disease. Yet most of the common killing and disabling diseases are more likely to have a complex variety of causes, including perhaps several genes each of which has some predictive relationship with the disease. These risk-oriented genetic predictors potentially are very interesting to employers and insurers.

Genetic information, in fact, is used now by insurers. There may be considerable genetic information in one's medical record. If your policy is being individually underwritten, that entire record can be copied and shipped to the prospective insurer and that information used to justify increasing the price or denying health insurance altogether. But this begs a prior question: should information about genetic differences be used at all in health insurance?

One argument against paying any special attention to genetic predictors of risk is that insurers already use risk predictors that have genetic components. Coronary artery disease is an example. It is well known that people with higher levels of cholesterol, especially the low-density-lipoprotein component, are at higher risk of coronary artery disease and subsequent heart attacks. It also seems clear that an individual's cholesterol level is at least in part determined by genetics. Variations in individual metabolism can have a substantial impact on a person's cholesterol level, such that two people can be equally virtuous (or careless) in diet and exercise and yet have very different cholesterol levels, and, presumably, very different risks for coronary artery disease and heart attack.

In time it is likely that researchers will discover a number of genes that affect cholesterol metabolism and, presumably, cholesterol level, arterial disease, and the risk of a heart attack. We may be able to construct a genetic profile of an individual's risk of heart disease. Does such a predictive index differ in any ethically significant way from today's cholesterol test, which has not evoked similar objections?

Genetic tests differ from a cholesterol test in that the latter, even if significantly influenced by genetics, is still in some measure under the individual's control. The risk of heart attack is affected by a variety of health-related behaviors including diet, exercise, stress, and smoking. To the extent that people can be held responsible for their behavior, their cholesterol level is something for which they have some responsibility. On the other hand, people cannot be said to be responsible for their genes. An old maxim in ethics is "Ought implies can." You should not be held morally accountable for that which you were powerless to influence.

Genetic tests may also have more direct distributional consequences. Alleles occur in different frequencies in different ethnic groups; it would not be surprising to find that an allele associated with an epidemiologically significant disease such as coronary artery disease was more prevalent in some ethnic groups than in others. Alpha-1 antitrypsin deficiency, associated with lung disease, appears to be more common among people of Scandinavian ancestry. If the group in which the allele occurs more often was not historically a target of discrimination, we might not be particularly concerned. If, however, the allele was more common in a group that continues to suffer discrimination, such as sickle-cell trait in people of African descent, we would have good reason for concern. The mere fact that genetic predictors have the potential to affect differentially ethnic groups that experience discrimination does not uniquely distinguish them from other risk predictors. Hypertension, for example, is more prevalent among Americans of African heritage. But the immediate and direct tie between genetics and ethnicity may make genetic testing a more blatant use of a potentially explosive and discriminatory social classification scheme.

A third response to the claim that we need not worry about genetic risk testing because it is essentially similar to things like cholesterol testing is to question the premise that people know about the genetic component of cholesterol. Discussions of cholesterol in the media emphasize the things people can do to lower it. Reminders that cholesterol level is also significantly affected by genetics appear less frequently, and it may well be that most people are unaware that cholesterol level has a substantial genetic component. If people did understand that, perhaps they would be less tolerant of the widespread use of cholesterol testing to determine insurance eligibility, precisely because it was to that extent outside of individuals' control.

There is yet another possibility: that the central notion underlying commercial health insurance underwriting—the greater the likelihood of illness, the more one should pay for coverage—is morally unsound.

ACTUARIAL FAIRNESS

Insurers take a particular view of fairness: actuarial fairness. Actuarial fairness claims that "policyholders with the same expected risk of loss should be treated equally. . . . An insurance company has the responsibility to treat all its policyholders fairly by establishing premiums at a level consistent with the risk represented by each individual policyholder."[2] This definition of fairness begs the question: Why should we count differences in risk of disease as an ethically relevant justification for treating people differently in their access to health insurance and health care?

Actuarial fairness does have a realm of application in which it seems reasonable. Call it the Lloyds of London model: if two oil tanker companies ask to have their cargoes and vessels insured, one for a trip up the Atlantic to a U.S. port, the other for a voyage through the Arabian Gulf during the height of the war in Kuwait and Iraq, the owner of the first ship would cry foul if she were charged the same extraordinarily high rate as the owner of the second. Most of us, I suspect, would agree that charging the two owners the same rate would be unfair. What makes it so?

For one thing, the two ships are exposed to vastly different risks, and it seems only fair to charge them accordingly. (The process of assessing risks is called underwriting.) Furthermore, the risks were assumed voluntarily. Third, the goal of both owners is profit, and it seems reasonable to ask them to bear the expense of voluntarily assumed risks. We could also ask how commercial insurance divides up the world. In this hypothetical it divides it into those who prefer prudent business ventures and those willing to take great risks. That does not seem to be an objectionable way to parse the world for the purpose of insuring oil tankers.

In practice, insurers do not behave as if actuarial fairness were an ironclad moral rule. Valid predictors may not be used for a variety of reasons, typically having to do with other notions of fairness—for example, not discriminating on the basis of race, sex, class, or locale, even though these characteristics are related to the likelihood of insurance claims. Deborah Stone, who has studied insurance practices for HIV infection, dismisses the idea of actuarial fairness and argues instead that:

> insurability is the set of policy decisions by insurers about whom to accept. It is not a trait, but a concept of *membership*. . . . Treated as a scientific fact about individuals, the notion of insurability disguises fundamentally political decisions about membership in a community of mutual responsibility.[3]

In a related vein, Norman Daniels points out that:

> we allow many considerations, both of justice and of other goals of social policy, to *override* appeals to actuarial fairness, suggesting that we do not treat it as a basic requirement of distributive justice in insurance contexts after all.[4]

According to actuarial fairness —the Lloyds of London model—insurers would be justified in using genetic tests that predicted who was likely to file a claim. But is actuarial fairness an adequate criterion of fairness in health insurance?

UNDERWRITING AND THE SOCIAL PURPOSES OF INSURANCE

The threat genetic testing poses to the future of insurance for health-related risks—including health, life, and disability insurance—compels us to reexamine the social purposes served by insurance. Two points are obvious: first, that different types of insurance can have different purposes; and second, that the purpose of a particular form of insurance must be understood within its social context.

Life insurance, for example, is meant to provide financial security for one's dependents in the event that one dies. In the contemporary United States we must evaluate the role of such insurance in the context of a not particularly generous social welfare system that would otherwise leave the surviving dependents of a deceased breadwinner in very poor financial condition. The typical purchaser is an individual with one or more dependents who are unlikely to become financially independent in the immediate future. The benefits from life insurance are intended to tide survivors over until they can become financially self-sufficient, or live out their lives decently; they are not meant to provide windfalls to friends of the deceased. To the extent that life insurance is perceived as serving a need rather than being merely a commodity, we are likely to regard it as something that ought to be available to all. Our public policies toward life insurance suggest we view it otherwise, however. We prohibit certain actuarially valid distinctions such as ethnicity in setting life insurance rates. But we do not require that all persons, whatever their age, employment, or health, be permitted to buy life insurance at identical prices or at all. In consequence, the financial dependents of a person unable to obtain life insurance may suffer devastating changes in their life prospects if the principal earner dies.

Does the Lloyds of London model fit health care? Despite the current enthusiasm for tying voluntary behavior to health, most illness and disability is neither chosen nor in any sense "deserved," distinguishing it from the risks of shipping oil in a war zone. Neither is the goal of health care for those who seek it profit. Daniels argues that "justice requires that we protect *fair equality of opportunity* for individuals in a society." Reasonable access to health care in the contemporary United States is a necessary condition for fair equality of opportunity to pursue other goods that life affords. The social purpose of health insurance, understood in this way, is to provide access to the health care that people need to have a fair opportunity in life.

Lastly, how does underwriting in health insurance divide the world? It sets off the well from the ill and those likely to become ill. For insurers, the concept of actuarial fairness provides a rationale for charging much higher rates or declining to insure persons with a substantial possibility of illness or disability, reasoning that such persons should bear the costs associated with their particular risks. Persons at risk could find it difficult to obtain insurance at affordable rates, or at all.

Because most persons with insurance get it through their employer rather than through individual policies, the impact of such individual underwriting by commercial insurers would be diminished. The Office of Technology Assessment estimated that 14.5 million individual or family policies are written for people under age sixty-five. This is a considerable number, to be sure, and people denied coverage from this source of insurance are greatly disadvantaged. But a far greater number of privately insured persons will be affected by what employers and group insurers do.

The pressure on employers to reduce costs may affect the insurance opportunities of employees. Although individual underwriting is still the exception rather than the rule in group policies, a recent OTA survey showed that 82 percent of commercial health insurers used some form of individual underwriting in their small group policies, and 48 percent did the same with late applicants in their large group policies. Blue Cross/Blue Shield plans used similar measures less frequently: 57 percent in small groups and 34 percent with late enrollees in large groups. It is reasonable to assume that such individual underwriting in group policies may continue to increase as a response to cost containment pressures. Another possibility is that self-insuring employers, who are largely exempt from state regulation, may use such testing to limit the employee to a policy that covers the employee alone, or the employee and spouse, but not an affected child.

IMPLICATIONS FOR POLICY

The era of predictive genetic testing coincides with a period of grave public concern about health care. In a recent survey, 82 percent of the public expressed such concern. For the first time, health care is the number two political issue in the United States. Some unfamiliar numbers help account for this intense and growing worry: an estimated 22 million people are refused care in each year and some 63 million people were without health insurance for at least part of the year—more than one in four Americans. Many others are afraid to change jobs because of waiting periods, exclusions, or other penalties for changing insurers.

Much has been made of the alleged distaste Americans have for government involvement in health care. Yet a recent survey shows that 60 percent of the people want the government to take the primary role in health care. There is little doubt that the current ragged system of private and public programs, with its many holes and frayed edges, must be changed. The conviction that health care ought to be available to those who need it seems to be widely shared. That conviction, together with a growing sense that the current patchwork is failing, may be strong enough to overcome the citizenry's hesitations about government inefficiency. Indeed, it seems likely that private health insurance would not have survived this long if not for government intervention. Tax subsidies for employer-sponsored health insurance programs amounted to $39.5 billion in 1991. In addition, we provide direct government coverage for the health needs of people that commercial insurers want to avoid. Medicare, for those much more likely to need health care; and Medicaid, for some of those unable to pay for their own insurance.

Public programs such as Medicare and Medicaid tell us something important about our moral convictions on health care. They suggest that we are not content to allow the old and the poor simply to languish without access to care. Had we not passed such legislation, we well might have overturned or radically restructured the existing system of commercial health insurance decades ago.

There are good reasons to doubt that actuarial fairness is an adequate description of genuine fairness in health insurance. It may be a sufficient principle for commercial insurance against losses of ships at sea, but even a brief inquiry into the social purpose of health insurance suggests that apportioning by risks, as actuarial fairness dictates, fails to accomplish the primary social goals of health insurance. Genetic tests, like other predictors of the need for health care, are not good reasons for treating people differently with respect to access to health insurance.

REFERENCES

1. Michael Walzer, *Spheres of Justice: A Defense of Pluralism and Equality* (New York: Basic Books, 1983).
2. Karen A. Clifford and R. P. Iuculano, "AIDS and Insurance: The Rationale for AIDS-Related Testing," *Harvard Law Review* 100 (1987): 1806–24
3. Deborah A. Stone, "AIDS and the Moral Economy of Insurance," *American Prospect* 1 (1990): 62–73.
4. Norman Daniels, "Insurability and the HIV Epidemic: Ethical Issues in Underwriting." *Milbank Quarterly* 68, no. 4 (1990): 497–525.

PATIENT AUTONOMY AND VALUE-NEUTRALITY IN NONDIRECTIVE GENETIC COUNSELING

Robert Wachbroit and David Wasserman

In recent years, medical scientists have identified a large number of genetic mutations associated with disease. This research has focused on a broad range of disorders, from rare conditions like Huntington's disease to certain forms of breast and colon cancer. With the use of genetic testing, mutations linked to such diseases are now or will soon be detectable long before the appearance of any symptoms. Often, these tests are used to detect mutations in germ cells and fetuses—mutations associated with disease in the patient's offspring, or potential offspring, as well as in the patient herself. The proliferation of genetic tests, and their significance for individuals beyond the patient tested, have increased the importance of genetic counseling—the effort to enable patients to understand and respond appropriately to genetic test results and diagnoses.

Despite some occasional dissents, the standard view of genetic counseling is that it must be "nondirective." Yet there has been a great deal of confusion over what "nondirective" means. Seymour Kessler, a leading writer on genetic counseling, observes: "[t]he terms "directiveness" and "nondirectiveness" have been part of the lexicon of genetic counseling for many decades. Yet one has little confidence that

Reprinted with permission of the authors and publisher from *Stanford Law & Policy Review 6:* 2(1995): 103–111.

Editor's note: Some footnotes have been deleted. Students who want to follow up on sources should consult the original article.

a consensus exists about the meaning given to these terms."[1]

One reason for the lack of consensus, we will argue, is that two distinct concerns fall under the rubric of "nondirectiveness"—value-neutrality and respect for patient autonomy. Much of the literature on genetic counseling does not regard these concerns as independent. The Institute of Medicine's (IOM) report on *Assessing Genetic Risks,* for example, asserts that "[t]he commitment to nondirectiveness in genetic counseling arises from respect for the patient's autonomy in decision making."[2] The report urges counselors to suppress the expression of "the values and biases they bring to their work" in order to respect their patients' autonomy. Other commentators have likewise understood nondirective genetic counseling to require a style of communication in which the counselor affects a complete neutrality about the moral issues raised by genetic diagnosis.

In this paper, we will argue that respect for patient autonomy is central to nondirective counseling, and that it does not require value-neutrality. Although rarely made explicit, the assumption linking the two concerns is a belief that the expression of the counselor's values undermines patients' abilities to make decisions for themselves. We will argue that this assumption is unwarranted: respect for autonomy in genetic counseling does not require any greater circumspection about values than in any other form of health care counseling.

Value-neutrality, we will argue, is neither desirable nor possible. Its appeal arises largely from a conception of values as less objective, and less suitable for public discourse, than scientific claims. Nondirectiveness, properly understood, does not demand such circumspection; it requires the counselor to adopt whatever method is most effective in ensuring that the patient's choices about genetic testing are informed and voluntary. This is an enormously difficult task, which the demand for value-neutrality only complicates.

DISTINGUISHING PATIENT AUTONOMY AND VALUE-NEUTRALITY

In order to understand why patient autonomy is central to nondirective genetic counseling, we must return to the generally agreed upon *aim* of genetic counseling: enabling patients to understand and appropriately respond to genetic test results and diagnoses. The phrase "appropriately respond" is crucial, for it generates the main disagreements about the proper role of the genetic counselor. The nondirective approach insists that the appropriate response is the one decided upon by the patient herself. Whatever she decides is "appropriate," as long as it results from her understanding of the facts and truly reflects her values. Whether or not the counselor agrees with this decision is irrelevant.

This understanding of what constitutes an "appropriate response" to genetic diagnosis is relatively new. In the first half of this century, it was widely agreed that the appropriate response was the one that promoted genetic health and reduced genetic disease. Any other response reflected ignorance or selfishness, indicating that the patient needed to be educated, bribed, or coerced to serve the greater good. This understanding of "appropriate response" was driven by the assimilation of genetic health into public health. Combating genetic disease was regarded as a public health problem: someone who failed to promote genetic health not only risked her own well-being but that of the "race" as well. This approach soon led to notorious abuses, from the practice of forced sterilization in the United States to the comprehensive eugenic programs in Nazi Germany. Policies whose aim was to promote "genetic hygiene" did so at the expense of individual liberties and, often, lives.

Nondirective genetic counseling is a reaction to this history of abuse. It rejects genetic hygiene as its primary objective, and it seeks to distance itself from the abuses committed in the name of genetic hygiene by ensuring that the patient's decisions about testing and intervention are well-informed and fully voluntary. Its goal is to make the patient aware not only of genetic risks, but of her freedom to choose whether or not to get tested and how to respond to positive test results.

More broadly, the history of eugenics helps explain why we have a profession of genetic counseling. There is no counseling profession associated with other medical testing: we do not have cardiac counselors or oncology counselors. The special need for genetic counseling cannot arise from the complexity of genetic tests or the etiology of genetic diseases—they are no more difficult to understand than an EKG or the etiology of a cancer. Nor can the need arise from the psychological impact of a positive genetic test result—that impact is no more severe than that of a positive result for a heart condition or cancer. The critical difference is that cardiac or oncological testing has no comparable history of being used against the patient's will and against her interests.

With the emergence of a separate genetic counseling profession in the late 1960s, the commitment to nondirectiveness went beyond the mere rejection of coercive means and public health objectives. Individualistic, client-centered therapy became the orthodoxy of the new profession—its goal was to strengthen the patient's decision-making processes and clarify the patient's preferences and value.

The concern with value-neutrality reflects a different history. The controversy over the scientific status of values—about whether there could be a science of values—reached a fever pitch at the end of the nineteenth century. By the early part of this century, the standard view was that scientific results neither confirmed nor refuted value claims, so that when someone made a value claim, she was exceeding the authority of science. Even now, scientists writing about values tend to treat them as merely psychological or social phenomena; they often use "values" and "biases" interchangeably. In genetic counseling, a commitment to value-neutrality is meant to ensure the objective and scientific character of the counselor's communications.

Clearly, respecting autonomy and maintaining value-neutrality are distinct concerns.[3] Respect for autonomy requires the counselor to ensure that the patient's choices concerning genetic diagnoses are informed and voluntary, reflecting her own values and interests. In contrast, value-neutrality requires the counselor to suppress any opinions she has about the value of the medical procedures the patient faces, or about the ethical issues the patient faces in making her choice. Value-neutrality is a constraint on the counselor's interaction with the patient. The question is whether this sort of constraint is necessary in order to respect the patient's autonomy. Why should genetic counselors be discouraged from giving the kind of advice that other health care professionals dispense so freely?

VALUE NEUTRALITY IN NONDIRECTIVE COUNSELING

The defender of value-neutrality might respond to this question in one of two ways. She might argue that value-neutrality was in fact necessary to dissociate genetic counseling from its eugenic legacy. Or she might argue that value-neutrality was required to respect patient autonomy in the context of genetic counseling.

Purging the Taint of Eugenics?

In order to develop the first response, we must distinguish somatic from reproductive genetic testing. A somatic test aims at detecting or diagnosing genetic conditions that are indicative of that individual's health status. Such tests might not only diagnose a current disease but also indicate future health problems or disease susceptibilities that the patient was unaware of. Tests for certain forms of breast cancer and colon cancer fall into this category. In contrast, reproductive genetic tests are performed to assess "genetic transmission" and thereby inform the patient's reproductive plans and decisions. Tests for whether the patient is a carrier of the genes associated with such conditions as Tay-Sachs, Cystic Fibrosis, or Fragile-X Syndrome fall into this category.

Reproductive testing yields information about the health status of individuals besides the proband (the person tested); it yields information about the proband's (possible) offspring. This gives reproductive counseling more of a public health aspect than somatic counseling. Moreover, it may raise questions about whether a particular life is worth living. For these reasons, reproductive counseling may evoke concerns about eugenics that nondirective genetic counseling seeks to dispel. While the counselor can offer opinions about somatic genetic testing as freely as any other health professional, she must be more circumspect in discussing reproductive genetic testing. If she does anything more than present the options in a value-neutral manner, she associates herself with the discredited but still dangerous legacy of coercive eugenics.

This response could be characterized as a concern about "dirty hands"—a concern that the counselor not associate herself in any way with the eugenic agenda of a Galton or Davenport. Even if we grant the dubious assumptions underlying this response, the fear of dirty hands seems misplaced. What distinguishes modern genetic practice from eugenics is the complete rejection of coercion as a method, not the complete abandonment of genetic health as an objective. A genetic counselor can more effectively distance herself from the eugenic legacy of her profession by encouraging her patients to make testing and termination decisions for themselves than by expression of her own beliefs.

Safeguarding Patient Autonomy?

Another general consideration supporting value-neutrality is the belief that respect for patient autonomy requires value-neutrality in the context of genetic counseling. There are several reasons for believing that respect for autonomy requires value-neutrality: 1) that the counselor's value judgments would enjoy a spurious scientific authority; 2) that the expression of such judgments would lead counselors down a slippery slope to coercive measures; 3) that the autonomy of patients considering genetic testing is especially fragile; and 4) that the social pressure on those patients is especially great. None of these reasons, we will argue, can withstand scrutiny.

It might be argued that because the counselor is seen by the patient as a medical authority, he must not present moral issues as matters of scientific judgment. The counselor would mislead the patient, and thereby violate her autonomy, if he gave the impression that the values he expressed had scientific authority. However, nothing compels him to give that false impression: if a counselor carefully disclaims special authority or expertise on matters of value, his expression of value may be compatible with a respect for the patient's autonomy.

The counselor's response to "what would *you* do?" questions illustrates this last point concretely. Those questions have mistakenly been regarded as presenting a litmus test for nondirectiveness. Kessler argues that it violates nondirectiveness to give a forthright answer to such a question, since "the counselor attempts to create the illusion that he/she has taken responsibility for the counselees' actions and decisions." Surely, then, the counselor would violate value-neutrality in giving a direct response, because he would express his own values. Yet such expression need not undermine the patient's autonomy. The counselor's willingness to express his own values need not suggest that he is willing to assume responsibility for the counselees' actions and decisions. Quite the contrary, by explaining how his values would inform his decision, while making it clear that he has no greater expertise in making moral judgments than the patient, the counselor might well emphasize the counselee's responsibility for a difficult choice.

A second concern, rarely asserted but often hinted at in discussions of nondirectiveness, is that value judgments represent the first step on a slippery slope towards blatantly coercive measures. While there may be little that is objectionable in the expression of values itself, it leads the counselor, or the counseling profession, on this fatal descent. This fear, however, seems groundless. It is a tenet of liberal society that the vigorous expression of opinion protects rather than endangers autonomy. Any plausibility in the fear of a slippery slope arises from the perception that value judgments made by genetic counselors will enjoy a spurious scientific authority, or that the autonomy of patients considering reproductive testing is unusually fragile or unusually threatened. We have already considered the first concern; we now turn to the latter two.

Proponents of value-neutrality might argue that there are some grounds for thinking that the autonomy of the patient seeking genetic counseling for reproductive or somatic testing is *especially* fragile. The patient in a genetic counseling session is apprehensive, anxious, and unsure, facing the possibility of receiving devastatingly bad news or good news alloyed with "survivor's guilt." In such circumstances, the patient is highly susceptible to any influence. If the genetic counselor expresses any value judgment, the patient will acquiesce since she has neither the strength nor self-confidence to disagree. The patient's autonomy is so fragile that *any* influence undermines it. Consequently, value-neutrality must be maintained in order to respect the patient's autonomy.

This "fragile autonomy" assumption is implausible. It is worth noting that no such assumption is generally made in other areas of medical practice. No one has suggested that physicians should be barred from giving advice. Indeed, it is a common part of medical practice to offer patients advice, recommendations, warnings, and encouragement—about lifestyle changes they should make, treatments they should undertake, exercise they should get, and foods they should avoid. All this would undermine the patient's autonomy if autonomy were too fragile to tolerate any influence. But such advice is not thought to threaten the patient's autonomy when it is properly dispensed—when the patient is fully informed of the situation, the need for the patient's consent in order to initiate certain procedures is acknowledged, and the patient's rational assessment of the diagnosis is supported. Indeed, this kind of advice can underscore the patient's autonomy by clarifying her responsibility for making treatment decisions.

Of course, because of anxiety and conflicting emotions, the patient considering genetic testing may be unusually impressionable. Yet the desperately ill patient deciding whether to undergo risky but potentially life-prolonging surgery also faces acute anxiety and emotional conflict. A cardiac or oncological surgeon who responded candidly to a patient's anxious inquiry about what she would do in his place might reveal strong values about health and risk. We would not, however, regard her candor as threatening to the patient's autonomy.

A final reason for thinking that respect for autonomy requires value-neutrality in the context of reproductive testing is that the autonomy of the patient faces a greater *threat* in that context than in other health care settings. One alleged difference between reproductive genetic testing and other medical testing lies in the social pressure to test for and abort "defective" fetuses in the interest of public health. Oliver Wendell Holmes' infamous remark that "three generations of imbeciles are enough"[4] may reflect an oppressive social consensus that a patient considering cardiac or oncological testing does not face. But there are other areas of health care where patients also face strong social pressure. Consider the massive social pressures facing an obese middle-aged man or a chain smoker. We hardly think these pressures compel the doctor treating the obese man or chain smoker to forgo his warnings to lose weight or stop smoking, lest those warnings infringe his patient's autonomy.

It might be claimed, however, that the pressure on the obese man and the chain smoker are essentially paternalistic, while the pressure on the prospective parent is not, and that paternalistic pressure is somehow less threatening to autonomy than non-paternalistic pressure. There is reason to doubt both these claims. But even assuming their validity, they do not distinguish prospective parents from other patients under considerable social pressure of a non-paternalistic sort. The patient with a communicable sexual disease faces great social pressure to refrain from sex or disclose the disease to his partners, and that pressure is clearly not paternalistic—it has at least as strong a public health focus as the pressure of to test for genetic disease. But we do not think a doctor undermines the autonomy of that patient by urging restraint or disclosure on him. There are, of course, significant moral differences between the reproductive and communicable disease contexts. However, the threat to autonomy from social pressure is not one of them.

THE POSSIBILITY OF VALUE-NEUTRALITY

We have doubtless overlooked some reasons for thinking that respect for autonomy requires value-neutrality. Possibly some of the reasons we have overlooked are more plausible than those we have considered. There is, however, a more conclusive ground for denying that respect for patient autonomy requires value-neutrality. In the context of genetic counseling, value-neutrality is impossible. This is so for two reasons. First, autonomy is itself a value about which the counselor cannot be neutral. Second, the promotion of genetic testing, especially reproductive testing, may be incompatible with value-neutrality.

Although respect for patient autonomy is the primary goal of genetic counseling, counselors and patients often differ as to the value of autonomy. Patients do not always regard reproductive decisions as theirs to make; they often defer uncritically to the judgments of their spouses, family, or religious leaders. Thus, the central principle of nondirectiveness—that the patient is to be treated as the decision maker—departs from neutrality with regard to a very controversial issue.

Moreover, respecting autonomy may conflict with other values. For example, Angus Clarke argues that the denigration of people with the genetic conditions tested for is an inevitable result of the development and promotion of those tests, so that the state should consider limiting genetic testing to the most severe and debilitating conditions:

> Adoption of criteria based on broader social considerations would restrict prenatal diagnosis to disorders where the affected individuals are either profoundly retarded (and hence socially unaware), very severely handicapped physically (as with Duchenne muscular dystrophy or Werdnig-Hoffman disease) or faced with prolonged physical suffering (e.g., Huntington's disease and Fabry's disease).[5]

Other genetic counselors respond that such restrictions would unfairly restrict the choices of patients already wrestling with the issues that trouble Clarke:

> Prenatal diagnosis and selective abortion provide the parents with an opportunity to plan a family without the risk of being responsible for bringing another affected child into the world. Most parents can reconcile the apparent inconsistency of love and protection of their handicapped child with the deliberate avoidance of the birth of a second, but I would be surprised if they need clinical geneticists to remind them that selective abortion throws into question their belief about the value of the life their handicapped child is living. These families would love extra help in giving their affected child, and even their whole family, a better life, as Clarke suggests, but I doubt if most would want to have their choice of what tests to have and how to act on the results curtailed on the grounds that their choice might be influenced by subtle pressures such as the very existence of the tests.[6]

One might argue that the genetic counselor should remain neutral about all values *except* the paramount value of patient autonomy. But this is not possible either. The very development and promotion of reproductive genetic testing conveys the impression that something should be done when an abnormal genetic condition is detected. The implicit assumption is that the condition should be eliminated, which, given the limitations of present technology, almost always means terminating the pregnancy. The genetic counselor may not share that view, but as the person who mediates the patient's encounter with this technology, he cannot stand apart from it. As Troy Duster observes about voluntary screening programs:

> Genetic counselors are probably, as professionals, indeed neutral, if this means they should do as much as possible not to communicate their personal prejudices and opinions about whether a couple should take a chance . . . etc. However, the individual neutrality of the counselor is not the issue. It is the fact of the machinery of a screen that has been erected. Even if one is neutral about whether one uses the advice or technology, etc., the simple fact that the screen is in place communicates a powerful message that something is wrong with the disorder for which the screen is in place.[7]

Clarke makes an even stronger claim:

> I contend that an offer of prenatal diagnosis implies a recommendation to accept that offer, which in turn entails a tacit recommendation to terminate a pregnancy if it is found to show any abnormality. I believe that this sequence is present irrespective of the counsellor's [*sic*] wishes, thoughts, or feelings, because it arises from the social context rather than the personalities involved—although naturally the counselor may reinforce these factors.[8]

We may recognize the force of these concerns if we imagine an expensive and risky test for fetal eye or hair color. Most of us would probably insist that a genetic counselor should not even offer his patients such a test, since eye or hair color should have no relevance to the patient's reproductive choices. To invite the patient to seriously consider a test with more than minimal costs and risks, is, at the very least, to suggest that the test has such relevance. This would be a significant departure from value-neutrality, and the values it implicitly endorses can be seen as eugenic ones. The genetic counselor can help to ensure that the patient makes her own decision about whether to accept those values, but he cannot proclaim his complete neutrality with respect to them.

There are also more general reasons for doubting the possibility of value-neutrality. One important function of the counselor is to provide information on risk, but the communication of risk cannot be neutral. The counselor must choose between characterizing a risk as a probability of a loss or as a probability of a gain. That choice is no more neutral than the choice between describing a glass as half-empty or as half-full. Such "framing" involves a departure from value-neutrality, and there is strong evidence that framing influences the patient's decision. As MacNeil found in a study of outcome framing and patient decisions, "surgery appeared to be much more attractive when the outcomes were framed in terms of the probability of survival rather than in terms of the probability of death."[9]

THE CHALLENGE OF RESPECTING PATIENT AUTONOMY

Our discussion so far might seem to suggest that respecting the patient's autonomy is not a challenging or problematic objective for the genetic counselor. In fact, it is an exceptionally difficult and important task. The decisions that patients make with respect to genetic testing not only have important consequences, they also test, and help define, the patient's most central values. The patient who must decide if she can unconditionally love and effectively nurture a profoundly retarded child, or can live with the knowledge that a Huntington's test will bestow, is making one of the most difficult decisions of her life. Respecting her autonomy is a daunting task, not because her autonomy is more fragile or threatened, but because the choices she must make will touch upon some of her deepest values.

Genetic testing, of course, is not the only area of health care to confront patients with such difficult choices. Patients considering passive euthanasia or high-risk surgery may also be forced to make decisions which reflect, or define, their central values. The success of genetic counselors in helping patients make such difficult choices may provide a model for the rest of the health care field.

The genetic counselor's role is further complicated because there is a great deal of uncertainty and controversy about how to respect the patient's autonomy in making such difficult choices. The counselor must confront two distinct sets of issues: empirical issues about the effect of tacit and expressed values on her patients' capacity to make a knowing and fully voluntary choice, and conceptual issues about the meaning of autonomy in the context of genetic testing. One empirical issue is whether the social values underlying the screening, testing, and counseling processes undermine autonomy more by being made explicit or by operating *sub rosa*. There is reason to suspect that the latter is more subversive than the former. Psychological research suggests that social pressures may have a greater effect on behavior when they are part of the unspoken background, and that, in fact, explicit attempts to control behavior often backfire, provoking autonomy-preserving defiance. Research also suggests that overtly directive counseling may not have a very coercive effect. Kessler cites studies from Eastern Europe, under communist rule, which found that "even under social and political conditions where directiveness is expected, nearly 40% of counselees with high genetic risk did not take the counselor's advice."

A second empirical issue is the importance of giving the patient an appreciation not only of the available options, but also of their viability. Genetic counselors might, for example, utilize support-group networks to establish contact between parents who receive positive results on a prenatal test and the parents of children who have the tested-for conditions. Exposure to parents who decided not to terminate, and who did not regret their decision, may act as a powerful corrective to the social pressure to terminate.[10] The conceptual issues are more difficult. As Diane Paul has observed: "Autonomy in respect to reproductive decisions has become a near-universal value. But this agreement masks fundamental conflicts about what it means for people to make their own decisions.[11] Many of the major debates in medical ethics involve questions about what autonomy means in particular contexts, what external factors threaten or subvert it, and what weight it should have in conflict with other values. For example, do we respect the autonomy of a dying patient of questionable mental capacity by mechanically executing his advance directive against life-extending treatment, or by deferring to any utterances that could even remotely be construed as requests for continued treatment? Is the patient who declines proffered information about a surgical procedure functioning in a truly autonomous manner when she consents to the operation? Can we be sure that a patient who decides to terminate her pregnancy following a private "family conference" has made an autonomous decision? Should we even worry about that? Based on such reservations, how should we modify our treatment approach?

One recurring issue is whether the counselor respects the patient's autonomy more by providing the patient with more information, or by letting her decide how much information to receive. On a view that associates autonomy with rationality, a patient's autonomy can only be enhanced by the receipt of accurate information; on a view that emphasizes the patient's control over the decision-making process, the communication of unsought information may violate her autonomy. Does the counselor respect or undermine the patient's autonomy by adopting the strategy, described by Barbara Katz Rothman, of urging women with misgivings about abortion to separate the decision to test from the decision to terminate, expecting or hoping that "once the woman actually knows she is carrying a fetus with Downs [*sic*] or some other disabling condition, she may think differently about abortion?"[12]

The counselor must also decide whether, or how, to inform the patient of her choice to receive or decline. If he describes her options, he unavoidably imparts some information the patient may not want to receive. But if he waits for a request from the patient, he risks keeping her in ignorance of information she would very much like but does not know enough to ask for.

Another set of difficult issues is raised by patients who accept, acquiesce in, or actively delegate the control of their reproductive decisions to others, such as spouses, parents, in-laws, or religious leaders. The counselor must decide if he respects his patient's autonomy more by deferring to the patient's willingness to let others (e.g., family members) make her decisions or by insisting that the patient regard the decision as her own. Does he let the patient decide *who* will take part in the counseling session? Does he intervene in the ensuing conversation to ensure that the patient's own views are expressed? Should the counselor distinguish between patients who voluntarily delegate decision making authority to others in order to escape responsibility, reduce anxiety, or circumvent weakness of will, from patients who fail to even recognize that the decision is theirs to delegate?

Perhaps the most familiar controversy over patient autonomy in the context of genetic testing concerns sex selection should the geneticist assist a patient in finding out whether her fetus has the "wrong" sex, or is the commitment to her autonomy outweighed by the objections to her decision criteria? Wertz and Fletcher have documented a shift among health professionals from rejection to compliance as patient autonomy has become more firmly entrenched as a dominant value in health care.[13] Although fetal sex selection involves sharp moral conflict, the rejection of value-neutrality offers the geneticist an option besides outright refusal and silent acquiescence; he can explore and challenge the reasons for his patient's sex selection preferences, even if he ultimately accepts the patient's decision.

But the conflict over sex selection also raises a broader, more difficult issue concerning the meaning and priority of patient autonomy in genetic counseling: individual reproductive decisions may, in the aggregate, have harmful social consequences, such as the denigration of women. The counselor must decide whether to urge his clients to consider those consequences. Sex selection is only the tip of the iceberg, deceptively unthreatening because of the broad consensus in this country against the practice and the negligible demand for it. As commentators like Diane Paul, Troy Duster, and Angus Clarke have observed, the real threat comes from the identification of an increasing number of genetic markers associated with conditions that are not life-threatening, but impairing or socially undesirable, such as hyperactivity, homosexuality, and obesity. The availability of prenatal tests for these conditions threatens to make pregnancy ever more tentative and to further stigmatize those with the conditions tested for.

Does the genetic counselor respect the patient's autonomy more by encouraging her to resist the social pressures to test for such conditions and terminate if the results are positive, or by blandly acquiescing in her decision to do so? Does it depend on the extent to which the patient has internalized, or identified with, the eugenic values that lie behind the social pressure? Should the counselor urge the patient to take account of the harmful impact of testing and termination, even if the patient seems committed to that course of action? These are critical issues in defining nondirectiveness, which require careful discussion about the meaning and weight of autonomy and other values central to counseling and health care. The demand for value-neutrality can only hinder their resolution.

NOTES

1. Seymour Kessler, *Psychological Aspects of Genetic Counseling. VII. Thoughts on Directiveness*, 1 Journal of Genetic Counseling 9 (1992).

2. INSTITUTE OF MEDICINE, ASSESSING GENETIC RISKS: IMPLICATIONS FOR HEALTH AND SOCIAL POLICY 154 (1994) (hereinafter, INSTITUTE OF MEDICINE).
3. We can illustrate the distinction between maintaining value-neutrality and respecting autonomy with the example of religious proselytizing, an activity in which communication is not merely value-laden but intended to bring about a change in the listener's values. Clearly, the proselytizer is not value-neutral: she seeks to promote a comprehensive system of values and beliefs. Yet proselytizers vary considerably in the extent to which they respect the autonomy of prospective converts. Some try to subvert or overwhelm the normal decision making processes with social pressure, brainwashing, or subtle manipulation; others show a scrupulous respect for those processes and do not regard a conversion as genuine unless it arises from careful, unpressured reflection. We do not suggest, of course, that genetic counselors become proselytizers; we merely wish to emphasize how distinct the concerns for value-neutrality and autonomy can be.
4. Buck v. Bell, 274 U.S. 200 (1927).
5. Angus Clarke, *Is Non-directive Genetic Counseling Possible?*, LANCET, Oct. 19, 1991, at 998, 1000.
6. Marcus Pembrey, *Letter to the Editor*, LANCET, Nov. 16, 1991, at 1266.
7. TROY DUSTER, BACK DOOR TO EUGENICS 76 (1990).
8. Clarke, *supra* note 5, at 1000. Barbara Katz Rothman has observed that many genetic counselors regard the reduction of genetic disease as a major goal of medical genetics and would themselves abort a fetus with relatively minor defects. She argues that even the most conscientious counselor can hardly keep such strong convictions from shaping her communication:

   > If the counselor thinks this woman sitting across from her is going to do something she will deeply regret for the rest of her life, how can she *not* influence her? Just what kind of person would she be if she saw someone heading off a cliff and sat back non-directively?

   BARBARA K. ROTHMAN, THE TENTATIVE PREGNANCY 47 (1986).
9. *On the Elicitation of Preferences for Alternative Therapies.* 306 New Eng. J. Med. 1259, 1262 (1982).
10. In this regard, it is instructive to consider the liberating effect of a single non-conforming confederate in Solomon Asch's classic study of conformity. *See* Solomon Asch, *Effects of Group Pressure Upon The Modification and Distortion of Judgment,* in GROUP DYNAMICS: RESEARCH and THEORY 189–200 (D. Cartwright & A. Zander eds., 1960).
11. Diane Paul, *Eugenic Anxieties, Social Realities, and Political Choices,* 59 SOC. RES. 663, 670 (1992).
12. ROTHMAN, *supra* note 8, at 44.
13. Dorothy Wertz & John Fletcher, *Ethical Problems in Prenatal Diagnosis: A Cross-Cultural Survey of Medical Geneticists in 18 Nations,* 9 PRENATAL DIAGNOSIS 145(1989).

ETHICAL ISSUES IN HUMAN GENE TRANSFER RESEARCH

Eric T. Juengst and LeRoy Walters

The autumn of 1995 celebrated a number of important anniversaries for the ethics of human gene-transfer research. October 1995 marked 30 years since R. D. Hotchkiss introduced the label "genetic engineering" in an essay entitled "Portents for a Genetic Engineering" that appeared in the *Journal of Heredity* (Hotchkiss 1965). December 1995 marked 20 years since the federal Guidelines for Recombinant DNA Research were developed to regulate genetic engineering, after scientists went public with their concerns in the early 1970s upon actually developing the tools to do what Hotchkiss anticipated (Krimsky 1985). November of 1995 was the tenth anniversary of the submission of the first formal protocol to conduct a clinical trial of gene therapy on a human being, and that trial began 5 years later, in September 1990 (Thomson 1994). Today, that first

Reprinted with permission from *The Development of Human Gene Therapy* © 1999 Cold Spring Harbor Laboratory Press 0-87969-528-5/99.

human gene therapy trial has been declared a success, more than 200 other trials are under way, and squadrons of molecular geneticists and biotechnologists now blithely call themselves "genetic engineers," oblivious to the ironic origins of the label.

One of the striking features of this 30-year history is the extent to which the discussion of human genetic engineering has been open to and influenced by concerns over social values and the public's voice. From the beginning, human gene transfer research seems to have been recognized to involve social value commitments that require the approval of the democratic process. Hotchkiss set the tone by concluding his prescient prediction of genetic interventions we are now capable of performing by prescribing that "The best preparation will be an informed and forewarned public, and a thoughtful body scientific. The teachers and the science writers can perform their historic duties by helping our public to recognize and evaluate these possibilities and avoid their abuses. For these things surely are on the way" (Hotchkiss 1965, p. 202).

In the early 1970s, prospective gene therapists such as W. French Anderson made this point the cornerstone of their arguments about how society should proceed, proposing that "This area holds such promise for alleviating human suffering, and yet is so basic to the needs and emotions of all men [*sic!*], that no individual or group of individuals should take it upon themselves to make the decisions. Only the conscience of an informed society as a whole should make these decisions" (Anderson 1972). This point of view found fertile ground in the nation's new interests in controlling the "biological revolution" in biomedicine, and the national public review process established through the Recombinant DNA Advisory Committee (RAC) was explicitly designed to help achieve that goal. In the years since, the ethos that has shaped the professional and public policy discussions of human gene-transfer research has remained grounded in the remarkably populist view that "the public review provided by the RAC assures both policymakers and the general public that they are well informed about developments in gene therapy and thus partners in the progress of this exciting new field" (Capron et al. 1993). With the development of local Institutional Biosafety Committees, the RAC's *Points to Consider* for the design of human gene-transfer research, and the process of open public discussion and national approval of all human gene-transfer protocols, the first 211 human gene-transfer trials in the United States have had the distinction of being the most thoroughly reviewed experiments in the history of biomedical research.

This populist tradition is important to recall, because it is the backdrop against which new professional ethical and social policy issues in gene-transfer research are and will be framed. There are four possible types of human gene-transfer interventions that can be performed on individuals. Such interventions can be targeted either toward an individual's somatic cells or toward the germ-line cells, and the goal of the intervention can be either the cure of disease or the enhancement of human capabilities. In this chapter, our goal is to review the ethical issues that arise with each of the four possible combinations of target cells and goals: somatic cell gene therapy, germ-line gene therapy, and the use of gene-transfer interventions to attempt to enhance normal human traits in either germ-line or somatic cells. In each case, our focus will be on the intersection of the ethos that guided the birth of gene therapy and the challenges that the field's future will bring, and on the implications of that intersection for professional practice and public policy.

ETHICAL ISSUES IN SOMATIC CELL GENE-TRANSFER RESEARCH

The literature that captures the public discussion of the ethics of human gene therapy displays an interesting metamorphosis between the early 1970s and the 1980s. The first wave of writing was characterized both by an awe in the face of the "New Biology" and by a sense of being ethically disoriented by its prospects. This period's response to these challenges was a sweeping reach of reflections that quickly took investigators to questions of philosophy and theology in search of moral bearings (Ramsey 1972). Much of this early work is still fresh and valuable at those deeper levels. But it was difficult to translate this work into practical policies for scientific research, and not much concrete policy development emerged from it.

In the early 1980s, driven by the news of Martin Cline's experiment (Kolata and Wade 1980) and lured by the prospect of coming clinical trials for somatic cell therapy at the National Institutes of Health (NIH) (Anderson and Fletcher 1980), the discussion rebounded. This second wave of discussion is captured best in the reports on human gene therapy by the President's Commission for Ethical Issues in Medicine and Biomedical and Behavioral Research (President's Commission 1982) and the congressional Office of Technology Assessment (U.S. Congress 1984), and culminates in the publication of the NIH's *Points to Consider* document in 1990 (Subcommittee on Human Gene Therapy 1990). In this literature, the community seems to have gained a moral compass that could allow policy to be developed without having to triangulate against deep questions of individual belief. As a result, commentators could thus write: "From the present vantage point, it may be hard to remember that in 1980, when the Commission began its work, critics (including respected religious groups) argued that 'fundamental dangers' were posed by any alteration of human genes" (Capron 1990).

This new sense of direction was the hybrid result of two sets of national ethical deliberations that occurred over the course of the 1970s: the discussion of biomedical research with human subjects and the debate over the use of recombinant DNA technology (Areen 1985). Neither of these discussions was conducted with human gene therapy in mind, but together they provided the investigators of the 1980s with a repertoire of widely recognized and well-grounded moral and policy considerations that was unavailable to the investigators of the first phase. With the formation of the RAC's Working Group on Human Gene Therapy, these two discussions came together. Collectively, through the RAC's *Points to Consider* document, their moral considerations now form the ethical framework against which protocols for human gene-transfer research are evaluated and the substantive principles for the next phase of deliberations.

The first important accomplishment of this second wave of discussion was to clarify and integrate into public policy the basic conceptual distinctions between the four possible types of human gene transfer introduced above (President's Commission 1982). This led to the recognition that somatic cell gene therapy, if it worked, would simply be an extension of traditional medical efforts to modulate the expression of genes (such as transplantation or gene-product therapy) and did not raise the special problems created by the other possible forms of gene transfer. Because the science required for successful germ-line interventions in humans was also undeveloped, this allowed the public discussion simply to table the most problematic issues until further notice and concentrate on helping to launch the first form of gene-transfer research in a responsible manner.

Framing somatic cell gene therapy as an extension of traditional medical approaches was progress, because it allowed the public review process to assess gene-transfer research protocols through the ethical questions that had already become normative within biomedical research with human subjects: questions that have to do with the anticipated benefits and risks of the intervention (including biosafety risks), the selection of research subjects, and the protection of the rights of research subjects and their proxies to informed consent, free withdrawal, and privacy. Ironically, however, framing somatic cell gene-transfer research as simply another form of innovative medical therapy also sowed the seeds of views that now challenge the need for any special societal oversight of investigators' ability to address these questions.

Risks and Benefits

Concerns about the relative risks and benefits of gene-transfer interventions reflect a commitment to the basic principle of research ethics that "risks to the subjects [must be] reasonable in relation to anticipated benefits, if any, to subjects, and the importance of the knowledge that may be reasonably expected to result." (45 CFR, Sec. 46.111a). Thus, the RAC says in the introduction to its *Points to Consider:*

> In their evaluation of proposals involving the transfer of recombinant DNA into human subjects, the RAC and its subcommittee will consider whether the design of such experiments offers adequate assurance that their consequences will not go beyond their purpose, which is the same as the traditional purpose of all clinical investigations, namely to protect the health and well-being of individual subjects being treated while at the same time gathering generalizable knowledge (Subcommittee on Human Gene Therapy 1990, p. 96).

In practice, this concern means that human gene-transfer researchers must have enough prior knowledge to believe that the probable benefits to the subject outweigh both the possible risks of the experiment and the known benefits of any alternative treatments available. Thus, it lies behind the RAC's questions about, and the community's discussion of, the safety and efficacy of somatic cell gene-therapy techniques, the adequacy of preliminary animal studies, and the relative value of emerging therapeutic alternatives (Brenner 1995).

Moreover, one of the striking legacies of the recombinant DNA debate in the public discussion of gene therapy is the acceptance of the need to prepare for the unforeseen as well as predictable risks in designing gene-transfer research. In the public review of gene-transfer protocols, this concern has concentrated primarily on the "biosafety" risks involved in gene transfer. Both the RAC and the scientific community have gone to unprecedented lengths to assess and minimize both the risks of "insertional mutagenesis" involved in the delivery and integration of exogenous DNA into the subject's cells and the risks that vectors may infect germ-line cells as well as their targets, even when the risks seem quite remote. In accepting this emphasis on safety, the community seems to agree with Howard Temin, when he writes that:

> There are often unexpected effects of new technologies. . . . The use of retrovirus vectors for somatic therapy of human genetic disease can be looked upon as either a novel improvement on present means of drug delivery or as the introduction of potentially dangerous technology. Although scientists and physicians may believe the first characterization is correct, I am convinced that we must act as if the second characterization is correct. We must design vector systems and protocols so that even quite unrealistic fears about safety are allayed (Temin 1990).

The Problem of "Compassionate Use" Unfortunately, one consequence of the public's preoccupation with the special risks of gene-transfer research has been its relative inattention to the issues involved in defining the benefits of gene-transfer research, and that is where issues are now emerging. Despite the fact that all initial gene-transfer experiments are ostensibly only Phase I investigations of the safety of a particular protocol, some patients and physicians seek to become involved in gene-transfer research out of hope of clinical benefit. In situations in which no alternative treatment exists and death is imminent, the risks of gene transfer pale, and any possibility of benefit, no matter how remote, seems worth attempting. Since little generalizable new knowledge can be expected from these situations, they raise a fundamental professional and public policy question: Are we ready to move beyond gene-transfer research, with its elaborate process of public review and approval, and to treat gene therapy as an "ordinary" innovative medical practice, performed at the discretion of clinicians and their patients? Given that the public review process was established, in part, in response to an attempt at human gene transfer defended on therapeutic grounds (the Martin Cline case), this question cuts to the heart of that process.

Our experience with this issue to date is instructive. In 1992, the NIH was asked to grant an exemption to the regular review process for gene-therapy protocols, on the basis of the clinical need of a particular patient. Borrowing the notion of "compassionate use" from the U.S. Food and Drug Administration (FDA), the investigator argued that a protocol involving the use of gene therapy for brain tumors that had not yet been approved by the RAC should be allowed to be performed on a terminally ill patient. After initially denying the request, the Director of the NIH granted the exemption on compassionate grounds and instructed the RAC to develop guidelines for the expedited review of such requests in the future (Thompson 1993).

In defending her decision to grant an exemption from public review for this intervention, the NIH Director offered an interesting response. She suggested that far from relinquishing public review of gene transfer, the time had come to expand that review beyond the research setting and to establish a public review mechanism that could oversee even the emergency clinical use of gene-transfer interventions (even if that meant bringing them to the public's attention after the fact) (Healy 1993). The RAC took that invitation seriously and developed an oversight process for the compassionate use of gene-transfer in "single-patient protocols" that makes such uses the single hardest form of clinical care to perform legitimately in modern medicine. By requiring Institutional Review Board and

Institutional Biosafety Committee (IBC) approval, declaring all gene-transfer interventions as "experimental," and advocating the use of the *Points to Consider* as review standards, the RAC essentially argues that emergency clinical uses of gene transfer should meet the same tests as research studies (Recombinant DNA Advisory Committee 1993). In essence, they suggest that no one should perform human gene transfer in a patient in hopes of therapeutic benefit that they would not do in hopes of simply learning something about the safety of the technique, regardless of the desperation of a particular patient's plight. This is a conservative standard: more conservative than that imposed by the FDA for the compassionate use of investigational drugs (Flannery 1986), and even more conservative than the standards used to implant the first artificial heart (Annas 1985).

Selection of Subjects

The development of national policies for research with human subjects in the 1970s was motivated in part by a concern that the burdens of participating in biomedical research were unfairly distributed among particularly vulnerable populations within society, including children and the seriously ill. Children have traditionally been viewed as vulnerable because of their inability to consent to research, and the seriously ill, like the parents of sick children, are capable of neglecting important risk considerations out of clinical desperation, to their own detriment. As a result, whenever it is possible, new biomedical interventions are usually first tested for their safety in healthy adult volunteers in phase I trials before being tested for efficacy in patient-subjects or children (Levine 1986). But both children and the seriously ill have been prominent among the initial subjects of human gene-transfer Phase I trials.

Children have been involved in gene-transfer trials when the diseases targeted are fatal in childhood, making their selection as initial subjects unavoidable. Seriously ill adult patients, however, have been typically selected as subjects against another rationale: Like cancer patients in chemotherapy trials, they are recruited because they are the least likely to suffer the consequences of any unanticipated harms from gene-transfer research, and they have the most to gain from any unanticipated benefits. This justification depends heavily on the assumption that, like chemotherapy, gene transfer involves serious potential "toxicities" that would not be appropriate to impose on healthy subjects with nothing to gain. If it were only a matter of distributing potential benefits, the argument would fail: The expectation of benefit from a Phase I study is by definition "unreasonable," and can only become a factor against the backdrop of the risks involved.

In this context, the new issues are the challenges presented by the lower expectations of risk from gene-transfer procedures. Here, the question is, as gene-transfer research becomes safer and our confidence in its techniques grows, when should it shift to the standard model for biomedical research and begin its work by testing the safety of its vectors with normal volunteers? This is the shift of ethical orientation that now confronts the public review process.

Respecting the Rights of Subjects

The need for informed consent by patient-subjects is one of the central tenets of research ethics. Thus, it is no surprise that this issue would be considered in ethical discussions of gene-transfer research, although the challenges in securing voluntary and informed participation do not differ in principle from other areas of biomedical research. Two complicating features of the gene-transfer context are worth noting. First, the proposed interventions in gene-transfer experiments are usually at the cutting edge of research and require that subjects or their proxies have at least a basic understanding of molecular biology. Effective techniques for conveying complex technical information to laypeople do exist and should be employed in the consent process for these research protocols. Second, to the extent that subjects are also patients, those securing their participation should be especially sensitive to the fact that prospective subjects will often be in relatively desperate clinical circumstances, which can exert a powerful influence on the motivations of the subjects, their families, and their physicians. One crucial precaution in this regard is to avoid fostering the "therapeutic misconception" that can be created when terms suggesting clinical benefit are used to describe basic research interventions. Thus, for many protocols, it is preferable to use the phrase "human gene transfer" rather than "gene therapy" to emphasize the remoteness of therapeutic benefit.

The protection of privacy and confidentiality for the subjects in gene transfer research has also been important. In other cases involving innovative therapy—for example, in the early heart transplants—a virtual media circus has surrounded both the subjects and the research team. Thus, the RAC's *Points to Consider* asks researchers to provide plans for dealing with the public disclosure of their research in responsible ways. A proper approach to subjects will not isolate them from public view, but will attempt to strike a balance between disclosure to an interested public and respect for the subject's privacy.

Protecting the privacy of research subjects, like the job of ensuring that research subjects participate in biomedical studies voluntarily and in an informed way, is in most areas of biomedical research the responsibility of the Institutional Review Boards that oversee research at the local level. Increasingly, concerns have been expressed that the additional public scrutiny of these protections at the national level by the RAC has become redundant and unnecessary. As a result, in 1998, on the basis of the recommendations of an external advisory panel, the NIH Director removed the RAC's authority to review and approve individual protocols for human gene-transfer research, effectively undercutting the public's ability to participate in the decision-making about gene-transfer research and the 30-year tradition of seeing gene therapy as very much the public's business.

In some respects, the national public review process that has overseen the development of human gene-transfer research has been the victim of its own success. With the widespread public acceptance of the idea of gene therapy and the successful review of over 200 pioneering protocols, the RAC and its process are often held up as a model of other scientific policy-making challenges (Wolf 1997). In sum, however, that very success has led to challenges on three fronts: (1) Some argue that the similarity between human gene transfer and other innovative medical therapies has become so strong that the prospects of clinical benefit from gene transfer interventions now justify decisions to apply gene-transfer techniques to seriously ill patients in the clinical setting without prior public discussion and review; (2) others argue that the risks of gene transfer have now been reduced to the point that it is time to shift into a more traditional biomedical research and development paradigm, and to test new interventions for safety on normal volunteers before recruiting seriously ill patients; and (3) still others argue that both the risks and benefits of somatic cell gene therapy are unremarkable enough to no longer need public discussion at the national level over and above the ordinary system of research review. As the field of human gene-transfer research matures and proliferates, each of these arguments is likely to be pressed further. At the same time, the next phase of our national conversation about the ethics of human gene transfer remains to be addressed.

ETHICAL ISSUES IN HUMAN GERM-LINE GENE TRANSFER

One of the problems that would be created by a premature dismantling of the public review process for human gene-transfer research is that the issues that were set aside during the development of criteria for assessing somatic-cell gene therapy would be left unaddressed at the national level. This would be an important loss, since these issues—the challenges raised by the prospect of germ-line gene-transfer interventions and the uses of gene transfer for enhancement purposes—were the ones that provoked the development of this process in the first place. As the discussion to date already shows, both of these categories raise fundamental social policy issues that require widespread public reflection and debate.

The major difference between somatic cell gene therapy and clinical techniques aimed at germ-line genetic intervention is that the latter would produce clinical changes that could be transmitted to the offspring of the person receiving the intervention. This simple difference is often the only consideration cited in the many official statements that endorse somatic cell gene therapy while proscribing or postponing research aimed at developing human germ-line gene therapy. Behind these official statements, however, lies a longer argument, revolving around four sets of concerns: scientific uncertainties, the need to use resources efficiently, social risks, and conflicting human rights concerns.

Scientific Uncertainties

Even the proponents of germ-line gene therapy agree that human trials under our current state of knowledge would be unacceptable. For gene-therapy techniques to be effective, the genes must be stably integrated, expressed correctly and only in the appropriate tissues, and reliably targeted to the correct location on a chromosome. If the intervention cannot eliminate the parents' risks of transmitting the alleles they carry or can only do so by substituting other genetic risks, its promise remains weak. Critics maintain that, given the complexity of gene regulation and expression during human development, germ-line gene-transfer experiments will always involve too many unpredictable long-term iatrogenic risks to the transformed subjects and their offspring to be justifiable (Council for Responsible Genetics 1993).

Proponents, however, respond that our current ignorance only justifies postponing human trials of germ-line therapy techniques until their promise can be improved. A more optimistic reading turns the argument around in that to the extent that the barriers to effective therapy can be overcome, its promise should encourage research to continue. Proponents add that by focusing on the obvious barriers to performing clinical trials today, critics of germ-line gene therapy ignore the fact that it will take future research to determine whether or not they are right. So the question remains as to whether current barriers should ultimately dissuade society from contemplating clinical trials in the future (Munson and Davis 1992).

Proponents bolster their technological optimism with an argument from medical utility: that germ-line gene therapy offers the only true cure for many diseases. If illnesses are understood to be, at root, "molecular diseases," then therapeutic interventions at any level above the causal gene can only be symptomatic. From this perspective, all gene therapies involving the simple addition of genes are palliative measures on the road to complete "gene-replacement surgery" in the germ line.

Allocation of Resources

One common criticism of the argument from medical utility is that it betrays a reductionistic attitude toward illness that fails to appreciate approaches that could achieve the same ends more efficiently. Since it must become possible to identify pre-embryos in need of therapy before their transformation, the argument goes, it would be more efficient simply to use the same techniques to identify healthy pre-embryos for implantation (Davis 1992). Many clinical geneticists argue that even our current methods of prenatal screening serve this function. Against these convenient, effective approaches, they conclude, germ-line gene therapy will never be cost-effective enough to merit high enough social priority to pursue.

One scientific rejoinder to this argument is that screening will not help with all cases. Presumably, for example, as more beneficiaries of somatic cell gene therapy survive to reproductive age, there will be more couples whose members are both afflicted with the same recessive disorders (Wivel and Walters 1993). Gene-therapy strategies that affect the germ line may also be the only effective ways of addressing some genetic diseases with origins very early in development. Moreover, by preventing the transmission of disease genes, germ-line gene therapy could obviate the need for screening and somatic cell gene therapy in subsequent generations of a family.

Social Risks

Proponents of germ-line gene-therapy research also point out that screening prevents genetic disease only by preventing the birth of the patients who would suffer from it. This, they point out, is a confusion of therapeutic goals that runs the long-term risk of encouraging coercive eugenic practices and tacitly fostering discrimination against those with genetic disease. By attempting to prevent disease in individuals rather than selecting against individuals according to genotype, germ-line gene therapy would allow us to maintain our commitment to the value of moral equality in the fact of our acknowledged biological diversity (Juengst 1995).

Critics reply to this that, to the contrary, it is germ-line therapy that has the more ominous social implications, by opening the door to genetic enhancement. One line of argument recalls the historical abuses of the eugenic movement to suggest that, to the extent that the line between gene therapy and enhancement would increasingly blur, germ-line interventions would be open to the same questions about the proper vision of human flourishing that eugenics faced. Even those who dispute the dangers of the "slippery slope" in this context take pains to defend the moral significance of the distinction "between uses that may relieve real suffering and those that alter characteristics that have little or nothing to do with disease" (Fletcher 1985, p. 303). Proponents must then argue that appropriate distinctions among these different uses can be confidently drawn (Anderson 1989) and point out that the same eugenic challenges already face those engaged in preimplantation screening or prenatal diagnosis (Fowler et al. 1989).

Human Rights Concerns

Finally, however, some critics argue that the focus of germ-line gene therapy on the embryonic patient has other implications that foreclose its pursuit. If the primary goal of the intervention is to address the health problems of the pre-embryo itself, germ-line gene therapy becomes an extreme case of fetal therapy, and the pre-embryo gains the status of a patient requiring protection. Germ-line gene-therapy experiments would involve research with early human embryos that would have effects on their offspring, effectively placing multiple human generations in the role of unconsenting research subjects (Lappe 1991). If pre-embryos are given the moral status of patients, it will be very hard to justify the risks of clinical research that would be necessary to develop the technique.

This objection to human germ-line gene-therapy research is framed in several ways. For European commentators, it is often interpreted as the right to one's genetic patrimony (Mauron and Thevoz 1991) in that germ-line gene-therapy interventions would violate the rights of subsequent generations to inherit a genetic endowment that has not been intentionally modified. For advocates of people with disabilities, this concern is interpreted in terms of the dangers of society's willingness to accept their differences (Buchanan 1996). Some feminists join this position as well, out of a concern for the impact on women of taking the pre-embryo too seriously as an object of medical care (Minden 1987).

Proponents can offer several responses to these concerns. First of all, some of these appeals, such as the appeals to the rights of future generations to an unmodified "genetic patrimony," can be criticized simply on scientific and conceptual grounds as incoherent (Juengst 1998a). Beyond that, proponents also argue that germ-line gene therapy is a reproductive health intervention aimed at the parents, not the embryo (Zimmerman 1991). Its goal is to allow the parents to address their reproductive risks and have a healthy baby, in cases in which the parents' own views prohibit preimplantation screening and embryo selection. In taking this position, proponents acknowledge the moral uncertainty over the status of the pre-embryo and defend parental requests for germ-line therapy as falling within the scope of their reproductive rights. Their argument is that, as a professional policy, medicine should continue to accept and respond to a wide range of interpretations of reproductive health needs by prospective parents, including requests for germ-line interventions (Fowler et al. 1989).

Germ-line gene transfer has traditionally been perceived as scientifically remote. However, the development of techniques in reproductive medicine, like in vitro ovum nuclear transfer (Rubenstein et al. 1995), makes the prospect of applying somatic cell gene-transfer techniques to preimplantation embryos a good bit more realistic. Although the application of gene-transfer techniques at that stage would still lack adequate background evidence of safety and efficacy, the relatively unregulated environment in which innovations in reproductive medicine are introduced increases the risks that such experimentation could occur. The danger of muting the public discussion of human gene transfer at the national level, of course, is the risk of creating a climate in which such experimentation could proceed without prior knowledge or review.

ENHANCEMENT USES OF HUMAN GENE-TRANSFER TECHNOLOGIES

The second distinction that has become standard in discussions of the ethics of human gene therapy contrasts the use of human gene-transfer techniques to treat health problems with their use to enhance or improve normal human traits. Whereas the somatic cell germ-line distinction is accused of lacking adequate ethical force (Moseley 1991), the conceptual line between those two classes of intervention is at least clear. The treatment–enhancement distinction, however, often seems in danger of evaporating entirely under its conceptual critiques and to that extent seems to pose the larger risk to our efforts at assessing human gene-transfer technology.

The Treatment–Enhancement Distinction

The treatment–enhancement distinction is usually used to argue that curative or therapeutic uses of genetic engineering fall within (and are protected by) the boundaries of medicine's traditional domain, whereas enhancement uses do not and to that extent are more problematic as a professional medical practice or a legitimate health-care need (Anderson 1989; Baird 1994). There are several interesting rejoinders to this argument. Some argue that medicine has no essential domain of practice, so that a coherent distinction between medical and nonmedical services can never be drawn in the first place (Engelhardt 1986). Others accept the distinction between treating and enhancing but take on the traditional values of medicine, by arguing that privileging treatment over enhancement is itself wrong (Silvers 1994). Others argue that, in any case, for psychological and economic reasons, the line between treatment and enhancement will be impossible to hold in practice (Gardner 1995).

There is another response to the treatment–enhancement distinction, however, that is particularly relevant to the immediate goals of gene-transfer research. This response criticizes the distinction by showing how it dissolves in the case of using human gene-transfer techniques to prevent disease when such interventions involve the enhancement of the body's health maintenance capacities. The argument is that, to the extent that disease prevention is a proper goal of medicine, and the use of gene-transfer techniques to strengthen or enhance human health maintenance capacities will help achieve that goal, then the treatment–enhancement distinction cannot confine or define the limits of the proper medical use of gene-transfer techniques (Walters and Palmer 1996). This argument is bolstered by the fact that the technical prospects for such preventive enhancement interventions already look good, given gene-therapy protocols now under way to treat ill patients in just those ways (Wilson et al. 1992). One gene therapist summarizes this current biomedical work by saying:

> Over the next few years, it appears that the greatest application will be in the treatment of cancer, where a number of genes that have been isolated have the potential to *empower* the immune system to eliminate cancer cells . . . Human gene therapy cancer trials have also been initiated for insertion of the tumor necrosis factor (TNF) gene into T-lymphocytes in an effort *to enhance the ability* of T-lymphocytes to kill tumors. Another approach has been to insert the TNF gene into tumor cells in an effort *to induce a more vigorous immune response* against the tumor (Culver 1993 [emphasis added]).

If human gene-therapy protocols like these are acceptable as forms of preventive medicine, the critics ask, how can we claim that we should be "drawing the line" at enhancement?

There have been a number of attempts to articulate the concept of "enhancement" in a way that will allow it to function as a necessary and sufficient criterion for drawing a boundary for medical practice that can include legitimate forms of preventive medicine. Some accounts use quasistatistical concepts of "normality" to argue that any intervention designed to restore or preserve a species-typical level of functioning for an individual should count as treatment, leaving only those that would give individuals capabilities beyond the range of normal human variation to fall outside the pale as enhancement (Daniels 1992). Others attempt to draw the line between interventions addressed to diagnosable pathologies and those aimed at improvements that do not bear on the individual's health (Juengst 1997). All of these efforts, however, face a fundamental practical challenge in that no matter how the line is drawn, most of the gene-transfer interventions that could become problematic as enhancement interventions would not have to cross that line to be developed and approved for clinical use, because they will also have legitimate therapeutic applications.

For example, consider the efforts to develop gene-transfer techniques for promoting the growth of blood vessels. As long as these techniques are developed and assessed as efforts to help treat coronary artery disease, the issues of their potential enhancement applications need not arise. However, once approved for use by the FDA and absent further public oversight or regulation, the same techniques could be used "off-label" to improve the oxygenation of the limb muscles of athletes as a permanent alternative to the various blood-doping schemes now used in competitive sport. Moreover, given the current regulatory vacuum surrounding the private practice of reproductive medicine, there is little to prohibit the application of these techniques to early human embryos as well, in hopes of effecting germ-line transformations.

These realities have pressed those who would use the treatment–enhancement distinction for policy purposes to articulate the moral dangers of genetic enhancement more clearly (Parens 1998). After all, personal improvement is praised in many spheres of human endeavor, and, as purely elective matter, biomedical interventions like cosmetic surgery are well accepted in our society as means to achieving personal improvement goals.

Enhancement as a Form of Cheating

There are two lines of thought that have emerged from this recent work. The first focuses on the idea that biomedical enhancements, unlike achievements, are a form of cheating. This is the view that taking the biomedical shortcut somehow cheats or undercuts the specific social practices that would make the analogous human achievement valuable in the first place. Thus, some argue that it defeats the purpose of the contest for the marathon runner to gain endurance chemically rather than through training, and it misses the point of meditation to gain Nirvana through psychosurgery. In both cases, the value of the improvements lie in the achievements they reward as well as the benefits they bring. The achievements—successful training or disciplined meditation—add value to the improvements because they are understood to be admirable social practices in themselves. Whenever a corporeal intervention is used to bypass an admirable social practice, then, the improvement's social value—the value of a runner's physical endurance or a mystic's visions—is weakened accordingly. If we are to preserve the value of the social practices we count as enhancing, it may be in society's interest to impose a means-based limit on biomedical enhancement efforts (Murray 1984).

Interpreting enhancement interventions as those that short-circuit admirable human practices in an effort to obtain some personal goal has special utility at two levels of ethical analysis. First, for individuals, it highlights the challenge that enhancement poses to their moral integrity. To what extent can they take credit for their accomplishments if they do not achieve them through the socially valued practices that have traditionally produced them? This question is not one about either causation or responsibility. Clearly, they are still the authors of their accomplishments. It would be a mistake for the student whose Ritalin-induced concentration yields a high exam grade from one night's cramming to think that it was literally the Ritalin that took the test and made the grade. The question is whether the student earned the grade, that is, whether the grade is serving its usual function of signaling the disciplined study and active learning that the practice of being a student is supposed to involve. If the grade is not serving that function, then, for that student, it is a hollow accomplishment, without the intrinsic value it would otherwise have.

Moreover, this interpretation of enhancement also has implications for the policies of the social institutions that maintain the practices we value. To the extent that biomedical shortcuts increasingly allow specific accomplishments, like test-taking, to be divorced from the admirable practices they were designed to signal, the social value of those accomplishments will be undermined. Not only will the intrinsic value be diminished for everyone that takes the shortcut, but the resulting disparity between the enhanced and unenhanced will call the fairness of the whole game (be it educational, recreational, or professional) into question. If the extrinsic value of being causally responsible for certain accomplishments is high enough (like professional sports salaries), the intrinsic value of the admirable practices that a particular institution was designed to foster may even start to be called into question. For institutions interested in continuing to foster the social values for which they have traditionally been the guardians, this has two alternative policy implications. Either they must redesign the game (of education, sports, etc.) to find new ways to evaluate excellence in the admirable practices that are not affected by available enhancements, or they must prohibit the use of the enhancing shortcuts. Which route an institution should take depends on the possibility and practicality of taking either, because ethically they are equivalent.

Enhancement as an Abuse of Medicine

Unfortunately, some of the social games we can play (and cheat in) do not turn on participants' achievements at all, but on traits over which individuals have little control, such as stature, shape, and skin color. The social games of stigmatization, discrimination, and exclusion use these traits in the same manner that other practices use achievements: as intrinsically valuable keys to extrinsic goods. Now it is becoming increasingly possible to seek biomedical help in changing these traits to short-circuit these games as well (Parens 1995). Here, the biomedical interventions involved, like skin lighteners or stature increasers, are enhancements because they serve to improve the recipient's social standing, but only by perpetuating the social bias under which they originally labored. Any normal medical tool that cured one patient by making other patients' problems worse would be considered medically perverse, and in this case, the perversion is compounded by the fact that the problem in question is social, not somatic. When enhancement is understood in this way, it warns of still another set of moral concerns.

With this interpretation, what makes the provision of human growth hormone to a short child a morally suspicious enhancement is not the absence of a diagnosable disease or the dictates of medical policy or the species-atypical hormone level that would result: Rather, it is the intent to improve the child's social status by changing the child rather than by changing her social environment. Enhancement interventions are almost always wrongheaded under this account, because the source of the social status they seek to improve is, by definition, the social group and not the individual. Attempting to improve that status in the individual without regard for its social nature amounts to a moral mistake akin to "blaming the victim": It misattributes causality, is ultimately futile, and can have harmful consequences. This is the interpretation of enhancement that seems to be at work when people argue that it inappropriately "medicalizes" a social problem to use Ritalin to induce cooperative behavior in the classroom or that breast augmentation surgery only exacerbates society's sexist vision of beauty (Morgan 1991). In each case, the critics dispute the assumption that the human need in question is one that is created by, and quenchable through, our bodies and assert that both its source and solution really lie in quite a different sphere of human experience.

This interpretation of the enhancement concept is useful to those interested in the ethics of personal improvement because it warns of a number of moral pitfalls beyond the base line considerations that the enhancement–treatment distinction provides. Attempting to improve social status by changing the individual risks being self-defeating (by exacerbating the individual's sense of inadequacy by inflating expectations), futile (if the individual's comparative gains are neutralized by the enhancement's availability to the whole social group), unfair (if the whole group does not have access to the enhancement), or complicitous with unjust social prejudices (by forcing people into a range of variation dictated by biases that favor one group over others). For those faced with decisions about whether to use performance-enhancing drugs in sports or to insert the leadership gene into embryos, this way of understanding enhancement is much more illuminating than attempts to distinguish it from medical treatment.

The medicalization of social problems, as opposed to merely assisting patients to cheat in specific social achievements, also has significant implications for the boundaries of medicine. Whereas stature or speed can at least be measured by medicine, there is a large class of traits, for example, loyalty and competitiveness, leadership and stewardship, aggression and altruism, that cannot even be perceived without a larger frame of reference. These latter are all traits that characterize our interactions with and evaluation by other people: the machinery of social flourishing. In fact, they are traits that are impossible to identify or evaluate without reference to the social context of the individuals who display them: The solitary shipwreck survivor does not display them. Thus, the improvement of these traits has traditionally been the domain of our social engineers (i.e., teachers, ministers, coaches, and counselors) supported by policymakers charged with creating environments in which such traits can be cultivated. When attempts are made to shift the improvement of these traits into the domain of the doctor, by working directly on the substrates for social capacities that our bodies provide, medicine runs up against a basic epistemic boundary. It is not clear how one would identify any optimum or even maximum conditions for social traits through medical means alone. For example, what dosage of human growth hormone will ensure optimum social advantage? This suggests a test for one kind of enhancement boundary. If criteria drawn from other spheres of experience seem like better measures of improvement than medical measures, then the intervention in question should probably count as an enhancement that goes beyond medicine's domain of expertise. Because of its own epistemic limits, the argument goes, biomedicine should restrict its ambitions to the sphere of bodily dynamics, which it knows something about, and leave the sphere of social dynamics in the hands of others (Juengst 1998b).

CONCLUSION

No other biomedical intervention in history has received as much international and interdisciplinary attention as human gene therapy (Fletcher 1990). Three points of striking consensus have emerged from that global discussion.

The first point is that somatic cell gene transfer research does not constitute a major break with medical therapeutics, but this technique still should be regulated through public review processes. The dangers of confusion over the therapeutic benefits of gene-transfer research, and the need for public discussion of the applications of gene-transfer techniques to the germ line and for enhancement purposes, all reinforce the importance of the unique populist tradition that governed the birth of the field. As somatic cell gene-therapy techniques mature into reliable clinical alternatives for different medical domains, this commitment will raise hard questions about how best to achieve public participation in this field.

The second point of consensus is that current concerns about clinical risks and biohazards make human experimentation with germ-line inventions unacceptable for the time being. Beyond that, discussion is flourishing about whether germ-line interventions could ever be ethically acceptable and, if so, under what circumstances.

The third point of consensus is the view that gene therapy, both somatic and germ line, should be evaluated as a clinical tool employed on behalf of the seriously ill, and not as a eugenic public-health tool designed to benefit the population nor as a shortcut to personal social advantage. In contemporary political argot, genetic medicine should continue to be an empowering, not exclusionary, science. It should be about helping living people address their individual health problems, not about protecting the "gene pool" from the ebb and flow of human alleles in populations or the social classifications that we impose our genetic differences.

ACKNOWLEDGMENTS

The research conducted for this chapter was supported in part by National Institutes of Health grant R01 HG-1446-02.

REFERENCES

Anderson F.W. 1972. Genetic therapy. In *The new genetics and the future of man* (ed. M. Hamilton), pp. 110–125. W.B. Eerdmans. Grand Rapids, Michigan.

——— 1989. Human gene therapy: Why draw a line? *J. Med. Philos.* **14:** 681–693

Anderson F.W. and Fletcher J. 1980. Gene therapy in human beings: When is it ethical to begin? *N. Eng. J. Med.* **303:** 1293–1297.

Annas G. 1985. The Phoenix heart: What we have to lose. *Hastings Cent. Rep.* **15:** 15–16.

Areen J. 1985. Regulating human gene therapy. *W Va. Law Rev.* **88:** 153.

Baird P. 1994. Altering human genes: Social, ethical and legal implications. *Perspect. Biol. Med.* 37: 566–575

Brenner M. *1995.* Human somatic gene therapy: Progress and problems. *J. Intern. Med.* **237:** 229–239.

Buchanan A. 1996. Choosing who will be disabled: Genetic intervention and the morality of inclusion. *Soc. Philos. Policy* **13:** 18–47.

Capron A. 1990. The impact of the report, Splicing Life. *Hum. Gene Ther* **1:** 69–73.

Capron A., Leventhal B., Post L., Walters L., and Zallen D. 1993. Requests for compassionate use of gene therapy:

Memorandum from the subcommittee to the RAC. *Hum Gene Ther* **4:** 199–200.
Council for Responsible Genetics. 1993. Position paper on human germ line manipulation (Fall, 1992). *Hum. Gene Ther.* **4:** 35–37.
Culver, K. 1993. Current status of human gene therapy research. In *The genetic resource.* vol. 7, pp. 5–10. New England Regional Genetics Group, Newton, Massachusetts.
Daniels N. 1992. Growth hormone therapy for short stature: Can we support the treatment/enhancement distinction? *Growth Genet. Horm.* (suppl. 1) **8:** 46–48.
Davis B. 1992. Germ-line gene therapy: Evolutionary and moral considerations. *Hum. Gene Ther* **3:** 361–365.
Engelhardt H.T. 1986. *The foundations of bioethics.* Oxford University Press, Oxford, United Kingdom.
Flannery E. 1986. Should it be easier or harder to use unapproved devices? *Hastings Cent.Rep.* **16:** 17–23.
Fletcher J. C. 1985. Ethical issues in and beyond prospective clinical trials of human gene therapy. *J. Med. Philos.* **10:** 293–309.
——— 1990. Evolution of ethical debate about human gene therapy. *Hum. Gene Ther.* **1:** 55–69.
Fowler G., Juengst E., and Zimmerman B. 1989. Germ-line gene therapy and the clinical ethos of medical genetics. *Theor. Med.* **10:** 151–165.
Gardner W. 1995. Can enhancement be prohibited? *J. Med. Philos.* **20:** 65–84.
Healy B. 1993. Remarks for the RAC regarding compassionate use exemption. *Hum. Gene Ther.* **4:** 195–197.
Hotchkiss R. 1965. Portents for a genetic engineering. *J. Hered.* **56:** 197–202.
Juengst E. 1995. "Prevention" and the goals of genetic medicine. *Hum. Gene Ther.* **6:** 1595–1605.
——— 1997. Can enhancement be distinguished from prevention in genetic medicine? *J. Med. Philos.* **22:** 125–142.
——— 1998a. Should we treat the human germ-line as a global human resource? In *Germ-line intervention and our responsibilities to future generations* (ed. E. Agius and S. Busuttil), pp. 85–102. Kluwer, Dordrecht, The Netherlands.
——— 1998b. The meanings of "enhancement" for biomedicine. In *Enhancing human traits: Conceptual complexities and ethical implications* (ed. E. Parens). Georgetown University Press, Washington D.C. (In press.)
Kolata G. and Wade N. 1980. Human gene treatment stirs new debate. *Science* **210:** 40.
Krimsky S. 1985. *Genetic alchemy: The social history of the recombinant DNA controversy.* MIT Press, Boston, Massachusetts.
Lappe M. 1991. Ethical issues in manipulating the human germ line. *J. Med. Philos.* **10:** 621–639.
Levine R. 1986. Ethics and regulation of clinical research. Urban and Schwarzenberg, New York.
Mauron A. and Thevoz J.-M. 1991. Germ-line engineering: A few European voices. *Med. Philos.* **16:** 649–666.
Minden S. 1987. Patriarchal designs: The genetic engineering of human embryo. *In Made to order: The myth of reproductive and genetic progress* (ed. P. Spallone and D. Steinberg), pp. 102–109. Pergamon Press, Oxford, United Kingdom.
Morgan K. 1991. Women and the knife: Cosmetic surgery and the colonization of women's bodies. *Hypatia* **6:** 25–53.
Moseley R. 1991. Maintaining the somatic/germ-line distinction: Some ethical drawbacks. *J Med. Philos.* **16:** 641–649.
Munson R. and Davis L. 1992. Germ-line gene therapy and the medical imperative. *Kennedy Inst. Ethics J.* **2:** 137–158.
Murray T. 1984. Drugs, sports and ethics. In *Feeling good and doing better: Ethics and nontherapeutic drug use* (ed. T. Murray et al.), pp. 107–129. Humana Press, Clifton, New Jersey.
Parens E. 1995. The goodness of fragility: On the prospect of genetic technologies aimed at the enhancement of human capabilities. *Kennedy Inst. Ethics J.* **5:** 151–153.
——— 1998. Is better always good? *Hastings Cent. Rep.* **28:** S1–S17.
President's Commission for the Study of Ethical Problems in Medicine and Biomedical and Behavioral Research. 1982. *Splicing life: A report on the social and ethical issues of genetic engineering with human beings.* U.S. Government Printing Office, Washington, D.C.
Ramsey P. 1972. Genetic therapy: A theologian's response. In *The new genetics and the future of man* (ed. M. Hamilton), pp. 157–179. W.B. Eerdmans, Grand Rapids, Michigan.
Recombinant DNA Advisory Committee. 1993. Procedures to be followed for expedited review of single patient protocols. *Hum. Gene Ther.* **4:** 307.
Rubenstein D.S., Thomasma D.C., Schon E.A., and Zinaman J. 1995. Germ-line gene therapy to cure mitochondrial disease: Protocol and ethics of in vitro ovum nuclear transplantation. *Camb. Q. Healthcare Ethics,* **4:** 316–339.
Silvers A. 1994. Defective agents: Equality, difference and the tyranny of the normal. *J. Soc. Philos.* **25:** 154–175.
Subcommittee on Human Gene Therapy (Recombinant DNA Advisory Committee National Institutes of Health). 1990. Points to consider in the design and submission of protocols for the transfer of recombinant DNA into the genome of human subjects *Hum. Gene Ther.* **1:** 93–103.
Temin H.M. 1990. Safety considerations in somatic gene therapy of human disease. *Hums Gene Ther.* **1:** 111–123.
Thompson L. 1993. Gene therapy: Healy approves an unproved treatment. *Science* **259:** 172.

——— 1994. *Correcting the code: Inventing the genetic cure for the human body*. Simon and Schuster, New York.
U.S. Congress (Office of Technology Assessment). 1984. *Human gene therapy*. U.S. Government Printing Office, Washington, D.C.
Walters L. and Palmer J. 1996. *The ethics of human gene therapy*. Oxford University Press, Oxford, United Kingdom.
Wilson J.M., Grossman M., Raper S.E., Baker Jr. J.R., Newton R.S., and Theone J.G. 1992. Ex vivo gene therapy for familial hypercholesterolemia. *Hum. Gene Ther.* **3:** 179–222.
Wivel N.A. and Walters L. 1993. Germ-line gene modification and disease prevention: Some medical and ethical perspectives. *Science* **262:** 533–538.
Wolf S.M. 1997. Ban cloning? Why NBAC is wrong. *Hastings Cent. Rep.* **27:** 12–15.
Zimmerman B.K. 1991. Human germ-line therapy: The case for its development and use. *J. Med. Philos.* **16:** 593–612.

GERM-LINE GENE THERAPY: ETHICALLY ACCEPTABLE IN PRINCIPLE

LeRoy Walters and Julie Gage Palmer

ETHICAL ISSUES

An Earlier Stage of the Discussion: *Muller* versus *Lederberg*

The ethical debate over intentionally introducing genetic changes into the human germ line through advanced biomedical techniques goes back at least to the 1920s and 1930s and the writings of classical geneticists J.B.S. Haldane and H. J. Muller. The discussion was renewed in the late 1950s and early 1960s, with two of the chief protagonists being H. J. Muller and molecular biologist Joshua Lederberg. Muller advocated the improvement of the gene pool through voluntary programs of assisted reproduction—specifically artificial insemination using semen from donors who had what Muller viewed as the best combination of physical, intellectual, and moral qualities. (Egg donation was not a technical possibility in the 1960s, as it is today. Given his general advocacy of women's rights, Muller would surely have approved the equal participation of women in this voluntary program for improving the human gene pool.) At a symposium held in London in November 1962, Joshua Lederberg criticized Muller's proposal for its lack of precision and for the very slow progress that Muller's plan for guided evolution would deliver. In Lederberg's words,

> The recent achievements of molecular biology strengthen our eugenic means to achieve [human survival]. But do they necessarily support proposals to transfer animal husbandry to man? My own first conclusion is that the technology of human genetics is pitifully clumsy, even by the standards of practical agriculture. Surely within a few generations we can expect to learn tricks of immeasurable advantage. Why bother now with somatic selection, so slow in its impact? Investing a fraction of the effort, we should soon learn how to manipulate chromosome ploidy [number of sets of chromosomes], homozygosis [the union of gametes that are identical for one or more pairs of genes], gametic selection, full diagnosis of heterozygotes, to accomplish in one or two generations of eugenic practice what would now take ten or one hundred.

Even 30+ years after Lederberg's statement there are many "tricks" that molecular biologists have not yet learned about genes, chromosomes,

From Chapter 3 in *The Ethics of Human Gene Therapy* by LeRoy Walters and Julie Gage Palmer (Oxford University Press, 1997). Reprinted by permission of the publisher.

and cells. The chief trick that remains elusive is guiding new genes to precise locations where they can replace malfunctioning genes. Also, in the 1990s we are less likely to *begin* our discussions of germ-line genetic intervention by thinking of global effects on human evolution. We are much more likely to begin by considering specific diseases and decisions that are likely to be faced by couples who are deciding whether or not to have children. The thinking of those couples will be focused, first and foremost, on the welfare of their children and perhaps on the welfare of their children's children as well.

A Preliminary Question: Should This Issue Be Discussed at All?

In September of 1992 a distinguished physician–scientist, Dr. James V. Neel, appeared before the NIH RAC [National Institutes of Health Recombinant DNA Advisory Committee] to discuss spontaneous and induced germ-line mutation. Dr. Neel argued that it would be premature for the RAC to discuss the scientific and ethical questions surrounding germ-line gene therapy. His precise message, as summarized in a 1993 editorial, was the following:

> The Committee's desire to prepare itself for future developments would under most circumstances be laudable, but for a Committee with this visibility and prestige to begin to consider the subject of germ-line therapy in an organized fashion at this time would send the wrong vibes to the scientific, ethical, and political communities. Such an action might appear to imply the belief that the Committee would be seriously considering this prospect within the terms of office of present Committee members. Given the tremendous issues at stake, and even with the utmost attempt on my part to anticipate the amazing speed of advances in the field of molecular genetics, I could not imagine serious organized discussions of this subject by such a group within the next 20 or 30 years. (Individuals will, of course, express their views as they please.)

Dr. Neel carefully avoids urging individuals, like the present authors, to refrain from discussing the topic of germ-line gene therapy. On the other hand, he clearly thinks that it would be a mistake for public advisory committees like the RAC to engage in anticipatory discussions of this subject. We respectfully disagree. In our view, the years from 1983 through 1988, during which the RAC looked ahead to the first hypothetical somatic-cell gene-therapy proposals, were very profitably devoted to anticipating what the new technology might mean and to developing "points to consider," or very general guidelines, for somatic cell therapy proposals. In a similar way, given the research advances outlined in the earlier part of this chapter, we think that both individuals and public advisory committees would be wise to begin the discussion of this important topic sooner rather than later. If proposals for human application of germ-line gene therapy are delayed because of technical obstacles, or if research moves in unanticipated directions that must then later be taken into account, the risks of premature discussion are low. On the other hand, if a technical breakthrough occurs that makes germ-line gene therapy feasible, the anticipatory discussion of the topic may turn out to have been essential for the calm formulation of rational oversight policies. . . .

Major Ethical Arguments in Favor of Germ-Line Gene Therapy

In this and the following section we will analyze the major ethical arguments for and against germ-line gene therapy. For this analysis we will make the optimistic assumption that germ-line intervention methods will gradually be refined until they reach the point where gene replacement or gene repair is technically feasible and able to be accomplished in more than 95% of attempted gene transfer procedures. Thus, the following analysis presents the arguments for and against germ-line intervention under the most favorable conditions for such intervention.

A first argument in favor of germ-line intervention is that it may be the only way to prevent damage to particular biological individuals when that damage is caused by certain kinds of genetic defects. . . . [O]nly genetic modifications introduced into preimplantation embryos are likely to be early enough to affect all of the important cell types (as in retinoblastoma), or to reach a large enough fraction of brain cells, or to be in time to prevent irreversible damage to the developing embryo. In these circumstances the primary intent of gene therapy would, or at least could, be to provide gene therapy for the early embryo. A side effect of the intervention would be that all of the embryonic cells, including reproductive cells that would later develop, would be genetically modified.

A second moral argument for germ-line genetic intervention might be advanced by parents. It is that they wish to spare their children and grandchildren from either (1) having to undergo somatic cell gene therapy if they are born affected with a genetic defect or (2) having to face difficult decisions regarding possibly transmitting a disease-related gene to their own children and grandchildren. In our first scenario, admittedly a rare case, two homozygous parents who have a genetic disease know in advance that all of their offspring are likely to be affected with the same genetic disease. In the second scenario, there is a certain probability that the parents' offspring will be affected or carriers. An assumption lying behind this second argument is that parents should enjoy a realm of moral and legal protection when they are making good-faith decisions about the health of their children. Only if their decisions are clearly adverse to the health interests of the children should moral criticism or legal intervention be considered.

A third moral argument for germ-line intervention is more likely to be made by health professionals, public-health officials, and legislators casting a waxy eye toward the expenditures for health care. This argument is that, from a social and economic point of view, germ-line intervention is more efficient than repeating somatic cell gene therapy generation after generation. From a medical and public health point of view, germ-line intervention fits better with the increasingly preferred model of disease prevention and health promotion. In the very long run, germ-line intervention, if applied to both affected individuals and asymptomatic carriers of serious genetic defects, could have a beneficial effect on the human gene pool and the frequency of genetic disease.

A fourth argument refers to the roles of researchers and health professionals. As a general rule, researchers deserve to have the freedom to explore new modes of treating and/or preventing human disease. To be sure, moral rules sets limits on how this research is conducted. For example, animals involved in the preclinical stages of the research should be treated humanely. In addition, the human subjects involved in the clinical trials should be treated with respect. When and if germ-line gene therapy is some day validated as a safe and effective intervention, health care providers should be free to, and may have a moral obligation to, offer it to their patients as a possible treatment. This freedom is based on the professional's general obligation to seek out and offer the best possible therapeutic alternatives to patients and society's recognition of a sphere in which health professionals are at liberty to exercise their best judgment on behalf of their patients.

A fifth and final argument in favor of germ-line gene therapy is that this kind of intervention best accords with the health professions' healing role and with the concern to protect rather than penalize individuals who have disabilities. This argument is not simply a plea for protecting all embryos and fetuses from the time of fertilization forward. Both authors of this book think that abortion is morally justifiable in certain circumstances. However, prenatal diagnosis followed by selective abortion and preimplantation diagnosis followed by selective discard seem to us to be uncomfortable and probably discriminatory halfway technologies that should eventually be replaced by effective modes of treatment. The options of selective abortion and selective discard essentially say to prospective parents, "There is nothing effective that the health care system has to offer. You may want to give up on this fetus or embryo and try again." To people with disabilities that are diagnosable at the prenatal or preimplantation stages of development the message of selective abortion and selective discard may seem more threatening. That message may be read as, "If we health professionals and prospective parents had known you were coming, we would have terminated your development and attempted to find or create a nondisabled replacement."

This argument is not intended to limit the legal access of couples to selective abortion in the case of serious health problems for the fetus. We support such access. Rather, it is an argument about what the long-term goal of medicine and society should be. In our view, that long-term goal should be to prevent disability and disease wherever possible. Where prevention is not possible, the second-best alternative is a cure or other definitive remedy. In cases where neither prevention nor cure is possible, our goal should be to help people cope with disability and disease while simultaneously seeking to find a cure.

Major Arguments Against Germ-Line Gene Therapy

First, if the technique has unanticipated negative effects, those effects will be visited not only on the recipient of the intervention himself or herself but also on all of the descendants of that recipient. This argument seems to assume that a mistake, once made, could not be corrected, or at least that the mistake might not become apparent until the recipient became the biological parent of at least one child. For that first child, at least, the negative effects could be serious, as well as uncorrectable.

Second, some critics of germ-line genetic intervention argue that this technique will never be necessary because of available alternative strategies for preventing the transmission of diagnosable genetic diseases. Specifically, critics of germ-line gene therapy have sometimes suggested that preimplantation diagnosis and the selective discard of affected embryos might be a reasonable alternative to the high-technology, potentially risky attempt to repair genetic defects in early human embryos. Even without in vitro fertilization and preimplantation diagnosis, the option of prenatal diagnosis and selective abortion is available for many disorders. According to this view, these two types of selection, before embryos or fetuses have reached the stage of viability, are effective means for achieving the same goal.

The third argument is closely related to the second: this technique will always be an expensive option that cannot be made available to most couples, certainly not by any publicly funded health care system. Therefore, like in vitro fertilization for couples attempting to overcome the problem of infertility, germ-line gene therapy will be available only to wealthy people who can afford to pay its considerable expense on their own.

The fourth argument builds on the preceding two: precisely because germ-line intervention will be of such limited utility in preventing disease, there will be strong pressures to use this technique for genetic enhancement at the embryonic stage, when it could reasonably be expected to make a difference in the future life prospects of the embryo. Again in this case, only the affluent would be able to afford the intervention. However, if enhancement interventions were safe and efficacious, the long-term effect of such germ-line intervention would probably be to exacerbate existing differences between the most-well-off and the least-well-off segments of society.

Fifth, even though germ-line genetic intervention aims in the long run to treat rather than to abort or discard, the issue of appropriate respect for preimplantation embryos and implanted fetuses will nonetheless arise in several ways. After thoroughgoing studies of germ-line intervention have been conducted in nonhuman embryos, there will undoubtedly be a stage at which parallel studies in human embryos will be proposed. The question of human embryo research was recently studied by a committee appointed by the director of the National Institutes of Health. Although the committee specifically avoided commenting on germ-line intervention, its recommendation that certain kinds of human embryo research should be continued and that such research should be funded by NIH provoked considerable controversy. Critics of the committee's position would presumably also oppose the embryo research that would be proposed to prepare the way for germ-line gene therapy in humans. Their principal argument would be that the destruction or other harming of preimplantation embryos in research is incompatible with the kind of respect that should be shown to human embryos.

Even after the research phase of germ-line genetic intervention is concluded, difficult questions about the treatment of embryos will remain. For example, preimplantation diagnosis may continue to involve the removal of one or two totipotential cells from a four- to eight-cell embryo. While the moral status of totipotential human embryonic cells has received scant attention in bioethical debates, there is, at least a plausible argument that a totipotential cell, once separated from the remainder of a preimplantation embryo, is virtually equivalent to a zygote; that is, under favorable conditions it could develop into an embryo, a fetus, a newborn, and an adult. This objection to the destruction of totipotential embryonic cells will only be overcome if a noninvasive genetic diagnostic test for early embryos (like an x-ray or a CT scan) can be developed. Further, even if a noninvasive diagnostic test is available, as we have noted above, a postintervention diagnostic test will probably be undertaken with each embryo to verify that the intervention has been successful. Health professionals and prospective parents will probably be at least open to the possibility of selective discard or selective abortion if something has gone radically wrong in the intervention procedure. Thus, germ-line genetic intervention may remain foreclosed as a moral option to those who are conscientiously opposed to any action that would directly terminate the life of a preimplantation embryo or a fetus.

The sixth argument points to potential perils of concentrating great power in the hands of human beings. According to this view, the technique of germ-line intervention would give human beings, or a small group of human beings, too much control over the future evolution of the human race. This argument does not necessarily attribute malevolent intentions to those who have the training that would allow them to employ the technique. It implies that there are built-in limits that humans ought not to exceed, perhaps for theological or metaphysical reasons, and at least hints that compatibility is an ever-present possibility for the very powerful.

The seventh argument explicitly raises the issue of malevolent use. If one extrapolates from Nazi racial hygiene programs, this argument asserts, it is likely the germ-line intervention will be used by unscrupulous dictators to produce a class of superior human beings. The same techniques could be also used in precisely the opposite way, to produce human-like creatures who would willingly perform the least-attractive and the most-dangerous work for a society. According to this view, Aldous Huxley's *Brave New World* should be updated, for modern molecular biology provides tyrants with tools for modifying human beings that Huxley could not have imagined in 1932.

The eighth and final argument against germ-line genetic intervention is raised chiefly by several European authors who place this argument in the context of human rights. According to these commentators, human beings have a moral right to receive from their parents a genetic patrimony that has not been subjected to artificial tampering. Although the term "tampering" is not usually defined, it seems to mean any intentional effort to introduce genetic changes into the germ line, even if the goal is to reduce the likelihood that a genetic disease will be passed on to the children and grandchildren of a particular couple. The asserted right to be protected against such tampering may be a slightly different formulation of the sixth argument noted above—namely, that there are built-in limits, embedded in the nature of things, beyond which not even the most benevolent human beings should attempt to go.

A Brief Evaluation of the Arguments

In our view, the effort to cure and prevent serious disease and premature death is one of the noblest of all human undertakings. For this reason the first pro argument—that germ-line intervention may be the only way to treat or prevent certain diseases—seems to us to be of overriding importance. We also find the third pro argument to be quite strong, that a germ-line correction, if demonstrated to be safe and effective, would be more efficient than repeated applications of somatic cell gene therapy. In addition, the final pro argument about the overall mission of the health professions and about society's approach to disabilities seems to us to provide a convincing justification for the germ-line approach, when gene replacement is available.

Our replies to the objections raised by critics of germ-line intervention are as follows:

1. *Irreversible Mistakes.* While we acknowledge that mistakes may be made in germ-line gene therapy, we think that the same sophisticated techniques that were employed to introduce the new genes will be able to be used to remove those genes or to compensate for their presence in some other way. Further, in any sphere of innovative therapy, a first step into human beings must be taken at some point.

2. *Alternative Strategies.* Some couples, perhaps even most couples, will choose the alternative strategies of selective abortion or selective discard. In our view, a strategy of attempting to prevent or treat potential disease or disability in the particular biological individual accords more closely with the mission of the health sciences and shows greater respect for children and adults who are afflicted with disease or disability.

3. *High Cost, Limited Availability.* It is too early to know what the relative cost of germ-line intervention will be when the technique is fully developed. In addition, the financial costs and other personal and social harms of preventable diseases will need to be compared with the financial costs of germ-line gene therapy. It is at least possible that this new technology could become widely diffused and available to many members of society.

4. *Use for Enhancement.* Prudent social policy should be able to set limits on the use of germ-line genetic intervention. Further, some enhancements of human capabilities may be morally justifiable, especially when those enhancements are health related. We acknowledge that the distribution of genetic enhancement is an important question for policy makers. . . .

5. *Human Embryos.* In our view, research with early human embryos that is directed toward the development of germ-line gene therapy is morally justifiable in principle. Further, we acknowledge the potential of a totipotential cell but think that the value of a genetic diagnosis outweighs the value of such a cell. We also accept that, if a serious error is made in germ-line gene therapy, terminating the life of the resulting embryo or fetus may be morally justifiable. In short, there is a presumption in favor of fostering the continued development of human embryos and fetuses, but that presumption can in our view be overridden by other considerations like serious harm to the developing individual or others and the needs of preclinical research.

6. *Concentration of Power.* We acknowledge that those who are able to use germ-line intervention will have unprecedented ability to introduce precise changes into the germ lines of particular individuals and families. However, in our view, it is better for human beings to possess this ability and to use it for constructive purposes like preventing disease in families than not to possess the ability. The central ethical question is public accountability by the scientists, health providers, and companies that will be involved with germ-line intervention. Such accountability presupposes transparency about the use of the technology and ongoing monitoring process aimed at preventing its misuse.

7. *Misuse by Dictators.* This objection focuses too much attention on technology and too little on politics. There is no doubt that bona fide tyrants have existed in the 20th century and that they have made use of all manner of technologies—whether the low-tech methods of surgical sterilization or the annihilation of concentration camp inmates with poison gas or high-tech weapons like nuclear warheads and long-range missiles—to terrify and to dominate. However, the best approach to preventing the misuse of genetic technologies may not be to discourage the development of the technologies but rather to preserve and encourage democratic institutions that can serve as an antidote to tyranny. A second possible reply to the tyrannical misuse objection is that germ-line intervention requires a long lead time, in order to allow the offspring produced to grow to adulthood. Tyrants are often impatient people and are likely to prefer the more instantaneous methods of propaganda, intimidation, and annihilation of enemies to the relatively slow pace of germ-line modification.

8. *Human Rights and Tampering.* It is a daunting task to imagine what the unborn and as-yet-unconceived generations of people coming after us will want. Even more difficult is the effort to ascribe rights to human beings. Insofar as we can anticipate the needs and wants of future generations, we think that any reasonable future person would prefer health to serious disease and would therefore welcome a germ-line intervention in his or her family line that effectively prevented cystic fibrosis from being transmitted to him or her. In our view, such a person would not regard this intervention as tampering and would regard as odd the claim that his or her genetic patrimony has been artificially tampered with. Cystic fibrosis was not a part of his or her family's heritage that the future person was eager to receive or to claim.

Would Germ-Line Gene Therapy Be, or Lead to, a Eugenics Program?

We can perhaps best approach this question by imagining a future world in which the global elimination of a genetic disease by means of germ-line gene therapy is technically feasible.

> The year is 2055, and a definitive genetic cure for the mutations that cause cystic fibrosis (CF) has recently been discovered, tested, and perfected. This target-specific mode of gene therapy takes a properly functioning gene to the site of the mutation, splices out and destroys the malfunctioning gene, and replaces it with the properly functioning gene. The new technique can be applied equally well to somatic and germ-line (sperm or egg) cells.
>
> The World Health Organization (WHO) has recently announced a global program to eradicate all CF mutations from the human gene pool. The program is modeled on the earlier campaign to eliminate smallpox. All at-risk persons will be required to undergo testing and, if found to be affected or heterozygous, to accept genetic treatment of both their somatic and reproductive cells. WHO estimates that the global campaign will succeed within 35 years, at the most, and that the effort, when completed, will save $40 billion annually (in 2050 dollars) in the world health budget.

This hypothetical situation is extrapolated from past and present programs aimed at controlling serious infectious diseases. These programs include the worldwide campaign that eliminated smallpox, as well as state-based programs of mandatory immunization against such diseases as measles and polio.

A first issue raised by this hypothetical is whether it is reasonable to draw an analogy between infectious disease and genetic disease. Proponents of the analogy point to the transmissibility of disease in both cases and argue that the mere direction or mode of transmission—horizontal or vertical—is less important than the spread of disease. Opponents of the analogy point out that, while some infectious diseases are transmitted by intimate behavior, all genetic disease transmission occurs in the context of reproduction, one of the most intensely personal and private spheres of human life.

Second, we are not told in the hypothetical whether a voluntary program of genetic screening and gene therapy for CF has been tried and has failed. If it has not been tried, the burden of proof for the proponent of a mandatory program is heavier. Yet there may be plausible arguments, based on cost or the number of decades required to reach the goal in a voluntary program, for the moral preferability of the mandatory approach in this case and all relevantly similar cases. If a voluntary program has been tried and has failed because of public inertia or unreasonable resistance, a mandatory program might seem to be morally justifiable in this case, even to a civil libertarian, as a reasonable means to a highly desirable end.

Here we as coauthors see no alternative to drawing a sharp, clear moral and public-policy line. In our view, state intervention in reproductive decisions by individuals and couples is virtually always wrong and virtually always counter-productive as a public policy. We would apply this strong preference for voluntary public-health programs to several current technologies, for example, maternal serum alpha-fetoprotein screening to detect neural tube disorders, prenatal testing of HIV-infected pregnant women and postnatal testing of their infants, and newborn screening for genetic disease. In the same way we would apply this preference to the future hypothetical possibility of germ-line genetic intervention. Thus, we would support the *offering* of diagnostic testing and germ-line gene therapy to all adults. In our view, the vast majority of individuals and couples would eagerly participate in such a program, just as the vast majority of parents consent to newborn testing in states where free choice in this matter is respected. However, we regard state intervention to compel people to accept germ-line genetic intervention in their reproduction as a violation of a basic human right.

Would a voluntary germ-line program that aimed to reduce the incidence of one or more genetic diseases in human populations be a eugenics program? Much depends on whether the term *eugenics* is employed as a morally neutral, descriptive term or as a term that already includes in its very meaning a negative moral judgment, like the words "murder" and "rape." The coercive and discriminatory eugenics programs adopted in the United States and Nazi Germany in the first half of the 20th century are rightly condemned as immoral. The question remains, however, whether there is a place for the notion of a morally justifiable eugenics program—one that is strictly voluntary and firmly based on reliable genetic technologies. In our view, the word "eugenics" has been so tainted by the discriminatory, coercive practices of multiple nations in this century that it cannot be rehabilitated. Thus, we would want to use a different and probably more cumbersome formulation to describe such a program, for example, "a voluntary program to reduce the incidence of genetic disease through germ-line genetic intervention."

Finally, we note that the kind of public-health program outlined in this scenario would only be feasible if safe, reliable methods for effecting precise genetic changes in human sperm (or sperm-producing) cells and human egg cells within the bodies of adults are developed. Any technique that depends on in vitro fertilization and in vitro gene repair will be much too expensive to be used on a population-wide basis.

The Continuing Relevance of "Points to Consider" and General Ethical Principles

The preceding chapter on somatic cell gene therapy discussed seven questions that are currently asked by the NIH RAC as it reviews somatic cell proposals. These questions are contained in a guidance document called the "Points to Consider." The questions can be summarized as follows:

1. What is the disease to be treated?
2. What alternative treatments are available?
3. What is the potential harm of the intervention?
4. What is the potential benefit of the intervention?
5. How will the selection of patients be conducted in a way that is fair to all candidates?
6. How will the voluntary and informed consent of patients (or their parents or guardians) be solicited?
7. How will the privacy and confidentiality of patients be preserved?

In our view, these questions will be relevant to germ-line gene therapy proposals, but their emphasis will shift in important ways. In answering question 2, future researchers may need to discuss not only alternative *treatments* but also alternative strategies to prevent the transmission of genetic disorders to future generations. The options of preimplantation diagnosis and selective discard and of prenatal diagnosis and selective abortion will surely be discussed in this context. Questions 3 and 4 will also be pertinent but with an important shift in emphasis. If germ-line gene therapy is performed on early human embryos, the principal risks will be to the embryo and the embryo's potential descendants, not to the genetic parents of the embryo. Even if the parents have their sperm and egg cells treated in vivo by means of gene therapy, it is more likely that something will go wrong in the offspring than in the parents themselves. Similarly, the benefits of germ-line intervention will accrue primarily to the genetically repaired embryo and the embryo's future children rather than to the parents. Thus, the focus of the benefit–harm calculus will be expanded to include multiple future generations within" a particular family, and both parents and researchers will know that their decisions will have long-term genetic effects.

The third and fourth questions will be broadened in another respect, as well. Some critics of germ-line genetic intervention have raised ethical objections to *ever* employing this technique on grounds of the serious social harm that might ensue. While the same critics have also been concerned about somatic cell gene therapy, their principal focus has been germ-line approaches. Thus, researchers proposing to undertake germ-line gene therapy, or at least the review bodies evaluating such proposals, will need to take into account a much broader range of nonmedical consequences. . . .

THE AUTHORS' CONCLUSION

Ultimately, the moral case for or against germ-line gene therapy must be established by good reasons. In our evaluation of the pro and con arguments and in our discussion of eugenics, we have attempted to indicate why we find voluntary programs of germ-line genetic intervention to be ethically acceptable in principle. We think that this strategy should be employed only when gene replacement or gene repair is a validated technique. In addition, we are hopeful that techniques will be developed for repairing sperm and egg cells in the bodies of prospective parents before fertilization occurs. Finally, we find both the goal of preventing disease in a particular individual and the goal of preventing the transmission of genetic disease to the individual's descendants to be worthy rationales for this intervention.

GERM-LINE GENE THERAPY: NO PLACE IN TREATMENT OF GENETIC DISEASE

David M. Danks

THE CIRCUMSTANCES OF THIS EDITORIAL

The recent publication of a discussion paper from the Council for Responsible Genetics (1993) moved me to ask the Editor to publish a letter commenting on the dubious utility of this form of therapy. He kindly asked me to expand the content of the letter for publication in this form. In the interim, the valuable contribution of Professor J. V. Neel appeared (1993). I admired his characteristically clear and efficient style of presentation so much that I have taken the liberty of copying the layout that he used.

MY POINT OF VIEW

I am surprised that so many people want to keep on talking about germ-line gene therapy and even more surprised that many of them seem to assume that it would be very valuable in the treatment of genetic disease and capable of correcting a defective gene in future generations, as well as in the initial patient. In fact, I believe that both these assumptions are wrong. I can see no significant place for germ-line gene therapy in the treatment of genetic disease, and it is quite wrong to suggest that the present methods of gene therapy would allow the correction to carry on through future generations.

In fact, the only application that I can really imagine for germ-line gene therapy would be in attempting to alter normal characteristics. I happen to believe that this would be quite inappropriate, but I cannot see much point in arguing about it at the moment. Like Professor Neel, I am aghast at the arrogance of those who think that we are close to understanding the genetic control of normal characteristics sufficiently to know how to enhance them. On the other hand, I think we would also be behaving in a most arrogant fashion if we were to presume to tell future generations how they should use this knowledge if it should ever become available.

Continuing discussion of germ-line gene therapy by ethicists and scientists only fuels media interest and thereby rouses community anxiety. It would be best if everyone were to forget about it and concentrate on discussing more useful aspects of modern genetics. Placing a ban on the procedure might help to allay public concern. Such a ban could always be reviewed if future new knowledge were to provide safe methods and useful applications.

THE BASIS FOR THIS POSITION

I have worked as a clinical geneticist for more than 30 years and have dealt with a very large number of couples facing genetic risks. For most of this time I have directed a research group involved in basic genetic research, latterly mainly molecular genetics.

No Logical Place for Germ-Line Gene Therapy Couples who face high risks of having children with serious genetic diseases face either a 1 in 2 (autosomal dominant) or 1 in 4 (autosomal recessive or X-linked recessive) risk. There are only two circumstances in which there is 100% risk to offspring—one is very rare and the other is quite unapproachable by present technology. The very rare circumstance concerns a man and a woman, both of whom have the same recessively inherited disease. Even if the frequency of survival of patients with diseases warranting gene therapy should increase in the future, the number of matings of this type will be very small indeed. The other situation with 100% risk to offspring is in maternally inherited mitochondrial gene defects,

Reprinted with permission of the author and publisher from *Human Gene Therapy* 5(1994): 151–152.

but we have no idea how to tackle these diseases at the gene level.

Germ-line gene therapy would require that fertilization should occur *in vitro.* The standard techniques involve superovulation and production of several fertilized ova. Among these will be some with the genotype that will result in an affected child and others with a genotype that allows the child to be healthy. It would surely be quite unacceptable to inject a correcting gene into a fertilized ovum that is already destined to produce a healthy child. Such a procedure could not possibly do any good and would carry some hazard.

Professor Neel has suggested that the hazard of germ-line gene therapy insertion is likely to be sufficient so that one could accept the procedure only if the DNA could be guaranteed to actually replace the defective part of the gene or the whole gene in its normal location. Even if this should become achievable, it is most unlikely that the process will be totally risk free.

It logically follows that one could not contemplate germ-line gene therapy until the available fertilized ova have been classified as "affected" or "unaffected" (meaning, leading to an affected or unaffected child, respectively). Assuming this is technically possible, we then come up against a logical absurdity. Are we to propose discarding those ova that are shown to be unaffected in order to correct an affected one and reimplant it? Surely one should discard the affected and reimplant one of the unaffected.

Some might argue that discarding any fertilized egg is unacceptable—surely this applies even more to discarding an unaffected fertilized egg than to discarding an affected one.

There is some risk that I may be interpreted as an advocate of preimplantation diagnosis of genetic diseases—I am not. At the present time, it is a ridiculously expensive way of achieving prenatal diagnosis. However, it would be essential if germline gene therapy were to be contemplated. What is more, the form of preimplantation diagnosis used would have to be genetic testing of a polar body, with all its intrinsic difficulties, because the therapy must be carried out at the one cell stage to gain the benefit of getting the inserted gene into all body cells.

Correction of Genetic Disease in Future Generations At first sight, it may seem that if germ-line gene therapy will deliver the correcting gene to all body cells it should also carry through into the next generation in the germ cells. However, this expectation ignores the random insertion of the injected DNA into a chromosome and the random assortment of different pairs of chromosomes during meiosis. The odds are at least 23 to 1 against the inserted DNA being incorporated into the chromosome that carries the mutant gene and more than 100 to 1 against the site of insertion being close enough to the disease-causing gene for both to be passed on together after genetic recombination has taken place. It is very unlikely that the corrective effect of the inserted gene would persist for more than one generation. To achieve heritable correction it will be necessary to achieve replacement of the effective gene by the inserted gene.

Genetic Enhancement We know very little about the genetic control of normal characteristics like intelligence, personality, temperament, behaviour, athletic ability, musical ability, etc. The little we do know tells us that there are many gene pairs involved in controlling any one of these complex characteristics.

Part of this knowledge comes from analyses of the distribution of abilities in communities and families. Genetic diseases give further strong clues about the numbers of genes involved. For instance, we know hundreds of different genetic diseases that cause mental retardation. Many of these are caused by defects in genes that control important aspects of the development of the brain and are therefore likely to be relevant to the determination of the variation in the intelligence of normal individuals. Gross defects in the function of these genes cause mental retardation. Slight variations in their function are likely to be involved in determining minor variations in normal people. (Not all genetic causes of mental retardation fit into this category—in some a metabolic abnormality in another organ causes toxic brain damage as in the hyperammonaemia of urea cycle defects.)

It requires an extraordinary combination of arrogance and ignorance to propose that we will soon understand these matters well enough to indulge in genetic manipulation to "improve the human race." Even the identification of all the human genes through the Human Genome Project will be but a tiny step towards a detailed understanding of the complex gene interactions underlying the normal human state.

I am not advocating that we should put a lot of effort into understanding the genetic basis of individuality. The range of gene combinations is likely to be so great as to defy analysis. I can think of few good uses to which such knowledge could be put and many potential misuses.

REFERENCES

Council for Responsible Genetics. (1993). Position paper on human germ-line manipulation. Hum. Gene Ther. **4,** 35–38.

Neel, J. V. (1993). Germ-line gene therapy: Another view. Hum. Gene Ther. **4,** 127–128.

ASSISTED REPRODUCTIVE TECHNOLOGIES

THE PRESUMPTIVE PRIMACY OF PROCREATIVE LIBERTY

John Robertson

Procreative liberty has wide appeal but its scope has never been fully elaborated and often is contested. The concept has several meanings that must be clarified if it is to serve as a reliable guide for moral debate and public policy regarding new reproductive technologies.

WHAT IS PROCREATIVE LIBERTY?

At the most general level, procreative liberty is the freedom either to have children or to avoid having them. Although often expressed or realized in the context of a couple, it is first and foremost an individual interest. It is to be distinguished from freedom in the ancillary aspects of reproduction, such as liberty in the conduct of pregnancy or choice of place or mode of childbirth.

The concept of reproduction, however, has a certain ambiguity contained within it. In a strict sense, reproduction is always genetic. It occurs by provision of one's gametes to a new person, and thus includes having or producing offspring. While female reproduction has traditionally included gestation, in vitro fertilization (IVF) now allows female genetic and gestational reproduction to be separated. Thus a woman who has provided the egg that is carried by another has reproduced, even if she has not gestated and does not rear resulting offspring. Because of the close link between gestation and female reproduction, a woman who gestates the embryo of another may also reasonably be viewed as having a reproductive experience, even though she does not reproduce genetically.[1]

In any case, reproduction in the genetic or gestational sense is to be distinguished from child rearing. Although reproduction is highly valued in part

---

From *Children of Choice: Freedom and the New Reproductive Technologies* by John Robertson, Princeton University Press, 1994.

Editors' note: Many of the notes in this chapter have been omitted; those wishing to follow up on sources should consult the original.

because it usually leads to child rearing, one can produce offspring without rearing them and rear children without reproduction. One who rears an adopted child has not reproduced, while one who has genetic progeny but does not rear them has.

In this book the terms "procreative liberty" and "reproductive freedom" will mean the freedom to reproduce or not to reproduce in the genetic sense, which may also include rearing or not, as intended by the parties. Those terms will also include female gestation whether or not there is a genetic connection to the resulting child.

Often the reproduction at issue will be important because it is intended to lead to child rearing. In cases where rearing is not intended, the value to be assigned to reproduction *tout court* will have to be determined. Similarly, when there is rearing without genetic or gestational involvement, the value of nonreproductive child rearing will also have to be assessed. In both cases the value assigned may depend on the proximity to reproduction where rearing is intended.

Two further qualifications on the meaning of procreative liberty should be noted. One is that "liberty" as used in procreative liberty is a negative right. It means that a person violates no moral duty in making a procreative choice, and that other persons have a duty not to interfere with that choice. However, the negative right to procreate or not does not imply the duty of others to provide the resources or services necessary to exercise one's procreative liberty despite plausible moral arguments for governmental assistance.

As a matter of constitutional law, procreative liberty is a negative right against state interference with choices to procreate or to avoid procreation. It is not a right against private interference, though other laws might provide that protection. Nor is it a positive right to have the state or particular persons providing the means or resources necessary to have or avoid having children. The exercise of procreative liberty may be severely constrained by social and economic circumstances. Access to medical care, child care, employment, housing, and other services may significantly affect whether one is able to exercise procreative liberty. However, the state presently has no constitutional obligation to provide those services. Whether the state should alleviate those conditions is a separate issue of social justice.

The second qualification is that not everything that occurs in and around procreation falls within liberty interests that are distinctively procreative. Thus whether the father may be present during childbirth, whether midwives may assist birth, or whether childbirth may occur at home rather than in a hospital may be important for the parties involved, but they do not implicate the freedom to reproduce (unless one could show that the place or mode of birth would determine whether birth occurs at all). Similarly, questions about a pregnant woman's drug use or other conduct during pregnancy . . . implicates liberty in the course of reproduction but not procreative liberty in the basic sense. Questions about whether the use of a technology is distinctively procreative recur throughout this book.

THE IMPORTANCE OF PROCREATIVE LIBERTY

Procreative liberty should enjoy presumptive primacy when conflicts about its exercise arise because control over whether one reproduces or not is central to personal identity, to dignity, and to the meaning of one's life. For example, deprivation of the ability to avoid reproduction determines one's self-definition in the most basic sense. It affects women's bodies in a direct and substantial way. It also centrally affects one's psychological and social identity and one's social and moral responsibilities. The resulting burdens are especially onerous for women, but they affect men in significant ways as well.

On the other hand, being deprived of the ability to reproduce prevents one from an experience that is central to individual identity and meaning in life. Although the desire to reproduce is in part socially constructed, at the most basic level transmission of one's genes through reproduction is an animal or species urge closely linked to the sex drive. In connecting us with nature and future generations, reproduction gives solace in the face of death. As Shakespeare noted, "nothing 'gainst Time's scythe can make defense/save breed."[2] For many people "breed"—reproduction and the parenting that usually accompanies it—is a central part of their life plan, and the most satisfying and meaningful experience they have. It also has primary importance as an expression of a couple's love or unity. For many persons, reproduction also has religious significance and is experienced as a "gift from God." Its denial—through infertility or governmental restriction—is experienced as a great loss, even if one has already had children or will have little or no rearing role with them.

Decisions to have or to avoid having children are thus personal decisions of great import that determine the shape and meaning of one's life. The person directly involved is best situated to determine whether that meaning should or should not occur. An ethic of personal autonomy as well as ethics of community or family should then recognize a presumption in favor of most personal reproductive choices. Such a presumption does not mean that reproductive choices are without consequence to others, nor that they should never be limited. Rather, it means that those who would limit procreative choice have the burden of showing that the reproductive actions at issue would create such substantial harm that they could justifiably be limited. Of course, what counts as the "substantial harm" that justifies interference with procreative choice may often be contested, as the discussion of reproductive technologies in this book will show.

A closely related reason for protecting reproductive choice is to avoid the highly intrusive measures that governmental control of reproduction usually entails. State interference with reproductive choice may extend beyond exhortation and penalties to gestapo and police state tactics. Margaret Atwood's powerful futuristic novel *The Handmaid's Tale* expresses this danger by creating a world where fertile women are forcibly impregnated by the ruling powers and their pregnancies monitored to replenish a decimated population.[3]

Equally frightening scenarios have occurred in recent years when repressive governments have interfered with reproductive choice. In Romania and China, men and women have had their most private activities scrutinized in the service of state reproductive goals. In Ceauşescu's Romania, where contraception and abortion were strictly forbidden, women's menstrual cycles were routinely monitored to see if they were pregnant. Women who did not become pregnant or who had abortions were severely punished. Many women nevertheless sought illegal abortions and died, leaving their children orphaned and subject to sale to Westerners seeking children for adoption.

In China, forcible abortion and sterilization have occurred in the service of a one-child-per-family population policy. Village cadres have seized pregnant women in their homes and forced them to have abortions. A campaign of forcible sterilization in India in 1977 was seen as an "attack on women and children" and brought Indira Gandhi's government down. In the United States, state-imposed sterilization of "mental defectives," sanctioned in 1927 by the United States Supreme Court in *Buck* v. *Bell,* resulted in 60,000 sterilizations over a forty-year period. Many mentally normal people were sterilized by mistake, and mentally retarded persons who posed little risk of harm to others were subjected to surgery. It is no surprise that current proposals for compulsory use of contraceptives such as Norplant are viewed with great suspicion.

TWO TYPES OF PROCREATIVE LIBERTY

To see how values of procreative liberty affect the ethical and public policy evaluation of new reproductive technologies, we must determine whether the interests that underlie the high value accorded procreative liberty are implicated in their use. This is not a simple task because procreative liberty is not unitary, but consists of strands of varying interests in the conception and gestation of offspring. The different strands implicate different interests, have different legal and constitutional status, and are differently affected by technology.

An essential distinction is between the freedom to avoid reproduction and the freedom to reproduce. When people talk of reproductive rights, they usually have one or the other aspect in mind. Because different interests and justifications underlie each and countervailing interests for limiting each aspect vary, recognition of one aspect does not necessarily mean that the other will also be respected; nor does limitation of one mean that the other can also be denied.

However, there is a mirroring or reciprocal relationship here. Denial of one type of reproductive liberty necessarily implicates the other. If a woman is not able to avoid reproduction through contraception or abortion, she may end up reproducing, with all the burdens that unwanted reproduction entails. Similarly, if one is denied the liberty to reproduce through forcible sterilization, one is forced to avoid reproduction, thus experiencing the loss that absence of progeny brings. By extending reproductive options, new reproductive technologies present challenges to both aspects of procreative choice.

AVOIDING REPRODUCTION: THE LIBERTY NOT TO REPRODUCE

One sense in which people commonly understand procreative liberty is as the freedom to avoid reproduction—to avoid begetting or bearing offspring and the rearing demands they make. Procreative liberty in this sense could involve several different choices, because decisions to avoid procreation arise at several different stages. A decision not to procreate could occur prior to conception through sexual abstinence, contraceptive use, or refusal to seek treatment for infertility. At this stage, the main issues concern freedom to refrain from sexual intercourse, the freedom to use contraceptives, and the freedom to withhold gametes for use in noncoital conception. Countervailing interests concern societal interests in increasing population, a partner's interest in sexual intimacy and progeny, and moral views about the unity of sex and reproduction.

Once pregnancy has occurred, reproduction can be avoided only by termination of pregnancy. Procreative freedom here would involve the freedom to abort the pregnancy. Competing interests are protection of embryos and fetuses and respect for human life generally, the most heated issue of reproductive rights. They may also include moral or social beliefs about the connectedness of sex and reproduction, or views about a woman's reproductive and work roles.

Once a child is born, procreation has occurred, and the procreators ordinarily have parenting obligations. Freeing oneself from rearing obligations is not strictly speaking a matter of procreative liberty, though it is an important personal interest. Even if parents relinquish the child for adoption, the psychological reality that one has reproduced remains. Opposing interests at this stage involve the need to provide parenting, nurturing, and financial support to offspring. The right to be free of those obligations, as well as the right to assume them after birth occurs, is not directly addressed in this book except to the extent that those rights affect reproductive decisions.

Technology and the Avoidance of Reproduction

Many reproductive technologies raise questions about the scope of the liberty interest in avoiding reproduction. New contraceptive, contragestive, and abortion technologies raise avoidance issues directly, though the issues raised are not always novel. For example, an important issue in voluntary use of long-lasting contraceptives concerns access by minors and the poor, an issue of justice in the distribution of medical resources that currently exists with other contraceptives. The more publicized issue of whether the state may require child abusers or women on welfare to use Norplant implicates the target group's right to procreate, not their liberty interest in avoiding reproduction.

Contragestive agents such as RU486, which prevent reproduction after conception has occurred, raise many of the current issues of the abortion debate. Because RU486 operates so early in pregnancy, however, it focuses attention on the moral status of very early abortions and the moral differences, if any, between postcoital contraceptives and abortifacients. Ethical assessment and legal rights to use contragestives will depend on the ethical and legal status of early prenatal stages of human life.

More novel avoidance issues will arise with IVF and embryo cryopreservation technology. IVF often produces more embryos than can be safely implanted in the uterus. If couples must donate rather than discard unwanted embryos, they will become biologic parents against their will. This prospect raises the question of whether the liberty interest in avoiding reproduction includes avoiding genetic offspring when no rearing obligations will attach—reproduction *tout court*. Is one's fundamental interest in avoiding reproduction seriously implicated if one will never know or have contact with one's offspring? The resulting moral and policy issue is how to balance the interest in avoiding genetic offspring *tout court* with respect for preimplantation stages of human life.

Technologies of quality control and selection through genetic screening and manipulation will also raise novel questions about the right to avoid reproduction. Prenatal screening enables couples to avoid reproduction because of the genetic characteristics of expected offspring. Are the interests that support protecting the freedom to avoid reproduction present when that freedom is exercised selectively? Because some reasons for rejecting fetuses are more appealing than others, would devising criteria for such choices violate the right not to procreate? For example, should law or morality permit abortion of a fetus with Tay-Sachs disease or Down's syndrome but not female fetuses or fetuses with a disease of varying expressivity such as cystic fibrosis?

Legal Status of Avoiding Reproduction

Legally, the negative freedom to avoid reproduction is widely recognized, though great controversy over abortion persists, and there is no positive constitutional right to contraception and abortion. The freedom to avoid reproduction is clearest for men and women prior to conception. In the United States and most developed countries, marriage and sexual intercourse are a matter of choice. However, rape laws do not always effectively protect women, and some jurisdictions do not criminalize marital rape. Legal access to contraception and sterilization is firmly established, though controversy exists over providing contraception to adolescents because of fears that it would encourage nonmarital sexual intercourse.

Constitutional recognition of the right to use contraceptives—to have sex and not reproduce—occurred in the 1965 landmark case of *Griswold* v. *Connecticut*. The executive director of Planned Parenthood and its medical director, a licensed physician, challenged a Connecticut law that made it a crime to use or distribute contraceptives. The United States Supreme Court found that the law violated a fundamental liberty right of married couples, which it later extended to unmarried persons, to use contraceptives as a matter of personal liberty or privacy. Although the Court alluded to the unsavory prospect of police searching the marital bedroom for evidence of the crime as a reason for invalidating the law, it is clear that the Court was protecting the right of persons who engage in sexual intimacy to avoid unwanted reproduction. The right to avoid reproduction through contraception is thus firmly protected, even where fornication laws remain in effect.

Legal protection also exists for other activities tied to avoiding reproduction prior to pregnancy. Thus both men and women are deemed owners of gametes within or outside their bodies, so that they may prevent them from being used for reproduction without their permission. Men and women also have rights to prevent extracorporeal embryos formed from their gametes from being placed in women and brought to term without their consent.

Once conception has occurred, the right to avoid reproduction differs for the woman and man involved. In the United States and most of Western Europe, abortion in early stages of the pregnancy is widely permitted. Under *Roe* v. *Wade*, whose central holding was reaffirmed in 1992 in *Planned Parenthood* v. *Casey*, women, whether single or married, adult or minor, have a right to terminate pregnancy up to viability. However, the state may inform them of its views concerning the worth of the fetus and require them to wait 24 hours before obtaining an abortion. Parental consent or notification requirements can be imposed on minors, as long as a judicial bypass is provided in cases in which the minor does not wish to inform her parents. Also, because the right to abortion is a negative right, the state has no obligation to fund abortions for indigent women.

Although pregnancy termination usually kills the fetus, the right to end pregnancy does not protect the right to cause the death of a fetus that has emerged alive from the abortion process, or even to choose a method of abortion that is most likely to cause fetal demise. Nor does it give a woman the right to engage in prenatal conduct that poses unreasonable risks to the health of future offspring when she is choosing to go to term. After birth occurs, the mother and father have obligations to the child until custody is formally relinquished or transferred to others.

The father, once conception through sexual intercourse has occurred, has no right to require or prevent abortion, and cannot avoid rearing duties of financial support once birth occurs. This is true even if the woman has lied to him about her fertility or her use of contraceptives. However, he is free to relinquish custody and give up for adoption. He is also free to determine whether IVF embryos formed from his sperm should be implanted in the uterus.

The law's recognition of a right to avoid reproduction both prior to and after conception provides the legal framework for resolving conflicts presented by new reproductive technologies that affect interests in avoiding reproduction. While many technologies raise the same issues confronted in *Griswold* and *Roe,* new twists will arise that directly challenge the scope of that right. To resolve those conflicts, the separate elements that comprise the interest in avoiding reproduction must be analyzed and evaluated against the competing interests affected by those technologies.

THE FREEDOM TO PROCREATE

In addition to freedom to avoid procreation, procreative liberty also includes the freedom to procreate—the freedom to beget and bear children if one chooses. As with avoiding reproduction, the right to reproduce is a negative right against public or private interference, not a positive right to the services or the resources needed to reproduce. It is an important freedom that is widely accepted as a basic, human right. But its various components and dimensions have never been fully analyzed, as technologies of conception and selection now force us to do.

As with avoiding reproduction, the freedom to procreate involves the freedom to engage in a series of actions that eventuate in reproduction and usually in child rearing. One must be free to marry or find a willing partner, engage in sexual intercourse, achieve conception and pregnancy, carry a pregnancy to term, and rear offspring. Social and natural barriers to reproduction would involve the unavailability of willing or suitable partners, impotence or infertility, and lack of medical and child-care resources. State barriers to marriage, to sexual intercourse, to conception, to infertility treatment, to carrying pregnancies to term, and to certain child-rearing arrangements would also limit the freedom to procreate. The most commonly asserted reasons for limiting coital reproduction are overpopulation, unfitness of parents, harm to offspring, and costs to the state or others. Technologies that treat infertility raise additional concerns that are discussed below.

The moral right to reproduce is respected because of the centrality of reproduction to personal identity, meaning, and dignity. This importance makes the liberty to procreate an important moral right, both for an ethic of individual autonomy and for ethics of community or family that view the purpose of marriage and sexual union as the reproduction and rearing of offspring. Because of this importance, the right to reproduce is widely recognized as a prima facie moral right that cannot be limited except for very good reason.

Recognition of the primacy of procreation does not mean that all reproduction is morally blameless, much less that reproduction is always responsible and praiseworthy and can never be limited. However, the presumptive primacy of procreative liberty sets a very high standard for limiting those rights, tilting the balance in favor of reproducing but not totally determining its acceptability. A two-step process of analysis is envisaged here. The first question is whether a distinctively procreative interest is involved. If so, the question then is whether the harm threatened by reproduction satisfies the strict standard for overriding this liberty interest.

The personal importance of procreation helps answer questions about who holds procreative rights and about the circumstances under which the right to reproduce may be limited. A person's capacity to find significance in reproduction should determine whether one holds the presumptive right, though this question is often discussed in terms of whether persons with such a capacity are fit parents. To have a liberty interest in procreating, one should at a minimum have the mental capacity to understand or appreciate the meanings associated with reproduction. This minimum would exclude severely retarded persons from having reproductive interests, though it would not remove their right to bodily integrity. However, being unmarried, homosexual, physically disabled, infected with HIV, or imprisoned would not disqualify one from having reproductive interests, though they might affect one's ability to rear offspring. Whether those characteristics justify limitations on reproduction is discussed later. Nor would already having reproduced negate a person's interest in reproducing again, though at a certain point the marginal value to a person of additional offspring diminishes.

What kinds of interests or harms make reproduction unduly selfish or irresponsible and thus could justifiably limit the presumptive right to procreate? To answer this question, we must distinguish coital and noncoital reproduction. Surprisingly, there is a widespread reluctance to speak of coital reproduction as irresponsible, much less to urge public action to prevent irresponsible coital reproduction from occurring. If such a conversation did occur, reasons for limiting coital reproduction would involve the heavy costs that it imposed on others—costs that outweighed whatever personal meaning or satisfaction the person(s) reproducing experienced. With coital reproduction, such costs might arise if there were severe overpopulation, if the persons reproducing were unfit parents, if reproduction would harm offspring, or if significant medical or social costs were imposed on others.

Because the United States does not face the severe overpopulation of some countries, the main grounds for claiming that reproduction is irresponsible is where the person(s) reproducing lack the financial means to raise offspring or will otherwise harm their children. As later discussions will show, both grounds are seriously inadequate as justifications for interfering with procreative choice. Imposing rearing costs on others may not rise to the level of harm that justifies depriving a person of a fundamental moral right. Moreover, protection of offspring from unfit parenting requires that unfit parents not rear, not that they not reproduce. Offspring could be protected by having others rear them without interfering with parental reproduction.

A further problem, if coital reproduction were found to be unjustified, concerns what action should then be taken. Exhortation or moral condemnation might be acceptable, but more stringent or coercive measures would act on the body of the person deemed irresponsible. Past experience with forced sterilization of retarded persons and the inevitable focus on the poor and minorities as targets of coercive policies make such proposals highly unappealing. Because of these doubts, there have been surprisingly few attempts to restrict coital reproduction in the United States since the era of eugenic sterilization, even though some instances of reproduction—for example, teenage pregnancy, inability to care for offspring—appear to be socially irresponsible.

An entirely different set of concerns arises with noncoital reproductive techniques. Charges that noncoital reproduction is unethical or irresponsible arise because of its expense, its highly technological character, its decomposition of parenthood into genetic, gestational, and social components, and its potential effects on women and offspring. To assess whether these effects justify moral condemnation or public limitation, we must first determine whether noncoital reproduction implicates important aspects of procreative liberty.

The Right to Reproduce and Noncoital Technology

If the moral right to reproduce presumptively protects coital reproduction, then it should protect noncoital reproduction as well. The moral right of the coitally infertile to reproduce is based on the same desire for offspring that the coitally fertile have. They too wish to replicate themselves, transmit genes, gestate, and rear children biologically related to them. Their infertility should no more disqualify them from reproductive experiences than physical disability should disqualify persons from walking with mechanical assistance. The unique risks posed by noncoital reproduction may provide independent justifications for limiting its use, but neither the noncoital nature of the means used nor the infertility of their beneficiaries means that the presumptively protected moral interest in reproduction is not present.

A major question about this position, however, is whether the noncoital or collaborative nature of the means used truly implicates reproductive interests. For example, what if only one aspect of reproduction—genetic transfer, gestation, or rearing—occurs, as happens with gamete donors or surrogates who play no rearing role? Is a person's procreative liberty substantially implicated in such partial reproductive roles? The answer will depend on the value attributed to the particular collaborative contribution and on whether the collaborative enterprise is viewed from the donor's or recipient's perspective.

Gamete donors and surrogates are clearly reproducing even though they have no intention to rear.

Because reproduction *tout court* may seem less important than reproduction with intent to rear, the donor's reproductive interest may appear less important. However, more experience with these practices is needed to determine the inherent value of "partial" reproductive experiences to donors and surrogates. Experience may show that it is independently meaningful, regardless of their contact with offspring. If not, then countervailing interests would more easily override their right to enter these roles.

Viewed from the recipient's perspective, however, the donor or surrogate's reproduction *tout court* does not lessen the reproductive importance of her contribution. A woman who receives an egg or embryo donation has no genetic connection with offspring but has a gestational relation of great personal significance. In addition, gamete donors and surrogates enable one or both rearing partners to have a biological relation with offspring. If one of them has no biological connection at all, they will still have a strong interest in rearing their partner's biologic offspring. Whether viewed singly through the eyes of the partner who is reproducing, or jointly as an endeavor of a couple seeking to rear children who are biologically related to at least one of the two, a significant reproductive interest is at stake. If so, noncoital, collaborative treatments for infertility should be respected to the same extent as coital reproduction is.

Questions about the core meaning of reproduction will also arise in the temporal dislocations that cryopreservation of sperm and embryos make possible. For example, embryo freezing allows siblings to be conceived at the same time, but born years apart and to different gestational mothers. Twins could be created by splitting one embryo into two. If one half is frozen for later use, identical twins could be born at widely different times. Sperm, egg, and embryo freezing also make posthumous reproduction possible.

Such temporally dislocative practices clearly implicate core reproductive interests when the ultimate recipient has no alternative means of reproduction. However, if the procreative interests of the recipient couple are not directly implicated, we must ask whether those whose gametes are used have an independent procreative interest, as might occur if they directed that gametes or embryos be thawed after their death for purposes of posthumous reproduction. In that case the question is whether the expectancy of posthumous reproduction is so central to an individual's procreative identity or life-plan that it should receive the same respect that one's reproduction when alive receives. The answer to such a question will be important in devising policy for storing and posthumously disposing of gametes and embryos. The answer will also affect inheritance questions and have implications for management of pregnant women who are irreversibly comatose or brain dead.

The problem of determining whether technology implicates a major reproductive interest also arises with technologies that select offspring characteristics. Some degree of quality control would seem logically to fall within the realm of procreative liberty. For many couples the decision whether to procreate depends on the ability to have healthy children. Without some guarantee or protection against the risk of handicapped children, they might not reproduce at all.

Thus viewed, quality control devices become part of the liberty interest in procreating or in avoiding procreation, and arguably should receive the same degree of protection. If so, genetic screening and selective abortion, as well as the right to select a mate or a source for donated eggs, sperm, or embryos should be protected as part of procreative liberty. The same arguments would apply to positive interventions to cure disease at the fetal or embryo stage. However, futuristic practices such as nontherapeutic enhancement, cloning, or intentional diminishment of offspring characteristics may so deviate from the core interests that make reproduction meaningful as to fall outside the protective canopy of procreative liberty.

Finally, technology will present questions of whether one may use one's reproductive capacity to produce gametes, embryos, and fetuses for nonreproductive uses in research or therapy. Here the purpose is not to have children to rear, but to get material for research or transplant. Are such uses of reproductive capacity tied closely enough to the values and interests that underlie procreative freedom to warrant similar respect? Even if procreative choice is not directly involved, other liberties may protect the activity.

Are Noncoital Technologies Unethical?

If this analysis is accepted, then procreative liberty would include the right to use noncoital and other technologies to form a family and shape the characteristics of offspring. Neither infertility nor the fact that one will only partially reproduce eliminates the existence of a prima facie reproductive experience for someone. However, judgments about the proximity of these partial reproductive experiences to the core meanings of reproduction will be required in balancing those claims against competing moral concerns.

Judgment about the reproductive importance of noncoital technologies is crucial because many people have serious ethical reservations about them, and are more than willing to restrict their use. The concerns here are not the fears of overpopulation, parental unfitness, and societal costs that arise with allegedly irresponsible coital reproduction. Instead, they include reduction of demand for hard-to-adopt children, the coercive or exploitive bargains that will be offered to poor women, the commodification of both children and reproductive collaborators, the objectification of women as reproductive vessels, and the undermining of the nuclear family.

However, often the harms feared are deontological in character. In some cases they stem from a religious or moral conception of the unity of sex and reproduction or the definition of family. Such a view characterizes the Vatican's strong opposition to IVF, donor sperm, and other noncoital and collaborative techniques. Other deontological concerns derive from a particular conception of the proper reproductive role of women. Many persons, for example, oppose paid surrogate motherhood because of a judgment about the wrongness of a woman's willingness to sever the mother-child bond for the sake of money. They also insist that the gestational mother is always morally entitled to rear, despite her preconception promise to the contrary. Closely related are dignitary objections to allowing any reproductive factors to be purchased, or to having offspring selected on the basis of their genes.

Finally, there is a broader concern that noncoital reproduction will undermine the deeper community interest in having a clear social framework to define boundaries of families, sexuality, and reproduction. The traditional family provides a container for the narcissism and irrationality that often drives human reproduction. This container assures commitments to the identifications and taboos that protect children from various types of abuse. The technical ability to disaggregate and recombine genetic, gestational, and rearing connections and to control the genes of offspring may thus undermine essential protections for offspring, couples, families, and society.

These criticisms are powerful ones that explain much of the ambivalence that surrounds the use of certain reproductive technologies. They call into question the wisdom of individual decisions to use them, and the willingness of society to promote or facilitate their use. Unless one is operating out of a specific religious or deontological ethic, however, they do not show that all individual uses of these techniques are immoral, much less that public policy should restrict or discourage their use.

These criticisms seldom meet the high standard necessary to limit procreative choice. Many of them are mere hypothetical or speculative possibilities. Others reflect moralisms concerning a "right" view of reproduction, which individuals in a pluralistic society hold or reject to varying degrees. In any event, without a clear showing of substantial harm to the tangible interests of others, speculation or mere moral objections alone should not override the moral right of infertile couples to use those techniques to form families. Given the primacy of procreative liberty, the use of these techniques should be accorded the same high protection granted to coital reproduction.

RESOLVING DISPUTES OVER PROCREATIVE LIBERTY

As this brief survey shows, new reproductive technologies will generate ethical and legal disputes about the meaning and scope of procreative liberty. Because procreative liberty has never been fully elaborated, the importance of procreative choice in many novel settings will be a question of first impression. The ultimate decision reached will reflect the value assigned to the procreative interest at stake in light of the effects causing concern. In an important sense, the meaning of procreative liberty will be created or constituted for society in the process of resolving such disputes.

If procreative liberty is taken seriously, a strong presumption in favor of using technologies that centrally implicate reproductive interests should be recognized. Although procreative rights are not absolute, those who would limit procreative choice should have the burden of establishing substantial harm. This is the standard used in ethical and legal analyses of restrictions on traditional reproductive decisions. Because the same procreative goals are involved, the same standard of scrutiny should be used for assessing moral or governmental restrictions on novel reproductive techniques.

In arbitrating these disputes, one has to come to terms with the importance of procreative interests relative to other concerns. The precise procreative interest at stake must be identified and weighed against the core values of reproduction. As noted, this will raise novel and unique questions when the technology deviates from the model of two-person coital reproduction, or otherwise disaggregates or alters ordinary reproductive practices. However, if an important reproductive interest exists, then use of the technology should be presumptively permitted. Only substantial harm to tangible interests of others should then justify restriction.

In determining whether such harm exists, it will be necessary to distinguish between harms to individuals and harms to personal conceptions of morality, right order, or offense, discounted by their probability of occurrence. As previously noted, many objections to reproductive technology rest on differing views of what "proper" or "right" reproduction is aside from tangible effects on others. For example, concerns about the decomposition of parenthood through the use of donors and surrogates, about the temporal alteration of conception, gestation and birth, about the alienation or commercialization of gestational capacity, and about selection and control of offspring characteristics do not directly affect persons so much as they affect notions of right behavior. Disputes over early abortion and discard or manipulation of IVF-created embryos also exemplify this distinction, if we grant that the embryo/previable fetus is not a person or entity with rights in itself.

At issue in these cases is the symbolic or constitutive meaning of actions regarding prenatal life, family, maternal gestation, and respect for persons over which people in a secular, pluralistic society often differ. A majoritarian view of "right" reproduction or "right" valuation of prenatal life, family, or the role of women should not suffice to restrict actions based on differing individual views of such preeminently personal issues. At a certain point, however, a practice such as cloning, enhancement, or intentional diminishment of offspring may be so far removed from even pluralistic notions of reproductive meaning that they leave the realm of protected reproductive choice. People may differ over where that point is, but it will not easily exclude most reproductive technologies of current interest.

To take procreative liberty seriously, then, is to allow it to have presumptive priority in an individual's life. This will give persons directly involved the final say about use of a particular technology, unless tangible harm to the interests of others can be shown. Of course, people may differ over whether an important procreative interest is at stake or over how serious the harm posed from use of the reproductive technology is. Such a focused debate, however, is legitimate and ultimately essential in developing ethical standards and public policy for use of new reproductive technologies.

THE LIMITS OF PROCREATIVE LIBERTY

The emphasis on procreative liberty that informs this book provides a useful but by no means complete or final perspective on the technologies in question. Theological, social, psychological, economic, and feminist perspectives would emphasize different aspects of reproductive technology, and might be much less sanguine about potential benefits and risks. Such perspectives might also offer better guidance in how to use these technologies to protect offspring, respect women, and maintain other important values.

A strong rights perspective has other limitations as well. Recognition of procreative liberty, whether in traditional or in new technological settings, does not guarantee that people will achieve their reproductive goals, much less that they will be happy with what they do achieve. Nature may be recalcitrant to the latest technology. Individuals may lack the will, the perseverance, or the resources to use effective technologies. Even if they do succeed, the results may be less satisfying than envisaged. In addition, many individual instances of procreative choice may cumulate into larger social changes that from our current vantage point seem highly undesirable. But these are the hazards and limitations of any scheme of individual rights.

Recognition of procreative liberty will protect the right of persons to use technology in pursuing their reproductive goals, but it will not eliminate the ambivalence that such technologies engender. Societal ambivalence about reproductive technology is recapitulated at the individual level, as individuals and couples struggle with whether to use the technologies in question. Thus recognition of procreative liberty will not eliminate the dilemmas of personal choice and responsibility that reproductive choice entails. The freedom to act does not mean that we will act wisely, yet denying that freedom may be even more unwise, for it denies individuals' respect in the most fundamental choices of their lives.

NOTES

1. Whether labeled reproductive or not, gestation is a central experience for women and should enjoy the special respect or protected status accorded reproductive activities. On this view, a woman who receives an embryo donation or who serves as a gestational surrogate is having a reproductive experience, whether or not she also rears.
2. Sonnet 12 ("When I do count the clock that tells the time/And see the brave day sunk in hideous night"). Sonnet 2 ("When forty winters shall besiege thy brow/ And dig deep trenches in thy beauty's field") also sings the praises of reproduction as an answer to death and old age.
3. Margaret Atwood, *The Handmaid's Tale* (Boston: Houghton Mifflin, 1986).

INSTRUCTION ON RESPECT FOR HUMAN LIFE IN ITS ORIGIN AND ON THE DIGNITY OF PROCREATION

Vatican, Congregation for the Doctrine of the Faith

BIOMEDICAL RESEARCH AND THE TEACHING OF THE CHURCH

The gift of life which God the Creator and Father has entrusted to man calls him to appreciate the inestimable value of what he has been given and to take responsibility for it: This fundamental principle must be placed at the center of one's reflection in order to clarify and solve the moral problems raised by artificial interventions on life as it originates and on the processes of procreation.

Thanks to the progress of the biological and medical sciences, man has at his disposal ever more effective therapeutic resources; but he can also acquire new powers, with unforeseeable consequences, over human life at its very beginning and in its first stages. Various procedures now make it possible to intervene not only in order to assist, but also to dominate the processes of procreation. These techniques can enable man to "take in hand his own destiny," but they also expose him "to the temptation to go beyond the limits of a reasonable dominion over nature." They might constitute progress in the service of man, but they also involve serious risks. Many people are therefore expressing an urgent appeal that in interventions on procreation the

Origins 16, No. 40, March 19, 1987. Abridged.

Editors' note: The notes have been omitted; those wishing to follow up on sources should consult the original article.

values and rights of the human person be safeguarded. Requests for clarification and guidance are coming not only from the faithful, but also from those who recognize the church as "an expert in humanity" with a mission to serve the "civilization of love" and of life.

The church's magisterium [asserts] . . . the criteria of moral judgment as regards the applications of scientific research and technology, especially in relation to human life and its beginnings . . . to be the respect, defense and promotion of man, his "primary and fundamental right" to life, his dignity as a person who is endowed with a spiritual soul and with moral responsibility and who is called to beatific communion with God. . . .

ANTHROPOLOGY AND PROCEDURES IN THE BIOMEDICAL FIELD

Which moral criteria must be applied in order to clarify the problems posed today in the field of biomedicine? The answer to this question presupposes a proper idea of the nature of the human person in his bodily dimension.

For it is only in keeping with his true nature that the human person can achieve self-realization as a "unified totality"; and this nature is at the same time corporal and spiritual. By virtue of its substantial union with a spiritual soul, the human body cannot be considered as a mere complex of tissues, organs and functions, nor can it be evaluated in the same way as the body of animals; rather, it is a constitutive part of the person who manifests and expresses himself through it.

The natural moral law expresses and lays down the purposes, rights and duties which are based upon the bodily and spiritual nature of the human person. Therefore this law cannot be thought of as simply a set of norms on the biological level; rather, it must be defined as the rational order whereby man is called by the Creator to direct and regulate his life and actions and in particular to make use of his own body.

A first consequence can be deduced from these principles: An intervention on the human body affects not only the tissues, the organs and their functions, but also involves the person himself on different levels. It involves, therefore, perhaps in an implicit but nonetheless real way, a moral significance and responsibility. . . .

Applied biology and medicine work together for the integral good of human life when they come to the aid of a person stricken by illness and infirmity and when they respect his or her dignity as a creature of God. No biologist or doctor can reasonably claim, by virtue of his scientific competence, to be able to decide on people's origin and destiny. This norm must be applied in a particular way in the field of sexuality and procreation, in which man and woman actualize the fundamental values of love and life.

God, who is love and life, has inscribed in man and woman the vocation to share in a special way in his mystery of personal communion and in his work as Creator and Father. For this reason marriage possesses specific goods and values in its union and in procreation which cannot be likened to those existing in lower forms of life. Such values and meanings are of the personal order and determine from the moral point of view the meaning and limits of artificial interventions on procreation and on the origin of human life. These interventions are not to be rejected on the grounds that they are artificial. As such, they bear witness to the possibilities of the art of medicine. But they must be given a moral evaluation in reference to the dignity of the human person, who is called to realize his vocation from God to the gift of love and the gift of life.

FUNDAMENTAL CRITERIA FOR A MORAL JUDGMENT

The fundamental values connected with the techniques of artificial human procreation are two: the life of the human being called into existence and the special nature of the transmission of human life in marriage. The moral judgment on such methods of artificial procreation must therefore be formulated in reference to these values.

Physical life, with which the course of human life in the world begins, certainly does not itself contain the whole of a person's value, nor does it represent the supreme good of man, who is called to eternal life. However it does constitute in a certain way the "fundamental" value of life precisely because upon this physical life all the other values of the person are based and developed. The inviolability of the innocent human being's right to life "from the moment of conception until death" is a sign and requirement of the very inviolability of the person to whom the Creator has given the gift of life.

By comparison with the transmission of other forms of life in the universe, the transmission of human life has a special character of its own, which derives from the special nature of the human person. "The transmission of human life is entrusted by nature to a personal and conscious act and as such is subject to the all-holy laws of God: immutable and inviolable laws which must be recognized and observed. For this reason one cannot use means and follow methods which could be licit in the transmission of the life of plants and animals."

Advances in technology have now made it possible to procreate apart from sexual relations through the meeting *in vitro* of the germ cells previously taken from the man and the woman. But what is technically possible is not for that very reason morally admissible. Rational reflection on the fundamental values of life and of human procreation is therefore indispensable for formulating a moral evaluation of such technological interventions on a human being from the first stages of his development. . . .

I. RESPECT FOR HUMAN EMBRYOS

What respect is due to the human embryo, taking into account his nature and identity?

The human being must be respected—as a person—from the very first instant of his existence. . . .

This congregation is aware of the current debates concerning the beginning of human life, concerning the individuality of the human being and concerning the identity of the human person. The congregation recalls the teachings found in the Declaration on Procured Abortion:

"From the time that the ovum is fertilized, a new life is begun which is neither that of the father nor of the mother; it is rather the life of a new human being with his own growth. It would never be made human if it were not human already. To this perpetual evidence . . . modern genetic science brings valuable confirmation. It has demonstrated that, from the first instant, the program is fixed as to what this living being will be: a man, this individual man with his characteristic aspects already well determined. Right from fertilization is begun the adventure of a human life, and each of its great capacities requires time . . . to find its place and to be in a position to act."

This teaching remains valid and is further confirmed, if confirmation were needed, by recent findings of human biological science which recognize that in the zygote (the cell produced when the nuclei of the two gametes have fused) resulting from fertilization the biological identity of a new human individual is already constituted.

Certainly no experimental datum can be in itself sufficient to bring us to the recognition of a spiritual soul; nevertheless, the conclusions of science regarding the human embryo provide a valuable indication for discerning by the use of reason a personal presence at the moment of this first appearance of a human life: How could a human individual not be a human person? The magisterium has not expressly committed itself to an affirmation of a philosophical nature, but it constantly reaffirms the moral condemnation of any kind of procured abortion. This teaching has not been changed and is unchangeable.

Thus the fruit of human generation from the first moment of its existence, that is to say, from the moment the zygote has formed, demands the unconditional respect that is morally due to the human being in his bodily and spiritual totality. The human being is to be respected and treated as a person from the moment of conception and therefore from that same moment his rights as a person must be recognized, among which in the first place is the inviolable right of every innocent human being to life. This doctrinal reminder provides the fundamental criterion for the solution of the various problems posed by the development of the biomedical sciences in this field: Since the embryo must be treated as a person, it must also be defended in its integrity, tended and cared for, to the extent possible, in the same way as any other human being as far as medical assistance is concerned. . . .

How is one to evaluate morally research and experimentation on human embryos and fetuses?

Medical research must refrain from operations on live embryos, unless there is a moral certainty of not causing harm to the life or integrity of the unborn child and the mother, and on condition that the parents have given their free and informed consent to the procedure. It follows that all research, even when limited to the simple observation of the embryo, would become illicit were it to involve risk to the embryo's physical integrity or life by reason of the methods used or the effects induced.

As regards experimentation, and presupposing the general distinction between experimentation for purposes which are not directly therapeutic and experimentation which is clearly therapeutic for the subject himself, in the case in point one must also distinguish between experimentation carried out on embryos which are still alive and experimentation carried out on embryos which are dead. *If the embryos are living, whether viable or not, they must be respected just like any other human person; experimentation on embryos which is not directly therapeutic is illicit.*

No objective, even though noble in itself such as a foreseeable advantage to science, to other human beings or to society, can in any way justify experimentation on living human embryos or fetuses, whether viable or not, either inside or outside the mother's womb. The informed consent ordinarily required for clinical experimentation on adults cannot be granted by the parents, who may not freely dispose of the physical integrity or life of the unborn child. Moreover, experimentation on embryos and fetuses always involves risk, and indeed in most cases it involves the certain expectation of harm to their physical integrity or even their death.

To use human embryos or fetuses as the object or instrument of experimentation constitutes a crime against their dignity as human beings having a right to the same respect that is due to the child already born and to every human person. . . .

In the case of experimentation that is clearly therapeutic, namely, when it is a matter of experimental forms of therapy used for the benefit of the embryo itself in a final attempt to save its life and in the absence of other reliable forms of therapy, recourse to drugs or procedures not yet fully tested can be licit.

The corpses of human embryos and fetuses, whether they have been deliberately aborted or not, must be respected just as the remains of other human beings. In particular, they cannot be subjected to mutilation or to autopsies if their death has not yet been verified and without the consent of the parents or of the mother. Furthermore, the moral requirements must be safeguarded that there be no complicity in deliberate abortion and that the risk of scandal be avoided. Also, in the case of dead fetuses, as for the corpses of adult persons, all commercial trafficking must be considered illicit and should be prohibited.

How is one to evaluate morally the use for research purposes of embryos obtained by fertilization "in vitro?"

Human embryos obtained *in vitro* are human beings and subjects with rights: Their dignity and right to life must be respected from the first moment of their existence. *It is immoral to produce human embryos destined to be exploited as disposable "biological material."*

In the usual practice of *in vitro* fertilization, not all of the embryos are transferred to the woman's body; some are destroyed. Just as the church condemns induced abortion, so she also forbids acts against the life of these human beings. *It is a duty to condemn the particular gravity of the voluntary destruction of human embryos obtained "in vitro" for the sole purpose of research, either by means of artificial insemination or by means of "twin fission." By acting in this way the researcher usurps the place of God; and, even though he may be unaware of this, he sets himself up as the master of the destiny of others inasmuch as he arbitrarily chooses whom he will allow to live and whom he will send to death and kills defenseless human beings.*

Methods of observation or experimentation which damage or impose grave and disproportionate risks upon embryos obtained *in vitro* are morally illicit for the same reasons. Every human being is to be respected for himself and cannot be reduced in worth to a pure and simple instrument for the advantage of others. *It is therefore not in conformity with the moral law deliberately to expose to death human embryos obtained "in vitro."* In consequence of the fact that they have been produced *in vitro*, those embryos which are not transferred into the body of the mother and are called "spare" are exposed to an absurd fate, with no possibility of their being offered safe means of survival which can be licitly pursued.

What judgment should be made on other procedures of manipulating embryos connected with the "techniques of human reproduction"?

Techniques of fertilization *in vitro* can open the way to other forms of biological and genetic manipulation of human embryos, such as attempts or plans for fertilization between human and animal gametes and the gestation of human embryos in the uterus of animals, or the hypothesis or project of constructing artificial uteruses for the human embryo. *These procedures are contrary to the human dignity proper to the embryo, and at the same time they are contrary to the right of every person to be conceived and to be born within marriage and from marriage. Also, attempts or hypotheses for obtaining a human being without any connection with sexuality through "twin fission," cloning or parthenogenesis are to be considered contrary to the moral law, since they are in opposition to the dignity both of human procreation and of the conjugal union.*

The freezing of embryos, even when carried out in order to preserve the life of an embryo—cryopreservation—*constitutes an offense against the respect due to human beings* by exposing them to grave risks of death or harm to their physical integrity and depriving them, at least temporarily, of maternal shelter and gestation, thus placing them in a situation in which further offenses and manipulation are possible.

Certain attempts to influence chromosomic or genetic inheritance are not therapeutic, but are aimed at producing human beings selected according to sex or other predetermined qualities. These manipulations are contrary to the personal dignity of the human being and his or her integrity and identity. . . .

II. INTERVENTIONS UPON HUMAN PROCREATION

. . . A preliminary point for the moral evaluation of [*in vitro* fertilization and artificial insemination] is constituted by the consideration of the circumstances and consequences which those procedures involve in relation to the respect due the human embryo. Development of the practice of *in vitro* fertilization has required innumerable fertilizations and destructions of human embryos. Even today, the usual practice presupposes a hyperovulation on the part of the woman: A number of ova are withdrawn, fertilized and then cultivated *in vitro* for some days. Usually not all are transferred into the genital tracts of the woman; some embryos, generally called "spare," are destroyed or frozen. On occasion, some of the implanted embryos are sacrificed for various eugenic, economic or psychological reasons. Such deliberate destruction of human beings or their utilization for different purposes to the detriment of their integrity and life is contrary to the doctrine on procured abortion already recalled.

The connection between *in vitro* fertilization and the voluntary destruction of human embryos occurs too often. This is significant: Through these procedures, with apparently contrary purposes, life and death are subjected to the decision of man, who thus sets himself up as the giver of life and death by decree. This dynamic of violence and domination may remain unnoticed by those very individuals who, in wishing to utilize this procedure, become subject to it themselves. The facts recorded and the cold logic which links them must be taken into consideration for a moral judgment on *in vitro* fertilization and embryo transfer: The abortion mentality which has made this procedure possible thus leads, whether one wants it or not, to man's domination over the life and death of his fellow human beings and can lead to a system of radical eugenics. . . .

A. Heterologous* Artificial Fertilization

Why must human procreation take place in marriage?

Every human being is always to be accepted as a gift and blessing of God. However, from the moral point of view a truly responsible procreation vis-a-vis the unborn child must be the fruit of marriage.

For human procreation has specific characteristics by virtue of the personal dignity of the parents and of the children: The procreation of a new person, whereby the man and the woman collaborate with the power of the Creator, must be the fruit and the sign of the mutual self-giving of the spouses, of their love and of their fidelity. *The fidelity of the spouses in the unity of marriage involves reciprocal respect of their right to become a father and a mother only through each other.*

---

*[Heterologous: involving sperm and egg from a man and woman who are not married to each other.]

The child has the right to be conceived, carried in the womb, brought into the world and brought up within marriage: It is through the secure and recognized relationship to his own parents that the child can discover his own identity and achieve his own proper human development.

The parents find in their child a confirmation and completion of their reciprocal self-giving: The child is the living image of their love, the permanent sign of their conjugal union, the living and indissoluble concrete expression of their paternity and maternity.

By reason of the vocation and social responsibilities of the person, the good of the children and of the parents contributes to the good of civil society; the vitality and stability of society require that children come into the world within a family and that the family be firmly based on marriage.

The tradition of the church and anthropological reflection recognize in marriage and in its indissoluble unity the only setting worthy of truly responsible procreation.

Does heterologous artificial fertilization conform to the dignity of the couple and to the truth of marriage?

Through *in vitro* fertilization and embryo transfer and heterologous artificial insemination, human conception is achieved through the fusion of gametes of at least one donor other than the spouses who are united in marriage. *Heterologous artificial fertilization is contrary to the unity of marriage, to the dignity of the spouses, to the vocation proper to parents, and to the child's right to be conceived and brought into the world in marriage and from marriage.*

Respect for the unity of marriage and for conjugal fidelity demands that the child be conceived in marriage; the bond existing between husband and wife accords the spouses, in an objective and inalienable manner, the exclusive right to become father and mother solely through each other. Recourse to the gametes of a third person in order to have sperm or ovum available constitutes a violation of the reciprocal commitment of the spouses and a grave lack in regard to that essential property of marriage which is its unity.

Heterologous artificial fertilization violates the rights of the child; it deprives him of his filial relationship with his parental origins and can hinder the maturing of his personal identity. Furthermore, it offends the common vocation of the spouses who are called to fatherhood and motherhood: It objectively deprives conjugal fruitfulness of its unity and integrity; it brings about and manifests a rupture between genetic parenthood, gestational parenthood and responsibility for upbringing. Such damage to the personal relationships within the family has repercussions on civil society: What threatens the unity and stability of the family is a source of dissension, disorder and injustice in the whole of social life.

These reasons lead to a negative moral judgment concerning heterologous artificial fertilization: Consequently, fertilization of a married woman with the sperm of a donor different from her husband and fertilization with the husband's sperm of an ovum not coming from his wife are morally illicit. Furthermore, the artificial fertilization of a woman who is unmarried or a widow, whoever the donor may be, cannot be morally justified.

The desire to have a child and the love between spouses who long to obviate a sterility which cannot be overcome in any other way constitute understandable motivations; but subjectively good intentions do not render heterologous artificial fertilization conformable to the objective and inalienable properties of marriage or respectful of the rights of the child and of the spouses.

Is "surrogate" motherhood morally licit?

No, for the same reasons which lead one to reject heterologous artificial fertilization: For it is contrary to the unity of marriage and to the dignity of the procreation of the human person. . . .

B. Homologous* Artificial Fertilization

Since heterologous artificial fertilization has been declared unacceptable, the question arises of how to evaluate morally the process of homologous artificial fertilization: *in vitro* fertilization and embryo transfer and artificial insemination between

*[Homologous: involving sperm and egg from a man and woman who are married to each other.]

husband and wife. First a question of principle must be clarified.

What connection is required from the moral point of view between procreation and the conjugal act?

(a) The church's teaching on marriage and human procreation affirms the "inseparable connection, willed by God and unable to be broken by man on his own initiative, between the two meanings of the conjugal act: the unitive meaning and the procreative meaning. Indeed, by its intimate structure the conjugal act, while most closely uniting husband and wife, capacitates them for the generation of new lives according to laws inscribed in the very being of man and of woman." . . . "By safeguarding both these essential aspects, the unitive and the procreative, the conjugal act preserves in its fullness the sense of true mutual love and its ordination toward man's exalted vocation to parenthood."

The same doctrine concerning the link between the meanings of the conjugal act and between the goods of marriage throws light on the moral problem of homologous artificial fertilization, since "it is never permitted to separate these different aspects to such a degree as positively to exclude either the procreative intention or the conjugal relation."

Contraception deliberately deprives the conjugal act of its openness to procreation and in this way brings about a voluntary dissociation of the ends of marriage. Homologous artificial fertilization, in seeking a procreation which is not the fruit of a specific act of conjugal union, objectively effects an analogous separation between the goods and the meanings of marriage.

Thus . . . *from the moral point of view procreation is deprived of its proper perfection when it is not desired as the fruit of the conjugal act, that is to say, of the specific act of the spouses' union.*

(b) The moral value of the intimate link between the goods of marriage and between the meanings of the conjugal act is based upon the unity of the human being, a unity involving body and spiritual soul. Spouses mutually express their personal love in the "language of the body," which clearly involves both "spousal meanings" and parental ones. The conjugal act by which the couple mutually express their self-gift at the same time expresses openness to the gift of life. It is an act that is inseparably corporal and spiritual. It is in their bodies and through their bodies that the spouses consummate their marriage and are able to become father and mother. In order to respect the language of their bodies and their natural generosity, the conjugal union must take place with respect for its openness to procreation; and the procreation of a person must be the fruit and the result of married love. The origin of the human being thus follows from a procreation that is "linked to the union, not only biological but also spiritual, of the parents, made one by the bond of marriage." Fertilization achieved outside the bodies of the couple remains by this very fact deprived of the meanings and the values which are expressed in the language of the body and in the union of human persons.

(c) Only respect for the link between the meanings of the conjugal act and respect for the unity of the human being make possible procreation in conformity with the dignity of the person. In his unique and irrepeatable origin, the child must be respected and recognized as equal in personal dignity to those who give him life. The human person must be accepted in his parents' act of union and love; the generation of a child must therefore be the fruit of that mutual giving which is realized in the conjugal act wherein the spouses cooperate as servants and not as masters in the work of the Creator, who is love.

In reality, the origin of a human person is the result of an act of giving. The one conceived must be the fruit of his parents' love. He cannot be desired or conceived as the product of an intervention of medical or biological techniques; that would be equivalent to reducing him to an object of scientific technology. No one may subject the coming of a child into the world to conditions of technical efficiency which are to be evaluated according to standards of control and dominion.

The moral relevance of the link between the meanings of the conjugal act and between the goods of marriage, as well as the unity of the human being and the dignity of his origin, demand that the procreation of a human person be brought about as the fruit of the conjugal act specific to the love between spouses. . . .

Is homologous "in vitro" fertilization morally licit?

The answer to this question is strictly dependent on the principles just mentioned. Certainly one cannot ignore the legitimate aspirations of sterile couples. For some, recourse to homologous *in vitro* fertilization and embryo transfer appears to be the only way of fulfilling their sincere desire for a child. The question is asked whether the totality of conjugal life in such situations is not sufficient to ensure the dignity proper to human procreation. It is acknowledged that *in vitro* fertilization and embryo transfer certainly cannot supply for the absence of sexual relations and cannot be preferred to the specific acts of conjugal union, given the risks involved for the child and the difficulties of the procedure. But it is asked whether, when there is no other way of overcoming the sterility which is a source of suffering, homologous *in vitro* fertilization may not constitute an aid, if not a form of therapy, whereby its moral licitness could be admitted.

The desire for a child—or at the very least an openness to the transmission of life—is a necessary prerequisite from the moral point of view for responsible human procreation. But this good intention is not sufficient for making a positive moral evaluation of *in vitro* fertilization between spouses. The process of *in vitro* fertilization and embryo transfer must be judged in itself and cannot borrow its definitive moral quality from the totality of conjugal life of which it becomes part nor from the conjugal acts which may precede or follow it. . . .

[E]ven in a situation in which every precaution were taken to avoid the death of human embryos, homologous *in vitro* fertilization and embryo transfer dissociates from the conjugal act the actions which are directed to human fertilization. For this reason the very nature of homologous *in vitro* fertilization and embryo transfer also must be taken into account, even abstracting from the link with procured abortion.

Homologous *in vitro* fertilization and embryo transfer is brought about outside the bodies of the couple through actions of third parties whose competence and technical activity determine the success of the procedure. Such fertilization entrusts the life and identity of the embryo into the power of doctors and biologists and establishes the domination of technology over the origin and destiny of the human person. Such a relationship of domination is in itself contrary to the dignity and equality that must be common to parents and children.

Conception *in vitro* is the result of the technical action which presides over fertilization. *Such fertilization is neither in fact achieved nor positively willed as the expression and fruit of a specific act of the conjugal union. In homologous "in vitro" fertilization and embryo transfer, therefore, even if it is considered in the context of de facto existing sexual relations, the generation of the human person is objectively deprived of its proper perfection: namely, that of being the result and fruit of a conjugal act* in which the spouses can become "cooperators with God for giving life to a new person." . . .

Although the manner in which human conception is achieved with *in vitro* fertilization and embryo transfer cannot be approved, every child which comes into the world must in any case be accepted as a living gift of the divine Goodness and must be brought up with love.

How is homologous artificial insemination to be evaluated from the moral point of view?

Homologous artificial insemination within marriage cannot be admitted except for those cases in which the technical means is not a substitute for the conjugal act but serves to facilitate and to help so that the act attains its natural purpose. . . .

"In its natural structure, the conjugal act is a personal action, a simultaneous and immediate cooperation on the part of the husband and wife, which by the very nature of the agents and the proper nature of the act is the expression of the mutual gift which, according to the words of Scripture, brings about union 'in one flesh.'" Thus moral conscience "does not necessarily proscribe the use of certain artificial means destined solely either to the facilitating of the natural act or to ensuring that the natural act normally performed achieves its proper end." If the technical means facilitates the conjugal act or helps it to reach its natural objectives, it can be morally acceptable. If, on the other hand, the procedure were to replace the conjugal act, it is morally illicit.

Artificial insemination as a substitute for the conjugal act is prohibited by reason of the voluntarily achieved dissociation of the two meanings of the conjugal act. Masturbation, through which the sperm is normally obtained, is another sign of this dissociation: Even when it is done for the purpose of procreation the act remains deprived of its unitive meaning: "It lacks the sexual relationship called for by the moral order, namely the relationship which realizes 'the full sense of mutual self-giving and human procreation in the context of true love.'". . .

What moral criterion can be proposed with regard to medical intervention in human procreation?

The medical act must be evaluated not only with reference to its technical dimension, but also and above all in relation to its goal, which is the good of persons and their bodily and psychological health. The moral criteria for medical intervention in procreation are deduced from the dignity of human persons, of their sexuality and of their origin.

Medicine which seeks to be ordered to the integral good of the person must respect the specifically human values of sexuality. The doctor is at the service of persons and of human procreation. He does not have the authority to dispose of them or to decide their fate. A medical intervention respects the dignity of persons when it seeks to assist the conjugal act either in order to facilitate its performance or in order to enable it to achieve its objective once it has been normally performed.

On the other hand, it sometimes happens that a medical procedure technologically replaces the conjugal act in order to obtain a procreation which is neither its result nor its fruit. In this case the medical act is not, as it should be, at the service of conjugal union, but rather appropriates to itself the procreative function and thus contradicts the dignity and the inalienable rights of the spouses and of the child to be born.

The humanization of medicine, which is insisted upon today by everyone, requires respect for the integral dignity of the human person first of all in the act and at the moment in which the spouses transmit life to a new person. It is only logical therefore to address an urgent appeal to Catholic doctors and scientists that they bear exemplary witness to the respect due to the human embryo and to the dignity of procreation. The medical and nursing staff of Catholic hospitals and clinics are in a special way urged to do justice to the moral obligations which they have assumed, frequently also, as part of their contract. Those who are in charge of Catholic hospitals and clinics and who are often religious will take special care to safeguard and promote a diligent observance of the moral norms recalled in the present instruction.

The suffering caused by infertility in marriage.

The suffering of spouses who cannot have children or who are afraid of bringing a handicapped child into the world is a suffering that everyone must understand and properly evaluate.

On the part of the spouses, the desire for a child is natural: It expresses the vocation to fatherhood and motherhood inscribed in conjugal love. This desire can be even stronger if the couple is affected by sterility which appears incurable. Nevertheless, marriage does not confer upon the spouses the right to have a child, but only the right to perform those natural acts which are per se ordered to procreation.

A true and proper right to a child would be contrary to the child's dignity and nature. The child is not an object to which one has a right nor can he be considered as an object of ownership: Rather, a child is a gift, "the supreme gift" and the most gratuitous gift of marriage, and is a living testimony of the mutual giving of his parents. For this reason, the child has the right as already mentioned, to be the fruit of the specific act of the conjugal love of his parents; and he also has the right to be respected as a person from the moment of his conception.

Nevertheless, whatever its cause or prognosis, sterility is certainly a difficult trial. The community of believers is called to shed light upon and support the suffering of those who are unable to fulfill their legitimate aspiration to motherhood and fatherhood. Spouses who find themselves in this sad situation are called to find in it an opportunity for sharing in a particular way in the Lord's cross, the source of spiritual fruitfulness. Sterile couples must not forget that "even when procreation is not possible, conjugal life does not for this reason lose its value. Physical sterility in fact can be for spouses the occasion for other important services to the life of the human person, for example, adoption, various forms of educational work and assistance to other families and to poor or handicapped children."...

III. MORAL AND CIVIL LAW

The Values and Moral Obligations That Civil Legislation Must Respect and Sanction in This Matter

The inviolable right to life of every innocent human individual and the rights of the family and of the institution of marriage constitute fundamental moral values because they concern the natural condition and integral vocation of the human person; at the same time they are constitutive elements of civil society and its order.

For this reason the new technological possibilities which have opened up in the field of biomedicine require the intervention of the political authorities and of the legislator, since an uncontrolled application of such techniques could lead to unforeseeable and damaging consequences for civil society. Recourse to the conscience of each individual and to the self-regulation of researchers cannot be sufficient for ensuring respect for personal rights and public order....

The intervention of the public authority must be inspired by the rational principles which regulate the relationships between civil law and moral law. The task of the civil law is to ensure the common good of people through the recognition of and the defense of fundamental rights and through the promotion of peace and of public morality....

As a consequence of the respect and protection which must be ensured for the unborn child from the moment of his conception, the law must provide appropriate penal sanctions for every deliberate violation of the child's rights. The law cannot tolerate—indeed it must expressly forbid—that human beings, even at the embryonic stage, should be treated as objects of experimentation, be mutilated or destroyed with the excuse that they are superfluous or incapable of developing normally.

The political authority is bound to guarantee to the institution of the family, upon which society is based, the juridical protection to which it has a right. From the very fact that it is at the service of people, the political authority must also be at the service of the family. Civil law cannot grant approval to techniques of artificial procreation which, for the benefit of third parties (doctors, biologists, economic or governmental powers), take away what is a right inherent in the relationship between spouses; and therefore civil law cannot legalize the donation of gametes between persons who are not legitimately united in marriage.

Legislation must also prohibit, by virtue of the support which is due to the family, embryo banks, post-mortem insemination and "surrogate motherhood."...

WHAT IS WRONG WITH COMMODIFICATION?

Ruth Macklin

What, if anything, is wrong with paying money to egg donors? Some people see nothing wrong, from an ethical point of view; it has even been argued that it would be wrong *not* to pay women who choose to provide oocytes for infertile women. Others are hesitant to endorse such payments, yet stop short of ethical condemnation. Still others are more critical, arguing that paying women for eggs, like paying women to be surrogates, amounts to commodification of the human body and therefore demeans women and degrades that which is distinctively human.

Underlying these different positions are arguments that appeal to different considerations: comparisons with paying men to be sperm donors; worries about a slippery slope that begins with paying for eggs, slides to paying for embryos, and lands at the bottom with paying for babies; the question of fairness in compensating women who provide this service; and worries about damage to the fabric of society when bodily products or services are commercialized. Arguments on both sides of the issue are persuasive, making it difficult to arrive at a clear resolution of the problem. Also underlying the different positions are moral sentiments, against which it is hard to mount a rational argument.

My own conclusion is that commodification of human beings for any purpose is unsavory and ought to be avoided whenever possible. Yet "unsavoriness" is not a category of moral disvalue strong enough to warrant prohibition. If commodification does not involve a violation of a moral principle or the rights of any person or group, then it would be unwarranted to ban such commercial transactions. The account that follows explores the arguments surrounding the practice of paying egg donors, and ends by opting for the "least worst" resolution.

The well-established tradition of paying sperm donors (making them vendors, properly speaking, rather than donors) leads some to argue that women who donate their ova should similarly be compensated. Another long-standing practice in the United States is that of commercial blood collection, which has been questioned in recent years more on grounds of the quality of the blood supply when paid donors are used than on the quite different premise that buying human body products is somehow wrong.

A great deal of criticism has been leveled at the practice of commercial surrogacy, wherein women are paid significant sums to bear a child for an infertile woman or couple. A number of states have enacted legislation prohibiting commercial surrogacy and assigning criminal penalties to brokers. Although payment to surrogates has been charged with being a form of "baby selling" and therefore against public policy, defenders—and even some critics—of commercial surrogacy deny that baby selling is a proper characterization. Paid surrogacy has been justified on the grounds that the money is for the surrogates' "time and inconvenience," not for the baby she eventually delivers and hands over. Payment for "time and inconvenience" is the same justification used for compensating normal, healthy volunteers to serve as subjects of biomedical or behavioral research. It is also the phrase that has been adopted to describe what ovum donors are being paid for.

The practice of surrogacy poses an array of ethical problems that go well beyond the issue of payment. For that reason, assisted reproduction using eggs from a third party is much more analogous to the use of donor sperm than it is to surrogacy. It is sufficient to note here that as a matter of

---

Reprinted with permission of the author and publisher from Cynthia B. Cohen, ed., *New Ways of Making Babies: The Case of Egg Donation*. Bloomington and Indianapolis: Indiana University Press, 1996.

Editors' note: Some footnotes have been deleted. Students who want to follow up on sources should consult the original article.

public policy, it would not be inconsistent to argue that commercial surrogacy ought to be prohibited but that commerce in gametes ought to be permitted.

WHAT ARE DONORS PAID FOR, AND DOES IT MATTER?

A presumption appears throughout the literature that although it would be wrong to pay donors for their eggs, it is ethically permissible, if not required, to compensate them for the time they spend, the risks they undergo, and the inconvenience they experience. However, nowhere is an explanation offered for why payment for eggs is ethically suspect but monetary compensation for these other things is not.

An ethical advisory committee report issued by the American Fertility Society (AFS) in 1990 stated that "there should be no compensation to the donor for the egg."[1] The sentence that followed asserted that "This does not exclude reimbursement for expenses, time, risk and associated inconvenience." The revised 1993 guidelines from AFS state that "Donors should be compensated for direct and indirect expenses associated with their participation, inconvenience, time, risk and discomfort." The implication of the wording is that it is at least suspect, if not ethically wrong , to pay women for their eggs. But it is not made clear just what is ethically problematic.

How can we tell if a woman is being paid for her eggs (and is thus a vendor) or for her inconvenience, time, risk, and discomfort? An interview with a woman who was an egg donor at an Austrian IVF clinic is revealing. The interviewers asked: "How much did you get paid per operation and how does the financial transaction take place?" The woman replied: "After the procedure I get os 10,000 (U.S. $800) no matter how many eggs they take out. If there are no matured eggs or they miss the ovulation I get no money except expenses like tramfare. But this has not happened to me so far. The doctors pay for the product 'egg.'"[2] In contrast, if a woman were paid the same amount of money whether or not any eggs are harvested, it would be reasonable to conclude that she is being paid for her time, inconvenience, and so on.

A report of the combined ethics committee of the Canadian Fertility and Andrology Society and the Society of Obstetricians and Gynaecologists of Canada includes the following recommendation: "The Societies endorse the payment of gamete donors to reimburse them in a reasonable fashion for the costs and inconvenience of donation and any screening procedures which are essential to the safe operation of donor gamete programs."[3] The combined ethics committee considered two other options. The first option was to permit no payment. The committee rejected this on grounds that it would likely result in shortages of donated gametes.

The second option was to permit unrestricted payment. This option was rejected on the grounds that an excessive financial incentive might tempt some individuals to lie about their medical or genetic history or previous gamete donations they had made. The committee's refusal to allow unrestricted payment was not based on the ethical consideration of protecting *donors* from exploitation that might result from coercive offers of money. Instead, the ethical justification rested on the "harm principle," that is, protection of gamete *recipients* who might be harmed as a result of transmission of infection or genetic disease.

The combined committee's reasoning makes clear why they rejected the two extreme options—permitting no payment to donors or permitting unrestricted payment. Yet the recommendation the committee did adopt is silent on the matter of paying for the eggs. The recommendation is phrased in terms of reimbursement to donors: "to reimburse them in a reasonable fashion for the costs and inconvenience of donation." This wording carefully avoids any implication that donors are being paid for the eggs.

Apparently uncomfortable with the commercial aspect, Sherman Elias and George Annas contend that "the Warnock and Waller Commissions may well be on the right track in discouraging commerce in gametes and in limiting payment to out-of-pocket and medical expenses."[4] Yet this recommendation is incomplete since it leaves open the question of how to characterize the egg donor's "time, inconvenience, and discomfort." Payment for medical expenses obviously does not cover these items. Payment for the woman's transportation, tolls, parking, and so on obviously does count as "out-of-pocket expenses." So we are left with the category of "time (other than lost wages), risk, discomfort, and inconvenience."

Even John Robertson, a staunch defender of payment to egg donors, avoids language implying that it is perfectly permissible to pay directly for the eggs: "Many persons would find payment for the egg donor's time and effort morally unobjectionable and appropriate, if not also obligatory."[5] In this passage and elsewhere, Robertson states that it would be unfair not to pay donors, but he is silent on the question of whether payment for the eggs would somehow be wrong.

The implication in all of these accounts seems to be that payment to people for their services is ethically permissible but paying them for bodily products is not. Payment to women for time and effort sounds like paying people for their work, surely an ethically acceptable if not obligatory social practice. Paying for risk and discomfort is like compensating normal, healthy volunteers of biomedical or behavioral research, also a widely accepted practice. Paying for human eggs begins to sound suspiciously like payment to live kidney donors, a transaction that gives rise to strong repugnance in many people.

It is, however, hard to find a basis for claiming that payment for the risks, discomfort, and inconvenience a donor undergoes is ethically sound but payment for the product extracted as a result of the process is ethically wrong. The only reason for subjecting women to these risks, discomforts, and inconvenience is to obtain the eggs. Perhaps it is the idea that paying for ova makes them into a commodity and that is somehow wrong. But it could equally well be maintained that payment for bodily services is also a form of "commodification." If there is something suspect about commodifying human reproductive products, it is similarly suspect to commodify human reproductive services.

GENDER PARITY: PAYMENT FOR SPERM AND EGGS

One argument in favor of paying ovum donors contends that a woman's eggs should be treated just like a man's sperm. Since there is a long tradition of paying men for sperm donations, why not pay women to be egg donors? Both male and female gametes that are donated are not needed by their owners. Sperm are continuously produced in men, and although women are born with their entire supply of eggs, that supply contains many more than a woman will ever need in her reproductive lifetime. It has been stated that paying sperm donors but not egg donors would unfairly discriminate against women, who undergo greater risk in order to donate eggs.

Others suggest that perhaps it is time to rethink the sale of sperm. For example, the Glover Report to the European Commission[6] offers several arguments against the established practice of paying semen donors. The report notes that "as with blood donation, payment may lead unsuitable people to apply, lying about their medical history (perhaps one of AIDS) in order to be paid." The reply to this objection in regard to semen donation has already occurred in the United States in the regulations governing licensed sperm banks. All semen donors are tested for HIV at the time of the donation, the sample is stored, and the donors retested after six months to ensure that they have not seroconverted in the interim. Since it is not (yet) possible to store frozen ova, egg donors can be tested only initially, leaving open the possibility the "unsuitable" people may choose to donate for the money.

There are other differences between sperm and egg donation, however, not in the nature of the products (both are human gametes) but in the nature of the process that yields the products. Sperm donors may undergo some inconvenience, but it could hardly be maintained that they are submitting themselves to considerable discomforts or undertaking substantial risks. The question whether sperm donors are paid for their sperm or compensated for their time and inconvenience seems never to have been addressed. The presumption seems to be that they are paid for the "product," but worries about commodification have not traditionally been expressed.

In contrast to sperm donors, women who become egg donors undergo a minor surgical procedure. Also, they take hormones prior to extraction of their eggs in order to make the eggs suitable for fertilization and subsequent implantation in the recipient. This difference between sperm and ovum donors in the level of risk, discomfort, and inconvenience has prompted some people to claim that women should not only be paid for their eggs, as men are for sperm, but that the increased risk and discomfort to these women justifies paying them a lot more. In a conversation in which the sum of $2,000 paid to egg donors was cited, a leading researcher in techniques of assisted reproduction remarked that these women ought to be paid even more than that, considering all that they undergo.

In one key respect, sperm and eggs are similar to one another and different from other bodily products. Gametes are human bodily materials from which other humans can be created. Whether this fact confers some distinct moral status on human gametes is unclear. It is surely true that people may care more about what happens to their donated gametes than to their donated blood. Yet the claim that their status as gametes makes it unethical to sell sperm or ova but permissible to donate them is puzzling without further argument.

EXPLOITATION OF WOMEN

The charge of "exploitation of women" has been leveled against paid surrogacy and payments for ovum donation. Since exploitation of human beings is, at least on one conception, a serious ethical wrong in violations of the Kantian imperative "never to treat persons merely as a means,"[7] it is important to determine whether paying egg donors can properly be charged with being a form of exploitation. This concern relates more to the amount of payment than to the simple fact of payment. The more money donors receive, the more it may become a coercive offer, one that is exploitive. If women were paid a nickel for their eggs, that could hardly be considered exploitation on the grounds that they are being paid *too much*, though it might be exploitive in paying *too little*. After all, when laborers are underpaid by their employers the latter are accused of exploiting the workers. This curious twist has occurred in the debates over paid surrogacy. It has been argued that the standard $10,000 fee paid to a surrogate is too *low*, that it is exploitive precisely because it is not a fair wage for services rendered. As an hourly wage, it comes to about $1.49 per hour. Whether egg donors are properly to be construed as "laborers" is one of the questions raised by the commodification argument.

Money is offered to men and women in order to induce them to be gamete donors. It can be assumed that without payment, the source of gametes from anonymous donors would dry up. The acceptability of this practice rests on the view that an inducement is ethically acceptable but an "undue" inducement is not. Whenever greater sums of money are involved, an undue inducement becomes elevated into a coercive offer. It can then be questioned whether the action is fully voluntary. Since voluntariness is a necessary condition for the ethical acceptability of a biomedical intervention such as egg retrieval, the more the voluntariness of the donor's decision can be questioned, the more ethically worrisome is the practice.

Here the contrast between the amount paid to sperm and egg donors is instructive. Intuitively, no one is likely to contend that $25 or $50 (the usual range) or even $100 paid to sperm donors is a coercive offer or undue inducement. That is partly because of the relatively low amount of money; and also because the donor is not being induced to engage in a form of behavior he might not do anyway. In contrast, $2,000 is a significant sum for students or for poor or lower-class women; and they are surely being induced to undergo something they would not otherwise be doing. This argument does not conclude that payment to donors is unethical, but simply that the amount to be paid is the important factor.

How can we determine when payment to egg donors is exploitive? John Harris identifies three issues: "The first involves the question of whether it is morally objectionable to use others as a means to our own ends, the second asks whether paying them for being such a means constitutes exploitation, and the third is of course whether in all the circumstances, exploitation is such a bad thing." Harris argues persuasively that it is not wrong to use others as a means to one's own ends when those others have autonomously accepted that project as their own and have not been coerced in some way into becoming instruments. Presumably, this reflects the Kantian notion that people must not be treated as a means *merely*. One may treat others as a means to one's own ends just so long as others' ends are also served in the process.

Harris proposes the following definition of exploitation: "Exploitation occurs when those exploited have not autonomously adopted their part in our projects as one of their own projects but have been coerced in some way into becoming instruments of ours." It does not follow from this that whenever financial interests are involved, the situation is then exploitive. The key ingredient in this conception of exploitation seems to be that of coercive pressure, or absence of genuine autonomy, rather than the fact of remuneration.

An antipaternalist line of argument leaves the decision whether to bear pain or undergo inconvenience in exchange for money up to the individual who is most affected, rather than seeking to regulate the practice by prohibiting or setting upper limits on payments. John Hoff[8] contends that people constantly make judgments balancing pain/inconvenience and money. The coal miner undertakes filth and danger for money; the nightshift employee receives a bonus. If the donor chooses to undertake the procedure despite the pain, is that coercion or the satisfaction of a need in a manner acceptable to the donor? Indeed, Hoff maintains, it could be argued there is more "coercion" where the donor gives eggs to a relative out of "guilt" rather than for money. The former donation does not benefit the donor, other than alleviation of guilt; the latter does.

All this is true enough. But it leads us to consider just which actions and transactions can reasonably be regulated and which cannot. No one would really want to regulate intrafamilial goings on, whereas providing professional guidelines or state health department regulations for acceptable limits that infertility programs may pay to egg donors would not interfere in any way with family privacy.

The exploitation line of argument takes a more specific form in relation to wealthier individuals or couples paying money to poorer women for use of their bodies. Here the argument does not focus on women generally, but rather on women of lower socioeconomic status. Taking an antipaternalist stance, John Hoff says it seems somewhat "matronizing" to deny poor people the opportunity to earn money by giving up "excess" body tissue (provided they are informed of the risk). Every service in our economy is sold: academics sell their minds; athletes sell the use of their bodies. The best art in the world is the subject of commodification. If a pretty actress can sell her body for television, why should a fecund woman be denied the ability to sell her eggs? Why is one more demeaning than the other? If anything, why is not the sale of eggs, which has a more socially useful purpose, a more appropriate transaction. Surely, Hoff asserts, we are beyond the point where the sale of a service by itself taints the service.

As a factual matter, it has been questioned whether paid egg donors do or are likely to come from the poorer socioeconomic class. John Robertson observes that "the recipient's desire to receive good genes will place a premium on women who are healthy and appear to be of good stock. Donors—even repeat donors—are as likely to be middle as well as lower class women." In addition, Robertson questions whether it follows that because donors are poorer than recipients, the arrangement therefore amounts to exploitation: "neither the risks nor the payments are so great that an unacceptable exploitation of poorer persons would occur."

All things considered, it is implausible to conclude that paying egg donors is exploitive. The facts surrounding the socioeconomic status of ovum donors show that they do not come from the poorest class of society. And there is nothing to suggest that these women are coerced, or do not autonomously choose to become donors. This is one way, among many others, of making money. Even if receiving compensation is the primary motive for choosing to become a donor, that does not imply that women are being exploited.

ETHICAL PRINCIPLES AND PAYING DONORS

An ethical analysis of any action or social practice is incomplete if it fails to address the question whether an ethical principle is violated. So, how about the practice of paying egg donors? The answer is not immediately evident because, as in almost all situations in which actions or practices are evaluated by appealing to ethical principles, the principles themselves must first be subjected to analysis and interpretation. The two leading principles of bioethics that are relevant in this context are respect for persons and justice.

Whether paying egg donors violates the principle of respect for persons depends on whether the principle is interpreted narrowly or broadly.

According to the narrow interpretation, if the subject of a biomedical intervention grants voluntary, informed consent to the procedure, the person is respected and the principle is not violated. Since prospective egg donors are fully informed (we may assume, or at least hope) of the purpose, procedures to be performed, the time involved, the risks, and the benefits, paying the donors does not violate the principle. Along the same lines, paying donors is not a violation of individuals' right to liberty or privacy if we assume that there are no coercive practices involved in commercial egg donation. Here again, there is no failure to respect persons. The principle of respect for persons would be violated if paying egg donors constitutes a form of exploitation. However, as John Harris argues convincingly, it is not plausible to say that women who autonomously agree to donate their eggs for a sum of money are being exploited in virtue of the payment.

Nevertheless, a broader interpretation of respect for persons might yield a different conclusion. This interpretation looks to the value that underlies and justifies the principle: the notion that human beings as such are uniquely valuable. This broader principle requires special respect not only for the informed choices of individuals, but for that which is human. It appears, then, that whether respect for persons is violated depends on whether the principle is given a narrow or a broad interpretation.

The same might be said for the principle of justice. In one respect, paying egg donors does not violate a principle of justice, since there appears to be no inequitable treatment of one group as opposed to another. Poorer women are paid for their eggs just like middle-class or wealthier women. If poorer and better-off women are paid the same amount for being donors, that seems fair since they are undergoing the same procedure and are thus subjected to the same risks, discomforts, and inconveniences. If payment is to be made as actual compensation for lost wages, working women who earn more would presumably get more money for the time they put in as donors than would women who earn less. That arrangement could be considered unjust because it violates the principle of "equal pay for equal work." To become clear about what is just in this realm seems to require a decision about precisely what women are being paid for: "the product egg"; risks, discomfort, and inconvenience; or what their time is worth on the labor market.

A different consideration of justice points to the fact that the pattern of commercial programs is one of better-off women as recipients and less-well-off women as donors, a pattern that results from the high cost of IVF and embryo implantation. That cost is beyond the reach of poorer women unless public funding for IVF becomes a matter of policy. According to this consideration, justice is violated because a wealthier class of women are the donors and a poorer class are the recipients. Here again, however, defenders of an interpretation of justice that allows the market to determine all transaction will view this class difference between donors and recipients as just another instance of the workings of the marketplace.

Appeals to ethical principles are thus quite complex, and argument employing them can cut both ways. Robertson observes that "objections to paying egg donors stem from a religious or moral view of human dignity that is not universally shared. . . . Indeed, refusing to pay donors for their efforts seems unfair and exploitative." So, contrary to the view that it is exploitive for wealthier women to pay poorer women for their reproductive products or services, Robertson argues that it is exploitive *not* to do so. This is what is required in order "to treat donors fairly."

COMMODIFICATION

If there is something wrong with paying money for bodily products or services, what is the nature of that wrong? One way of characterizing the wrong is *commodification* of the procreative process. The theory that there are some forms of exchange among human beings that should be prevented from being carried out for money has been put forth by a number of writers. For example, Michael Walzer has argued that some market exchanges should be blocked.[9] The fact that our society is capitalistic and is dominated by commercial transactions of all sorts does not compel the conclusion that therefore, anything whatsoever may be put up for sale. An illustration offered as uncontroversial is "the norm that citizens should be legally free to vote or not as they wish, but not to sell their votes or to vote a certain way for a price."[10] This general line of argument can be applied to the specific situation involving the sale of bodily parts and reproductive services.[11]

To quote an expression used by Leon Kass in discussing embryos produced by *in vitro* fertilization, the human body, its parts, and its reproductive product are not "mere meat."[12] Therefore, they should not be subject to the same market forces that govern the sale of pork bellies. Human organs are not like calves' livers or thymus glands, at least in the judgment of the U.S. Congress when it enacted a law prohibiting commercial procurement and distribution of organs for transplantation.[13]

Commercial traffic in frozen embryos would constitute another instance of unacceptable commodification, although it would surely be a mistake to characterize that as "baby-selling." Nevertheless, the line between selling babies and selling embryos is not sharp and distinct. Elias and Annas argue that "the problem with commerce in human embryos is that the sale of human embryos can become confused with the sale of human children. Accordingly, it seems reasonable to outlaw the sale of human embryos." Laws have been enacted in Florida, Louisiana, and Massachusetts banning the sale of embryos. John Robertson contends that the terms of these laws would not cover the sale of unfertilized eggs. Although Elias and Annas say that sale of sperm and ova does not present the same problem as the sale of human embryos, their remark quoted earlier suggests that they disapprove of commercial traffic in gametes.

Similarly, the Glover Report evinces a strong preference for a noncommercial ethos both for semen donation and for egg donation, but stops short of proposing a legal ban, "which would anyway probably be unenforceable." The report urges strong public campaigns for altruistic donation, "bringing the plight of the infertile to the front of public attention."

We are still left with the question whether paying egg donors constitutes an ethically suspect or unacceptable commercial traffic in human products. It is merely different from commercial traffic in organs, primarily because of the greater risks organ donors face from surgery and anesthesia as well as (in the case of kidney donors) their heightened risk of living with one rather than two kidneys. It is more like payment for blood, another bodily product, although blood donation requires less time and fewer risks and discomforts than egg retrieval.

Yet even the sale of blood, like other human bodily materials, is a form of commodification. The Glover Report offers arguments that weigh equally against payment to blood donors and to gamete donors. One is that payment is likely to incline donors to think less about the implications of what they are doing. A second is that payment "deprives donors of the chance of doing something purely for others." Citing the remark of some blood donors that "paying for blood would debase the value of the act," the Glover Report observes that payment and nonpayment seem to lead to two different conceptions of donation.

The reasons the Glover Report gives for favoring a noncommercial approach to semen donations rest on values quite different from those of a market economy. The idea that gamete donors should think about the implications of what they are doing, and that altruism is a good thing, are sound premises in an argument that questions payment but are not likely to move those who see nothing amiss in making everything subject to market forces.

A point made by John Harris is illustrative in this connection: "In the case of gamete donation, if it is acceptable to make voluntary donation of such things, then the addition of a financial interest does not necessarily add anything to the *morality* of the practice."

Although it seems correct to say that commodification does not violate any ethical principle, it can nevertheless be viewed as an unsavory feature of our society, a society in which almost everything is subject to market forces. Commodification is unsavory for the same sort of reason that public executions and public humiliation of criminals are unsavory. This is not an aesthetic judgment. It is a judgment about what kind of society we value.

THE FABRIC OF SOCIETY

Even if it can be convincingly argued that neither respect for person nor justice is violated, it can still be maintained that the practice of paying for reproductive services is somehow demeaning or degrading to us as a society, that it ruptures the very fabric of society. Although the fabric of society is a hard concept to define, and although it is difficult to determine empirically just when the fabric is being torn and when it remains intact, it is a useful concept for thinking about what is undesirable about certain sorts of human interactions and societal practices. A practice in which women are paid to ingest hormones and to have their eggs extracted may not contravene an ethical principle or violate anyone's rights. Still, it reflects the extent to which our society is willing to accept the idea that if people are prepared to receive money to have their bodies invaded, it is just like any other commercial transaction.

Margaret Jane Radin provides an analysis in terms of our conception of personhood and human flourishing: "In our understanding of personhood we are committed to an ideal of individual uniqueness that does not cohere with the idea that each person's attributes are fungible, that they have a monetary equivalent, and that they can be traded off against those of other people."[14] Radin argues that if market rhetoric were adopted by everyone in many contexts, it would transform "the texture of the modern world." That texture is another way of referring to the elusive concept of the fabric of society. Market rhetoric leads us to view "reproductive capacity as just a scarce good for which there is high demand." This way of talking and thinking fosters "an inferior conception of human flourishing." As an example of the "intuitive grasp of the injury to personhood involved in commodification of human beings," Radin cites baby selling and slavery. Her lengthy analysis of "market-inalienabilty" (not to be bought and sold on the market) and the wrongs involved in commodification of human beings cannot be replicated here, but it is sufficient to note that not everyone is likely to buy into her analysis.

Suppose one does not accept Radin's analysis and sees nothing wrong, in principle, with commodification. Is it acceptable to conclude, then, that the best public policy is simply to abandon any attempt to regulate the amount of money paid to egg donors? In that case, market forces would truly govern the practice, and clinics that perform the services would become truly competitive in this regard (if they are not already). Inevitably, this would raise the cost of the procedure to egg recipients, since the money to pay the donors will have to come from somewhere and it is unlikely to come out of the clinic's profit margin. Furthermore, we must recall the objection to unrestricted payment noted by the Canadian Combined Ethics Committee. The "harm principle" calls for protection of gamete recipients from transmission of infection or genetic disease by donors who are induced by excessive payments to lie about their medical or genetic history.

Those who argue for unrestricted payments to donors and letting the market govern egg donation have to face the question of consistency. Can an argument for prohibiting a commercial market in organs be consistent with an unregulated approach to commercial egg donation? Why not allow payment to kidney donors for their "risks, time, and inconvenience" and deny that payment is for the organ itself? If paying living persons for donation of one of their paired organs, or even for bone marrow, is ethically unacceptable but paying egg donors is ethically acceptable, wherein lies the difference?

One reply is that the difference lies in the degree of risk to the donor. The problem becomes one of drawing the line, with the need to specify where that line is and why it is appropriate to draw it there. If the reply is that blood and sperm are renewable resources, then we must contend with the fact that so, too, is bone marrow. Kidneys can certainly not be regenerated by the human body, but then neither can a woman's eggs. However, ova are plentiful and exist in much greater supply than any one woman could ever use. The same cannot be said of kidney, since a donor's remaining kidney might be damaged in an accident. Is that the grounds for a public policy that prohibits selling human kidneys but can permit selling human eggs?

There is little doubt that most people feel a repugnance at the idea of allowing commercial traffic in human organs. Repugnance is a moral emotion, and if moral emotions are ever a guide to reasoned ethical judgment,[15] this is a good case in point. It may well be the case that people who are opposed to paying egg donors experience a similar, albeit weaker, moral emotion. We are left with the puzzlement of whether the strength of a moral emotion provides a justifiable ground for drawing ethical lines governing matters of public policy.

CONSEQUENTIALISM: PROHIBITING VERSUS PERMITTING PAYMENT

With so many other concepts brought into play—exploitation, commodification, respect for persons, altruism, and justice—it is easy to overlook a fundamental approach to ethics and public policy. That approach calls for an assessment of the consequences of alternative courses of action, in this case prohibiting versus permitting payment to egg donors.

The leading consequentialist argument is that if women are not paid to donate eggs, who would do it? The source of eggs for donation would disappear, and fewer infertile women could then be assisted in this way. How great a loss this would be depends on one's assessment of the social and personal importance of enabling couples to have children who are biologically related to at least one parent, or of a woman's undergoing the experience of pregnancy and childbirth.

Recall that the Canadian Combined Ethics Committee rejected the option of permitting no payment to gamete donors on grounds that altruism would not encourage sufficient donors "to meet the need unless these individuals *at least* received fair compensation for their costs in terms of time and inconvenience." John Robertson uses the same justification, contending that "the ethical objection to payment must be balanced against the need to pay women to assure an egg supply for needy recipients. . . ." Indeed, Robertson goes further in surmising that moral objections to payment would not constitute "the compelling need necessary to justify interference with the reproductive freedom of infertile couples." "Moralistic" or symbolic reasons for prohibiting payment could not count as sufficient justification for interfering with a fundamental right, that is, the infertile couple's right to form families noncoitally.

One likely consequence of legally prohibiting payments to egg donors is to drive the practice underground. Private arrangements or transactions "off the books" might flourish, thereby making the practice more difficult to monitor or regulate. A system that could lead to a black market in human ova would create more ethical problems than one like the current practice of permitting payment to donors for their "time, risk, inconvenience, and discomfort."

It is hard to predict whether the consequences of prohibiting payment would be to encourage an underground economy in sale of gametes, to deny procreative rights to infertile couples, or to perpetuate the existing imbalance between poorer women as donors and wealthier women as recipients. One consequence of allowing payment is to increase the available options to poorer women, enabling them to earn money by a method that is no more degrading than alternative means they might choose.

Regulation, rather than prohibition, would likely lead to the best overall consequences. Regulatory measures should include at least three key elements. First, adequate screening safeguards need to be established to ensure that paying egg donors does not compromise the quality of the product, as has occurred in the case of paid blood donors. Second, an upper limit should be set on the amount of payment to guard against the possibility of exploitation. And third, women who agree to be donors must be paid for their time, risk, inconvenience, and discomfort regardless of whether eggs are successfully retrieved and regardless of the number of eggs obtained.

If, in the end, the consequences of prohibiting payment to egg donors would cause more damage to the fabric of society than allowing such payments, then as unsavory as commodification may be it remains the lesser of two evils. As an ethical conclusion, this is unsatisfying. It does not endorse payment to oocyte donors as a good thing. Nor does it dismiss the ethical concerns about degrading women, commodifying the human body, or perpetuating the unjust distribution whereby poorer women provide the eggs and wealthier women receive them. Opting for the "least worst" solution is the only sound way to resolve ethical debates about policy when reasonable people disagree. Regulation of the practice of paid egg donation is a reasonable middle ground between free-market commercialization and outright prohibition of payment.

CONCLUSION

The debate over the ethics of paying egg donors comes down to a disagreement over commodification. Some, like Radin, hold that treating reproduction capacity as just another market force leads to "an inferior conception of human flourishing" and is damaging to the texture of the modern world. Others, like Robertson, view these reasons for prohibiting payment as "moralistic" or symbolic'" and therefore find it appropriate to pay women "to assure an egg supply for needy recipients." The most serious ethical objections to paying egg donors are those that rest on the prospect of exploitation. Yet the facts relating to the relative wealth of egg donors and recipients do not support the contention that payment to donors is a form of exploitation of poor women by the rich.

Considerations of justice may still apply, however. Even though individual women may not be exploited in receiving payment for their oocytes, the class of women who are donors is, in general, less well-off financially than the class of women who receive the eggs. But, it is argued, this disparity is no different from that which obtains in a wide variety of other situations in a market-driven society. So we are left with the question of whether the values of market-driven societies should permeate every aspect of those societies, the debate over commodification. It is hard to find fault with the point made by Harris, noted above: ". . . if it is acceptable to make voluntary donations of [gametes], then the addition of a financial interest does not necessarily add anything to the morality of the practice."

My conclusion is that although commodification is not immoral, it is nonetheless "unsavory." This category of disvalue does not involve a violation of ethical principles; yet it rests on the conviction that not every human exchange ought to be subject to market forces. Although unsavoriness is not a full-blooded moral category, it serves to remind us that there are degrees of ethical value and that reasonable people disagree about the ethical acceptability of practices that fall in the middle of a continuum ranging from evil incarnate, at one end, to supreme moral virtue, at the other.

NOTES

1. Quoted in Machelle M. Seibel and Ann Kiessling, "Compensating Egg Donors: Equal Pay for Equal Time?" (letter), *New England Journal of Medicine,* 328 (1993):737.
2. Johanna Riegler and Aurelia Weikert, "Product Egg: Egg Selling in an Austrian IVF Clinic," *Reproductive and Genetic Engineering* 1 (1988):222.
3. A Report of the Combined Ethics Committee of the Canadian Fertility and Andrology Society and The Society of Obstetricians and Gynaecologists of Canada, "Ethical Considerations of the new Reproductive Technologies" (September 1990), p. 41.
4. Sherman Elias and George J. Annas, *Reproductive Genetics and the Law* (Chicago: Year Book Medical Publishers, 1987), p. 240.
5. John A. Robertson, "Technology and Motherhood: Legal and Ethical Issues in Human Egg Donation," *Case Western Reserve Law Review* 39 (1988–89):31.
6. Jonathan Glover and others, *The Glover Report to the European Commission* (DeKalb Northern Illinois University Press, 1989).
7. See John Harris, *Wonderwoman and Superman* (Oxford: Oxford University Press, 1992), p. 121, and Harris's citations of Feinberg and the Warnock Report.
8. These comments were made during discussion of an earlier draft of this paper by John Hoff, a member of NABER.
9. Michael Walzer, *Spheres of Justice* (New York: Basic Books, 1983).
10. Richard J. Arneson, "Commodification and Commercial Surrogacy," *Philosophy & Public Affairs* 21 (1992):133.
11. See generally, Margaret Jane Radin, "Market-Inalienability," *Harvard Law Review* 100 (1987): 1849–1937.
12. See Leon R. Kass, "'Making Babies' Revisited," *The Public Interest* 54 (1979):32–60.
13. National Organ Transplant Act of 1984, 42 U.S.C. Para. 274(e) (1982).
14. Radin, "Market-Inalienability," p. 177. Pages cited here are from an excerpt of Radin's original article, published in Kenneth D. Alpern (ed.), *The Ethics of Reproductive Technology* (New York: Oxford University Press, 1992).
15. See Sidney Callahan, *In Good Conscience: Reason and Emotion in Moral Decision Making* (New York: Harper Collins, 1991).

SELLING BABIES AND SELLING BODIES

Sara Ann Ketchum

The "Baby M" case has turned into something approaching a national soap opera, played out in newspapers and magazines. The drama surrounding the case tends to obscure the fact that the case raises some very abstract philosophical and moral issues. It forces us to examine questions about the nature and meaning of parenthood, of the limits of reproductive autonomy, of how the facts of pregnancy should affect our analysis of sexual equality, and of what counts as selling people and of what forms (if any) of selling people we should honor in law and what forms we should restrict. It is this last set of questions whose relevance I will be discussing here. One objection to what is usually called "surrogate motherhood" and which I will call "contracted motherhood" (CM) or "baby contracts" is that it commercializes reproduction and turns human beings (the mother and/or the baby) into objects of sale. If this is a compelling objection, there is a good argument for prohibiting (and/or not enforcing contracts for) commercial CM. Such a prohibition would be similar to laws on black market adoptions and would have two parts, at least: 1) a prohibition of commercial companies who make the arrangements and/or 2) a prohibition on the transfer of money to the birth mother for the transfer of custody (beyond expenses incurred) (Warnock 1985, 46–7). I will also argue that CM law should follow adoption law in making clear that pre-birth agreements to relinquish parental rights are not binding and will not be enforced by the courts (the birth mother should not be forced to give up her child for adoption).

Reprinted with permission from *Hypatia* vol. 4, no. 3 (Fall 1989).

Editor's note: All footnotes have been deleted. Students who want to follow up on sources should consult the original article.

CM AND AID: THE REAL DIFFERENCE PROBLEM

CM is usually presented as a new reproductive technology and, moreover, as the female equivalent of AID (artificial insemination by donor) and, therefore, as an extension of the right to privacy or the right to make medical decisions about one's own life. There are two problems with this description: 1) CM uses the same technology as AID—the biological arrangements are exactly the same—but intends an opposite assignment of custody. 2) No technology is necessary for CM as is evidenced by the biblical story of Abraham and Sarah who used a "handmaid" as a birth mother. Since artificial insemination is virtually uncontroversial it seems clear that what makes CM controversial is not the technology, but the social arrangements—that is, the custody assignment. CM has been defended on the ground that such arrangements enable fertile men who are married to infertile women to reproduce and, thus, are parallel to AID which enables fertile women whose husbands are infertile to have children. It is difficult not to regard these arguments as somewhat disingenuous. The role of the sperm donor and the role of the egg donor/mother are distinguished by pregnancy, and pregnancy is, if anything is, a "real difference" which would justify us in treating women and men differently. To treat donating sperm as equivalent to biological motherhood would be as unfair as treating the unwed father who has not contributed to his children's welfare the same as the father who has devoted his time to taking care of them. At most, donating sperm is comparable to donating ova; however, even that comparison fails because donating ova is a medically risky procedure, donating sperm is not.

Therefore, the essential morally controversial features of CM have to do with its nature as a social and economic institution and its assignment of family relationships rather than with any technological features. Moreover, the institution of CM requires of contracting birth mothers much more time commitment, medical risk, and social disruption than AID does of sperm donors. It also requires substantial male control over women's bodies and time, while AID neither requires nor provides any female control over men's bodies. Christine Overall (1987, 181–185) notes that when a women seeks AID, she not only does not usually have a choice of donor, but she also may be required to get her husband's consent if she is married. The position of the man seeking CM is the opposite; he chooses a birth mother and his wife does not have to consent to the procedure (although the mother's husband does). The contract entered into by Mary Beth Whitehead and William Stern contains a number of provisions regulating her behavior, including: extensive medical examinations, an agreement about when she may or may not abort, an agreement to follow doctors' orders, and agreements not to take even prescription drugs without the doctor's permission. Some of these social and contractual provisions are eliminable. But the fact that CM requires a contract and AID does not reflects the differences between pregnancy and ejaculation. If the sperm donor wants a healthy child (a good product), he needs to control the woman's behavior. In contrast, any damage the sperm-donor's behavior will have on the child will be present in the sperm and could, in principle, be tested for before the woman enters to AID procedure. There is no serious moral problem with discarding defective sperm; discarding defective children is a quite different matter.

COMMODIFICATION

There are three general categories of moral concern with commercializing either adoption (baby selling) or reproductive activities. The three kinds of argument are not always separated and they are not entirely separable:

1) There is the Kantian argument, based on a version of the Second Formulation of the Categorical Imperative. On this argument, selling people is objectionable because it is treating them as means rather than as ends, as objects rather than as persons. People who can be bought and sold are being treated as being of less moral significance than are those who buy and sell. Allowing babies to be bought and sold adds an extra legal wedge between the status of children and that of adults, and allowing women's bodies to be bought and sold (or "rented" if you prefer) adds to the inequality between men and women. Moreover, making babies and women's bodies available for sale raises specters of the rich "harvesting" the babies of the poor. 2) Consequentialist objections are fueled by concern for what may happen to the children and women who are bought and sold, to their families, and to the society as a whole if we allow an area of this magnitude and traditional intimacy to become commercialized. 3) Connected to both 1 and 2, are concerns about protecting the birth mother and the mother-child relationship from the potential coerciveness of commercial transactions. These arguments apply slightly differently depending on whether we analyze the contracts as baby contracts (selling babies) or as mother contracts (as a sale of women's bodies) although many of the arguments will be very similar for both.

Selling Babies The most straightforward argument for prohibiting baby-selling is that it is selling a human being and that any selling of a human being should be prohibited because it devalues human life and human individuals. This argument gains moral force from its analogy with slavery. Defenders of baby contracts argue that baby selling is unlike selling slaves in that it is a transfer of parental rights rather than of ownership of the child—the adoptive parents cannot turn around and sell the baby to another couple for profit (Landes and Posner 1978, 344). What the defenders of CM fail to do is provide an account of the wrongness of slavery such that baby-selling (or baby contracts) do not fall under the argument. Landes and Posner, in particular, would, I think, have difficulty establishing an argument against slavery because they are relying on utilitarian arguments. Since one of the classic difficulties with utilitarianism is that it cannot yield an argument that slavery is wrong in principle, it is hardly surprising that utilitarians will find it difficult to discover within that theory an argument against selling babies. Moreover, their economic argument is not even utilitarian because it only counts people's interest to the extent that they can pay for them.

Those who, unlike Landes and Posner, defend CM while supporting laws against baby-selling, distinguish CM from paid adoptions in that in CM the person to whom custody is being transferred is the biological (genetic) father. This suggests a parallel to custody disputes, which are not obviously any more appropriately ruled by money than is adoption. We could argue against the commercialization of either on the grounds that child-regarding concerns should decide child custody and that using market criteria or contract considerations would violate that principle by substituting another, unrelated, and possibly conflicting, one. In particular, both market and contract are about relations between the adults involved rather than about the children or about the relationship between the child and the adult.

Another disanalogy cited between preadoption contracts and CM is that, in preadoption contracts the baby is already there (that is, the preadoption contract is offered to a woman who is already pregnant, and, presumably, planning to have the child), while the mother contract is a contract to create a child who does not yet exist, even as an embryo. If our concern is the commodificaiton of children, this strikes me as an odd point for the defenders of CM to emphasize. Producing a child to order for money is a paradigm case of commodifying children. The fact that the child is not being put up for sale to the highest bidder, but is only for sale to the genetic father, may reduce some of the harmful effects of an open market in babies but does not quiet concerns about personhood.

Arguments for allowing CM are remarkably similar to the arguments for legalizing black-market adoption in the way they both define the problem. CM, like a market for babies, is seen as increasing the satisfaction and freedom of infertile individuals or couples by increasing the quantity of the desired product (there will be more babies available for adoption) and the quality of the product (not only more white healthy babies, but white healthy babies who are genetically related to one of the purchasers). These arguments tend to be based on the interest of infertile couples and obscure the relevance of the interests of the birth mothers (who will be giving the children up for adoption) and their families, the children who are produced by the demands of the market, and (the most invisible and most troubling group) needy children who are without homes because they are not "high-quality" products and because we are not, as a society, investing the time and money needed to place the hard to adopt children. If we bring these hidden interests to the fore, they raise a host of issues about consequences—both utilitarian issues and issues about the distribution of harms and benefits.

Perhaps the strongest deontological argument against baby selling is an objection to the characterization of the mother-child relationship (and, more generally, of the adult-child relationship) that it presupposes. Not only does the baby become an object of commerce, but the custody relationship of the parent becomes a property relationship. If we see parental custody rights as correlates of parental responsibility or as a right to maintain a relationship, it will be less tempting to think of them as something one can sell. We have good reasons for allowing birth-mothers to relinquish their children because otherwise we would be forcing children into the care of people who either do not want them or feel themselves unable to care for them. However, the fact that custody may be waived in this way does not entail that it may be sold or transferred. If children are not property, they cannot be gifts either. If a mother's right is a right to maintain a relationship, (see Ketchum 1987) it is implausible to treat it as transferable; having the option of terminating a relationship with A does not entail having the option of deciding who A will relate to next—the right to a divorce does not entail the right to transfer one's connection to one's spouse to someone else. Indeed, normally, the termination of a relationship with A ends any right I have to make moral claims on A's relationships. Although in giving up responsibilities I may have a responsibility to see to it that someone will shoulder them when I go, I do not have a right to choose that person.

Selling Women's Bodies Suppose we do regard mother contracts as contracts for the sale or rental of reproductive capacities. Is there good reason for including reproductive capacities among those things or activities that ought not to be bought and sold? We might distinguish between selling reproductive capacities and selling work on a number of grounds. A conservative might argue against commercializing reproduction on the grounds that it disturbs family relationships, or on the grounds that there are some categories of human activities that should not be for sale. A Kantian might argue that there are some activities that are close to our personhood and that a commercial traffic in these activities constitutes treating the person as less than an end (or less than a person).

One interpretation of the laws prohibiting baby selling is that they are an attempt to reduce or eliminate coercion in the adoption process, and are thus based on a concern for the birth mother rather than (or as well as) the child. All commercial transactions are at least potentially coercive in that the parties to them are likely to come from unequal bargaining positions and in that, whatever we have a market in, there will be some people who will be in a position such that they have to sell it in order to survive. Such concerns are important to arguments against an open market in human organs or in the sexual use of people's bodies as well as arguments against baby contracts of either kind.

As Margaret Radin suggests (1987, 1915–1921), the weakness of arguments of this sort—that relationships or contracts are exploitative on the grounds that people are forced into them by poverty—is that the real problem is not in the possibility of commercial transactions, but in the situation that makes these arrangements attractive by comparison. We do not end the feminization of poverty by forbidding prostitution or CM. Indeed, if we are successful in eliminating these practices, we may be reducing the income of some women (by removing ways of making money) and, if we are unsuccessful, we are removing these people from state protection by making their activities illegal. Labor legislation which is comparably motivated by concern for unequal bargaining position (such as, for example, minimum wage and maximum hours laws, and health and safety regulations) regulates rather than prevents that activity and is thus less vulnerable to this charge. Radin's criticism shows that the argument from the coerciveness of poverty is insufficient as a support for laws rejecting commercial transactions in personal services. This does not show that the concern is irrelevant. The argument from coercion is still an appropriate response to simple voluntarist arguments—those that assume that these activities are purely and freely chosen by all those who participate in them. Given the coerciveness of the situation, we cannot assume that the presumed or formal voluntariness of the contract makes it nonexploitative.

If the relationship of CM is, by its nature, disrespectful of personhood, it can be exploitative despite short-term financial benefits to some women. The disrespect for women as persons that is fundamental to the relationship lies in the concept of the woman's body (and of the child and mother-child relationship) implicit in the contract. I have argued elsewhere (1984), that claiming a welfare right to another person's body is to treat that person as an object:

> An identity or intimate relation between persons and their bodies may or may not be essential to our metaphysical understanding of a person, but it is essential to a minimal moral conceptual scheme. Without a concession to persons' legitimate interests and concerns for their physical selves, most of our standard and paradigm moral rules would not make sense; murder might become the mere destruction of the body; assault, a mere interference with the body . . . and so on. We cannot make sense out of the concept of assault unless an assault on S's body is ipso facto an assault on S. By the same token, treating another person's body as part of my domain—as among the things that I have a rightful claim to—is, if anything is, a denial that there is a person there. (1984, 34–35)

This argument is, in turn, built on the analysis of the wrongness of rape developed by Marilyn Frye and Carolyn Shafer in "Rape and Respect" (1977):

> The use of a person in the advancement of interest contrary to its own is a limiting case of disrespect. It reveals the perception of the person simply as an object which can serve some purpose, a tool or a bit of material, and one which furthermore is dispensable or replaceable and thus of little value even as an object with a function. (341)

We can extend this argument to the sale of persons. To make a person or a person's body an object of commerce is to treat the person as part of another person's domain, particularly if the sale of A to B gives B rights to A or to A's body. What is objectionable is a claim—whether based on welfare or on contract—to a right to another person such that that person is part of my domain. The assertion of such a right is morally objectionable even without the use of force. For example, a man who claims to have a *right* to sexual intercourse with his wife, on the grounds of the marriage relationship, betrays a conception of her body, and thus her person, as being properly within his domain, and thus a conception of her as an object rather than a person.

Susan Brownmiller, in *Against Our Will* (1975) suggests that prostitution is connected to rape in that prostitution makes women's bodies into consumer goods that might—if not justifiably, at least understandably—be forcibly taken by those men who see themselves as unjustly deprived.

> When young men learn that females may be bought for a price, and that acts of sex command set prices, then how should they not also conclude that that which may be bought may also be taken without the civility of a monetary exchange? . . . legalized prostitution institutionalizes the concept that it is a man's monetary right, if not his divine right, to gain access to the female body, and that sex is a female service that should not be denied the civilized male. (391, 392)

The same can be said for legalized sale of women's reproductive services. The more hegemonic this commodification of women's bodies is, the more the woman's lack of consent to sex or to having children can present itself as unfair to the man because it is arbitrary.

A market in women's bodies—whether sexual prostitution or reproductive prostitution—reveals a social ontology in which women are among the things in the world that can be appropriately commodified—bought and sold and, by extension, stolen. The purported freedom that such institutions would give women to enter into the market by selling their bodies is paradoxical. Sexual or reproductive prostitutes enter the market not so much as *agents* or subjects, but as commodities or objects. This is evidenced by the fact that the pimps and their counterparts, the arrangers of baby contracts make the bulk of the profits. Moreover, once there is a market for women's bodies, all women's bodies will have a price, and the woman who does not sell her body becomes a hoarder of something that is useful to other people and is financially valuable. The market is a hegemonic institution; it determines the meanings of actions of people who choose not to participate as well as of those who choose to participate.

Contract The immediate objection to treating the Baby M case as a contract dispute is that the practical problem facing the court is a child custody problem and to treat it as a contract case is to deal with it on grounds other than the best interests of the child. That the best interests of the child count need not entail that contract does not count, although it helps explain one of the reasons we should be suspicious of this particular contract. There is still the question of whether the best interests of the child will trump contract considerations (making the contract nonbinding) or merely enter into a balancing argument in which contract is one of the issues to be balanced. However, allowing contract to count at all raises some of the same Kantian objections as the commodification problem. As a legal issue, the contract problem is more acute because the state action (enforcing the contract) is more explicit.

Any binding mother contract will put the state in the position of enforcing the rights of a man to a women's body or to his genetic offspring. But this is to treat the child or the mother's body as objects of the sperm donor's rights, which, I argued above, is inconsistent with treating them as persons. This will be clearest if the courts enforce specific performance and require the mother to go through with the pregnancy (or to abort) if she chooses not to or requires the transfer of custody to the contracting sperm-donor on grounds other than the best interests of the child. In those cases, I find it hard to avoid the description that what is being awarded is a person and what is being affirmed is a right to a person. I think the Kantian argument still applies if the court refuses specific performance but awards damages. Damages compensate for the loss of something to which one has a right. A judge who awards damages to the contracting sperm donor for having been deprived of use of the contracting woman's reproductive capacities or for being deprived of custody of the child gives legal weight to the idea that the contracting sperm donor had a legally enforceable right to them (or, to put it more bluntly, to those commodities or goods).

The free contract argument assumes that Mary Beth Whitehead's claims to her daughter are rights (rather than, for example, obligations or a more complex relationship), and, moreover, that they are alienable, as are property rights. If the baby is not something she has an alienable right to, then custody of the baby is not something she can transfer by contract. In cases where the state is taking children away from their biological parents and in custody disputes, we do not want to appeal to some rights of the parents. However, I think it would be unfortunate to regard these rights as rights to the child, because that would be to treat the child as the object of the parent's rights and violate the principles that persons and persons' bodies cannot be the objects of other people's rights. The parents' rights in these cases should be to consideration, to non-arbitratiness and to respect for the relationship between the parent and the child.

CONCLUDING REMARKS

The Kantian, person-respecting arguments I have been offering do not provide an account of all of the moral issues surrounding CM. However, I think that they can serve as a counter-balance to arguments (also Kantian) for CM as an expression of personal autonomy. They might also add some weight to the empirical arguments against CM that are accumulating. There is increasing concern that women cannot predict in advance whether or not they and their family will form an attachment to the child they will bear nor can they promise not to develop such feelings (as some on the contracts ask them to do). There is also increasing concern for the birth-family and for the children produced by the arrangement (particularly where there is a custody dispute). A utilitarian might respond that the problems are outweighed by the joys of the adopting/sperm donor families, but, if so, we must ask: are we simply shifting the misery from wealthy (or wealthier) infertile couples to poorer fertile families and to the "imperfect" children waiting for adoption?

These considerations provide good reason for prohibiting commercialization of CM. In order to do that we could adopt new laws prohibiting the transfer of money in such arrangements or simply extend existing adoption laws, making the contracts non-binding as are pre-birth adoption contracts (Cohen 1984, 280–284) and limiting the money that can be transferred. There are some conceptual problems remaining about what would count as prohibiting commodification. I find the English approach very attractive. This approach has the following elements 1) it strictly prohibits third parties from arranging mother contracts; 2) if people arrange them privately, they are allowed, 3) the contracts are not binding. If the birth-mother decides to keep the baby, her decision is final (*and* the father may be required to pay child-support; that may be too much for Americans). 4) Although, in theory, CM is covered by limitations on money for adoption, courts have approved payments for contracted motherhood, and there is never criminal penalty on the parents for money payments.

REFERENCES

Brownmiller, Susan. 1975. *Against our will: Men, women, and rape*. New York: Simon and Schuster.

Cohen, Barbara. 1984. Surrogate mothers: Whose baby is it? *American Journal of Law and Medicine* 10: 243–285.

Frye, Marilyn and Carolyn Shafer. 1977. Rape and respect. In *Feminism and philosophy*. Mary Vetterling-Braggin, Frederick A. Elliston and Jane English, eds. Totowa, N.J.: Littlefield, Adams and Co.

Ketchum, Sara Ann. 1987. New reproductive technologies and the definition of parenthood: A feminist perspective. Presented at Feminism and legal theory: Women and intimacy, a conference sponsored by the Institute for Legal Studies at the University of Wisconsin-Madison.

Landes, Elizabeth A. and Richard M. Posner. 1978. The economics of the baby shortage. *Journal of Legal Studies* 7.

Overall, Christine. 1987. *Ethics and human reproduction*. Boston: Allen & Unwin.

Radin, Margaret. 1987. Market-Inalienability. *Harvard Law Review* 100: 1849–1937.

Warnock, Mary. 1985. *A question of life: The Warnock report on human fertilization and embryology*. Oxford: Basil Blackwell.

HUMAN CLONING AND STEM CELL RESEARCH

CLONING HUMAN BEINGS: AN ASSESSMENT OF THE ETHICAL ISSUES PRO AND CON

Dan W. Brock

INTRODUCTION

The world of science and the public at large were both shocked and fascinated by the announcement in the journal *Nature* by Ian Wilmut and his colleagues that they had successfully cloned a sheep from a single cell of an adult sheep. Scientists were in part surprised because many had believed that after the very early stage of embryo development at which differentiation of cell function begins to take place it would not be possible to achieve cloning of an adult mammal by nuclear transfer. In this process the nucleus from the cell of an adult mammal is inserted into an enucleated ovum, and the resulting embryo develops following the complete genetic code of the mammal from which the inserted nucleus was obtained. But some scientists and much of the public were troubled or apparently even horrified at the prospect that if adult mammals such as sheep could be cloned, then cloning of adult humans by the same process would likely be possible as well. Of course, the process is far from perfected even with sheep—it took 276 failures by Wilmut and his colleagues to produce Dolly, their one success, and whether the process can be successfully replicated in other mammals, much less in humans, is not now known. But those who were horrified at the prospect of human cloning were not assuaged by the fact that the science with humans is not yet there, for it looked to them now perilously close.

The response of most scientific and political leaders to the prospect of human cloning, indeed of

---

Reprinted with permission from *Cloning Human Beings: Report and Recommendations of the National Bioethics Advisory Commission*, Rockville, MD, 1997.

Editors' note: This article has been edited and most of the notes omitted. Readers who wish to follow up on sources should consult the original.

Dr. Wilmut as well, was of immediate and strong condemnation. In the United States President Clinton immediately banned federal financing of human cloning research and asked privately funded scientists to halt such work until the newly formed National Bioethics Advisory Commission could review the "troubling" ethical and legal implications. The Director-General of the World Health Organization characterized human cloning as "ethically unacceptable as it would violate some of the basic principles which govern medically assisted reproduction. These include respect for the dignity of the human being and the protection of the security of human genetic material." Around the world similar immediate condemnation was heard as human cloning was called a violation of human rights and human dignity. Even before Wilmut's announcement, human cloning had been made illegal in nearly all countries in Europe and had been condemned by the Council of Europe.

A few more cautious voices were heard both suggesting some possible benefits from the use of human cloning in limited circumstances and questioning its too quick prohibition, but they were a clear minority. In the popular media, nightmare scenarios of laboratory mistakes resulting in monsters, the cloning of armies of Hitlers, the exploitative use of cloning for totalitarian ends as in Huxley's *Brave New World*, and the murderous replicas of the film *Blade Runner*, all fed the public controversy and uneasiness. A striking feature of these early responses was that their strength and intensity seemed far to outrun the arguments and reasons offered in support of them—they seemed often to be "gut level" emotional reactions rather than considered reflections on the issues. Such reactions should not be simply dismissed, both because they may point us to important considerations otherwise missed and not easily articulated, and because they often have a major impact on public policy. But the formation of public policy should not ignore the moral reasons and arguments that bear on the practice of human cloning—these must be articulated in order to understand and inform people's more immediate emotional responses. This paper is an effort to articulate, and to evaluate critically, the main moral considerations and arguments for and against human cloning. Though many people's religious beliefs inform their views on human cloning, and it is often difficult to separate religious from secular positions, I shall restrict myself to arguments and reasons that can be given a clear secular formulation and will ignore explicitly religious positions and arguments pro or con. I shall also be concerned principally with cloning by nuclear transfer, which permits cloning of an adult, not cloning by embryo splitting, although some of the issues apply to both.

I begin by noting that on each side of the issue there are two distinct kinds of moral arguments brought forward. On the one hand, some opponents claim that human cloning would violate fundamental moral or human rights; while some proponents argue that its prohibition would violate such rights. On the other hand, both opponents and proponents also cite the likely harms and benefits, both to individuals and to society, of the practice. While moral and even human rights need not be understood as absolute, that is, as morally requiring people to respect them no matter how great the costs or bad consequences of doing so, they do place moral restrictions on permissible actions that an appeal to a mere balance of benefits over harms cannot justify overriding. For example, the rights of human subjects in research must be respected even if the result is that some potentially beneficial research is more difficult or cannot be done, and the right of free expression prohibits the silencing of unpopular or even abhorrent views; in Ronald Dworkin's striking formulation, rights trump utility (Dworkin 1978). I shall take up both the moral rights implicated in human cloning, as well as its more likely significant benefits and harms, because none of the rights as applied to human cloning is sufficiently uncontroversial and strong to settle decisively the morality of the practice one way or the other. But because of their strong moral force, the assessment of the moral rights putatively at stake is especially important. A further complexity here is that it is sometimes controversial whether a particular consideration is merely a matter of benefits and harms, or is instead a matter of moral or human rights. I shall begin with the arguments in support of permitting human cloning, although with no implication that it is the stronger or weaker position.

MORAL ARGUMENTS IN SUPPORT OF HUMAN CLONING

A. Is There a Moral Right to Use Human Cloning?

What moral right might protect at least some access to the use of human cloning? Some commentators have argued that a commitment to individual liberty, as defended by J.S. Mill, requires that individuals be left free to use human cloning if they so choose and if their doing so does not cause significant harms to others, but liberty is too broad in scope to be an uncontroversial moral right. Human cloning is a means of reproduction (in the most literal sense) and so the most plausible moral right at stake in its use is a right to reproductive freedom or procreative liberty. Reproductive freedom includes not only the familiar right to choose not to reproduce, for example, by means of contraception or abortion, but also the right to reproduce. The right to reproductive freedom is properly understood to include as well the use of various artificial reproductive technologies, such as in vitro fertilization (IVF), oocyte donation, and so forth. The reproductive right relevant to human cloning is a negative right, that is, a right to use assisted reproductive technologies without interference by the government or others when made available by a willing provider. The choice of an assisted means of reproduction, such as surrogacy, can be defended as included within reproductive freedom even when it is not the only means for individuals to reproduce, just as the choice among different means of preventing conception is protected by reproductive freedom. However, the case for permitting the use of a particular means of reproduction is strongest when that means is necessary for particular individuals to be able to procreate at all. Sometimes human cloning could be the only means for individuals to procreate while retaining a biological tie to the child created, but in other cases different means of procreating would also be possible.

It could be argued that human cloning is not covered by the right to reproductive freedom because whereas current assisted reproductive technologies and practices covered by that right are remedies for inabilities to reproduce sexually, human cloning is an entirely new means of reproduction; indeed, its critics see it as more a means of manufacturing humans than of reproduction. Human cloning is a different means of reproduction than sexual reproduction, but it is a means that can serve individuals' interest in reproducing. If it is not covered by the moral right to reproductive freedom, I believe that must be not because it is a new means of reproducing, but instead because it has other objectionable moral features, such as eroding human dignity or uniqueness; we shall evaluate these other ethical objections to it below.

When individuals have alternative means of procreating, human cloning typically would be chosen because it replicates a particular individual's genome. The reproductive interest in question then is not simply reproduction itself, but a more specific interest in choosing what kind of children to have. The right to reproductive freedom is usually understood to cover at least some choice about the kind of children one will have; for example, genetic testing of an embryo or fetus for genetic disease or abnormality, together with abortion of an affected embryo or fetus, is now used to avoid having a child with that disease or abnormality. Genetic testing of prospective parents before conception to determine the risk of transmitting a genetic disease is also intended to avoid having children with particular diseases. Prospective parents' moral interest in self-determination, which is one of the grounds of a moral right to reproductive freedom, includes the choice about whether to have a child with a condition that is likely to place severe burdens on them, and to cause severe burdens to the child itself.

The more a reproductive choice is not simply the determination of oneself and one's own life but the determination of the nature of another, as in the case of human cloning, the more moral weight the interests of that other person, that is, the cloned child, should have in decisions that determine its nature. But even then parents are typically taken properly to have substantial, but not unlimited, discretion in shaping the persons their children will become, for example, through education and other childrearing decisions. Even if not part of reproductive freedom, the right to raise one's children as one sees fit, within limits mostly determined by the interests of the children, is also a right to determine within limits what kinds of persons one's children will become. This right includes not just preventing certain diseases or harms to children, but selecting and shaping desirable features and traits in one's children. The use of human cloning is one way to exercise that right.

It is worth pointing out that current public and legal policy permits prospective parents to conceive, or to carry a conception to term, when there is a significant risk, or even certainty that the child will suffer from a serious genetic disease. Even when others think the risk or presence of genetic disease makes it morally wrong to conceive, or to carry a fetus to term, the parents' right to reproductive freedom permits them to do so. Most possible harms to a cloned child that I shall consider below are less serious than the genetic harms with which parents can now permit their offspring to be conceived or born.

I conclude that there is good reason to accept that a right to reproductive freedom presumptively includes both a right to select the means of reproduction, as well as a right to determine what kind of children to have, by use of human cloning. However, the particular reproductive interest of determining what kind of children to have is less weighty than other reproductive interests and choices whose impact falls more directly and exclusively on the parents rather than the child. Accepting a moral right to reproductive freedom that includes the use of human cloning does not settle the moral issue about human cloning, however, since there may be other moral rights in conflict with this right, or serious enough harms from human cloning to override the right to use it; this right can be thought of as establishing a serious moral presumption supporting access to human cloning. . . .

B. What Individual or Social Benefits Might Human Cloning Produce?

Largely Individual Benefits The literature on human cloning by nuclear transfer, as well as the literature on embryo splitting where it is relevant to the nuclear transfer case, contain a few examples of circumstances in which individuals might have good reasons to want to use human cloning. However, a survey of that literature strongly suggests that human cloning is not the unique answer to any great or pressing human need and that its benefits would at most be limited. What are the principal benefits of human cloning that might give persons good reasons to want to use it?

1. Human cloning would be a new means to relieve the infertility some persons now experience. Human cloning would allow women who have no ova or men who have no sperm to produce an offspring that is biologically related to them. Embryos might also be cloned, either by nuclear transfer or embryo splitting, in order to increase the number of embryos for implantation and improve the chances of successful conception. While the moral right to reproductive freedom creates a presumption that individuals should be free to choose the means of reproduction that best serves their interests and desires, the benefits from human cloning to relieve infertility are greater the more persons there are who cannot overcome their infertility by any other means acceptable to them. I do not know of data on this point, but they should be possible to obtain or gather from national associations concerned with infertility.

It is not enough to point to the large number of children throughout the world possibly available for adoption as a solution to infertility, unless we are prepared to discount as illegitimate the strong desire many persons, fertile and infertile, have for the experience of pregnancy and for having and raising a child biologically related to them. While not important to all infertile (or fertile) individuals, it is important to many and is respected and met through other forms of assisted reproduction that maintain a biological connection when that is possible; there seems no good reason to refuse to respect and respond to it when human cloning would be the best or only means of overcoming individuals' infertility.

2. Human cloning would enable couples in which one party risks transmitting a serious hereditary disease, a serious risk of disease, or an otherwise harmful condition to an offspring, to reproduce without doing so. Of course, by using donor sperm or egg donation, such hereditary risks can generally be avoided now without the use of human cloning. These procedures may be unacceptable to some couples, however, or at least considered less desirable than human cloning because they introduce a third party's genes into their reproduction, instead of giving their offspring only the genes of one of them. Thus, in some cases human cloning would be a means of preventing genetically transmitted harms to offspring. Here too, there are not data on the likely number of persons who would wish to use human cloning for this purpose instead of either using other available means of avoiding the risk of genetic transmission of the harmful condition or accepting the risk of transmitting the harmful condition.

3. Human cloning a later twin would enable a person to obtain needed organs or tissues for transplantation. Human cloning would solve the problem of finding a transplant donor who is an acceptable organ or tissue match and would eliminate, or drastically reduce, the risk of transplant rejection by the host. The availability of human cloning for this purpose would amount to a form of insurance policy to enable treatment of certain kinds of medical needs. Of course, sometimes the medical need would be too urgent to permit waiting for the cloning, gestation and development of the later twin necessary before tissues or organs for transplant could be obtained. In other cases, the need for an organ that the later twin would him- or herself need to maintain life, such as a heart or a liver, would preclude cloning and then taking the organ from the later twin.

Such a practice has been criticized on the ground that it treats the later twin not as a person valued and loved for his or her own sake, as an end in itself in Kantian terms, but simply as a means for benefiting another. This criticism assumes, however, that only this one motive would determine the relation of the person to his or her later twin. The well-known case some years ago in California of the Ayalas, who conceived in the hopes of obtaining a source for a bone marrow transplant for their teenage daughter suffering from leukemia illustrates the mistake in this assumption. They argued that whether or not the child they conceived turned out to be a possible donor for their daughter, they would value and love the child for itself, and treat it as they would treat any other member of their family. That one reason it was wanted was as a means to saving their daughter's life did not preclude its also being loved and valued for its own sake; in Kantian terms, it was treated as a possible means to saving their daughter, but not *solely as a means*, which is what the Kantian view proscribes.

Indeed, when people have children, whether by sexual means or with the aid of assisted reproductive technologies, their motives and reasons for doing so are typically many and complex, and include reasons less laudable than obtaining lifesaving medical treatment, such as having a companion like a doll to play with, enabling one to live on one's own, qualifying for public or government benefit programs, and so forth. While these other motives for having children sometimes may not bode well for the child's upbringing and future, public policy does not assess prospective parents motives and reasons for procreating as a condition of their doing so.

One commentator has proposed human cloning for obtaining even lifesaving organs. After cell differentiation some of the brain cells of the embryo or fetus would be removed so that it could then be grown as a brain dead body for spare parts for its earlier twin. This body clone would be like an anencephalic newborn or presentient fetus, neither of whom arguably can be harmed because of their lack of capacity for consciousness. Most people would likely find this practice appalling and immoral, in part because here the cloned later twin's capacity for conscious life is destroyed *solely as a means* for the benefit of another. Yet if one pushes what is already science fiction quite a bit further in the direction of science fantasy, and imagines the ability to clone and grow in an artificial environment only the particular lifesaving organ a person needed for transplantation, then it is far from clear that it would be morally impermissible to do so.

4. Human cloning would enable individuals to clone someone who had special meaning to them, such as a child who had died. There is no denying that if human cloning were available, some individuals would want to use it in order to clone someone who had special meaning to them, such as a child who had died, but that desire usually would be based on a deep confusion. Cloning such a child would not replace the child the parents had loved and lost, but rather would create a new different child with the same genes. The child they loved and lost was a unique individual who had been shaped by his or her environment and choices, not just his or her genes, and more importantly who had experienced a particular relationship with them. Even if the later cloned child could have not only the same genes but also be subjected to the same environment, which of course is in fact impossible, it would remain a different child than the one they had loved and lost because it would share a different history with them. Cloning the lost child might help the parents accept and move on from their loss, but another already existing sibling or another new child that was not a clone might do this equally well; indeed, it might do so better since the appearance of the cloned later twin would be a constant reminder of the child they had lost. Nevertheless, if human cloning enabled some individuals to clone a person who had special meaning to them and doing so gave them deep satisfaction, that would be a benefit to them even if their reasons for wanting to do so, and the satisfaction they in turn received, were based on a confusion.

Largely Social Benefits

5. Human cloning would enable the duplication of individuals of great talent, genius, character, or other exemplary qualities. The first four reasons for human cloning considered above all looked to benefits to specific individuals, usually parents, from being able to reproduce by means of human cloning. This reason looks to benefits to the broader society from being able to replicate extraordinary individuals—a Mozart, Einstein, Gandhi, or Schweitzer. Much of the appeal of this reason, like much thinking both in support of and in opposition to human cloning, rests on a confused and mistaken assumption of genetic determinism, that is, that one's genes fully determine what one will become, do, and accomplish. What made Mozart, Einstein, Gandhi, and Schweitzer the extraordinary individuals they were was the confluence of their particular genetic endowments with the environments in which they were raised and lived and the particular historical moments they in different ways seized. Cloning them would produce individuals with the same genetic inheritances (nuclear transfer does not even produce 100% genetic identity, although for the sake of exploring the moral issues I have followed the common assumption that it does), but neither by cloning, nor by any other means, would it be possible to replicate their environments or the historical contexts in which they lived and their greatness flourished. We do not know, either in general or with any particular individual, the degree or specific respects in which their greatness depended on their "nature" or their "nurture," but we do know in all cases that it depended on an interaction of them both. Thus, human cloning could never replicate the extraordinary accomplishments for which we admire individuals like Mozart, Einstein, Gandhi, and Schweitzer.

If we make a rough distinction between the extraordinary capabilities of a Mozart or an Einstein and how they used those capabilities in the particular environments and historical settings in which they lived, it would also be a mistake to assume that human cloning could at least replicate their extraordinary capabilities, if not the accomplishments they achieved with them. Their capabilities too were the product of their inherited genes and their environments, not of their genes alone, and so it would be a mistake to think that cloning them would produce individuals with the same capabilities, even if they would exercise those capabilities at different times and in different ways. In the case of Gandhi and Schweitzer, whose extraordinary greatness lies more in their moral character and commitments, we understand even less well the extent to which their moral character and greatness were produced by their genes.

None of this is to deny that Mozart's and Einstein's extraordinary musical and intellectual capabilities, nor even Gandhi's and Schweitzer's extraordinary moral greatness, were produced in part by their unique genetic inheritances. Cloning them might well produce individuals with exceptional capacities, but we simply do not know how close their clones would be in capacities or accomplishments to the great individuals from whom they were cloned. Even so, the hope for exceptional, even if less and different, accomplishment from cloning such extraordinary individuals might be a reasonable ground for doing so.

I have used examples above of individuals whose greatness is widely appreciated and largely uncontroversial, but if we move away from such cases we encounter the problem of whose standards of greatness would be used to select individuals to be cloned for the benefit of society or mankind at large. This problem inevitably connects with the important issue of who would control access to and use of the technology of human cloning, since those who controlled its use would be in a position to impose their standards of exceptional individuals to be cloned. This issue is especially worrisome if particular groups or segments of society, or if government, controlled the technology for we would then risk its use for the benefit of those groups, segments of society, or governments under the cover of benefiting society or even mankind at large.

6. Human cloning and research on human cloning might make possible important advances in scientific knowledge, for example about human development. While important potential advances in scientific or medical knowledge from human cloning or human cloning research have frequently been cited in some media responses to Dolly's cloning there are at least three reasons why these possible benefits are highly uncertain. First, there is always considerable uncertainty about the nature and importance of the new scientific or medical knowledge that a dramatic new technology like human cloning will lead to; the road to that new knowledge is never mapped in advance and takes many unexpected turns. Second, we also do not know what new knowledge from human cloning or human cloning research could also be gained by other methods and research that do not have the problematic moral features of human cloning to which its opponents object. Third, what human cloning research would be compatible with ethical and legal requirements for the use of human subjects in research is complex, controversial, and largely unexplored. For example, in what contexts and from whom would it be necessary, and how would it be possible, to secure the informed consent of parties involved in human cloning? No human cloning should ever take place without the consent of the person cloned and the woman receiving a cloned embryo, if they are different. But we could never obtain the consent of the cloned later twin to being cloned, so research on human cloning that produces a cloned individual might be barred by ethical and legal regulations for the use of human subjects in research. Moreover, creating human clones solely for the purpose of research would be to use them solely for the benefit of others without their consent, and so unethical. Of course, once human cloning was established to be safe and effective, then new scientific knowledge might be obtained from its use for legitimate, non-research reasons. How human subjects regulations would apply to research on human cloning needs much more exploration than I can give it here in order to help clarify how significant and likely the potential gains are in scientific and medical knowledge from human cloning research and human cloning.

Although there is considerable uncertainty concerning most of the possible individual and social benefits of human cloning that I have discussed above, and although no doubt it may have other benefits or uses that we cannot yet envisage, I believe it is reasonable to conclude that human cloning at this time does not seem to promise great benefits or uniquely to meet great human needs. Nevertheless, a case can be made that scientific freedom supports permitting research on human cloning to go forward and that freedom to use human cloning is protected by the important moral right to reproductive freedom. We must therefore assess what moral rights might be violated, or harms produced, by research on or use of human cloning.

MORAL ARGUMENTS AGAINST HUMAN CLONING

A. Would the Use of Human Cloning Violate Important Moral Rights?

Many of the immediate condemnations of any possible human cloning following Wilmut's cloning of an adult sheep claimed that it would violate moral or human rights, but it was usually not specified precisely, or often even at all, what the rights were that would be violated. I shall consider two possible candidates for such a right: a right to have a unique identity and a right to ignorance about one's future or to an open future. The former right is cited by many commentators, but I believe even if any such a right exists, it is not violated by human cloning. The latter right has only been explicitly defended to my knowledge by two commentators, and in the context of human cloning, only by Hans Jonas; it supports a more promising, even if in my view ultimately unsuccessful, argument that human cloning would violate an important moral or human right. . . .

We need not pursue what the basis or argument in support of a moral or human right to a unique identity might be—such a right is not found among typical accounts and enumerations of moral or human rights—because even if we grant that there is such a right, sharing a genome with another individual as a result of human cloning would not violate it. The idea of the uniqueness, or unique identity, of each person historically predates the development of modern genetics and the knowledge that except in the case of homozygous twins each individual has a unique genome. A unique genome thus could not be the ground of this long-standing belief in the unique human identity of each person.

I turn now to whether human cloning would violate what Hans Jonas called a right to ignorance, or what Joel Feinberg called a right to an open future (Feinberg 1980). Jonas argued that human cloning in which there is a substantial time gap between the beginning of the lives of the earlier and later twin is fundamentally different from the simultaneous beginning of the lives of homozygous twins that occur in nature. Although contemporaneous twins begin their lives with the same genetic inheritance, they also begin their lives or biographies at the same time, and so in ignorance of what the other who shares the same genome will by his or her choices make of his or her life. To whatever extent one's genome determines one's future, each begins ignorant of what that determination will be and so remains as free to choose a future, to construct a particular future from among open alternatives, as are individuals who do not have a twin. Ignorance of the effect of one's genome on one's future is necessary for the spontaneous, free, and authentic construction of a life and self.

A later twin created by human cloning, Jonas argues, knows, or at least believes he or she knows, too much about him- or herself. For there is already in the world another person, one's earlier twin, who from the same genetic starting point has made the life choices that are still in the later twin's future. It will seem that one's life has already been lived and played out by another, that one's fate is already determined, and so the later twin will lose the spontaneity of authentically creating and becoming his or her own self. One will lose the sense of human possibility in freely creating one's own future. It is tyrannical, Jonas claims, for the earlier twin to try to determine another's fate in this way. And even if it is a mistake to believe the crude genetic determinism according to which one's genes determine one's fate, what is important for one's experience of freedom and ability to create a life for oneself is whether one thinks one's future is open and undetermined, and so still to be determined by one's own choices. . . .

In a different context, and without applying it to human cloning, Joel Feinberg has argued for a child's right to an open future. This requires that others raising a child not so close off the future possibilities that the child would otherwise have as to eliminate a reasonable range of opportunities for the child to choose autonomously and construct his or her own life. One way this right to an open future would be violated is to deny even a basic education to a child, and another way might be to create it as a later twin so that it will believe its future has already been set for it by the choices made and the life lived by its earlier twin.

A central difficulty in evaluating the implications for human cloning of a right either to ignorance or to an open future, is whether the right is violated merely because the later twin may be likely to *believe* that its future is already determined, even if that belief is clearly false and supported only by the crudest genetic determinism. I believe that if the twin's future in reality remains open and his to freely choose, then someone's acting in a way that unintentionally leads him to believe that his future is closed and determined has not violated his right to ignorance or to an open future. Likewise, suppose I drive down the twin's street in my new car that is just like his knowing that when he sees me he is likely to believe that I have stolen his car, and therefore to abandon his driving plans for the day. I have not violated his property right to his car even though he may feel the same loss of opportunity to drive that day as if I had in fact stolen his car. In each case he is mistaken that his open future or car has been taken from him, and so no right of his to them has been violated. If we know that the twin will believe that his open future has been taken from him as a result of being cloned, even though in reality it has not, then we know that cloning will cause him psychological distress, but not that it will violate his right. Thus, I believe Jonas' right to ignorance, and our employment of Feinberg's analogous right of a child to an open future, turns out not to be violated by human cloning, though they do point to psychological harms that a later twin may be likely to experience and that I will take up below.

The upshot of our consideration of a moral or human right either to a unique identity or to ignorance and an open future, is that neither would be violated by human cloning. Perhaps there are other possible rights that would make good the charge that human cloning is a violation of moral or human rights, but I am unsure what they might be. I turn now to consideration of the harms that human cloning might produce.

B. What Individual or Social Harms Might Human Cloning Produce?

There are many possible individual or social harms that have been posited by one or another commentator and I shall only try to cover the more plausible and significant of them.

Largely Individual Harms

1. Human cloning would produce psychological distress and harm in the later twin. This is perhaps the most serious individual harm that opponents of human cloning foresee, and we have just seen that even if human cloning is no violation of rights, it may nevertheless cause psychological distress or harm. No doubt knowing the path in life taken by one's earlier twin may in many cases have several bad psychological effects. The later twin may feel, even if mistakenly, that his or her fate has already been substantially laid out, and so have difficulty freely and spontaneously taking responsibility for and making his or her own fate and life. The later twin's experience or sense of autonomy and freedom may be substantially diminished, even if in actual fact they are diminished much less than it seems to him or her. Together with this might be a diminished sense of one's own uniqueness and individuality, even if once again these are in fact diminished little or not at all by having an earlier twin with the same genome. If the later twin is the clone of a particularly exemplary individual, perhaps with some special capabilities and accomplishments, he or she may experience excessive pressure to reach the very high standards of ability and accomplishment of the earlier twin. All of these psychological effects may take a heavy toll on the later twin and be serious burdens under which he or she would live. One commentator has also cited special psychological harms to the first, or first few, human clones from the great publicity that would attend their creation. While public interest in the first clones would no doubt be enormous, medical confidentiality should protect their identity. Even if their identity became public knowledge, this would be a temporary effect only on the first few clones and the experience of Louise Brown, the first child conceived by IVF, suggests this publicity could be managed to limit its harmful effects.

While psychological harms of these kinds from human cloning are certainly possible, and perhaps even likely, they do remain at this point only speculative since we have no experience with human cloning and the creation of earlier and later twins. With naturally occurring identical twins, while they sometimes struggle to achieve their own identity, a struggle shared by many people without a twin, there is typically a very strong emotional bond between the twins and such twins are, if anything, generally psychologically stronger and better adjusted than non-twins (Robertson 1994b). Scenarios are even possible in which being a later twin confers a psychological benefit on the twin; for example, having been deliberately cloned with the specific genes the later twin has might make the later twin feel especially wanted for the kind of person he or she is. Nevertheless, if experience with human cloning confirmed that serious and unavoidable psychological harms typically occurred to the later twin, that would be a serious moral reason to avoid the practice.

In the discussion above of potential psychological harms to a later twin, I have been assuming that one later twin is cloned from an already existing adult individual. Cloning by means of embryo splitting, as carried out and reported by Hall and colleagues at George Washington University in 1993, has limits on the number of genetically identical twins that can be cloned. Nuclear transfer, however, has no limits to the number of genetically identical

questionable if we are logical, rational ppl. most of us would know this is not true.

Same as children feeling they need to follow in their parents footsteps.

individuals who might be cloned. Intuitively, many of the psychological burdens and harms noted above seem more likely and serious for a clone who is only one of many identical later twins from one original source, so that the clone might run into another identical twin around every street corner. This prospect could be a good reason to place sharp limits on the number of twins that could be cloned from any one source. . . .

2. Human cloning procedures would carry unacceptable risks to the clone. One version of this objection to human cloning concerns the research necessary to perfect the procedure, the other version concerns the later risks from its use. Wilmut's group had 276 failures before their success with Dolly, indicating that the procedure is far from perfected even with sheep. Further research on the procedure with animals is clearly necessary before it would be ethical to use the procedure on humans. But even assuming that cloning's safety and effectiveness is established with animals, research would need to be done to establish its safety and effectiveness for humans. Could this research be ethically done? There would be little or no risk to the donor of the cell nucleus to be transferred, and his or her informed consent could and must always be obtained. There might be greater risks for the woman to whom a cloned embryo is transferred, but these should be comparable to those associated with IVF procedures and the woman's informed consent too could and must be obtained.

What of the risks to the cloned embryo itself? Judging by the experience of Wilmut's group in their work on cloning a sheep, the principal risk to the embryos cloned was their failure successfully to implant, grow, and develop. Comparable risks to cloned human embryos would apparently be their death or destruction long before most people or the law consider it to be a person with moral or legal protections of its life. Moreover, artificial reproductive technologies now in use, such as IVF, have a known risk that some embryos will be destroyed or will not successfully implant and will die. It is premature to make a confident assessment of what the risks to human subjects would be of establishing the safety and effectiveness of human cloning procedures, but there are no unavoidable risks apparent at this time that would make the necessary research clearly ethically impermissible.

Could human cloning procedures meet ethical standards of safety and efficacy? Risks to an ovum donor (if any), a nucleus donor, and a woman who receives the embryo for implantation would likely be ethically acceptable with the informed consent of the involved parties. But what of the risks to the human clone if the procedure in some way goes wrong, or unanticipated harms come to the clone; for example, Harold Varmus, director of the National Institutes of Health, has raised the concern that a cell many years old from which a person is cloned could have accumulated genetic mutations during its years in another adult that could give the resulting clone a predisposition to cancer or other diseases of aging. Moreover, it is impossible to obtain the informed consent of the clone to his or her own creation, but, of course no one else is able to give informed consent for their creation either.

I believe it is too soon to say whether unavoidable risks to the clone would make human cloning unethical. At a minimum, further research on cloning animals, as well as research to better define the potential risks to humans, is needed. For the reasons given above, we should not set aside risks to the clone on the grounds that the clone would not be harmed by them since its only alternative is not to exist at all; I have suggested that is a bad argument. But we should not insist on a standard that requires risks to be lower than those we accept in sexual reproduction, or in other forms of assisted reproduction. It is not possible now to know when, if ever, human cloning will satisfy an appropriate standard limiting risks to the clone.

Largely Social Harms

3. Human cloning would lessen the worth of individuals and diminish respect for human life. Unelaborated claims to this effect in the media were common after the announcement of the cloning of Dolly. Ruth Macklin has explored and criticized the claim that human cloning would diminish the value we place on, and our respect for, human life because it would lead to persons being viewed as replaceable (Macklin 1994). As I argued above concerning a right to a unique identity, only on a confused and indefensible notion of human identity is a person's identity determined solely by their genes. Instead, an individual's identity is determined by the interaction of his or her genes over time with his or her environment, including the choices the individual makes and the important relations he or she forms with other persons. This means in turn that no individual could be fully replaced by a later clone possessing the same genes. Ordinary people recognize this clearly. For example, parents of a 12-year-old child dying of a fatal disease would consider it insensitive and ludicrous if someone told them they should not grieve for their coming loss because it is possible to replace him by cloning him; it is *their child who is dying* whom they love and value, and that child and his importance to them could never be replaced by a cloned later twin. Even if they would also come to love and value a later twin as much as their child who is dying, that would be to love and value that *different child* who could never replace the child they lost. Ordinary people are typically quite clear about the importance of the relations they have to distinct, historically situated individuals with whom over time they have shared experiences and their lives, and whose loss to them would therefore be irreplaceable.

A different version of this worry is that human cloning would result in persons' worth or value seeming diminished because we would now see humans as able to be manufactured or "handmade." This demystification of the creation of human life would reduce our appreciation and awe of it and of its natural creation. It would be a mistake, however, to conclude that a human being created by human cloning is of less value or is less worthy of respect than one created by sexual reproduction. It is the nature of a being, not how it is created, that is the source of its value and makes it worthy of respect. Moreover, for many people gaining a scientific understanding of the extraordinary complexity of human reproduction and development increases, instead of decreases, their awe of the process and its product.

A more subtle route by which the value we place on each individual human life might be diminished could come from the use of human cloning with the aim of creating a child with a particular genome, either the genome of another individual especially meaningful to those doing the cloning or an individual with exceptional talents, abilities, and accomplishments. The child might then be valued only for its genome, or at least for its genome's expected phenotypic expression, and no longer be recognized as having the intrinsic equal moral value of all persons, simply as persons. For the moral value and respect due all persons to come to be seen as resting only on the instrumental value of individuals, or of individuals' particular qualities, to others would be to fundamentally change the moral status accorded to persons. Everyone would lose their moral standing as full and equal members of the moral community, replaced by the different instrumental value each of us has to others.

Such a change in the equal moral value and worth accorded to persons should be avoided at all costs, but it is far from clear that such a change would take place from permitting human cloning. Parents, for example, are quite capable of distinguishing their children's intrinsic value, just as individual persons, from their instrumental value based on their particular qualities or properties. The equal moral value and respect due all persons just as persons is not incompatible with the different instrumental value of people's particular qualities or properties; Einstein and an untalented physics graduate student have vastly different value as scientists, but share and are entitled to equal moral value and respect as persons. It would be a mistake and a confusion to conflate the two kinds of value and respect. Making a large number of clones from one original person might be more likely to foster this mistake and confusion in the public, and if so that would be a further reason to limit the number of clones that could be made from one individual.

4. Human cloning would divert resources from other more important social and medical needs. As we saw in considering the reasons for, and potential benefits from, human cloning, in only a limited number of uses would it uniquely meet important human needs. There is little doubt that in the United States, and certainly elsewhere, there are more pressing unmet human needs, both medical or health needs and other social or individual needs. This is a reason for not using public funds to support human cloning, at least if the funds actually are redirected to more important ends and needs. It is not a reason, however, either to prohibit other private individuals or institutions from using their own resources for research on human cloning or for human cloning itself, or to prohibit human cloning or research on human cloning.

The other important point about resource use is that it is not now clear how expensive human cloning would ultimately be, for example, in comparison with other means of relieving infertility. The procedure itself is not scientifically or technologically extremely complex and might prove not to require a significant commitment of resources.

5. Human cloning might be used by commercial interests for financial gain. Both opponents and proponents of human cloning agree that cloned embryos should not be able to be bought and sold. In a science fiction frame of mind, one can imagine commercial interests offering genetically certified and guaranteed embryos for sale, perhaps offering a catalogue of different embryos cloned from individuals with a variety of talents, capacities, and other desirable properties. This would be a fundamental violation of the equal moral respect and dignity owed to all persons, treating them instead as objects to be differentially valued, bought, and sold in the marketplace. Even if embryos are not yet persons at the time they would be purchased or sold, they would be being valued, bought, and sold for the persons they will become. The moral consensus against any commercial market in embryos, cloned or otherwise, should be enforced by law whatever public policy ultimately is on human cloning. It has been argued that the law may already forbid markets in embryos on grounds that they would violate the thirteenth amendment prohibiting slavery and involuntary servitude (Turner 1981).

6. Human cloning might be used by governments or other groups for immoral and exploitative purposes. In *Brave New World,* Aldous Huxley imagined cloning individuals who have been engineered with limited abilities and conditioned to do, and to be happy doing, the menial work that society needed done. Selection and control in the creation of people was exercised not in the interests of the persons created, but in the interests of the society and at the expense of the persons created. Any use of human cloning for such purposes would exploit the clones solely as means for the benefit of others, and would violate the equal moral respect and dignity they are owed as full moral persons. If human cloning is permitted to go forward, it should be with regulations that would clearly prohibit such immoral exploitation.

Fiction contains even more disturbing and bizarre uses of human cloning, such as Mengele's creation of many clones of Hitler in Ira Levin's *The Boys from Brazil,* Woody Allen's science fiction cinematic spoof *Sleeper* in which a dictator's only remaining part, his nose, must be destroyed to keep it from being cloned, and the contemporary science fiction film *Blade Runner.* Nightmare scenarios like Huxley's or Levin's may be quite improbable, but their impact should not be underestimated on public concern with technologies like human cloning. Regulation of human cloning must assure the public that even such farfetched abuses will not take place.

7. Human cloning used on a very widespread basis would have a disastrous effect on the human gene pool by reducing genetic diversity and our capacity to adapt to new conditions. This is not a realistic concern since human cloning would not be used on a wide enough scale, substantially replacing sexual reproduction, to have the feared effect on the gene pool. The vast majority of humans seem quite satisfied with sexual means of reproduction; if anything, from the standpoint of worldwide population, we could do with a bit less enthusiasm for it. Programs of eugenicists like Herman Mueller earlier in the century to impregnate thousands of women with the sperm of exceptional men, as well as the more recent establishment of sperm banks of Nobel laureates, have met with little or no public interest or success. People prefer sexual means of reproduction and they prefer to keep their own biological ties to their offspring.

CONCLUSION

Human cloning has until now received little serious and careful ethical attention because it was typically dismissed as science fiction, and it stirs deep, but difficult to articulate, uneasiness and even revulsion in many people. Any ethical assessment of human cloning at this point must be tentative and provisional. Fortunately, the science and technology of human cloning are not yet in hand, and so a public and professional debate is possible without the need for a hasty, precipitate policy response.

The ethical pros and cons of human cloning, as I see them at this time, are sufficiently balanced and uncertain that there is not an ethically decisive case either for or against permitting it or doing it. Access to human cloning can plausibly be brought within a moral right to reproductive freedom, but the circumstances in which its use would have significant benefits appear at this time to be few and infrequent. It is not a central component of a moral right to reproductive freedom and it serves no major or pressing individual or social needs. On the other hand, contrary to the pronouncements of many of its opponents, human cloning seems not to be a violation of moral or human rights. But it does risk some significant individual or social harms, although most are based on common public confusions about genetic determinism, human identity, and the effects of human cloning. Because most moral reasons against doing human cloning remain speculative they seem insufficient to warrant at this time a complete legal prohibition of either research on or later use of human cloning. Legitimate moral concerns about the use and effects of human cloning, however, underline the need for careful public oversight of research on its development, together with a wider public debate and review before cloning is used on human beings.

REFERENCES

Dworkin, R. (1978). *Taking Rights Seriously.* London: Duckworth.

Feinberg, J. (1980). "The Child's Right to an Open Future," in *Whose Child? Children's Rights, Parental Authority, and State Power,* ed. W. Aiken and H. LaFollette. Totowa, NJ: Rowman and Littlefield.

Macklin, R. (1994). "Splitting Embryos on the Slippery Slope: Ethics and Public Policy." *Kennedy Institute of Ethics Journal* 4: 209–226.

PREVENTING A BRAVE NEW WORLD: WHY WE SHOULD BAN HUMAN CLONING NOW

Leon R. Kass

I.

The urgency of the great political struggles of the twentieth century, successfully waged against totalitarianisms first right and then left, seems to have blinded many people to a deeper and ultimately darker truth about the present age: all contemporary societies are traveling briskly in the same utopian direction. All are wedded to the modern technological project; all march eagerly to the drums of progress and fly proudly the banner of modern science; all sing loudly the Baconian anthem, "Conquer nature, relieve man's estate." Leading the triumphal procession is modern medicine, which is daily becoming ever more powerful in its battle against disease, decay, and death, thanks especially to astonishing achievements in biomedical science and technology—achievements for which we must surely be grateful.

Yet contemplating present and projected advances in genetic and reproductive technologies, in neuroscience and psychopharmacology, and in the development of artificial organs and computerchip implants for human brains, we now clearly recognize new uses for biotechnical power that soar beyond the traditional medical goals of healing disease and relieving suffering. Human nature itself lies on the operating table, ready for alteration, for eugenic and psychic "enhancement," for wholesale re-design. In leading laboratories, academic and

Reprinted with permission from *The New Republic,* May 21, 2001: 30–39.

industrial, new creators are confidently amassing their powers and quietly honing their skills, while on the street their evangelists are zealously prophesying a post-human future. For anyone who cares about preserving our humanity, the time has come to pay attention.

Some transforming powers are already here. The Pill. In vitro fertilization. Bottled embryos. Surrogate wombs. Cloning. Genetic screening. Genetic manipulation. Organ harvesting. Mechanical spare parts. Chimeras. Brain implants. Ritalin for the young, Viagra for the old, Prozac for everyone. And, to leave this vale of tears, a little extra morphine accompanied by Muzak.

Years ago Aldous Huxley saw it coming. In his charming but disturbing novel, *Brave New World* (it appeared in 1932 and is more powerful on each rereading), he made its meaning strikingly visible for all to see. Unlike other frightening futuristic novels of the past century, such as Orwell's already dated *Nineteen Eighty-Four,* Huxley shows us a dystopia that goes with, rather than against, the human grain. Indeed, it is animated by our own most humane and progressive aspirations. Following those aspirations to their ultimate realization, Huxley enables us to recognize those less obvious but often more pernicious evils that are inextricably linked to the successful attainment of partial goods.

Huxley depicts human life seven centuries hence, living under the gentle hand of humanitarianism rendered fully competent by genetic manipulation, psychoactive drugs, hypnopaedia, and high-tech amusements. At long last, mankind has succeeded in eliminating disease, aggression, war, anxiety, suffering, guilt, envy, and grief. But this victory comes at the heavy price of homogenization, mediocrity, trivial pursuits, shallow attachments, debased tastes, spurious contentment, and souls without loves or longings. The Brave New World has achieved prosperity, community, stability, and nigh-universal contentment, only to be peopled by creatures of human shape but stunted humanity. They consume, fornicate, take "soma," enjoy "centrifugal bumble-puppy," and operate the machinery that makes it all possible. They do not read, write, think, love, or govern themselves. Art and science, virtue and religion, family and friendship are all passè. What matters most is bodily health and immediate gratification: "Never put off till tomorrow the fun you can have today." Brave New Man is so dehumanized that he does not even recognize what has been lost.

Huxley's novel, of course, is science fiction. Prozac is not yet Huxley's "soma"; cloning by nuclear transfer or splitting embryos is not exactly "Bokanovskification"; MTV and virtual-reality parlors are not quite the "feelies"; and our current safe and consequenceless sexual practices are not universally as loveless or as empty as those in the novel. But the kinships are disquieting, all the more so since our technologies of bio-psycho-engineering are still in their infancy, and in ways that make all too clear what they might look like in their full maturity. Moreover, the cultural changes that technology has already wrought among us should make us even more worried than Huxley would have us be.

In Huxley's novel, everything proceeds under the direction of an omnipotent—albeit benevolent—world state. Yet the dehumanization that he portrays does not really require despotism or external control. To the contrary, precisely because the society of the future will deliver exactly what we most want—health, safety, comfort, plenty, pleasure, peace of mind and length of days—we can reach the same humanly debased condition solely on the basis of free human choice. No need for World Controllers. Just give us the technological imperative, liberal democratic society, compassionate humanitarianism, moral pluralism, and free markets, and we can take ourselves to a Brave New World all by ourselves—and without even deliberately deciding to go. In case you had not noticed, the train has already left the station and is gathering speed, but no one seems to be in charge.

Some among us are delighted, of course, by this state of affairs: some scientists and biotechnologists, their entrepreneurial backers, and a cheering claque of sci-fi enthusiasts, futurologists, and libertarians. There are dreams to be realized, powers to be exercised, honors to be won, and money—big money—to be made. But many of us are worried, and not, as the proponents of the revolution self-servingly claim, because we are either ignorant of science or afraid of the unknown. To the contrary, we can see all too clearly where the train is headed, and we do not like the destination. We can distinguish cleverness about means from wisdom about ends, and we are loath to entrust the future of the race to those who cannot tell the difference. No friend of humanity cheers for a post-human future.

Yet for all our disquiet, we have until now done nothing to prevent it. We hide our heads in the sand because we enjoy the blessings that medicine keeps supplying, or we rationalize our inaction by declaring that human engineering is inevitable and we can do nothing about it. In either case, we are complicit in preparing for our own degradation, in some respects more to blame than the biozealots who, however misguided, are putting their money where their mouth is. Denial and despair, unattractive outlooks in any situation, become morally reprehensible when circumstances summon us to keep the world safe for human flourishing. Our immediate ancestors, taking up the challenge of their time, rose to the occasion and rescued the human future from the cruel dehumanizations of Nazi and Soviet tyranny. It is our more difficult task to find ways to preserve it from the soft dehumanizations of well-meaning but hubristic biotechnical "recreationism"—and to do it without undermining biomedical science or rejecting its genuine contributions to human welfare.

Truth be told, it will not be easy for us to do so, and we know it. But rising to the challenge requires recognizing the difficulties. For there are indeed many features of modern life that will conspire to frustrate efforts aimed at the human control of the biomedical project. First, we Americans believe in technological automatism: where we do not foolishly believe that all innovation is progress, we fatalistically believe that it is inevitable ("If it can be done, it will be done, like it or not"). Second, we believe in freedom: the freedom of scientists to inquire, the freedom of technologists to develop, the freedom of entrepreneurs to invest and to profit, the freedom of private citizens to make use of existing technologies to satisfy any and all personal desires, including the desire to reproduce by whatever means. Third, the biomedical enterprise occupies the moral high ground of compassionate humanitarianism, upholding the supreme values of modern life—cure disease, prolong life, relieve suffering—in competition with which other moral goods rarely stand a chance. ("What the public wants is not to be sick," says James Watson, "and if we help them not to be sick, they'll be on our side.")

There are still other obstacles. Our cultural pluralism and easygoing relativism make it difficult to reach consensus on what we should embrace and what we should oppose; and moral objections to this or that biomedical practice are often facilely dismissed as religious or sectarian. Many people are unwilling to pronounce judgments about what is good or bad, right and wrong, even in matters of great importance, even for themselves—never mind for others or for society as a whole. It does not help that the biomedical project is now deeply entangled with commerce: there are increasingly powerful economic interests in favor of going full steam ahead, and no economic interests in favor of going slow. Since we live in a democracy, moreover, we face political difficulties in gaining a consensus to direct our future, and we have almost no political experience in trying to curtail the development of any new biomedical technology. Finally, and perhaps most troubling, our views of the meaning of our humanity have been so transformed by the scientific-technological approach to the world that we are in danger of forgetting what we have to lose, humanly speaking.

But though the difficulties are real, our situation is far from hopeless. Regarding each of the aforementioned impediments, there is another side to the story. Though we love our gadgets and believe in progress, we have lost our innocence regarding technology. The environmental movement especially has alerted us to the unintended damage caused by unregulated technological advance, and has taught us how certain dangerous practices can be curbed. Though we favor freedom of inquiry, we recognize that experiments are deeds and not speeches, and we prohibit experimentation on human subjects without their consent, even when cures from disease might be had by unfettered research; and we limit so-called reproductive freedom by proscribing incest, polygamy, and the buying and selling of babies.

Although we esteem medical progress, biomedical institutions have ethics committees that judge research proposals on moral grounds, and, when necessary, uphold the primacy of human freedom and human dignity even over scientific discovery. Our moral pluralism notwithstanding, national commissions and review bodies have sometimes reached moral consensus to recommend limits on permissible scientific research and technological application. On the economic front, the patenting of genes are life forms and the rapid rise of genomic commerce have elicited strong concerns and criticisms, leading even former enthusiasts of the new biology to recoil from the impending commodification of human life. Though we lace political institutions experienced in setting limits on biomedical innovation, federal agencies years ago rejected the development of the plutonium-powered artificial heart, and we have nationally prohibited commercial traffic in organs for transplantation, even though a market would increase the needed supply. In recent years, several American states and many foreign countries have successfully taken political action, making certain practices illegal and placing others under moratoriums (the creation of human embryos solely for research; human germline genetic alteration). Most importantly, the majority of Americans are not yet so degraded or so cynical as to fail to be revolted by the society depicted in Huxley's novel. Though the obstacles to effective action are significant, they offer no excuse for resignation. Besides, it would be disgraceful to concede defeat even before we enter the fray.

Not the least of our difficulties in trying to exercise control over where biology is taking us is the fact that we do not get to decide, once and for all, for or against the destination of a post-human world. The scientific discoveries and the technical powers that will take us there come to us piecemeal, one at a time and seemingly independent from one another, each often attractively introduced as a measure that will "help [us] not to be sick." But sometimes we come to a clear fork in the road where decision is possible, and where we know that our decision will make a world of difference—indeed, it will make a permanently different world. Fortunately, we stand now at the point of such a momentous decision. Events have conspired to provide us with a perfect opportunity to seize the initiative and to gain some control of the biotechnical project. I refer to the prospect of human cloning, a practice absolutely central to Huxley's fictional world. Indeed, creating and manipulating life in the laboratory is the gateway to a Brave New World, not only in fiction but also in fact.

"To clone or not to clone a human being" is no longer a fanciful question. Success in cloning sheep, and also cows, mice, pigs, and goats, makes it perfectly clear that a fateful decision is now at hand: whether we should welcome or even tolerate the cloning of human beings. If recent newspaper reports are to be believed, reputable scientists and physicians have announced their intention to produce the first human clone in the coming year. Their efforts may already be under way.

The media, gawking and titillating as is their wont, have been softening us up for this possibility by turning the bizarre into the familiar. In the four years since the birth of Dolly the cloned sheep, the tone of discussing the prospect of human cloning has gone from "Yuck" to Oh?" to "Gee whiz" to Why not?" The sentimentalizers, aided by leading bioethicists, have downplayed talk about eugenically cloning the beautiful and the brawny or the best and the brightest. They have taken instead to defending clonal reproduction for humanitarian or compassionate reasons: to treat infertility in people who are said to "have no other choice," to avoid the risk of severe genetic disease, to "replace" a child who has died. For the sake of these rare benefits, they would have us countenance the entire practice of human cloning, the consequences be damned.

But we dare not be complacent about what is at issue, for the stakes are very high. Human cloning, though partly continuous with previous reproductive technologies, is also something radically new in itself and in its easily foreseeable consequences—especially when coupled with powers for genetic "enhancement" and germline genetic modification that may soon become available, owing to the recently completed Human Genome Project. I exaggerate somewhat, but in the direction of the truth: we are compelled to decide nothing less than whether human procreation is going to remain human, whether children are going to be made to order rather than begotten, and whether we wish to say yes in principle to the road that leads to the dehumanized hell of *Brave New World*.

Four years ago I addressed this subject in these pages, trying to articulate the moral grounds of our repugnance at the prospect of human cloning ("The Wisdom of Repugnance," TNR, June 2, 1997). Subsequent events have only strengthened my conviction that cloning is a bad idea whose time should not come; but my emphasis this time is more practical. To be sure, I would still like to persuade undecided readers that cloning is a serious evil, but I am more interested in encouraging those who oppose human cloning but who think that we are impotent to prevent it, and in mobilizing them to support new and solid legislative efforts to stop it. In addition, I want readers who may worry less about cloning and more about the impending prospects of germline genetic manipulation or other eugenic practices to realize the unique practical opportunity that now presents itself to us.

For we have here a golden opportunity to exercise some control over where biology is taking us. The technology of cloning is discrete and well defined, and it requires considerable technical know-how and dexterity; we can therefore know by name many of the likely practitioners. The public demand for cloning is extremely low, and most people are decidedly against it. Nothing scientifically or medically important would be lost by banning clonal reproduction; alternative and non-objectionable means are available to obtain some of the most important medical benefits claimed for (non-reproductive) human cloning. The commercial interests in human cloning are, for now, quite limited; and the nations of the world are actively seeking to prevent it. Now may be as good a chance as we will ever have to get our hands on the wheel of the runaway train now headed for a post-human world and to steer it toward a more dignified human future.

II.

What is cloning? Cloning, or asexual reproduction, is the production of individuals who are genetically identical to an already existing individual. The procedure's name is fancy—somatic cell nuclear transfer—but its concept is simple. Take a mature but unfertilized egg; remove or deactivate its nucleus; introduce a nucleus obtained from a specialized (somatic) cell of an adult organism. Once the egg begins to divide, transfer the little embryo to a woman's uterus to initiate a pregnancy. Since almost all the hereditary material of a cell is contained within its nucleus, the re-nucleated egg and the individual into which it develops are genetically identical to the organism that was the source of the transferred nucleus.

An unlimited number of genetically identical individuals—the group, as well as each of its members, is called "a clone"—could be produced by nuclear transfer. In principle, any person, male or female, newborn or adult, could be cloned, and in any quantity; and because stored cells can outlive their sources, one may even clone the dead. Since cloning requires no personal involvement on the part of the person whose genetic material is used it could easily be used to reproduce living or deceased persons without their consent—a threat to reproductive freedom that has received relatively little attention.

Some possible misconceptions need to be avoided. Cloning is not Xeroxing: the clone of Bill Clinton, though his genetic double, would enter the world hairless, toothless, and peeing in his diapers, like any other human infant. But neither is cloning just like natural twinning: the cloned twin will be identical to an older, existing adult: and it will arise not by chance but by deliberate design; and its entire genetic makeup will be pre-selected by its parents and/or scientists. Moreover, the success rate of cloning, at least at first, will probably not be very high: the Scots transferred two hundred seventy-seven adult nuclei into sheep eggs, implanted twenty-nine clonal embryos, and achieved the birth of only one live lamb clone.

For this reason, among others, it is unlikely that, at least for now, the practice would be very popular; and there is little immediate worry of mass-scale production of multicopies. Still, for the tens of thousands of people who sustain more than three hundred assisted-reproduction clinics in the United States and already avail themselves of in vitro fertilization and other techniques, cloning would be an option with virtually no added fuss. Panos Zavos, the Kentucky reproduction specialist who has announced his plans to clone a child, claims that he has already received thousands of e-mailed requests from people eager to clone, despite the known risks of failure and damaged off-spring. Should commercial interests develop in "nucleus-banking," as they have in sperm-banking, and egg-harvesting; should famous athletes or other celebrities decide to market their DNA the way they now market their autographs and nearly everything else; should techniques of embryo and germline genetic testing and manipulation arrive as anticipated, increasing the use of laboratory assistance in order to obtain "better" babies—should all this come to pass, cloning, if it is permitted, could become more than a marginal practice simply on the basis of free reproductive choice.

What are we to think about this prospect? Nothing good. Indeed, most people are repelled by nearly all aspects of human cloning: the possibility of mass production of human beings, with large clones of look-alikes, compromised in their individuality; the idea of father-son or mother-daughter "twins"; the bizarre prospect of a woman bearing and rearing a genetic copy of herself, her spouse, or even her deceased father or mother; the grotesqueness of conceiving a child as an exact "replacement" for another who has died; the utilitarian creation of embryonic duplicates of oneself, to be frozen away or created when needed to provide homologous tissues or organs for transplantation; the narcissism of those who would clone themselves, and the arrogance of others who think they know who deserves to be cloned; the Frankensteinian hubris to create a human life and increasingly to control its destiny; men playing at being God. Almost no one finds any of the suggested reasons for human cloning compelling , and almost everyone anticipates its possible misuses and abuses. And the popular belief that human cloning cannot be prevented makes the prospect all the more revolting.

Revulsion is not an argument; and some of yesterday's repugnances are today calmly accepted—not always for the better. In some crucial cases, however, repugnance is the emotional expression of deep wisdom, beyond reason's power completely to articulate it. Can anyone really give an argument fully adequate to the horror that is father-daughter incest (even with consent), or bestiality, or the mutilation of a corpse, or the eating of human flesh, or the rape or murder of another human being? Would anybody's failure to give full rational justification for his revulsion at those practices make that revulsion ethically suspect?

I suggest that our repugnance at human cloning belongs in this category. We are repelled by the prospect of cloning human beings not because of the strangeness or the novelty of the undertaking, but because we intuit and we feel, immediately and without argument, the violation of things that we rightfully hold dear. We sense that cloning represents a profound defilement of our given nature as procreative beings, and of the social relations built on this natural ground. We also sense that cloning is a radical form of child abuse. In this age in which everything is held to be permissible so long as it is freely done, and in which our bodies are regarded as mere instruments of our autonomous rational will, repugnance may be the only voice left that speaks up to defend the central core of our humanity. Shallow are the souls that have forgotten how to shudder.

III.

Yet repugnance need not stand naked before the bar of reason. The wisdom of our horror at human cloning can be at least partially articulated, even if this is finally one of those instances about which the heart has its reasons that reason cannot entirely know. I offer four objections to human cloning: that it constitutes unethical experimentation; that it threatens identity and individuality; that it turns procreation into manufacture (especially when understood as the harbinger of manipulations to come); and that it means despotism over children and perversion of parenthood. Please note: I speak only about so-called reproductive cloning, not about the creation of cloned embryos for research. The objections that may be raised against creating (or using) embryos for research are entirely independent of whether the research embryos are produced by cloning. What is radically distinct and radically new is reproductive cloning.

Any attempt to clone a human being would constitute an unethical experiment upon the resulting child-to-be. In all the animal experiments, fewer than two to three percent of all cloning attempts succeeded. Not only are there fetal deaths and stillborn infants, but many of the so-called "successes" are in fact failures. As has only recently become clear, there is a very high incidence of major disabilities and deformities in cloned animals that attain live birth. Cloned cows often have heart and lung problems; cloned mice later develop pathological obesity; other live-born cloned animals fail to reach normal developmental milestones.

The problem, scientists suggest, may lie in the fact that an egg with a new somatic nucleus must re-program itself in a matter of minutes or hours (whereas the nucleus of an unaltered egg has been prepared over months and years). There is thus a greatly increased likelihood of error in translating the genetic instructions, leading to developmental defects some of which will show themselves only much later. (Note also that these induced abnormalities may also affect the stem cells that scientists hope to harvest from cloned embryos. Lousy embryos, lousy stem cells.) Nearly all scientists now agree that attempts to clone human beings carry massive risks of producing unhealthy, abnormal, and malformed children. What are we to do with them? Shall we just discard the ones that fall short of expectations? Considered opinion is today nearly unanimous, even among scientists: attempts at human cloning are irresponsible and unethical. We cannot ethically even get to know whether or not human cloning is feasible.

If it were successful, cloning would create serious issues of identity and individuality. The clone may experience concerns about his distinctive identity not only because he will be, in genotype and in appearance, identical to another human being, but because he may also be twin to the person who is his "father" or his "mother"—if one can still call them that. Unaccountably, people treat as innocent the homey case of intrafamilial cloning—the cloning of husband or wife (or single mother). They forget about the unique dangers of mixing the twin relation with the parent-child relation. (For this situation, the relation of contemporaneous twins is no precedent; yet even this less problematic situation teaches us how difficult it is to wrest independence from the being for whom one has the most powerful affinity.) Virtually no parent is going to be able to treat a clone of himself or herself as one treats a child generated by the lottery of sex. What will happen when the adolescent clone of Mommy becomes the spitting image of the woman with whom Daddy once fell in love? In case of divorce, will Mommy still love the clone of Daddy, even though she can no longer stand the sight of Daddy himself?

Most people think about cloning from the point of view of adults choosing to clone. Almost nobody thinks about what it would be like to be the cloned child. Surely his or her new life would constantly be scrutinized in relation to that of the older version. Even in the absence of unusual parental expectations for the clone—say, to live the same life, only without its errors—the child is likely to be ever a curiosity, ever a potential source of déjà vu. Unlike "normal" identical twins, a cloned individual—copied from whomever—will be saddled with a genotype that has already lived. He will not be fully a surprise to the world: people are likely always to compare his doings in life with those of his alter ego, especially if he is a clone of someone gifted or famous. True, his nurture and his circumstance will be different; genotype is not exactly destiny. But one must also expect parental efforts to shape this new life after the original—or at least to view the child with the original version always firmly in mind. For why else did they clone from the star basketball player, the mathematician, or the beauty queen—or even dear old Dad—in the first place?

Human cloning would also represent a giant step toward the transformation of begetting into making, of procreation into manufacture (literally, "handmade"), a process that has already begun with in vitro fertilization and genetic testing of embryos. With cloning, not only is the process in hand, but the total genetic blueprint of the cloned individual is selected and determined by the human artisans. To be sure, subsequent development is still according to natural processes; and the resulting children will be recognizably human. But we would be taking a major step into making man himself simply another one of the man-made things.

How does begetting differ from making? In natural procreation, human beings come together to give existence to another being that is formed exactly as we were, by what we are—living, hence perishable, hence aspiringly erotic, hence procreative human beings. But in clonal reproduction, and in the more advanced forms of manufacture to which it will lead, we give existence to a being not by what we are but by what we intend and design.

Let me be clear. The problem is not the mere intervention of technique, and the point is not that "nature knows best." The problem is that any child whose being, character, and capacities exist owing to human design does not stand on the same plane as its makers. As with any product of our making, no matter how excellent, the artificer stands above it, not as an equal but as a superior, transcending it by his will and creative prowess. In human cloning, scientists and prospective "parents" adopt a technocratic attitude toward human children: human children become their artifacts. Such an arrangement is profoundly dehumanizing, no matter how good the product.

Procreation dehumanized into manufacture is further degraded by commodification, a virtually inescapable result of allowing baby-making to proceed under the banner of commerce. Genetic and reproductive biotechnology companies are already growth industries, but they will soon go into commercial orbit now that the Human Genome Project has been completed. "Human eggs for sale" is already a big business, masquerading under the pretense of "donation." Newspaper advertisements on elite college campuses offer up to $50,000 for an egg "donor" tall enough to play women's basketball and with SAT scores high enough for admission to Stanford; and to nobody's surprise, at such prices there are many young coeds eager to help shoppers obtain the finest babies money can buy. (The egg and womb-renting entrepreneurs shamelessly proceed on the ancient, disgusting, misogynist premise that most women will give you access to their bodies, if the price is right.) Even before the capacity for human cloning is perfected, established companies will have invested in the harvesting of eggs from ovaries obtained at autopsy or through ovarian surgery, practiced embryonic genetic alteration, and initiated the stockpiling of prospective donor tissues. Through the rental of surrogate-womb services, and through the buying and selling of tissues and embryos priced according to the merit of the donor, the commodification of nascent human life will be unstoppable.

Finally, the practice of human cloning by nuclear transfer—like other anticipated forms of genetically engineering the next generation—would enshrine and aggravate a profound misunderstanding of the meaning of having children and of the parent-child relationship. When a couple normally chooses to procreate, the partners are saying yes to the emergence of new life in its novelty—are saying yes not only to having a child, but also to having whatever child this child turns out to be. In accepting our finitude, in opening ourselves to our replacement, we tacitly confess the limits of our control.

Embracing the future by procreating means precisely that we are relinquishing our grip in the very activity of taking up our own share in what we hope will be the immortality of human life and the human species. This means that our children are not our children: they are not our property, they are not our possessions. Neither are they supposed to live our lives for us, or to live anyone's life but their own. Their genetic distinctiveness and independence are the natural foreshadowing of the deep truth that they have their own, never-before-enacted life to live. Though sprung from a past, they take an uncharted course into the future.

Much mischief is already done by parents who try to live vicariously through their children. Children are sometimes compelled to fulfill the broken dreams of unhappy parents. But whereas most parents normally have hopes for their children, cloning parents will have expectations. In cloning, such overbearing parents will have taken at the start a decisive step that contradicts the entire meaning of the open and forward-looking nature of parent-child relations. The child is given a genotype that has already lived, with full expectation that this blueprint of a past life ought to be controlling the life that is to come. A wanted child now means a child who exists precisely to fulfill parental wants. Like all the more precise eugenic manipulations that will follow in its wake, cloning is thus inherently despotic, for it seeks to make one's children after one's own image (or an image of one's choosing) and their future according to one's will.

Is this hyperbolic? Consider concretely the new realities of responsibility and guilt in the households of the clones. No longer only the sins of the parents, but also the genetic choices of the parents, will be visited on the children—and beyond the third and fourth generation; and everyone will know who is responsible. No parent will be able to blame nature or the lottery of sex for an unhappy adolescent's big nose, dull wit, musical ineptitude, nervous disposition, or anything else that he hates about himself. Fairly or not, children will hold their cloners responsible for everything, for nature as well as for nurture. And parents, especially the better ones, will be limitlessly liable to guilt. Only the truly despotic souls will sleep the sleep of the innocent.

IV.

The defenders of cloning are not wittingly friends of despotism. Quite the contrary. Deaf to most other considerations, they regard themselves mainly as friends of freedom: the freedom of individuals to reproduce, the freedom of scientists and inventors to discover and to devise and to foster "progress" in genetic knowledge and technique, the freedom of entrepreneurs to profit in the market. They want large-scale cloning only for animals, but they wish to preserve cloning as a human option for exercising our "right to reproduce"—our right to have children, and children with "desirable genes." As some point out, under our "right to reproduce" we already practice early forms of unnatural, artificial, and extra-marital reproduction, and we already practice early forms of eugenic choice. For that reason, they argue, cloning is no big deal.

We have here a perfect example of the logic of the slippery slope. The principle of reproductive freedom currently enunciated by the proponents of cloning logically embraces the ethical acceptability of sliding all the way down: to producing children wholly in the laboratory from sperm to term (should it become feasible), and to producing children whose entire genetic makeup will be the product of parental eugenic planning and choice. If reproductive freedom means the right to have a child of one's own choosing by whatever means, then reproductive freedom knows and accepts no limits.

Proponents want us to believe that there are legitimate uses of cloning that can be distinguished from illegitimate uses, but by their own principles no such limits can be found. (Nor could any such limits be enforced in practice: once cloning is permitted, no one ever need discover whom one is cloning and why.) Reproductive freedom, as they understand it, is governed solely by the subjective wishes of the parents-to-be. The sentimentally appealing case of the childless married couple is on these grounds, indistinguishable from the case of an individual (married or not) who would like to clone someone famous or talented, living or dead. And the principle here endorsed justifies not only cloning but also all future artificial attempts to create (manufacture) "better" or "perfect" babies.

The "perfect baby," of course, is the project not of the infertility doctors, but of the eugenic scientists and their supporters, who, for the time being, are content to hide behind the skirts of the partisans of reproductive freedom and compassion for the infertile. For them, the paramount right is not the so-called right to reproduce, it is what the biologist Bentley Glass called, a quarter of a century ago, "the right of every child to be born with a sound physical and mental constitution, based on a sound genotype . . . the inalienable right to a sound heritage." But to secure this right, and to achieve the requisite quality control over new human life, human conception and gestation will need to be brought fully into the bright light of the laboratory, beneath which the child-to-be can be fertilized, nourished, pruned, weeded, watched, inspected, prodded, pinched, cajoled, injected, tested, rated, graded, approved, stamped, wrapped, sealed, and delivered. There is no other way to produce the perfect baby.

If you think that such scenarios require outside coercion or governmental tyranny, you are mistaken. Once it becomes possible, with the aid of human genomics, to produce or to select for what some regard as "better babies"—smarter, prettier, healthier, more athletic—parents will leap at the opportunity to "improve" their off-spring. Indeed, not to do so will be socially regarded as a form of child neglect. Those who would ordinarily be opposed to such tinkering will be under enormous pressure to compete on behalf of their as yet unborn children—just as some now plan almost from their children's birth how to get them into Harvard. Never mind that, lacking a standard of "good" or "better," no one can really know whether any such changes will truly be improvements.

Proponents of cloning urge us to forget about the science-fiction scenarios of laboratory manufacture or multiple-copy clones, and to focus only on the sympathetic cases of infertile couples exercising their reproductive rights. But why, if the single cases are so innocent, should multiplying their performance be so off-putting? (Similarly, why do others object to people's making money from that practice if the practice itself is perfectly acceptable?) The so-called science-fiction cases—say, *Brave New World*—make vivid the meaning of what looks to us, mistakenly, to be benign. They reveal that what looks like compassionate humanitarianism is, in the end, crushing dehumanization.

V.

Whether or not they share my reasons, most people, I think, share my conclusion: that human cloning is unethical in itself and dangerous in its likely consequences, which include the precedent that it will establish for designing our children. Some reach this conclusion for their own good reasons, different from my own: concerns about distributive justice in access to eugenic cloning; worries about the genetic effects of asexual "inbreeding"; aversion to the implicit premise of genetic determinism; objections to the embryonic and fetal wastage that must necessarily accompany the efforts; religious opposition to "man playing God." But never mind why: the overwhelming majority of our fellow Americans remain firmly opposed to cloning human beings.

For us, then, the real questions are: What should we do about it? How can we best succeed? These questions should concern everyone eager to secure deliberate human control over the powers that could re-design our humanity, even if cloning is not the issue over which they would choose to make their stand. And the answer to the first question seems pretty plain. What we should do is work to prevent human cloning by making it illegal.

We should aim for a global legal ban, if possible, and for a unilateral national ban at a minimum—and soon, before the fact is upon us. To be sure, legal bans can be violated; but we certainly curtail much mischief by outlawing incest, voluntary servitude, and the buying and selling of organs and babies. To be sure, renegade scientists may secretly undertake to violate such a law, but we can deter them by both criminal sanctions and monetary penalties, as well as by removing any incentive they have to proudly claim credit for their technological bravado.

Such a ban on clonal baby-making will not harm the progress of basic genetic science and technology. On the contrary, it will reassure the public that scientists are happy to proceed without violating the deep ethical norms and intuitions of the human community. It will also protect honorable scientists from a public backlash against the brazen misconduct of the rogues. As many scientists have publicly confessed, free and worthy science probably has much more to fear from a strong public reaction to a cloning fiasco than it does from a cloning ban, provided that the ban is judiciously crafted and vigorously enforced against those who would violate it.

Five states—Michigan, Louisiana, California, Rhode Island, and Virginia—have already enacted a ban on human cloning, and several others are likely to follow suit this year. Michigan, for example, has made it a felony, punishable by imprisonment for not more than ten years or a fine of not more than $10 million, or both, to "intentionally engage in or attempt to engage in human cloning," where human cloning means "the use of human somatic cell nuclear transfer technology to produce a human embryo." Internationally, the movement to ban human cloning gains momentum. France and Germany have banned cloning (and germline genetic engineering), and the Council of Europe is working to have it banned in all of its forty-one member countries, and Canada is expected to follow suit. The United Nations, UNESCO, and The Group of Seven have called for a global ban on human cloning. Given the decisive actions of the rest of the industrialized world, the United States looks to some observers to be a rogue nation. A few years ago, soon after the birth of Dolly, President Clinton called for legislation to outlaw human cloning, and attempts were made to produce a national ban. Yet none was enacted, despite general agreement in Congress that it would be desirable to have such a ban. One might have thought that it would be easy enough to find clear statutory language for prohibiting attempts to clone a human being (and other nations have apparently not found it difficult). But, alas, in the last national go-around, there was trouble over the apparently vague term "human being," whether it includes the early (pre-implantation) embryonic stages of human life. Learning from this past failure, we can do better this time around. Besides, circumstances have changed greatly in the intervening three years, making a ban both more urgent and less problematic.

Two major anti-cloning bills were introduced into the Senate in 1998. The Democratic bill (Kennedy-Feinstein) would have banned so-called reproductive cloning by prohibiting transfer of cloned embryos into women to initiate pregnancy. The Republican bill (Frist-Bond) would have banned *all* cloning by prohibiting the creation even of embryonic human clones. Both sides opposed "reproductive cloning," the attempt to bring to birth a living human child who is the clone of someone now (or previously) alive. But the Democratic bill sanctioned creating cloned embryos for research purposes, and the Republican bill did not. The pro-life movement could not support the former, whereas the scientific community and the biotechnology industry opposed the latter; indeed, they successfully lobbied a dozen Republican senators to oppose taking a vote on the Republican bill (which even its supporters now admit was badly drafted). Owing to a deep and unbridgeable gulf over the question of embryo research, we did not get the congressional ban on reproductive cloning that nearly everyone wanted. It would be tragic if we again failed to produce a ban on human cloning because of its seemingly unavoidable entanglement with the more divisive issue of embryo research.

To find a way around this impasse, several people (myself included) advocated a legislative "third way," one that firmly banned only reproductive cloning but did not legitimate creating cloned embryos for research. This, it turns out, is hard to do. It is easy enough to state the necessary negative disclaimer that would set aside the embryo-research question: "Nothing in this act shall be taken to determine the legality of creating cloned embryos for research; this act neither permits nor prohibits such activity." It is much more difficult to state the positive prohibition in terms that are unambiguous and acceptable to all sides. To indicate only one difficulty: indifference to the creation of embryonic clones coupled with a ban (only) on their transfer would place the federal government in the position of demanding the destruction of nascent life, a bitter pill to swallow even for pro-choice advocates.

Given both these difficulties, and given the imminence of attempts at human cloning, I now believe that what we need is an all-out ban on human cloning, including the creation of embryonic clones. I am convinced that all halfway measures will prove to be morally, legally, and strategically flawed, and—most important—that they will not be effective in obtaining the desired result. Anyone truly serious about preventing human reproductive cloning must seek to stop the process from the beginning. Our changed circumstances, and the now evident defects of the less restrictive alternatives, make an all-out ban by far the most attractive and effective option.

Here's why. Creating cloned human children ("reproductive cloning") necessarily begins by producing cloned human embryos. Preventing the latter would prevent the former, and prudence alone might counsel building such a "fence around the law." Yet some scientists favor embryo cloning as a way of obtaining embryos for research or as sources of cells and tissues for the possible benefit of others. (This practice they misleadingly call "therapeutic cloning" rather than the more accurate "cloning for research" or "experimental cloning," so as to obscure the fact that the clone will be "treated" only to exploitation and destruction, and that any potential future beneficiaries and any future "therapies" are at this point purely hypothetical.)

The prospect of creating new human life solely to be exploited in this way has been condemned on moral grounds by many people—including *The Washington Post,* President Clinton, and many other supporters of a woman's right to abortion—as displaying a profound disrespect for life. Even those who are willing to scavenge so-called "spare embryos"—those products of in vitro fertilization made in excess of people's reproductive needs, and otherwise likely to be discarded—draw back from creating human embryos explicitly and solely for research purposes. They reject outright what they regard as the exploitation and the instrumentalization of nascent human life. In addition, others who are agnostic about the moral status of the embryo see the wisdom of not needlessly offending the sensibilities of their fellow citizens who are opposed to such practices.

But even setting aside these obvious moral first impressions, a few moments of reflection show why an anti-cloning law that permitted the cloning of embryos but criminalized their transfer to produce a child would be a moral blunder. This would be a law that was not merely permissively "pro-choice" but emphatically and prescriptively "anti-life." While permitting the creation of an embryonic life, it would make it a federal offense to try to keep it alive and bring it to birth. Whatever one thinks of the moral status or the ontological status of the human embryo, moral sense and practical wisdom recoil from having the government of the United States on record as requiring the destruction of nascent life and, what is worse, demanding the punishment of those who would act to preserve it by (feloniously!) giving it birth).

But the problem with the approach that targets only reproductive cloning (that is, the transfer of the embryo to a woman's uterus) is not only moral but also legal and strategic. A ban only on reproductive cloning would turn out to be unenforceable. Once cloned embryos were produced and available in laboratories and assisted-reproduction centers, it would be virtually impossible to control what was done with them. Biotechnical experiments take place in laboratories, hidden from public view, and, given the rise of high-stakes commerce in biotechnology, these experiments are concealed from the competition. Huge stockpiles of cloned human embryos could thus be produced and bought and sold without anyone knowing it. As we have seen with in vitro embryos created to treat infertility, embryos produced for one reason can be used for another reason: today "spare embryos" once created to begin a pregnancy are now used in research, and tomorrow clones created for research will be used to begin a pregnancy.

Assisted reproduction takes place within the privacy of the doctor-patient relationship, making outside scrutiny extremely difficult. Many infertility experts probably would obey the law, but others could and would defy it with impunity, their doings covered by the veil of secrecy that is the principle of medical confidentiality. Moreover, the transfer of embryos to begin a pregnancy is a simple procedure (especially compared with manufacturing the embryo in the first place), simple enough that its final steps could be self-administered by the woman, who would thus absolve the doctor of blame for having "caused" the illegal transfer. (I have in mind something analogous to Kevorkian's suicide machine, which was designed to enable the patient to push the plunger and the good "doctor" to evade criminal liability).

Even should the deed become known, governmental attempts to enforce the reproductive ban would run into a swarm of moral and legal challenges, both to efforts aimed at preventing transfer to a woman and—even worse—to efforts seeking to prevent birth after transfer has occurred. A woman who wished to receive the embryo clone would no doubt seek a judicial restraining order, suing to have the law overturned in the name of a constitutionally protected interest in her own reproductive choice to clone. (The cloned child would be born before the legal proceedings were complete.) And should an "illicit clonal pregnancy" be discovered, no governmental agency would compel a woman to abort the clone, and there would be an understandable storm of protest should she be fined or jailed after she gives birth. Once the baby is born, there would even be sentimental opposition to punishing the doctor for violating the law—unless, of course, the clone turned out to be severely abnormal.

For all these reasons, the only practically effective and legally sound approach is to block human cloning at the start, at the production of the embryo clone. Such a ban can be rightly characterized not as interference with reproductive freedom, nor even as interference with scientific inquiry, but as an attempt to prevent the unhealthy, unsavory, and unwelcome manufacture of and traffic in human clones.

VI.

Some scientists, pharmaceutical companies, and bio-entrepreneurs may balk at such a comprehensive restriction. They want to get their hands on those embryos, especially for their stem cells, those pluripotent cells that can in principle be turned into any cells and any tissues in the body, potentially useful for transplantation to repair somatic damage. Embryonic stem cells need not come from cloned embryos, of course; but the scientists say that stem cells obtained from clones could be therapeutically injected in the embryo's adult "twin" without any risk of immunological rejection. It is the promise of rejection-free tissues for transplantation that so far has been the most successful argument in favor of experimental cloning. Yet new discoveries have shown that we can probably obtain the same benefits without embryo cloning. The facts are much different than they were three years ago, and the weight in the debate about cloning for research should shift to reflect the facts.

Numerous recent studies have shown that it is possible to obtain highly potent stem cells from the bodies of children and adults—from the blood, bone marrow, brain, pancreas, and, most recently, fat. Beyond all expectations, these non-embryonic stem cells have been shown to have the capacity to turn into a wide variety of specialized cells and tissues. (At the same time, early human therapeutic efforts with stem cells derived from embryos have produced some horrible results, the cells going wild in their new hosts and producing other tissues in addition to those in need of replacement. If an in vitro embryo is undetectably abnormal—as so often they are—the cells derived from it may also be abnormal.) Since cells derived from our own bodies are more easily and cheaply available than cells harvested from specially manufactured clones, we will almost surely be able to obtain from ourselves any needed homologous transplantable cells and tissues, without the need for egg donors or cloned embryonic copies of ourselves. By pouring our resources into *adult* stem cell research (or, more accurately, "non-embryonic" stem cell research), we can also avoid the morally and legally vexing issues in embryo research. And more to our present subject, by eschewing the cloning of embryos, we make the cloning of human beings much less likely.

A few weeks ago an excellent federal anti-cloning bill was introduced in Congress, sponsored by Senator Sam Brownback and Representative David Weldon. This carefully drafted legislation seeks to prevent the cloning of human beings at the very first step, by prohibiting somatic cell nuclear transfer to produce embryonic clones, and provides substantial criminal and monetary penalties for violating the law. The bill makes very clear that there is to be no interference with the scientific and medically useful practices of cloning DNA fragments (molecular cloning), with the duplication of somatic cells (or stem cells) in tissue culture (cell cloning), or with whole-organism or embryo cloning of non-human animals. If enacted, this law would bring the United States into line with the current or soon-to-be-enacted practices of many other nations. Most important, it offers us the best chance—the only realistic chance—that we have to keep human cloning from happening, or from happening much.

Getting this bill passed will not be easy. The pharmaceutical and biotech companies and some scientific and patient-advocacy associations may claim that the bill is the work of bio-Luddites: anti-science, a threat to free inquiry, an obstacle to obtaining urgently needed therapies for disease. Some feminists and pro-choice groups will claim that this legislation is really only a sneaky device for fighting *Roe* v. *Wade,* and they will resist anything that might be taken even to hint that a human embryo has any moral worth. On the other side, some right-to-life purists, who care not how babies are made as long as life will not be destroyed, will withhold their support because the bill does not take a position against embryo twinning or embryo research in general.

All of these arguments are wrong, and all of them must be resisted. This is not an issue of pro-life versus pro-choice. It is not about death and destruction, or about a woman's right to choose. It is only and emphatically about baby design and manufacture: the opening skirmish of a long battle against eugenics and against a post-human future. As such, it is an issue that should not divide "the left" and "the right"; and there are people across the political spectrum who are coalescing in the efforts to stop human cloning. (The prime sponsor of Michigan's comprehensive anti-cloning law is a pro-choice Democratic legislator.) Everyone needs to understand that, whatever we may think about the moral status of embryos, once embryonic clones are produced in the laboratories the eugenic revolution will have begun. And we shall have lost our best chance to do anything about it.

As we argue in the coming weeks about this legislation, let us be clear about the urgency of our situation and the meaning of our action or inaction. Scientists and doctors whose names we know, and probably many others whose names we do not know, are today working to clone human beings. They are aware of the immediate hazards, but they are undeterred. They are prepared to screen and to destroy anything that looks abnormal. They do not care that they will not be able to detect most of the possible defects. So confident are they in their rectitude that they are willing to ignore all future consequences of the power to clone human beings. They are prepared to gamble with the well-being of any live-born clones, and, if I am right, with a great deal more, all for the glory of being the first to replicate a human being. They are, in short, daring the community to defy them. In these circumstances, our silence can only mean acquiescence. To do nothing now is to accept the responsibility for the deed and for all that follows predictably in its wake.

I appreciate that a federal legislative ban on human cloning is without American precedent, at least in matters technological. Perhaps such a ban will prove ineffective; perhaps it will eventually be shown to have been a mistake. (If so, it could later be reversed.) If enacted, however, it will have achieved one overwhelmingly important result, in addition to its contribution to thwarting cloning: it will place the burden of practical proof where it belongs. It will require the proponents to show very clearly what great social or medical good can be had only by the cloning of human beings. Surely it is only for such a compelling case, yet to be made or even imagined, that we should wish to risk this major departure—or any other major departure—in human procreation.

Americans have lived by and prospered under a rosy optimism about scientific and technological progress. The technological imperative has probably served us well, though we should admit that there is no accurate method for weighing benefits and harms. And even when we recognize the unwelcome outcomes of technological advance, we remain confident in our ability to fix all the "bad" consequences—by regulation or by means of still newer and better technologies. Yet there is very good reason for shifting the American paradigm, at least regarding those technological interventions into the human body and mind that would surely effect fundamental (and likely irreversible) changes in human nature, basic human relationships, and what it means to be a human being. Here we should not be willing to risk everything in the naïve hope that, should things go wrong, we can later set them right again.

Some have argued that cloning is almost certainly going to remain a marginal practice, and that we should therefore permit people to practice it. Such a view is shortsighted. Even if cloning is rarely undertaken, a society in which it is tolerated is no longer the same society—any more than is a society that permits (even small-scale) incest or cannibalism or slavery. A society that allows cloning, whether it knows it or not, has tacitly assented to the conversion of procreation into manufacture and to the treatment of children as purely the projects of our will. Willy-nilly, it has acquiesced in the eugenic re-design of future generations. The humanitarian superhighway to a Brave New World lies open before this society.

But the present danger posed by human cloning is, paradoxically, also a golden opportunity. In a truly unprecedented way, we can strike a blow for the human control of the technological project, for wisdom, for prudence, for human dignity. The prospect of human cloning, so repulsive to contemplate, is the occasion for deciding whether we shall be slaves of unregulated innovation, and ultimately its artifacts, or whether we shall remain free human beings who guide our powers toward the enhancement of human dignity. The humanity of the human future is now in our hands.

HUMAN CLONING: MYTHS, MEDICAL BENEFITS AND CONSTITUTIONAL RIGHTS

Mark D. Eibert

This article discusses three topics. The first is what cloning is, how it's done, what is going on in cloning today, and most importantly, what cloning is not. The second is the potential medical benefits of cloning, especially in the treatment of infertility and the prevention of genetic disease and defects. My third topic is the current state of the law on cloning, and what constitutional questions those laws raise, especially with respect to reproductive and scientific freedom.

WHAT CLONING IS AND HOW IT IS DONE

Cloning is a method of producing a baby—whether animal or human—that has almost the same genetic

---

This article is adapted from a speech and multimedia presentation on cloning given by Mark D. Eibert, Esq., at the annual joint meeting of the San Bernardino County Medical Society, the Riverside County Medical Society, and the San Bernardino County Bar Association, on September 23, 1999. It is being reprinted by the permission of the author, makeup as its parent. In very simple terms, it works like this.

You take an egg, and remove the nucleus, thereby removing nearly all of the egg's DNA or genes. You throw that nucleus away, because you don't need it anymore.

Then, you take a nucleus from a cell belonging to the adult parent. (Ian Wilmut used a mammary cell—that's why he named his sheep "Dolly" after Dolly Parton.)

You insert this cell nucleus into the egg, either by fusing the adult cell with the enucleated egg, or by a more sophisticated nuclear transfer.

You then stimulate the reconstructed egg, either electrically or chemically, to trick it into behaving like a fertilized egg—into dividing and becoming an embryo. The embryo is then cultured, and when it reaches the appropriate stage, you transfer it to the uterus of a surrogate mother. There it follows the usual course of any embryo. It becomes a fetus, gestates for the usual time, and is then born in the usual way, looking and acting just like any other newborn of its species. That's how Dolly the sheep was created.

Today Dolly is a normal, healthy sheep, who has had four lambs of her own, one single lamb followed by a set of triplets, all the result of ordinary sexual reproduction.

Now you may have heard that Dolly was born already the age of the sheep that she was cloned from—which is six years old. This assertion is based on an experiment that attempted to measure Dolly's "telomeres"—structures within cells that become shorter with each cell division. But that experiment has been widely criticized for technical reasons (it seems that the telomere measurements were within both the margin of error of the study and the normal variation for sheep), and also because on the same day that Ian Wilmut announced the "telomere problem," the company he works for announced that it had found the solution to the problem—a substance called telomerase.

There is a more fundamental reason not to worry about Dolly's telomeres. If Dolly were really born 6 years old, then she was 9 years old when she had her triplets. Since virtually all Poll Dorset sheep are dead by the age of 9, that would make her the "fertile octogenarian" of sheep. I don't think so. Not only does Dolly show no signs of premature aging, she is doing things—like having triplets—that would be impossible if she were prematurely aged. The truth is that Dolly is a healthy young sheep.

Now, I hate to start with badly outdated science, but before I tell you where cloning is today I need to dispel one of the great cloning myths. People seem to almost universally believe that because it took "277 tries" to make Dolly, that means there were 276 miscarriages or deformed or dead lambs along the road to Dolly. The *Washington Post* reported exactly that shortly after Dolly was born, and we've been reading it in the newspapers ever since. But that's not true. What really happened is this:

Dr. Wilmut started with 277 reconstructed eggs—eggs that had their nucleus removed and were then fused with an adult cell. That's what the number 277 refers to.

The eggs were then cultured in sheep oviducts, and of the 277, only 29 divided and became embryos. All 29 embryos were transferred to the uteruses of 13 sheep—some got one, some got two, and some got three.

When Wilmut later performed an ultrasound, he learned that only one of the 13 sheep had become pregnant. That pregnancy proceeded normally and produced Dolly. There were no dead or deformed lambs, no miscarriages, and no discarded embryos in this particular experiment.

More importantly, let's put this in perspective—the perspective of fertility treatments involving in vitro fertilization (IVF).

IVF doctors and the federal government measure the success rate of IVF clinics by the ratio of live births to uterine transfers. IVF with humans began in 1978, but it wasn't until 1990, after 12 years of worldwide human clinical practice, that the average success rate for IVF in humans got to be as good as one live birth out of 13 uterine transfers—the Dolly success rate. (Today the average IVF success rate is about one out of four, but it took 20 years of human clinical practice and research to get it there.)

And in the year Dolly was conceived, 1995, the largest IVF clinic in my area, the San Francisco Bay Area, was creating thirty human embryos for every one that made it to the delivery room, compared with 29 for the Dolly experiment.

The only part of the Dolly experiment that was out of line with IVF success rates of either today or the recent past was the large number of eggs it took. It was very inefficient.

WHERE CLONING TECHNOLOGY IS TODAY (SEPTEMBER 1999)

But the second cloning experiment to be reported in a peer review journal, the cloning of 50 mice in Hawaii, had an efficiency rate (measured by number of eggs per live birth) that was ten times higher than the Dolly experiment['s].

The third published adult cell cloning experiment, using cows in Japan, was seventeen times more efficient than the Dolly experiment in terms of the number of eggs needed to get each live birth. Furthermore, if you go back to the measurement of success that IVF clinics use—live births per uterine transfer—the Japanese transferred two embryos into each of 5 cows and ended up with 8 calves—all five cows gave birth to at least one calf, which is better than any IVF clinic in the world can do today.

And cloning has continued with a variety of other species, like goats and pigs. There are now literally hundreds of animals in the world who were conceived through adult cell cloning.

Most importantly, scientists are already using cloning technology to create cloned human embryos. The first cloned human embryo was created by a pair of IVF doctors at a fertility clinic in South Korea. They used the egg and body cells of an infertile woman patient. Unfortunately, they only allowed the embryo to reach the two-cell stage before stopping the experiment.

In addition, a biotechnology company on the East Coast is currently mass producing cloned human embryos for medical research on stem cells. According to BBC-TV, they are producing them in batches of 600 at a time. They use cow eggs to hold the human DNA, but the cloned embryos they produce are quite human.

I'm not saying that cloning is sufficiently developed and safe enough for human clinical use right now. It probably isn't—not just yet. Nor do I advocate trying it before there is evidence of reasonable safety from animal studies.

What I am saying is that cloning is not nearly as dangerous as the press makes it out to be—in fact, when compared with early IVF success rates, the current success rates with cloning look very promising indeed. I'm also saying that the process is improving very rapidly. And most of the scientists involved in cloning research that I talk to report that their success rates are steadily increasing, and that they're optimistic that improvements in efficiency and safety will continue with more research, just as you would expect with any new treatment—just as occurred with IVF and heart transplants, for example.

In other words, if "safety" is your main argument against cloning, you'd better have a backup, because if the current trend of research continues, that may not be an issue for very much longer.

WHAT CLONING IS NOT—THE "XEROX COPY" MYTH

If you've been watching television and movies and reading popular fiction for the last 30 years, you've learned a lot about cloning. Unfortunately, almost everything you learned about cloning was scientifically false.

For example, in "The Boys From Brazil," starring Gregory Peck as the evil cloning expert Dr. Joseph Mengele, you learned—or thought you learned—that cloning could be used to "replicate" Adolph Hitler, and the Third Reich along with him—unless the good guys could stop him in time. They did stop him, but it was a real cliffhanger.

In less serious movies like "Mulitplicity" with Michael Keaton, you learned—or thought you learned—that "clones" would be "Xerox copies" of the original person, born fully grown and with all the memories and feelings of the original—but if you copied one too many times, it was like making a Xerox of a Xerox of a Xerox, and you might end up with a fuzzy copy, like Michael Keaton number four, the gibbering idiot.

But the problem with these and other cloning fiction is that the whole idea of cloning as copying or replicating people is just plain false. Even the National Bioethics Advisory Commission, which is no friend of cloning, admits that the vision of cloning portrayed by popular fiction is "based on gross misunderstandings of human biology and psychology." Let me explain some of the reasons why.

Yes, children conceived with the aid of cloning technology will be genetic twins—or almost genetic twins—of the person who is the cell donor. But we already have 1.5 million genetic twins walking around the United States. We call them "identical twins" but it would be just as accurate to call them naturally occurring clones.

We know a lot about these natural clones. An entire branch of academia is devoted to the study of identical twins. There is a "Twin Studies" department at Cal State Fullerton, another at the University of Minnesota. Physicians, psychologists, sociologists, people who study family relationships, all just love to study twins. And the one thing we know for sure after decades of research is that so-called identical twins are not identical.

Physically, twins have different fingerprints and different organic brain structures, among many other examples.

Intellectually, twins have different IQs—a recent analysis of 212 separate studies of twins concluded that genes are only responsible for about 48% of a person's IQ.

And of course, twins have different personalities. If you have ever known "identical" twins you know that each member of the pair is a separate and different person. That's why the law and society and everyone who knows twins treat them as unique individuals.

And children conceived with the aid of cloning technology will be even more different from their genetic parents than natural twins are.

Most of their genes will come from the adult cell donor. However, a small percentage of the child's genes will come from the mitochondria of the egg donated for the procedure. This mitochondrial DNA primarily affects how cells process energy. Thus, the child will have almost—but not quite—the same genes as the adult cell donor.

The child will grow in a different uterus. Uterine environment has an enormous impact on many different aspects of fetal development. That's why doctors tell you not to smoke and drink during pregnancy, for example.

Most importantly, these children will be born into different families, have different parents and siblings, go to different schools, have different friends, have different experiences from the day they are born, be raised in a different culture—surfing the Web rather than watching "Leave It to Beaver" after school, for example. The nurture part of the "nature versus nurture" equation will be completely different.

But even that's not all.

I have a beautiful calico cat named Tribble. What if I used cloning technology to give Tribble kittens—what would they look like?

Interestingly, they would not look like Tribble. Like all calicos, Tribble has patches and splotches of different colored fur—black, orange and white. If I cloned Tribble, the kitten would also have patches of different colored fur—but they wouldn't be the same size or shape or location as they are on Tribble. Where Tribble has a mostly black back with a few patches of orange fur, her cloned kitten might have a mostly orange back with patches of black. Instead of a face that was half black and half orange, like Tribble, the cloned kitten's face might be all one color. And so on.

The reason for that is a phenomenon known as "random inactivation of the X chromosome."

Chromosomes are structures that carry genes. The X chromosome of a cat, for example, has about 5,000 genes on it. Male mammals—human and tomcats—have one X chromosome and one Y chromosome. Female humans and cats have two X chromosomes—they inherited one from their mother and the other from their father, so the genes on the two X chromosomes are all different.

What happens when you have two sets of blueprints for the same 5,000 genetic traits in the same mammal? Which one gets used? Well, nature decides in a very fair way. Randomly. In every cell in Tribble's body, one of the two X chromosomes is switched off. And which of the two is switched off—the one from mom or the one from dad—is completely random.

What genes are on the X chromosome? Well in cats, the genes that determine fur color are among those located on the X chromosome. The reason that the patches and splotches of color on a calico's coat look random is because they are random, thanks to random inactivation of the X chromosome. In other words, you can make a million clones of Tribble, and not one of them will look exactly like Tribble, or exactly like any of the other Tribble clones. Although it wouldn't be as visual and dramatic, the same principle would apply to humans.

A related concept, called gene expression, would also apply equally to male and female "clones."

Basically, two identical twins could have the same gene, but they might express that genetic trait differently—or one might not express it at all. That's because whether and how a specific genetic trait or characteristic is expressed depends on very complex interactions both among genes and between genes and the environment. People who have all the same genes can and do turn out differently, even with respect to genetic traits.

In other words, every "clone" is different.

My final example is Chang and Eng Bunker. They were the original "Siamese Twins," what we now call conjoined twins. They were joined at the chest, and they shared one liver between them.

Chang and Eng were identical twins, with identical nuclear and mitochondrial DNA. They grew in the same uterine environment. They were born at the same moment. That had the same parents and family. And from the moment they were born, they had as close to the same experiences—as close to the same nurture in the nature versus nurture sense—as any two humans could possibly have. When they got married, they even married sisters.

In spite of all that, Chang and Eng turned out to have radically different personalities.

Chang was an alcoholic, a moody introvert who hated people and was verbally and physically abusive.

Eng was a lifelong teetotaler, an extrovert who loved parties and children and was generally liked by everyone who knew him—everyone who could stand being around Chang long enough to get to know him.

But enough examples. The point I'm trying to make is this: anybody who thinks their child conceived through cloning technology is going to be a little copy of himself is going to be hugely disappointed. You can't copy or replicate a human. That is scientifically impossible, even with cloning.

The truth is this: children conceived with the aid of cloning technology will be ordinary children who will grow up to be unique individuals, just like everyone else.

Once you understand that scientific fact, over 90 percent of the arguments—including most of the "ethical" arguments—against human cloning evaporate like fog when the sun comes up.

Of course you can't replicate Hitler, or an army of Arnold Schwarzenegger soldiers, or a factory full of compliant zombie workers. Cloning by itself has no more potential to do those things that IVF does.

Nor are the children going to be burdened or restricted by how they were conceived. These children will not be freaks leading second-hand lives; they will be unique individuals who have as much of an open future as anyone does. And there is no scientifically valid reason for these children to think of themselves as mere copies, or to be treated like copies by anyone else, or to be psychologically harmed by such an absurd thought.

MEDICAL USES OF CLONING

Now we're ready to answer the next question: who in their right mind would want to be "cloned"?

Now that you understand that cloning has nothing to do with copying people, you can eliminate dictators, narcissists, megalomaniacs, ruthless employers, people who want to bring Hitler or Christ or Elvis back to life, and so on. There's nothing in cloning for them. People like that will find cloning totally useless.

The only thing cloning is really good for is building families, families composed of genetically related but unique individuals—a lot like the families we have now.

And the largest group of people who would be interested in that, once the technology is reasonably safe, is infertile people. About 10 to 15 percent of the population is infertile—physically unable to have children.

Medically, infertility is classified as a disease, according to the American Society for Reproductive Medicine and the American College of Obstetricians and Gynecologists.

Legally, infertility is a disability—the kind that entitles people to protection from discrimination under the Americans with Disabilities Act. That's based on both a recent U.S. Supreme Court case called *Bragdon* v. *Abbott* and on a recent decision of the EEOC in New York.

Psychologically, infertility is a devastating condition. It frustrates a basic and very powerful biological drive, one that is an intimate part of the will to survive. One analogy that you hear over and over again from infertile people is that learning that you are incurably infertile is not like having your child die. It's like having all your children die, and all your grandchildren as well. Infertile people are so motivated to find a cure that many of them spend year after year undergoing painful and expensive treatments that are not covered by health insurance and that, for many of them, have a very low chance of success.

Now everybody knows that in vitro fertilization (IVF) is one way that infertility is treated. The first so-called "test-tube baby," Louise Brown, was born in 1978. She's a college student now.

But IVF doesn't work for everyone. For a 21-year-old woman who's infertile because of blocked fallopian tubes, IVF will probably be a miracle cure. But for a woman who can't produce viable eggs or a man who can't produce viable sperm, IVF isn't much help. To get a good embryo out of the dish, you have to put good ingredients into the dish. There are literally millions of women who can't produce viable eggs no matter how big a dose of infertility drugs you give them—that's why they're infertile.

What makes cloning so revolutionary as an infertility treatment is that it does not require the patient to produce viable eggs or viable sperm. If they can spare a few cells scraped from inside of their cheeks, they can have genetically related children.

Now for a little historical footnote: twenty years ago, when the idea of IVF was first being discussed, most people had a strong visceral reaction against the idea of "manufacturing babies in test tubes." At first they thought it was weird and disgusting and it reminded them of "Frankenstein." And there was a debate about whether so-called "test-tube babies" should be outlawed.

All the same arguments now used against cloning were used against IVF. IVF would be "unsafe," the babies would be born deformed or with birth defects, they would be psychologically harmed when they found out that they were only "test-tube babies" rather than "real" babies, family structures and relationships would be radically altered, and so on. Part of the reason the arguments were the same is that the people making them were the same—some of the current leaders of the anti-cloning movement were also leaders of the movement to outlaw IVF 20 years ago. And before Louise Brown was born, 85 percent of the American public agreed with them and thought that IVF should be outlawed, which is about the same percentage that think cloning should be outlawed today. If you know your history, this cloning debate is just what Yogi Berra called "deja vu all over again."

But then along came Louise Brown, the world's first "test-tube baby," whose face graced the front pages of almost every newspaper in the world for awhile. People looked at those pictures and said "that just looks like an ordinary baby, ten fingers, ten toes, mom is grinning from ear to ear—what's so terrible about that?" And the movement to outlaw IVF faded away.

Today it's 21 years later. The public has forgotten its horror and now accepts IVF, which so far has brought children, families and happiness to over 150,000 disabled couples. And we now know that all the arguments against IVF were wrong. The same thing will happen with cloning. And it will happen a lot sooner than most people expect.

The second biggest group of people who will be interested in the use of cloning to create children is people who know, from family history or genetic testing or counseling, that they have a high risk of producing children with serious genetic diseases or defect.

As explained by Dr. Lee Silver in his excellent book "Remaking Eden: Cloning and Beyond in a Brave New World," the vast majority of genetic diseases and defects are caused one of two ways. The first is errors that occur during meiosis, which is part of the process of sexual reproduction. These types of errors cause problems like Down Syndrome.

The second major way to get a serious genetic disease is by inheriting it from a parent who is a carrier. That's how children get born with such serious and often lethal conditions as Tay Sachs disease, sickle cell anemia, cystic fibrosis, hemophilia, and so on—there's a long list of horribles.

Cloning should make all of these kinds of diseases and defects extremely rare, if not impossible. There is no reduction of genetic material in cloning, so there is no opportunity for the kinds of errors that cause Down Syndrome to occur.

And a child conceived with the aid of cloning technology shouldn't get a genetic disease that his genetic parent didn't have—if the parent is a carrier the child will be a carrier too, but he typically won't actually get the disease.

For a lot of people who are at risk of having seriously ill or defective children, cloning technology may soon be a safer way to have children, and a more certain way of having normal, healthy children, than sex is.

So-called "reproductive cloning" isn't the only medical use of the technology. There are also some exciting and important medical uses that don't require the production of whole human beings.

For example, cloning could be used to create embryonic stem cells, which could be used to make tissues, and perhaps even organs, for transplant. Not only would this relieve the serious shortage of tissues and organs for transplant, but if you use cells from the patient who needs the tissue or organ, you could virtually eliminate the danger that the patient's body would reject it. Examples would include creating bone marrow for transplants for leukemia victims, islet cells to return to the pancreas of a diabetic, heart or liver tissue to repair the damage caused by heart attacks or hepatitis, healthy skin for grafts to burn victims, and so on.

Cloning can also be used to create animals that excrete therapeutic human proteins, like insulin, in their milk. You do this by inserting selected human genes into animal embryos during the process of cloning, thereby turning cows into walking drug factories providing an endless supply of cheap and plentiful human medicines. This is already being done.

Cloning may even help to find a cure for cancer by teaching us how to reprogram cells. Cancer cells grow uncontrollably; perhaps they could be reprogrammed.

These are just a few examples of the many exciting medical breakthroughs that should be possible with cloning technology.

CLONING AND THE CONSTITUTION—THE STATE OF THE LAW

Now let's talk about law. What is the current state of the law about human cloning?

First of all, by Executive Order signed by President Clinton, you can't use federal funds for human cloning research. But since there's already a ban on the use of federal funds for embryo research, that doesn't add very much—it was a purely political gesture.

Beyond that, human cloning is currently illegal in three—and only three—states.

California is one of the three, with a moratorium that automatically expires after five years (about 3 years from now) on using cloning to create a child. In the meantime, the penalty for using cloning to create a child in California is a fine of up to $1 million for an organization and $250,000 for an individual—it's not at all clear that the fine wouldn't apply to the patient as well as the doctors involved—and the doctor could lose his medical license. Rhode Island has a similar law, also with a five-year sunset clause. Michigan has an even more radical law, which permanently outlaws not just the conception of children, but also the creation of cloned embryos for laboratory research on, say, curing diseases. The penalty is up to 10 years in prison, and that applies whether you are a laboratory researcher trying to cure cancer, a doctor helping an infertile patient, or an infertile woman who uses cloning to have children.

Human cloning is legal in the other 47 states. It's also legal in most countries, Western Europe being the major exception.

And there is no federal law on cloning. Last year, Congress debated various anti-cloning bills, but they got bogged down in a debate over abortion and couldn't agree on a law. The Republicans wanted a Michigan-style law forbidding the creation of all cloned human embryos. The Democrats filibustered that because it would end almost all cloning research and prevent the technology from being used for all the important non-reproductive medical purposes I mentioned. They proposed a law more like California's, but the Republicans wouldn't go along with it because they thought it was the moral equivalent of abortion—"clone then kill" they called it. Of course, both sides wanted to outlaw "clone then love," but because they couldn't agree on the "clone then kill" issue they fought themselves to a standstill and no law got passed. And now it seems very unlikely that they will be able to agree on a federal law anytime in the foreseeable future.

The last piece to the legal puzzle is kind of confusing. When it became clear that Congress couldn't agree on a law, the Food and Drug Administration announced that it had authority to regulate cloning. Not to ban it exactly, but to make researchers go through a lot of hoops to prove to the FDA that cloning is safe and effective before they use it on patients.

What's confusing is that nothing in the Food, Drug and Cosmetics Act or any other piece of relevant legislation gives the FDA jurisdiction over cloning or anything that could even arguably include cloning. As most doctors know, the FDA has no authority to regulate the practice of medicine, and as one of the most vehemently anti-cloning members of Congress (Rep. Ron Ehlers) put it, "it's hard to argue that a cloning procedure is a drug." Moreover, the FDA has for years totally ignored reproductive medicine, including procedures like ICSI and cytoplasm transfer that have a lot in common with cloning.

So far, I have yet to find a lawyer on either side of this debate who thinks the FDA really has statutory authority to regulate cloning, and when I called the FDA myself to find out what statute they were relying on, even they couldn't tell me.

So that's the state of the law. Human cloning is legal in 47 out of 50 states, and in about 175 of 200 countries, and the FDA may or may not be able to enforce safety and efficacy standards. The courts will have to decide that.

CONSTITUTIONAL RIGHTS: REPRODUCTIVE FREEDOM

What I personally find most interesting about this topic is the profound questions raised by anti-cloning laws.

Can the state really ban cloning? I'm going to suggest that under current constitutional principles, it probably cannot.

Let's start with a few highlights of the legal arguments of infertile people for whom cloning technology, once it's reasonably safe, will be the only way possible to have biologically related children and families.

Reproductive freedom means a lot more than just the right to an abortion. The Supreme Court has said many times that every American has a constitutional right to have children, and to make all sorts of reproductive decisions without government interference. That right stems from the constitutional right to privacy, because reproductive decisions are some of the most private and personal and life-changing decisions an individual can make.

The statement that is quoted over and over again in cases discussing reproductive freedom comes originally from a Supreme Court case about the right to contraception, *Eisenstadt* v. *Baird*. There the Supreme Court said that "if the right of privacy means anything, it is the right of the individual, married or single, to be free from unwarranted governmental intrusion into matters so fundamentally affecting a person as the decision whether to bear or beget a child."

Now, some people argue, "that only applies to sex. People who need high-tech medical help to have children don't have the same right to reproductive freedom that healthy people do." Well there isn't a lot of case law on that yet, but what there is says just opposite.

In 1990, for example, the state of Illinois tried to outlaw a variety of reproductive technologies and tests, some of which were related to IVF and could be used to treat infertility. In a decision that was later affirmed on appeal, a federal district court struck down that law, explaining that "[i]t takes no great leap of logic to see that within the cluster of constitutionally protected choices that includes the right to have access to contraceptives, there must be included within that cluster the right to submit to a medical procedure that may bring about, rather than prevent, pregnancy."

So it looks like you have a constitutional right to high-tech baby-making too, at least if you're infertile. And notice the progression. In 1978, 85 percent of the American people thought "test-tube babies" were terrible and ought to be outlawed. Just 12 years later, in 1990, courts were starting to rule that IVF was a constitutional right. But the right to privacy isn't the only constitutional principle that protects people from government interference with their reproductive decisions. There's also equal protection—the principle that you can't deny basic rights to some people and not to others without a very good reason.

In 1942, for example, the state of Oklahoma had a law requiring the sterilization of convicted criminals. It was a eugenics law, based on the idea that criminal tendencies could be passed down genetically to children.

The Supreme Court analyzed the case under the equal protection clause of the Fourteenth Amendment, and unanimously ruled that "procreation involves one of the fundamental rights of man" and that even a convicted criminal who is sterilized "is forever deprived of a basic liberty."

Because the Oklahoma law affected a fundamental constitutional right—which the Supreme Court described as the "right to have offspring"—the court applied what is known as "strict scrutiny." That means that the Supreme Court placed the burden of proof on Oklahoma to justify its discriminatory law. And strict scrutiny is the highest and toughest burden of proof there is. The state couldn't carry that burden, so the Supreme Court struck the law down. There are a number of other more recent cases that reaffirm that having children is a fundamental right and that laws that interfere with that right are subject to strict scrutiny.

This is my favorite reproductive freedom case because it means that sometime soon—certainly before the current anti-cloning law sunsets—lawyers for the state of California will have to explain to a court, under a strict scrutiny standard, why legally disabled citizens should have less of a right to have children and families than convicted rapists and child molesters do.

Now it's time for a second historical footnote, a legal one this time.

The case I just told you about struck down a state "eugenics law." Oklahoma was just one of 36 American states that passed eugenics laws in the early part of this century. Those laws required the sterilization of people who were thought likely to produce seriously defective children. People with leprosy and other dread diseases, mentally retarded people, mentally ill people, habitual criminals and others were sterilized, mostly because the best science of their day said that such people would probably produce children with the same defects.

Supporters of eugenics laws argued that they were necessary to protect the safety and welfare of children. It was said to be in the best interests of children who might be born with defects that they never be born at all. It wasn't until the Vietnam war that our military came up with an accurate characterization of this brand of logic—it's called "destroying the village in order to save it."

The most successful—if you want to call it that—state eugenics law was California's. During the early part of this century, our state government rendered more than 30,000 of its sick and disabled citizens unable to have children. So when the Nazis were drafting their own eugenics law, they modeled it in part on the eugenics law that came out of Sacramento.

But during World War II, Americans got a graphic demonstration of what politicians could do when given the power to decide who was and was not "perfect" enough to be born, and attitudes about eugenics began to change. By the 1960s almost all of our state eugenics laws had either been repealed, struck down as unconstitutional, or fallen into disuse, and states got out of the business of regulating their citizens' reproduction.

Until now. Two years ago, California passed the first anti-cloning law in the nation. Once again, the state of California has singled out a class of disabled Californians and forbidden them by law to have children. Once again, the state has defined a class of children that it says are so likely to be born "imperfect" that the state won't allow them to be born or to live at all. Once again, California has a reproductive police charged with stopping unauthorized breeding by California citizens. Once again, the politicians in Sacramento have a chance to play God. And once again California has a eugenics law.

What our legislature has done is radical all right, but it's not unprecedented. We've been here before.

SCIENTIFIC FREEDOM AND THE FIRST AMENDMENT

Reproductive freedom isn't the only constitutional value that anti-cloning laws infringe on.

For instance, there's a lot of Supreme Court dictum to suggest that scientific freedom might have some constitutional protection, and some lower courts and about a million legal scholars have said that scientific freedom does or should have constitutional protection. That protection is based on the First Amendment right to free speech. In science, it's not enough to argue for your theory, or to publish your theory. You and others —including those who disagree with you—have to be able to test your theory through experimentation. That's how science works and how it finds the truth.

Now the Supreme Court hasn't directly addressed that question yet. But cloning may not be such a bad case to try to determine the extent of constitutional protection for science. After all, as one member of the National Bioethics Advisory Commission observed, anti-cloning laws like California's moratorium are the first time in American history that an entire field of medical research has been outlawed. That's a very radical thing to do. And in Michigan today, a scientist who clones cells in a dish to try to find a cure for cancer can get up to 10 years in prison—that's even more radical. In Michigan, the ACLU is considering challenging their anti-cloning law on both scientific freedom and reproductive freedom grounds, and perhaps we will get some new case law on scientific freedom as well.

THE REAL QUESTION

Now I want to conclude by telling you that I think there is only one question of lasting social significance that cloning presents to us. That question is this: Who decides?

Who should decide whether and how a particular individual can have children—the individual, or the government?

Who should decide which classes of children are likely to be perfect enough, or happy enough, or socially desirable enough, or politically popular enough, to be born—the prospective parents or the politicians?

Who should decide which treatment is medically best for a particular patient, the physician acting with the informed consent of his patient, or the bureaucrat? Aren't doctors regulated enough already? Do they really need to have the reproductive police looking over their shoulder along with everyone else?

Who should decide how much risk is acceptable for a prospective mother and her unborn child, the mother, with the advice of her physician, or the legislature, making one risk-benefit calculation for all patients at all times, no matter what their personal medical condition is, no matter what their personal religious and moral beliefs may be, and no matter how the technology may have changed during the three or five years since the politician last debated appropriate treatment protocols? You know, for 200 years American women have been free to make decisions that pose much greater risks to their unborn children than cloning possibly could.

And who should decide what subjects scientists can investigate, or what truths the general public is ready for them to uncover—the scientist or the platform committees at political conventions?

If the word "copy" is the scientific fallacy of the anti-cloning argument, the word "we" is the legal fallacy. The opponents of cloning are always wringing their hands and asking what should "we" do about cloning, and whether "we" should allow it. But "we" don't decide whether John and Mary Smith can have children, they do. That's a private decision, not a political one. And I don't think there is anything so horrible or horrifying about twins that would justify changing that.

This question—"who decides"—is the real heart of the cloning debate. And the Constitution, supported by over 200 years of American tradition and culture, permits only one answer.

EVEN IF IT WORKED, CLONING WOULDN'T BRING HER BACK

Thomas H. Murray

Eleven days ago, as I awaited my turn to testify at a congressional hearing on human reproductive cloning, one of five scientists on the witness list took the microphone. Brigitte Boisselier, a chemist working with couples who want to use cloning techniques to create babies, read aloud a letter from "a father, (Dada)." The writer, who had unexpectedly become

Reprinted with permission from *The Washington Post*, April 8, 2001.

a parent in his late thirties, describes his despair over his 11-month-old son's death after heart surgery and 17 days of "misery and struggle." The room was quiet as Boisselier read the man's words: "I decided then and there that I would never give up on my child. I would never stop until I could give his DNA—his genetic make-up—a chance.

I listened to the letter writer's refusal to accept the finality of death, to his wish to allow his son another opportunity at life through cloning, and I was struck by the futility and danger of such thinking. I had been asked to testify as someone who has been writing and teaching about ethical issues in medicine and science for more than 20 years; but I am also a grieving parent. My 20-year-old daughter's murder, just five months ago, has agonizingly reinforced what I have for years argued as an ethicist: Cloning can neither change the fact of death nor deflect the pain of grief.

Only four years have passed since the birth of the first cloned mammal—Dolly the sheep—was announced and the possibility of human cloning became real. Once a staple of science fiction, cloning was now the stuff of scientific research. A presidential commission, of which I am a member, began to deliberate the ethics of human cloning; scientists disavowed any interest in trying to clone people; and Congress held hearings but passed no laws. A moratorium took hold, stable except for the occasional eruption of self-proclaimed would-be cloners such as Chicago-based physicist Richard Seed and a group led by a man named Rael who claims that we are all clones of alien ancestors.

Recently, Boisselier, Rael's chief scientist, and Panos Zavos, an infertility specialist in Kentucky, won overnight attention when they proclaimed that they would indeed create a human clone in the near future. The prospect that renegade scientists might try to clone humans reignited the concern of lawmakers, which led to the recent hearings before the House Energy and Commerce subcommittee on oversight and investigations.

Cloning advocates have had a difficult time coming up with persuasive ethical arguments. Indulging narcissism—so that someone can create many Mini-Me's—fails to generate much support for their cause. Others make the case that adults should have the right to use any means possible to have the child they want. Their liberty trumps everything else; the child's welfare barely registers, except to avoid a life that would be worse than never being born, a standard akin to dividing by zero—no meaningful answer is possible. The strategy that has been the most effective has been to play the sympathy card—and who evokes more sympathy than someone who has lost a child?

Sadly, I'm in a position to correct some of these misunderstandings. I'm not suggesting that my situation is the same as that of the letter's author. Not better. Not worse. Simply different. His son was with him for less than a year, our daughter for 20; his son died of disease in a hospital; Emily, daughter to Cynthia and me, sister to Kate and Matt, Nicky and Pete, was reported missing from her college campus in early November. Her body was found more than five weeks later. She had been abducted and shot.

As I write those words, I still want to believe they are about someone else, a story on the 11 o'clock news. Cynthia and I often ask each other, how can this be our life? But it is our life and Emily, as a physical, exuberant, loving presence, is not in the same way a part of it anymore. Death changes things and, I suspect, the death of a child causes more wrenching grief than any other death. So I am told; so my experience confirms.

I want to speak, then, to the author of that letter, father to father, grieving parent to grieving parent; and to anyone clinging to unfounded hope that cloning can somehow repair the arbitrariness of disease, unhappiness and death. I have nothing to sell you, I don't want your money, and I certainly don't want to be cruel. But there are hard truths here that some people, whether through ignorance or self-interest, are obscuring.

The first truth is that cloning does not result in healthy, normal offspring. The two scientific experts on animal cloning who shared the panel with Boisselier reported the results of the cattle, mice and other mammals cloned thus far: They have suffered staggering rates of abnormalities and death; some of the females bearing them have been injured and some have died. Rudolf Jaenisch, an expert on mouse cloning at MIT's Whitehead Institute for Biomedical Research, told the subcommittee that he did not believe there was a single healthy cloned mammal in existence—not even Dolly, the sheep that started it all, who is abnormally obese.

Scientists do not know why cloning fails so miserably. One plausible explanation begins with what we already know—that as the cells of an embryo divide and begin to transform into the many varieties of tissue that make up our bodies, most of the genes in each cell are shut down, leaving active only those that the cell needs to perform its specific role. A pancreatic islet cell, for example, needs working versions of the genes that recognize when a person needs the hormone insulin, then cobble it together and shunt it into the bloodstream. All of that individual's other genetic information is in that islet cell, but most of it is chemically locked, like an illegally parked car immobilized by a tire boot.

To make a healthy clone, scientists need to unlock every last one of those tire boots in the cell that is to be cloned. It is not enough to have the genes for islet cells; every gene will be needed sometime, somewhere. Unless and until scientists puzzle out how to restore all the genes to their original state, we will continue to see dead, dying and deformed clones.

You do not need to be a professional bioethicist, then, to see that trying to make a child by cloning, at this stage in the technology, would be a gross violation of international standards protecting people from overreaching scientists, a blatant example of immoral human experimentation.

Some scientists claim they can avoid these problems. Zavos, who spoke at the hearing, has promised to screen embryos and implant only healthy ones. But Zavos failed to give a single plausible reason to believe that he can distinguish healthy from unhealthy cloned embryos.

Now for the second truth: Even if cloning produced a healthy embryo, the result would not be the same person as the one whose genetic material was used. Each of us is a complex amalgam of luck, experience and heredity. Where in the womb an embryo burrows, what its mother eats or drinks, what stresses she endures, her age—all these factors shape the developing fetus. The genes themselves conduct an intricately choreographed dance, turning on and off, instructing other genes to do the same in response to their interior rhythms and to the pulses of the world outside. How we become who we are remains a mystery.

About the only thing we can be certain of is that we are much more than the sum of our genes. As I said in my testimony, perhaps the best way to extinguish the enthusiasm for human cloning would be to clone Michael Jordan. Michael II might well have no interest in playing basketball but instead long to become an accountant. What makes Michael I great is not merely his physical gifts, but his competitive fire, his determination, his fierce will to win.

Yet another hard truth: Creating a child to stand in for another—dead—child is unfair. No child should have to bear the oppressive expectation that he or she will live out the life denied to his or her idealized genetic avatar. Parents may joke about their specific plans for their children; I suspect their children find such plans less amusing. Of course, we should have expectations for our children: that they be considerate, honest, diligent, fair and more. But we cannot dictate their temperament, talents or interest. Cloning a child to be a reincarnation of someone else is a grotesque, fun-house mirror distortion of parental expectations.

Which brings me to the final hard truth: There is no real escape from grief.

Cynthia and I have fantasized about time running backward so that we could undo Emily's murder. We would give our limbs, our organs, our lives to bring her back, to give her the opportunity to live out her dream of becoming an Episcopal priest, of retiring as a mesmerizing old woman sitting on her porch on Cape Cod, surrounded by her grandchildren and poodles.

But trying to recreate Emily from her DNA would be chasing an illusion. Massive waves of sorrow knock us down, breathless; we must learn to live with them. When our strength returns we stagger to our feet, summon whatever will we can, and do what needs to be done. Most of all we try to hold each other up. We can no more wish our grief away than King Canute could stem the ocean's tide.

So I find myself wanting to say to the letter writer, and to the scientists who offer him and other sorrowing families false hope: There are no technological fixes for grief; cloning your dear dead son will not repair the jagged hole ripped out of the tapestry of your life. Your letter fills me with sadness for you and you wife, not just for the loss of your child but also for the fruitless quest to quench your grief in a genetic replica of the son you lost.

It would be fruitless even—especially—if you succeeded in creating a healthy biological duplicate. But there is little chance of that.

Emily lived until a few months shy of her 21st birthday. In those years our lives became interwoven in ways so intricate that I struggle for words to describe how Cynthia and I now feel. We were fortunate to have her with us long enough to see her become her own person, to love her wholeheartedly and to know beyond question that she loved us. Her loss changes us forever. Life flows in one direction; science cannot reverse the stream or reincarnate the dead.

The Emily we knew and loved would want us to continue to do what matters in our lives, to love each other, to do good work, to find meaning. Not to forget her, ever: We are incapable of that. Why would we want to? She was a luminous presence in our family, an extraordinary friend, a promising young philosopher. And we honor her by keeping her memory vibrant, not by trying to manufacture a genetic facsimile. And that thought makes me address the letter's author once more: I have to think that your son, were he able to tell you, would wish for you the same.

RESPECT FOR HUMAN EMBRYOS

Bonnie Steinbock

How ought we to think about human embryos? Are they due the respect owed to any human person? Do they have the same human rights? These questions are crucial to diverse topics, from abortion and contraception (because some forms of contraception, such as the intrauterine device, work by preventing implantation of a very early embryo) to embryo research, assisted reproductive technology (ART), and germ-line genetic manipulation, in which early embryos are genetically changed, without, it hardly needs to be said, their consent, informed or otherwise. . . . Most recently, the topic of stem cell research has raised the question of the moral status of embryos, since a promising source of stem cells is embryos either left over from fertility treatment or created for the purpose of deriving stem cells.

. . . What are the implications of the interest view for areas like assisted reproductive technology, embryo research, germ-line engineering, and cloning? In particular, does the interest view imply that it is morally permissible to do anything you like to embryos? Or are there limits to the ways in which embryos may be treated? In particular, can we make sense of the idea of having respect for embryos if we deny that they have interests, rights, and moral status?

The view that embryo research, while acceptable in principle, should nevertheless be restricted to demonstrate "profound respect" for embryos as a form of human life has been taken by several important official bodies, including the Ethics Advisory Board (EAB) in the United States and the Warnock Committee in Great Britain. This was also the position taken in 1994 by the Human Embryo Research Panel of the National Institutes of Health (NIH) in its report on the ex utero preimplantation embryo. It concluded that the preimplantation embryo "deserves special respect" and "serious moral consideration as a developing form of human life."

Giving meaning to this concept of "special respect" or "serious moral consideration," however, remains problematic. As John Robertson[1] incisively describes the difficulty: "If the embryo has no rights or interest, how can it be owed 'special respect'? On the other hand, if the embryo is owed special

Reprinted with permission from Paul Lauritzen, ed., *Cloning and the Future of Human Embryo Research* (New York: Oxford University Press, 2001), pp. 21–33.

Editor's note: Most footnotes have been deleted. Students who want to follow up on sources should consult the original article.

respect, is it not then a holder of rights, including the right not to be the subject of research? What does 'special respect' mean?"

Unless we can give a convincing account of "special respect," the suspicion will remain in many minds that this phrase merely allows us to kill embryos and not feel so bad about it.

If giving embryos "serious moral consideration" meant taking seriously their interests or advancing their welfare, then it would be impossible to show them serious moral consideration because, on the view I have been advancing (the interest view), embryos do not have interests or a welfare of their own.

There is another sense of showing "serious moral consideration," however, which does not imply that the entity in question has interests or rights or a welfare of its own. Consider, for example, a proposal to build a shopping center or a baseball field on a sacred burial ground. Most people would find this morally offensive, not because the piece of land is harmed or wronged by this usage (which is absurd) or even because the bodies buried there would be harmed or wronged. Rather, the wrongness is explained by saying that the interest served by building a shopping center or baseball field—that is, commercial and entertainment purpose—are insufficiently important to justify the destruction of a place that has solemn religious significance.

It might be objected that it is wrong to say, in advance, that commercial or entertainment purposes are inevitably "trumped" by things that have religious significance. After all, a shopping center may employ hundreds of people and contribute significantly to their welfare and the welfare of the community. Why should we think that this is less important than preserving burial grounds, however sacred they may be to some?

I readily concede that economic interests may be pressing and, indeed, more important than religious interests. Insofar as the conflict is between two sets of interests, there is no guarantee that one set of interests will prevail. The point of the example of a burial ground is not that symbolic or religious significance is always more important than other kinds of interests. Rather, it is intended to show that things that lack moral status can nevertheless have moral value. It makes no sense to talk about the interest or rights of a burial ground, but perfectly good sense to talk about its moral significance, which stems from its connection with a value that is clearly moral, namely, respect for the dead.

Respect for the dead is a moral value in virtually every culture. It seems likely that it is also what Ronald Dworkin[2] calls an *intrinsic* value. That is, the value of respecting the dead is independent of what people happen to enjoy or want or need or of what is good for them. Dworkin suggests that great paintings, wilderness areas, human cultures, languages, some species, traditional crafts, and human life itself all have intrinsic value. Respect for the dead also seems to fall into this category. If a culture lacked respect for its dead (had no death rituals, for example) we would probably regard it as considerably less evolved, even not quite human. As Feinberg[3] explains:

> It would be wrong, for example, to hack up Grandfather's body after he has died a natural death, and dispose of his remains in the trash can on a cold winter's morning. That would be wrong not because it violates Grandfather's rights; he is dead and no longer has the same sort of rights as the rest of us, and we can make it part of the example that he was not offended while alive at the thought of such posthumous treatment and indeed even consented to it in advance. Somehow acts of this kind if not forbidden would strike at our respect for living human persons (without which organized society would be impossible) in the most keenly threatening way.

Just as disrespect for dead bodies can strike at our respect for living human persons, so, too, I want to suggest, an inappropriate treatment or use of embryos. Embryos, as much as dead bodies, are a "potent symbol of human life"[4] and for that reason have moral value and deserve respect, even though they lack interests, rights, and (therefore) moral status. Let us consider the implications of this for research and disposition of frozen embryos.

Respect for embryos as a form of human life does not rule out using embryos in important medical research, for example, in reproductive medicine, genetics, or cancer and other diseases, as these are endeavors with the potential for enormous human benefit. What would be impermissible is frivolous or trivial research on human embryos, such as using embryos to teach high school science classes, to test the safety of new cosmetics,[5] or to create jewelry. These are situations in which there is no pressing need to use human embryos, and their use displays contempt rather than respect for human life.

Daniel Callahan has charged that the NIH Human Embryo Research Panel, while paying lip service to the idea of respect for embryos, failed to support this with a clear demonstration that progress in scientific research depends on using human embryos. Instead, its members simply gave a blank check to scientific research. He writes:

> Duly reverential, the panel satisfied itself with simply listing all the research possibilities, including the improvement and increased safety of IVF, the creation of cell lines that might someday be useful for bone marrow transplantation, repair of spinal cord injuries, skin replacement and, naturally, the hint of a greater understanding of cancer.[6]

Callahan thinks that more skepticism was called for, including a more thorough examination of the ways in which knowledge might be gained without using human embryos.

Callahan's point, I take it, is not that respect for embryos entails that they never be destroyed or used in research. Rather, it is that the interests or goals to be accomplished by using human embryos in research must be shown to be compelling and unreachable by other means. For if any purposes can justify the destruction of embryos, in what sense are they being shown "profound respect"? The very idea appears hollow.

Although Callahan's point is a good one, it is surely too stringent to ask that researchers know what results embryo research will yield before the research is done. A lot of research is promissory in the sense that it is impossible to predict which research will have beneficial results. Advances in reproductive medicine are, however, hard to envisage if researchers are not permitted to use human embryos. In any event, the principle elaborated by the panel is the correct one: that research using human embryos should be limited to research likely to result in significant benefit to people, as only such research demonstrates respect. Callahan would have liked to see more evidence of the benefit and of the fact that this research could not be done without using human embryos. Because the panel was not charged with determining which specific research projects should be permitted or funded, the criticism seems misapplied.

Another area in which the question of respect for embryos occurs is in the disposition of frozen embryos no longer needed or wanted for reproduction by the individuals who created them. Tens of thousands of embryos are steadily accumulating in tanks of liquid nitrogen in the United States alone. Ideally, their progenitors should decide what to do with them, whether, once they are no longer needed for reproduction, they should be discarded, used in research, or donated (if they are still viable) to other couples. Some couples are unwilling to make this decision, however, preferring to keep the embryos frozen indefinitely rather than discard them. In some cases, the clinic loses touch with the gamete donors.

In August 1996, scientists at fertility clinics in Great Britain "reluctantly destroyed several thousand abandoned human embryos"[7] under the Human Fertilization and Embryology Act, which limits storage to 5 years. The destruction of the embryos was greeted with outrage in some quarters; some officials in the Catholic Church referred to the event as "a prenatal massacre."[8] Italian doctors offered to pay to "adopt" the embryos, with the intention of bringing them to Italy to implant them in women there. Some Catholics argued that the embryos be given a proper funeral and others that the embryos be allowed to die naturally.

It seems to me that these attitudes make sense only if one thinks of preimplantation embryos as human persons who deserve the same respect in death as any other person. (Even if one does take this view of pre-embryos, it is hard to imagine how such respect would be shown. How does one give a proper funeral to something smaller than the period at the end of a sentence?) But suppose one does not regard embryos as very tiny human persons, but instead takes the view that, while not persons, they are forms of human life and, as such, deserving of respect. What would be required to show respect for embryos no longer wanted by their progenitors for reproduction? In particular, may they be discarded? It is hard to see why keeping them frozen in perpetuity shows more respect than discarding them or using them in valuable research. Of course, they could be donated to other couples wishing to use them to reproduce. This certainly should be an option for the individuals who created the embryos. To use them in this way without the knowledge or consent of the gamete donors would, however, violate the principles of informed consent and procreative autonomy. This idea was forcefully expressed by Ruth Deech, chairman of the Human Fertilization and Embryology Authority (HFEA). She writes.

> It would not be appropriate to either human dignity or the autonomy of the individual to give these embryos away or use them for research without the informed consent of the parents.
>
> I would not regard letting them perish as a waste of human life as Life [a British antiabortion organization] does, because an embryo is not a little baby in the freezer.[9]

It might be objected that even if preimplantation embryos are not "babies in the freezer," nevertheless their destruction is a waste of human life and that it is intrinsically bad when human life, once begun, is deliberately ended.[10] This could be so even though embryos have no stake in their own existence and cannot be harmed or wronged or deprived of anything if they are discarded, killed, or allowed to die. In response, I suggest that this intrinsic badness is heavily outweighed by the wrongness of using people's embryos for procreative purposes without their consent. Respect for embryos does not justify violating the rights of persons. Respect is demonstrated by placing limits on the uses to which human embryos may be put, not on the methods for disposing of them when such use is no longer possible. . . .

What then are the implications for debates about human cloning of treating early embryos as forms of life that deserve respect? To answer this question, we need to keep in mind that somatic cell nuclear transfer (SCNT) has applications other than creation of human beings. For example, SCNT cloning might provide knowledge about how cells grow, divide, and become specialized, which not only has intrinsic interest but also may have implications for cancer therapies and other disease treatments. Additionally, SCNT cloning might be used to create organs for transplant and skin for burn victims. These applications would involve cloning human cells, but not the cloning of a human being. The report of the National Bioethics Advisory Commission (NBAC)[11] was careful to direct its recommendations for a moratorium only to cloning human beings, not to other kinds of human cloning.

The objections to cloning human beings rest largely on the possibility of harm to them. Although this remains controversial because of an ongoing debate about whether a person can be harmed by a technique on which his or her very existence depends,[12] most people would regard the risk of serious defects in offspring as an obvious reason to ban a technique. Yet, this concern about cloning refers to harm to future persons and has nothing to do with respect for embryos.

Some critics argue that the very idea of creating a human clone reflects narcissism, obsession with control, loss of the capacity for awe, and "Frankensteinian hubris."[13] Like respect for dead bodies and human embryos, these are symbolic concerns, ones about which reasonable people can differ. Is creating a child by cloning necessarily any more narcissistic than ordinary reproduction? Would developing cloning reflect hubris any more than any other novel branch of medicine? These questions are no less important for being extremely difficult to answer, perhaps being unanswerable. Even if we agree that human embryos deserve respect, we may not be able to come to consensus on the appropriate ways of showing that respect or on how to balance the good of scientific and medial research, or the reproductive interests of individuals, against that respect. Our only hope is to continue to formulate, as precisely as possible, our views on these symbolic, intangible issues and to listen carefully to those who have opposing views.

NOTES

1. John A. Robertson, "Symbolic Issues in Embryo Research," *Hastings Center Report* 25, no. 1 (1995): 37–38.
2. Ronald Dworkin, *Life's Dominion* (New York: Knopf, 1993), pp. 71–84.
3. Joel Feinberg, *Freedom and Fulfillment*, (Princeton University Press, 1992), p. 53.
4. Robertson, "Symbolic Issues in Embryo Research," p. 37.
5. *Ibid.*, p. 38.
6. Daniel Callahan, "The Puzzle of Profound Respect," *Hastings Center Report* 25, no. 1 (1995): 39–40.

7. "British Clinics, Obeying Law, End Embryos By Thousands," *New York Times*, August 2, 1996, p. A3.
8. Youssef M. Ibrahim, "Ethical Furor Erupts in Britain: Should Unclaimed Embryos Die?" *New York Times*, August 1, 1996, p. A1.
9. Annabel Ferriman, "2,500 'orphan embryos' to be destroyed within days" *Independent on Sunday*, July 7, 1996, p. 1.
10. See Dworkin, *Life's Dominion*, p. 84.
11. *Cloning Human Beings: Report and Recommendations of the National Bioethics Advisory Commission* (Rockville, MD: National Bioethics Advisory Commission, June 1997).
12. See John Robertson, "Liberty, Identity, and Human Cloning," *Texas Law Review* 76, no. 6 (1998): 1371–456, esp. pp. 1405–09.
13. Leon Kass, "The Wisdom of Repugnance: Why We Should Ban the Cloning of Humans," *The New Republic*, June 2, 1997. Excerpted and reprinted in John D. Arras and Bonnie Steinbock, eds., *Ethical Issues in Modern Medicine*, 5th Ed. (Mountain View, CA: Mayfield Publishing Company, 1998), pp. 496–510.

CREATING EMBRYOS FOR RESEARCH: ON WEIGHING SYMBOLIC COSTS

Maura A. Ryan

Much of the controversy surrounding the release of the report of the Human Embryo Research Panel (HERP) in September 1994 concerned its approval of federal funding for research involving embryos created expressly for experimental use. Critics as diverse as the Ramsey Colloquium and Daniel Callahan joined in accusing the panel of going a step too far; the *Washington Post* pronounced the creation of research embryos "unconscionable" and President Clinton promptly declared his intention to block the appropriation of federal funds for research of this kind.

For those who object to the experimental use of human embryos under any circumstances, there is no point in asking whether it is ethical to create embryos solely for the purpose of experimentation. If it is wrong to use embryos as experimental subjects, it is wrong to create them so that you can use them. If experimentation on human embryos cannot be conducted without violating obligations of informed consent or violating a human life, as theologian Paul Ramsey argued almost 30 years ago, it makes little difference whether we are contemplating the use of "spare" embryos (embryos generated in the course of assisted reproduction) or embryos created expressly for that purpose. If human potential in itself obliges us to act so as to bring it to fruition, any experiment that entails the destruction of early embryos will be immoral.

Alternatively, what if we hold that at least some kinds of embryo research can be justified? Suppose that we agree with the conclusion of the HERP that embryos in the earliest stages of development ought to be respected as a form of potential human life, but that they are not yet persons and that, therefore, at least under some circumstances, experimentation on the preimplantation embryo should be permitted up to the appearance of the primitive streak.

In that case, is there any reason to object to the production of embryos for research use? Are we doing anything different, in a moral sense, when we initiate embryonic life for research use than when we use embryos that exist as by-products of medically assisted reproduction? Does the creation of

Reprinted with permission of the author and publisher from Paul Lauritzen, ed., *Cloning and the Future of Human Embryo Research* (New York: Oxford University Press, 2001).

Editor's note: Many footnotes have been deleted. Students who want to follow up on sources should consult the original article.

research embryos weaken or insult our communal respect for the sanctity of human life or the integrity of human reproduction in some way that in vitro fertilization (IVF) or the experimental use of "spare embryos" does not?

In this chapter, I argue that it is possible to draw a valid distinction between research involving the deliberate creation of embryos and research involving by-products of medically assisted reproduction. I argue, further, that we should find the former deeply troubling even if we accept the latter. My position does not rest on claims about the moral status of the preimplantation embryo or assertions concerning the "rights" of embryos. Rather, I show that the most persuasive argument offered in defense of the deliberate creation of embryos for experimental use neglects fundamental questions concerning the proper or just use of procreative technologies. The power to remove conception from women's bodies is hardly a neutral power. Rather, it is a power that poses material risks to women's health and contains the potential to alter profoundly the practices of reproduction and parenthood. I argue that reproductive interventions are justified only insofar as they serve the goals of responsible and human reproduction: the bringing forth of new life in loving and nurturing relationship. Creating embryos for research is incompatible with the goals that legitimate and should direct reproductive interventions.

I take as my starting point the defense of research embryos offered by Bonnie Steinbock in *Life Before Birth.* Her analysis is useful for at least two reasons. First, Steinbock provides the deep theoretical background for the position taken by the HERP. Here, for example, we see laid out the important distinction between moral status and moral value assumed in the panel's report as well as the justification for marginalizing "symbolic issues" in the development of public policy. Second, and more important, anyone who wishes to object to the creation of research embryos on grounds other than the special moral status of the preimplantation embryo must reckon with the "interest view" Steinbock defends.

If, as Steinbock and the HERP would have us accept, the only serious question is whether the preimplantation embryo is harmed by being brought into existence solely to serve research goals, it is difficult indeed to see how those who hold a developmental view of personhood can offer any rational objection to the use of research embryos. If we want to argue that initiating human embryonic life with the sole intention of producing material for research is morally objectionable even if we accept such a view of personhood, we have to be able to show that there are morally important considerations neglected in the interest view.

Although this chapter is concerned with the conduct of embryo research, the questions it raises have implications for our thinking about reproductive and genetic technologies in general. Debates about human cloning, genetic engineering, and collaborative reproduction turn, in large part, on disagreements about the moral status of the embryo and the limits of procreative liberty. As with embryo research, however, a preoccupation with competing rights and interest, especially in policy debate, obscures crucial questions about the ends we are pursuing in developing and employing reproductive and genetic technologies as well as the means. Whether we are dealing with the deliberate creation of embryos for experimentation or the cloning of a deceased child, narrow assumptions about what is morally important blind us to what we really should be asking: What are we doing when we fertilize in vitro or manipulate genetic material or clone a human being? What is the price and for what ends should we be willing to pay it?

STEINBOCK AND THE INTEREST VIEW

According to Bonnie Steinbock, "We may choose to respect embryos and preconscious fetuses as powerful symbols of human life, but we cannot protect them for their sake (p. 10). It is the failure to acknowledge the distinction between choosing to protect embryos and preconscious fetuses because of what they represent to us and claiming to protect the interests of embryos and preconscious fetuses, argues Steinbock, that accounts for a persistent confusion and inconsistency in our approach to the treatment of the unborn. That we can find the same voices decrying the use of research embryos and insisting on the right to abortion testifies to the fact that we do not have a single or clear sense of what we mean by "respect" for embryonic or fetal life.

It is true that the manipulation or destruction of human embryos awakens deep moral impulses, even in those who wish to remain agnostic on the question of when an embryo or a fetus becomes a person. Protectiveness toward potential human life is a common and reasonable impulse. But there is an important and, in Steinbock's view, frequently neglected difference between acknowledging the moral and social value of human embryos and according embryos moral standing. To have moral standing is to count morally, to be the sort of being whose interests must be considered, whose interest exert a claim on the behavior of others (Steinbock, p. 10). Following Joel Feinberg, Steinbock argues that a "being can have interests only if it can matter to the being what is being done to it . . ." and ". . . if nothing at all can possibly matter to a being, then that being has no interests." Human embryos have the potential to develop into "the kind of being that will have interests," but, lacking conscious awareness, embryos and even presentient fetuses lack interests of their own; that is, they exist—at this stage—as the sort of being "to whom nothing at all can possibly matter. . . ." (p. 15). Because a human embryo or a presentient fetus has no interests, its interests need not, indeed cannot, be taken into account; thus, human embryos and presentient fetuses lack moral status.

In the interest view, sentience is both a necessary and a sufficient condition for moral standing. Only a being that is conscious and aware of its own experience can have a stake in what is or is not done to it. Having interests (and thus moral status) does not, however, depend on a capacity for "higher order consciousness" (e.g., the ability to use language). According to Steinbock, "[s]o long as a being is sentient—that is, capable of experiencing pleasure and pain—it has an interest in not feeling pain, and its interest provides moral agents with *prima facie* reasons for acting" (p. 24). Sentience acts, therefore, as a threshold as well as a dividing line for the interest view: "mere things and nonconscious living things fall below the moral status line; animals and people lie above it."

She grants that there are good reasons to be concerned about what happens to human embryos and fetuses. As potential persons, embryos and fetuses have a symbolic value that precludes, for example, using them in unnecessary experiments or for purely commercial gain (p. 41). In the interest view, however, it does not make sense to talk about moral obligations to avoid harm to or promote the welfare of preconscious or presentient embryos or fetuses or to object to research using preimplantation human embryos on the ground that we are "experimenting on unconsenting human subjects." Embryos do not have moral status. "[I]t is more accurate to acknowledge their importance for us by ascribing to them moral value" (p. 209).

What exactly is the difference between moral status and moral value? As we have seen, to have moral status is to possess interests that exert claims on the behavior of others. To accord moral status is to recognize the interests of a being as morally obligating. When we acknowledge the moral value of an entity, however, we are simply admitting that there are "moral reasons why [that entity] ought to be preserved." We resist the careless destruction of trees or flags or fine art, argues Steinbock, not because protection is in their interests, but because protection is in our interests. In other words, the moral reasons we give for protecting a flowering tree or a Picasso or a national flag have to do not with obligating features of the thing in question but with the symbolic or material value we have conferred on it. In the same way, when Steinbock argues that embryos or presentient fetuses should not be used in frivolous research or for crassly commercial purposes, it is not because to do so violates the interest of the embryo or presentient fetus or causes harm to them but because of the potentially brutalizing effect of such use on society—the possibility of undermining "commonly held fundamental values" such as respect for human life.

It does not follow that embryos and even presentient fetuses should not be used in the conduct of legitimate research or that it is wrong to create embryos expressly for research. We respect the moral or symbolic value of human embryonic life when we "choose to treat the embryo differently than other human tissue" (p. 209). In determining the boundaries of permissible research, however, the moral reasons for pursuing certain kinds of research must be weighed against the moral reasons for deciding not to pursue them. Obviously, support for frivolous or unnecessary research does not weigh very heavily against the importance of fostering cultural attitudes of respect for human life;

neither does simply furthering the financial gain of certain individuals or groups. Yet when we are "likely to be able to use what we learn from [research on human embryos or presentient fetuses] to save many lives and ameliorate many conditions which make life miserable," the reasons for proceeding are far more compelling, in Steinbock's view, than the reasons for not proceeding (p. 209).[1] Whatever the social or symbolic value of the embryo or presentient fetus, it does not outweigh the interests of real persons in access to goods and services they need and desire. Moreover, respect for human life is hardly expressed when embryos or presentient fetuses are protected at the expense of the "vital human interests" of already existing persons.

Steinbock's conclusion is the same whether she is considering the creation of embryos for research purposes or the use of spare embryos. For obvious reasons she rejects arguments for banning the practice based on appeals to the interests of the preimplantation embryo in being brought to viability. She dismisses, as well, "slippery slope" anxieties about the expansion of the practice into routine and invalid research. She grants that the prospect of human embryos being created merely to provide a plentiful and ready source of material for research, no matter what the research, is distasteful. Yet, in the absence of evidence that the practice cannot be regulated effectively, such anxieties are mere conjecture. Invoking "slippery slope" scenarios is rhetorically powerful, but the argument begs the question (p. 210).

Neither is she persuaded by the claim that it is repugnant to treat the preimplantation embryo merely as a means to research ends (p. 211). She rejects the suggestion that there is an important difference between conducting research on embryos that cannot be used for the purpose for which they were created (to establish a pregnancy) and would otherwise be discarded and creating embryos in order to provide material for research.

It is no more repugnant, in the interest view, to create embryos for use in research than to create embryos for use in medically assisted reproduction. It simply makes no sense, according to Steinbock, to argue that having been created merely for research objectifies the preimplantation embryo in a way that being created for implantation does not (p. 210). Embryos and presentient fetuses have no interests. Therefore, they are neither benefited by being brought into existence for the purpose of establishing a pregnancy nor harmed or demeaned by being brought into existence merely to serve research goals. In both cases, embryos are created to serve the purposes of the initiating parties. The only important question, then, is what purposes are legitimate. Surely, argues Steinbock, "saving lives and preventing misery" is no less legitimate than establishing pregnancies.

The argument Steinbock advances is very persuasive. The HERP, through similar logic, overcame (at least in part) the reluctance of panel members to recommend funding for the creation of research embryos. As we will see, however, when we move beyond the narrow issue of whether the preimplantation embryo has interests that can be served or frustrated in embryo research, an additional set of questions emerges: Beyond whether embryos can be harmed is the question of what we are doing when we intervene in the process of reproduction, what we are affirming or denying when we create embryos for research purposes.

WEIGHING THE SYMBOLIC

The debate about acceptable limits to embryo research is often cast as a "fight over symbolic issues."[2] At least for those who agree that fertilized ova and early embryos are not fully persons in a moral sense, the controversy over experimentation on human embryos is about what it means to display respect for embryos not as persons but as potent symbols of human life.

Concerns about the implications of embryo research or cloning on deep symbolic understandings of the sanctity of life or the integrity of human reproduction are quickly dismissed as unimportant or inappropriate for public debate in a pluralistic society into which is admitted only the "objective" language of rights and interests. As Gilbert Meilaender reminds us in *Body, Soul and Bioethics,* however, it is a serious mistake to ignore such concerns as "merely symbolic." Human thought and language is inescapably symbolic. Symbols express and shape the deepest levels of human experience, the most crucial matters of human society. To overlook or dismiss the symbolic is to "cut ourselves off from what is most important in the life of human beings who are, after all, symbol-making animals."[3]

In the case of embryo research or human cloning, overlooking or dismissing the symbolic evades what is really at stake in conflicts over where to draw the line. It is only when we recognize our anxieties about what we are doing when we fertilize human eggs in vitro or reproduce asexually as acknowledgments that we are close to and may be violating, some of the deepest and most basic of human matters—procreation, kinship, marital intimacy—and our unwillingness to pay disrespect to human embryos as a powerful statement of our societal commitment to the value of human life generally that we come to the important questions: What practices, what acceptable harms, are ultimately consistent with such a commitment? What research goals are we willing to sacrifice to sustain it? If we believe that there is some risk on both sides, are we endangering respect for the sanctity of human life more immediately in permitting the creation of embryos for research or in slowing the pace at which we address the needs and wants of existing human beings?

For Steinbock this last question is easily decided in favor of advancing the goals of research. As we have seen, she take it as obvious that we have an interest in opposing frivolous or crassly commercial uses of human embryos, but equally obvious that symbolic commitments to human life ought to give way when embryo research makes it possible "to save many lives and ameliorate many conditions which make life miserable." With a speed reminiscent of John Robertson's treatment of symbolic issues in the defense of reproductive liberty, Steinbock gives the "vital interests of real persons" trump over all other moral considerations. Indeed, so obvious is the importance of embryo research vis-à-vis symbolic commitments to the sanctity of life or the integrity of reproduction to Steinbock that it seems to require no proof. That is, she merely assumes rather than argues for the importance of the information to be gained through embryo research: Possible goals of embryo research include "developing more adequate contraception, determining causes of infertility, investigating the development and potential transformation of moles into malignant tumors, evaluating the effects of teratogens on the early embryo and understanding normal and abnormal cell growth and differentiation." Embryo research "may be particularly valuable for understanding, preventing, and treating cancers, and for studying and treating genetic disease" (p. 204). Given the present state of embryo research and the limits of Steinbock's own professional competence, a certain humility in expressing anticipated benefits is appropriate. Still, because the force of her position depends on convincing us that the human interest to be served by embryo research are compelling enough to override widespread moral and religious anxieties about the production of research embryos, one expects more evidence than she offers.

This very objection was raised by several critics in response to the report of the HERP. Central to the panel's defense of federal funding for embryo research is the claim that withholding public funds or banning the fertilization of oocytes for research purposes impedes research of "great scientific and therapeutic value." As Daniel Callahan points out, however, the report gives us simply a list of research possibilities rather than a substantive argument for proceeding at this time. Although it contains an extensive discussion of the moral status of the preimplantation embryo, there is no discussion of what he calls "the moral status of the proposed research." Although the panel rigorously acknowledges the need to balance the respect owed the preimplantation embryo against the imperatives of research, the report is "utterly silent on how research claims and possibilities should be evaluated for their moral weight and benefit" or what criteria are necessary to establish proportionality. Despite invoking the history of embryo research in the private sector and in countries where federal support exists, the HERP report makes no mention of results achieved or benefits gained.

Sheldon Krimsky and Ruth Hubbard[4] contend that the panel conflates "scientific interest" and "human benefit." There is no question that research into the processes of fertilization, early cell division, implantation, and embryonic development is of immediate scientific interest and that it holds some therapeutic promise (e.g., for improving the safety and efficacy of assisted reproduction). Why assume, however, that advancing the state of procreative technology should be a research priority or that overcoming infertility should lay a serious claim on medical resources and public funds? Why even assume that better technology is the best way to address infertility? Embryo research holds promise for improving techniques in preimplantation genetic diagnosis and developing more adequate methods of contraception. Yet why think that the ability to identify susceptibility to a range of genetic disorders is obviously and transparently beneficial or that introducing more effective artificial contraception obviously serves "vital human interests"?

Of course, a case can be made for the place of medically assisted reproduction in the allocating of health care resources and for research aimed at improving outcomes in reproductive medicine, just as a case can be made for developing safe and effective methods for understanding and addressing genetic disorders or preventing unplanned pregnancies. The claim to be seeking a balance between respect for the human embryo as a potential form of life and the imperatives of research, however, risks being disingenuous, where the importance of the research in question is merely taken for granted and where no serious attention is given to the existence of genuine conflicts between competing and qualitatively different interests. It may be that embryo research will allow us to "save lives and prevent misery." We might come to agree that saving lives and preventing the sorts of misery that can be prevented through embryo research are worth overriding religious and moral reticence about the manipulation and destruction of embryonic life. We might even come to agree that they are important enough to warrant suspending current limits on the use of embryos for research, for example, suspending limits on research after the appearance of the primitive streak. Any argument that treats these conclusions as self-evident, however, begs the question.

Thus, one objection we can raise to the argument in favor of permitting research embryos advanced by Steinbock and reflected in the report of the HERP concerns the sincerity of the commitment to respect for the human embryo and the adequacy of the criteria used in weighing competing values. In addition, Steinbock's distinction between moral status and moral value is problematic. She takes it as obvious that we should find the creation of human embryos for crassly commercial purposes or for use in frivolous research distasteful. Equally distasteful is the prospect of human embryos generated merely to have an ample supply of research material.

It is not at all clear, however, why this should be obvious, particularly why we should find the latter so obviously distasteful. On her own account, there is nothing intrinsically valuable or obligating about the human embryo. Without interests, she argues, a being "can have no claim to our moral attention and concern" (p. 68). Rather, we choose to confer value on the embryo just as we choose to value trees, national flags, and fine art. Although we can and sometimes do choose to value and therefore protect trees as works of nature, however, more often we do not, and trees in an arboretum have a distinctly different value than trees in an area slated for commercial development. National flags are both objects of reverence and articles of clothing depending on fashion trends, and what will count as fine art depends on the sensibilities of a given culture's elites. If we do not recognize the human embryo as potential life, as laying some claim on us morally that distinguishes it from a tree, as having a significance independent of our bestowal, what prevents us from producing as many embryos as we need for research just as we grow trees for furniture or auction art for charity? As a potential human being, the embryo or presentient fetus "is a powerful symbol of human life" argues Steinbock. "This is enough of a reason not to treat it as a mere commodity or convenient tool for research" (p. 167). Yet is not the embryo or presentient fetus "a powerful symbol of human life" precisely when it is recognized as having a transcendent value, a moral standing that, even if not equivalent to full personhood, distinguishes it from things and non-human forms of life?

The questions raised earlier point to a still deeper but related objection to the interest view. There is no doubt that the moral status of the preimplantation embryo is a fundamental issue in the assessment of embryo research. A narrow focus on the question of whether the preimplantation embryo ought to be shown the same respect as an infant or a child, whether or not the preimplantation embryo has interests that could be violated in the course of research, however, neglects critical questions about the setting, as well as the character and conduct, of embryo research. As Mary Mahowald[5] argues, moral status language abstracts the question of how we ought to treat human embryos from "the social context in which decisions about disposition of embryos, zygotes or gametes are made."

One consequence is that, for the most part, the debate about acceptable limits for embryo research ignores the question of who is really likely to benefit from embryo research. Improving success rates for medically assisted reproduction serves those who have access to specialized infertility treatments. Developing better methods for preimplantation genetic testing benefits those who are able to take advantage of opportunities for preimplantation diagnosis. Discovering safer and more effective contraception is useful to those who are able to choose from the full range of available methods. The high cost of specialized fertility services in the United States makes medically assisted reproduction and preimplantation screening genuine options only for those who have the financial resources. Despite the higher incidence of primary infertility among young African Americans with low income, the typical infertility patient is white, middle to upper income, and over 30 years of age. In developing countries around the world, one-third or more of all couples lack access to reliable methods of contraception already available elsewhere. According to a recent report of the United Nations Population Fund, lack of access to desired methods of contraception results in 75 million unwanted pregnancies a year. Many women turn to unsafe abortion as their only option, resulting in more than 70,000 deaths a year. Even a cursory look at the history of international population policy suggests that the existence or even the availability of contraceptives is much less important in the success or failure of family planning programs than cultural, political, and economic factors. It is not unreasonable to ask: Whose interests or what interests are at stake in funding embryo research? Whose lives are we really interested in saving, whose misery in preventing? What role will scientific or medical advancements actually play in the amelioration of those human miseries that concern us?

It might be argued that the potential clinical applications of embryo research are broader than I have indicated, that research into cell growth and differentiation holds promise for understanding how to prevent and treat cancer and other diseases that occur across populations—the prevention and treatment of which are in everyone's interest. It might also be argued that it is not unjust for infertility patients to benefit from the immediate clinical applications of embryo research if they also bear the primary burden as research subjects. Fair enough. But there is nothing in the argument from moral status that requires us even to ask whether embryo research or the creation of embryos for research is just or responsible under existing social, cultural, economic, or political conditions. In much the same way as appeals to moral status in the abortion debate have the effect of isolating decisions about continuing or ending pregnancy from the physical and social contexts that mediate and constrain the experience of pregnancy, appeals to the moral status of the preimplantation embryo isolate judgments about how far we can go in research from the institutional and social conditions under which scientific goals are defined and resources allocated.

THE DEEP CONTEXT: MEDICALLY ASSISTED REPRODUCTION

There is a more immediate and even more important "social context" that is obscured in arguments from moral status. It should seem obvious that we cannot separate the business of embryo research from its setting in the practice of medically assisted reproduction. It almost goes without saying, as Krimsky and Hubbard observe, that

> without the medicalization of infertility and the public acceptance of IVF as a proper scientific and medical response, there would be no way to justify the collection of eggs and their fertilization outside a woman's body. Societal acceptance of IVF constitutes the essential port of entry into all forms of human embryo research.

In vitro fertilization is the "port of entry" for human embryo research in both a practical and a conceptual sense. The most immediate applications of embryo research are in reproductive medicine and the clinical treatment of infertility. Current methods for recruiting and harvesting ova and techniques for effecting fertilization outside the body were developed for IVF programs. In the short term, women undergoing assisted reproduction are likely to be the major source of research ova. More important, the mainstreaming of IVF as a treatment for infertility signified a radical shift in personal, social, and scientific relationships to reproduction. As Lee Silver[6] argues, the birth of the first IVF baby represented a "singular movement in human evolution," a moment in which it became possible "in a very literal sense . . . to hold the future of our species in our own hands." Although developed for the treatment of infertility, IVF undeniably opens up possibilities for reproductive and genetic manipulations far beyond assisted reproduction. By "bringing the embryo out of the darkness of the womb and into the light of day," IVF allows for and makes acceptable the manipulation of the embryo on the cellular level, the transfer of embryos from "one maternal venue to another," and the ability to access and alter genetic material.

Yet, the debate over the limits of embryo research prescinds unselfconsciously from judgments about goals and methods in reproductive technology. In this sense, the debate is "disembodied." It is as if eggs did not come from within particular women or embryos were not formed from the gametes of particular individuals. That is not to say that issues of informed consent or worries about harms to donors do not arise. Rather, the problem is that the question of how we ought to treat the preimplantaiton embryo is abstracted from the larger question of what we are doing when we intervene in the process of reproduction. More important, the problem of determining the scope of embryo research is addressed as though it had no relation to the rationale for introducing IVF into the clinical setting.

It is precisely when we resituate embryo research within the practice of medically assisted reproduction that we see why the creation of embryos for research purposes is troubling. By "re-embodying" the debate, we raise up what the moral status or interest view neglects: the ambiguity attached to our expanding power to alter the conditions under which fertilization and gestation occur; and the relationship between the expansion of reproductive technologies and the social meanings of sexuality, procreation, and parenthood. It is only against the backdrop of a technological capacity that has the potential to be alienating as well as generative, destructive as well as creative, that we can fairly weigh the cost of severing the act of initiating human embryonic life from intentions and commitments to care for and sustain it.

Elsewhere I have joined with feminists and others in arguing for caution in the development and clinical application of reproductive technologies. There is no doubt that advances in reproductive medicine expand treatment options for couples struggling with infertility and provide new possibilities for biological reproduction. The ability to intervene in the process of reproduction gives new hope for overcoming both female and male factor infertility as well as for preventing and treating genetic diseases. Worldwide, IVF has already resulted in more than 150,000 live births, most of which would not have been possible without medical assistance. Just as the introduction of effective oral contraceptives gave women greater freedom in determining when they would reproduce, the advent of collaborative reproduction opens unprecedented possibilities for deciding how we will reproduce.

Yet medically assisted reproduction is not without risks. Drug regimes used to provide multiple ova for therapies such as IVF, GIFT, and ZIFT pose both long-term and short-term threats to women's health, including the immediate risk of hyperstimulation and the possibility of slightly increased risk of ovarian and breast cancer. Although studies show no increased incidence of birth defects associated with the use of reproductive technology, the long-range effects of the drugs used to initiate and sustain assisted pregnancies on the reproductive capacities of offspring are still unknown. Women conceiving through IVF and IVF-related therapies experience higher rates of ectopic pregnancy, miscarriage, and multiple gestation.

Perhaps more important and more relevant for our purposes are the emotional, relational, and social costs. Specialized treatment for infertility can be invasive, intrusive, emotionally draining, and financially exhausting. The turn to reproductive technologies can provide new avenues of possibility; it can also draw patients deeper into the repeated cycles of hope and despair that characterize the experience of infertility. The appearance of highly sophisticated therapies "ups the ante" for the infertile, creating the new burden of "not trying hard enough." Often, patients cannot even begin to resolve the crisis of involuntary childlessness until they have sought every possible treatment and exhausted all medical options.

In addition, the advent of procreative technologies furthers the medicalization of infertility, constraining options for resolving the crisis of involuntary childlessness (e.g., adoption) and drawing attention away from the medical and social causes of infertility. While expanding possibilities for biological parenting, assisted reproduction also severs connections long thought important between sexuality, procreation, and parenthood. To many, new ways of configuring the family are welcome; still, doubts linger about the extent to which primary biological and genetic relationships can be refashioned without ultimately harming children.

Perhaps most troubling for feminists is the capacity of procreative technologies to "disembody" reproduction. As Margaret Farley[7] observes, "for many feminists the sundering of the power and process of reproduction from the bodies of women constitutes a loss of major proportions." Women's previous experience with reproductive technologies suggests that women's own agency is likely to be submerged in the network of multiple experts needed to achieve IVF. Far from this accomplishing a liberation from childbearing responsibilities, it can entail "further alienation of our life processes."

For feminists such as Patricia Spallone and Gena Corea, the submersion of women's agency to the "experts" has frightening social and political implications. "Scientist-controlled, technological reproduction offers solutions," argues Spallone, but in ways that ultimately disempower women and at the cost of forcing women to hand over their very "life power" to the (primarily male) medical establishment. "Women's struggle for sexual, reproductive, economic and social autonomy," she warns, "is undermined by the proliferation of a kind of reproduction which necessitates interference from the state and its institutions, especially medical science professionals."[8]

Still, I believe that reproductive technologies can be used justly and responsibly and without "making women redundant," as feminists rightly fear. Along with Christian ethicist Lisa Sowle Cahill, I take the view that the human ideal for procreation and parenthood is biological and relational partnership: a couple "committed to one another, as well as to the child-to-be, and who initiate their parental project with a loving sexual act."[9] It is a view that I would defend ultimately on theological grounds, although I believe it is defensible on nontheological grounds. The question posed by reproductive technologies concerns what exceptions to the ideal are justifiable. If the union of sexual intimacy, procreation, and parenthood cannot always be realized—indeed, if sometimes it ought not be—what possibilities for procreation and parenthood are consistent with a commitment to the value of biological and relational partnership?

Also with Cahill, I support the view that reproductive interventions are defensible to the degree that they maintain "the crucial biological relations that undergird the personal and social relations of spousehood, parenthood and childhood." In vitro fertilization using gametes from within a marriage is more easily defended from this position, therefore, than IVF using donor gametes; in the former, procreation remains a shared biological endeavor, growing out of a sexual and marital relationship. That the sexual act "in which these physical relations are united and by which they are symbolized" is not realized can be justified, as Cahill argues, "by achievement of higher values: shared parenthood as part of the partnership of a couple committed to one another . . . and by the ability to maintain the important biological values. . . ."

Reproductive interventions are defensible also insofar as they respect the well-being of offspring as well as the needs and rights of adult parties. They are defensible insofar as they honor individual women's agency in creating, sustaining, and bringing forth life. They are defensible to the extent that their use meets the norms of justice, that is, that they are used in a way that is socially responsible and in a way that respects obligations to offspring through the relationship of procreation. Reproductive technologies open the opportunity of biological parenting to those for whom it would be impossible, but not without a price; the technologies are both justified and properly constrained by the goal to which they aspire: the bringing forth of new life in loving and nurturing relationship.

It is in light of this account of the goals of reproductive technologies that it becomes possible to say what is troubling about the creation of embryos for research purposes. Although it is reasonable to argue that we do not harm very early embryos by bringing them into existence merely to use them for experimental purposes, to initiate human life in the absence of intentions to care for and sustain it is nonetheless an assault on the character of procreation. It is an extension of the power to remove conception from the body, to manipulate the basic material of reproduction, that moves outside the most compelling justifications for developing and exercising it. As I have argued, reproductive interventions can serve the goods of intimacy, generativity, and commitment to nurture, but interventions carry with them the risk of "further alienation from our life processes" and loss of regard for the embodied and relational character of reproduction. To initiate human embryonic life with the intention of bringing it to fruition is consistent with the best reasons for "paying the price" of intervening in biological reproduction. This remains so even if the well-being of procreators or potential offspring dictates that implantation not be attempted or if embryos that would otherwise be destroyed are later donated for research. To initiate human embryonic life in the absence of intentions to care for and nurture it is, however, inconsistent with the goals I have argued justify and ought to constrain reproductive interventions.

In excluding as oocyte donors women who are not scheduled to undergo a surgical procedure, the Human Embryo Research Panel itself recognized a distinction between the intention to initiate a pregnancy and the pursuit of research goals, however important. The panel argued that "women who are not scheduled to undergo a surgical procedure are not a permissible source of oocytes for research at this time, even if they wish to volunteer to donate their oocytes":

> The Panel is concerned about the risks that current methods of oocyte retrieval pose to the health of donors. In order to obtain a number of fertilizable oocytes, hormonal stimulation and an invasive procedure are now required. Because alternative sources of oocytes are available, the Panel believes that such risks to donor cannot be justified. The Panel, however, is willing to allow such volunteers to donate oocytes if the intent is to transfer the resulting embryo for the purpose of establishing a pregnancy. . . . Absent the goal of establishing a pregnancy for an infertile couple, however, the lack of direct therapeutic benefit to the donor and the dangers of commercial exploitation do not justify exposing women to such risks.

Although I have drawn the risks involved differently from the panel, it seems to me that we agree on at least this much: The goal of bringing about a pregnancy provides a rationale for accepting a degree of risk, for allowing certain kinds of harms to occur, that other goals do not.

Someone might argue that creating embryos for research does not undermine the relational and embodied significance of procreation as long as research embryos are not transferred for implantation. To sever the initiation of human life from intentions to care for and sustain it is only problematic, someone might say, if children are brought into the world within instrumental rather than nurturing relationships. Fertilizing oocytes for research is not the same as procreating; it does not violate the moral character of procreation to create embryos that will never develop into human personhood. To be sure, to bring a child to life in the absence of anyone committed to his or her well-being or merely for the use of others would be indefensible in light of the position I have defended. Yet initiating human embryonic life with the sole intention of obtaining research material is the appropriation of the power of procreation divorced from the context in which it finds its meaning and focus, whether or not the embryo is brought to personhood. I have argued that it is precisely the intention to create life for the purposes of establishing a parental relationship that provides the primary justification for intervening in the procreative process; it is therefore also the intention to create embryonic life for research purposes that is problematic.

Of course, the very meaning of *procreation* is no longer clear. Is the activation of eggs to begin development without fertilization, as in parthenogenesis, a "procreative act"? Is human cloning by nuclear transfer "procreation" or "replication"? The question of what ought to count as "reproduction" or "procreation" in the face of expanding possibilities is far too complex to answer here. We have only begun to debate the meanings of sexuality, reproduction, and parenthood under the radically different circumstance introduced by IVF. Yet, if cloning by nuclear transfer or parthenogenesis or fertilizing ova for research purposes are not properly called *procreative* acts, it is fair to ask whether they should be held to the moral standard for procreation I have invoked.

Even if only a preliminary response can be given, it should be obvious why, in this account, cloning by nuclear transfer would violate the moral character of reproduction. I have defended a view of the significance of reproduction that underscores the integrity of its relational and biological dimensions. In addition to the risks of commercial exploitation that attend human cloning by nuclear transfer, it introduces the initiation of human life through a single progenitor. From a biological sense, cloning fails to honor the ideal of embodied partnership that I defended earlier.

Parthenogenesis is a more difficult case. As described in the report of the Human Embryo Research Panel, ova that are activated to begin cleavage and development without fertilization lack the genes necessary to develop as viable human embryos. Unlike the research embryo, the parthenote intrinsically lacks the potentiality for development. Thus, it is reasonable to argue that the concerns about the conditions under which it is moral to initiate human life that I have raised with respect to the research embryo would not apply in the same way to parthenogenesis, just as it is reasonable to argue that concerns about the morality of human cloning would not apply directly to the use of cloning in initiating nonreproductive cell lines. Throughout this chapter, however, my primary interest has been with justifications for intervening in the normal or "natural" process of reproduction. Rather than taking the removal of eggs from women's bodies and fertilization in vitro as routine or morally neutral and asking only "What are we permitted to do with gametes or embryos now that we have them?" I have insisted that we must continue to ask "Why are we doing this in the first place?" Taking seriously the risks to women's health and reproductive agency posed by reproductive technologies as well as the potential to undermine important connections between sexuality, procreation and parenthood, I have maintained that the intention to bring forth offspring in responsible and loving relationships provides the most compelling justification.

Finally, it might be argued that the creation of research embryos is not incompatible with the rationale for reproductive interventions if the research in question seeks to advance the goal of biological parenthood. If the availability of research embryos has the potential to improve the safety and efficacy of IVF, are not the goals of research in such a case consonant with the good of reproduction? On the face of it, this objection seems persuasive. If the achievement of biological parenthood drives our willingness to accept the risks of assisted reproduction, why not do anything necessary to advance that cause? It is not, however, only the ends of reproduction that are important in this analysis, but also the means. It is not only opening possibilities for biological parenting that is morally important, but also opening possibilities that are responsible to the goods at stake, that is, the embodied and relational character of procreation. It is only when we resist the temptation to split ends from means, when we reject the assumption that an end state can be clearly demarcated from the processes that lead up to it, that we see why creating research embryos is incompatible with commitments to maintaining the relational significance of procreation and why it remains so even when the research in question serves the overall goal.

CONCLUSION

In her statement of dissent, panel member Patricia King stated that "fertilization marks a significant point in the process of human development, and the prospect of disconnecting fertilization from the rest of the procreative process in which there is an intent to produce a child is profoundly unsettling." I have tried to suggest here why, indeed, we might find the prospect of severing fertilization from the rest of the procreative process, or, more accurately, from the rest of the parenting project, profoundly unsettling. In the end, King was persuaded that the benefits to be gained though embryo research outweighed the anxieties, although she approved the use of research embryos only where the information needed could not be gained in any other way. Assessing the risks and benefits somewhat differently than King did, I remain unsettled.

Disagreements over the use of research embryos have centered, on the one hand, on conflicting assessments of the moral status of the preimplantation embryo and, on the other hand, on differing judgments about how to weigh moral anxieties over the treatment of human embryos against the social importance of the research.

I have argued that a narrow focus on moral status abstracts the question of acceptable limits to embryo research from its larger setting. Beyond the question of whether embryos can be harmed is the deeper question of how we justify interventions into the procreative process. Severing fertilization from reproduction, in the full sense, is problematic precisely because it stands outside of the goods and values that medically assisted reproduction most directly and appropriately serves. The risks to be weighed, therefore, involve not only the "interests" of the preimplantation embryo, but also societal interests in women's health and in the integrity of sexuality, reproduction, and parenthood.

I have left an important issue unaddressed. The argument I have offered rests on a particular account of the intrinsic relationship between sexuality, procreation, and parenthood, an account with which many in this society may disagree and one with important theological influences. It is not unfair to ask what weight such arguments should have in public and policy-oriented debates. Should arguments for banning the use of research embryos be accepted that depend on what may constitute a minority position on the goals of medically assisted reproduction?

The limits of this essay make an adequate answer impossible, although it does seem to me that there is an important place in public debate for perspectives that challenge the dominant research ethos, particularly when it concerns issues of such human importance as the limits of research and the nature of reproduction. Here, however, I share Lisa Sowle Cahill's conclusion: The important thing is not how to prevent embryo research or cloning from occurring. Indeed, given the vast commercial potential in reproductive and genetic technologies, I am not optimistic that it will be possible even to contain them well, let alone prevent them from being introduced. What is important is how to open up public discussion to values beyond unexamined scientific progress or self-determination.[10] For now, the important thing is to expand the range of what is taken to be morally important in the debate over the creation of embryos for research or the introduction of human cloning, to resituate the question of what it means to respect human embryos in our ongoing reflection about the meaning of intervention into human reproduction.

NOTES

1. Here Steinbock is quoting John Harris, "Embryos and Hedgehogs: On the Moral Status of the Embryo," in *Experiments on Embryos* eds. Anthony Dyson and John Harris (London: Routledge, 1990), pp. 65–81.
2. John A. Robertson, "Symbolic Issues in Embryo Research," Hastings Center Report 25, no. 1 (January–February 1995): 37–38.
3. Gilbert C. Meilaender, *Body, Soul and Bioethics* (Notre Dame, IN: University of Notre Dame Press, 1995), p. 87.
4. Sheldon Krimsky and Ruth Hubbard, "The Business of Research." *Hastings Center Report* 25, no. 1 (1995): 41–43.
5. Mary Briody Mahowald, *Women and Children in Health Care: An Unequal Majority* (New York: Oxford University Press, 1993), p. 119.
6. Lee M. Silver, *Remaking Eden: Cloning and Beyond in a Brave New World* (New York: Avon Books, 1997), p. 75.
7. Margaret A. Farley, "Feminist Theology and Bioethics," in *Women's Consciousness, Women's Conscience,* eds. Barbara Hilkert Andolsen, Christine E. Gudorf, and Mary D. Pellauer (Minneapolis, MN: Winston Press, 1985), pp. 285–305.
8. Patricia Spallone, *Beyond Conception: The New Politics of Reproduction* (Granby, MA: Bergin and Garvey Publishers, Inc., 1989), p. 183. See also Gina Corea, *The Mother Machine* (New York: Harper and Row, 1985).
9. Lisa Sowle Cahill, "Women, Marriage, Parenthood: What Are Their 'Natures'?" *Logos* 9 (1988): 31.
10. Lisa Sowle Cahill, *Sex, Gender and Christian Ethics* (Cambridge: Cambridge University Press, 1996), p. 254.

RECOMMENDED SUPPLEMENTARY READING

GENERAL WORKS

Alpern, Kenneth D., ed. *The Ethics of Reproductive Technology.* New York: Oxford University Press, 1992.

Andrews, Lori B. *The Clone Age: Adventures in the New World of Reproductive Technology*. New York: Henry Holt and Company, 1999.

Andrews, Lori B., Fullarton, Jane E., Holtzman, Neil A., and Motulsky, Arno G., eds., *Assessing Genetic Risks: Implications for Health and Social Policy.* Washington, DC: National Academy Press, 1994.

Bartels, Dianne M., et al., eds. *Beyond Baby M: Ethical Issues in the New Reproductive Technologies.* Clifton, NJ: Humana Press, 1990.

Buchanan, Allen, Brock, Dan W., Daniels, Norman, & Wikler, Daniel. *From Chance to Choice: Genetics & Justice*. Cambridge: Cambridge University Press, 2000.

Callahan, Joan C., ed. *Reproduction, Ethics, and the Law.* Bloomington: Indiana University Press, 1995.

Caulfield, Timothy A., Williams-Jones, Bryn, eds., *The Commercialization of Genetic Research: Legal, Ethical, and Policy Issues.* Dordrecht, The Netherlands: Kluwer Academic Publishers, 1999.

Cohen, Sherrill, and Taub, Nadine. *Reproductive Laws for the 1990s.* Clifton, NJ: Humana Press, 1989.

Cranor, Carl F. *Are Genes Us? The Social Consequences of the New Genetics.* New Brunswick, New Jersey: Rutgers University Press, 1994.

Davis, Dena S. *Genetic Dilemmas: Reproductive Technology, Parental Choices, and Children's Futures.* New York and London: Routledge, 2001.

Dyson, Anthony, and Harris, John, eds. *Ethics and Biotechnology.* London: Routledge, 1994.

Elias, Sherman, and Annas, George J. *Reproductive Genetics and the Law*. Chicago: Year Book Medical Publishers, 1987.

Fotion, Nich, and Heller, Jan, eds. *Contingent Future Persons: On the Ethics of Deciding Who Will Live, or Not, in the Future*. Dordrecht, Holland: Kluwer Academic Publishers, 1997.

Glover, Jonathan. *What Sort of People Should There Be?* New York: Random House, 1977.

Harris, John. *Wonderwoman and Superman: The Ethics of Human Biotechnology*. Oxford: Oxford University Press, 1992.

———. *Clones, Genes, and Immortality: Ethics and the Genetic Revolution*. New York: Oxford University Press, 1998.

Harris, John, and Holm, Soren, eds. *The Future of Human Reproduction*. Oxford: Clarendon Press, 1998.

Heyd, David. *Genethics: Moral Issues in the Creation of People*. Berkeley: University of California Press, 1992.

Kelves, Daniel J. *In the Name of Eugenics: Genetics and the Uses of Human Heredity*. New York: Alfred A. Knopf, 1985.

Kitcher, Philip. *The Lives to Come: The Genetic Revolution and Human Possibilities*. New York: Simon & Schuster, 1996.

McCullough, Laurence B., and Chervenak, Frank A. *Ethics in Obstetrics and Gynecology*. New York: Oxford University Press, 1994.

Mehlman, Maxwell J. and Botkin, Jeffrey R. *Access to the Genome: The Challenge to Equality*. Washington, DC: Georgetown University Press, 1998.

Murray, Thomas H. *The Worth of a Child*. Berkeley: University of California Press, 1996.

Murray, Thomas H. and Mehlman, Maxwell J., eds., *Encyclopedia of Ethical, Legal, and Policy Issues in Biotechnology*, Vols. 1 and 2. New York: John Wiley & Sons, Inc., 2000.

Parfit, Derek. *Reasons and Persons*. Oxford: Clarendon Press, 1984.

Purdy, Laura. *Reproducing Persons: Issues in Feminist Bioethics*. Ithaca, New York: Cornell University Press, 1996.

Reilly, Philip. *The Surgical Solution: A History of Involuntary Sterilization in the United States.* Baltimore: Johns Hopkins University Press, 1991.

Roberts, Melinda. *Child versus Childmaker: Future Persons and Present Duties in Ethics and the Law.* Rowman & Littlefield, 1998.

Robertson, John A. *Children of Choice: Freedom and the New Reproductive Technologies*. Princeton: Princeton University Press, 1994.

Rothman, Barbara Katz. *Recreating Motherhood: Ideology and Technology in a Patriarchal Society*. New York: W. W. Norton, 1989.

———. *The Tentative Pregnancy. How Amniocentesis Changes the Experience of Motherhood*. New York: W. W. Norton, 1993.

Silver, Lee M. *Remaking Eden: How Genetic Engineering and Cloning Will Transform the American Family*. New York: Avon Books, Inc., 1997.

Singer, Peter. *Animal Liberation*. New York: Avon Books, 1975.

Singer, Peter, and Wells, Deane. *Making Babies: The New Science and Ethics of Conception*. New York: Charles Scribner's Sons, 1985.

Steinbock, Bonnie. *Life Before Birth: The Moral and Legal Status of Embryos and Fetuses*. New York: Oxford University Press, 1992.

———, ed. *Legal and Ethical Issues in Human Reproduction*. Hampshire, UK: Ashgate Publishing Ltd., 2002.

Strong, Carson. *Ethics in Reproduction and Perinatal Medicine. A New Framework*. New York: Oxford University Press, 1997.

Warren, Mary Anne. *Moral Status: Obligations to Persons and Other Living Things*. New York: Oxford University Press, 1997.

Wolf, Susan M., ed. *Feminism and Bioethics*. New York: Oxford University Press, 1996.

THE MORALITY OF ABORTION

Bassen, Paul. "Present Stakes and Future Prospects: The Status of Early Abortion." *Philosophy and Public Affairs* 11:4 (1982): 314–337.

Bavertz, Kurt, ed. *Sanctity of Life and Human Dignity*. Dordrecht, Holland: Kluwer Academic Publishers, 1996.

Boonin, David. *A Defense of Abortion*. Cambridge: Cambridge University Press, forthcoming, 2002.

Callahan, Sidney, and Callahan, Daniel, eds. *Abortion: Understanding Differences*. New York: Plenum Press, 1984.

Davis, Nancy Ann. "The Abortion Debate: The Search for Common Ground." 2 parts. *Ethics* 103 (April/July 1993): 731–778.

———. "Abortion and Self-Defense." *Philosophy and Public Affairs* 13, no. 3 (Summer 1984): 516–539.

Dworkin, Ronald. *Life's Dominion: An Argument about Abortion, Euthanasia, and Individual Freedom*. New York: Alfred A. Knopf, 1993.

Dwyer, Susan, and Feinberg, Joel, eds. *The Problem of Abortion*. 3rd ed. Belmont, CA: Wadsworth Publishing Co., 1997.

Feinberg, Joel. "Abortion." In *Matters of Life and Death*, edited by Tom Regan. 2nd ed. New York: Random House, 1986.

Garrow, David J. *Liberty and Sexuality: The Right to Privacy and the Making of Roe v. Wade*. New York: Macmillan Publishing Company, 1994.

Gorney, Cynthia. *Articles of Faith: A Frontline History of the Abortion Wars*. New York: Simon & Schuster, 1998.

Graber, Mark A. *Rethinking Abortion: Equal Choice, the Constitution, and Reproductive Politics*. Princeton, NJ: Princeton University Press, 1996.

Hursthouse, Rosalind. *Beginning Lives*. Oxford: Basil Blackwell, 1987.

———. "Virtue Theory and Abortion." *Philosophy and Public Affairs* 20, no. 3 (Summer 1991): 223–246.

Kamm, Frances Myrna. *Creation and Abortion: A Study in Moral and Legal Philosophy*. New York: Oxford University Press, 1992.

Little, Margaret. "Abortion, Intimacy, and the Duty to Gestate," *Ethical Theory and Moral Practice* 2 (1999): 295–312.

———. *Abortion, Intimacy, and the Duty to Gestate*. Oxford: Clarendon Press, forthcoming, 2002.

Luker, Kristin. *Abortion and the Politics of Motherhood*. Berkeley: University of California Press, 1984.

Marquis, Don. "Why Most Abortions Are Wrong," in Rem B. Edwards and E. Edward Bittar, eds., *Advances in Bioethics*, Vol. 5. Stamford, Connecticut: JAI Press, Inc., 1999, 215–244.

McDonaugh, Eileen. *Breaking the Abortion Deadlock*. New York: Oxford University Press, 1996.

Norcross, Alastair. "Killing, Abortion, and Contraception: A Reply to Marquis." *Journal of Philosophy* (1990): 268–278.

Petchesky, Rosalind P. *Abortion and Woman's Choice: The State, Sexuality and Reproductive Freedom*. Revised ed. Boston, MA: Northeastern Press, 1990.

Regan, Donald. "Rewriting *Roe v. Wade*." *Michigan Law Review* 77 (1979).

Robertson, John A. "*Casey* and the Resuscitation of *Roe v. Wade*." *Hastings Center Report* 22, no. 5 (1992): 24–29.

Sumner, L. W. *Abortion and Moral Theory*. Princeton, NJ: Princeton University Press, 1981.

Tooley, Michael. *Abortion and Infanticide*. New York: Oxford University Press, 1983.

Tribe, Laurence. *Abortion: The Clash of Absolutes*. New York: W. W. Norton, 1990.

CARRIER SCREENING, PRENATAL TESTING, AND REPRODUCTIVE DECISIONS

Andre, Judith, Fleck, Leonard M., and Tomlinson, Tom. "On Being Genetically 'Irresponsible.'" *Kennedy Institute of Ethics Journal* 10 (2000): 129–146.

Annas, George J. "Noninvasive Prenatal Diagnostic Technology: Medical, Market, or Regulatory Model?" *Annals of the New York Academy of Sciences* 731 (1994): 262–268.

Botkin, Jeffrey R. "Fetal Privacy and Confidentiality." *Hastings Center Report* (Sept.–Oct.1995): 32–39.

———. "Prenatal Screening: Professional Standards and the Limits of Parental Choice." *Obstetrics and Gynecology* 75, no. 5 (1990): 328–329.

Brock, Dan. "The Non-Identity Problem and Genetic Harms—The Case of Wrongful Handicaps." *Bioethics*, 9, no. 2 (1995): 269–276.

Buchanan, Allen. "Choosing Who Will Be Disabled: Genetic Manipulation and the Morality of Inclusion." *Social Philosophy and Policy* 13, no. 2 (1996): 18–46.

Chadwick, Ruth, Shickle, Darren, ten Have, Henk, and Wiesing, Urban, eds., *The Ethics of Genetic Screening*. Dordrecht, The Netherlands: Kluwer Academic Publishers (1999).

Cohen, Cynthia B., "The Morality of Knowingly Conceiving Children With Serious Conditions: An Expanded "Wrongful Life" Standard," in Nick Fotion and Jan C. Heller, eds., *Contingent Future Persons*. Dordrecht, The Netherlands: Kluwer Academic Publishers, 1997.

Cohen, Cynthia B., and McCloskey, Elizabeth L., eds., Special Issue: Genetic Testing. *Kennedy Institute of Ethics Journal* 8, no. 2 (June 1998): 111–200.

Davis, Dena. "Genetic Dilemmas and the Child's Right to an Open Future." *Hastings Center Report* (Mar.–Apr. 1997): 7–15.

Fost, Norman. "Ethical Implications of Screening Asymptomatic Individuals." *FASEB Journal* 6 (1992): 2813–2817.

Feinberg, Joel. "Wrongful Life and The Counterfactual Element in Harming," *Social Philosophy & Policy* 4:1 (1987): 174.

Glover, Jonathan. "Future People, Disability and Screening." In Peter Laslett and James Fishkin, eds., *Justice Between Age Groups and Generations*. New Haven, CT: Yale University Press, 1992.

Green, Ronald M. "Paternal Autonomy and the Obligation Not to Harm One's Child Genetically." *Journal of Law, Medicine and Ethics* 25 (1997): 5–15.

Lippman, Abby. "Prenatal Genetic Testing and Screening: Constructing Needs and Reinforcing Inequities." *American Journal of Law and Medicine* 17 (1991): 15–50.

Murphy, Timothy. "Abortion and the Ethics of Genetic Sexual Orientation Research." *Cambridge Quarterly of Healthcare Ethics* 4 (1995): 340–350.

Peters, Philip G. "Protecting the Unconceived: Nonexistence, Avoidability, and Reproductive Technology." *Arizona Law Review* 31, no. 3 (1989): 487–548.

———. "Rethinking Wrongful Life: Bridging the Boundary Between Tort and Family Law," *Tulane Law Review* 67, no. 2 (1992): 397–454.

———. "Harming Future Persons: Obligations to the Children of Reproductive Technology," *Southern California Interdisciplinary Law Journal* 8 (1999): 375–400.

President's Commission for the Study of Ethical Problems in Medicine and Biomedical and Behavioral Research. *Screening and Counseling for Genetic Conditions: The Ethical, Social, and Legal Implications of Genetic Screening, Counseling, and Education Programs*. Washington, DC: U.S. Government Printing Office, 1983.

Robertson, John A. "Ethical and Legal Issues in Preimplantation Genetic Screening." *Fertility and Sterility* 57 (1992): 1–11.

———. "Genetic Selection of Offspring Characteristics." *Boston University Law Review* 76 (1996): 421–482.

Rothenberg, Karen H. and Thomson, Elizabeth J., eds. *Women & Prenatal Testing: Facing the Challenges of Genetic Technology*. Columbus, OH: Ohio State University Press, 1994.

Savulescu, J. "Procreative Beneficence: Why We Should Select the Best Children." *Bioethics* 15 nos. 5/6 (2001): 413–426.

Schuklenk, Udo, Stein, Edward, Kerin, Jacinta, and Byrne, William. "The Ethics of Genetic Research on Sexual Orientation." *Hastings Center Report* 27, no. 4 (July/August 1997): 6–13.

Stein, Edward. "Choosing the Sexual Orientation of Children." *Bioethics* 12, no. 1 (1998).

Steinbock, Bonnie. "The Logical Case for 'Wrongful Life,'" *Hastings Center Report* 16, no. 2 (April 1986): 15–20.

Steinbock, Bonnie and McClamrock, Ron. "When Is Birth Unfair to the Child?" *Hastings Center Report* 24, no. 6 (November 1994): 15–21.

Warren, Mary Anne. *Gendercide: The Implications of Sex Selection*. Totowa, NJ: Rowman and Allenheld, 1985.

Wertz, Dorothy C. and Fletcher, John C. "A Critique of Some Feminist Challenges to Prenatal Diagnosis." *Journal of Women's Health* 2 (1993): 173–188.

MAPPING THE HUMAN GENOME: Implications for Genetic Testing, Genetic Counseling, and Genetic Interventions

Anderson, W. French. "Genetic Engineering and our Humanness," *Human Gene Therapy* 5 (1994): 755–759.

Anderson, W. French and Friedmann, Theodore. "Gene Therapy: Strategies for Gene Therapy." In Warren T. Reich, ed., *Encyclopedia of Bioethics*, Vol. 2. New York: MacMillan, 1995: 907–914.

Annas, George J. "Reforming Informed Consent to Genetic Research." *JAMA* 286, no. 18 (2001): 2326–2328.

Annas, George J., and Elias, Sherman, eds. *Gene Mapping: Using Law and Ethics as Guides*. New York: Oxford University Press, 1992.

Baird, Patricia A. "Altering Human Genes: Social, Ethical, and Legal Implications." *Perspectives in Biology and Medicine* 37, no. 4 (Summer 1994): 566–575.

Bartels, Dianne M., et al. *Prescribing Our Future: Ethical Challenges in Genetic Counseling*, New York: Aldine de Gruyter, 1993.

Bernhardt, Barbara A. "Empirical Evidence That Genetic Counseling Is Directive: Where Do We Go from Here? *American Journal of Human Genetics* 60 (1997): 17–20.

Beskow, L. M. et al. "Informed Consent for Population-Based Research Involving Genetics." *JAMA* 286, no. 18 (2001): 2315–2321.

Billings, Paul. "Genetic Discrimination and Behavioral Genetics: The Analysis of Sexual Orientation." In *Intractable Neurological Disorders, Human Genome, Research and Society*. Edited by Norio Fujiki and Darryl Macer. Christchurch and Tsukuba: Eubios Ethics Institute (1992): 114–117.

Bonnicksen, Andrea L. "National and International Approaches to Human Germ-Line Gene Therapy." *Politics and the Life Sciences* 13, no. 1 (February 1994): 39–49.

Brenner, M.K. "Human Somatic Gene Therapy: Progress and Problems," *Journal of Internal Medicine*, Vol. 237 (1995): 229–239.

Carson, Sandra A., and Buster, John E. "Diagnosis and Treatment Before Implantation: The Ultimate Prenatal Medicine," *Contemporary OB/GYN* (December 1995): 71–85.

Collins, Francis S. and Guttmacher, A.E. "Genetics Moves Into the Medical Mainstream." *JAMA* 286 no. 18 (2001): 2322–2324.

Collins, Francis S. and McKusick, Victor A. "Implications of the Human Genome Project for Medical Science." *JAMA* 285, no. 5 (February 7, 2001): 540–544.

Cook-Deegan, Robert Mullan. "Germ-Line Gene Therapy: Keep the Window Open a Crack." *Politics and the Life Sciences* 13, no. 2 (August 1994): 217–220.

Coutts, Mary Carrington. "Human Gene Therapy: Scope Note 24." *Kennedy Institute of Ethics Journal* 4 (1994): 63–83.

de Wachter, M.A.M. "Ethical Aspects of Human Germ-Line Therapy." *Bioethics* 7 (1993): 166–177.

Fletcher, John C. "Germ-Line Gene Therapy: The Costs of Premature Ultimates." *Politics and the Life Sciences* 13, no. 2 (August 1994): 225–227.

Fletcher, John C., and Anderson, W. French. "Germ-Line Gene Therapy: A New Stage of Debate." *Law, Medicine & Health Care* 20, nos. 1–2 (1992): 26–39.

Fost, Norman, "Ethical Issues in Genetics." *Pediatric Clinics of North America* 39, no. 1 (1992): 79–89.

———. "Genetic Diagnosis and Treatment." *AJDC* 147 (1993): 1190–1195.

Frankel, Mark S. & Chapman, Audrey R. *Human Inheritable Genetic Modifications*. American Association for the Advancement of Science (2000).

Gardner, William. "Can Human Genetic Enhancement be Prohibited?" *The Journal of Medicine and Philosophy* 20, no. 1 (1995): 65–84.

Gostin, Lawrence O. "National Health Information Privacy: Regulations Under the Health Insurance Portability and Accountability Act." *JAMA* 285 (2001): 3015–3021.

Gostin, Lawrence O., Hodge, James G. Jr, Calvo, Cheye M. "Genetics Policy and Law: A Report for Policymakers." National Conference of State Legislatures (2001).

Gustafson, James M. "Genetic Therapy: Ethical and Religious Reflections." *Journal of Contemporary Health Law and Policy* 8 (1992): 183–2001.

Holtug, Nils. "Does Justice Require Genetic Enhancements?" *Journal of Medical Ethics* 25 (1999): 137–143.

———. "Human Gene Therapy: Down the Slippery Slope?" *Bioethics* 7 (1993): 402–419.

Juengst, Eric T. "Germ-line Gene Therapy: Back to Basics." *Journal of Medicine and Philosophy* 16 (1991): 587–592.

———. "'Prevention' and the Goals of Genetic Medicine." *Human Gene Therapy* 6 (1995): 1595–1605.

———. "Can Enhancement Be Distinguished from Prevention in Genetic Medicine?" *The Journal of Medicine and Philosophy* 22, no. 2 (1997): 125–142.

———. "Caught in the Middle Again: Professional Ethical Considerations in Genetic Testing for Health Risks," *Genetic Testing*, Vol. 1, no. 3 (1997/98): 189–200.

———. "Concepts of Disease After the Human Genome Project." In Stephen Wear, James J. Bono, Gerald Logue and Adrianne McEvoy (eds.) *Ethical Issues in Health Care on the Frontiers of the Twenty-First Century*. Great Britain: Kluwer Academic Publishers (2000): 127–154.

Kaji, Eugene H. and Leiden, Jeffrey M. "Gene and Stem Cell Therapies." *JAMA* 285 (February 7, 2001): 545–550.

Kodish, Eric D. "Testing Children for Cancer Genes: The Rule of Earliest Onset," *Journal of Pediatrics* 135 (1999): 390–395.

Lancaster, Johnathan M., Wiseman, Roger W., and Berchuck, Andres. "An Inevitable Dilemma: Prenatal Testing for Mutations in the BRCA1 Breast-Ovarian Cancer Susceptibility Gene." *Obstetrics & Gynecology* 87 (1996): 306–309.

McGee, Glenn. *The Perfect Baby: A Pragmatic Approach to Genetics*. Lanham, PA: Rowman & Littlefield, 1997.

McKusick, V.A. "The Anatomy of the Human Genome: A Neo-Vesalian Basis for Medicine in the 21st Century." *JAMA* 286, no. 18 (2001): 2289–2295.

Mehlman, Maxwell. "The Law of Above Averages: Leveling the New Genetic Enhancement Playing Field." *Iowa Law Review* 85 (2000): 517–593.

Merz, Beverly. "The Human Genome Project." (2001) http://www.hhmi.org/Genetic.

Munson, Ronald, and Davis, Lawrence. "Germ-Line Gene Therapy and the Medical Imperative." *Kennedy Institute of Ethics Journal* 2, no. 2 (1992): 137–158.

Murphy, Timothy F., and Lappe, Marc A., eds. *Justice and the Human Genome Project*. Berkeley, CA: University of California Press, 1994.

New York State Task Force on Life and the Law. *Genetic Testing and Screening in the Age of Genomic Medicine*. November 2000.

Parens, Erik. "Should We Hold the (Germ) Line?" *Journal of Law, Medicine and Ethics* 23, no. 2 (1995): 173–176.

———. "The Goodness of Fragility: On the Prospect of Genetic Technologies Aimed at the Enhancement of Human Capacities." *Kennedy Institute of Ethics Journal* 5 (1996): 141–153.

———. "Taking Behavioral Genetics Seriously." *Hastings Center Report* (July–Aug. 1996): 13–22.

———, ed. *Enhancing Human Traits: Ethical and Social Implications*. Washington, DC: Georgetown University Press, 1998.

Pokorski, Robert J. "Insurance Underwriting in the Genetic Era," *American Journal of Human Genetics*, Vol. 60 (1997): 205–216.

Press, Nancy, Fishman, Jennifer R. and Koenig, Barbara A. "Collective Fear, Individualized Risk: The Social and Cultural Context of Genetic Testing for Breast Cancer," *Nursing Ethics*, Vol. 7, no 3 (2000): 237–249.

Reilly, Philip R., Boshar, Mark F., and Holtzman, Steven H. "Ethical Issues in Genetic Research: Disclosure and Informed Consent." *Nature Genetics* 15 (1997): 16–20.

Ross, Gail et al. "Gene Therapy in the United States: A Five-Year Status Report," *Human Gene Therapy*, Vol. 7 (September 10, 1996): 1781–1790.

Scott, W.K. et al. "Complete Genomic Screen in Parkinson Disease: Evidence for Multiple Genes." *JAMA* 286, no. 18 (2001): 2239–2244.

Stock, Gregory and Campbell, John, eds. *Engineering the Human Germline: An Exploration of the Science and Ethics of Altering the Genes We Pass to Our Children*. New York: Oxford University Press, 2000.

Subramanian, G. et al. "Implications of the Human Genome for Understanding Human Biology and Medicine." *JAMA* 286, no. 18 (2001): 2296–2307.

Symposium. "Regulating Germ-Line Gene Therapy." *Politics and the Life Sciences* 13, no. 2 (August 1994): 217–248.

Symposium. "The Genome Imperative." *Journal of Law, Medicine and Ethics* 23, no. 4 (1995).

Symposium. "The Genetic Privacy Act Roundtable Commentary." *Journal of Law, Medicine and Ethics* 23, no. 4 (1995).

Walters, LeRoy. "Gene Therapy: Overview." In Murray, Thomas H. and Mehlman, Maxwell J., eds., *Encyclopedia of Ethical, Legal, and Policy Issues in Biotechnology*, Vol. 1. New York: John Wiley & Sons, Inc., 2000.

Wertz, Dorothy C. "Leave the Door Open to Research." *Politics and the Life Sciences* 13, no. 2 (August 1994): 235–236.

———. "Society and the Not-So-New Genetics: What Are We Afraid Of? Some Future Predictions from a Social Scientist." *The Journal of Contemporary Health Law and Policy* 13 (1997): 299–346.

Wertz, Dorthy C., and Fletcher, John C., eds. *Ethics and Human Genetics: A Cross-Cultural Perspective*. New York: Springer-Verlag, 1989.

Winston, Robert M. L. "Germ-Line Gene Therapy: An Exaggerated Threat." *Politics and the Life Sciences* 13, no. 2 (August 1994): 237–238.

Wivel, Nelson A., and Walters, LeRoy. "Germ-Line Gene Modification and Disease Prevention: Some Medical and Ethical Perspectives." *Science* 262 (October 22, 1993).

ASSISTED REPRODUCTIVE TECHNOLOGIES

Anderson, Elizabeth. "Is Women's Labor a Commodity? *Philosophy and Public Affairs* 19, no. 1 (Winter 1990).

Annas, George J. "Baby M: Babies (and Justice) for Sale." *Hastings Center Report* 17, no. 3 (1987).

Arneson, Richard J. "Commodification and Commercial Surrogacy." *Philosophy and Public Affairs* 21, no. 2 (Spring 1992).

Charo, R. Alta. "And Baby Makes Three—Or Four, Or Five, Or Six: Redefining the Family After the Reprotech Revolution." *Wisconsin Women's Law Journal* 7 (1992–93): 1–23.

Callahan, Daniel. "Bioethics and Fatherhood." *Utah Law Review* (1992): 735–746.

Cohen, Cynthia B. "Give Me Children or I Shall Die!" New Reproductive Technologies and Harm to Children." *Hastings Center Report* (March–April 1996): 19–29.

———, ed. *New Ways of Making Babies*. Bloomington: Indiana University Press, 1996.

———. "Unmanaged Care: The Need to Regulate New Reproductive Technologies in the United States." *Bioethics* 11, no. 3&4 (1997): 348–365.

Congregation for the Doctrine of the Faith. "Instruction on Respect for Human Life in Its Origin and on the Dignity of Procreation: Replies to Certain Questions of the Day." Rome, Italy: The Vatican, March 10, 1987.

Corea, Gena. *The Mother Machine: Reproductive Technologies from Artificial Insemination to Artificial Wombs*. New York: Harper, 1985.

Field, Martha A. *Surrogate Motherhood: The Legal and Human Issues*. Cambridge, MA: Harvard University Press, 1988.

Glover, Jonathan. *Ethics of New Reproductive Technologies: The Glover Report to the European Commission*. DeKalb, IL: Northern Illinois University Press, 1989.

Gorovitz, Samuel. "Progeny, Progress, and Primrose Paths." In Gorovitz, *Doctors' Dilemmas: Moral Conflict and Medical Care*. New York: Oxford University Press, 1982.

Gostin, Laurence O., ed. *Surrogate Motherhood: Politics and Privacy*. Bloomington: Indiana University Press, 1990.

Holland, Suzanne, and Davis, Dena S., Guest Editors. Special Issue: Who's Afraid of Commodification? *Kennedy Institute of Ethics Journal* 11, no. 3 (September 2001).

Holland, Suzanne. "Contested Commodities at Both Ends of Life: Buying and Selling Gametes, Embryos, and Body Tissues." *Kennedy Institute of Ethics Journal* 11, no. 3 (2001).

Kalfoglou, Andrea, and Geller, Gail. "Navigating Conflict of Interest in Oocyte Donation: an Analysis of Donors' Experiences. *Women's Health Issues* 10, no. 5 (2000): 226–239.

Lauritzen, Paul. *Pursuing Parenthood: Ethical Issues in Assisted Reproduction*. Bloomington: Indiana University Press, 1993.

Macklin, Ruth. "Artificial Means of Reproduction and Our Understanding of the Family." *Hastings Center Report* 21, no. 1 (1991): 5–11.

Mahoney, Julia D., "The Market for Human Tissue." *Virginia Law Review* 86, no. 2 (March 2000): 163–223.

New York State Task Force on Life and the Law. *Surrogate Parenting*, 1988.

———. *Assisted Reproductive Technologies: Analysis and Recommendations for Public Policy*, 1998.

Radin, Margaret Jane. "Market-Inalienability." *Harvard Law Review* 100 (1987): 1839–1947.

Robertson, John A. "Posthumous Reproduction," *Indiana Law Journal* 69, no. 4 (1994): 1027–1065.

———. "Legal Issues in Human Egg Donation and Gestational Surrogacy." *Seminars in Reproductive Endocrinology* 13, no. 3 (1995): 210–218.

Satz, Debra. "Markets in Women's Reproductive Labor," *Philosophy and Public Affairs* 21 (1992): 107–131.

Seibel, Michelle M., and Crockin, Susan, eds. *Family Building Through Egg and Sperm Donation: Medical, Legal and Ethical Issues*. Sudbury, MA: Jones and Bartlett, 1996.

Steinbock, Bonnie. "Surrogate Motherhood as Prenatal Adoption." *Law, Medicine and Health Care* 16 (1988): 44–50.

———. "Payment to Egg Donors." *Mount Sinai Journal of Medicine* (forthcoming).

Wertheimer, Alan. "Two Questions about Surrogacy and Exploitation." *Philosophy and Public Affairs* 21, no. 3 (Summer 1992): 211–239.

HUMAN CLONING AND STEM CELL RESEARCH

Allmers, H., and Kenwright, S. "Ethics of Cloning." *Lancet* 349 no. 9062 (May 10, 1997): 1401.

Annas, George J. "Regulatory Models for Human Embryo Cloning: The Free Market, Professional Guidelines, and Government Restrictions." *Kennedy Institute of Ethics Journal* 4 (1994): 235–249.

Andrews, Lori B. "Mom, Dad, Clone: Implications for Reproductive Privacy." *Cambridge Quarterly of Healthcare Ethics*, vol. 7, no. 2 (1998): 176–186.

Brannigan, Michael C., ed., *Ethical Issues in Human Cloning*. New York and London: Seven Bridges Press, 2001.

Callahan, Daniel. "The Puzzle of Profound Respect," *Hastings Center Report* 25 (1995): 39–40.

Capron, Alexander Morgan. "Inside the Beltway Again: A Sheep of a Different Feather." *Kennedy Institute of Ethics Journal* 7 (1997): 171–179.

Charo, R. Alta. "The Hunting of the Snark: The Moral Status of Embryos, Right-to-lifers, and Third World Women." *Stanford Law & Policy Review* 6 (1995): 11–37.

"Cloning Human Beings: Responding to the National Bioethics Advisory Commission's Report." *Hastings Center Report* (September–October 1997).

Cloning Symposium, *Jurimetrics* 38, no. 1 (1997).

Doerflinger, Richard. "The Ethics of Funding Embryonic Stem Cell Research: A Catholic Viewpoint." *Kennedy Institute of Ethics Journal* 9, no. 2 (1999): 137–150.

Green, Ronald M. *The Human Embryo Research Debates: Bioethics in the Vortex of Controversy*. New York: Oxford University Press, 2001.

Holland, Suzanne, Lebacqz, Karen, and Zoloth, Laurie, eds. *The Human Embryonic Stem Cell Debate*. Cambridge, MA: The MIT Press, 2001.

Humber, James M., and Almeder, Robert. *Human Cloning*. Totowa, NJ: Humana, 1998.

Juengst, Eric and Fossel, Michael. "The Ethics of Embryonic Stem Cells—Now and Forever, Cells Without End," *JAMA*, Vol. 284, no. 24 (December 27, 2000): 3180–3184.

Kass, Leon. "The Wisdom of Repugnance: Why We Should Ban the Cloning of Humans." *The New Republic* (June 2, 1997): 17–26.

Klotzko, Arlene Judith. *The Cloning Sourcebook*. New York: Oxford University Press, 2001.

Kolata, Gina. *Clone: The Road to Dolly and the Path Ahead*. New York: William Morrow & Co., 1998.

Lauritzen, Paul, ed., *Cloning and the Future of Human Embryo Research*. New York: Oxford University Press, 2001.

Lester, Lane P., and Hefley, James C. *Human Cloning*. Ada, MI: Baker, 1998.

Lewontin, Richard. "The Confusion over Cloning." *New York Review of Books* 44 (October 23, 1997).

Lewontin, Richard; with Harold T. Shapiro; James F. Childress; and Thomas H. Murray. "'The Confusion over Cloning': An Exchange" *New York Review of Books* 45, no. 4 (March 5, 1998): 46–47.

Mackinnon, Barbara, ed., *Human Cloning: Science, Ethics, and Public Policy*. University of Illinois Press, 2000.

Macklin, Ruth. "Splitting Embryos on the Slippery Slope: Ethics and Public Policy." *Kennedy Institute of Ethics Journal* 4, no. 3 (September 1994): 209–225.

McConnick, R.A. "Should We Clone Humans?" *The Christian Century* 17–24 (November 1993): 1148–1149.

McGee, Glenn. *The Human Cloning Debate*. Berkeley, CA: Berkeley Hills Books, 1998.

McGee, Glenn and Caplan, Arthur. "The Ethics and Politics of Small Sacrifices in Stem Cell Research." *Kennedy Institute of Ethics Journal* 9 (1999): 151–158.

Meilaender, Gilbert. "The Point of a Ban." *Hastings Center Report* 31, no. 1 (2001): 9–16.

National Bioethics Advisory Commission. *Cloning Human Beings: Report and Recommendations*. Rockville, MD, 1997.

National Bioethics Advisory Commission. *Ethical Issues in Human Stem Cell Research*. Vol. I–III. Rockville, MD, 2000.

Nussbaum, Martha C., and Sunstein, Cass R., eds., *Clones and Clones: Facts and Fantasies about Human Cloning*. New York: W. W. Norton & Company, 1998.

Parens, Erik. "What Has the President Asked of NBAC? On the Ethics and Politics of Embryonic Stem Cell Research." In *Ethical Issues in Human Stem Cell Research*, Vol. II Rockville, Maryland, 2000.

Pence, Gregory. *Flesh of My Flesh: The Ethics of Cloning—A Reader*. Lanham, PA: Littlefield, 1998.

———. *Who's Afraid of Human Cloning?* Lanham, Md: Rowman & Littlefield, 1998.

Rantala, M. L., and Milgram, Arthur J., eds., *Cloning: For and Against*. Chicago: Open Court, 1999.

Rhodes, Rosamond. "Clones, Harms, and Rights." *Cambridge Quarterly of Healthcare Ethics* 4 (1995): 285–290.

Roberts, Melinda. "Human Cloning: A Case of No Harm Done?" *Journal of Medicine and Philosophy* 21 (1996): 537–554.

Robertson, John A. "The Question of Human Cloning." *Hastings Center Report* 24, no. 2 (Mar./Apr. 1994): 6–14.

———. "Liberty, Identity, and Human Cloning." *Texas Law Review* 76, no. 6 (1998).

———. "Ethics and Policy in Embryonic Stem Cell Research." *Kennedy Institute of Ethics Journal* 9 (1999): 109–136.

———. "Two Models of Human Cloning." *Hofstra Law Review* 27 (1999): 609–638.

Verhey, A. "Cloning: Revisiting an Old Debate." *Kennedy Institute of Ethics Journal* 4, no. 3 (September 1994): 227–234.

———. "Playing God and Invoking a Prespective." *Journal of Medicine and Philosophy* 20 (1995): 347–364.

Winters, Paul A. *Cloning*. San Diego, CA: Greenhaven, 1998.

PART FIVE

EXPERIMENTATION ON HUMAN SUBJECTS

Self-conscious scientific experimentation is a relatively new phenomenon in the long history of medicine. For centuries, the introduction of innovative medical procedures was regarded with suspicion. Anyone who deviated from the established norms of medical practice was likely to be regarded as an upstart medical heretic and could even be charged with the tort of negligence, or "malpractice." But the advent of properly scientific medicine in the nineteenth and twentieth centuries transformed controlled scientific investigation into the driving force behind the spectacular successes of modern medicine. With the impressive advances in medical care that have been generated by contemporary medical science, what previous centuries had regarded with fear and distrust has now become a scientific, and even an ethical, imperative.

But here, as elsewhere in the field of biomedicine, success has not been unalloyed: Ethical problems of the greatest magnitude have been posed by the methods of scientific medicine. With the development of ever more advanced research methods has come the ability to use the bodies of ordinary men and women as complex laboratories in which can be found the answers to questions of profound importance. At times, the zeal to unlock these mysteries has blinded researchers to the fact that these amazing engines of scientific progress are also individual people whose dignity and moral worth are equal to their own. In the worst of such cases, intolerable wrongs have been committed under the otherwise noble banner of medical science and regard for the welfare of future patients. The exposure of such cases to public scrutiny, and the controversies this exposure has engendered, have played a crucial role in shaping the development of research ethics in the United States.

Part 5 begins with some of the high-profile cases that have shaped the ethical response to, and regulation of, human-subjects research in the United States. The uproar over flagrant abuses of the rights of human subjects both abroad and at home led to the establishment of serious protections both at the national level, through the Food and Drug Administration, and at the local level, through institutional review boards (IRBs). This new era of biomedical research was defined by several important assumptions. It was assumed, for example, that participation in research was both risky and burdensome; that the maintenance of high ethical standards justified a slower rate of progress in finding effective medical interventions; and that populations that may be more vulnerable to exploitation—such as minority groups, women, and children—should be either shielded or excluded altogether from participation in research studies.

This view began to change in the 1980s, however, as it came under fire from a coalition of unlikely partners. One particularly effective force for change was composed of conservative libertarians and liberal AIDS activists who challenged the bureaucratic obstacles that hindered the public's access to innovative therapies. For conservatives, the lengthy review process that slowed the introduction of medical innovations represented a stumbling block to free enterprise, on the one hand, and to the liberty of consumers to make their own judgments about when they were ready to accept the risks associated with novel interventions, on the other. Alternatively, watching their family and friends die of AIDS while the nation's government and research establishment responded at glacial speed, a new generation of activists claimed that participation in research is a benefit and that it was unjustifiably paternalistic for governmental agencies to protect persons with AIDS from the very medical research that might stave off the death they were already facing from their disease. Soon, similar challenges were lodged by women whose exclusion from clinical trials was intended to safeguard their potential children from harmful effects of experimental agents and to protect pharmaceutical companies from lawsuits. While this exclusion may have been well intended, it was becoming clear that it had resulted in a gap in knowledge about how to diagnose and to treat common diseases in women. The legacy of this decade was the realization that protecting "vulnerable" groups from participating in research could have detrimental effects on the quality of the health care those groups received.

In the 1980s, the protectionism of previous decades gave way to an effort to include what were once perceived as vulnerable populations in research as a matter of health care equity. Although it is true that exclusion from medical research can have important social and individual consequences, it remains true that the ends of clinical research and the ends of therapeutic treatment often diverge. How can these ends be reconciled in an ethically and clinically responsible way? Under what circumstances is it acceptable to conduct clinical research? To Kantians, for instance, no research question is so important that it could justify treating persons as mere means to the ends of science—no matter how noble or important the objective. By what mechanisms, then, can we ensure that the dignity of individual subjects is properly respected without compromising the integrity of important research? Is it ethical to enroll subjects in research who are not capable of giving free and fully informed consent, such as children, people with significant cognitive impairments, or institutionalized populations such as prisoners or elderly nursing home residents? Disparities in health and access to health care often track disparities in social and economic status. What role, if any, should research play in addressing health problems that are largely caused by circumstances of social and economic deprivation? Should different standards apply to research that crosses national boundaries if the social and economic circumstances of the target population are significantly different from those of the research sponsors?

BORN IN SCANDAL: THE ORIGINS OF U.S. RESEARCH ETHICS

At the end of World War II, the most gruesomely spectacular examples of unethical research were showcased at the trials of Nazi doctors at Nuremberg. During the war, physicians sympathetic to Nazi ideology conducted or participated in a range of medical experiments in which victims of the Nazi concentration camps were subjected to cruel, humiliating, and often lethal procedures in the name of medical research. At the Buchenwald camp, for example, homosexual men, Jews, Gypsies, and other prisoners were divided into study groups; subjects in the experimental arm were given an experimental vaccine against typhus and members of the control group were injected with typhus-infected blood. Nearly all of the unimmunized controls, and many who received the experimental vaccines, died as a result of the infections they contracted. At Revensbrück, bones were transplanted from one prisoner to another in order to study the regeneration of nerves, muscle, and bone. In other experiments, prisoners in the camps were shot in order to study the ballistics of bullets, starved in order to observe the physiology of malnutrition, or infected with gangrene so that the efficacy of different treatments could be studied.

In order to study the length of time that a downed pilot could survive in freezing water, Jewish and Russian prisoners were submerged in tubs of freezing water until they froze to death. Others were removed at various points and different methods for reviving them were tested, including the use of naked Jewish women who were forced to revive the near frozen subject with the warmth of their bare flesh. In order to study the effect of high altitude on pilots, camp prisoners were put into pressure chambers that subjected them to lethal extremes in atmospheric pressure. All the while researchers observed through a window, documenting the readouts of their instruments and the state of the agonized subject.

At the end of the war, twenty-three Nazi physicians and bureaucrats were placed on trial and sixteen were subsequently convicted of war crimes. Of these, seven were sentenced to death. In an effort to support and explicate the tribunal's judgment that the Nazi medical experiments were monstrosities masquerading as medical science, the judges enunciated a set of principles that would make explicit the ethical requirements for acceptable human-subjects research. The product of that effort, the Nuremberg Code, is the opening reading of Section 1.

In unambiguous and unqualified language the Nuremberg Code states as the first of its ten principles that:

> 1. The voluntary consent of the human subject is absolutely essential. This means that the person involved should have legal capacity to give consent; should be so situated as to be able to exercise free power of choice, without the intervention of any element of force, fraud, deceit, duress, over-reaching, or other ulterior form of constraint or coercion; and should have sufficient knowledge and comprehension of the elements of the subject matter involved as to enable him to make an understanding and enlightened decision. . . .

Although the tribunal appeared to believe that the principles they articulated were already widely accepted by the medical and scientific community, one of the very reasons the trial of the Nazi doctors was so protracted was the ability of defense lawyers to show striking parallels to medical experiments that had been performed by American doctors. Far from merely codifying what was already common knowledge among allied medical researchers, the principles of the Nuremberg Code together set out stringent and revolutionary ethical constraints on human-subjects research.

In the immediate aftermath of World War II, the principles of the Nuremberg Code appear to have had little direct impact on the way public medical research was conducted in the United States. In part this was due to the fact that these principles had been enunciated in the context of the Nazi war crimes trials, and it was widely believed that the atrocities of the concentration camps had no parallel in civilized and scientifically sound medical research. Often what the Nazi doctors characterized as research had little or no scientific value and merely provided an excuse to brutalize people who were regarded as inferior. Additionally, however, it is precisely because the principles of the code were not widely accepted and the restrictions that they imposed were so severe that many researchers viewed them as applicable to monsters and mad men but not to legitimate medical researchers.

Until only fairly recently, when clinical research in the United States involved people who were already patients, the conduct of research was generally subsumed under the norms of the prevailing paternalistic model. This is poignantly illustrated in the material in "The Jewish Chronic Disease Hospital Case," compiled by Jay Katz. Here, the validity of the research question, and the quality of the research date were not an issue. Because previous studies had shown that people with cancer take longer to expel foreign cancer cells than do otherwise healthy people, Dr. Chester Southam and his colleagues wanted to measure the rate at which foreign cancer cells would be rejected from the bodies of people who were suffering from illnesses other than cancer. To do this, they injected foreign cancer cells into the skin of twenty-two debilitated residents of the Jewish Chronic Disease Hospital in Brooklyn, New York.

In order to ensure sufficient enrollment in their study, the researchers did not inform subjects of the nature of the injections—that they contained live cancer cells—because they wanted to avoid irrational fears about the word *cancer.* To the researchers, the importance of the research and the low probability of harm provided sufficient reason to justify the use of chronically debilitated hospital patients without further burdening them with irrational worries about contracting cancer. To members of the Board of Regents of the University of the State of New York, however, these considerations could not obviate the fact that the researchers subjected vulnerable individuals to nontherapeutic procedures without their informed consent, thereby violating the subjects' rights to control the disposition of their person and to be free from unwanted molestation.

This case thus represents the hub in which a range of important issues intersect. Here the research question is important and the risk of harm to participants very low. But should these considerations override the right of individuals to control their persons and safeguard their own bodily integrity? The trust that marks the foundation of the doctor-patient relationship is predicated on the idea that both parties are working towards the same goal—attending to the best interests of the patient. Is it ethical to exploit that trust for nontherapeutic purposes? Dr. Southam and his colleagues did not see their conduct as falling outside of the doctor-patient relationship, even though the reasons they offer to justify their conduct focus entirely on the importance of the research for society, since this research was not intended to benefit the individual subjects. Moreover, the fear and skepticism engendered by the revelation of such experiments has a corrosive effect on the very trust upon which they are predicated.

Additionally, the subjects of the research at the Jewish Chronic Disease Hospital were chronically ill, long-term residents of the facility whose compromised decisional capacity made them vulnerable targets. In contrast to the exhortations of the Nuremberg Code, the practice of using the most vulnerable as subjects of research has a long tradition in the United States. Consider the research that was conducted from 1956 to 1971 on the mentally retarded children housed at the Willowbrook State School in New York.

As described by David J. Rothman and Sheila M. Rothman in "The Willowbrook Hepatitis Studies," researchers at Willowbrook, lead by Dr. Saul Krugman, intentionally infected children at the institution with hepatitis in the search for an effective vaccine. Here again, the quality of the data generated by the research was not in question, but the methods used were the subject of heated controversy. Hepatitis was one of a number of infectious diseases that spread easily through the unsanitary conditions of the overcrowded institution. After discovering that immunity could be generated by injections of gamma globulin, Krugman opened a separate unit at the school where children between three and eleven were divided into groups, some of whom were inoculated with gamma globulin and then fed live hepatitis virus while controls were merely fed the live virus.

As Saul Krugman argues in "The Willowbrook Hepatitis Studies Revisited: Ethical Aspects," the researchers reasoned that residents in the overcrowded institution would inevitably contract the virus on the ward and that the social will did not exist to clean up the unsanitary conditions responsible for the underlying problem. By infecting some children with a milder strain of the virus than the one they might contract on the ward, the researchers reasoned that the children themselves were better off for participating in the research and that the results of the research would provide invaluable results to future patients as well. Without the research, both the present children and future patients would have been worse off.

As Rothman notes, however, the consent form provided to parents painted a deceptively sanitized picture of the research carried out at Willowbrook, and the fact that participation in research was condition for being admitted to the hospital exerted a coercive influence on parents. More important, however, is Rothman's skepticism about the claim that being infected with hepatitis could be seen as a benefit of participating in research. The retarded children of Willowbrook were under the care of the state and, as such, it was the state's responsibility to look after their welfare. Is it accurate to say that the children in the institution would *inevitably* be infected with the virus, given that the conditions through which the virus is spread *could have been ameliorated?* The school could have been closed or its conditions publicized in an effort to clean up the conditions that threatened residents and staff alike. At the very least, every resident could have been inoculated with gamma globulin in an effort to provide some positive benefit to all alike.

Critics of the Willowbrook studies argue that where a harm can be avoided, and the failure for preventing harm is someone's fault, that person or those persons are at least partly causally and morally responsible for the harm's occurring. Additionally, they worry about using the unsanitary conditions at Willowbrook as a laboratory because it creates a disincentive to undertake any actions that might disturb the laboratory environment. If this sounds incredible, consider what is perhaps the most profound case in unethical research in the United States history. As recounted by historian Allan M. Brandt in "Racism and Research: The Case of the Tuskegee Syphilis Study," this project involved the systematic deception and abuse of poor African American men from 1932 to 1972. Undertaken in part to determine the effects of untreated syphilis in this population, the study recruited its 400 subjects by lying to them outright about providing treatment for "bad blood." As Brandt observes, "deceit was integral to the study." In addition to this flagrant disregard for the principles of veracity and informed consent, the Tuskegee researchers, drawn largely from the U.S. Public Health Service, also withheld all medical treatments that were considered standard therapy for syphilis at the time, including penicillin when it became widely available at the end of World War II. There can be no doubt that this failure to treat led to the premature deaths of many subjects, their spouses and sexual partners, and their children.

Brandt concludes that "the Tuskegee study revealed more about the pathology of racism than it did about the pathology of syphilis; more about the nature of scientific inquiry than the nature of the disease process." Like many of the Nazi experiments judged at Nuremberg, the revelation of the Tuskegee study shocked the public. In both cases: (1) The experiments were scientifically pointless or redundant; (2) their design was shoddy, precluding meaningful results; (3) subjects were either coerced or deceived into participating; and (4) research subjects were drawn from socially deprived groups.

Although the Tuskegee syphilis study was initiated before World War II, it was not until the summer of 1997 that President Clinton finally apologized on behalf of the United States to a handful of aged survivors and their relatives. In spite of this long overdue gesture of repentance and reconciliation, much damage had already been done both to the human beings involved in the study and to the fabric of trust between the enterprise of medical science and the African American community.

By the time the details of the Tuskegee syphilis study came to light in 1972, broader social reform movements were already scrutinizing the prevailing norms of American medicine. In 1974 the National Commission for the Protection of Human Subjects of Biomedical and Behavioral Research was formed and given the task of identifying the basic principles that ought to govern ethically responsible human-subjects research. After four years of study they produced what has come to be known as "The Belmont Report." This seminal document has played a fundamental role in shaping contemporary ethical and regulatory standards for acceptable research.

The Belmont Report begins by distinguishing the practice of medicine from clinical research. Here, the principal difference lies in the ends around which the physician/researcher's activities are coordinated. In treatment, the goal is to enhance the well-being of an individual patient, whereas in medical research the primary goal is to generate generalizable knowledge. While these goals can support and enhance one another, they can also diverge and come into conflict. Next, the report articulates the general ethical principles that ought to govern medical research: respect for persons, beneficence, and justice. In order to illustrate the implications of these general principles for actual practice, they suggest mechanisms for ensuring that these requirements are met. Respect for persons requires the voluntary and informed consent of the subject. Beneficence requires a favorable assessment of the risks and benefits involved in research, and justice requires that equitable procedures for selecting subjects be employed so that vulnerable populations do not bear disproportionate burdens of research.

THE ETHICS OF RANDOMIZED CLINICAL TRIALS

The Hippocratic tradition and recent codes of medical ethics speak clearly and emphatically concerning the physician's duty to individual patients. The tradition has emphasized the physician's covenantal duty of undivided loyalty to the patient, as opposed to what Paul Ramsey has called "that celebrated non-patient—the future of medical science." This traditional duty of exclusive personal care for the individual patient is expressed in a number of applicable codes. For example, the AMA Principles of Medical Ethics state, "Physicians should merit the confidence of patients entrusted to their care, rendering to each a full measure of service and devotion . . ." while the AMA's Ethical Guidelines for Clinical Investigation declare, "In conducting clinical investigation, the investigator should demonstrate the same concern and caution for the welfare, safety, and comfort of the person involved as is required of a physician who is furnishing medical care to a patient independent of any clinical investigation."

This traditional posture of undivided loyalty to the patient-subject was easy to maintain when clear-cut distinctions could be made between "therapeutic" and "nontherapeutic" experimentation—that is, between trials performed primarily for the benefit of patient-subjects and those designed primarily for the purpose of gaining valuable knowledge for future patients. Although this distinction is still useful in some contexts, the boundaries between these different kinds of experimentation have become blurred in the conduct of modern biomedical research.

Physicians plausibly maintain that they have a *moral obligation* to employ the most effective means for combating disease and disability, regardless of the time-honored status of standard procedures, many of which often turn out to be quite useless or even harmful. The duty, grounded in the physician's Hippocratic commitment to "do no harm," is expressed in Section 3 of the AMA Principles of Medical Ethics, which states that "a physician should practice a method of healing founded on a scientific basis. . . ." The vexing ethical problem posed by this kind of clinical research is that it places the physician's traditional duty of personal care in direct opposition to his or her duty to practice scientific medicine. Whereas the horrors of Nuremberg and Tuskegee invited spontaneous moral outrage, the dilemmas posed by research today demand nuanced ethical reflection and creative thinking about experimental design.

One of the most problematic features of scientific research design is the common practice of "randomizing" patients—i.e., assigning them by chance—to one of several competing treatments or to a control group receiving no treatment. Section 2 begins with a discussion of three case studies of morally troubling randomizations, presented by Maurie Markman, a prominent cancer researcher. According to the advocates of so-called randomized clinical trials (RCTs), there are both scientific and ethical advantages to assigning research subjects to treatment groups by chance. By eliminating bias in the selection and care of patient-subjects, randomization helps generate scientifically reliable data that will enable future patients to receive better care. Indeed, some defenders of RCTs claim that this disciplined procedure is *more ethical* than introducing new procedures on the informal basis of clinical impressions and historical comparisons.

The critics of RCTs, including Dr. Markman, are less sanguine about the prospects of reconciling the imperatives of hard science with the physician's duty to provide personal care. Samuel Hellman and Deborah S. Hellman, in "Of Mice but Not Men," object to the fact that in an RCT, the individual's therapy is determined not simply by an investigation into his or her physical needs and personal values, but also by consideration of the needs of the experimental design. Randomization for the sake of future patients, they claim, thus supersedes the individualized treatment of present patients. Does this not amount to a sacrifice of the individual for the sake of society at large? Samuel and Deborah Hellman conclude that it does, and they therefore condemn RCTs for violating the central tenet of Kantian ethics: that the personhood of the individual should not be submerged in utilitarian calculations of social benefit. The Hellmans urge the medical community to develop and use less morally problematic techniques for gaining reliable knowledge.

Defenders of RCTs attempt to counter these objections by noting that in order to be ethically justified, the two (or more) arms of study—e.g., comparing two different drugs, or one drug against a placebo—must be in "equipoise." That is, the researchers must not have any scientifically sound reason for preferring one arm to another. But what is to count as "scientific soundness" here?

Some critics of RCTs argue that such studies are problematic if the researchers have formed a "treatment preference" either before or after the initiation of the trial. In one of his case studies, for example, Markman contends that a physician who has a strong opinion in favor of a new cancer drug, taxol, cannot ethically advise his or her patients about a trial comparing taxol to the standard treatment.

According to this view, if researchers develop a "strong hunch" about the comparative effectiveness of a new drug, either at the beginning or in the midst of a trial, it is unethical to continue an RCT.

Benjamin Freedman, in his "Response" to Markman, claims that such worries are based on a flawed conception of equipoise. Instead of insisting that the evidence on behalf of two treatments be exactly balanced and that the researchers develop no treatment preferences throughout the duration of the trial—both seemingly impossible requirements—Freedman argues for a concept of equipoise based on the existence of honest, professional disagreement within the scientific community. So long as there exists a genuine dispute among clinicians, Freedman contends, RCTs are ethically permissible even if a particular physician has a decided preference for one treatment over others. Indeed, he adds, the original and overriding purpose of RCTs is to dispel precisely this kind of professional disagreement. Many a strong hunch has become standard practice in medicine, not by virtue of meeting rigorous scientific standards, but rather by dint of the investigator's passionate commitment, charisma, or professional standing. When this has happened, patients have often been subjected to unnecessary risk and harm for extended periods of time.

ETHICAL ISSUES IN INTERNATIONAL RESEARCH

The moral tension between ensuring access to important medical research while safeguarding the welfare of individual trial participants is particularly acute when we turn to internationally sponsored research in developing countries. Collaborative international research often poses special challenges to researchers because of differences in language, custom, and culture. In many cases, these differences converge in the context of informed consent. Members of a host population may speak a language different from that of the researchers. They may differ in their level of formal education or familiarity with Western medicine or science, and they may have different beliefs about the relative importance of individual, rather than collective decision making. In such cases, researchers must struggle to negotiate these differences in ways that are respectful of the host population without compromising their own commitments to ethically responsible human-subjects research.

Equally troubling are differences that are rooted not in culture and custom, but in social and economic circumstance. Every day an estimated 1600 children are infected with HIV and 90 percent of these infections occur in countries of the developing world. In economically and technologically developed countries such as the United States the rate of HIV infection passed from mothers to children can be dramatically reduced (from roughly 30 percent to 8 percent) by giving pregnant women several doses of the drug AZT during pregnancy and at birth, followed by the administration of the drug to the infants themselves after delivery. This particular regimen (called the "076 protocol") has been hailed as a major breakthrough and quickly became the accepted standard of medical practice throughout the United States. But what of the plight of the millions of HIV-infected women in foreign countries too poor to afford AZT for everyone? What can and should be done for them?

This question led health officials in Africa and Asia to join forces with researchers at the U.S. National Institutes of Health (NIH) and Centers for Disease Control and Prevention (CDC) in an effort to test a lower and less-expensive dose of AZT in pregnant women. A wide variety of studies, examining a wide variety of doses and drugs, were subsequently initiated throughout Africa. With few exceptions, however, these studies exhibited a very controversial design element: Almost all of them compared the new, less-expensive drug regimens against a placebo group. In effect, a set proportion of the women in each study intentionally received an inert substance, while their more fortunate counterparts received a lesser (experimental) amount of the active drug; meanwhile, the truly fortunate inhabitants of Europe and North America receive a standard dose that is known to effect a dramatic reduction in the rate of infection from mothers to children.

While agreeing with these researchers that the discovery of a less-expensive preventive treatment for HIV-infected pregnant women is an important goal, critics have charged them and their sponsoring institutions with exploiting the vulnerable people of impoverished, postcolonial societies in a manner reminiscent of the infamous Tuskegee study (Angell 1997). Peter Lurie and Sidney M. Wolfe in "Unethical Trials of Interventions to Reduce Perinatal Transmission of the Human Immunodeficiency Virus in Developing Countries" charge that the use of the placebo controls following the discovery of an effective treatment constitutes a blatant violation of human rights and codes of research ethics that would never have been contemplated, let alone implemented, in developed countries. They contend that researchers from developed countries should apply the same high ethical standards and norms of appropriate treatment that they observe at home while collaborating with their counterparts in poorer nations. If, as Benjamin Freedman would put it, protocol 076 has upset "clinical equipoise" in Boston, researchers in Zaire cannot pretend that it exists there merely because governments and drug companies have decided not to make an effective drug available. Lurie and Wolfe conclude that sufficient information about these new drugs and doses may be obtained by pitting them in trials against the standard dose of the 076 protocol.

In "AZT Trials and Tribulations," Robert A. Crouch and John D. Arras offer a more charitable evaluation of the short-course AZT trials. They begin by arguing that the design of these studies should be evaluated in light of the purpose of the proposed research and the requirements of sound trial design. Here, they present a cautious defense of the placebo-controlled design as the most reliable method for conducting research that is tailored to the specific circumstances of developing world populations. With these considerations in place, they then consider whether there might be other factors in virtue of which the subjects in such trials would be morally entitled to a higher standard of care than they currently receive—that is, nothing. Drawing on what they refer to as the "liberal consensus view" of justice in health care, they argue that there are no grounds for such an entitlement. Together, these considerations provide a powerful argument in support of the claim that it was ethically permissible to use placebo controls in the short-course AZT studies.

Crouch and Arras recognize that the short-course AZT trials may have been morally problematic for other reasons, in particular, because it was not clear that the local populations that participated in the research would receive an effective treatment after the completion of the trial. We will return to these worries in a moment. For now, it is important to consider more carefully the relationship between the standard of care to which participants in clinical research are entitled, the demands of sound trial design, and the economic background conditions that limit the health care options of developing world populations.

In "The Ambiguity and the Exigency: Clarifying 'Standard of Care' Arguments in International Research," Alex John London takes a detailed look at the standard of care to which participants in international trials are entitled. He begins by arguing that the widespread focus on the question of whether the standard of care ought to be "local" or "global" is less important than the more fundamental question of whether the standard ought to be "de facto" or "de jure." Whereas de facto standards are set by the level of care that is *actually* available in the relevant population, the de jure standard is set by what the expert medical community knows to be effective for treating the relevant illness in the relevant population. He then argues that a de jure standard is the most ethically and scientifically defensible standard, and in doing so he links the standard of care to the requirement that clinical trials begin in and be designed to disturb equipoise.

Perhaps most importantly, London stresses that what we know about the effectiveness of possible interventions within a population cannot be separated from the issue of whether the interventions in question can be implemented and sustained over time within the relevant community (see London 2001). As a result, he argues that it is possible that equipoise would not exist between two interventions in a wealthy, developed nation with a robust health care infrastructure, but that it would exist in a developing country with only a rudimentary health care infrastructure. He also argues, however, that in addition to the existence of equipoise, researchers need to provide reasons for thinking that running a clinical trial will be a responsible means of meeting the health care needs of the population in question rather than attempting to ameliorate the conditions that cause equipoise to exist in their community when it does not exist in others.

In "Research in Developing Countries: Taking 'Benefit' Seriously," Leonard H. Glanz, George J. Annas, Michael A. Grodin and Wendy K. Mariner take up in detail the requirement that medical research must be responsive to the needs of the host population. They note that the purpose of research is to gather generalizable data, not to treat large numbers of people, and that research will not provide a real benefit to host populations unless the resources are committed to make the fruits of that research reasonably available. As a result, they argue that before internationally sponsored research like the short-course AZT trials is approved, funding agreements must be in place to ensure that members of the host population will in fact be provided with an effective treatment developed out of the research. Making such funding agreements a condition for the approval of international research has met with resistance from many who view the proposal as a serious impediment to potentially valuable research. After all, such funding commitments are not required for domestic research and many worry that governmental and nongovernmental funding sources will refuse to commit significant resources to a treatment program without reliable data on the effectiveness of the proposed interventions.

RESEARCH ON CHILDREN AND OTHER "VULNERABLE" POPULATIONS

As we saw earlier, by the 1980s it was becoming clear that unmitigated protectionist attitudes toward vulnerable populations threatened to create, or to further exacerbate, significant disparities in medical knowledge about the distinctive health care needs of those populations. In some cases, however, the drive to ensure health care equity among these groups is in tension with the need to ensure that genuinely vulnerable individuals are not exploited for the benefit of future subjects. In Section 4 we examine two populations in which this tension is particularly acute, children and psychiatric patients.

The vast majority of drugs prescribed to children in the United States has not been specifically evaluated for use in pediatric populations. Pediatricians prescribe these drugs by extrapolating information about dosage and effects that has been gained from trials in adults. In a 1997 report, the FDA listed the following ten drugs that are prescribed to children on an outpatient basis over five million times a year despite inadequate pediatric drug labeling:

Albuterol inhalation solution for nebulization for treatment of asthma (prescribed 1,626,000 times to pediatric patients under 12);

Phenergan for treatment of allergic reactions (prescribed 663,000 times to pediatric patients under 2); ampicillin injections for treatment of infection (prescribed 639,000 times to pediatric patients under 12);

Auralgan otic solution for treatment of ear pain (prescribed 600,000 times to pediatric patients under 16);

Lotrisone cream for treatment of topical infections (prescribed 325,000 times to pediatric patients under 12);

Prozac for treatment of depression and obsessive compulsive disorder (prescribed 349,000 times to pediatric patients under 16, including 3,000 times to infants under 1);

Intal for treatment of asthma (solution prescribed 109,000 times to pediatric patients under 2; aerosol prescribed 399,000 times to pediatric patients under 5);

Zoloft for treatment of depression (prescribed 248,000 times to pediatric patients under 16);

Ritalin for treatment of attention deficit disorders and narcolepsy (prescribed 226,000 times to pediatric patients under 6);

Alupent for treatment of asthma (184,000 times to pediatric patients under 6).[1]

In response to such findings, since 1994, federal agencies like the FDA and the NIH and the U.S. Congress have initiated policy changes aimed at increasing the inclusion of pediatric populations in medical research. These changes require pediatric populations to be included in federally funded research and in the evaluation of new drugs, unless researchers or their sponsors can provide a justification for their exclusion.

When new pharmaceuticals are not tested in pediatric populations under controlled conditions, children are exposed to greater risks than their adult counterparts when they receive these drugs in a clinical setting. Nevertheless, as we have seen, the ends of treatment and the ends of research can diverge, and expanding the mandate to include children in research means that more healthy children will be asked to participate in research that does not hold out the prospect of direct benefit to

1. Food and Drug Administration. Regulations Requiring Manufacturers to Assess the Safety and Effectiveness of New Drugs and Biological Products in Pediatric Patients. 1997. Http://www.fda.gov/cder/guidance/pedrule.htm.

the individual child. Furthermore, unlike their adult counterparts, children are not capable of giving informed consent to participate in medical research. Instead, the task of looking after their welfare is entrusted to their parents or legal guardian. Under what circumstances is it permissible to enroll an individual child in a clinical trial in which there is little or no prospect of a direct benefit to that child?

In "Children and 'Minimal Risk' Research: The Kennedy-Krieger Lead Paint Study," Alex John London explores a recent case in which some of these issues were cast into stark relief. In order to quantify the effectiveness of several different methods for removing or controlling lead paint in low-income inner city housing units, researchers from the Johns Hopkins–affiliated Kennedy Krieger Institute (KKI) conducted a study in which families with small children were recruited to live in, or encouraged to remain living in, homes that received varying degrees of lead abatement. Although many of these units were not as safe as newly constructed suburban homes, they were probably significantly safer than alternative low-income housing that had not received any degree of lead removal or containment. To researchers from the KKI, this study provided a benefit to the individual participants, as well as to the group of impoverished inner city families whose poverty often restricts them to poor quality housing.

Others have taken a less sanguine view of this case. The Maryland Court of Appeals was skeptical about the claim that exposure to known levels of lead dust could constitute a benefit to study participants. They were also critical of the trial's informed consent process, and they went so far as to argue that in Maryland a parent, appropriate relative, or other applicable surrogate, cannot consent to the participation of a child or other person under legal disability in nontherapeutic research or studies in which there is *any risk* of injury or damage to the health of the subject. While it is unlikely that this ruling will change the legal requirement for conducting pediatric research, the court's reaction to this case enunciates a standard for nontherapeutic pediatric research that found its most ardent proponent in the theologian and ethicist Paul Ramsey.

In his popular and influential book *The Patient as Person,* Ramsey argued that parents violate the trust in which they hold the interests and welfare of their children if they attempt to consent for the child's participation in research that does not hold out the prospect of a direct benefit to the child. Ramsey was an early and vocal critic of the hepatitis studies at the Willowbrook State School and a staunch defender of the idea that the free and fully informed consent of research participants is a necessary condition for ethical research. In this respect, for Ramsey, the first principle of the Nuremberg Code had gotten it right; he thus viewed nontherapeutic research on children as abrogating the parents' most basic and profound duty.

In "Research on Children and the Scope of Responsible Parenthood," Thomas H. Murray confronts Ramsey's challenge head on. He begins by describing another controversial case of pediatric medical research, the NIH sponsored trials of artificial human growth hormone in children. In this study, children were randomized either to an investigational arm that would receive between 600 and 1,100 injections of artificial human growth hormone over a seven-year period or to a control group that would receive the same number of injections of saline solution. Although Murray is sensitive to some of the potentially problematic assumptions in which this trial was predicated, he nevertheless argues that enrolling a child in this study would not necessarily fall outside of the boundaries of responsible parenthood. Murray is dubious of the attempt to funnel all acceptable parental decisions through the condition of informed consent, and he notes that responsible parents often involve their children in activities that further worthwhile goals but which also pose some degree of risk to their children without the promise of direct benefit. He therefore defends the permissibility of enrolling children into research that poses only a minor increment over minimal risk on the ground that exposing one's children to such risks in the pursuit of a worthwhile goal is perfectly consistent with the trust in which parents hold the interest and welfare of their children.

In making this move, however, we are forced to grapple with one of the thornier issues raised by the Kennedy-Krieger lead paint study. In the federal regulations governing human-subjects research in the United States, it is considered acceptable to subject children to a minor increment over minimal risk, where *minimal risk* is defined as: "the probability and magnitude of harm or discomfort anticipated in the research are not greater in and of themselves than those ordinarily encountered in daily life or during the performance of routine physical or psychological examinations or tests." As the KKI lead paint study illustrates, however, children in different areas may experience different degrees of risk in their daily lives. How are we to set the baseline against which risks are to be measured in a clinical trial?

This standard is the focus of "*In Loco Parentis:* Minimal Risk as an Ethical Threshold for Research upon Children," by Benjamin Freedman, Abraham Fuks, and Charles Weijer. These authors argue that although it is not possible to give a precise quantification of this standard, minimal risks are the ones to which we are exposed all the time. They thus suggest that the more uncertainty there is about whether a particular case meets this standard, the more likely it is that it does not. If norms differ across communities about the level of risk to which it is acceptable to expose children, they appear to endorse what they call a "both-and" approach in which the standards of both communities are applied. While this standard may remain fuzzy around the edges, they argue that it is clear enough to assist in the case by case examination of particular clinical trials.

We close this section with a case study and critical reflections on a persistent problem in research with psychiatric patients. The problem concerns the fate of severely schizophrenic patients who are taking powerful drugs to control such symptoms as hallucinations, delusions, disorganized thinking, social withdrawal, and, most seriously, suicide. Current antipsychotic medications generally work well, but at the cost of serious side effects, such as tardive dyskinesia, a syndrome characterized by involuntary muscle ticks. Researchers are thus keenly interested in learning which patients might be able to quit taking these drugs without suffering a relapse of their psychotic symptoms. To answer this important question, researchers at UCLA designed a controversial protocol described by psychiatrist Paul S. Appelbaum in "Drug-Free Research in Schizophrenia." The UCLA study called for a period of withdrawal from all drugs; a standard dose of a standard drug for all patients, instead of individualized treatment; and for the use of placebo controls at various phases of the experiment. Some of the test subjects relapsed with very disconcerting results and one committed suicide; charges of unethical research and calls for federal investigation followed shortly thereafter.

In his comprehensive and thoughtful assessment, Paul Appelbaum notes that many schizophrenics are at elevated risk of having impaired capacity for giving informed consent. Although he is sensitive to the many risks and ethical difficulties surrounding such research, Appelbaum suggests several ways in which such clearly important and desirable research might be carried out with increased protections for such a vulnerable position. In his case commentary, Jay Katz notes several shortcomings in the informed consent form used in the UCLA study, including the understatement of some serious risks involved with schizophrenic relapse. Katz also observes that many patients in this study had difficulty understanding the difference between clinical treatment and research designed primarily to gain generalizable knowledge, and he criticizes the UCLA team for their apparent reluctance to emphasize their research orientation in discussions with potential subjects. This so-called therapeutic misconception is widespread in the area of clinical research (Appelbaum 1987) and might be particularly problematic when dealing with patients who are mentally ill.

We are thus confronted with the essential tension haunting all research with so-called vulnerable populations. In spite of recent crusades for increased access to the fruits of research to benefit HIV-infected patients, women, and others, some groups of patients, such as the schizophrenics enrolled in the UCLA study, remain particularly vulnerable to abuse and/or neglect and may well require an enhanced level of protection in the design and conduct of medical research. On the other hand, such enhanced protection always carries the potential for excessive and misguided paternalism. As we protect such patients from overreaching on the part of researchers, we must guard against a failure to acknowledge their capacity, when present, for meaningful participation in, and consent to, research of the utmost importance.

BORN IN SCANDAL: THE ORIGINS OF U.S. RESEARCH ETHICS

THE NUREMBERG CODE

(1) The voluntary consent of the human subject is absolutely essential.

This means that the person involved should have legal capacity to give consent; should be so situated as to be able to exercise free power of choice, without the intervention of any element of force, fraud, deceit, duress, over-reaching, or other ulterior form of constraint or coercion; and should have sufficient knowledge and comprehension of the elements of the subject matter involved as to enable him to make an understanding and enlightened decision. This latter element requires that before the acceptance of an affirmative decision by the experimental subject there should be made known to him the nature, duration, and purpose of the experiment; the method and means by which it is to be conducted; all inconveniences and hazards reasonably to be expected; and the effects upon his health or person which may possibly come from his participation in the experiment.

The duty and responsibility for ascertaining the quality of the consent rests upon each individual who initiates, directs or engages in the experiment. It is a personal duty and responsibility which may not be delegated to another with impunity.

(2) The experiment should be such as to yield fruitful results for the good of society, unprocurable by other methods or means of study, and not random and unnecessary in nature.

(3) The experiment should be so designed and based on the results of animal experimentation and a knowledge of the natural history of the disease or other problem under study that the anticipated results will justify the performance of the experiment.

(4) The experiment should be so conducted as to avoid all unnecessary physical and mental suffering and injury.

(5) No experiment should be conducted where there is an *a priori* reason to believe that death or disabling injury will occur; except, perhaps, in those experiments where the experimental physicians also serve as subjects.

From "Permissible Medical Experiments," *Trials of War Criminals before the Nuernberg Military Tribunals under Control Council Law No. 10: Nuernberg, October 1946–April 1949* (Washington: U.S. Government Printing Office, n.d., vol. 2), 181–182.

(6) The degree of risk to be taken should never exceed that determined by the humanitarian importance of the problem to be solved by the experiment.

(7) Proper preparations should be made and adequate facilities provided to protect the experimental subject against even remote possibilities of injury, disability, or death.

(8) The experiment should be conducted only by scientifically qualified persons. The highest degree of skill and care should be required through all stages of the experiment of those who conduct or engage in the experiment.

(9) During the course of the experiment the human subject should be at liberty to bring the experiment to an end if he has reached the physical or mental state where continuation of the experiment seems to him to be impossible.

(10) During the course of the experiment the scientist in charge must be prepared to terminate the experiment at any stage, if he has probable cause to believe, in the exercise of the good faith, superior skill and careful judgment required of him that a continuation of the experiment is likely to result in injury, disability, or death to the experimental subject.

THE JEWISH CHRONIC DISEASE HOSPITAL CASE

Jay Katz

In July 1963, three doctors, with approval from the director of medicine of the Jewish Chronic Disease Hospital in Brooklyn, New York, injected "live cancer cells" subcutaneously into twenty-two chronically ill and debilitated patients. The doctors did not inform the patients that live cancer cells were being used or that the experiment was designed to measure the patients' ability to reject foreign cells—a test unrelated to their normal therapeutic program.

The cancer experiment engendered a heated controversy among the hospital's doctors and led to an investigation by the hospital's grievance committee and board of directors. William A. Hyman, a member of the board who disapproved of the experiment, took the hospital to court to force disclosure of the hospital's records, claiming that the directors' approval of the experiment had not been properly obtained. As Hyman *v.* Jewish Chronic Disease Hospital *wound its way up from the trial court through two appellate tribunals, it became clear that the legal issue involved in the suit, whether a hospital director is entitled to look at patients' medical records, only provided the backdrop for the questions really at issue which concerned the duties and obligations that the various participants in the human experimentation process should have toward one another.*

Subsequently, these issues were confronted more directly when the Board of Regents of the University of the State of New York heard charges brought by the attorney general against two of the doctors involved. The board imposed sanctions, under the authority given it by New York Education Law § 6514(2) to revoke, suspend, or annul the license of a practitioner of medicine upon determining "after due hearing . . . that a physician . . . is guilty of fraud or deceit in the practice of medicine [or] that a physician is or has been guilty of unprofessional conduct.". . .

Jay Katz, "The Jewish Chronic Disease Hospital Case," in *Experimentation with Human Beings.*

REBUTTAL AFFIDAVITS FOR RESPONDENT

Chester M. Southam, M.D.—February 4, 1964

I address myself first to the question of the measure of risk of bodily harm to the patients who were the subject of the procedures in question at the Jewish Chronic Disease Hospital. At the outset I should say that in clinical procedures neither I nor any scientist or doctor can deal in absolutes. We are always limited, at least when dealing with the human body, to speaking in terms of measurable risks. Thus while no doctor or scientist can say as to any clinical procedure, even the simplest, that there is *no possibility* of untoward results, we are constantly required, both in therapeutic and in investigative procedures, to make judgments as to whether there is any unusual risk of untoward results, and if so, the degree of that risk. In terms of this standard I unhesitatingly assert that on the basis of present biological knowledge supplemented by clinical experience to date there was no practical possibility of untoward results to the patients who received injections of homotransplants in the form of tissue-cultured cells derived from other patients. The probability of any unforeseen deleterious consquences [*sic*] of this test is so extremely small as to be comparable to numerous other procedures used routinely in clinical medicine for therapeutic, diagnostic, or investigative purposes, e.g., blood transfusions, intravenous pyelograms (kidney x-rays), or tuberculin tests. The fact that these cells were tissue-cultured cancer cells did not measurably increase any risk inherent in the procedure because, being foreign to the recipient (the person injected), they bring about an immunologic reaction (defense reaction, rejection reaction) that ultimately causes their destruction and elimination.

It has been known for many years that a human being will reject cells transplanted from another human being unless both are of precisely the same genetic makeup (i.e., identical twins). In fact, intensive clinical studies are now being carried on at many research centers attempting to find methods (such as treatment with certain drugs or x-ray) to overcome this rejection reaction in the hope that diseased organs, such as kidneys, might be successfully replaced. While the precise mechanisms of cell rejection are not yet known, the fact that such mechanisms exist is beyond question. The efficiency of this type of immunological reaction can be measured in terms of the time required for complete rejection of homotransplanted cells. As yet no other method of measuring this reaction has been found, and tissue-cultured cancer cells are the only kind of cells which provide sufficient reproducibility for comparison of results in different individuals at different times.

The three lines of cells derived from human cancer which were used in the studies at the Jewish Chronic Disease Hospital were derived from tumor tissues of three patients, from 4 to 12 years ago. Since that time these cells have been cultivated in sterile bottles in the laboratory in a solution of nutrients which include salts, vitamins and blood serum. This is the process called tissue culture. After such years of growth under these artificial laboratory conditions each line of cultured cells has a high degree of uniformity and, consequently, the reaction which it will produce is highly predictable. I have had an extensive experience with each of these three cell lines in homotransplantation studies in cancer patients and in healthy volunteers during the past several years.

In the early 1950's it began to appear that the defense mechanisms (i.e., the mechanism of rejection of homotransplants) of those persons who develop cancer might be in some way impaired. The most striking indication of this was the result of clinical tests on a limited number of patients with terminal cancer as reported over the signatures of myself and Drs. Rhoads and Moore in *Science.* These were all patients suffering from advanced stages of widely disseminated cancer for whom there was no known method of treatment to either inhibit their disease or prolong their lives, each of whom died as the result of his own cancer within a relatively short time. In view of the then state of knowledge the precise details of the procedure were explained and the patients freely and readily consented.

The significant result of the test was that the rate of rejection of the foreign transplants was in all cases slower than would have been expected, indicating that there was some impairment of their immunological reaction. Because these patients had far advanced cancer before the homotransplants were injected, they did not survive for long after the tests were performed. Obviously this was not the result of the test, but rather was the reason that these particular patients were selected for these earliest tests. In no case was the patient deleteriously affected by the implants. Several patients in this initial group and in subsequent groups had not rejected their transplants in the brief interval between the start of the test and their death. In fact, at autopsy a lymph node from the armpit of one of these patients contained unrejected cancer cells of the type used for the test. (These lymph nodes are in the natural route of drainage from the forearm where the test was made in this patient.)

Prior to the publication of the article in question tests were made on a number of volunteer healthy human beings in the Ohio Penitentiary. In all such cases the foreign transplants were quickly and completely rejected, as would have been expected.

After the initial tests reported in *Science*, intensive studies were undertaken, designed to increase our body of knowledge as to the immunological reaction both of normal healthy persons and those with cancer, to homotransplants of tissue-cultured lines of human cells derived from normal and tumor tissues. Between the time of the initial tests and July 16, 1963 (the date on which the injections were made in Jewish Chronic Disease Hospital) approximately 600 persons had been studied by means of the techniques employed at Jewish Chronic Disease Hospital, approximately 300 of whom were patients with cancer and 300 healthy, normal persons. In every healthy recipient of tissue-cultured cells, these foreign transplants were rejected with uniform promptness. Some patients with cancer rejected the cells less rapidly and after significantly varying intervals of time. Patients in the earlier stages of neoplastic disease showed normal or only slightly impaired rejection reaction. Patients in the terminal stages of cancer showed the greatest deficiency in these immunological defense mechanisms (as measured by the length of time to effect rejection) and in several such persons rejection had not been accomplished in the few weeks or months that elapsed between injection of the test cells and the patient's death from his own cancer. These patients died from the effects of their own cancer before the expected ultimate rejection of the implants. The studies also demonstrated a correlation between the rate of rejection of homotransplanted cancer cells and the patient's apparent ability to restrain his own disease, thus providing additional direct evidence that patients may have immunological (defense) mechanisms to restrain their own cancer. These results, of course, give hope that, through further clinical research, methods of stimulating such mechanisms to greater efficacy can be developed.

The studies of healthy, normal persons at the Ohio Penitentiary, aside from demonstrating that the normal body will reject cancer cell homotransplants with the same efficiency as other types of homotransplants, further indicated the potentially highly significant fact that the body's rate of rejection increased with successive implantations of foreign cancer cells, suggesting long-run possibilities of building up the immunological mechanisms where deficiencies now occur. At present, studies are being continued to verify these scientific observations and to investigate their possible applicability to the treatment and prevention of human cancer. Such studies of human cancer can be accomplished only through the cooperation of patients and healthy volunteers.

Until the investigation conducted at the Jewish Chronic Disease Hospital, there was no direct clinical evidence that the impairment of the immunologic responses in patients with advanced cancer (as measured by the slow rate at which they rejected homotransplants) was associated with the fact that they had cancer rather than with the fact that they were in a debilitated state. This study provided direct clinical evidence that indeed the impairment was associated with the fact of cancer rather than general debilitation. The patients at Jewish Chronic Disease Hospital reacted in essentially the same manner as normal, healthy human beings. I want to make perfectly clear that the question in this investigation was not whether the patients would reject the tissue-cultured cancer cell homotransplants. The only question was how fast would the body mobilize its resources of rejection. Three patients known to have cancer were also included in these tests. It was expected that rejection in the three cancer patients might be delayed, consistent with our previous experience in cancer patients, but that rejection would occur after the predicted delay unless these patients succumbed very rapidly to their own cancer.

I next turn to the question of procedures. In the early stages of this clinical research and, indeed, until the last few years a full explanation was given to the patient or healthy volunteer, including the fact that the techniques employed were not designed for his own therapy, the nature of the cultured cells involved, the general purposes of the test and the expected reactions. More recently, as our body of knowledge has increased and the course of reaction to the injections became predictable, we have simply explained that the procedure was a test which had nothing to do with treatment, that it involved the injection of foreign material, described the expected course of reaction, and that its purpose was to determine the rate at which the expected nodules would develop and then regress. In all instances in which the test was done the patients have readily given their consent, and the tests were not performed if such consent was not readily given. Unless the patient inquired, we refrained from describing the precise nature of the human cells (i.e., that they had originally been derived from tumors and then grown in tissue culture) for the reason that in my own professional judgment as well as that of my professional colleagues who had followed the course of these experiments, the precise nature of the foreign cells was irrelevant to the bodily reactions which could be expected to occur.

This course was followed, I submit, not out of any disregard for the rights or best interests of the patient nor of my responsibilities as a practitioner of medicine. It was a sincere professional judgment, based upon extensive scientific and clinical experience, that the procedures involved only the same low degree of risk inherent in many routine clinical test procedures, the patient in all such cases being informed only of the facts which are important from his standpoint. I submit that but for the highly emotion-charged term "cancer cells," this conclusion would be unquestioned by those in the medical profession who are fully cognizant of the present stage of knowledge with respect to immunological reactions.

Furthermore, in my own clinical judgment—based on fifteen years of clinical management of advanced cancer patients—to use the dreaded word "cancer" in connection with any clinical procedure on an ill person is potentially deleterious to that patient's well-being because it may suggest to him (rightly or wrongly) that his diagnosis is cancer or that his prognosis is poor. Some cancer patients do not know that their diagnosis is cancer, and even those who have been informed rarely discuss it and may even deny it. It is seldom possible for the physician to be full cognizant of the cancer patient's extent of knowledge of and his attitude toward his disease. The doctor's choice of words in discussions with the patient has a great influence upon the patient's mental attitude. Since the initial neoplastic source of the test material employed was not germane to the reaction being studied and not, in my opinion, a cause of increased risk to the patient, I believe that such revelation is generally contraindicated in the best consideration of the patient's welfare and therefore to withhold such emotionally disturbing but medically nonpertinent details (unless requested by the patient) is in the best tradition of responsible clinical practice.

On these questions concerning procedure, I will readily submit to the judgment of my colleagues after they are fully informed. . . .

Emanuel E. Mandel, M.D.—February 4, 1964

The method of obtaining the consents to the Sloan-Kettering tests, outlined in the answering papers, must be evaluated in relation to the basic medical principle that the extent of information to be imparted to the patient must be left to the judgment of the responsible physician. There are many standard techniques used by physicians for the purpose of diagnosis and treatment which may result in injury, or even death, to patients. Yet, in the interest of the patient, they are not normally preceded by any thoroughgoing explanations, or even by any written or oral consents (e.g., penicillin injections, the obtaining of intravenous pyelograms, "BSP" tests, X-ray treatment for non-cancerous patients, the administration of radioactive substances (iodine and phosphorus), etc.).

It must be patent that the investigative team of Sloan-Kettering and JCDH acted in full compliance with conventional procedure accepted by the medical profession at large. The injections of cell suspensions in question here were no more hazardous than any of the above named routine tests, and, indeed, far safer than most of them or perhaps all of them. In fact, consideration was being given at the outset of this study to the possibility of adopting those injections as routine tests to uncover hidden (subclinical) cancer, since it was regarded as a routine test at Memorial Hospital (see minutes of the hearing in the offices of the New York State Education Department on December 19, 1963). For even advanced (metastatic) cancer can escape the physician's attention in a patient suffering from other chronic and debilitating disease, and even advanced cancer can, at times, be treated with success. There is no basis for the argument of Dr. Strauss and other medical witnesses that the tests were "dissociated" from the "patient's ailment and condition.". . .

HOW AND BY WHOM SHOULD THE CONSEQUENCES OF RESEARCH BE REVIEWED?

1. INFORMING THE BOARD OF REGENTS GRIEVANCE COMMITTEE FOR DECISION

A. LOUIS J. LEFKOWITZ, ATTORNEY GENERAL OF THE STATE OF NEW YORK PETITIONER'S POST-HEARING MEMORANDUM

In the Matter of the

Application for the revocation of the authorization and license heretofore granted to Emanuel Mandel, M.D. and Chester Southam, M.D. to practice medicine in the State of New York, and for the cancellation of their registrations as such, and for such other relief as the premises warrant.

The Statutes

The applicable provisions of the Education Law are as follows:

Section 6514. Revocation of Certificates.

2. The license or registration of a practitioner of medicine . . . may be revoked, suspended or annulled or such practitioner reprimanded or disciplined in accordance with the provisions and procedure of this article upon decision after due hearing in any of the following cases:

2 (a) That a physician . . . is guilty of fraud or deceit in the practice of medicine. . . .

2 (g) That a physician is or has been guilty of unprofessional conduct. As implemented and defined by the Rules of the Commissioner, filed pursuant to Statute in the Office of the Secretary of State under Title 8, part 60.1, subd. (d) 7 of the Official Compilation Codes, Rules and Regulations of the State of New York, i.e. "immoral conduct of a physician in his practice as a physician."

1. A Valid and Informed Consent Was Not Obtained Since the Patients Were Not Fully Informed of the Nature and Details of the Experiment

At the outset, it should be firmly understood that while we are dealing with 22 patients in a hospital, what was done to them, in the experimentation involved herein, was not done in the care or treatment of whatever illnesses or infirmities they had; and the respondents so admit.

It should also be remembered that, [all patients] had a right to expect and to demand from those charged with the administration of the hospital in its care and treatment of patients, that only those procedures and administrations of drugs that were a necessary part of their care and treatment be given and administered.

. . . An analysis of the patients selected amply illustrates that a substantial number of them had not sufficient mental or physical ability to comprehend what was being told to them or what was being done to them; and those who may have had the capacity to understand were not given the full and true nature of the experiment.

As to Patient #18: Leichter had testified this patient had Parkinsons [*sic*]; developed lung abscess; was always running and falling against wall; had difficulty in communicating; that patient did not understand what was being explained and his speech was unintelligible. Leichter had treated this patient during the years from 1959 to 1963 and stated the patient's condition worsened with respect to July 16th. He further stated as his opinion this patient was unable to understand what an experiment of the type performed would mean.

Rosenfeld testified this patient was in a vegetative state and incommunicative the last year at the hospital; and could not have given a consent.

Southam testified this patient was in complete possession of his senses to extent he nodded agreement to permit examination at site of injection; that each time Southam saw the patient he was ambulatory, had marked shuffling gait, drooled considerably; that he did not regard the patient to be in a vegetative state, but was fully capable of understanding.

This testimony of Southam's is based upon observations made *after* injections were given. An examination of the record of this patient reveals Southam saw patient first time July 19th, then August 13, August 20 and finally October 1st.

Further, what probative weight should be given to Southam's testimony—based as it is on four visits—when it is compared to that of Leichter or Rosenfeld, doctors who have been constantly in attendance at Blumberg Building for many years prior to date of injections, and who have seen this patient countless numbers of times, examined him and treated him? . . .

It is respectfully urged, with respect to this patient, that Leichter and Rosenfeld, because of their length of service in Blumberg Building, were in a much better position to see, examine and observe this patient than were Southam (who never saw the patient before July 16th), Mandel and Custodio. . . .

It is submitted that the testimony of Leichter and Rosenfeld as to this patient should be accepted by the committee, and that a finding be made declaring this patient was incapable of understanding and thus could not have given a valid consent to participate in this experiment.

While only the records and testimony pertaining to a few patients have been shown to illustrate that the believable and probative proof established the absence of ability to understand fully the scope of the experimentation and thus give valid consent, it is by no means conceded that, in those patients not shown, there was present ability to understand and give consent.

The procedures adopted by the respondents in their conduct in pursuing the same give rise to certain compelling and important questions. . . .

Why wasn't a careful screening done by both Mandel and Custodio, with a careful scrutiny of the hospital records which were available to them prior to July 16th? Why wasn't, prior to July 16th, a detailed statement prepared concerning the test, detailing each and every step of the procedures, the purposes for which the test was to be given and the names of the patients to be selected to participate? And, most important of all, why wasn't each patient informed that the injectable material was cancer cells? Why all the secrecy concerning cancer cells being injected if Mandel and Southam were so sure no deleterious effect could befall the patients? Yet Mandel had the gall to state in an affidavit submitted to the Supreme Court that everything was open and above-board!

Where was consideration shown to the patients with respect to their comfort; their freedom from unnecessary molestation and their absolute right to expect only such procedures and administrations necessary to their care and treatment? How dared Mandel introduce strangers to his hospital and to his patients and to permit these strangers to go through the various wards of the hospital, in open view of other patients? Oh, yes, those strangers were dressed like doctors—they had the long white coat commonly worn by visiting doctors; this then perhaps justified the intrusion as far as Mandel was concerned!

The haphazard method of selecting patients; the almost complete disregard of their comfort; the slipshod manner in which the entire project was conceived and conducted, is evident throughout the record.

Southam was not concerned with whether Mandel had the right to proceed with this project without sanction or authority. Nor was he concerned with what patients were selected; whether they were informed, and whether they were capable of giving consent. Mandel was evidently flattered that his hospital had been selected; he made no independent investigation concerning Southam or the project: he took Southam's word that no risk was involved, *although this was the first time they were engaged in performing this test upon debilitated patients;* he failed or refused to select a more capable and experienced participator than Custodio; and failed to assist and supervise the selection of patients.

And the greatest sin of all was the deliberate and willful failure on the part of the respondents herein, to inform each of the 22 patients that they were going to be injected with live cancer cells.

We are dealing with a project which admittedly was in no way therapeutic. It was, rather, an experiment relating to cancer research which had as its ultimate intention the benefit of humanity. This being the fact, it was then incumbent upon the respondents to have seen to it that ALL information connected with the experiment was given, since the patients at JCDH were being asked to become volunteers.

Respondents both admit they sanctioned and counseled the withholding from each patient the fact that the cell suspension to be used was indeed "live cancer cells." Their reasoning? They state that to release this information to the patients would cause a phobia, make them frightened, cause fear and anxiety—and this they wanted to avoid!

Every human being has an inalienable right to determine what shall be done with his own body. These patients then had a right to know what was being planned—not just the bald statement that an injection was to be given, but also the contents of the syringe: and if this knowledge was to cause fear and anxiety or make them frightened, they had a right to be fearful and frightened and thus say NO to the experiment.

Petitioner's exhibit #19, an article entitled "Problems of Informed Consent May Be Unsolvable" cites that Nuremberg Code—"the voluntary consent of the human subject is absolutely essential."

Petitioner's exhibit #6 and Resp. Southam's exhibit AA are entitled "The Normal Volunteer Program of the NIH Clinical Center" and is published by the U.S. Department of Health, Education and Welfare. Under the heading "Definitions" a distinction is made between the "normal volunteer"—a person who is judged to be in excellent health, etc., and "volunteer"—one who offers himself for a service of his own free will. Concededly, the patients at JCDH would come under the second classification. "Informed Consent" is defined as follows:

> A formal, explicit, free expression of willingness to serve as a subject for research after the values and effects of such participation have been explained by the investigator and are sufficiently understood for the Volunteer to make a mature judgment.

At page 3 of the exhibit, under "Informed Consent" appears the following language:

> The principal investigator *personally* provides the assigned volunteer, *in lay language* and at the level of his comprehension, with information about the proposed research project. He outlines its purpose, method, demands, inconveniences and discomforts, to enable the volunteer to make a *mature judgment* as to his willingness and ability to participate. When he is fully cognizant of all that is entailed, the volunteer gives his *signed consent* to take part in it. (Emphasis supplied.)

It should be remembered that one of the sponsors for Southam's project and experimentation was the NIH!

How then did Southam discharge his duties and obligations to the volunteers as the principal and chief investigator in this experiment? Again, do we not see the careless and absolute disregard for the rights of the patients who were chosen to participate? While it may be argued that Southam was a stranger to JCDH and its patients and therefore relied upon Mandel, it nevertheless remains the undisputed fact that the 22 patients selected were volunteers in this project, and as to them in that capacity, Southam owed them every consideration and obligation as described by the NIH (supra). His was the duty *personally* to provide the volunteer *in lay language* at the level of his comprehension with information about the proposed research project; outlining its purpose; methods; demands; inconveniences and discomforts; so as to enable the volunteer to make a mature judgment as to his willingness and ability to participate; and only when the volunteer is fully cognizant of *all that is entailed,* does he give Southam his *signed* consent. And how did Southam discharge this duty and obligation? First, he said he left it to Mandel to decide the question of "consent" and the manner by which it was to be obtained, albeit he stressed to Mandel the method of obtaining oral consents at Memorial which, in Southam's opinion, were sufficient although the recipient of the injection was not told that cancer cells were being injected. Secondly, he said he was satisfied to have Custodio as his collaborator, despite the fact that he saw Custodio for the first time on the day of the experiment and knew nothing whatever of the latter's ability, experience or knowledge in projects of this kind. This, it is strongly urged, Southam had no right to do. As a scientist engaged in research he had the duty and responsibility for ascertaining the quality of the consent, which may not be delegated to another with impunity. This was his project, and, if it was to serve any useful purpose he should have taken and assumed full and complete authority; by having carefully screened, with Mandel, the patients that were to be selected; by having, with Mandel, spoken, in advance of the injections, to each patient, explaining in lay language at the level of the patient's comprehension, the purpose, methods, demands, inconveniences and discomforts of the proposed project.

For the record is replete with contradictory statements as to the manner by which "consents" were obtained; Mandel wasn't sure whether he had obtained so-called oral consents from one or two patients; he wasn't sure of the language he used in speaking of the project. Custodio likewise is not sure of just what words were used when speaking to the patients stating that interchangeably he used words as "immunity," "resistance" or "immunological response."

But the salient factor remains that at *no time* and to *no volunteer patient* was information given that in truth and in fact the cell suspension mentioned contained *live cancer cells.*

This then is the nub of the entire case. These volunteers, the 22 debilitated patients at JCDH, were not each made *"fully cognizant of ALL that is entailed"* in the proposed project. There was *missing,* deliberately and willfully so, any statement to the effect that the injectable material contained live cancer cells. As was stated in SCIENCE, petitioner's exhibit #9, in the article entitled "Medical Ethics" and that portion under the chapter heading "Procedures not of direct benefit to the individual" found on page 1025 of the exhibit:

> The common feature of this type of investigation is that it is of no direct benefit to the particular individual and that, in consequence, if he is to submit to it he must volunteer in the full sense of the word.
>
> It should be clearly understood that the possibility or probability that a particular investigation will be of benefit to humanity or to posterity would afford no defense in the event of legal proceedings. The individual has rights that the law protects and nobody can infringe those rights for the public good. In investigations of this type it is, therefore, always necessary to ensure that the true consent of the subject is explicitly obtained.

It is therefore respectfully submitted that the respondents herein failed to secure a valid and informed consent from each of the 22 patient-volunteers to participate in the experimentation conducted at JCDH.

2. The Respondents Are Each Guilty of Each Specification of the Charges

The failure of each respondent to reveal ALL that was entailed in the experimentation to each of the volunteer debilitated patients that were selected to participate was fraudulent and deceitful. As illustrated supra, the licensees herein had no right, moral or legal, to withhold any information relating to the experimentation. By so doing they violated the absolute right of each patient to determine what shall be done with his own body. By withholding the fact that live cancer cells were to be injected in this experiment, they deprived each patient of their inalienable right to refuse such an injection. *No choice* was given to these volunteers.

The conduct of each respondent was unprofessional, immoral and shocking to one's sense of fairness. Mandel has testified that patients do not question procedures that are done to them in a hospital because they have confidence in the doctors and that patients tend to accept what doctors say to them. It is submitted this confidence was misplaced; that all of these patient-volunteers were duped and misled by Southam and Mandel. Surely, the image of the medical profession must be sullied in the eyes of the public, if the conduct of the respondents herein was to be sanctioned and blessed with innocence.

Again and again it must be repeated and emphasized that a human being has rights and privileges that may not be trespassed upon to any degree. How shocking indeed it would be if a person were to realize that he had no rights or privileges as to what should be done to his body, and that he was a mere "guinea pig" in the eyes of any doctor, whether scientist or researcher, who desired to perform some experimentation on him!

Such a fantastic and gruesome thought could never withstand the indignation and denial of the public.

Upon the entire case therefore it is respectfully submitted each licensee is guilty of each specification contained in the charges.

B.
MORRIS PLOSCOWE, ESQ. BRIEF ON BEHALF OF DR. EMANUEL E. MANDEL

The Charge that Dr. Mandel Is Guilty of Fraud and Deceit Because the Patients Were Not Advised "That Live Cancer Cells Were To Be Injected In Their Bodies" Cannot Be Sustained

The reasons why the patients were not told that the injections contained tissue cultured cancer cells are not found in fraud or deceit. This is apparent from the following:

Dr. Southam was asked why he deliberately refrained from describing (the injected cells) as "cancer cells." He testified as follows:

> For two reasons really. First, I saw no reason why we should use such a word because it is not pertinent to the phenomenon which is going to follow. We are not doing something which is going to induce cancer. We are not going to do something which is going to cause them any harm; it is not going to produce a transplanted cancer. We are going to observe the growth and rejection of these transplanted cancer cells.
>
> The fact then that they are cancer cells does not mean that there is any risk of cancer to this patient.
>
> Now, the second point is simply that the word, "cancer," has a tremendous emotive value, disvalue, to everybody, not only to the cancer patients but to you and me. What the ordinary patient, what the non-medical person, and even many doctors whose competence in clinical medicine is great but whose knowledge of the basic science behind transplantation is not great—to them the use of a cancer cell might imply a risk that it will grow and produce cancer, and the fear that this word strikes in people is great, and I don't think I have to argue the point to make the point. I think we all recognize it. If we use words like neoplastic; if we use words like tumor, we have no problem.
>
> . . . Many of these patients undoubtedly know deep down that they have cancer, but the great majority of them have either suppressed this knowledge from the surface or at least they are not talking about it and they don't welcome conversation that brings it up. So, it is our firmly established and I feel very sound policy *not to use the word "cancer"* with the cancer patients. . . .

The position taken by Dr. Mandel and Dr. Southam in not mentioning the fact that the injections contained cancer cells is justified by medical ethics and current medical practice. Medical ethics do not require the full disclosure to a patient of all conceivable risks and all relevant information as a basis for obtaining patients' consent to a medical procedure. The amount of information imparted to a patient must bear some relation to the risk of a particular procedure. Where there is no substantial risk of harm to a patient, the information imparted to him may be kept at a minimum. We submit that in the instant case it was not necessary to tell the patient that the injections involved tissue cultured cancer cells since there was no possibility that harm could come to the patients from the said cells.[*]

It should also be noted that the amount of information which should be imparted to a patient as a prerequisite for consent to a medical or surgical procedure may be left to the sound discretion of a conscientious physician.[†] This is the import of the rules concerning the testing of drugs which is in evidence as respondent's Exhibit B, and which state that while consent should be obtained for testing of investigational drugs, the laws and the regulations

---

[*] CROSS-EXAMINATION OF DR. CHESTER M. SOUTHAM BY MR. CALANESE.

Q: Doctor, in Vol. 143 of *Science* which is issued February 1964 at page 551 you wrote that there was no theoretical likelihood that the injections would produce cancer. Yet, in the same article, Doctor, you stated that you were unwilling to inject yourself or your colleagues, and you stated, and I quote, "But, let's face it, there are relatively few skilled cancer researchers, and it seemed stupid to take even the little risk."

A: I deny the quote. I am sure I didn't say, "let's face it."

Q: Did you make any statement similar to that?

A: I think the philosophy is an accurate statement.

Q: What was your statement, do you recall?

A: What I am objecting to is the phrase, "let's face it." The statement that I see no reason why a doctor should necessarily serve as a recipient, this is valid, that is, this statement may validly be attributed to me.

Q: The statement, Doctor, was published by Elinor Langer in *Science* of February 7, 1964, Vol. 143, and I quote from her statement that I want to find out from you whether or not what she is quoting as coming from you is correct or not. "Southam, however, who ought to know, said in an interview with *Science* that, although there was no theoretical likelihood that the injections would produce cancer, he had nonetheless been unwilling to inject himself or his colleagues, when there was a group of normal volunteers at the Ohio Penitentiary fully informed about the experiment and its possible risks and nonetheless eager to take part in it. 'I would not have hesitated' Southam said, 'if it would have served a useful purpose. But,' he continued, 'to me it seemed like false heroism, like the old question whether the General should march behind or in front of his troops. I do not regard myself as indispensable—if I were not doing this work someone else would be—and I did not regard the experiments as dangerous. But, let's face it, there are relatively few skilled cancer researchers, and it seemed stupid to take even the little risk.' "

Did you make that statement?

A: As I said before, the philosophy is correct. I do not know if I made that statement. This is reported—I remember the interview very well. I am still saying that the quotes are not necessarily correct; the philosophy is correct.

Q: That part of the quoting concerning the, "stupid to take even the little risk," do you recall that?

A: No, I don't, and this is one of the reasons that I question whether it is a true quote.

Q: Do you recall the statement that you made that there was no theoretical likelihood that injections would produce cancer?

A: This is, in other words, exactly what I have said earlier this afternoon. [From transcript of proceedings before a Subcommittee of the Committee on Grievances, Department of Education of the State of New York, September, 1964, pp. 636–638.]

[†] EXAMINATION OF DR. EMANUEL E. MANDEL BY MR. RASHKIS, INVESTIGATOR, NEW YORK STATE DEPARTMENT OF EDUCATION.

Q: Each patient was told that an experiment to determine his immunity was to be conducted. Was each patient told that cell tissue was to be injected?

A: Yes, cell suspension was to be injected.

Q: Each patient was told this?

A: Yes, each patient was told.

Q: Did any patient ask you what a cell suspension is?

MR. PLOSCOWE: If you can recall.

A: I can't.

Q: No one asked you?

A: (No response.)

Q: Did you actually have a conversation with the patients that you spoke to them and they answered you?

A: Yes.

Q: Every patient?

A: Every patient. I asked them if they have—each and every one of them has any objection to doing the test and they said no.

Q: Did any patient answer anything other than yes or no; that he would agree—

A: No.

Q: No patient questioned any of the terms that you used?

A: I don't remember. I don't think anyone asked.

DR. MANDEL: May I add to that?

MR. RASHKIS: Yes.

DR. MANDEL: I will say almost every day doctors come into situations where they have to ask a patient for permission to do a certain procedure, say a bone marrow aspiration, a spinal tap, what not.

Most patients don't question these procedures; the patients have confidence in the doctors.

MR. RASHKIS: What is the purpose for the tests?

DR. MANDEL: Diagnostic nature.

MR. RASHKIS: For that particular patient?

DR. MANDEL: For that particular patient.

(continued on page 716)

make it clear that if in the professional judgment of the investigator "it is not feasible or in the best interests of the subject to obtain permission, *the investigational nature of the drug need not be disclosed.*" This concept of patient consent is not new, but has been part of the Code of Ethics of the American Medical Association for many years.

If, in the judgment of a conscientious physician, the investigational nature of a drug need not be disclosed, when it is tested, then there appears to be no reason why the nature of the injected material should have been disclosed to the patients at JCDH, since there was no hazard to the patients from the injections.

The following statements made by distinguished physicians in affidavits submitted on behalf of Dr. Southam, support our contention that a proper consent was obtained from the patients at JCDH in the tests conducted at JCDH and that it was not fraud or deceit not to tell the patients that the injected material contained cancer cells:

Dr. Michael J. Brennan, physician in charge of the division of oncology, Henry Ford Hospital, Detroit, Michigan, stated as follows:

> . . . The need to enter into detailed description of the source and nature of a test material cannot be shown to be a part of our moral and legal duty unless it would be objectively helpful to the patient in coming to a rational and knowledgeable conclusion about the real risks of the procedure to his health.
>
> . . . He [Southam] did not speak to these patients of giving them a treatment. He asked permission to do a test of considerable scientific import. He then faithfully explained to them the sequence of reactions which they could expect and rightly and correctly assured them of their innocuous character. He hid nothing from the patients which would have been useful to them in making a rational decision regarding the real risks of the test.
>
> He did not mention that the test solutions were made from tissue cultures of cancer cells. This now proves to have been imprudent because of the emotional character of the response which followed revelation of that fact and the opening it gave for accusations of dishonesty and duplicity on his part. There is a difference between withholding information and giving false information but it is often overlooked. However, *the information he withheld was not needed by the patients for judging rightly that his test was safe.*
>
> The real test of the adequacy of his description to the patients of what would happen is whether it corresponded with what did in fact happen.
>
> It was the compassion of the good physician, not the deceit of the charlatan or the calculation of the cold experimentalist, which has laid him open to his present troubles. . . .

(continued from page 715)

MR. RASHKIS: Would these patients have understood these tests were to be diagnostic in nature?

DR. MANDEL: No.

MR. RASHKIS: Is there any relevancy in the statement you made about the bone-marrow test?

DR. MANDEL: Only in terms of conversation with patients. Ordinarily they listen and tend to accept what the doctor says to them. [From transcript of proceedings before a Subcommittee of the Committee on Grievances, Department of Education of the State of New York, September, 1964, pp. 96–100.]

4. THE BOARD OF REGENTS DECIDES

BOARD OF REGENTS OF THE UNIVERSITY OF THE STATE OF NEW YORK LICENSES SUSPENDED, SUSPENSIONS STAYED, RESPONDENTS PLACED ON PROBATION*

Upon the report of the Regents Committee on Discipline, made in accordance with the provisions of section 211 of the Education Law, it was

Voted, That the determination of the Medical Committee on Grievances in the matter of Chester M. Southam . . . and Emanuel E. Mandel . . . be accepted, but that the recommendation of said

* 34 *Journal of a Meeting of the Board of Regents of the University of the State of New York* 787 (1965). [The Board of Regents consists of 15 individuals elected by joint resolution of the two houses of New York's legislature for terms of 15 years. The Regents have jurisdiction over all education in the state, public and private, and over all licensed professions excluding the law. The three Regents most intimately involved in this decision were the three members of a special committee on discipline: Joseph W. McGovern, a lawyer; Joseph T. King, a lawyer; and Carl H. Pforzheimer, Jr., an investment banker. The remaining Regents, who concurred in the decision, are drawn from a variety of business and professional interests, including law, banking, education, and philanthropy.]

Committee be modified and license No. 71055 and license No. 37359 respectively, issued under date of March 21, 1951, to said Dr. Southam and December 1, 1939, to said Dr. Mandel, and their registration or registrations as physicians, wherever they may appear, be suspended for a period of 1 year on each specification, said suspensions to run concurrently from the date of the service of the order effecting such suspensions, but that the execution of such suspensions be stayed, and each respondent be placed on probation for a period of 1 year upon the following terms and conditions:

1. That each respondent shall conduct himself in all ways in a manner befitting his professional status and shall conform fully to the moral and professional standards of conduct imposed by law and by his profession;
2. That so long as there is no indication of any further misconduct, each respondent may continue to practice as a physician, but the Department, upon receipt of satisfactory evidence of any such further misconduct, may forthwith terminate the stay of execution and order that the stay be vacated and the medical license of the respondent or respondents involved be suspended for a period of 1 year from the date of said order;
3. That any such action by the Department vacating the stay of the suspension as to either or both respondents shall in no way bar further disciplinary action based upon additional misconduct;
4. That each respondent shall notify the Department of any change of address or employment;
5. That upon full compliance with these conditions for a period of 1 year each respondent may apply to the Department for discharge from probation; and that the Commissioner of Education be empowered to execute, for and on behalf of the Board of Regents, all orders necessary to carry out the terms of this vote.

NOTE

AMERICAN ASSOCIATION FOR CANCER RESEARCH MINUTES OF THE 59TH ANNUAL MEETING*

The Annual Business Meeting of Members was called to order at 5:10 P.M., April 12, 1968, at Haddon Hall, Atlantic City, New Jersey by Vice-President Southam. . . .

* * *

Dr. Southam announced that the tellers had informed him that Dr. Abraham Cantarow had been selected as the Vice-President of the Association for 1968–69. The Secretary-Treasurer said that the Board recommended that Dr. Chester M. Southam be elected President for 1968–69. When no additional nominations were made from the floor, it was moved that these two officers be declared duly elected. . . .

* 10 *Proceedings of the American Association for Cancer Research* 110–111 (1969). Copyright 1969 by Cancer Research, Inc. Reprinted by permission.

THE WILLOWBROOK HEPATITIS STUDIES

David J. Rothman and Sheila M. Rothman

The attempt to bar Willowbrook's hepatitis carriers from the public schools had a special irony to it, for from 1956 through 1971, researchers fed live viruses to children in Willowbrook in order to study the disease and attempt to create a vaccine against it.

The head of the team was Saul Krugman. In appearance, he borders on the colorless, but controversy surrounds him. Krugman's research at Willowbrook brought him fame and power. He has chaired national committees on hepatitis, directed

Reprinted with permission from *The Willowbrook Wars* (New York: Harper and Row, 1984).

huge federally funded projects, been the subject of laudatory editorials in the *Journal of the American Medical Association,* and won the John Russell Award of the Markle Foundation (which read, in part: "In all his work Dr. Krugman proceeded quietly and cautiously. . . . He has zealously guarded the rights and sensibilities of patients and their families. . . . Dr. Krugman has provided an example of how [good clinical research] should be done"). Yet in April 1972, when Dr. Krugman received a prize from the American College of Physicians, a line of police surrounded the podium while 150 protesters denounced his research as grossly unethical.

Saul Krugman's interest in infectious diseases began when, as a physician with the armed forces in the South Pacific, he treated many patients who contracted malaria or jungle parasites. Upon discharge, Krugman took a residency at New York's public hospital for infectious diseases, Willard Parker, which in several ways prepared him to work at Willowbrook. Krugman recalled entering a pavilion where some sixty children lay one next to the other "with every complication of measles—encephalitis, pneumonia, everything. I could go to another area and see dozens of children with diphtheria.... Every summer the Parker Hospital would admit at least 50 and sometimes more than 100 children with paralytic poliomyelitis."

In such a setting, Krugman became convinced that even the most diligent efforts at treatment were not likely to bring benefits. "Therapeutics," he once remarked, "was a slender reed in those days." Rather, the goal had to be prevention, which to Krugman meant not cleaning up a water supply or sewer system, but finding vaccines.

In 1947, Krugman moved to Bellevue Hospital and joined the NYU faculty, and in 1954 he became consulting physician to the newly opened Willowbrook facility. He immediately conducted an epidemiological survey, which disclosed an amazing variety of infectious diseases: measles, hepatitis, respiratory infections, shigella, and assorted intestinal parasites.

If Willowbrook was a hell for its residents, it could be a paradise for a researcher. On these disease-ridden wards, the line between treatment and experimentation seemed to vanish. A researcher could select his disease and enjoy substantial freedom to experiment, believing that he was serving both society and the residents.

Events in 1960 confirmed the validity of these presumptions for Krugman. Every two years or so, New York City experienced a measles epidemic, and new admissions to Willowbrook invariably brought in the disease. The results were usually disastrous, with hundreds of cases and fatality rates as high as 10 percent. At the start of 1960, Dr. John Enders, working in Boston, had succeeded in growing measles virus in culture and had managed to attenuate it to the point where it might be an effective vaccine. Krugman wanted to run trial tests at Willowbrook. The disease struck there so often and so hard that findings could be obtained quickly; and if the vaccine offered protection, the Willowbrook residents would obviously benefit. Krugman contacted Enders, received twenty samples of the limited number of doses available, and vaccinated the residents of one ward.

A measles epidemic soon struck at Willowbrook, but no one among the vaccinated children contracted the disease. "Willowbrook's children," observed Dr. Krugman, "enabled us to acquire in a short time solid information about Dr. Enders's vaccine." By 1963, before the vaccine was officially licensed, 90 percent of Willowbrook's residents had been inoculated, and measles was never again a threat. The use of an experimental vaccine at Willowbrook, Krugman concluded, "was obviously beneficial to the children."

The measles study was a sideshow at Willowbrook. It was hepatitis that held center stage. Soon after completing his initial epidemiological survey, Dr. Krugman decided to explore this widespread but little understood disease. Its symptoms had been recognized for centuries, but not until World War II did medical researchers suspect that the disease was infectious and occurred in two varieties: the short, thirty-day-incubation type that we now label hepatitis A and commonly associate with eating contaminated shellfish; and the long, ninety-day-incubation type that we now label hepatitis B and commonly associate with blood transfusions. Beyond these simple categories, little was known about causes, cure, or prevention.

In this vacuum Dr. Krugman began his experiments. Between 1953 and 1957, Willowbrook had

had about 350 cases of hepatitis among the residents and 76 among the staff; in 1955 alone (the year before his research began), the disease rate was 25 per thousand among the residents, 40 per thousand among the staff. (In New York State, the rate was 25 per *one hundred thousand* of the population.) And these figures included only the observable, acute cases of patients with jaundice; the number of milder, subclinical cases was still greater. To Dr. Krugman, these conditions called for an active research strategy. Scientists had not yet found a nonhuman host for the virus or succeeded in growing it in a laboratory culture. Thus experiments would have to be carried out on live subjects, and what better subjects than the Willowbrook children? The high rate of contagion in the institution meant that they were bound to get the disease and the effectiveness of intervention could be measured almost immediately.

Krugman's experiments had a logic, a simplicity, and, one would dare to add, an elegance about them. His initial project was to determine whether injections of gamma globulin, that part of the blood plasma which is rich in antibodies, protected recipients against hepatitis. The literature suggested that gamma globulin offered temporary, "passive" immunity; the antibodies in the fluid would be able to counteract the disease for some six weeks. The critical question was whether injections of gamma globulin in the presence of the virus would lead recipients to produce their own antibodies, thereby acquiring permanent immunity that would last for years.

The team first administered varying doses of gamma globulin to one group of new admissions to Willowbrook and withheld it from another. Then, eight to ten months later, it tallied the numbers from each group who had contracted the illness. The results were clear: of 1,812 residents who had been inoculated, only two cases of hepatitis occurred (a rate of 1.7 per 1,000); of the 1,771 residents who were not inoculated, forty-one contracted the disease (22.5 per 1,000). Thus Krugman confirmed that gamma globulin did protect against hepatitis and the finding "pointed the way to the practical method for the control of infectious hepatitis at this institution."

But had the gamma globulin injection stimulated active immunity? Those inoculated were protected against the disease for almost a year, but no one understood how this protection was acquired or how long it would last. Had the gamma globulin first provided a passive immunity, which then turned active when recipients came in contact with the live virus from other residents? Could permanent active immunity be acquired by injecting patients with gamma globulin and live virus at the same time?

To answer these questions, Krugman opened a separate unit on the Willowbrook grounds. Staffed by its own personnel, it admitted children between the ages of three and eleven, directly from their own homes; when their role in the research was completed, weeks or months later, they moved onto the general wards. The experiments typically involved injecting some of the unit residents with gamma globulin and feeding them the live hepatitis virus (obtained from the feces of Willowbrook hepatitis patients). At the same time, other unit residents served as "controls"; they were fed the live virus without the benefit of gamma globulin, to ascertain that the virus was actually "live," capable of transmitting the disease, and to measure the different responses. Then Krugman would calculate how many of those who had received both gamma globulin and live virus, as compared with controls, initially came down with hepatitis; six or nine or twelve months later, he would again feed both groups another dose of live virus and measure how many of those who had earlier received the gamma globulin contracted the disease as against those who had not.

As is often the case in scientific research, Dr. Krugman's most important observation came by chance. In keeping track of the hepatitis rates in the institution, he noted that 4 to 8 percent of those who contracted hepatitis went on to suffer a second attack within a year. The second attack might possibly have been caused by a very heavy exposure to the virus, which overwhelmed the immunity the body had built up after the first attack. But Dr. Krugman believed that the etiology of the disease was more complicated than researchers had recognized. The repeat attack indicated that more than one type of virus could be causing hepatitis.

To investigate this "very attractive hypothesis," Dr. Krugman in 1964 started a new series of experiments, and within three years he helped to clarify the distinction between hepatitis A and B. In this round, the Krugman team admitted new Willowbrook residents to its special unit and fed them a dose of pooled Willowbrook virus, that is, a mixture that came from a large number of hepatitis victims and, therefore, contained all the hepatitis viruses within the institution. In short order, these First Trial subjects contracted the disease and recovered from it. The team then reinfected these children with the same pooled virus in a Second Trial, and a number of them again contracted the disease. In the course of these procedures, the team drew a sample of blood from one of the boys during his first illness (and labeled it MS-1), and then another sample from him in his second illness (labeled MS-2). Next, the researchers admitted a new group of fourteen children to the unit and infected these Third Trial subjects with the MS-1 virus. Within thirty-one to thirty-eight days, all but one came down with hepatitis. Simultaneously, the team admitted still another fourteen children to the unit, and injected this Fourth Trial group with the MS-2 virus. Within forty-one to sixty-nine days, all but two contracted the illness. Now the stage was set for the final procedure. The team gave all the hepatitis victims in the third (MS-1) group and fourth (MS-2) group the MS-1 virus. It turned out that not one child in the Third Trial group came down with hepatitis a second time; six of the eight children in the Fourth Trial group again contracted the disease.

With these findings in hand, Krugman announced that hepatitis was caused by at least two distinct viruses. There was hepatitis A, MS-1, of short incubation and highly contagious (all of the controls who lived with the Third Trial group but were not fed the virus directly came down with the disease). And there was hepatitis B, MS-2, of long incubation and lower contagion (only two of the five controls living with the Fourth Trial group caught the disease). In short, the Krugman research established the distinctive features of two strains of hepatitis.

The findings met with acclaim, and Krugman was praised not only for his results but for his methods. The *Journal of the American Medical Association* credited Krugman's "judicious use of human beings"; Franz Inglefinger, later the editor of the *New England Journal of Medicine,* went further: "By being allowed to participate in a carefully supervised study and by receiving the most expert attention available for a disease of basically unknown nature, the patients themselves benefited. . . . How much better to have a patient with hepatitis, accidentally or deliberately acquired, under the guidance of a Krugman than under the care of a [rights-minded] zealot."

Underlying these attempts at justification, and those that Krugman himself made, was the notion that the Willowbrook experiments were, in the words of Claude Bernard, the nineteenth-century French physician who was among the first to address the ethics of research, "experiments in nature." Researchers who studied the course and spread of a disease that had no known antidote were acting ethically, for no intervention on their part could have altered the outcome. But how could feeding live hepatitis viruses to children be considered the equivalent of observing a disease? Krugman's answer was that if he had not infected the children, they still would have contracted hepatitis. Had he never come to Willowbrook, the likelihood was overwhelming that entering residents would have suffered the disease. Thus his feeding them the virus did not really change anything and was an experiment in nature. Krugman also noted that he had obtained permission from the parents of all his subjects, and he had signed consent forms to prove it.

Many parents of children accepted at Willowbrook but still awaiting actual admission—a wait that could last for several years—did receive the following letter from Dr. H. H. Berman, then Willowbrook's director:

> November 15, 1958
>
> Dear Mrs. ———:
>
> We are studying the possibility of preventing epidemics of hepatitis on a new principle. Virus is introduced and gamma globulin given later to some, so that either no attack or only a mild attack of hepatitis is expected to follow. This may give the children immunity against this disease for life. We should like to give your child this new form of prevention with the hope that it will afford protection.
>
> Permission form is enclosed for your consideration. If you wish to have your child given the benefit of this new preventive, will you so signify by signing the form.

Almost every phrase in this particular letter encourages parents to commit their children to the unit. The team is "studying" hepatitis, not doing research. The virus "is introduced," in the passive voice, rather than the team's being said to feed the child a live virus. Gamma globulin is given "to some," but the letter does not explicitly state that it is withheld from others. "No attack" or a "mild attack" of the disease "is expected to follow," but absent gamma globulin, a claim of "no attack" was false and left unsaid was that in some cases the attack would not be mild. Finally, the letter twice described introducing the live virus as a "new form of prevention," but feeding a child hepatitis hardly amounted to prevention. In truth, the goal of the experiment was to *create*, not deliver, a new form of protection.

To send such a letter over the signature of Willowbrook's director appeared coercive. These parents wanted to please the man who would be in charge of their child. Moreover, an especially raw form of coercion may have occasionally intruded. When overcrowding at Willowbrook forced a close in regular admissions, an escape hatch was left—admission via Krugman's unit. A parent wanting to institutionalize a retarded child had a choice: Sign the form or forgo the placement.

What of Krugman's contention that his research was an experiment in nature? The claim ignores the fact that the underlying problem was not ignorance about a disease but an unwillingness to alter the social environment. Had Krugman wished to, he could have insisted that hygienic measures be introduced to decrease the spread of the virus. Should the facility resist carrying out the necessary cleanup, he might have asked the Department of Health to close the place down as a health hazard, which it surely was. Furthermore, Krugman had at hand an antidote of some efficacy. His own findings demonstrated that gamma globulin provided some protection, and yet he infected control groups with the virus and withheld the serum from them in order to fulfill the requirements of his research design.

Finally, to introduce one more irony to this account: While Krugman was trying to discover the etiology of hepatitis at Willowbrook, Dr. Baruch Blumberg was actually solving the puzzle in his laboratory, without conducting experiments on humans. In the course of his research on the body's immunological reaction to transfused blood, Blumberg observed that a strange band occurred when he mixed a vial of blood drawn from a hemophiliac with that drawn from an Australian aborigine. Labeling the band the Australia antigen, he investigated its properties; like a detective on the trail of a culprit, he followed several false leads and then the true one, discovering that the Australia antigen was the infective agent in hepatitis B. His first published report appeared in 1967 and Krugman confirmed the finding (the Australia antigen was in the blood of the MS-2 children but not the MS-1 children). Thus those with a utilitarian bent, who might be prepared to give Krugman leeway with his means because his ends were important, will have to consider that, however accidentally, we would have learned almost everything we needed to know about hepatitis B in the laboratory.

THE WILLOWBROOK HEPATITIS STUDIES REVISITED: ETHICAL ASPECTS

Saul Krugman

During the first half of this century, outbreaks of various infectious diseases were prevalent in orphanages, military barracks, and institutions for mentally retarded children. These outbreaks involved highly susceptible populations living in conditions of overcrowding and poor hygiene. Certain infectious diseases, such as influenza and measles, occurred as epidemics at variable intervals. Other infections, such as shigellosis and hepatitis, were generally endemic in nature.

During the mid-1950s my colleague, Dr. Robert Ward, and I were invited to join the staff of Willowbrook State School as consultants in infectious diseases. This institution for mentally retarded children had been plagued by the occurrence of such epidemic and endemic diseases as measles and hepatitis. Our efforts during the next two decades were devoted to the control of these infectious diseases.

In 1960 an epidemic of measles swept through Willowbrook, leaving 60 children dead. The studies that we initiated with the live attenuated measles vaccine developed by Dr. John Enders and his colleagues culminated in the eradication of measles from the institution by the end of 1963.

Hepatitis, which affected virtually every child in Willowbrook as well as many employees, proved to be a more difficult problem. It was essential to acquire new knowledge about the natural history of this disease knowledge that might lead to its ultimate control.

The studies during the subsequent two decades were perceived by some critics to be unethical. As a matter of fact, in recent years the name "Willowbrook" has become synonymous with medical research gone astray. With time, facts have become distorted or forgotten, leaving only emotions.

Thirty years have elapsed since the Willowbrook hepatitis studies were initiated in the mid-1950s. I am as convinced today as I was at that time that our studies were ethical and justifiable. This judgment is based on knowledge of the extraordinary conditions that existed in the institution as well as on an assessment of the potential risks and benefits for the participants. The purpose of this article is to discuss the ethical aspects of our studies, within their appropriate historical context. It is hoped that this information will enable the reader to make an independent, objective judgment as to the ethics of the Willowbrook studies.

ESTABLISHMENT OF THE WILLOWBROOK STATE SCHOOL

In 1938 the New York state legislature perceived the need for an additional institution for the care of mentally retarded children. It allocated funds to purchase 375 acres of land located at Willowbrook on Staten Island and authorized the construction of facilities to care for 3,000 mentally retarded children from the greater–New York metropolitan area. The institution, completed in 1942 and designated Willowbrook State School, was taken over by the federal government to meet an urgent need for an army hospital to care for disabled military personnel from World War II. The U.S. Army Medical Corps renamed it the Halloran General Hospital in honor of the late Colonel Paul Stacey Halloran, a U.S. Army medical corpsman.

After the war ended in 1945, there was considerable political pressure to retain Halloran General Hospital as a Veterans Administration hospital. The conflict between the needs of the Veterans Administration and the needs of the New York State Department of Mental Hygiene was described in the following letter sent by Governor Thomas Dewey to General Omar Bradley, who was director of the Veterans Administration at that time.

> Every year in the State of New York, thousands of children come into this world who are mentally and

Reprinted with permission from *Review of Infectious Disease,* 8, no. 1 (1986): 157–162.

> physically defective and feeble minded, who never can become members of society. They require constant care, both medically and physically, and in many cases, for social, psychological and economic reasons, few parents can afford to place them in private institutions. Even if such institutions existed in sufficient quantity, the result is that the state must take responsibility for the care of these children and do so with a high degree of tenderness and attention.
>
> At present, the State of New York operates two downstate institutions for the care of such infants and children. One is the Wassaic State School in Duchess and the other is Letchworth Village in Rockland County. There are several other state schools for mental defectives but they are too overcrowded and none is or can be equipped for the additional care of infants.
>
> Hundreds of infants and children unable to care for themselves are sleeping on mattresses on floors of these institutions. What is more serious is that there are eight to nine hundred infants on the waiting list for admission and the State Commission of Mental Hygiene daily must deal with distracted parents who seek to have their children placed in state institutions. The mail of the Commissioner of Mental Hygiene is filled with letters from such parents, many of whom are veterans.
>
> It seems to me that we are now confronted with these two conflicting obligations at Willowbrook. The first is that of the Federal Government to provide hospital care for its veterans after they are discharged from service. The second is the obligation of the State of New York to provide care for permanently helpless infants. Obviously, Willowbrook cannot be used for both.

Finally, on October 24, 1947, after a delay of five years, 10 patients from Wassaic State School and 10 patients from Letchworth Village were transferred to Willowbrook State School. Initially, patients were both transferred from other institutions and admitted from the community. In retrospect, it is apparent that the infectious diseases endemic in Wassaic State School and Letchworth Village were introduced into Willowbrook by patients who were transferred from these institutions.

RECOGNITION OF HEPATITIS AS AN ENDEMIC DISEASE

The occurrence of so-called infectious hepatitis was first observed in 1949. Later, in response to extraordinary pressure from many parents, the patient population increased rapidly in subsequent years; it exceeded 3,000 in 1953, 4,000 in 1955, and eventually it exceeded 6,000. In his report to a joint legislative committee on mental and physical handicap, the late Dr. Jack Hammond, director of Willowbrook State School stated:

> The overcrowded conditions in the buildings make care, treatment, supervision and possible training of the patients difficult, if not impossible. When the patients are up and in the day rooms, they are crowded together, soiling, attacking each other, abusing themselves and destroying their clothing. At night in many of the dormitories the beds must be placed together in order to provide sufficient space for all patients. Therefore, except for one narrow aisle, it is virtually necessary to climb over beds in order to reach the children.

The residents of Willowbrook State School were the most severely retarded, the most handicapped, and the most helpless of those being cared for in the New York state system. The population of about 6,000 included 77% who were severely or profoundly retarded, 60% who were not toilet trained, 39% who were not ambulatory, 30% who had convulsive seizures, and 64% who were incapable of feeding themselves. Thus, the conditions were optimal for the transmission of hepatitis, shigellosis, respiratory infections, and parasitic infections.

By the early 1950s the director of Willowbrook and his staff were convinced that serious overcrowding and an inadequate staff were in great part responsible for the increasing hepatitis problem. Their statistics indicated that the annual attack rate of hepatitis with jaundice was 25 per 1,000 among the children and 40 per 1,000 among the adults. Efforts to correct this intolerable situation were unsuccessful. Society had created a problem, but it provided no solution. It was during that period that my colleague, the late Dr. Robert Ward, and I were asked to join the staff of Willowbrook as consultants in infectious diseases. We were not qualified to deal with the societal problems, but we believed that we could help control the existing medical problem of hepatitis.

IDENTIFICATION OF THE HEPATITIS PROBLEM IN WILLOWBROOK

Our first objective in 1955 was to carry out an extensive epidemiologic survey. We were fortunate because new tests to detect hepatic dysfunction were described that year, namely, serum glutamic oxaloacetic transaminase (SGOT) and serum glutamic pyruvic transaminase (SGPT). These sensitive assays enabled us to detect the presence of hepatitis without jaundice (anicteric hepatitis). Today, SGOT is called alanine aspartate transaminase (AST), and SGPT is called alanine aminotransferase (ALT).

Our colleague, the late Dr. Joan P. Giles, joined us during this period. During the course of our epidemiologic surveys and the performance of routine physical examinations, she collected many thousands of serum specimens. Instead of discarding them—the usual practice in most laboratories—we store them in an increasing number of deep freezers. The scientific dividends of this serum bank proved to be incalculable in later years.

After the results of the SGOT and SGPT assays were reviewed, it was obvious that the detected cases of icteric hepatitis represented the tip of a hepatitis iceberg. The results of these highly sensitive tests of liver dysfunction convinced us that most newly admitted children were destined to contract hepatitis infection under the conditions that existed in the institution. The occurrence of hepatitis among Willowbrook children was as predictable and inevitable as the occurrence of respiratory infections among children in day care centers.

During the course of our epidemiologic survey in 1955, all of the evidence indicated that the endemic disease was so-called infectious or type A hepatitis, an infection that spread via the fecal-oral route. The disease was mild and there were no deaths. Although the same disease was more severe and more debilitating in the adult employees, they, too, recovered completely. Previous experience of various investigators had revealed that hepatitis A was much milder in children than in adults. Efforts to reduce the overcrowded conditions at Willowbrook continued to be unsuccessful. In a desperate attempt the director mailed letters to about 5,000 parents, requesting that they return a questionnaire that contained the statement, "I wish to discuss the possibility and advisability of removing my child from Willowbrook State School so that he/she can live at home." A total of 24 parents responded, and only two children were taken home at that time!

THE WILLOWBROOK HEPATITIS STUDIES

After one year of careful observation and study in 1955, we concluded that the control of hepatitis in Willowbrook could be achieved if it were possible to devise and conduct well-designed studies to shed new light on the natural history and prevention of the disease—new knowledge that could conceivably lead to the development of a vaccine. Thus, our decision to propose the exposure of a small number of newly admitted children to the endemic Willow-brook strain of hepatitis virus was reached after serious consideration of the following factors and assumptions:

(1) As indicated previously, under the conditions existing in the institution, most newly admitted children would contract hepatitis. This empiric impression was confirmed in the 1970s when newly developed serologic tests revealed that >90% of the residents of the institution had hepatitis A and B markers of past infection.
(2) Hepatitis was known to be especially mild in the three- to 10-year age group that would participate in the studies. Our extensive survey confirmed that most infections were inapparent or benign and there were no deaths.
(3) The artificially induced infection would induce immunity to the endemic strain of hepatitis virus and, we hoped, to other strains that might be introduced by new admissions or transfers to Willowbrook. Studies in the 1940s had revealed that hepatitis A infection was followed by homologous immunity. Therefore, the artificially induced infection would be prophylactic.
(4) The children would be admitted to a specially equipped, specially staffed unit where they would be isolated from exposure to other endemic infectious diseases occurring in the institution—namely, shigellosis, respiratory infections, and parasitic infections.
(5) Only children whose parents gave consent would be included. Our method of obtaining informed consent changed progressively

during the course of the studies. In 1956 the information was conveyed to individual parents by letter or personal interview. Later, we adopted a group technique of obtaining consent. First, a psychiatric social worker discussed the project with parents during a preliminary interview. Those who were interested were invited to attend a group session at the institution to discuss the project in greater detail. These sessions were conducted by our staff responsible for the program, including Dr. Giles, the supervising nurse, staff attendants, and psychiatric social workers. Meetings were often attended by outside physicians who had expressed interest. Parents, in groups of six to eight, were given a tour of the facilities. The purposes, potential benefits, and potential hazards of the program were discussed with them, and they were encouraged to ask questions. Thus, all parents could hear the response to questions posed by the more articulate members of the group. After leaving this briefing session, parents had an opportunity to talk with their private physicians, who could call Dr. Giles for more information. Approximately two weeks after the visit, the psychiatric social worker contacted the parents for their decision. If the decision was in the affirmative, the consent was signed, but parents were informed that consent could be withdrawn at any time. It was clear that the group method enabled us to obtain a more thorough informed consent. Children who were wards of the state or children without parents were never included in our studies.

From 1956 the protocols were reviewed and sanctioned by various local, state, and federal agencies. These studies were reviewed and approved by the New York University and Willowbrook State School committees on human experimentation after their formation in February 1967. Prior to this date, the functions of the present Institutional Review Board were performed by the Executive Faculty of the School of Medicine for studies of this type. The initial proposal in 1956 was reviewed and approved by the following groups: Executive Faculty, New York University School of Medicine; New York State Department of Mental Hygiene; New York State Department of Health; and Armed Forces Epidemiological Board. It is of interest that the guidelines that were adopted for the hepatitis studies at their inception in 1956 conformed to the World Medical Association's draft Code of Ethics on Human Experimentation, which was presented to its general assembly in September 1961, five years later. It is also of interest that our established policy of informed consent was instituted at least 10 years before it was mandated by most research institutes and medical centers in the United States.

During the period 1956–1967, we believed that we were dealing with endemicity of hepatitis A, an infection that should be followed by lasting immunity. However, by 1967 it was obvious that many children had had two attacks of hepatitis. Our studies of this phenomenon revealed that one attack was caused by the so-called MS-1 strain of hepatitis virus and the second attack, by the MS-2 strain. Thus, it became apparent that two types of hepatitis were endemic in Willowbrook—MS-1, resembling hepatitis A, and MS-2, resembling hepatitis B. By 1969, after Blumberg discovered the Australia antigen, the new technology enabled us to confirm that Willowbrook MS-2 serum contained hepatitis B antigen.

Our serum bank contained specimens obtained from most patients who contracted naturally acquired hepatitis during the period 1956–1969. When we tested these serum specimens in the 1970s, using the newly developed serologic assays, it was obvious that both hepatitis A (MS-1) and hepatitis B (MS-2) had been endemic in the institution since 1956. It was also apparent that hepatitis B, like hepatitis A, was generally a mild or inapparent infection in Willowbrook children. A retrospective diagnosis was made by testing the sera for the presence of hepatitis B antigen and abnormal serum transaminase values. During the course of this new survey, we found that most children had markers of present or past hepatitis B infection. Thus, it was likely that newly admitted children would be intensely exposed to both types of hepatitis. When this new information was presented to the members of the Commission on Viral Infections of the Armed

Forces Epidemiological Board in 1969, they agreed that the studies should be continued.

It should be emphasized that the studies were conducted in Willowbrook State School because hepatitis was a severe problem in this institution and not, as some charged, because we were looking for a facile "guinea pig" population. The fact that the children were mentally retarded was relevant only to the extent that society placed them in an institution where hepatitis was prevalent. The primary objective of our studies was to protect the children and employees while acquiring new knowledge in the process.

SUMMARY OF CONTRIBUTIONS OF WILLOWBROOK HEPATITIS STUDIES

The accomplishments of the Willowbrook studies are well documented in the medical literature. . . . They include:

(1) *Identification of two distinctive clinical, epidemiologic, and immunologic types of hepatitis, MS-1 (type A) and MS-2 (type B).* The serum specimens collected from patients with MS-1 and MS-2 infection provided many investigators with "pedigreed" sera known to be specific for hepatitis A or B. After the discovery of Australia antigen by Blumberg and colleagues, the use of these clinical samples by various investigators established the association between Australia antigen, and hepatitis B virus.

(2) *Demonstration that hepatitis B infection is transmitted by intimate contact and oral as well as parenteral exposure.* Previously, it was believed that percutaneous inoculation with contaminated needles, blood, or blood products was essential for the transmission of hepatitis B. It is well recognized today that hepatitis B is a sexually transmitted infection and it is spread by intimate physical contact and transfer of body fluids.

(3) *Demonstration that hepatitis B immune globulin is effective for the prevention of type B hepatitis.* The results of this study led to the initiation of several large multicenter trials to determine the efficacy of HBIG in preventing hepatitis B among such high-risk individuals as hemodialysis staff and patients, newborns of HBsAg-positive mothers, sexual contacts of patients with acute hepatitis B, and persons accidentally inoculated with HBsAg-positive blood by needle-stick exposures.

(4) *Development of the first prototype inactivated hepatitis B vaccine.* It was demonstrated that a boiled 1:10 dilution of MS-2 serum in distilled water was not infectious, but it was immunogenic and protective. These studies, published in 1970, clearly demonstrated the feasibility of developing a hepatitis B vaccine and stimulated various investigators to prepare inactivated vaccines from the plasma of chronic hepatitis B carriers.

CONCLUSION

While I agree with the critics of medical research who state that the ends (successful accomplishments) do not justify the means, I believe that this generalization does not apply to our Willowbrook studies. Under the conditions that existed in the institution, all children were constantly exposed to the naturally acquired hepatitis viruses. Moreover, the overall risk for children in our special isolation unit was less than the risk for other children who were admitted to buildings in the institution where shigellosis and respiratory infections, as well as hepatitis, were endemic.

A century ago Claude Bernard defined the limits of human experimentation. He stated that

> it is our duty and our right to perform an experiment on man whenever it can save life, cure him, or gain some potential benefit. The principle of medical and surgical morality, therefore, consists in never performing on man an experiment which might be harmful to him to any extent, even though the result may be highly advantageous to science or to the health of others. But performing experiments and operations exclusively from the point of view of the patient's own advantage does not prevent their turning out profitably to science.

My colleague, the late Dr. Joan P. Giles, expressed it beautifully and succinctly in her letter to the *Lancet,* published May 29, 1971, in which she said, "A farmer may pull up corn seedlings to destroy them or he may pull them up to set them in better hills for better growing. How then does one judge the deed without the motive?" This describes the motivation for our studies at Willowbrook State School.

I am greatly indebted to many collaborators, colleagues, and organizations for support and encouragement during the course of our Willowbrook hepatitis studies:

To the late Dr. Robert Ward, who was the principal investigator of our studies from 1956 to 1958. He was an outstanding investigator and a colleague who had exceptional human qualities.

To the late Dr. Joan P. Giles, who died of cancer in 1973 after devoting 17 years of her life to the care of the children in our hepatitis unit. She was a highly ethical physician and a person of great humanity and integrity.

To Harriet Friedman and Cass Lattimer, research associates, for more than 25 years of competent and meticulous work in our laboratory.

To the late Dr. Jack Hammond, director of Willowbrook State School. He and his dedicated staff labored under the most difficult circumstances. They were subjected to incredible abuse by certain representatives of the news media and by publicity-seeking legislators who criticized them for the horrible conditions in the institution. Their morale was devastated because they knew that the pressures of society (distraught parents and their legislators) were responsible for increasing the census to more than 6,000 in a 3,000-bed institution. It was "society" that was responsible for the overcrowded, unhygienic conditions in Willowbrook, not the dedicated people who worked there under stressful conditions.

To the late Dr. John R. Paul and Dr. Robert McCollum of Yale University for their encouragement and wise counsel during the 1950s and 1960s.

To the Armed Forces Epidemiological Board and the U.S. Army Medical Research and Development Command for 25 consecutive years of financial support.

And, finally, to many loyal and devoted colleagues and friends whose support helped ease the pain inflicted by many vicious attacks during the late 1960s and early 1970s. We were especially grateful to the parents of the Willowbrook chapter of the Benevolent Society of Retarded Children for the plaque that they presented to us at their 1967 annual meeting. The inscription on the plaque stated, "In recognition of distinguished, pioneering, humanitarian research in the prevention of infectious diseases and their resultant complication in children, born and unborn."

RACISM AND RESEARCH: THE CASE OF THE TUSKEGEE SYPHILIS STUDY

Allan M. Brandt

In 1932 the U.S. Public Health Service (USPHS) initiated an experiment in Macon County, Alabama, to determine the natural course of untreated, latent syphilis in black males. The test comprised 400 syphilitic men, as well as 200 uninfected men who served as controls. The first published report of the study appeared in 1936 with subsequent papers issued every four to six years, through the 1960s. When penicillin became widely available by the early 1950s as the preferred treatment for syphilis,

---

Hastings Center Report, December 1978, pp. 21–29.

Editors' note: Many notes have been omitted. Readers who wish to follow up on sources should consult the original article.

the men did not receive therapy. In fact on several occasions, the USPHS actually sought to prevent treatment. Moreover, a committee at the federally operated Center for Disease Control decided in 1969 that the study should be continued. Only in 1972, when accounts of the study first appeared in the national press, did the Department of Health, Education and Welfare halt the experiment. At that time seventy-four of the test subjects were still alive; at least twenty-eight, but perhaps more than 100, had died directly from advanced syphilitic lesions.[1] In August 1972, HEW appointed an investigatory panel which issued a report the following year. The panel found the study to have been "ethically unjustified," and argued that penicillin should have been provided to the men.[2]

This article attempts to place the Tuskegee Study in a historical context and to assess its ethical implications. Despite the media attention which the study received, the HEW *Final Report,* and the criticism expressed by several professional organizations, the experiment has been largely misunderstood. The most basic questions of *how* the study was undertaken in the first place and *why* it continued for forty years were never addressed by the HEW investigation. Moreover, the panel misconstrued the nature of the experiment, failing to consult important documents available at the National Archives which bear significantly on its ethical assessment. Only by examining the specific ways in which values are engaged in scientific research can the study be understood.

RACISM AND MEDICAL OPINION

A brief review of the prevailing scientific thought regarding race and heredity in the early twentieth century is fundamental for an understanding of the Tuskegee Study. By the turn of the century, Darwinism had provided a new rationale for American racism. Essentially primitive peoples, it was argued, could not be assimilated into a complex, white civilization. Scientists speculated that in the struggle for survival the Negro in America was doomed. Particularly prone to disease, vice, and crime, black Americans could not be helped by education or philanthropy. Social Darwinists analyzed census data to predict the virtual extinction of the Negro in the twentieth century, for they believed the Negro race in America was in the throes of a degenerative evolutionary process.

The medical profession supported these findings of late nineteenth- and early twentieth-century anthropologists, ethnologists, and biologists. Physicians studying the effects of emancipation on health concluded almost universally that freedom had caused the mental, moral, and physical deterioration of the black population. They substantiated this argument by citing examples in the comparitive [*sic*] anatomy of the black and white races. As Dr. W. T. English wrote: "A careful inspection reveals the body of the negro a mass of minor defects and imperfections from the crown of the head to the soles of the feet. . . ."[3] Cranial structures, wide nasal apertures, receding chins, projecting jaws, all typed the Negro as the lowest species in the Darwinian hierarchy.

Interest in racial differences centered on the sexual nature of blacks. The Negro, doctors explained, possessed an excessive sexual desire, which threatened the very foundations of white society. As one physician noted in the *Journal of the American Medical Association,* "The negro springs from a southern race, and as such his sexual appetite is strong; all of his environments stimulate this appetite, and as a general rule his emotional type of religion certainly does not decrease it." Doctors reported a complete lack of morality on the part of blacks:

> Virtue in the negro race is like angels' visits—few and far between. In a practice of sixteen years I have never examined a virgin negro over fourteen years of age.[4]

A particularly ominous feature of this overzealous sexuality, doctors argued, was the black males' desire for white women. "A perversion from which most races are exempt," wrote Dr. English, "prompts the negro's inclination towards white women, whereas other races incline towards females of their own."[5] Though English estimated the "gray matter of the negro brain" to be at least a thousand years behind that of the white races, his genital organs were overdeveloped. As Dr. William Lee Howard noted:

> The attacks on defenseless white women are evidences of racial instincts that are about as amenable to ethical culture as is the inherent odor of the race. . . . When education will reduce the size of the negro's penis as well as bring about the sensitiveness of the terminal fibers

> which exist in the Caucasian, then will it also be able to prevent the African's birthright to sexual madness and excess.[6]

One southern medical journal proposed "Castration Instead of Lynching," as retribution for black sexual crimes. "An impressive trial by a ghost-like kuklux klan [*sic*] and a 'ghost' physician or surgeon to perform the operation would make it an event the 'patient' would never forget," noted the editorial.[7]

According to these physicians, lust and immorality, unstable families, and reversion to barbaric tendencies made blacks especially prone to venereal diseases. One doctor estimated that over 50 percent of all Negroes over the age of twenty-five were syphilitic.[8] Virtually free of disease as slaves, they were now overwhelmed by it, according to informed medical opinion. Moreover, doctors believed that treatment for venereal disease among blacks was impossible, particularly because in its latent stage the symptoms of syphilis become quiescent. As Dr. Thomas W. Murrell wrote:

> They come for treatment at the beginning and at the end. When there are visible manifestations or when they are harried by pain, they readily come, for as a race they are not averse to physic; but tell them not, though they look well and feel well, that they are still diseased. Here ignorance rates science a fool. . . .[9]

Even the best educated black, according to Murrell, could not be convinced to seek treatment for syphilis. Venereal disease, according to some doctors, threatened the future of the race. The medical profession attributed the low birth rate among blacks to the high prevalence of venereal disease which caused stillbirths and miscarriages. Moreover, the high rates of syphilis were thought to lead to increased insanity and crime. One doctor writing at the turn of the century estimated that the number of insane Negroes had increased thirteen-fold since the end of the Civil War. Dr. Murrell's conclusion echoed the most informed anthropological and ethnological data:

> So the scourge sweeps among them. Those that are treated are only half cured and the effort to assimilate a complex civilization driving their diseased minds until the results are criminal records. Perhaps here, in conjunction with tuberculosis, will be the end of the negro problem. Disease will accomplish what man cannot do.[10]

This particular configuration of ideas formed the core of medical opinion concerning blacks, sex, and disease in the early twentieth century. Doctors generally discounted socioeconomic explanations of the state of black health, arguing that better medical care could not alter the evolutionary scheme. These assumptions provide the backdrop for examining the Tuskegee Syphilis Study.

THE ORIGINS OF THE EXPERIMENT

In 1929, under a grant from the Julius Rosenwald Fund, the USPHS conducted studies in the rural South to determine the prevalence of syphilis among blacks and explore the possibilities for mass treatment. The USPHS found Macon County, Alabama, in which the town of Tuskegee is located, to have the highest syphilis rate of the six counties surveyed. The Rosenwald Study concluded that mass treatment could be successfully implemented among rural blacks.[11] Although it is doubtful that the necessary funds would have been allocated even in the best economic conditions, after the economy collapsed in 1929, the findings were ignored. It is, however, ironic that the Tuskegee Study came to be based on findings of the Rosenwald Study that demonstrated the possibilities of mass treatment.

Three years later, in 1932, Dr. Taliaferro Clark, Chief of the USPHS Venereal Disease Division and author of the Rosenwald Study report, decided that conditions in Macon County merited renewed attention. Clark believed the high prevalence of syphilis offered an "unusual opportunity" for observation. From its inception, the USPHS regarded the Tuskegee Study as a classic "study in nature,"* rather than an experiment.[12] As long as syphilis was so prevalent in Macon and most of the blacks went

---

*In 1865, Claude Bernard, the famous French physiologist, outlined the distinction between a "study in nature" and experimentation. A study in nature required simple observation, an essentially passive act, while experimentation demanded intervention which altered the original condition. The Tuskegee Study was thus clearly not a study in nature. The very act of diagnosis altered the original condition. "It is on this very possibility of acting or not acting on a body," wrote Bernard, "that the distinction will exclusively rest between sciences called sciences of observation and sciences called experimental."

untreated throughout life, it seemed only natural to Clark that it would be valuable to observe the consequences. He described it as a "ready-made situation." Surgeon General H. S. Cumming wrote to R. R. Moton, Director of the Tuskegee Institute:

> The recent syphilis control demonstration carried out in Macon County, with the financial assistance of the Julius Rosenwald Fund, revealed the presence of an unusually high rate in this county and, what is more remarkable, the fact that 99 per cent of this group was entirely without previous treatment. This combination, together with the expected cooperation of your hospital, offers an unparalleled opportunity for carrying on this piece of scientific research which probably cannot be duplicated anywhere else in the world.

Although no formal protocol appears to have been written, several letters of Clark and Cumming suggest what the USPHS hoped to find. Clark indicated that it would be important to see how disease affected the daily lives of the men:

> The results of these studies of case records suggest the desirability of making a further study of the effect of untreated syphilis on the human economy among people now living and engaged in their daily pursuits.

It also seems that the USPHS believed the experiment might demonstrate that antisyphilitic treatment was unnecessary. As Cumming noted: "It is expected the results of this study may have a marked bearing on the treatment, or conversely the non-necessity of treatment, of cases of latent syphilis."

The immediate source of Cumming's hypothesis appears to have been the famous Oslo Study of untreated syphilis. Between 1890 and 1910, Professor C. Boeck, the chief of the Oslo Venereal Clinic, withheld treatment from almost two thousand patients infected with syphilis. He was convinced that therapies then available, primarily mercurial ointment, were of no value. When arsenic therapy became widely available by 1910, after Paul Ehrlich's historic discovery of "606," the study was abandoned. E. Bruusgaard, Boeck's successor, conducted a follow-up study of 473 of the untreated patients from 1925 to 1927. He found that 27.9 percent of these patients had undergone a "spontaneous cure," and now manifested no symptoms of the disease. Moreover, he estimated that as many as 70 percent of all syphilitics went through life without inconvenience from the disease.[13] His study, however, clearly acknowledged the dangers of untreated syphilis for the remaining 30 percent.

Thus every major textbook of syphilis at the time of the Tuskegee Study's inception strongly advocated treating syphilis even in its latent stages, which follow the initial inflammatory reaction. In discussing the Oslo Study, Dr. J. E. Moore, one of the nation's leading venereologists wrote, "This summary of Bruusgaard's study is by no means intended to suggest that syphilis be allowed to pass untreated."[14] If a complete cure could not be effected, at least the most devastating effects of the disease could be avoided. Although the standard therapies of the time, arsenical compounds and bismuth injection, involved certain dangers because of their toxicity, the alternatives were much worse. As the Oslo Study had shown, untreated syphilis could lead to cardiovascular disease, insanity, and premature death.[15] Moore wrote in his 1933 textbook:

> Though it imposes a slight though measurable risk of its own, treatment markedly diminishes the risk from syphilis. In latent syphilis, as I shall show, the probability of progression, relapse, or death is reduced from a probable 25-30 percent without treatment to about 5 percent with it; and the gravity of the relapse if it occurs, is markedly diminished.[16]

"Another compelling reason for treatment," noted Moore, "exists in the fact that every patient with latent syphilis may be, and perhaps is, infectious for others."[17] In 1932, the year in which the Tuskegee Study began, the USPHS sponsored and published a paper by Moore and six other syphilis experts that strongly argued for treating latent syphilis.

The Oslo Study, therefore, could not have provided justification for the USPHS to undertake a study that did not entail treatment. Rather, the suppositions that conditions in Tuskegee existed "naturally" and that the men would not be treated anyway provided the experiment's rationale. In turn, these two assumptions rested on the prevailing medical attitudes concerning blacks, sex, and disease. For example, Clark explained the prevalence of venereal disease in Macon County by emphasizing promiscuity among blacks:

> This state of affairs is due to the paucity of doctors, rather low intelligence of the Negro population in this

> section, depressed economic conditions, and the very common promiscuous sex relations of this population group which not only contribute to the spread of syphilis but also contribute to the prevailing indifference with regard to treatment.

In fact, Moore, who had written so persuasively in favor of treating latent syphilis, suggested that existing knowledge did not apply to Negroes. Although he had called the Oslo Study "a never-to-be-repeated human experiment," he served as an expert consultant to the Tuskegee Study:

> I think that such a study as you have contemplated would be of immense value. It will be necessary of course in the consideration of the results to evaluate the special factors introduced by a selection of the material from negro males. Syphilis in the negro is in many respects almost a different disease from syphilis in the white.

Dr. O. C. Wenger, chief of the federally operated venereal disease clinic at Hot Springs, Arkansas, praised Moore's judgment, adding, "This study will emphasize those differences." On another occasion he advised Clark, "We must remember we are dealing with a group of people who are illiterate, have no conception of time, and whose personal history is always indefinite."

The doctors who devised and directed the Tuskegee Study accepted the mainstream assumptions regarding blacks and venereal disease. The premise that blacks, promiscuous and lustful, would not seek or continue treatment, shaped the study. A test of untreated syphilis seemed "natural" because the USPHS presumed the men would never be treated; the Tuskegee Study made that a self-fulfilling prophecy.

SELECTING THE SUBJECTS

Clark sent Dr. Raymond Vonderlehr to Tuskegee in September 1932 to assemble a sample of men with latent syphilis for the experiment. The basic design of the study called for the selection of syphilitic black males between the ages of twenty-five and sixty, a thorough physical examination including x-rays, and finally, a spinal tap to determine the incidence of neuro-syphilis. They had no intention of providing any treatment for the infected men.[18] The USPHS originally scheduled the whole experiment to last six months; it seemed to be both a simple and inexpensive project.

The task of collecting the sample, however, proved to be more difficult than the USPHS had supposed. Vonderlehr canvassed the largely illiterate, poverty-stricken population of sharecroppers and tenant farmers in search of test subjects. If his circulars requested only men over twenty-five to attend his clinics, none would appear, suspecting he was conducting draft physicals. Therefore, he was forced to test large numbers of women and men who did not fit the experiment's specifications. This involved considerable expense since the USPHS had promised the Macon County Board of Health that it would treat those who were infected, but not included in the study. Clark wrote to Vonderlehr about the situation: "It never once occured to me that we would be called upon to treat a large part of the county as return for the privilege of making this study. . . . I am anxious to keep the expenditures for treatment down to the lowest possible point because it is the one item of expenditure in connection with the study most difficult to defend despite our knowledge of the need therefor." Vonderlehr responded: "If we could find from 100 to 200 cases . . . we would not have to do another Wassermann on useless individuals . . ."

Significantly, the attempt to develop the sample contradicted the prediction the USPHS had made initially regarding the prevalence of the disease in Macon County. Overall rates of syphilis fell well below expectations; as opposed to the USPHS projection of 35 percent, 20 percent of those tested were actually diseased. Moreover, those who had sought and received previous treatment far exceeded the expectations of the USPHS. Clark noted in a letter to Vonderlehr:

> I find your report of March 6th quite interesting but regret the necessity of Wassermanning [*sic*] . . . such a large number of individuals in order to uncover this relatively limited number of untreated cases.

Further difficulties arose in enlisting the subjects to participate in the experiment, to be "Wassermanned," and to return for a subsequent series of examinations. Vonderlehr found that only the offer of treatment elicited the cooperation of the men. They were told they were ill and were promised free care. Offered therapy, they became willing subjects.[19] The USPHS did not tell the men that they were participants in an experiment; on the contrary, the subjects believed they were being treated for "bad blood"—the rural South's colloquialism for syphilis. They thought they were participating in a public health demonstration similar to the one that had been conducted by the Julius Rosenwald Fund in Tuskegee several years earlier. In the end, the men were so eager for medical care that the number of defaulters in the experiment proved to be insignificant.

To preserve the subjects' interest, Vonderlehr gave most of the men mercurial ointment, a noneffective drug, while some of the younger men apparently received inadequate dosages of neoarsphenamine. This required Vonderlehr to write frequently to Clark requesting supplies. He feared the experiment would fail if the men were not offered treatment.

> It is desirable and essential if the study is to be a success to maintain the interest of each of the cases examined by me through to the time when the spinal puncture can be completed. Expenditure of several hundred dollars for drugs for these men would be well worth while if their interest and cooperation would be maintained in so doing. . . . It is my desire to keep the main purpose of the work from the negroes in the county and continue their interest in treatment. That is what the vast majority wants and the examination seems relatively unimportant to them in comparison. It would probably cause the entire experiment to collapse if the clinics were stopped before the work is completed.

On another occasion he explained:

> Dozens of patients have been sent away without treatment during the past two weeks and it would have been impossible to continue without the free distribution of drugs because of the unfavorable impression made on the negro.

The readiness of the test subjects to participate of course contradicted the notion that blacks would not seek or continue therapy.

The final procedure of the experiment was to be a spinal tap to test for neuro-syphilis. The USPHS presented this purely diagnostic exam, which often entails considerable pain and complications, to the men as a "special treatment." Clark explained to Moore:

> We have not yet commenced the spinal punctures. This operation will be deferred to the last in order not to unduly disturb our field work by any adverse reports by the patients subjected to spinal puncture because of some disagreeable sensations following this procedure. These negroes are very ignorant and easily influenced by things that would be of minor significance in a more intelligent group.

The letter to the subjects announcing the spinal tap read:

> Some time ago you were given a thorough examination and since that time we hope you have gotten a great deal of treatment for bad blood. You will now be given your last chance to get a second examination. This examination is a very special one and after it is finished you will be given a special treatment if it is believed you are in a condition to stand it. . . .
>
> REMEMBER THIS IS YOUR LAST CHANCE FOR SPECIAL FREE TREATMENT. BE SURE TO MEET THE NURSE.[20]

The HEW investigation did not uncover this crucial fact: the men participated in the study under the guise of treatment.

Despite the fact that their assumption regarding prevalence and black attitudes toward treatment had proved wrong, the USPHS decided in the summer of 1933 to continue the study. Once again, it seemed only "natural" to pursue the research since the sample already existed, and with a depressed economy, the cost of treatment appeared prohibitive—although there is no indication it was ever considered. Vonderlehr first suggested extending the study in letters to Clark and Wenger:

> At the end of this project we shall have a considerable number of cases presenting various complications of syphilis, who have received only mercury and may still be considered untreated in the modern sense of therapy. Should these cases be followed over a period of from five to ten years many interesting facts could be learned regarding the course and complications of untreated syphilis.

"As I see it," responded Wenger, "we have no further interest in these patients until they die." Apparently, the physicians engaged in the experiment believed that only autopsies could scientifically confirm the findings of the study. Surgeon General Cumming explained this in a letter to R. R. Moton, requesting the continued cooperation of the Tuskegee Institute Hospital:

> This study which was predominantly clinical in character points to the frequent occurrence of severe complications involving the various vital organs of the body and indicates that syphilis as a disease does a great deal of damage. Since clinical observations are not considered final in the medical world, it is our desire to continue observation on the cases selected for the recent study and if possible to bring a percentage of these cases to autopsy so that pathological confirmation may be made of the disease processes.

Bringing the men to autopsy required the USPHS to devise a further series of deceptions and inducements. Wenger warned Vonderlehr that the men must not realize that they would be autopsied:

> There is one danger in the latter plan and that is if the colored population become aware that accepting free hospital care means a post-mortem, every darkey will leave Macon County and it will hurt [Dr. Eugene] Dibble's hospital.

"Naturally," responded Vonderlehr, "it is not my intention to let it be generally known that the main object of the present activities is the bringing of the men to necropsy." The subjects' trust in the USPHS made the plan viable. The USPHS gave Dr. Dibble, the Director of the Tuskegee Institute Hospital, an interim appointment to the Public Health Service. As Wenger noted:

> One thing is certain. The only way we are going to get post-mortems is to have the demise take place in Dibble's hospital and when these colored folks are told that Doctor Dibble is now a Government doctor too they will have more confidence.*

After the USPHS approved the continuation of the experiment in 1933, Vonderlehr decided that it would be necessary to select a group of healthy, uninfected men to serve as controls. Vonderlehr, who had succeeded Clark as Chief of the Venereal Disease Division, sent Dr. J. R. Heller to Tuskegee to gather the control group. Heller distributed drugs (noneffective) to these men, which suggests that they also believed they were undergoing treatment. Control subjects who became syphilitic were simply transferred to the test group—a strikingly inept violation of standard research procedure.[21]

The USPHS offered several inducements to maintain contact and to procure the continued cooperation of the men. Eunice Rivers, a black nurse, was hired to follow their health and to secure approval for autopsies. She gave the men noneffective medicines—"spring tonic" and aspirin—as well as transportation and hot meals on the days of their examinations.[22] More important, Nurse Rivers provided continuity to the project over the entire forty-year period. By supplying "medicals," the USPHS was able to continue to deceive the participants, who believed that they were receiving therapy from the government doctors. Deceit was integral to the study. When the test subjects complained about spinal taps one doctor wrote:

> They simply do not like spinal punctures. A few of those who were tapped are enthusiastic over the results but to most, the suggestion causes violent shaking of the head; others claim they were robbed of their procreative powers (regardless of the fact that I claim it stimulates them).

Letters to the subjects announcing an impending USPHS visit to Tuskegee explained: "[The doctor]

---

*The degree of black cooperation in conducting the study remains unclear and would be impossible to properly assess in an article of this length. It seems certain that some members of the Tuskegee Institute staff such as R. R. Moton and Eugene Dibble understood the nature of the experiment and gave their support to it. There is, however, evidence that some blacks who assisted the USPHS physicians were not aware of the deceptive nature of the experiment. Dr. Joshua Williams, an intern at the John A. Andrew Memorial Hospital (Tuskegee Institute) in 1932, assisted Vonderlehr in taking blood samples of the test subjects. In 1973 he told the HEW panel: "I know we thought it was merely a service group organized to help the people in the area. We didn't know it was a research project at all at the time." (See, "Transcript of Proceedings," Tuskegee Syphillis Study Ad Hoc Advisory Panel, February 23, 1973, Unpublished typescript. National Library of Medicine, Bethesda, Maryland.) It is also apparent that Eunice Rivers, the black nurse who had primary responsibility for maintaining contact with the men over the forty years, did not fully understand the dangers of the experiment. In any event, black involvement in the study in no way mitigates the racial assumption of the experiment, but rather, demonstrates their power.

wants to make a special examination to find out how you have been feeling and whether the treatment has improved your health." In fact, after the first six months of the study, the USPHS had furnished no treatment whatsoever.

Finally, because it proved difficult to persuade the men to come to the hospital when they became severely ill, the USPHS promised to cover their burial expenses. The Milbank Memorial Fund provided approximately $50 per man for this purpose beginning in 1935. This was a particularly strong inducement as funeral rites constituted an important component of the cultural life of rural blacks. One report of the study concluded, "Without this suasion it would, we believe, have been impossible to secure the cooperation of the group and their families."

Reports of the study's findings, which appeared regularly in the medical press beginning in 1936, consistently cited the ravages of untreated syphilis. The first paper, read at the 1936 American Medical Association annual meeting, found "that syphilis in this period [latency] tends to greatly increase the frequency of manifestations of cardiovascular disease." Only 16 percent of the subjects gave no sign of morbidity as opposed to 61 percent of the controls. Ten years later, a report noted coldly, "The fact that nearly twice as large a proportion of the syphilitic individuals as of the control group has died is a very striking one." Life expectancy, concluded the doctors, is reduced by about 20 percent.

A 1955 article found that slightly more than 30 percent of the test group autopsied had died *directly* from advanced syphilitic lesions of either the cardiovascular or the central nervous system.[23] Another published account stated, "Review of those still living reveals that an appreciable number have late complications of syphilis which probably will result, for some at least, in contributing materially to the ultimate cause of death."[24] In 1950, Dr. Wenger had concluded, "We now know, where we could only surmise before, that we have contributed to their ailments and shortened their lives." As black physician Vernal Cave, a member of the HEW panel, later wrote, "They proved a point, then proved a point, then proved a point."

During the forty years of the experiment the USPHS had sought on several occasions to ensure that the subjects did not receive treatment from other sources. To this end, Vonderlehr met with groups of local black doctors in 1934, to ask their cooperation in not treating the men. Lists of subjects were distributed to Macon County physicians along with letters requesting them to refer these men back to the USPHS if they sought care. The USPHS warned the Alabama Health Department not to treat the test subjects when they took a mobile VD unit into Tuskegee in the early 1940s. In 1941, the Army drafted several subjects and told them to begin antisyphilitic treatment immediately. The USPHS supplied the draft board with a list of 256 names they desired to have excluded from treatment, and the board complied.

In spite of these efforts, by the early 1950s many of the men had secured some treatment on their own. By 1952, almost 30 percent of the test subjects had received some penicillin, although only 7.5 percent had received what could be considered adequate doses.[25] Vonderlehr wrote to one of the participating physicians, "I hope that the availability of antibiotics has not interfered too much with this project." A report published in 1955 considered whether the treatment that some of the men had obtained had "defeated" the study. The article attempted to explain the relatively low exposure to penicillin in an age of antibiotics, suggesting as a reason: "the stoicism of these men as a group; they still regard hospitals and medicines with suspicion and prefer an occasional dose of time-honored herbs or tonics to modern drugs." The authors failed to note that the men believed they were already under the care of the government doctors and thus saw no need to seek treatment elsewhere. Any treatment which the men might have received, concluded the report, had been insufficient to compromise the experiment.

When the USPHS evaluated the status of the study in the 1960s they continued to rationalize the racial aspects of the experiment. For example, the minutes of a 1965 meeting at the Center for Disease Control recorded:

> Racial issue was mentioned briefly. Will not affect the study. Any questions can be handled by saying these people were at the point that therapy would no longer help them. They are getting better medical care than they would under any other circumstances.

A group of physicians met again at the CDC in 1969 to decide whether or not to terminate the study. Although one doctor argued that the study should be stopped and the men treated, the consensus was to continue. Dr. J. Lawton Smith remarked, "You will never have another study like this; take advantage of it." A memo prepared by Dr. James B. Lucas, Assistant Chief of the Venereal Disease Branch, stated: "Nothing learned will prevent, find, or cure a single case of infectious syphilis or bring us closer to our basic mission of controlling venereal disease in the United States." He concluded, however, that the study should be continued "along its present lines." When the first accounts of the experiment appeared in the national press in July 1972, data were still being collected and autopsies performed.

THE HEW FINAL REPORT

HEW finally formed the Tuskegee Syphilis Study Ad Hoc Advisory Panel on August 28, 1972, in response to criticism that the press descriptions of the experiment had triggered. The panel, composed of nine members, five of them black, concentrated on two issues. First, was the study justified in 1932 and had the men given their informed consent? Second, should penicillin have been provided when it became available in the early 1950s? The panel was also charged with determining if the study should be terminated and assessing current policies regarding experimentation with human subjects. The group issued their report in June 1973.

FROM THE HEW FINAL REPORT (1973)

1. In retrospect, the Public Health Service Study of Untreated Syphilis in the Male Negro in Macon County, Alabama, was ethically unjustified in 1932. The judgment made in 1973 about the conduct of the study in 1932 is made with the advantage of hindsight acutely sharpened over some forty years, concerning an activity in a different age with different social standards. Nevertheless, one fundamental ethical rule is that a person should not be subjected to avoidable risk of death or physical harm unless he freely and intelligently consents. There is no evidence that such consent was obtained from the participants in this study.

2. Because of the paucity of information available today on the manner in which the study was conceived, designed and sustained, a scientific justification for a short term demonstration study cannot be ruled out. However, the conduct of the longitudinal study as initially reported in 1936 and through the years is judged to be scientifically unsound and its results are disproportionately meager compared with known risk to human subjects involved. . . .

By focusing on the issues of penicillin therapy and informed consent, the *Final Report* and the investigation betrayed a basic misunderstanding of the experiment's purposes and design. The HEW report implied that the failure to provide penicillin constituted the study's major ethical misjudgment; implicit was the assumption that no adequate therapy existed prior to penicillin. Nonetheless medical authorities firmly believed in the efficacy of arsenotherapy for treating syphilis at the time of the experiment's inception in 1932. The panel further failed to recognize that the entire study had been predicated on nontreatment. Provision of effective medication would have violated the rationale of the experiment—to study the natural course of the disease until death. On several occasions, in fact, the USPHS had prevented the men from receiving proper treatment. Indeed, there is no evidence that the USPHS ever considered providing penicillin.

The other focus of the *Final Report*—informed consent—also served to obscure the historical facts of the experiment. In light of the deceptions and exploitations which the experiment perpetrated, it is an understatement to declare, as the *Report* did, that the experiment was "ethically unjustified," because it failed to obtain informed consent from the subjects. The *Final Report's* statement, "Submitting voluntarily is not informed consent," indicated that the panel believed that the men had volunteered *for the experiment.*[26] The records in the National Archives make clear that the men did not submit voluntarily to an experiment; they were told and they believed that they were getting free treatment from expert government doctors for a serious disease. The failure of the HEW *Final Report* to expose this critical fact—that the USPHS lied to the subjects—calls into question the thoroughness and credibility of their investigation.

Failure to place the study in a historical context also made it impossible for the investigation to deal with the essentially racist nature of the experiment. The panel treated the study as an aberration, well-intentioned but misguided.[27] Moreover, concern that the *Final Report* might be viewed as a critique of human experimentation in general seems to have severely limited the scope of the inquiry. The *Final Report* is quick to remind the reader on two occasions: "The position of the Panel must not be construed to be a general repudiation of scientific research with human subjects."[28] The Report assures us that a better designed experiment could have been justified:

> It is possible that a scientific study in 1932 of untreated syphilis, properly conceived with a clear protocol and conducted with suitable subjects who fully understood the implications of their involvement, might have been justified in the prepenicillin era. This is especially true when one considers the uncertain nature of the results of treatment of late latent syphilis and the highly toxic nature of therapeutic agents then available.[29]

This statement is questionable in view of the proven dangers of untreated syphilis known in 1932.

Since the publication of the HEW *Final Report,* a defense of the Tuskegee Study has emerged. These arguments, most clearly articulated by Dr. R. H. Kampmeier in the *Southern Medical Journal,* center on the limited knowledge of effective therapy for latent syphilis when the experiment began. Kampmeier argues that by 1950, penicillin would have been of no value for these men.[30] Others have suggested that the men were fortunate to have been spared the highly toxic treatments of the earlier period. Moreover, even these contemporary defenses assume that the men never would have been treated anyway. As Dr. Charles Barnett of Stanford University wrote in 1974, "The lack of treatment was not contrived by the USPHS but was an established fact of which they proposed to take advantage."[31] Several doctors who participated in the study continued to justify the experiment. Dr. J. R. Heller, who on one occasion had referred to the test subjects as the "Ethiopian population," told reporters in 1972:

> I don't see why they should be shocked or horrified. There was no racial side to this. It just happened to be in a black community. I feel this was a perfectly straightforward study, perfectly ethical, with controls. Part of our mission as physicians is to find out what happens to individuals with disease and without disease.[32]

These apologies, as well as the HEW *Final Report,* ignore many of the essential ethical issues which the study poses. The Tuskegee Study reveals the persistence of beliefs within the medical profession about the nature of blacks, sex, and disease—beliefs that had tragic repercussions long after their alleged "scientific" bases were known to be incorrect. Most strikingly, the entire health of a community was jeopardized by leaving a communicable disease untreated.[33] There can be little doubt that the Tuskegee researchers regarded their subjects as less than human.[34] As a result, the ethical canons of experimenting on human subjects were completely disregarded.

The study also raises significant questions about professional self-regulation and scientific bureaucracy. Once the USPHS decided to extend the experiment in the summer of 1933, it was unlikely that the test would be halted short of the men's deaths. The experiment was widely reported for forty years without evoking any significant protest within the medical community. Nor did any bureaucratic mechanism exist within the government for the periodic reassessment of the Tuskegee experiment's ethics and scientific value. The USPHS sent physicians to Tuskegee every several years to check on the study's progress, but never subjected the morality or usefulness of the experiment to serious scrutiny. Only the press accounts of 1972 finally punctured the continued rationalizations of the USPHS and brought the study to an end. Even the HEW investigation was compromised by fear that it would be considered a threat to future human experimentation.

In retrospect the Tuskegee Study revealed more about the pathology of racism than it did about the pathology of syphilis; more about the nature of scientific inquiry than the nature of the disease process. The injustice committed by the experiment went well beyond the facts outlined in the press and the HEW *Final Report.* The degree of deception and damages have been seriously underestimated. As this history of the study suggests, the notion that science is a value-free discipline must be rejected. The need for greater vigilance in assessing the specific ways in which social values and attitudes affect professional behavior is clearly indicated.

NOTES

1. The best general account of the study is James Jones, *Bad Blood*, 2nd ed. (New York: The Free Press, 1993).
2. *Final Report* of the Tuskegee Syphilis Study Ad Hoc Advisory Panel, Department of Health, Education, and Welfare (Washington, D.C.: GPO, 1973). (Hereafter, HEW *Final Report*).
3. W. T. English, "The Negro Problem from the Physician's Point of View," *Atlanta Journal-Record of Medicine* 5 (October 1903), 461.
4. Daniel David Quillian. "Racial Peculiarities: A Cause of the Prevalence of Syphilis in Negroes," *American Journal of Dermatology and Genito-Urinary Diseases* 10 (July 1906), p. 277.
5. English, p. 463.
6. William Lee Howard. "The Negro as a Distinct Ethnic Factor in Civilization," *Medicine* (Detroit) 9 (June 1903), 424.
7. "Castration Instead of Lynching," *Atlanta Journal-Record of Medicine* 8 (October 1906), 457.
8. Searle Harris, "The Future of the Negro from the Standpoint of the Southern Physician." *Alabama Medical Journal* 14 (January 1902), 62.
9. Thomas W. Murrell, "Syphilis in the Negro: Its Bearing on the Race Problem," *American Journal of Dermatology and Genito-Urinary Diseases* 10 (August 1906), 307.
10. Murrell, "Syphilis in the Negro; Its Bearing on the Race Problem," p. 307.
11. Taliaferro Clark, *The Control of Syphilis in Southern Rural Areas* (Chicago: Julius Rosenwald Fund, 1932), 53–58. Approximately 35 percent of the inhabitants of Macon County who were examined were found to be syphilitic.
12. See Claude Bernard, *An Introduction to the Study of Experimental Medicine* (New York: Dover, 1865, 1957), pp. 5–26.
13. The best discussion of the Boeck-Bruusgaard data is E. Gurney Clark and Niels Danbolt, "The Oslo Study of the Natural History of Untreated Syphilis," *Journal of Chronic Diseases* 2 (September 1955), 311–44.
14. Joseph Earl Moore, *The Modern Treatment of Syphilis* (Baltimore: Charles C. Thomas, 1933), p. 24.
15. Moore, pp. 231–47.
16. Moore, p. 237.
17. Moore, p. 236.
18. As Clark wrote: "You will observe that our plan has nothing to do with treatment. It is purely a diagnostic procedure carried out to determine what has happened to the syphilitic Negro who has had no treatment." Clark to Paul A. O'Leary, September 27, 1932, NA-WNRC.
19. Vonderlehr later explained: The reason treatment was given to many of these men was twofold: First, when the study was started in the fall of 1932, no plans had been made for its continuation and a few of the patients were treated before we fully realized the need for continuing the project on a permanent basis. Second it was difficult to hold the interest of the group of Negroes in Macon County unless some treatment was given." Vonderlehr to Austin V. Diebert, December 5, 1938, Tuskegee Syphilis Study Ad Hoc Advisory Panel Papers, Box 1, National Library of Medicine, Bethesda, Maryland (Hereafter, TSS-NLM). This collection contains the materials assembled by the HEW investigation in 1972.
20. Macon County Health Department, "Letter to Subjects," n.d., NA-WNRC.
21. Austin V. Diebert and Martha C. Bruyere, "Untreated Syphilis in the Male Negro, III." *Venereal Disease Information* 27 (December 1946), 301–14.
22. Eunice Rivers, Stanley Schuman, Lloyd Simpson, Sidney Olansky, "Twenty-Years of Followup Experience In a Long-Range Medical Study," *Public Health Reports* 68 (April 1953), 391–95. In this article Nurse Rivers explains her role in the experiment. She wrote: "Because of the low educational status of the majority of the patients, it was impossible to appeal to them from a purely scientific approach. Therefore, various methods were used to maintain their interest. Free medicines, burial assistance or insurance (the project being referred to as 'Miss Rivers' Lodge'), free hot meals on the days of examination, transportation to and from the hospital, and an opportunity to stop in town on the return trip to shop or visit with friends on the streets all helped. In spite of these attractions, there were some who refused their examinations because they were not sick and did not see that they were being benefited." (p. 393).
23. Jesse J. Peters, James H. Peers, Sidney Olansky, John C. Cutler, and Geraldine Gleeson, "Untreated Syphilis in the Male Negro: Pathologic Findings in Syphilitic and Non-Syphilitic Patients," *Journal of Chronic Diseases* 1 (February 1955), 127–48.
24. Sidney Olansky, Stanley H. Schuman, Jesse J. Peters, C. A. Smith, and Dorothy S. Rambo, "Untreated Syphilis in the Male Negro, X. Twenty Years of Clinical Observation of Untreated Syphilitic and Presumably Nonsyphilitic Groups," *Journal of Chronic Diseases* 4 (August 1956), 184.
25. Stanley H. Schuman, Sidney Olansky, Eunice Rivers, C. A. Smith, and Dorothy S. Rambo, "Untreated

Syphilis in the Male Negro: Background and Current Status of Patients in the Tuskegee Study," *Journal of Chronic Diseases* 2 (November 1955), 550–53.
26. HEW *Final Report*, p. 7.
27. The notable exception is Jay Katz's eloquent "Reservations About the Panel Report on Charge 1," HEW *Final Report*, pp. 14–15.
28. HEW *Final Report*, pp. 8, 12.
29. HEW *Final Report*, pp. 8, 12.
30. See R. H. Kampmeier, "The Tuskegee Study of - Untreated Syphilis," Southern Medical Journal 65 (October 1972), 1247–51; and "'Final Report on the 'Tuskegee Syphilis Study,'" *Southern Medical Journal* 67 (November 1974), 1349–53.
31. Quoted in "Debate Revives on the PHS Study," *Medical World News* (April 19, 1974), p. 37.
32. Heller to Vonderlehr, November 28, 1933, quoted in *Medical Tribune* (August 23, 1972), p. 14.
33. Although it is now known that syphilis is rarely infectious after its early phase, at the time of the study's inception latent syphilis was thought to be communicable. The fact that members of the control group were placed in the test group when they became syphilitic proves that at least some infectious men were denied treatment.
34. When the subjects are drawn from minority groups, especially those with which the researcher cannot identify, basic human rights may be compromised. Hans Jonas has clearly explicated the problem in his "Philosophical Reflections on Experimentation," *Daedalus* 98 (Spring 1969), 234–37. As Jonas writes: "If the properties we adduced as the particular qualifications of the members of the scientific fraternity itself are taken as general criteria of selection, then one should look for additional subjects where a maximum of identification, understanding, and spontaneity can be expected—that is, among the most highly motivated, the most highly educated, and the least 'captive' members of the community."

THE BELMONT REPORT: ETHICAL PRINCIPLES AND GUIDELINES FOR THE PROTECTION OF HUMAN SUBJECTS OF RESEARCH

April 18, 1979

The National Commission for the Protection of Human Subjects of Biomedical and Behavioral Research

ETHICAL PRINCIPLES AND GUIDELINES FOR RESEARCH INVOLVING HUMAN SUBJECTS

Scientific research has produced substantial social benefits. It has also posed some troubling ethical questions. Public attention was drawn to these questions by reported abuses of human subjects in biomedical experiments, especially during the Second World War. During the Nuremberg War Crime Trials, the Nuremberg code was drafted as a set of standards for judging physicians and scientists who had conducted biomedical experiments on concentration camp prisoners. This code became the prototype of many later codes intended to assure that research involving human subjects would be carried out in an ethical manner.

The codes consist of rules, some general, others specific, that guide the investigators or the reviewers of research in their work. Such rules often are inadequate to cover complex situations; at times they come into conflict, and they are frequently difficult to interpret or apply. Broader ethical principles will provide a basis on which specific rules may be formulated, criticized and interpreted.

From http://ohrp.osophs.dhhs.gov/humansubjects/guidance/belmont.htm.22October2001.

Editor's note: Some footnotes have been deleted. Students who want to follow up on sources should consult the original article.

Three principles, or general prescriptive judgments, that are relevant to research involving human subjects are identified in this statement. Other principles may also be relevant. These three are comprehensive, however, and are stated at a level of generalization that should assist scientists, subjects, reviewers and interested citizens to understand the ethical issues inherent in research involving human subjects. These principles cannot always be applied so as to resolve beyond dispute particular ethical problems. The objective is to provide an analytical framework that will guide the resolution of ethical problems arising from research involving human subjects.

This statement consists of a distinction between research and practice, a discussion of the three basic ethical principles.

PART A: BOUNDARIES BETWEEN PRACTICE & RESEARCH

It is important to distinguish between biomedical and behavioral research, on the one hand, and the practice of accepted therapy on the other, in order to know what activities ought to undergo review for the protection of human subjects of research. The distinction between research and practice is blurred partly because both often occur together (as in research designed to evaluate a therapy) and partly because notable departures from standard practice are often called "experimental" when the terms "experimental" and "research" are not carefully defined.

For the most part, the term "practice" refers to interventions that are designed solely to enhance the well-being of an individual patient or client and that have a reasonable expectation of success. The purpose of medical or behavioral practice is to provide diagnosis, preventive treatment or therapy to particular individuals.[1] By contrast, the term "research" designates an activity designed to test an hypothesis, permit conclusions to be drawn, and thereby to develop or contribute to generalizable knowledge (expressed, for example, in theories, principles, and statements of relationships). Research is usually described in a formal protocol that sets forth an objective and a set of procedures designed to reach that objective.

When a clinician departs in a significant way from standard or accepted practice, the innovation does not, in and of itself, constitute research. The fact that a procedure is "experimental," in the sense of new, untested or different, does not automatically place it in the category of research. Radically new procedures of this description should, however, be made the object of formal research at an early stage in order to determine whether they are safe and effective. Thus, it is the responsibility of medical practice committees, for example, to insist that a major innovation be incorporated into a formal research project.

Research and practice may be carried on together when research is designed to evaluate the safety and efficacy of a therapy. This need not cause any confusion regarding whether or not the activity requires review; the general rule is that if there is any element of research in an activity, that activity should undergo review for the protection of human subjects.

PART B: BASIC ETHICAL PRINCIPLES

The expression "basic ethical principles" refers to those general judgments that serve as a basic justification for the many particular ethical prescriptions and evaluations of human actions. Three basic principles, among those generally accepted in our cultural tradition, are particularly relevant to the ethics of research involving human subjects: the principles of respect [for] persons, beneficence and justice.

1. Respect for Persons Respect for persons incorporates at least two ethical convictions: first, that individuals should be treated as autonomous agents, and second, that persons with diminished autonomy are entitled to protection. The principle of respect for persons thus divides into two separate moral requirements: the requirement to acknowledge autonomy and the requirement to protect those with diminished autonomy.

An autonomous person is an individual capable of deliberation about personal goals and of acting under the direction of such deliberation. To respect autonomy is to give weight to autonomous persons' considered opinions and choices while refraining from obstructing their actions unless they are clearly detrimental to others. To show lack of respect for an autonomous agent is to repudiate that person's considered judgments, to deny an individual the freedom to act on those considered judgments, or to withhold information necessary to make a considered judgment, when there are no compelling reasons to do so.

However, not every human being is capable of self-determination. The capacity for self-determination matures during an individual's life, and some individuals lose this capacity wholly or in part because of illness, mental disability, or circumstances that severely restrict liberty. Respect for the immature and the incapacitated may require protecting them as they mature or while they are incapacitated.

Some persons are in need of extensive protection, even to the point of excluding them from activities which may harm them; other persons require little protection beyond making sure they undertake activities freely and with awareness of possible adverse consequence. The extent of protection afforded should depend upon the risk of harm and the likelihood of benefit. The judgment that any individual lacks autonomy should be periodically reevaluated and will vary in different situations.

In most cases of research involving human subjects, respect for persons demands that subjects enter into the research voluntarily and with adequate information. In some situations, however, application of the principle is not obvious. The involvement of prisoners as subjects of research provides an instructive example. On the one hand, it would seem that the principle of respect for persons requires that prisoners not be deprived of the opportunity to volunteer for research. On the other hand, under prison conditions they may be subtly coerced or unduly influenced to engage in research activities for which they would not otherwise volunteer. Respect for persons would then dictate that prisoners be protected. Whether to allow prisoners to "volunteer" or to "protect" them presents a dilemma. Respecting persons, in most hard cases, is often a matter of balancing competing claims urged by the principle of respect itself.

2. Beneficence Persons are treated in an ethical manner not only by respecting their decisions and protecting them from harm, but also by making efforts to secure their well-being. Such treatment falls under the principle of beneficence. The term "beneficence" is often understood to cover acts of kindness or charity that go beyond strict obligation. In this document, beneficence is understood in a stronger sense, as an obligation. Two general rules have been formulated as complementary expressions of beneficent actions in this sense: (1) do not harm and (2) maximize possible benefits and minimize possible harms.

The Hippocratic maxim "do no harm" has long been a fundamental principle of medical ethics. Claude Bernard extended it to the realm of research, saying that one should not injure one person regardless of the benefits that might come to others. However, even avoiding harm requires learning what is harmful; and, in the process of obtaining this information, persons may be exposed to risk of harm. Further, the Hippocratic Oath requires physicians to benefit their patients "according to their best judgment." Learning what will in fact benefit may require exposing persons to risk. The problem posed by these imperatives is to decide when it is justifiable to seek certain benefits despite the risks involved, and when the benefits should be foregone because of the risks.

The obligations of beneficence affect both individual investigators and society at large, because they extend both to particular research projects and to the entire enterprise of research. In the case of particular projects, investigators and members of their institutions are obliged to give forethought to the maximization of benefits and the reduction of risk that might occur from the research investigation. In the case of scientific research in general, members of the larger society are obliged to recognize the longer term benefits and risks that may result from the improvement of knowledge and from the development of novel medical, psychotherapeutic, and social procedures.

The principle of beneficence often occupies a well-defined justifying role in many areas of research involving human subjects. An example is found in research involving children. Effective ways of treating childhood diseases and fostering healthy development are benefits that serve to justify research involving children—even when individual research subjects are not direct beneficiaries. Research also makes it possible to avoid the harm that may result from the application of previously accepted routine practices that on closer investigation turn out to be dangerous. But the role of the principle of beneficence is not always so unambiguous. A difficult ethical problem remains, for example, about research that presents more than minimal risk without immediate prospect of direct benefit to the children involved. Some have argued that such research is inadmissible, while others have pointed out that this limit would rule out much research promising great benefit to children in the future. Here again, as with all hard cases, the different claims covered by the principle of beneficence may come into conflict and force difficult choices.

3. Justice Who ought to receive the benefits of research and bear its burdens? This is a question of justice, in the sense of "fairness in distribution" or "what is deserved." An injustice occurs when some benefit to which a person is entitled is denied without good reason or when some burden is imposed unduly. Another way of conceiving the principle of justice is that equals ought to be treated equally. However, this statement requires explication. Who is equal and who is unequal? What considerations justify departure from equal distribution? Almost all commentators allow that distinctions based on experience, age, deprivation, competence, merit and position do sometimes constitute criteria justifying differential treatment for certain purposes. It is necessary, then, to explain in what respects people should be treated equally. There are several widely accepted formulations of just ways to distribute burdens and benefits. Each formulation mentions some relevant property on the basis of which burdens and benefits should be distributed. These formulations are (1) to each person an equal share, (2) to each person according to individual need, (3) to each person according to individual effort, (4) to each person according to societal contribution, and (5) to each person according to merit.

Questions of justice have long been associated with social practices such as punishment, taxation and political representation. Until recently these questions have not generally been associated with scientific research. However, they are foreshadowed even in the earliest reflections on the ethics of research involving human subjects. For example, during the 19th and early 20th centuries the burdens of serving as research subjects fell largely upon poor ward patients, while the benefits of improved medical care flowed primarily to private patients. Subsequently, the exploitation of unwilling prisoners as research subjects in Nazi concentration camps was condemned as a particularly flagrant injustice. In this country, in the 1940's the Tuskegee syphilis study used disadvantaged, rural black men to study the untreated course of a disease that is by no means confined to that population. These subjects were deprived of demonstrably effective treatment in order not to interrupt the project, long after such treatment became generally available.

Against this historical background, it can be seen how conceptions of justice are relevant to research involving human subjects. For example, the selection of research subjects needs to be scrutinized in order to determine whether some classes (e.g., welfare patients, particular racial and ethnic minorities, or persons confined to institutions) are being systematically selected simply because of their easy availability, their compromised position, or their manipulability, rather than for reasons directly related to the problem being studied. Finally, whenever research supported by public funds leads to the development of therapeutic devices and procedures, justice demands both that these not provide advantages only to those who can afford them and that such research should not unduly involve persons from groups unlikely to be among the beneficiaries of subsequent applications of the research.

PART C: APPLICATIONS

Applications of the general principles to the conduct of research leads to consideration of the following requirements: informed consent, risk/benefit assessment, and the selection of subjects of research.

1. Informed Consent Respect for persons requires that subjects, to the degree that they are capable, be given the opportunity to choose what shall or shall not happen to them. This opportunity is provided when adequate standards for informed consent are satisfied.

While the importance of informed consent is unquestioned, controversy prevails over the nature and possibility of an informed consent. Nonetheless, there is widespread agreement that the consent process can be analyzed as containing three elements: information, comprehension and voluntariness.

Information Most codes of research establish specific items for disclosure intended to assure that subjects are given sufficient information. These items generally include: the research procedure, their purposes, risks and anticipated benefits, alternative procedures (where therapy is involved), and a statement offering the subject the opportunity to ask questions and to withdraw at any time from the research. Additional items have been proposed, including how subjects are selected, the person responsible for the research, etc.

However, a simple listing of items does not answer the question of what the standard should be for judging how much and what sort of information should be provided. One standard frequently invoked in medical practice, namely the information commonly provided by practitioners in the field or in the locale, is inadequate since research takes place precisely when a common understanding does not exist. Another standard, currently popular in malpractice law, requires the practitioner to reveal the information that reasonable persons would wish to know in order to make a decision regarding their care. This, too, seems insufficient since the research subject, being in essence a volunteer, may wish to know considerably more about risks gratuitously undertaken than do patients who deliver themselves into the hand of a clinician for needed care. It may be that a standard of "the reasonable volunteer" should be proposed: the extent and nature of information should be such that persons, knowing that the procedure is neither necessary for their care nor perhaps fully understood, can decide whether they wish to participate in the furthering of knowledge. Even when some direct benefit to them is anticipated, the subjects should understand clearly the range of risk and the voluntary nature of participation.

A special problem of consent arises where informing subjects of some pertinent aspect of the research is likely to impair the validity of the research. In many cases, it is sufficient to indicate to subjects that they are being invited to participate in research of which some features will not be revealed until the research is concluded. In all cases of research involving incomplete disclosure, such research is justified only if it is clear that (1) incomplete disclosure is truly necessary to accomplish the goals of the research, (2) there are no undisclosed risks to subjects that are more than minimal, and (3) there is an adequate plan for debriefing subjects, when appropriate, and for dissemination of research results to them. Information about risks should never be withheld for the purpose of eliciting the cooperation of subjects, and truthful answers should always be given to direct questions about the research. Care should be taken to distinguish cases in which disclosure would destroy or invalidate the research from cases in which disclosure would simply convenience the investigator.

Comprehension The manner and context in which information is conveyed is as important as the information itself. For example, presenting information in a disorganized and rapid fashion, allowing too little time for consideration or curtailing opportunities for questioning, all may adversely affect a subject's ability to make an informed choice.

Because the subject's ability to understand is a function of intelligence, rationality, maturity and language, it is necessary to adapt the presentation of the information to the subject's capacities. Investigators are responsible for ascertaining that the subject has comprehended the information. While there is always an obligation to ascertain that the information about risk to subjects is complete and adequately comprehended, when the risks are more serious, that obligation increases. On occasion, it may be suitable to give some oral or written tests of comprehension.

Special provision may need to be made when comprehension is severely limited—for example, by conditions of immaturity or mental disability. Each class of subjects that one might consider as incompetent (e.g., infants and young children, mentally disabled patients, the terminally ill and the comatose) should be considered on its own terms. Even for these persons, however, respect requires giving them the opportunity to choose to the extent they are able, whether or not to participate in research. The objections of these subjects to involvement should be honored, unless the research entails providing them a therapy unavailable elsewhere. Respect for persons also requires seeking the permission of other parties in order to protect the subjects from harm. Such persons are thus respected both by acknowledging their own wishes and by the use of third parties to protect them from harm.

The third parties chosen should be those who are most likely to understand the incompetent subject's situation and to act in that person's best interest. The person authorized to act on behalf of the subject should be given an opportunity to observe the research as it proceeds in order to be able to withdraw the subject from the research, if such action appears in the subject's best interest.

Voluntariness An agreement to participate in research constitutes a valid consent only if voluntarily given. This element of informed consent requires conditions free of coercion and undue influence. Coercion occurs when an overt threat of harm is intentionally presented by one person to another in order to obtain compliance. Undue influence, by contrast, occurs through an offer of an excessive, unwarranted, inappropriate or improper reward or other overture in order to obtain compliance. Also, inducements that would ordinarily be acceptable may become undue influences if the subject is especially vulnerable.

Unjustifiable pressures usually occur when persons in positions of authority or commanding influence—especially where possible sanctions are involved—urge a course of action for a subject. A continuum of such influencing factors exists, however, and it is impossible to state precisely where justifiable persuasion ends and undue influence begins. But undue influence would include actions such as manipulating a person's choice through the controlling influence of a close relative and threatening to withdraw health services to which an individual would otherwise be entitled.

2. Assessment of Risks and Benefits The assessment of risks and benefits requires a careful arrayal of relevant data, including, in some cases, alternative ways of obtaining the benefits sought in the research. Thus, the assessment presents both an opportunity and a responsibility to gather systematic and comprehensive information about proposed research. For the investigator, it is a means to examine whether the proposed research is properly designed. For a review committee, it is a method for determining whether the risks that will be presented to subjects are justified. For prospective subjects, the assessment will assist the determination whether or not to participate.

The Nature and Scope of Risks and Benefits The requirement that research be justified on the basis of a favorable risk/benefit assessment bears a close relation to the principle of beneficence, just as the moral requirement that informed consent be obtained is derived primarily from the principle of respect for persons. The term "risk" refers to a possibility that harm may occur. However, when expressions such as "small risk" or "high risk" are used, they usually refer (often ambiguously) both to the chance (probability) of experiencing a harm and the severity (magnitude) of the envisioned harm.

The term "benefit" is used in the research context to refer to something of positive value related to health or welfare. Unlike, "risk," "benefit" is not a term that expresses probabilities. Risk is properly contrasted to probability of benefits, and benefits are properly contrasted with harms rather than risks of harm. Accordingly, so-called risk/benefit assessments are concerned with the probabilities and magnitudes of possible harm and anticipated benefits. Many kinds of possible harms and benefits need to be taken into account. There are, for example, risks of psychological harm, physical harm, legal harm, social harm and economic harm and the corresponding benefits. While the most likely types of harms to research subjects are those of psychological or physical pain or injury, other possible kinds should not be overlooked.

Risks and benefits of research may affect the individual subjects, the families of the individual subjects, and society at large (or special groups of subjects in society). Previous codes and federal regulations have required that risks to subjects be outweighed by the sum of both the anticipated benefit to the subject, if any, and the anticipated benefit to society in the form of knowledge to be gained from the research. In balancing these different elements, the risks and benefits affecting the immediate research subject will normally carry special weight. On the other hand, interests other than those of the subject may on some occasions be sufficient by themselves to justify the risks involved in the research, so long as the subjects' rights have been protected. Beneficence thus requires that we protect against risk of harm to subjects and also that we be concerned about the loss of the substantial benefits that might be gained from research.

The Systematic Assessment of Risks and Benefits It is commonly said that benefits and risks must be "balanced" and shown to be "in a favorable ratio." The metaphorical character of these terms draws attention to the difficulty of making precise judgments. Only on rare occasions will quantitative techniques be available for the scrutiny of research protocols. However, the idea of systematic, nonarbitrary analysis of risks and benefits should be emulated insofar as possible. This ideal requires those making decisions about the justifiability of research to be thorough in the accumulation and assessment of information about all aspects of the research, and to consider alternatives systematically. This procedure renders the assessment of research more rigorous and precise, while making communication between review board members and investigators less subject to misinterpretation, misinformation and conflicting judgments. Thus, there should first be a determination of the validity of the presuppositions of the research; then the nature, probability and magnitude of risk should be distinguished with as much clarity as possible. The method of ascertaining risks should be explicit, especially where there is no alternative to the use of such vague categories as small or slight risk. It should also be determined whether an investigator's estimates of the probability of harm or benefits are reasonable, as judged by known facts or other available studies.

Finally, assessment of the justifiability of research should reflect at least the following considerations: (i) Brutal or inhumane treatment of human subjects is never morally justified. (ii) Risks should be reduced to those necessary to achieve the research objective. It should be determined whether it is in fact necessary to use human subjects at all. Risk can perhaps never be entirely eliminated, but it can often be reduced by careful attention to alternative procedures. (iii) When research involves significant risk of serious impairment, review committees should be extraordinarily insistent on the justification of the risk (looking usually to the likelihood of benefit to the subject—or, in some rare cases, to the manifest voluntariness of the participation). (iv) When vulnerable populations are involved in research, the appropriateness of involving them should itself be demonstrated. A number of variables go into such judgments, including the nature and degree of risk, the condition of the particular population involved, and the nature and level of the anticipated benefits. (v) Relevant risks and benefits must be thoroughly arrayed in documents and procedures used in the informed consent process.

3. Selection of Subjects Just as the principle of respect for persons finds expression in the requirements for consent, and the principle of beneficence in risk/benefit assessment, the principle of justice gives rise to moral requirements that there be fair procedures and outcomes in the selection of research subjects.

Justice is relevant to the selection of subjects of research at two levels: the social and the individual. Individual justice in the selection of subjects would require that researchers exhibit fairness: thus, they should not offer potentially beneficial research only to some patients who are in their favor or select only "undesirable" persons for risky research. Social justice requires that distinction be drawn between classes of subjects that ought, and ought not, to participate in any particular kind of research, based on the ability of members of that class to bear burdens and on the appropriateness of placing further burdens on already burdened persons. Thus, it can be considered a matter of social justice that there is an order of preference in the selection of classes of subjects (e.g., adults before children) and that some classes of potential subjects (e.g., the institutionalized mentally infirm or prisoners) may be involved as research subjects, if at all, only on certain conditions.

Injustice may appear in the selection of subjects, even if individual subjects are selected fairly by investigators and treated fairly in the course of research. Thus injustice arises from social, racial, sexual and cultural biases institutionalized in society. Thus, even if individual researchers are treating their research subjects fairly, and even if IRBs are taking care to assure that subjects are selected fairly within a particular institution, unjust social patterns may nevertheless appear in the overall distribution of the burdens and benefits of research. Although individual institutions or investigators may not be able to resolve a problem that is pervasive in their social setting, they can consider distributive justice in selecting research subjects.

Some populations, especially institutionalized ones, are already burdened in many ways by their infirmities and environments. When research is proposed that involves risks and does not include a therapeutic component, other less burdened classes of persons should be called upon first to accept these risks of research, except where the research is directly related to the specific conditions of the class involved. Also, even though public funds for research may often flow in the same directions as public funds for health care, it seems unfair that populations dependent on public health care constitute a pool of preferred research subjects if more advantaged populations are likely to be the recipients of the benefits.

One special instance of injustice results from the involvement of vulnerable subjects. Certain groups, such as racial minorities, the economically disadvantaged, the very sick, and the institutionalized may continually be sought as research subjects, owing to their ready availability in settings where research is conducted. Given their dependent status and their frequently compromised capacity for free consent, they should be protected against the danger of being involved in research solely for administrative convenience, or because they are easy to manipulate as a result of their illness or socioeconomic condition.

NOTE

1. Although practice usually involves interventions designed solely to enhance the well-being of a particular individual, interventions are sometimes applied to one individual for the enhancement of the well-being of another (e.g., blood donation, skin grafts, organ transplants) or an intervention may have the dual purpose of enhancing the well-being of a particular individual, and, at the same time, providing some benefit to others (e.g., vaccination, which protects both the person who is vaccinated and society generally). The fact that some forms of practice have elements other than immediate benefit to the individual receiving an intervention, however, should not confuse the general distinction between research and practice. Even when a procedure applied in practice may benefit some other person, it remains an intervention designed to enhance the well-being of a particular individual or groups of individuals; thus, it is practice and need not be reviewed as research.

THE ETHICS OF RANDOMIZED CLINICAL TRIALS

ETHICAL DIFFICULTIES WITH RANDOMIZED CLINICAL TRIALS INVOLVING CANCER PATIENTS: EXAMPLES FROM THE FIELD OF GYNECOLOGIC ONCOLOGY

Maurie Markman

In a recent issue of the *New England Journal of Medicine*, two prominent clinical investigators took opposite sides in a debate on the need for and the ethics of randomized clinical trials.[1] The basic argument in support of randomized clinical trials is that in the absence of such studies it is not possible to be certain that a new drug or clinical intervention is actually beneficial to patients with a particular disease or condition, compared either to a "standard" (accepted or approved) therapeutic strategy or to no treatment at all (an untreated control population). The major argument against the performance of randomized clinical trials is that the individual physician's principal ethical responsibility is to the *individual patient* that he or she is treating, and *not* to future patients who may benefit from the potentially important information gained through a well-designed and well-conducted randomized trial. If one accepts this argument, a physician should only recommend that an individual patient participate in a randomized trial if he or she is convinced that neither one of the treatment programs is superior based on previous data available in the medical literature. If it is the *physician's best judgment*—based on his or her interpretation of this data, personal experience, and knowledge of the individual patient's specific medical condition—that one regimen would be preferred over the other(s), then the physician should not recommend that the patient participate in this trial, no matter how important the information gained may be to society.

Physicians working with cancer patients have frequently been able to avoid the difficult ethical dilemma presented above, as experimental (not FDA-approved) antineoplastic agents have traditionally

Journal of Clinical Ethics, 3, No. 3 (Fall 1992): 193–195.

only been available to patients who are willing to participate in a clinical trial. Drug development of new agents has followed a logical sequence: toxicity/dose finding studies (phase 1), followed by single-arm efficacy trials in specific disease settings (phase 2), followed by randomized trials to define the "true benefit" of the new therapy (phase 3). In the toxicity studies, the major goal of the treatment is to define the appropriate dose that produces acceptable toxicity, while in the efficacy studies, the aim is to determine if the agent is effective in a particular disease setting. Thus, the physician who believes, based on previously reported clinical data (usually from phase-2 drug trials), that a new drug is potentially superior to the standard therapy would have no choice but to recommend that the patient participate in the trial. In this way, the patient would have a 50 percent chance of receiving the new therapy (and a 50 percent chance of being placed in the control group), compared to a 0 percent chance if he or she does not participate in the study.

We are currently witnessing this process with the new antineoplastic agent, taxol. The drug, which has a unique mechanism of cytotoxic activity, has recently been demonstrated to cause temporary regression of tumor in approximately 20 to 30 percent of patients with advanced ovarian cancer who have previously failed standard therapy for their disease.[2] At the present time, there is absolutely no evidence that the drug is curative when used in the advanced refractory disease setting, and most responses last less than six to nine months. However, the response rate observed in this particular patient population is superior to what has been demonstrated with other commercially available drugs.

Interest in, and praise for, the effectiveness of taxol has spread far beyond the confines of medical meetings and the peer-reviewed medical literature. This is partly due to the fact that the agent is a natural product, and obtaining sufficient quantities of the drug requires the sacrifice of a large number of endangered trees in the Pacific Northwest. A number of scientists and biomedical companies, as well as the National Cancer Institute, are actively seeking to find new sources of taxol so as to make the drug more widely available to patients with ovarian cancer and other malignancies.

Currently, the Gynecologic Oncology Group, a national multi-institutional cooperative group devoted to the study of cancers involving gynecologic organs, is conducting a randomized trial of a standard chemotherapy regimen (without taxol) compared to a program that includes taxol, in patients with ovarian cancer who have not previously received chemotherapy. This is an important trial, as it should determine what role, if any, taxol should play in the initial management of a patient with advanced ovarian cancer.

A physician hoping to give a patient taxol, in the belief that a regimen that includes this drug may be superior to the current standard regimen, would have to attempt to enter the patient into this randomized trial. But what if the drug, still considered an experimental agent, were made more widely available from the National Cancer Institute? Would a physician who wanted a woman with ovarian cancer to receive taxol be justified in placing the individual on a randomized trial when there were other methods to obtain the drug without randomization? Or, as is frequently asked of cancer specialists when they discuss treatment options with patients, would they recommend this trial to their wife, sister, or mother? This question, perhaps the most difficult one addressed to oncologists concerning experimental clinical trials, gets to the fundamental core of the issue: Is the physician acting *solely* in the best interest of the patient, or are other considerations (such as the scientific or societal need to know whether one treatment program is superior) playing a role in the doctor's deliberations?

A second example of the physician's dilemma over whether to recommend that a patient participate in a randomized trial—one that is more complex, as it does not involve the use of experimental drugs whose access can be controlled—concerns the current status of chemotherapy for advanced metastatic cancer of the uterus (endometrial cancer). Unfortunately, chemotherapy has only demonstrated limited activity in this disease, with partial responses of short durations being observed in approximately 20 percent of treated patients.

Recently, clinical investigators at the Mayo Clinic reported the results of a nonrandomized trial of a combination chemotherapy regimen in twenty-five patients with advanced cancer of the uterus that employed four commercially available cytotoxic agents.[3] The investigators observed a 60 percent objective response rate, and the authors of the report concluded that the regimen "is highly active in advanced endometrial carcinoma and results in improved survival compared to literature controls."[4] The Mayo Clinic investigators are noted for the quality of their work. In addition, they are generally conservative in the interpretation of their own data. Thus, the results of this trial are quite interesting and encouraging. However, this was a nonrandomized trial, and it is possible that unintentional selection bias may have accounted for the results observed. The only method available to determine definitively if the more toxic, multidrug combination regimen is superior in efficacy to a standard single-agent program would be to conduct a randomized clinical trial.

One can be fairly certain that a randomized trial comparing these two treatment programs will be forthcoming. Should patients be entered into such a trial? Again, the ethical issue for the individual physician comes down to how he or she interprets the results of this investigative program compared to a standard chemotherapy regimen in cancer of the uterus. If the physician cannot accept the results as providing reasonable evidence for superiority of the newer regimen over standard therapy, then he or she is justified in entering patients into such a trial. But if the physician believes that the results suggest increased efficacy with acceptable toxicity, it is difficult to agree with the argument that the physician is acting in the *patient's* best interest if he recommends entry into the randomized trial. The question must be asked again: If this were your wife, mother, or sister, what would you recommend?

A final example illustrates the potential for serious ethical conflict between the importance of obtaining information to define management options for future patients with malignancy, and the critical need to safeguard the patient's best interest. Standard treatment of patients with advanced cancer of the ovary involves an attempt to remove surgically as much tumor as possible from the abdominal cavity (tumor "debulking") prior to the institution of chemotherapy.[5] This is a unique management strategy. In almost all other malignancies, surgery is employed in the initial management of the disease only when it is believed possible that all macroscopic tumor can be removed. However, in patients with ovarian cancer, this surgery is a standard management strategy, even though physicians know that the approach cannot cure patients with disease disseminated throughout the abdominal cavity. What, then, is the justification for this therapeutic strategy?

Multiple retrospective and prospective studies have demonstrated that patients with ovarian cancer who start chemotherapy after surgical resection with small-volume residual disease respond better to the chemotherapy and survive longer than patients with large-volume residual disease.[6] This has led to the conclusion that the surgical removal of tumor increases the effectiveness of chemotherapy, presumably resulting from improved blood supply and delivery of the cytotoxic drug to the remaining tumor, or removal of a large portion of cells that may be resistant to the effects of the anticancer agents. However, this hypothesis has *never* been tested in a randomized trial. It is certainly possible that the surgeon's ability to remove bulky intra-abdominal tumor and leave the patient with small-volume residual disease may simply select patients who would have done well with chemotherapy even if surgery were not performed. Perhaps the factors that permit invasiveness and interfere with a surgeon's ability to debulk tumor are the same factors that lead to a tumor having an enhanced ability to develop drug-resistant cells rapidly and escape the effects of the antineoplastic agents.

Thus, the only way to answer this important biological and clinical question would be to randomize women with ovarian cancer *who would otherwise be able to undergo debulking surgery* either to have the procedure performed or to start the treatment program with chemotherapy but without surgery. In this way, the role of a major surgical procedure could be evaluated definitively. Unfortunately, the conduct of such a trial leads to serious ethical difficulties. A woman who is randomized to debulking surgery, followed by chemotherapy, will be receiving standard therapy, and her ultimate clinical outcome will be unaffected by the conduct of the trial. However, a woman randomized to receive chemotherapy without surgery cannot be given such a guarantee. While that patient may experience less morbidity by not undergoing the debulking surgery, there is no reason to believe her ultimate outcome will be favorably influenced by participating in this trial. And if it is subsequently determined that surgery does, in fact, play an important role in the management of this condition, *her* survival may have been compromised by participating in the study. Clinical science may have benefited greatly from the conduct of this study, but individual patients may have paid dearly for their participation. Thus, unless another method can be found to address the question of the role of debulking surgery in patients with cancer of the ovary, this procedure must remain a major part of the management of individuals with the disease.

In this article, I have attempted to present examples of the ethical difficulties with randomized clinical trials experienced by physicians caring for real patients with malignant disease. Above all, the physician's responsibility is to the individual patient, and the need to increase knowledge to improve the lot of future patients must always take second place.

NOTES

1. S. Hellman and D. Hellman, "Of Mice but Not Men: Problems of the Randomized Clinical Trial," *New England Journal of Medicine* 324 (1991): 1585–89; E. Passamani, "Clinical Trials: Are They Ethical?" *New England Journal of Medicine* 324 (1991): 1589–92.
2. W.P. McGuire, E.K. Rowinsky, N.B. Rosenshein, *et al.*, "Taxol: A Unique Antineoplastic Agent with Significant Activity in Advanced Ovarian Epithelial Neoplasms," Annals of Internal Medicine 111 (1989): 273–79.
3. H.J. Long, R.M. Langdon, and H.S. Wieand, "Phase II Trial of Methotrexate, Vinblastine, Doxorubicin, and Cisplatin in Women with Advanced Endometrial Carcinoma," *Proceedings of the American Society of Clinical Oncology* 10 (1991): 184.
4. *Ibid.*
5. R.C. Young, Z. Fuks, and W.J. Hoskins, "Cancer of the Ovary," in *Cancer: Principles and Practice of Oncology*, ed. V.T. DeVita, Jr., S. Hellman, and S.A. Rosenberg (Philadelphia: J.B. Lippincott, 1989), 1162–96.
6. *Ibid.*

OF MICE BUT NOT MEN: PROBLEMS OF THE RANDOMIZED CLINICAL TRIAL

Samuel Hellman and Deborah S. Hellman

As medicine has become increasingly scientific and less accepting of unsupported opinion or proof by anecdote, the randomized controlled clinical trial has become the standard technique for changing diagnostic or therapeutic methods. The use of this technique creates an ethical dilemma.[1,2] Researchers participating in such studies are required to modify their ethical commitments to individual patients and do serious damage to the concept of the physician as a practicing, empathetic professional who is primarily concerned with each patient as an individual. Researchers using a randomized clinical trial can be described as physician-scientists, a term that expresses the tension between the two roles. The physician, by entering into a relationship with an individual patient, assumes certain obligations, including the commitment always to act in the patient's best interests. As Leon Kass has rightly maintained, "the physician must produce unswervingly the virtues of loyalty and fidelity to his patient."[3] Though the ethical requirements of this relationship have been modified by legal obligations to report wounds of a suspicious nature and certain

---

New England Journal of Medicine 324, No. 22, May 30, 1991: 1589–1592.

infectious diseases, these obligations in no way conflict with the central ethical obligation to act in the best interests of the patient medically. Instead, certain nonmedical interests of the patient are preempted by other social concerns.

The role of the scientist is quite different. The clinical scientist is concerned with answering questions—i.e., determining the validity of formally constructed hypotheses. Such scientific information, it is presumed, will benefit humanity in general. The clinical scientist's role has been well described by Dr. Anthony Fauci, director of the National Institute of Allergy and Infectious Diseases, who states the goals of the randomized clinical trial in these words: "It's not to deliver therapy. It's to answer a scientific question so that the drug can be available for everybody once you've established safety and efficacy."[4] The demands of such a study can conflict in a number of ways with the physician's duty to minister to patients. The study may create a false dichotomy in the physician's opinions; according to the premise of the randomized clinical trial, the physician may only know or not know whether a proposed course of treatment represents an improvement; no middle position is permitted. What the physician thinks, suspects, believes, or has a hunch about is assigned to the "not knowing" category, because knowing is defined on the basis of an arbitrary but accepted statistical test performed in a randomized clinical trial. Thus, little credence is given to information gained beforehand in other ways or to information accrued during the trial but without the required statistical degree of assurance that a difference is not due to chance. The randomized clinical trial also prevents the treatment technique from being modified on the basis of the growing knowledge of the physicians during their participation in the trial. Moreover, it limits access to the data as they are collected until specific milestones are achieved. This prevents physicians from profiting not only from their individual experience, but also from the collective experience of the other participants.

The randomized clinical trial requires doctors to act simultaneously as physicians and as scientists. This puts them in a difficult and sometimes untenable ethical position. The conflicting moral demands arising from the use of the randomized clinical trial reflect the classic conflict between rights-based moral theories and utilitarian ones. The first of these, which depend on the moral theory of Immanuel Kant (and seen more recently in neo-Kantian philosophers, such as John Rawls[5]), asserts that human beings, by virtue of their unique capacity for rational thought, are bearers of dignity. As such, they ought not to be treated merely as means to an end; rather, they must always be treated as ends in themselves. Utilitarianism, by contrast, defines what is right as the greatest good for the greatest number—that is, as social utility. This view, articulated by Jeremy Bentham and John Stuart Mill, requires that pleasures (understood broadly, to include such pleasures as health and well-being) and pains be added together. The morally correct act is the act that produces the most pleasure and the least pain overall.

A classic objection to the utilitarian position is that according to that theory, the distribution of pleasures and pains is of no moral consequence. This element of the theory severely restricts physicians from being utilitarians, or at least from following the theory's dictates. Physicians must care very deeply about the distribution of pain and pleasure, for they have entered into a relationship with one or a number of individual patients. They cannot be indifferent to whether it is these patients or others that suffer for the general benefit of society. Even though society might gain from the suffering of a few, and even though the doctor might believe that such a benefit is worth a given patient's suffering (i.e., that utilitarianism is right in the particular case), the ethical obligation created by the covenant between doctor and patient requires the doctor to see the interests of the individual patient as primary and compelling. In essence, the doctor-patient relationship requires doctors to see their patients as bearers of rights who cannot be merely used for the greater good of humanity.

As Fauci has suggested,[4] the randomized clinical trial routinely asks physicians to sacrifice the interests of their particular patients for the sake of the study and that of the information that it will make available for the benefit of society. This practice is ethically problematic. Consider first the initial formulation of a trial. In particular, consider the case of a disease for which there is no satisfactory therapy—for example, advanced cancer or the acquired immunodeficiency syndrome (AIDS). A new agent that promises more effectiveness is the subject of the study. The control group must be given either an unsatisfactory treatment or a placebo. Even though the therapeutic value of the new agent is unproved, if physicians think that it has promise, are they acting in the best interests of their patients in allowing them to be randomly assigned to the control group? Is persisting in such an assignment consistent with the specific commitments taken on in the doctor-patient relationship? As a result of interactions with patients with AIDS and their advocates, Merigan[6] recently suggested modifications in the design of clinical trials that attempt to deal with the unsatisfactory treatment given to the control group. The view of such activists has been expressed by Rebecca Pringle Smith of Community Research Initiative in New York: "Even if you have a supply of compliant martyrs, trials must have some ethical validity."[4]

If the physician has no opinion about whether the new treatment is acceptable, then random assignment is ethically acceptable, but such lack of enthusiasm for the new treatment does not augur well for either the patient or the study. Alternatively, the treatment may show promise of beneficial results but also present a risk of undesirable complications. When the physician believes that the severity and likelihood of harm and good are evenly balanced, randomization may be ethically acceptable. If the physician has no preference for either treatment (is in a state of equipoise[7,8]), then randomization is acceptable. If, however, he or she believes that the new treatment may be either more or less successful or more or less toxic, the use of randomization is not consistent with fidelity to the patient.

The argument usually used to justify randomization is that it provides, in essence, a critique of the usefulness of the physician's beliefs and opinions, those that have not yet been validated by a randomized clinical trial. As the argument goes, these not-yet-validated beliefs are as likely to be wrong as right. Although physicians are ethically required to provide their patients with the best available treatment, there simply is no best treatment yet known.

The reply to this argument takes two forms. First, and most important, even if this view of the reliability of a physician's opinions is accurate, the ethical constraints of an individual doctor's relationship with a particular patient require the doctor to provide individual care. Although physicians must take pains to make clear the speculative nature of their views, they cannot withhold these views from the patient. The patient asks from the doctor both knowledge and judgment. The relationship established between them rightfully allows patients to ask for the judgment of their particular physicians, not merely that of the medical profession in general. Second, it may not be true, in fact, that the not-yet-validated beliefs of physicians are as likely to be wrong as right. The greater certainty obtained with a randomized clinical trial is beneficial, but that does not mean that a lesser degree of certainty is without value. Physicians can acquire knowledge through methods other than the randomized clinical trial. Such knowledge, acquired over time and less formally than is required in a randomized clinical trial, may be of great value to a patient.

Even if it is ethically acceptable to begin a study, one often forms an opinion during its course—especially in studies that are impossible to conduct in a truly double-blinded fashion—that makes it ethically problematic to continue. The inability to remain blinded usually occurs in studies of cancer or AIDS, for example, because the therapy is associated by nature with serious side effects. Trials attempt to restrict the physician's access to the data in order to prevent such unblinding. Such restrictions should make physicians eschew the trial, since their ability to act in the patient's best interests will be limited. Even supporters of randomized clinical trials, such as Merigan, agree that interim findings should be presented to patients to ensure that no one receives what seems an inferior treatment.[6] Once physicians have formed a view about the new treatment, can they continue randomization? If random assignment is stopped, the study may be lost and the participation of the previous patients wasted. However, if physicians continue the randomization when they have a definite opinion about the efficacy of the experimental drug, they are not acting in accordance with the requirements of the doctor-patient relationship. Furthermore, as their opinion becomes more firm, stopping the randomization may not be enough. Physicians may be ethically required to treat the patients formerly placed in the control group with the therapy that now seems probably effective. To do so would be

What if...

faithful to the obligations created by the doctor-patient relationship, but it would destroy the study.

To resolve this dilemma, one might suggest that the patient has abrogated the rights implicit in a doctor-patient relationship by signing an informed-consent form. We argue that such rights cannot be waived or abrogated. They are inalienable. The right to be treated as an individual deserving the physician's best judgment and care, rather than to be used as a means to determine the best treatment for others, is inherent in every person. This right, based on the concept of dignity, cannot be waived. What of altruism, then? Is it not the patient's right to make a sacrifice for the general good? This question must be considered from both positions—that of the patient and that of the physician. Although patients may decide to waive this right, it is not consistent with the role of a physician to ask that they do so. In asking, the doctor acts as a scientist instead. The physician's role here is to propose what he or she believes is best medically for the specific patient, not to suggest participation in a study from which the patient cannot gain. Because the opportunity to help future patients is of potential value to a patient, some would say physicians should not deny it. Although this point has merit, it offers so many opportunities for abuse that we are extremely uncomfortable about accepting it. The responsibilities of physicians are much clearer; they are to minister to the current patient.

Moreover, even if patients could waive this right, it is questionable whether those with terminal illness would be truly able to give voluntary informed consent. Such patients are extremely dependent on both their physicians and the health care system. Aware of this dependence, physicians must not ask for consent, for in such cases the very asking breaches the doctor-patient relationship. Anxious to please their physicians, patients may have difficulty refusing to participate in the trial the physicians describe. The patients may perceive their refusal as damaging to the relationship, whether or not it is so. Such perceptions of coercion affect the decision. Informed-consent forms are difficult to understand, especially for patients under the stress of serious illness for which there is no satisfactory treatment. The forms are usually lengthy, somewhat legalistic, complicated, and confusing, and they hardly bespeak the compassion expected of the medical profession. It is important to remember that those who have studied the doctor-patient relationship have emphasized its empathetic nature.

> [The] relationship between doctor and patient partakes of a peculiar intimacy. It presupposes on the part of the physician not only knowledge of his fellow men but sympathy. . . . This aspect of the practice of medicine has been designated as the art; yet I wonder whether it should not, most properly, be called the essence.[9]

How is such a view of the relationship consonant with random assignment and informed consent? The Physician's Oath of the World Medical Association affirms the primacy of the deontologic view of patients' rights: "Concern for the interests of the subject must always prevail over the interests of science and society."[10]

Issue

Furthermore, a single study is often not considered sufficient. Before a new form of therapy is generally accepted, confirmatory trials must be conducted. How can one conduct such trials ethically unless one is convinced that the first trial was in error? The ethical problems we have discussed are only exacerbated when a completed randomized clinical trial indicates that a given treatment is preferable. Even if the physician believes the initial trial was in error, the physician must indicate to the patient the full results of that trial.

3rd?

The most common reply to the ethical arguments has been that the alternative is to return to the physician's intuition, to anecdotes, or to both as the basis of medical opinion. We all accept the dangers of such a practice. The argument states that we must therefore accept randomized, controlled clinical trials regardless of their ethical problems because of the great social benefit they make possible, and we salve our conscience with the knowledge that informed consent has been given. This returns us to the conflict between patients' rights and social utility. Some would argue that this tension can be resolved by placing a relative value on each. If the patient's right that is being compromised is not a fundamental right and the social gain is very great, then the study might be justified. When the right is fundamental, however, no amount of social gain, or almost none, will justify its sacrifice. Consider, for example, the experiments on humans done by physicians under the Nazi regime. All would agree that these are unacceptable regardless of the value

As well

of the scientific information gained. Some people go so far as to say that no use should be made of the results of those experiments because of the clearly unethical manner in which the data were collected. This extreme example may not seem relevant, but we believe that in its hyperbole it clarifies the fallacy of a utilitarian approach to the physician's relationship with the patient. To consider the utilitarian gain is consistent neither with the physician's role nor with the patient's rights.

It is fallacious to suggest that only the randomized clinical trial can provide valid information or that all information acquired by this technique is valid. Such experimental methods are intended to reduce error and bias and therefore reduce the uncertainty of the result. Uncertainty cannot be eliminated, however. The scientific method is based on increasing probabilities and increasingly refined approximations of truth.[11] Although the randomized clinical trial contributes to these ends, it is neither unique nor perfect. Other techniques may also be useful.[12]

Randomized trials often place physicians in the ethically intolerable position of choosing between the good of the patient and that of society. We urge that such situations be avoided and that other techniques of acquiring clinical information be adopted. For example, concerning trials of treatments for AIDS, Byar et al.[13] have said that "some traditional approaches to the clinical-trials process may be unnecessarily rigid and unsuitable for this disease." In this case, AIDS is not what is so different; rather, the difference is in the presence of AIDS activists, articulate spokespersons for the ethical problems created by the application of the randomized clinical trial to terminal illnesses. Such arguments are equally applicable to advanced cancer and other serious illnesses. Byar et al. agree that there are even circumstances in which uncontrolled clinical trials may be justified: when there is no effective treatment to use as a control, when the prognosis is uniformly poor, and when there is a reasonable expectation of benefit without excessive toxicity. These conditions are usually found in clinical trials of advanced cancer.

The purpose of the randomized clinical trial is to avoid the problems of observer bias and patient selection. It seems to us that techniques might be developed to deal with these issues in other ways. Randomized clinical trials deal with them in a cumbersome and heavy-handed manner, by requiring large numbers of patients in the hope that random assignment will balance the heterogeneous distribution of patients into the different groups. By observing known characteristics of patients, such as age and sex, and distributing them equally between groups, it is thought that unknown factors important in determining outcomes will also be distributed equally. Surely, other techniques can be developed to deal with both observer bias and patient selection. Prospective studies without randomization, but with the evaluation of patients by uninvolved third parties, should remove observer bias. Similar methods have been suggested by Royall.[12] Prospective matched-pair analysis, in which patients are treated in a manner consistent with their physician's views, ought to help ensure equivalence between the groups and thus mitigate the effect of patient selection, at least with regard to known covariates. With regard to unknown covariates, the security would rest, as in randomized trials, in the enrollment of large numbers of patients and in confirmatory studies. This method would not pose ethical difficulties, since patients would receive the treatment recommended by their physician. They would be included in the study by independent observers matching patients with respect to known characteristics, a process that would not affect patient care and that could be performed independently any number of times.

This brief discussion of alternatives to randomized clinical trials is sketchy and incomplete. We wish only to point out that there may be satisfactory alternatives, not to describe and evaluate them completely. Even if randomized clinical trials were much better than any alternative, however, the ethical dilemmas they present may put their use at variance with the primary obligations of the physician. In this regard, Angell cautions, "If this commitment to the patient is attenuated, even for so good a cause as benefits to future patients, the implicit assumptions of the doctor-patient relationship are violated."[14] The risk of such attenuation by the randomized trial is great. The AIDS activists have brought this dramatically to the attention of the academic medical community. Techniques appropriate to the laboratory may not be applicable to humans. We must develop and use alternative methods for acquiring clinical knowledge.

NOTES

1. Hellman S. Randomized clinical trials and the doctor-patient relationship: an ethical dilemma. *Cancer Clin Trials* 1979; 2:189–93.
2. *Idem*. A doctor's dilemma: the doctor-patient relationship in clinical investigation. In: Proceedings of the Fourth National Conference on Human Values and Cancer, New York, March 15–17, 1984. New York: American Cancer Society, 1984:144–6.
3. Kass LR. *Toward a more natural science: biology and human affairs*. New York: Free Press, 1985:196.
4. Palca J. AIDS drug trials enter new age. *Science* 1989; 246:19–21.
5. Rawls J. *A theory of justice.* Cambridge, Mass.: Belknap Press of Harvard University Press, 1971:183–92, 446–52.
6. Merigan TC. You *can* teach an old dog new tricks—how AIDS trials are pioneering new strategies. *N Engl J Med* 1990; 323: 1341–3.
7. Freedman B. Equipoise and the ethics of clinical research. *N Engl J Med* 1987; 317:141–5.
8. Singer PA, Lantos JD, Whitington PF, Broelsch CE, Siegler M. Equipoise and the ethics of segmental liver transplantation. *Clin Res* 1988; 36:539–45.
9. Longcope WT. Methods and medicine. *Bull Johns Hopkins Hosp* 1932; 50:4–20.
10. Report on medical ethics. *World Med Assoc Bull* 1949; 1:109, 111.
11. Popper K. The problem of induction. In: Miller D, ed., *Popper selections*. Princeton, N.J.: Princeton University Press, 1985: 101–17.
12. Royall RM. Ethics and statistics in randomized clinical trials. *Stat Sci* 1991; 6(1):52–62.
13. Byar DP, Schoenfeld DA, Green SB, et al. Design considerations for AIDS trials. *N Engl J Med* 1990; 323: 1343–8.
14. Angell M. Patients' preferences in randomized clinical trials. *N Engl J Med* 1984; 310:1385–7.

A RESPONSE TO A PURPORTED ETHICAL DIFFICULTY WITH RANDOMIZED CLINICAL TRIALS INVOLVING CANCER PATIENTS

Benjamin Freedman

In recent years, for a variety of reasons, the mainstay of clinical investigation—the randomized controlled clinical trial (RCT)—has increasingly come under attack. Since Charles Fried's influential monograph,[1] the opponents of controlled trials have claimed the moral high ground. They claim to perceive a conflict between the medical and scientific duties of the physician-investigator, and between the conduct of the trial and a patient's rights. Samuel and Deborah Hellman write, for example, that "the randomized clinical trial routinely asks physicians to sacrifice the interests of their particular patients for the sake of the study and that of the information that it will make available for the benefit of society."[2] Maurie Markman's attraction to this point of view is clear when he writes that "the individual physician's principal ethical responsibility is to the *individual patient* that he or she is treating, and *not* to future patients [emphases in original]." In the interests of returning Markman to the fold, I will concentrate on resolving this central challenge to the ethics of RCTs.

Journal of Clinical Ethics 3, No. 3, Fall 1992: 231–234.

It is unfortunately true that the most common responses from pro-trialists, by revealing fundamental misunderstandings of basic ethical concepts, do not inspire confidence in the ethics of human research as it is currently conducted. Proponents of clinical trials will commonly begin their apologia by citing benefits derived from trials—by validating the safety and efficacy of new treatments, and, at least as important, by discrediting accepted forms of treatment. So far so good. But they often go on to argue that there is a need to balance the rights of subjects against the needs of society. By this tactic, the proponents of clinical trials have implicitly morally surrendered, for to admit that something is a right is to admit that it represents a domain of action protected from the claims or interests of other individuals or of society itself. A liberal society has rightly learned to look askance at claims that rights of individuals need to yield to the demands of the collective. Patients' claims, then, because of their nature as rights, supersede the requirements of the collectivity.

Sometimes, indeed, the surrender is explicit. At the conclusion of a symposium on the ethics of research on human subjects, Sir Colin Dollery, a major figure in clinical trials, complained to the speaker: "You assume a dominant role for ethics—I think to the point of arrogance. Ethical judgments will be of little value unless the scientific innovations about which they are made . . . are useful."[3] But it is the nature of ethical judgments that they are, indeed, "dominant" as normative or accepted guides to action. One may say, "I know that *X* is the ethical thing to do, but I won't *X*." That expresses no logical contradiction, but simply weakness of will. But it is, by contrast, plainly contradictory to admit that *X* is ethical, yet to deny or doubt that one ought to *X*.

Closer examination and finer distinctions reveal, however, that the conflict between patients' rights and social interests is not at all at issue in controlled clinical trials. There is no need for proponents of clinical trials to concede the moral high ground.

What is the patient right that is compromised by clinical trials? The fear most common to patients who are hesitant about enrolling is that they would not receive the best care, that their right to treatment would be sacrificed in the interests of science. This presumes, of course, that the patient has a right to treatment. Such a right must in reason be grounded in patient need (a patient who is not ill has no right to treatment) and in medical knowledge and capability (a patient with an incurable illness has rights to be cared for, but no right to be cured).

That granted, we need to specify the kind of treatment to which a patient might reasonably claim a right. It was in this connection that I introduced the concept of *clinical equipoise* as critical to understanding the ethics of clinical trials.[4] Clinical equipoise is a situation in which there exists (or is pending) an honest disagreement in the expert clinical community regarding the comparative merits of two or more forms of treatment for a given condition. To be ethical, a controlled clinical trial must begin and be conducted in a continuing state of clinical equipoise—as between the arms of the study—and must, moreover, offer some reasonable hope that the successful conclusion of the trial will disturb equipoise (that is, resolve the controversy in the expert clinical community).

This theory presumes that a right to a specific medical treatment must be grounded in a professional judgment, which is concretized in the term *clinical equipoise*. A patient who has rights to medical treatment has rights restricted to, though not necessarily exhaustive of, those treatments that are understood by the medical community to be appropriate for his condition. A patient may eccentrically claim some good from a physician that is not recognized by the medical community as appropriate treatment. A physician may even grant this claim; but in so doing, he must realize that he has not provided medical treatment itself. Contrariwise, by failing to fulfill this request, the physician has not failed to satisfy the patient's right to medical treatment.

Provided that a comparative trial is ethical, therefore, it begins in a state of clinical equipoise. For that reason, by definition, nobody enrolling in the trial is denied his or her right to medical treatment, for no medical consensus for or against the treatment assignment exists.

(The modern climate requires that I introduce two simple caveats. First, I am ignoring economic and political factors that go into the grounding of a right to treatment. This is easy enough for one in Canada to write, but may be difficult for someone in the United States to read. Second, when speaking of treatment that is recognized to be condition-appropriate by the medical community, I mean to include only those judgments grounded in medical knowledge rather than social judgments. I would hope to avoid the current bioethical muddle over "medical futility," but if my claims need to be translated into terms appropriate to that controversy, "physiological futility" is close but not identical to what I mean by "inappropriate." For simplicity's sake, the best model to have in mind is the common patient demand for antibiotic treatment of an illness diagnosed as viral.)

Two errors are commonly committed in connection with the concept of clinical equipoise. The first mistake is in thinking that clinical equipoise (or its disturbance) relates to a single endpoint of a trial—commonly, efficacy. As a function of expert clinical judgment, clinical equipoise must incorporate all of the many factors that go into favoring one regimen over its competitors. Treatment *A* may be favored over *B* because it is more effective; or, because it is almost as effective but considerably less toxic; or, because it is easier to administer, allowing, for example, treatment on an outpatient basis; or, because patients are more compliant with it; and so forth.

Just as equipoise may be based upon any one or a combination of these or other factors, it may be disturbed in the same way. Markman's second example, which discusses the efficacy of a multidrug combination chemotherapy regimen, seems vulnerable to this objection. Even were the results of the Mayo trial convincing with regard to the efficacy of this approach, it has not disturbed clinical equipoise in its favor unless other issues, such as toxicity, have been resolved as well. It is well worth pointing out that the endpoints of trials, particularly in cancer treatment, are far too narrow to disturb clinical equipoise in and of themselves, but they are necessary steps along a seriatim path. For that matter, in ignoring the compendious judgment involved in ascertaining equipoise, some studies spuriously claim that all of their arms are in equipoise on the basis of one variable (such as five-year survival rates), when they are clearly out of equipoise because of other factors (such as differences in pain and disfigurement).

The second mistake occurs in identifying clinical equipoise with an individual physician's point of indifference between two treatments. Citing the article in which I developed the concept and another article applying it, for example, the Hellmans write, "If the physician has no preference for either treatment (is in a state of equipoise), then randomization is acceptable."[5] But an individual physician is not the arbiter of appropriate or acceptable medical practice.

There are numerous occasions outside of clinical trials where outsiders need to determine whether the treatment provided was appropriate to the patient's condition. Regulators, as well as third-party payers—private or governmental—need to answer the question, as do health planners and administrators of health-care facilities. Disciplinary bodies of professional associations, and, most tellingly, courts judging allegations of malpractice, have to ascertain this as well. It is never the case that the judgment of an individual physician concerning whether a treatment is condition-appropriate (that is, whether it belongs within the therapeutic armamentarium) is sufficient. In all of these instances, however varied might be their rules of investigation and procedure, the ultimate question is: Does the expert professional community accept this treatment as appropriate for this condition? Since clinical equipoise and its disturbance applies to putative medical treatments for given conditions, this is a matter that is determined legally, morally, and reasonably by that medical community with the recognized relevant expertise.

Markman may have fallen into this error, writing repeatedly of the judgment of the treating or enrolling physician (and, in the first page, of the responsibility of "the individual physician") with respect to the clinical trial. There is, however, another way of looking at this. Whereas the status of a putative treatment within the medical armamentarium must be settled by the medical *community*, the application of that judgment *vis-à-vis* a given patient is, of course, the judgment (and the responsibility) of the *individual physician*. This individual clinical judgment must be exercised when enrolling a subject, rather than subjugated to the judgment of those who constructed the trial. Indeed, many studies will list this as a criterion of exclusion: "Those subjects who, in the judgment of the accruing physician, would be put at undue risk by participating."

Another point: the Hellmans write of a physician's duty in treating a patient to employ what he "thinks, suspects, believes, or has a hunch about."[6] This is clearly overstated as a duty: why not add to the list the physician's hopes, fantasies, fond but dotty beliefs, and illusions? Yet patients do choose physicians, in part, because of trust in their tacit knowledge and inchoate judgment, and not merely their sapient grasp of the current medical consensus. It would be a disservice to patients for a physician to see his or her role simply as a vehicle for transmitting the wisdom received from the expert medical community in all cases (though when a departure is made, this is done at the legal peril of the doctor!).

But what follows from this inalienable duty of the treating physician? Not as much as the opponents of trials would have us believe. A physician certainly has the right to refuse to participate in a trial that he believes places some participants at a medical disadvantage. Moreover, if he or she is convinced of that, he or she has a *duty* to abstain from participating. But that only speaks to the physician, and does not necessarily affect the patient. What opponents of trials forget is that the patient—the subject—is the ultimate decision maker—in fact, in law, and in ethics. In at least some cases, the fact that there is an open trial for which a patient meets the eligibility criteria needs to be disclosed as one medical alternative, to satisfy ethical norms of informed consent. A physician with convictions that the trial will put subjects at undue risk should inform the prospective subject of that conviction and the reasons for it, and may well recommend to the subject to decline participation. It will then be up to the patient whether to seek enrollment via another physician.

Most commonly at issue, though, is a physician's preference rather than conviction. In such cases, it is perfectly ethical—and becomingly modest—for a physician to participate in a trial, setting aside private misgivings based upon anecdote as overbalanced by the medical literature.

Finally, something should be said about the underlying philosophical buttress on which antitrialists rely. Following Kant, the Hellmans argue that the underlying issue is that persons "ought not to be treated merely as means to an end; rather, they must always be treated as ends in themselves."[7] Clinical trials, however, are designed to yield reliable data and to ground scientifically valid inferences. In that sense, the treatments and examinations that a subject of a clinical trial undergoes are means to a scientific end, rather than interventions done solely for the subject's own benefit.

But the Kantian formulation is notoriously rigoristic, and implausible in the form cited. We treat others as means all the time, in order to achieve ends the others do not share, and are so treated in return. When buying a carton of milk or leaving a message, I am treating the cashier or secretary as means to an end they do not share. Were this unvarnished principle to hold, all but purely altruistic transactions would be ethically deficient. Clinical trials would be in very good (and, indeed, very bad) company. Those who follow the Kantian view are not concerned about treating another as a means, but rather about treating someone in a way that contradicts the other's personhood itself—that is, in a way that denies the fact that the person is not simply a means but is also an end. A paradigm case is when I treat someone in a way that serves my ends but, at the same time, is contrary to the other's best interests. It is true that a subject's participation in a clinical trial serves scientific ends, but what has not been shown is that it is contrary to the best interests of the subject. In cases where the two equipoise conditions are satisfied, this cannot be shown.

However, in some cases we are uncertain about whether an intervention will serve the best interests of the other, and so we ask that person. That is one reason for requiring informed consent to studies. There is another. By obtaining the consent of the other party to treat him as an end to one's own means, in effect, an identity of ends between both parties has been created. Applying this amended Kantian dictum, then, we should ask: Is there anything about clinical trials that necessarily implies that subjects are treated contrary to their personhood? And the answer is, of course, no—provided a proper consent has been obtained.

There remain many hard questions to ask about the ethics of controlled clinical studies. Many talents will be needed to address those questions and to reform current practice. Since those questions will only be asked by those who understand that such studies rest upon a sound ethical foundation, I am hopeful that Markman and others will reconsider their misgivings.

NOTES

1. C. Fried, *Medical Experimentation: Personal Integrity and Social Policy* (New York: Elsevier, 1974).
2. S. Hellman and D.S. Hellman, "Of Mice but Not Men," *New England Journal of Medicine* 324 (1991): 1585–89, at 1586.
3. Comment by Sir Colin Dollery in discussion following H.-M. Sass, "Ethics of Drug Research and Drug Development," *Arzneimittel Forschung/Drug Research* 39 (II), Number 8a (1989): 1041–48, at 1048.
4. B. Freedman, "Equipoise and the Ethics of Clinical Research," *New England Journal of Medicine* 317 (1987): 141–45.
5. Hellman and Hellman, "Of Mice," 1586.
6. *Ibid.*
7. *Ibid.*

ETHICAL ISSUES IN INTERNATIONAL RESEARCH

UNETHICAL TRIALS OF INTERVENTIONS TO REDUCE PERINATAL TRANSMISSION OF THE HUMAN IMMUNODEFICIENCY VIRUS IN DEVELOPING COUNTRIES

Peter Lurie and Sidney M. Wolfe

It has been almost three years since the *Journal*[1] published the results of AIDS Clinical Trials Group (ACTG) Study 076, the first randomized, controlled trial in which an intervention was proved to reduce the incidence of human immunodeficiency virus (HIV) infection. The antiretroviral drug zidovudine, administered orally to HIV-positive pregnant women in the United States and France, administered to the newborn infants, reduced the incidence of HIV infection by two thirds.[2] The regimen can save the life of one of every seven infants born to HIV infected women.

Because of these findings, the study was terminated at the first interim analysis and within two months after the results had been announced, the Public Health Service had convened a meeting and concluded that the ACTG 076 regimen should be recommended for all HIV-positive pregnant women without substantial prior exposure to zidovudine and should be considered for other HIV-positive pregnant women on a case-by-case basis.[3] The standard of care for HIV-positive pregnant women thus became the ACTG 076 regimen.

In the United States, three recent studies of clinical practice report that the use of the ACTG 076 regimen is associated with decreases of 50 percent or more in perinatal HIV transmission.[4–6] But in developing countries, especially in Asia and sub-Saharan Africa, where it is projected that by the year 2000, 6 million pregnant women will be infected with HIV,[7] the potential of the ACTG 076 regimen remains unrealized primarily because of the drug's exorbitant cost in most countries.

New England Journal of Medicine 337, September 18, 1997, 853–856.

Clearly, a regimen that is less expensive than ACTG 076 but as effective is desirable, in both developing and industrialized countries. But there has been uncertainty about what research design to use in the search for a less expensive regimen. In June 1994, the World Health Organization (WHO) convened a group in Geneva to assess the agenda for research on perinatal HIV transmission in the wake of ACTG 076. The group, which included no ethicists, concluded, "Placebo-controlled trials offer the best option for a rapid and scientifically valid assessment of alternative antiretroviral drug regimens to prevent [perinatal] transmission of HIV.[8] This unpublished document has been widely cited as justification for subsequent trials in developing countries. In our view, most of these trials are unethical and will lead to hundreds of preventable HIV infections in infants.

Primarily on the basis of documents obtained from the Centers for Disease Control and Prevention (CDC), we have identified 18 randomized, controlled trials of interventions to prevent perinatal HIV transmission that either began to enroll patients after the ACTG 076 study was completed or have not yet begun to enroll patients. The studies are designed to evaluate a variety of interventions: antiretroviral drugs such as zidovudine (usually in regimens that are less expensive or complex than the ACTG 076 regimen), vitamin A and its derivatives, intrapartum vaginal washing, and HIV immune globulin, a form of immunotherapy. These trials involve a total of more than 17,000 women.

In the two studies being performed in the United States, the patients in all the study groups have unrestricted access to zidovudine or other antiretroviral drugs. In 15 of the 16 trials in developing countries, however, some or all of the patients are not provided with antiretroviral drugs. Nine of the 15 studies being conducted outside the United States are funded by the U.S. government through the CDC or the National Institutes of Health (NIH), 5 are funded by other governments, and 1 is funded by the United Nations AIDS Program. The studies are being conducted in Côte d'Ivoire, Uganda, Tanzania, South Africa, Malawi, Thailand, Ethiopia, Burkina Faso, Zimbabwe, Kenya, and the Dominican Republic. These 15 studies clearly violate recent guidelines designed specifically to address ethical issues pertaining to studies in developing countries. According to these guidelines, "The ethical standards applied should be no less exacting than they would be in the case of research carried out in [the sponsoring] country."[9] In addition, U.S. regulations governing studies performed with federal funds domestically or abroad specify that research procedures must "not unnecessarily expose subjects to risk."[10]

The 16th study is noteworthy both as a model of an ethically conducted study attempting to identify less expensive antiretroviral regimens and as an indication of how strong the placebo-controlled trial orthodoxy is. In 1994, Marc Lallemant, a researcher at the Harvard School of Public Health, applied for NIH funding for an equivalency study in Thailand in which three shorter zidovudine regimens were to be compared with a regimen similar to that used in the ACTG 076 study. An equivalency study is typically conducted when a particular regimen has already been proved effective and one is interested in determining whether a second regimen is about as effective but less toxic or expensive.[11] The NIH study section repeatedly put pressure on Lallemant and the Harvard School of Public Health to conduct a placebo-controlled trial instead, prompting the director of Harvard's human subjects committee to reply, "The conduct of a placebo-controlled trial for [zidovudine] in pregnant women in Thailand would be unethical and unacceptable, since an active-controlled trial is feasible."[12] The NIH eventually relented, and the study is now under way. Since the nine studies of antiretroviral drugs have attracted the most attention, we focus on them in this article.

ASKING THE WRONG RESEARCH QUESTION

There are numerous areas of agreement between those conducting or defending these placebo-controlled studies in developing countries and those opposing such trials. The two sides agree that perinatal HIV transmission is a grave problem meriting concerted international attention; that the ACTG 076 trial was a major breakthrough in perinatal HIV prevention; that there is a role for research on this topic in developing countries; that identifying less expensive, similarly effective interventions would be of enormous benefit, given the limited resources for medical care in most developing countries; and that randomized studies can help identify such interventions.

The sole point of disagreement is the best comparison group to use in assessing the effectiveness of less-expensive interventions once an effective intervention has been identified. The researchers conducting the placebo-controlled trials assert that such trials represent the only appropriate research design, implying that they answer the question, "Is the shorter regimen better than nothing?" We take the more optimistic view that, given the finding of ACTG 076 and other clinical information, researchers are quite capable of designing a shorter antiretroviral regimen that is approximately as effective as the ACTG 076 regimen. The proposal for the Harvard study in Thailand states the research question clearly: "Can we reduce the duration of prophylactic [zidovudine] treatment without increasing the risk of perinatal transmission of HIV, that is, without compromising the demonstrated efficacy of the standard ACTG 076 [zidovudine] regimen?"[13] We believe that such equivalency studies of alternative antiretroviral regimens will provide even more useful results than placebo-controlled trials, without the deaths of hundreds of newborns that are inevitable if placebo groups are used.

At a recent congressional hearing on research ethics, NIH director Harold Varmus was asked how the Department of Health and Human Services could be funding both a placebo-controlled trial (through the CDC) and a non-placebo-controlled equivalency study (through the NIH) in Thailand. Dr. Varmus conceded that placebo-controlled studies are "not the only way to achieve results."[14] If the research can be satisfactorily conducted in more than one way, why not select the approach that minimizes loss of life?

INADEQUATE ANALYSIS OF DATA FROM ACTG 076 AND OTHER SOURCES

The NIH, CDC, WHO, and the researchers conducting the studies we consider unethical argue that differences in the duration and route of administration of antiretroviral agents in the shorter regimens, as compared with the ACTG 076 regimen, justify the use of a placebo group.[15–18] Given that ACTG 076 was a well-conducted, randomized, controlled trial, it is disturbing that the rich data available from the study were not adequately used by the group assembled by WHO in June 1994, which recommended placebo-controlled trials after ACTG 076, or by the investigators of the 15 studies we consider unethical.

In fact, the ACTG 076 investigators conducted a subgroup analysis to identify an appropriate period for prepartum administration of zidovudine. The approximate median duration of prepartum treatment was 12 weeks. In a comparison of treatment for 12 weeks or less (average, 7) with treatment for more than 12 weeks (average, 17), there was no univariate association between the duration of treatment and its effect in reducing perinatal HIV transmission ($P = 0.99$) (Gelber R: personal communication). This analysis is somewhat limited by the number of infected infants and its post hoc nature. However, when combined with information such as the fact that in non–breast-feeding populations an estimated 65 percent of cases of perinatal HIV infection are transmitted during delivery and 95 percent of the remaining cases are transmitted within two months of delivery,[19] the analysis *suggests* that the shorter regimens may be equally effective. This finding should have been explored in later studies by randomly assigning women to longer or shorter treatment regimens.

What about the argument that the use of the oral route for intrapartum administration of zidovudine in the present trials (as opposed to the intravenous route in ACTG 076) justifies the use of a placebo? In its protocols for its two studies in Thailand and Côte d'Ivoire, the CDC acknowledged that previous "pharmacokinetic modeling data suggest that [zidovudine] serum levels obtained with this [oral] dose will be similar to levels obtained with an intravenous infusion."[20]

Thus, on the basis of the ACTG 076 data, knowledge about the timing of perinatal transmission, and pharmacokinetic data, the researchers should have had every reason to believe that well-designed shorter regimens would be more effective than placebo. These findings seriously disturb the equipoise (uncertainty over the likely study result) necessary to justify a placebo-controlled trial on ethical grounds.[21]

DEFINING PLACEBO AS THE STANDARD OF CARE IN DEVELOPING COUNTRIES

Some officials and researchers have defended the use of placebo-controlled studies in developing countries by arguing that the subjects are treated at least according to the standard of care in these countries, which consists of unproven regimens or no treatment at all. This assertion reveals a fundamental misunderstanding of the concept of the standard of care. In developing countries, the standard of care (in this case, not providing zidovudine to HIV-positive pregnant women) is not based on a consideration of alternative treatments or previous clinical data, but is instead an economically determined policy of governments that cannot afford the prices set by drug companies. We agree with the Council for International Organizations of Medical Sciences that researchers working in developing countries have an ethical responsibility to provide treatment that conforms to the standard of care in the sponsoring country, when possible.[9] An exception would be a standard of care that required an exorbitant expenditure, such as the cost of building a coronary care unit. Since zidovudine is usually made available free of charge by the manufacturer for use in clinical trials, excessive cost is not a factor in this case. Acceptance of a standard of care that does not conform to the standard in the sponsoring country results in a double standard in research. Such a double standard, which permits research designs that are unacceptable in the sponsoring country, creates an incentive to use as research subjects those with the least access to health care.

What are the potential implications of accepting such a double standard? Researchers might inject live malaria parasites into HIV-positive subjects in China in order to study the effect on the progression of HIV infection, even though the study protocol had been rejected in the United States and Mexico. Or researchers might randomly assign malnourished San (bushmen) to receive vitamin-fortified or standard bread. One might also justify trials of HIV vaccines in which the subjects were not provided with condoms or state-of-the-art counseling about safe sex by arguing that they are not customarily provided in the developing countries in question. These are not simply hypothetical worst-case scenarios; the first two studies have already been performed,[22–23] and the third has been proposed and criticized.[24]

Annas and Grodin recently commented on the characterization and justification of placebos as a standard of care: "'Nothing' is a description of what happens; 'standard of care' is a normative standard of effective medical treatment, whether or not it is provided to a particular community."[25]

JUSTIFYING PLACEBO-CONTROLLED TRIALS BY CLAIMING THEY ARE MORE RAPID

Researchers have also sought to justify placebo-controlled trials by arguing that they require fewer subjects than equivalency studies and can therefore be completed more rapidly. Because equivalency studies are simply concerned with excluding alternative interventions that fall below some preestablished level of efficacy (as opposed to establishing which intervention is superior), it is customary to use one-sided statistical testing in such studies.[25] The numbers of women needed for a placebo-controlled trial and an equivalency study are similar.[26] In a placebo-controlled trial of a short course of zidovudine, with rates of perinatal HIV transmission of 25 percent in the placebo group and 15 percent in the zidovudine group, an alpha level of 0.05 (two-sided), and a beta level of 0.2, 500 subjects would be needed. An equivalency study with a transmission rate of 10 percent in the group receiving the ACTG 076 regimen, a difference in efficacy of 6 percent (above the 10 percent), an alpha level of 0.05 (one-sided), and a beta level of 0.2 would require 620 subjects (McCarthy W: personal communication).

TOWARD A SINGLE INTERNATIONAL STANDARD OF ETHICAL RESEARCH

Researchers assume greater ethical responsibilities when they enroll subjects in clinical studies, a precept acknowledged by Varmus recently when he insisted that all subjects in an NIH-sponsored needle-exchange trial be offered hepatitis B vaccine.[27] Residents of impoverished, postcolonial countries, the majority of whom are people of color, must be protected from potential exploitation in research. Otherwise, the abominable state of health care in these countries can be used to justify studies that could never pass ethical muster in the sponsoring country.

With the increasing globalization of trade, government research dollars becoming scarce, and more attention being paid to the hazards posed by "emerging infections" to the residents of industrialized countries, it is likely that studies in developing countries will increase. It is time to develop standards of research that preclude the kinds of double standards evident in these trials. In an editorial published nine years ago in the *Journal,* Marcia Angell stated, "Human subjects in any part of the world should be protected by an irreducible set of ethical standards."[28] Tragically, for the hundreds of infants who have needlessly contracted HIV infection in the perinatal-transmission studies that have already been completed, any such protection will have come too late.

REFERENCES

1. Conner EM, Sperling RS, Gelber R, et al. Reduction of maternal–infant transmission of immunodeficiency virus type 1 with zidovudine treatment. N Engl J Med 1994;331:1173–80.
2. Sperling KS, Shapiro DE, Coombs RW, et al. Maternal viral load, zidovudine treatment, and the risk of transmission of human immunodeficiency virus type 1 from mother to infant. N Engl J Med 1996;33i:1621–9.
3. Recommendations of the U.S. Public Health Service Task Force on the use of zidovudine to reduce perinatal transmission of human immunodeficiency virus. MMWR Morb Mortal Wkly Rep 1994;43(RR-11):1–20.
4. Fiscus SA, Adimora AA, Schoenbach VJ, et al. Perinatal HIV infection and the effect of zidovudine therapy on transmission in rural and urban counties. JAMA 1996; 275;1483–8.
5. Cooper E, Diaz C, Pitt J, et al. Impact of ACTG 076: use of zidovudine during pregnancy and changes in the rate of HIV vertical transmission. In: Program and abstracts of the Third Conference on Retroviruses and Opportunistic Infections, Washington, D.C., January 28–February 1, 1996. Washington, D.C.: Infectious Diseases Society of America, 1996:57.
6. Simonds RJ, Nesheim 5, Matheson P. et al. Declining mother to child HIV transmission following perinatal ZDV recommendations. Presented at the 11th International Conference on AIDS, Vancouver, Canada, July 7–12, 1996. abstract.
7. Scarlatti C, Paediatric HIV infection. Lancet 1996;348: 863–8.
8. Recommendations from the meeting on mother-to-infant transmission of HIV by use of antiretrovirals, Geneva, World Health Organization, June 23–25, 1994.
9. World Health Organization. International ethical guidelines for biomedical research involving human subjects. Geneva: Council for International Organizations of Medical Sciences, 1993.
10. 45 CFR 46.111(a)(1).
11. Testing equivalence of two binomial proportions. In: Machin D, Campbell MJ. Statistical tables for the design of clinical trials. Oxford, England: Blackwell Scientific, 1987:35–53.
12. Brennan TA, Letter to Gilbert Meier. NIH Division of Research Ethics, December 28, 1994.
13. Lallemant M, Vithayasai V. A short ZDV course to prevent perinatal HIV in Thailand. Boston: Harvard School of Public Health, April 28, 1995.
14. Varmus H. Testimony before the Subcommittee on Human Resources, Committee on Government Reform and Oversight, U.S. House of Representatives, May 8, 1997.
15. Draft talking points: responding to Public Citizen press conference. Press release of the National Institutes of Health, April 22, 1997.
16. Questions and answers: CDC studies of AZT to prevent mother-to-child HIV transmission in developing countries. Press release of the Centers for Disease Control and Prevention, Atlanta. (undated document.)
17. Questions and answers on the UNAIDS sponsored trials for the prevention of mother-to-child transmission: background brief to assist in responding to issues raised by the public and the media. Press release of the United Nations AIDS Program. (undated document.)
18. Halsey NA, Meinert CL, Ruff AJ., et al. Letter to Harold Varmus, Director of National Institutes of Health. Baltimore: Johns Hopkins University, May 6, 1997.
19. Wiktor SZ, Ehounou E. A randomized placebo-controlled intervention study to evaluate the safety and effectiveness of oral zidovudine administered in late pregnancy to reduce the incidence of mother-to-child transmission of HIV-1 in Abidjan, Côte D'Ivoire. Atlanta: Centers for Disease Control and Prevention. (undated document.)
20. Rouzioux C, Costagliola D, Burgard M, et al. Timing of mother-to-child HIV-1 transmission depends on maternal status. AIDS 1993; 7: Suppl 2: S49-S52.
21. Freedman B. Equipoise and the ethics of clinical research. N Engl J Med 1987; 317:141–5.
22. Heimlich HJ, Chen XP, Xiao BQ et al. CD4 response in HIV-positive patients treated with malaria therapy.

Presented at the 11th International Conference on AIDS, Vancouver, B.C., July 7–12, 1996. abstract.
23. Bishop WB, Laubscher I, Labadarios D, Rehder P. Louw ME, Fellingham SA. Effect of vitamin-enriched bread on the vitamin status of an isolated rural community—a controlled clinical trial. S Afr Med J 1996;86: Suppl:458–62.
24. Lurie P, Bishaw M, Chesney MA, et al. Ethical, behavioral, and social aspects of HIV vaccine trials in developing countries. JAMA 1994;271:295–301.
25. Annas G, Grodin M. An apology is not enough. Boston Globe. May 18, 1997:C1–C2.
26. Freedman B, Weijer C, Glass KC. Placebo orthodoxy in clinical research. I. Empirical and methodological myths. J Law Med Ethics 1996; 24:243–51.
27. Varmus H. Comments at the meeting of the Advisory Committee to the Director of the National Institutes of Health, December 12, 1996.
28. Angell M. Ethical imperialism? Ethics in international collaborative clinical research. N Engl J Med 1988; 319:1061–3.

AZT TRIALS AND TRIBULATIONS

Robert A. Crouch and John D. Arras

With the successful completion of a placebo-controlled trial of zidovudine (AZT) in pregnant women in Thailand—a study designed to determine the safety and efficacy of a short course of AZT in the prevention of maternal-infant HIV transmission—the Centers for Disease Control and Prevention have announced the suspension or modification of all similar trials involving placebos elsewhere in the world. The CDC has claimed victory, asserting that its hotly contested placebo-driven methodology has been vindicated by the study's impressive results. But the critics of this controversial research remain unmoved. For them, the moral of the CDC/Thailand study is a rueful "Better late than never." Both sides can agree on one thing, however: they are glad it's over.

But our society and research communities in fact have yet to definitively resolve some crucial questions posed by these studies. Are placebo-controlled trials justified in the developing world when a proven treatment already exists in developed countries? Must the same ethical standards be used to judge research conducted at home or abroad, in Rochester or Rwanda? We must try to come to terms with these crucial questions bearing on the ethical conduct of international trials because they will soon recur, either in the form of studies on AIDS vaccines, the effects of breastfeeding on HIV transmission, or any number of other pressing issues on the horizon of biomedical research.

THE CONTROVERSY: ARE PLACEBO-CONTROLLED TRIALS JUSTIFIED?

While HIV-infected women and their newborns in industrialized nations can look forward to receiving the AIDS Clinical Trials Group (ACTG) 076 study treatment, the largest public health burden associated with perinatal HIV transmission is to be found in the developing world, where the vast majority of the approximately 1,000 babies born HIV-infected each day reside. Given such grim facts, it is imperative that an alternative safe and effective therapy be established for use in the developing world, where, it has been argued, the intensive 076 protocol could not realistically be implemented. First, the regimen

Reprinted with permission from *Hastings Center Report* 28, no. 6 (1998): 26–34.

Editor's note: Most footnotes have been deleted. Students who want to follow up on sources should consult the original article.

of antenatal, intrapartum, and neonatal AZT requires that women present to the clinic early in their pregnancy for HIV testing and counseling; that they follow the rigorous 076 protocol, which includes five pills per day for at least twelve weeks, and intravenous administration of AZT during delivery; and that the neonates follow a six-week, four-times-per-day, oral AZT regimen, during which time the women are required to abstain from breastfeeding. Unfortunately, however, pregnant women in many developing world settings do not turn up for prenatal care until very late in their pregnancy if indeed at all; many health care clinics in such locales are not equipped to administer intravenous AZT or, generally, to deliver the fastidious care required by the treatment protocol; and, finally, almost all women in the developing world breastfeed because of the established health benefits for their children and the prohibitive expense of baby formula, thus making adherence to the treatment protocol all but impossible. Second, the 076 regimen has been variously estimated to cost as much as $1,000 to $1,500, but certainly no less than $800 per mother and infant—a sum that makes it unaffordable for most of the developing world.

Consequently, U.S. researchers, in cooperation with researchers and public health officials in eleven developing world nations, designed and planned to carry out clinical trials that would compare a shorter, less intensive regimen of AZT to placebo, in the hope of demonstrating that the short course AZT was safe and effective in preventing perinatal HIV transmission in local populations, and that it would be affordable to most developing nations. Though these goals are laudable and endorsed by all, the proposed means to achieve them have engendered fierce criticism, as well as analogies to the infamous Tuskegee syphilis study, from those who believe that the planned means to achieve these results—in particular, the inclusion of a placebo arm in the studies—are unethical.

Three main lines of argument are advanced against the ethical permissibility of the clinical trials planned for the developing world. First, as Peter Lurie and Sidney Wolfe argue, the main point of conflict revolves around the choice of an appropriate comparison group. As against the study designers, Lurie and Wolfe claim that the short course AZT should be compared not to placebo, but rather to the 076 regimen itself, because an equivalency study will yield "even more useful results than placebo-controlled trials, without the deaths of hundreds of newborns that are inevitable if placebo groups are used.[1]

Second, according to Lurie and Wolfe, a subgroup analysis within the 076 protocol indicates that short course AZT (treatment no longer than twelve weeks) is as effective as long course AZT (treatment longer than twelve weeks), suggesting an affirmative answer to the research question implied by the placebo-controlled design—"Is the shorter regimen better than nothing?"—and thereby rendering the studies unnecessary and, thus, unethical.[2]

Finally, as Lurie and Wolfe and Marcia Angell have stated, Western researchers in the studies are shirking their duties to their research subjects on two accounts. First, as set out in the Declaration of Helsinki (Article II.3), all research subjects, including those in the control group, should be assured of the "best proven diagnostic and therapeutic method."[3] Thus in conditions of genuine uncertainty as to the comparative merits of the two AZT regimens, enrolled subjects have a right to, and researchers a correlative duty to provide, either the short course AZT or the 076 regimen, thereby making the use of a placebo arm in the international studies unethical. Second, Lurie and Wolfe interpret guideline 15 of the *International Ethical Guidelines for Biomedical Research Involving Human Subjects* promulgated by the Council for International Organizations of Medical Sciences (CIOMS) as mandating that researchers have "an ethical responsibility to provide treatment that conforms to the standard of care in the sponsoring country, when possible."[4] Since this standard of care would include access to AZT for all participants, to rest the justification for the placebo-controlled design on the fact that the standard of care in most developing world countries consists of no treatment is to fail to recognize a prior duty and to endorse a potentially dangerous double standard for research.

CLARIFYING THE ISSUES

It is well established that for a clinical trial to be ethical, a state of genuine uncertainty as to the comparative merits of the treatments under study must exist within the expert clinical community. Given the uncertainty regarding the study treatments—in other words, given that a state of clinical equipoise exists—trials must be conducted with the aim of removing this uncertainty. The aim of the study must be to disturb equipoise and, thus, alter clinical practice. This means, *inter alia,* that conduct of a clinical trial requires that the "compendious effect of a treatment, a portmanteau measure including all the elements that contribute to the acceptance of a drug within clinical practice," rather than one discrete measure of a treatment's effect should be the focus of the research.[5] And, because clinical trials are responsive to and centrally concerned with the realities of clinical practice, it is crucial for the clinical trialists to take the study context into account when designing and conducting such studies. Recognition of these considerations has several consequences for this discussion.

Given the widespread poverty and lack of resources endemic to much of the developing world, to be understood properly the proposed trials must be analyzed within a framework of extreme fiscal scarcity. Within such a framework, clinical trialists should be concerned with a compendious evaluation of the AZT regimen's effects: reduction of HIV transmission, safety, ease of administration, and, importantly, cost.

In these studies, therefore, the question is not merely whether short course AZT is better than nothing. Rather, the study question is whether the shorter AZT regimen is safe in these populations, and, if so, whether the demonstrated efficacy is large enough, as compared to the placebo group, to make it affordable to the governments in question. For government officials in the developing world to make sound public health policy decisions regarding a treatment to reduce perinatal HIV transmission, trials must demonstrate that AZT is safe for women and their infants and offer convincing evidence about the treatment difference that exists between short course AZT and placebo.

Unanswered questions about the safety of AZT for populations among whom anemia is prevalent, as is well documented among pregnant women in Africa, and whose immune status is compromised by malnutrition argue against use of the 076 regimen as a control arm in these efficacy studies, as does the real possibility that zidovudine-resistant HIV variants may develop in the mother and be passed on to the fetus.

Further, the use of the 076 regimen (or, indeed, another less intensive AZT regimen) as a comparison would yield less informative results because there is ample evidence to suggest that the mother-to-infant HIV transmission rate is highly variable within the developing world (as well as between developed and developing worlds) and that determinants of this variation are not fully understood and hence cannot easily be predicted. Thus part of the information to be gleaned from a placebo-controlled study is the background rate of perinatal HIV transmission in a particular population, which will give researchers a more definite baseline against which to assess AZT efficacy.

This leaves us with the final charge raised by critics of the trials: that it is simply unjust for researchers to operate according to a double standard with regard to the developed and developing worlds. There are two distinct issues here: Are the subjects in placebo-controlled trials morally entitled to more than nothing? And, are these trials unjust because they exploit poor, deprived, developing world subjects largely for the benefit of the more affluent populations of sponsoring countries?

THE CLAIM OF ENTITLEMENT

The critics of placebo-controlled AZT studies assume, either implicitly or explicitly, that all research subjects are morally entitled to receive the prevailing standard of care in more developed countries. One possible source of such an entitlement would be a theory of health care justice as applied to the host countries in question. Importantly, this approach does not rely on any special research-related features of the situation. Although there are many competing theories of equitable access to health care, the account we present here for illustrative purposes embodies several elements common to a variety of leading theories. According to what we will call "the liberal consensus view," justice is equivalent to the kind and amounts of health care that informed, rational, and prudent individuals would choose for themselves against a background entitlement to a fair share of their society's resources. Realizing that they have a limited but fair amount of resources to spend on health care—and that they have many competing needs both within the health care sphere and in such areas as education, housing, employment, and leisure—individuals would no doubt abandon their usual "spare no cost" attitude toward health care in favor of a much more discriminating, cost effective approach. Would they opt for a good, solid basic package of health care benefits? Most likely. Would they pay thousands of extra dollars to insure continuing care for years in a persistent vegetative state? Surely not. According to the liberal consensus view, then, health care justice simply is what such real or hypothetical persons would choose against a backdrop of basic equity.

Applying the liberal consensus view to the situation of individuals in developing countries, we must first ask whether their present standard of living would qualify as a fair share of societal resources. If their present shares were deemed to constitute a reasonably just baseline situation, the citizens of most, if not all, developing countries would clearly not choose to purchase and thus would have no right to expensive antiretroviral therapies. Given the extreme shortages of goods, services, infrastructure, and personnel across a wide spectrum of basic needs, individuals and governments would realize that they simply don't have the money to invest in such treatments, and that the meager amount of money that they do control would be better spent on cheaper, more effective interventions that could reach many more people and save many more lives. Instead of the 076 protocol at $800 per person—or even the CDC/Thailand protocol at $50—in a country that currently spends $5 per person per year on health care, they might favor more modest public health measures, such as improved nutrition or water systems. According to this analysis, research subjects randomized to placebos in the recent short course trials were not deprived of anything to which they were already justly entitled.

It is highly debatable, however, whether the current holdings of citizens in most developing countries satisfy the condition of background fairness required by the liberal consensus view. Agreeing with Judith Shklar's perceptive observation that it is always "easier to see misfortune rather than injustice in the afflictions of other people,"[6] we are loathe to conclude that the current plight of these impoverished peoples is unfortunate but not unjust. Their misery must be due in no small measure to the flagrantly unjust behavior of the former colonial powers, which plundered their natural resources and subjugated their peoples; in many subsequent cases to the rapacious behavior of their home-grown military dictators, who treated their country's natural resources as their own private stock; and more recently to global economic policies that often stifle economic growth under huge debt-servicing policies. In a more just world, the citizens of the developing world would have a more equitable share of their country's resources, and the colonial powers and the generals would have a lot less. Recalculating their social and economic baseline to reflect the demands of compensatory justice, would these people have a just claim to expensive antiretroviral therapy, a claim denied by placebo-driven AIDS trials?

Although we support any and all efforts to narrow the huge economic gap separating developing from more developed countries, we doubt that even taking past injustices into account would yield a moral entitlement to expensive antiretroviral treatments. In the first place, many of these countries are so poor and underdeveloped that even the best efforts at compensatory redistribution would not take them very far. Under the rosiest of estimates, such countries might be able to afford the $50 CDC/Thailand protocol, but certainly not the hugely expensive 076 regimen.

Second, even if compensatory redistribution were required by justice, it will usually be impossible to tell who owes what kind and amount of compensation to whom, and there are currently no authoritative international bodies that could legitimately adjudicate such compensatory claims. As a result, the citizens of these impoverished countries may indeed have a moral right to a better standard of living, but this is almost certainly a claim that will go unredeemed for the foreseeable future. Hence the desirability and feasibility of choosing to pay for expensive antiretroviral therapies must be gauged against the backdrop of their present, admittedly unjust, baseline.

Third, claiming and *per impossibile* securing such a right would surely generate new injustices, as more numerous people with equally pressing needs would be passed over in favor of HIV-infected pregnant women and their children. The families of children and adults dying from diarrhea, malnutrition, and malaria could reasonably claim a higher priority on public funds. Their numbers are greater and it would cost far less to mount effective preventive programs in such areas.

Perhaps most importantly, the plausibility of a claimed right to antiretroviral treatment fundamentally depends upon the successful completion of the contested placebo-controlled trials. Even if we assume that the potential subjects' current baseline situation is unjust, any set of more just holdings will perforce be limited, they will have many competing (and expensive) needs, and they will thus be extremely sensitive to the opportunity costs of spending money on expensive AIDS therapies rather than on less expensive and more cost-effective lifesaving interventions. To tell whether they would reasonably choose to spend large sums of money on AIDS therapies, reliable scientific data on their costs, risks, and benefits must first be accumulated so that reasonable and prudent investment comparisons might be made. Thus until we know just how safe and effective the short course of AZT is in these host countries, it makes little sense to say that people there independently have a right to it.

A second approach to justifying an entitlement would focus not on theories of health care justice, but rather on certain role-specific duties of researchers. Whether or not potential subjects have a preexisting right to antiretroviral therapies, it might be claimed that researchers have a duty to provide it to them based upon their special relationship. One might claim, for example, that participating subjects assume additional burdens by participating in a drug trial and are therefore owed special treatment. Or one could argue that researchers have special fiduciary responsibilities for all those who are placed in their care, responsibilities that include providing all subjects in the control group with the highest standard of care in the world (that is, with the 076 protocol).

Although both of these arguments contain a large grain of truth, neither succeeds in justifying a claim to the 076 protocol for subjects in the control group. Even if subjects do assume additional burdens by participating in a trial, they also become eligible for important benefits not normally available off study, especially if they end up receiving a safe and efficacious active drug. And even if they end up in the placebo group, they will probably receive better basic medical care than would have been available to them otherwise. Moreover, there are other more realistic ways of compensating them for burdens incurred, especially when this proposed method of compensation would have the undesirable effect of preventing researchers from answering the most meaningful questions that motivated the research in the first place.

This last point is crucial for determining the scope of researchers' fiduciary responsibilities to subjects entrusted to their care. Although researchers undeniably have such role-specific duties, we doubt that they would include enticements to kinds and amounts of health care services that, first, are unavailable elsewhere in the host country and to which its citizens have no independent right of access, and second, would arguably preclude the timely and successful completion of desperately needed clinical trials. As we argued above, the point of running a clinical trial is to disturb equipoise and thereby potentially change clinical practice. Researchers must therefore show that the proposed short course AZT intervention is both safe and sufficiently effective to warrant large-scale investments on the part of host governments, developed nations, and pharmaceutical companies. In the absence of reliable information on the background vertical HIV transmission rate—information that can only be gained via a placebo group—researchers will be unable to meet this burden of demonstration. Neither the assumption of special burdens nor the enhanced fiduciary responsibilities of researchers for their subjects can ground an entitlement to the best treatment available anywhere. . . .

REFERENCES

1. Peter Lurie and Sidney M. Wolfe, "Unethical Trials of Interventions to Reduce Perinatal Transmission of the Human Immunodeficiency Virus in Developing Countries," *NEJM* 337 (1997): 853–56, at 854.
2. Lurie and Wolfe, "Unethical Trials"; Sidney M. Wolfe and Peter Lurie, letter to Donna Shalala, Secretary of Health and Human Services, 23 October 1997.
3. Wolfe and Lurie, letter to Donna Shalala; Marcia Angell, "The Ethics of Clinical Research in the Third World," *NEJM* 337 (1997): 847–49.

4. Lurie and Wolfe, "Unethical Trials," p. 855.
5. Benjamin Freedman, "Placebo-Controlled Trials and the Logic of Clinical Purpose," *IRB: A Review of Human Subjects Research* 12, no. 6 (1990): 1–6, at 5.
6. Judith N. Shklar, *The Faces of Injustice* (New Haven: Yale University Press, 1990), p. 15.

THE AMBIGUITY AND THE EXIGENCY: CLARIFYING "STANDARD OF CARE" ARGUMENTS IN INTERNATIONAL RESEARCH

Alex John London

I. INTRODUCTION

For some time now, the medical and bioethics communities have been struggling with a number of difficult and sometimes divisive issues concerning the ethics of international research. Many of these issues were raised in the recent controversy over the decision to use placebo control groups in clinical trials designed to test the efficacy of a short-course of zidovudine (AZT) for the prevention of maternal-infant HIV infection in sixteen countries in sub-Saharan Africa, Southeast Asia, and the Caribbean. The studies, sponsored by the National Institutes of Health (NIH) and the Centers for Disease Control and Prevention (CDC), became the topic of a heated debate when a pair of articles published in the *New England Journal of Medicine* (Angell, 1997; Lurie and Wolfe, 1997) charged that the use of a placebo control group made them unethical. Even though subsequent studies involving placebos were either suspended or modified after the completion of a CDC-sponsored study in Thailand, the controversy has continued and the ethical and scientific debate has intensified. Now, however, the dispute surrounding some of these issues could have far-reaching implications for the whole of international human subjects research. Plans are underway to revise key guidelines governing the ethical conduct of international medical research, and several of the most controversial issues at the heart of the short-course AZT trials are playing a central role in the debate over some of the proposed revisions.

Rather than attempting a wholesale appraisal of the diverse and complex array of issues involved in this debate, the present paper will focus instead on one prominent, and highly controversial, issue. From the outset of the controversy over the short-course AZT studies, both proponents and critics of the placebo-controlled design supported their positions with what I will call the 'standard of care' argument. Critics argued that the placebo driven trial design was unethical, at least in part, because it failed to provide the current standard of care to all members of the clinical trial. In support of their position they pointed to article II.3 of the Declaration of Helsinki which states that "In any medical study, every patient—including those of a control group, if any—should be assured of the best proven diagnostic and therapeutic method." They also pointed to the fact that in technologically developed countries such as France and the U.S., the standard treatment used for preventing the transmission of HIV from seropositive pregnant women to their infant children, known as the AIDS Clinical Trials Group (ACTG) regimen 076, had been shown to cut maternal-infant HIV transmission rates by more

Reprinted with permission from *Journal of Medicine and Philosophy* 2000, Vol. 25, No. 4, pp. 379–397.

Editor's note: All footnotes have been deleted. Students who want to follow up on sources should consult the original article.

than half. To adopt a standard of care for developing nations that falls below the standard of care in the sponsoring countries, it was argued, was to adopt an unacceptable double standard in international research.

Proponents of the placebo design countered by pointing out that the 076 protocol was unavailable in the countries that would host the short-course trials because, at $800 per dose, it far outstripped the $10 average per-capita health budgets of the developing countries in which the trials had been proposed. As a result, they argued, the standard of care that governs the citizens of those countries is no treatment at all. Because they believed that the local standard of care was the most relevant, they concluded that the placebo design was not unethical. Now, current proposals would amend the Declaration of Helsinki so as to reflect this view. Instead of requiring that subjects receive the "best proven diagnostic and therapeutic method," one proposed revision would require only that subjects "not be denied access to the best proven diagnostic, prophylactic, or therapeutic method that would otherwise be available to him or her."

In what follows, I will argue that this debate has been complicated by some unrecognized ambiguities in the notion of a standard of care. In particular, I will argue that this concept is ambiguous along two different axes, with the result that there are at least four possible standard of care arguments that must be clearly distinguished. Without a clear map of the normative terrain it has been difficult to assess the implications of opposing standard of care arguments, to recognize important differences in their supporting rationales, and even to locate the crux of the disagreement in some instances. The goal of this discussion, therefore, is to disambiguate the concept of a standard of care and to make the areas of genuine disagreement among different standards salient. This kind of conceptual cartography is fundamentally important for assessing the relevance and validity of the arguments in question and I will argue that it highlights important ways in which one of these arguments in particular may be more complex than it originally appears.

Because the goal of this paper is to provide a careful examination of the concept of a standard of care and the normative arguments that it supports, it does not attempt to provide an overall evaluation of the short-course AZT studies. As a result, it also will not present an overall evaluation of the importance of standard of care arguments relative to these broader concerns. This is important because it may be the case that there are other issues raised by these trials that carry sufficient moral weight to trump the standard of care argument. Before we can know whether this is so, however, we need to carry out the necessary conceptual and ethical analysis of the standard of care arguments that will enable this larger conversation to proceed more carefully, and hopefully, more fruitfully as well.

II. WHAT IS (ARE) THE STANDARD OF CARE ARGUMENTS(S)?

In order to tease out some important ambiguities in the concept of a standard of care, it will be helpful to look carefully at one prominent way in which the debate over the standard of care has been framed. Consider the following claims:

> When Helsinki calls for the "best proven therapeutic method" does it mean [A] the best therapy available anywhere in the world? Or does it mean [B] the standard that prevails in the country in which the trial is conducted? Helsinki is not clear about this. But I think that [1] a careful analysis of this document and its history suggests that the best proven therapy standard was intended primarily as a standard of medical practice. A consideration of that conclusion yields a second conclusion: that [2] the best proven therapy standard must necessarily mean the standard that prevails in the country in which the clinical trial is carried out (Levine, R.J., 1998, p. 6; letters and numbers added).

In part, interpretations A and B differ over what I will call the question of the *relevant reference point.* Emphasizing this disagreement makes it appear as though the dispute hinges on the question of whose medical practice constitutes the relevant medical practice. Interpretation A holds that the relevant standard of care is the one determined by the best therapeutic methods available anywhere in the world. Call this the *global* reference point. Interpretation B holds that the relevant standard of care is determined by the standard that prevails in the country in which the trial is conducted. Call this the *local* reference point. So understood, the sides of this debate are divided into proponents of a local standard of care and critics who champion a global standard of care.

Framing the debate as a question of the relevant reference point, however, effectively obscures a more fundamental and largely unarticulated source of disagreement. To see this, consider a crucial assumption that lies behind the following argument. It is sometimes claimed that (1) because the content of the standard of care is fixed by the local reference point and (2) because the prevailing treatment for preventing maternal-infant HIV transmission in the countries where the short-course AZT trials were conducted was no treatment at all, that (3) the use of a placebo does not fall below the established standard of care. It is important to see, however, that in order for (3) to follow from (1) and (2), we have to do more than simply adopt the local reference point for the standard of care. For the argument to be valid it must also employ what I will call a *de facto* interpretation of the concept of the standard of care. Let me explain.

Let's grant the claim that the standard of care is intended to be a standard of medical practice. The above argument tacitly assumes a *de facto* interpretation of the standard of care according to which the standards of medical practice for a community are set by the actual medical practices of that community. It is only under this interpretation that the use of a placebo does not fall below the standard of care in countries where there is no effective treatment for maternal-infant transmission of HIV. For the sake of clarity, the argument from the *local de facto* interpretation of the standard of care can be stated as follows:

(A) **1.** It is unethical to conduct a clinical trial in which some subjects receive a level of care that falls below the established standard of care.

2. The established standard of care is to be determined by the local *de facto* practices of the host community.

3. In the countries where the short-course AZT trials were conducted the local *de facto* clinical practice for preventing maternal-infant HIV transmission was no treatment at all.

4. The use of a placebo control group in these countries does not fall below the established standard of care.

5. Therefore, the use of a placebo control group is not unethical on the ground that it fails to provide the established standard of care.

If we assume that the crux of the debate hinges on the question of the relevant reference point then we must also assume that critics of this argument accept the *de facto* interpretation but opt instead for a more global reference point. So understood, they would be making a *global de facto* argument:

(B) **1.** It is unethical to conduct a clinical trial in which some subjects receive a level of care that falls below the established standard of care.

2. The established standard of care is to be determined by the broader *de facto* practices of the sponsoring nations.

3. The *de facto* clinical practice for preventing maternal-infant HIV transmission in the countries of the developed world sponsoring the short-course AZT trials is the 076 protocol.

4. The use of a placebo control group in the countries where short-course AZT trials were proposed falls below the established standard in the developed world.

5. Therefore, the use of a placebo control group is unethical on the ground that it fails to provide the established standard of care.

This may represent a common way of framing the debate over the standard of care, but it obscures the fact that the *de facto* interpretation of the standard is itself highly contentious. As a result, it fails to capture a more fundamental area of disagreement. If we return to the language of the Declaration of Helsinki, for example, we see that it speaks of providing the best *proven* diagnostic and therapeutic interventions. This seems to indicate that the idea of a standard of care is what I will call a *de jure* standard in that it is set, not by what physicians in some locality actually do, but by the judgment of experts in the medical community as to which diagnostic and therapeutic practices have proven most effective against the illness in question. This is the interpretation embraced by Marcia Angell when she argues that the investigators conducting a trial "would be guilty of knowingly giving inferior treatment to some participants of the trial," unless subjects in the control group "receive the best known treatment." For critics like Angell, the question of the relevant reference point is irrelevant because adopting the *de jure* interpretation of the standard of care allows them to argue that a placebo control is unjustified even relative to the local point of reference. To see how this might be so, consider the argument from the *local de jure* standard of care:

(C) **1.** It is unethical to conduct a clinical trial in which some subjects receive a level of care that falls below the established standard of care.
2. The established standard of care is to be determined by the judgment of medical experts in the host community as to which diagnostic and therapeutic interventions have been proven most effective.
3. Medical experts in the relevant host communities know the 076 protocol has been shown to cut the maternal-infant HIV transmission rate by more than half in developed nations such as the United States.
4. The use of a placebo control group in the developing countries where the short-course AZT trials were proposed falls below the established standard in those very countries.
5. Therefore, the use of a placebo control group is unethical on the ground that it fails to provide the established standard of care.

A global version of this argument can be constructed by substituting the following for premise C2:

(D) **2.** The established standard of care is to be determined by the judgment of medical experts in some larger medical community as to which diagnostic and therapeutic interventions have been proven most effective.

Below, I will suggest that this argument is more complex than even its proponents may realize and that its implications have yet to be clearly explored. For the moment, however, I simply want to note that the choice of reference points does not affect the conclusion of the argument. As a result, it looks like the real crux of the dispute may hinge, not on the question of the relevant reference point, but on the way we interpret the standard of medical practice that is embodied in the standard of care: is it a *de facto* or a *de jure* standard?

When the crux of the argument is understood this way, it becomes absolutely essential not to confuse the argument from the global *de facto* standard (B) with the argument from the local *de jure* standard (C). In part, this is because arguments (B) and (C) themselves differ over the question of the relevant reference point. As a result, objections that tell against the use of a global reference point may carry weight against argument (B) and not militate against—and may even support—argument (C). Furthermore, given that these arguments embody different conceptions of the standard of care, each of which has a substantially different supporting rationale, we must not assume that they will have the same implications for the conduct of international research. In the following section I will suggest that a failure to differentiate arguments (B) and (C) may have led to the acceptance of a false dilemma: either we accept the local *de facto* standard of care or we accept a higher standard that rules out altogether the international research that could be most important for populations of the developing world. In order to appreciate this, however, and to evaluate the merits of the local *de facto* and local *de jure* arguments, it will be necessary to look more carefully at the differences between the *de facto* and *de jure* interpretations of the standard of care.

III. THE LOCAL *DE FACTO* STANDARD OF CARE

One fairly simple reason that we might be inclined to accept the local *de facto* standard of care is that it appears to be more reasonable than the global *de facto* standard. Consider, for instance, some of the problems with the latter argument (B). On its face it appears to place arbitrary restrictions on important international research. Critics can easily question why the practices of some wealthy, technologically developed groups with sophisticated and well-entrenched healthcare infrastructures should also govern people who live under conditions of extreme fiscal scarcity, without a robust healthcare infrastructure, under different cultural and social conditions. Isn't this arbitrary? Might it not be ethical, rather than social or cultural, imperialism?

In contrast, proponents of the narrow *de facto* argument (A) argue that it will foster the research that will ultimately lead to the kinds of interventions that will best address the healthcare concerns of developing populations. The local *status quo* frames the appropriate clinical question and enables us to design a study that will demonstrate the effectiveness of an intervention when compared to the current treatment situation (in the case of the short-course trials, nothing) (Levine, R. J., 1998, p. 7). This difference in the treatment situation is what makes it permissible to conduct a placebo-controlled trial in a developing country when it could not be conducted ethically in the U.S. Furthermore, it is argued, the use of a placebo does not deny subjects of developing countries care that they would otherwise receive, since they aren't currently receiving any beneficial care, and it does not inflict new or additional health burdens on research subjects. In fact, it is likely that in many cases research subjects would receive a net benefit from participating in this kind of research since they would probably receive routine health care, otherwise unavailable, as a part of the clinical trial.

When the alternative is the global *de facto* argument (B), we may be inclined to support the local *de facto* argument (A) simply out of the desire to help developing countries conduct the research that will answer the healthcare questions that best address their substantial and urgent healthcare needs. This way of thinking, however, may also keep us from recognizing the substantial shortcomings of the local *de facto* standard of care. For many, the most appealing aspect of this standard of care is the fact that it allows us to design clinical trials that will answer the right experimental questions. In the case of the short-course AZT trials, for instance, the relevant question was not how a short-course of AZT compared to the 076 regimen but how much better it would be than nothing. Unfortunately, however, it is precisely because the *status quo* is what sets research into motion that it cannot also function as an independent test of the moral acceptability of a clinical trial. Let me be clear about what this means. The research questions that are relevant to a particular community are, to a large degree, a function of the needs of the people in that community relative to the level of healthcare they actually receive. It is also true that acceptable clinical trials should produce results that will be relevant to a community's healthcare needs. But it doesn't follow from this that all research that would be relevant to a community's healthcare needs is morally acceptable research. Relevance, elegance, efficiency, these are all virtues that morally acceptable trials should possess. But not all relevant, elegant, and efficient trials are morally acceptable.

It is important to recognize, therefore, that the local *de facto* standard of care does not receive independent support from the claim that subjects who would not receive medical care outside of a clinical trial are not denied care when they are given a placebo. Rather than providing independent support for the *de facto* standard of care, this is simply an alternative formulation of the very standard in question. As a result, the truth of this claim itself presupposes the truth of the argument from the local *de facto* standard of care. Those who reject the latter argument would rightly reject this claim on the grounds that it simply assumes the conclusion that is in dispute. This means that proponents of a different standard of care could make an equally valid claim that subjects of medical research *are* being denied medical care to which they are entitled if, for example, they do not receive the same level of care that the researchers or their sponsoring agencies normally provide to people with their condition. I will return to this point in a moment.

For now, consider some of problems that argument (A) faces in its own right. For example, the scope of this argument is more comprehensive than its proponents may be willing to accept. In particular, we want to know whether there are non-arbitrary reasons for keeping this argument, and its supporting rationale, from applying to sub-groups within established political borders. After all, if the standard of care is set by a community's *de facto* medical practices, and if the actual practices of doctors differ within ethnic, cultural, or economic subgroups, shouldn't those subgroups be governed by different standards of care in research? This is a powerful and potentially damning objection, because most proponents of the placebo design appear to believe that it would be genuinely unethical to conduct short-course AZT trials with a placebo control in the U.S. If this objection cannot be met, it would mean that the members of marginalized or oppressed subgroups, even within a developed nation like the U.S., would be governed by a lower standard of care in medical research than their wealthier counterparts precisely because they have been socially and economically marginalized or oppressed. This, however, is antithetical to the very idea of ethically sound human subjects research. As a result, anyone who is inclined to accept this argument takes on the increased burden of providing non-arbitrary reasons for limiting its scope of applicability.

This is also a powerful objection because it highlights the degree to which the narrow *de facto* standard of care appears to be out of step with the rationale for protecting human subjects in research within the U.S. This way of formulating the standard of care trades on the assumption that the level of care research subjects receive should be determined by factors that are extrinsic to the researcher/subject relationship. Another way of putting this is to say that, on this view, the terms of the researcher/subject relationship are to be determined by circumstances that are largely independent of the existence of that relationship. In order to know what standard of care subjects are entitled to, researchers, on this view, have to look at the circumstances in which those subjects live. In order to know whether subjects in Tanzania should be subject to the same standards of care as subjects in Tucson, we have to look at the socio-economic circumstances in which they live. Traditionally, however, the debate about the protections that human research subjects should receive has been formulated largely in terms of problems that are inherent to the nature of medical research and the researcher/subject relationship. Socio-economic factors were important but largely because they marked out vulnerable populations where an increased sensitivity to issues of exploitation and competence was warranted. As such, Lurie and Wolfe (1997) were right to argue that this interpretation of the standard of care marks a change in the way research protections are conceived—a double standard for medical research.

Not only is this a different standard, it is a dangerous standard because it fails to take account of the context in which a community's *de facto* medical practices originate. By simply elevating the status quo to the level of a normative standard it does not distinguish between situations of scarcity that are the result of exploitation, force or fraud and those that are not. This leaves it open to exploitation and the danger of being manipulated in unscrupulous ways, on the international level by the economic or military interference of an outside group on the availability of medicines, medical personnel, or medical training within a particular nation, and on an *intra*-national level by these same activities on the part of dominant power groups.

The fact that argument (A) unreflectively embraces the status quo may sometimes be overlooked because of an ambiguity in the notion of a 'practice.' As it has come to be used by some (communitarians, for example), a practice is a norm-governed activity in which people engage, in part at least, for the sake of goods that are internal to the practice. On this view, a practice is an activity through which people pursue certain goods and understand themselves, their community, and perhaps their larger world. Because practices of this kind can play an integral part in the identity of individuals or communities, they may deserve special protections or carry special normative weight. However, the *de facto* 'practice' of physicians in Thailand, for example, is not such a practice. Thai physicians understand that they are unable to effectively prevent maternal-infant transmission of HIV and are themselves calling for the international help required to change this. As Lurie and Wolfe rightly point out, "In developing countries, the standard of care . . . is not based on a consideration of alternative treatments or previous clinical data, but is instead an economically determined policy of governments that cannot afford the prices set by drug companies" (1997, p. 855). So we must be careful not to confuse this kind of *de facto* practice with the more normatively weighty sense of "practice" favored by communitarians.

IV. THE LOCAL *DE JURE* STANDARD OF CARE

When the crux of the debate over the standard of care is framed, not as a question of the relevant reference point, but as hinging on the choice between the local *de facto* and local *de jure* interpretations, many of these problems with argument (A) become salient. For the proponents of a *de jure* standard, the local *de facto* standard is formulated in response to the wrong question. The latter standard answers the question of what research subjects may be entitled to outside of the research context, what they would be entitled to if research were not taking place (with the dubious assumption that their current situation is unfortunate and not unjust). But this is not what is at issue. What is at issue is what subjects are entitled to within the context of research itself, given the nature of scientific research and the fact that the researchers studying them have the knowledge and training—and often work for governments or institutions with the resource—to prevent some of the harms they encounter as a result of their vast, unmet healthcare needs. It may be true that the use of analogies with past research scandals has not generally helped to advance the present debate, but critics of this position are right to point out that this idea—that research subjects are only entitled to what they would otherwise receive outside of the research context and that researchers are under no independent obligation to prevent outcomes that would occur outside of the research context anyway—was also used to support the studies at Tuskegee and Willowbrook. It may also be true that the proposed short-course trials were crucially different from these scandalous studies. But this point only highlights the need for those who defend the former studies to reject a moral justification that would also license the latter. After all, the claim that roughly the same states of affairs would likely have obtained even if no research had been conducted does not obviate the fact that, in the actual case, the state of affairs that actually obtains is at least partially a product of the explicit choices and activities of specific individuals and agencies.

For this reason, the *de jure* standard is founded upon the researchers' obligation to ensure that subjects of clinical trials are not knowingly exposed to foreseeable and preventable harms. Clinical trials are not the products of natural events or inevitable processes; they are the result of deliberation and choice on the part of actual individuals and agencies. The *de jure* requirement that researchers provide the treatment that has been shown to be most effective against the relevant illness is itself a corollary of the requirement that equipoise exist in order for a clinical trial to be morally permissible.

Clinical equipoise exists when there is genuine uncertainty among experts as to whether a proposed intervention is as good as or better than the current, known beneficial treatment for the illness at issue (Freedman, 1987 and 1990). A trial of a short course of AZT that used a placebo control group within the United States would be unethical because the 076 protocol has been shown to cut maternal-infant HIV transmission rates by more than half. In order for clinical equipoise to exist, the short course would have to be tried against the 076 regimen *and* there would have to be reason to believe that the short-course of AZT might be equally or more effective than its established counterpart.

By linking the standard of care to the knowledge and abilities of researchers, argument (C) highlights the fact that medical research is a human activity, the terms of which are fundamentally shaped by human agency and choice. The fundamental goal of medical research is not to provide health care but to gather medical knowledge which, it is hoped, will result in the development or perfection of interventions that will benefit future patients. Because the design of a trial is the result of the exercise of such agency and choice, the researchers and agencies that sponsor clinical trials are responsible for the ramifications that trial designs have on the welfare of the people who submit themselves to scientific study. The requirement that clinical equipoise obtain is essential to the conduct of acceptable medical research because it ensures that researchers do not undertake trials in which the welfare of some individuals is knowingly sacrificed in exchange for knowledge, and ultimately, the welfare of future patients. By providing the *de jure* standard of care, researchers and their sponsoring agencies ensure that the subjects of clinical research are not exploited, even for what we can all agree is a noble end.

Now that the rationale for the *de jure* standard is clear, it remains to elucidate the implications of this standard for international medical research. I suggested above that, to some degree, support for the local *de facto* interpretation may be rooted in the perception that a higher standard of care would place unduly stringent restrictions on the use of placebos in international research. Although this may be true for the global *de facto* standard, is it true for the local *de jure* standard as well?

V. THE COMPLEXITY OF THE *DE JURE* FRAMEWORK

I want to suggest that the local *de jure* standard of care does not yield as unequivocal a restriction on the use of placebo controls as one might think and that answering this question will be more complicated than it may first appear. In particular, because this standard is built around the concept of clinical equipoise, the severity of the restriction that it does yield will depend in large part on the nature of the conception of clinical equipoise that we embrace. This is an important claim, because it points to a way in which we might formulate the debate over the moral legitimacy of the use of placebo controls in international research from within the framework of the local *de jure* standard of care itself. In order to see how this is so, and why it might be desirable, let me explain how some placebo controls might be justified according to the local *de jure* standard of care.

In her original article in the *New England Journal of Medicine,* Marcia Angell argued for what I am calling a *de jure* standard of care. However, it is not clear how sweeping a restriction she takes this standard to yield. At one point, for instance, she says that "only when there is no known effective treatment is it ethical to compare a potential new treatment with a placebo" (1997, p. 847). This has encouraged some to frame the debate as a question of what I call the local *de facto* standard versus the best therapy available anywhere in the world (e.g., Levine, R.J., 1998, p. 6). But Angell's claim can be interpreted in two different ways:

I1. Only when there is no known effective treatment for illness x anywhere in the world is it ethical to compare a potential new treatment with a placebo.

I2. Only when there is no known effective treatment anywhere in the world for illness x within a population p is it ethical to compare a potential new treatment with a placebo in population p.

Although the local *de facto* standard is often contrasted with interpretation I1—the more restrictive standard—this interpretation is itself out of step with the rationale of the *de jure* conception of the standard of care. The reason is simply that such substantial differences between treatment populations can exist as to warrant genuine and credible doubts in the medical community about whether a treatment that is effective in one population will be effective in another. As a result, interpretation I2 most accurately reflects the *de jure* standard of care. It yields a more reasonable and defensible standard because it recognizes that the same standard can yield different conclusions if it is applied the same way in sufficiently different contexts. It is also less restrictive than its critics, and perhaps its proponents, may recognize.

Exactly how restrictive I2 is, however, will depend on our conception of clinical equipoise. If we embrace a narrow conception of clinical equipoise according to which effectiveness is measured solely by the brute biological impact of an intervention on the illness in question relative to some end point, then the resulting standard of care will likely permit the use of a placebo only in cases where the biological differences between populations are substantial enough to cast credible doubt on the intervention's ability to function effectively in the trial population.

If we subscribe to a more robust concept of clinical equipoise, however, the ability to effect beneficial healthcare outcomes within a population will be measured as a product of a wider range of factors. For instance, Freedman (1990) has argued that the attractiveness of a drug in comparison to its alternatives should always be determined by a "compendious measure of a drug's net therapeutic advantage" (p. 2). Here, however, the concept of "net therapeutic advantage" is conceived of as a "*portmanteau* measure including all the elements that contribute to the acceptance of a drug within clinical practice" (p. 5). In addition to concerns about relative toxicity, this sort of robust conception of clinical equipoise will include factors such as ease of administration and availability. Some recent commentators have argued for the importance of relying on this conception of clinical equipoise when evaluating the short-course AZT trials (Crouch and Arras, 1998, p. 27). But their arguments have mainly emphasized the fact that doing so enables researchers to design trials that will change clinical practice. This is an important point, but one which also supports the local *de facto* standard of care and whose implications I criticized above. What needs to be stressed, instead, is that the rationale for including such broader factors in our concept of clinical equipoise can be supported by the epistemological concerns central to the *de jure* standard of care itself. The reason is that in order to know whether a treatment will be effective within a specific population we need to know whether it can be successfully administered in that context. This, however, will likely depend on a variety of social, cultural, and economic factors.

Consider, for instance, a treatment protocol that required frequent and prolonged hospital stays. Such a protocol might fail to have a significant health impact in a nomadic population if compliance required what members of that population viewed as unacceptable changes to their way of life. The same might be true for a highly diffuse and largely immobile population with few hospitals if the travel that would be required for compliance required unacceptable social or economic sacrifices. Likewise, consider the case of an illness that can only be treated by a surgical procedure that requires sophisticated equipment, an extended intensive care stay, and frequent, sophisticated follow up treatments. This procedure is the *de jure* standard of care in wealthy nations with well-established, high-tech healthcare infrastructures, because it can be safely and effectively administered in such a setting. In a country that lacks this kind of setting it may be practically impossible to establish the conditions under which it could be effectively implemented even for a small group of people.

These examples are put forth as suggestive instances of cases in which equipoise could exist in one population even though it is disturbed in more developed nations, for other than purely biological reasons. The point of sketching them is to suggest that, in instances such as these, a *prima facie* case can be made—on the very grounds that support the *de jure* standard of care—for the legitimacy of a placebo control when testing a more portable intervention (assuming that one does not already exist). This kind of argument does not rest solely on the need to design a clinical trial that will provide a clear answer to a clinical question, although it ensures that all morally acceptable trials will have this feature. Nor does it rest on the claim that the subjects of such trials are not denied care that they would not otherwise receive. Instead, it rests on the claim that it may be ethically permissible to answer this particular question with a placebo-controlled trial because, in doing so, researchers would not knowingly be denying subjects *care that has proven effective for their illness in their population.*

As I said earlier, the implications of this position are far from clear and it may in fact raise more questions than it answers. For my present purposes, it is sufficient simply to note (a) that there are compelling reasons to treat equipoise as a broad measure of a treatment's effectiveness, and (b) that as we broaden our measure of an intervention's effectiveness the use of a placebo control may become acceptable in a wider variety of situations. Unlike the global *de facto* argument, this standard pays greater attention to substantive differences in social, cultural, and economic contexts and their impact on the permissibility of international research. Unlike the local *de facto* argument, however, it would prohibit the use of a placebo control in cases of international research where an intervention is known to be effective (where effectiveness is broadly construed) for illness x in population p, even if it is not currently available in population p.

Nevertheless, difficult questions would need to be resolved in order to make this a workable standard. We still need to know, for example, which social, cultural, and economic factors should bear on the question of equipoise and how much weight different factors should be afforded. For instance, what if we had a safe, effective, easily administered treatment that was simply so expensive that it could not be reasonably supplied to significant numbers of a developing population? Should this fact alone be sufficient to establish equipoise in the relevant population? What should we do in situations where the *de jure* standard in one population can be administered to members of the control group in another population, even though it could not be made available to members of the larger population?

Those who are familiar with the debate over the short course AZT trials will recognize many of these questions. The fact that they can be raised from within the framework of the local *de jure* argument testifies to its complexity. I believe that it also testifies to the fact that we can retain some of the most substantive areas of genuine dispute over the standards that should govern international research even if we agree that the local *de facto* standard of care is a bad, if not a perfidious, standard. In itself this is an important point because it may help us to reorient the current debate in a way that makes the actual lines of dispute salient. Not only might this allow both sides to agree on the values that structure the problem and then to recognize the operative areas of genuine dispute, it might make it possible to find a way towards building a more stable and sustainable consensus on these issues.

One thing that we can say, even from this admittedly terse sketch, is that relocating the debate within the context of the local *de jure* standard of care will provide a more coherent framework for relating technical questions that concern the conduct of specific clinical trials to ethical issues that arise at a broader social and political level. At the trial level, for instance, this standard requires researchers to ensure that their choice of trial design does not allow some participants to suffer harms that could be foreseen and prevented with reasonable care. At the policy level, however, this standard requires researchers, their sponsoring agencies, and relevant political bodies to ensure that conducting a clinical trial represents a responsible means of addressing the healthcare priorities of the population in question. In cases where equipoise exists in one country but not in another we will have to consider whether equally or more profound healthcare outcomes could be achieved, perhaps with the imposition of fewer burdens, by altering some of the conditions that cause equipoise to exist in the one case when it does not exist in the other. In other words, not only is it necessary that morally acceptable clinical trials be effective and efficient, it must also be the case that conducting a clinical trial represents the most effective and efficient means of addressing the healthcare needs of a particular population.

The short course AZT trials have generated a lengthy and trenchant debate because they are open to reasonable challenges on a variety of fronts at both of these levels. As a result, I agree with those who remind us that tough cases generally make bad policy. The local *de facto* standard of care may be attractive for the way it promises a simple solution to this complex debate, but this simplicity is purchased at the price of important ethical principles. I have tried to argue that the local *de jure* standard of care may not yield as simple a solution as either its proponents or its critics may think, but that this is itself an exciting discovery. The possibility that both sides of this debate may be able to articulate their concerns within a shared framework holds out the possibility of moving beyond the present state of affairs in which the proponents of different standards of care appear only to be entrenching and fortifying their positions. I hope that the present study is sufficient to show that the work it will take to explore the complexities of the *de jure* standard, and its implications for the short-course AZT studies and future international research, is important, and remains to be done.

REFERENCES

Angell, M. (1997). 'The ethics of clinical research in the third world,' *New England Journal of Medicine* 337, 847–849.

Crouch, R.A. and J.D. Arras (1998). 'AZT trials and tribulations,' *Hastings Center Report* 28, 26–34.

Freedman, B. (1990). 'Placebo-controlled trials and the logic of clinical purpose,' *IRB: A Review of Human Subjects Research* 12, 1–6.

Freedman, B. (1987). 'Equipoise and the ethics of clinical research,' *New England Journal of Medicine* 317, 141–145.

Levine, R.J. (1999). 'The need to revise the Declaration of Helsinki,' *The New England Journal of Medicine* 341, 531–534.

Levine, R.J. (1998). 'The "best proven therapeutic method" standard in clinical trials in technologically developing countries,' *IRB: A Review of Human Subjects Research* 20, 5–9.

Lurie, P. and S.M. Wolfe (1997). 'Unethical trials of interventions to reduce perinatal transmission of the Human Immunodeficiency Virus in developing countries,' *New England Journal of Medicine* 337, 853–856.

RESEARCH IN DEVELOPING COUNTRIES: TAKING "BENEFIT" SERIOUSLY

Leonard H. Glantz, George J. Annas, Michael A. Grodin and Wendy K. Mariner

An April 1998 *New York Times Magazine* article described Ronald Munger's efforts to obtain blood samples from a group of extremely impoverished people in the Philippine island of Cebu.[1] Munger sought the blood to study whether there was a genetic cause for this group's unusually high incidence of cleft lip and palate. One of many obstacles to the research project was the need to obtain the cooperation of the local health officer. It was not clear to Munger, or the reader, whether the health officer had a bona fide interest in protecting the populace or was looking for a bribe. The health officer asked Munger a few perfunctory questions about informed consent and the study's ethical review in the United States, which Munger answered. Munger also explained the benefits that mothers and children would derive from participating in the research. The mothers would learn their blood types (which they apparently desired) and whether they were anemic. If they were anemic, they would be given iron pills. Lunch would be served, and raffles arranged so that families could win simple toys and other small items.

Munger told the health officer that if his hypotheses were correct, the research would benefit the population of Cebu: if the research shows that increased folate and vitamin B6 reduces the risk of cleft lip and palate, families could reduce the risk of facial deformities in their future offspring. The reporter noted that the health officer "laughs aloud at the suggestion that much of what is being discovered in American laboratories will make it back to Cebu any time soon." Reflecting on his experience with another simple intervention, iodized salt, the health officer said that when salt was iodized, the price rose threefold "so those who need it couldn't afford it and those who didn't need it are the only ones who could afford it."

The simple blood collecting mission to Cebu illustrates almost all the issues presented by research in developing countries. First is the threshold question of the goal of the research and its importance to the population represented by the research subjects. Next is the quality of informed consent including whether the potential subjects thought that participation in the research was related to free surgical care that was offered in the same facility (although it clearly was not) and whether one could adequately explain genetic hypotheses to an uneducated populace. Finally, there is the question whether the population from which subjects were drawn could benefit from the research. This research intervention is very low risk—the collection of 10 drops of blood from affected people and their family members. The risk of job or insurance discrimination that genetic research poses in this country did not exist for the Cebu population; ironically, they were protected from the risk of economic discrimination by the profound poverty in which they lived.

Even this simple study raises the most fundamental question: "Why is it acceptable for researchers in developed countries to use citizens of developing countries as research subjects?" A cautionary approach to permitting research with human subjects in underdeveloped countries has been recommended because of the risk of their inadvertent or deliberate exploitation by researchers from developed countries. This cautionary approach generally is invoked when researchers propose to use what are considered "vulnerable populations," such as prisoners and children, as research subjects. Vulnerable populations are those that are less able to protect themselves, either because they are not capable of making their own decisions or because

Reprinted with permission from *Hastings Center Report* 28, no. 6 (1998): 38–42.

Editor's note: Some footnotes have been deleted. Students who want to follow up on sources should consult the original article.

they are particularly susceptible to mistreatment. For example, children may be incapable of giving informed consent or of standing up to adult authority, while prisoners are especially vulnerable to being coerced into becoming subjects. Citizens of developing countries are often in vulnerable situations because of their lack of political power, lack of education, unfamiliarity with medical interventions, extreme poverty, or dire need for health care and nutrition. It is the dire need of these populations that may make them both appropriate subjects of research and especially vulnerable to exploitation. This combination of need and vulnerability has led to the development of guidelines for the use of citizens of developing countries as research subjects.

CIOMS GUIDELINES

In 1992, the Council for International Organizations of Medical Sciences (CIOMS), in collaboration with the World Health Organization, published guidelines for the appropriate use of research subjects from "underdeveloped communities."

Like other human research codes, the CIOMS guidelines combine the protection of subjects' rights with protection of their welfare; as subjects become less able to protect their own rights (and therefore become more vulnerable), researchers and reviewers must increase their efforts to protect the welfare of subjects. Perhaps the most important statement in these guidelines is what appears to be the injunction against using subjects in developing countries if the research could be carried out reasonably well in developed countries. Commentary to guideline 8 notes, for example, that there are diseases that rarely or never occur in economically developed countries, and that prevention and treatment research therefore needs to be conducted in the countries at risk for those diseases. The conclusion to be drawn from the substance of these guidelines is that in order for research to be ethically conducted, it must offer the potential of actual benefit to the inhabitants of that developing country.

In order for underdeveloped communities to derive potential benefit from research, they must have access to the fruits of such research. The CIOMS commentary to guideline 8 states that, "as a general rule, the sponsoring agency should ensure that, at the completion of successful testing, any product developed *will* be made reasonably available to inhabitants of the underdeveloped community in which the research was carried out: exceptions to this general requirement should be justified, and agreed to by all concerned parties before the research is begun." This statement is directed at minimizing exploitation of the underdeveloped community that provides the research subjects. If developed countries use inhabitants of underdeveloped countries to create new products that would be beneficial to both the developed and the underdeveloped country, but the underdeveloped country cannot gain access to the product because of expense, then the subjects in the underdeveloped countries have been grossly exploited. As written, however, this CIOMS guideline is not strong or specific enough to prevent exploitation. Exemplifying this problem are recent short course zidovudine (AZT) studies in Africa that were approved and conducted despite the existence of the CIOMS guidelines.

THE AFRICAN MATERNAL-FETAL HIV TRANSMISSION STUDIES

The goal of the short course AZT studies was to see if lower doses of the drug AZT than those used in the United States could reduce the rate of maternal-child transmission of HIV. It was well established that doses of AZT that cost $800 (not taking into account screening and other related costs) reduced maternal-fetal transmission of HIV by as much as two-thirds in the United States. If the developed countries had been willing to subsidize the cost of this regimen in Africa, no additional research would have been needed. But because many African countries could not afford this expense, the decision was made to attempt to see if lower (and therefore cheaper) doses would prevent maternal-fetal HIV transmission. Several impoverished countries were chosen as research sites. The justification for conducting research in those countries was not that they suffered from a disease that did not afflict people in developed countries, and not because no treatment existed, but because their impoverishment made an existing therapy unavailable to them (as long as developed countries refused to subsidize the costs).

The issue, as always, is to determine the ethical acceptability of the proposed research *before* it is conducted. In a case like this, where the researchable problem exists *solely* because of economic reasons, the research hypothesis must contain an economic component. The research question should be formulated as follows:

1. We know that a given regimen of AZT will reduce the rate of maternal-child transmission of HIV.
2. Maternal-child transmission of HIV in many African countries is a serious problem but the effective AZT regimen is not available because it is too expensive.
3. If an effective AZT regimen costs $X, then it will be made available in the country in which it is to be studied.
4. Therefore, we will conduct trials in certain African countries to see if $X worth of AZT will effectively reduce maternal-child transmission of HIV in those countries.

The most important part of the development of this research question is number 3. Without knowing what dollar amount X actually represents, it is impossible to formulate a research question that can lead to any benefit to the citizens of the country in which the research is to be conducted. There is no way to determine what $X represents in the absence of committed funding. Therefore, an essential prerequisite to designing ethical research in underdeveloped countries is identifying the source and amount of funding for providing the fruits of the research to the people of the developing country in which it is to be studied as a condition of the research being approved.

If a study found, for example, that $50 worth of AZT has the same effect as $800 worth of AZT, it would greatly benefit the developed world. Developed countries, which currently spend $800 per case on drugs alone, could pay substantially less for this preventive measure, and, because the research was conducted elsewhere, none of their citizens would have been put at any risk. At the same time, if the underdeveloped country could not afford to spend $50 any more than it could spend $800, then it could not possibly derive information that would be of any benefit to its population. This is the definition of exploitation.[2]

It is only now that an effort is being made to determine how to raise the money to actually provide AZT to prevent maternal-child HIV transmission (as well as the other costly services that go with the appropriate administration of the drug) to the impoverished African countries that provided the human subjects. These efforts began after parallel studies conducted in Thailand reported that lower doses of AZT reduced maternal-fetal transmission of HIV. The Thai government had committed to providing the AZT before its trials began. In the African trials, however, no one "ensured" that at the completion of successful testing the product would be made reasonably available, thereby violating the CIOMS guidelines. The guidelines say that there can be exceptions to this general requirement, but that exceptions must be "justified" and "agreed to by all concerned parties." It is not clear to whom the exception must be "justified" or on what grounds. Moreover, if the "concerned parties" are the sponsor and/or the investigator and the host country, they may not adequately represent the interests of the research subjects. The fact that representatives of the research community and officials of the host countries agree to exploit the population does not make the research any less exploitive.

RULES FOR ETHICAL RESEARCH IN DEVELOPING COUNTRIES

We believe the standards for research in developing countries should include the following.

There should be a rebuttable presumption that researchers from developed countries will not conduct research in developing countries unless it can be shown that a direct benefit *will* be bestowed upon the residents of that country if the research proves to be successful. The person or entities proposing to conduct the study must demonstrate that there is a realistic plan, which includes identified funding, to provide the newly proven intervention to the population from which the potential pool of research subjects is to be recruited. In the absence of a realistic plan and identified funding, the population from which the research subjects will be drawn cannot derive benefit from the research. Therefore, the benefits cannot outweigh the risks, because there are, and will be, no benefits. Only by having committed funding and a plan to make a successful intervention available can it be determined that there will be sufficient benefit to justify conducting research on the target population. The distribution plan must be realistic. Where the health care infrastucture is so undeveloped that it would be impossible to deliver the intervention even if it were free, research would be unjustified in the absence of a plan to improve that country's health care delivery capabilities.

Some might argue that this standard is too strict and that it would reduce the amount of research that could be conducted in certain countries. The answer, of course, is that if the benefits of the research are not made available to the inhabitants of that country, they have lost nothing by the lack of such research. Others might argue that research in underdeveloped countries is justified if it might benefit the individual research subjects, even if it will not benefit anyone else in the population. However, research is, by definition, designed to create generalizable knowledge, and is legitimate in a developing country only if its purpose is to create generalizable knowledge that will benefit the citizens of that country. If the research only has the potential to benefit the limited number of individuals who participate in the study, it cannot offer the benefit to the underdeveloped country that legitimizes the use of its citizens as research subjects. It should be emphasized that research whose goal is to prevent or treat large populations is fundamentally public health research, and public health research makes no sense (and thus should not be done) if its benefits are limited to the small population of research subjects.

It might be argued that there is no requirement that such a plan be devised prior to conducting research in the United States, and, therefore, that by adopting such a requirement we would be imposing a higher standard for research conducted in developing countries than we do for research conducted in the United States.

This argument only further demonstrates the differences between wealthy and poor countries. The reality in the United States is that regardless of the very significant gaps in insurance and Medicaid coverage and the health care discrepancies between the rich and poor, medical interventions are relatively widely available, especially when compared to developing countries. Upon the successful completion of the research that demonstrated the effectiveness of the 076 regimen in reducing maternal-child transmission, the primary beneficiaries of this new preventive intervention in the United States were poor women and their newborns. Unlike the United States, absent a plan to pay for a new intervention and lacking the infrastructure to deliver an intervention, it is virtually guaranteed that the intervention will not be generally available in a developing country.

The more accurate analogy to the African AIDS trials would be if investigators proposed the 076 protocol in the United States knowing that only poor women would be recruited as research subjects and that, if successful, the intervention would not be made generally available to poor women. Such research would be clearly unethical. Not only would this be a gross violation of the ethical principle of distributive justice, it would be a violation of the regulatory obligation of the equitable selection of subjects.

A further objection is that one cannot always trust what a government or another potential funder promises. What is to prevent the promisor from reneging? The answer is, nothing. One can try to expose the funder to embarrassment and other pressures that might cause it to live up to the promise upon which researchers and subjects relied. However, the potential unethical behavior in the future by the funder is no excuse for not having a realistic plan at the outset. Furthermore, if we take this obligation seriously, this should only occur once per funder. After reneging once, they cannot be relied upon again to justify research in the future.

An additional objection to our position is that it will restrict access to new interventions because once a new intervention is developed, the price will come down and therefore the intervention will become available to the people of the impoverished country. The answer is to ask those who control the pricing of interventions if this will be the case in any particular instance. One could have asked Glaxo if it would reduce its price once it was shown that lower doses of AZT were effective. If the answer is yes, one can proceed. If the answer is no, or "we have not decided," there seems to be no justification to proceed if the current price would significantly restrict availability. There is nothing magical about pricing. Pricing is in the absolute control of manufacturers and there is no need to guess or speculate about what will happen to price. Indeed, this objection to our argument would justify conducting the full 076 trial itself in developing countries. The price *might* come down enough so that determining the efficacy of short course AZT regimens might not be needed at all. Such speculation should not be sufficient to put subjects at risk.

Finally, it might be argued that there are diseases that only affect people in developing countries for which there are no effective treatments, but that the treatments that might be discovered could be expensive. The argument continues that it is not right to fail to develop treatments that could benefit some affected people because it will not be available to most affected people. This objection raises quite a different issue from the one addressed in this article. The impetus for such research is the absence of effective treatment and not the absence of economic resources. We have discussed research intended to determine whether effective but unaffordable interventions would work if used in lower, less expensive dosages. The researchable issue arises from an economic circumstance. The only way such research could offer any benefit is by "curing" the economic problem by establishing that the less expensive form of the intervention will be affordable and available. Absent knowledge of financial resources, one might well be creating a new unaffordable, and therefore useless, intervention. In contrast, in the case in which one is developing a new intervention, not because of poverty; but because no known effective intervention exists, and the disease is prevalent in a particular geographic area, the issue is quite different. In such a case one is not conducting research to try to "cure" the effects of poverty but rather because of the need to create new knowledge to treat a currently untreatable disease. However, even this case may raise problems similar to the ones addressed here. If one were to try to develop an intervention for such a condition and chose research subjects from impoverished segments of a society, knowing that only the richest segment of that society could benefit from that intervention, such subject selection would be unethical for many of the reasons we have discussed.

Our proposal to require researchers and their funders to develop realistic plans to make their interventions available to the relevant population of the developing country in which the research is proposed should not be controversial. It is well accepted in principle not only by groups like CIOMS, but by the funders of many of the African HIV trials, including the Centers for Disease Control and Prevention and the National Institutes of Health. The principle is often honored in the breach, however. Research funders who hope that their studies will yield beneficial knowledge may neglect the steps necessary to ensure that the benefits will be made available. Ethical codes have not been sufficiently specific or enforceable to protect research subjects from exploitation. It is essential to replace vague promises with realistic plans that must be reviewed and approved before the research commences.

In at least one other instance it has been suggested that economic issues be addressed in the review of proposed research projects. The U.S. National Research Council's Committee on Human Genome Diversity recommended that "Arrangements regarding financial interests in the products or outcomes of the research should be negotiated *as part of the original project review* and informed-consent process."[3]

It is essential that the wealthier countries of the world use their resources, both financial and technological, to help resolve the health problems that afflict the poor of the world. Doing so will undoubtedly require research. But research is a means to solving health problems, not an end in itself. The goal must be to create interventions that will benefit the people of the countries in which the research is conducted. They will benefit only if the knowledge gained produces interventions that are affordable and accessible. This needs to be determined as a condition of approval before research is conducted so that limited research funds are not wasted, and research subjects are not drawn from populations that will not be able to benefit from the research.

REFERENCES

1. Lisa Belkin, "The Clues Are in the Blood," *New York Times Magazine*, 26 April 1998.
2. The per capita health care expenditures of most of the African countries involved in mother-to-child HIV

transmission prevention trials range from $5 to $22 U.S. *World Bank Sector Strategy Health Nutrition and Population*, 1997.

3. Committee on Human Genetic Diversity, *Evaluating Human Genetic Diversity* (Washington, D.C.: National Academy Press, 1997), pp. 55–68, 65.

RESEARCH ON CHILDREN AND OTHER "VULNERABLE" POPULATIONS

CHILDREN AND "MINIMAL RISK" RESEARCH: THE KENNEDY-KRIEGER LEAD PAINT STUDY

Alex John London

In 1993 the Kennedy Krieger Institute (KKI), a Johns Hopkins affiliated children's hospital and research center, received a $200,000 grant from the U.S. Environmental Protection Agency to study the short and long-term efficacy of several different strategies for removing or containing lead-paint in residential housing units in Baltimore City. For researchers at the prestigious research center, the grant represented an important step in the KKI's ongoing fight to encourage a more proactive approach to preventing lead poisoning in children. In August of 2001, however, less than a decade after the study's inception, the Maryland Court of Appeals would compare the study to some of the darkest and most troubling abuses of human subjects in history, including the Tuskegee Syphilis Study and the typhus experiments at Buchenwald concentration camp during World War II.[1]

Unlike many industrialized nations that banned the use of lead paint for interior use at the dawn of the twentieth century, it was not until 1978 that the U.S. outlawed its use. As a result, even in early 1990's it was estimated that 35–40% of children from low-income inner-city neighborhoods nationwide had dangerous levels of lead in their blood, compared to only 5% of non-Hispanic white children living outside of city centers. In some urban areas the prevalence of lead paint in low-income housing was particularly high. Researchers from the KKI estimated that as many as 95% of the low-income housing units in Baltimore's inner city neighborhoods were contaminated with lead paint and the number of children from those neighborhoods with elevated blood lead levels was estimated to be as high as two thirds. Children are at special risk for lead poisoning because their high

1. *Erika Grimes* v. *Kennedy Krieger Institute, Inc. Myron Higgins, a minor, etc., et al.* v. *Kennedy Krieger Institute, Inc.* No. 128, No. 129 Court Appeals of Maryland, 2001 Md. August 16,2001, Filed.

rate of hand-to-mouth activity increases the likelihood that they will ingest the lead-contaminated dust generated by deteriorating paints. When lead is absorbed into their bodies it can adversely affect their cognitive development, behavior, and growth. In fact, extremely high levels of lead can precipitate seizures, coma, and even death.

Safely removing lead paint from home interiors poses special challenges. In the late 1980's researchers at the KKI helped to show that traditional methods of removing lead paint—burning or scraping it off—actually generated large amounts of contaminated dust, thereby exacerbating the hazard for the children who would occupy those homes. New methods of abatement would have to be developed that would provide safer methods of removing or containing the hazard posed by the poisonous paint. In addition, in urban settings where affordable low-income housing is at a premium, the cost of removing lead from rental units frequently exceeds the value of the properties themselves. When faced with the financial burdens of abating what are often only marginally profitable properties in the first place, many landlords chose simply to close their properties and leave them unoccupied. In 1990 the Department of Housing and Urban Development estimated the cost of complete lead abatement nationwide at roughly $500 billion.

Prior to the 1993 study, researchers at the KKI had shown that several more economical strategies for removing or controlling lead paint could effectively reduce the amount of lead-contaminated dust in empty houses. In order to know whether these strategies would translate into a similar reduction of lead poisoning in children, researchers wanted to measure the effectiveness of these strategies in terms of their impact on the blood lead levels of children who would occupy such units. The 1993 study would therefore measure lead levels in household dust and in the blood of children residing in housing units involved in the study.

The study included 75 housing units that were divided into five groups. Group I houses received a minimal level of repair and maintenance costing approximately $1,650. Group II houses received a greater level of repair and maintenance costing approximately $3,500. Repair and maintenance in Group III houses was more extensive and cost between $6,000 and $7,000. The study also included two control groups. Group IV properties consisted of houses that had been fully abated by the city under a local government program. Because of the extent of this previous abatement, these properties received no additional repair or maintenance. Finally, Group V properties were modern units constructed after 1980 in which it could reasonably be assumed that no lead paints had been used.

Researchers from the KKI worked with landlords to obtain grants and loans to fund these repairs. In many cases the properties were already occupied by families prior to the inception of the study, but when properties were vacant, landlords were encouraged to rent to families with small children. In all cases, researchers were looking for families with healthy children between 5 and 48 months old who did not have plans to leave the properties before the study was completed. Parents were asked to sign consent forms in which they were informed that the purpose of the study was to measure the effectiveness of repairs that were intended to reduce, but not to completely remove, the lead exposure in their home. In return for their participation they received small payments of $5 and $15 and they were told that the KKI would provide them with the results of the periodic blood lead testing.

To the researchers conducting the study, this was a win-win situation.[2] Every property in the study had received what they believed was a significant level of lead abatement and, as a result, the families residing in those properties faced lower risks than they would have experienced if they had lived in comparable properties that had not been so repaired. Additionally, the data generated by this study would provide valuable information about the efficacy of more affordable measures of reducing and controlling lead exposure for reducing child lead poisoning. If successful, these measures would offer significant and affordable means of reducing a widespread public health hazard that disproportionately affects the poorest and most vulnerable populations of children in the U.S.

---

2. See the "Lead-Based Paint Study Fact Sheet" published on the Johns Hopkins School of Medicine web page at: http://www.hopkinsmedicine.org/press/2001/SEPTEMBER/leadfactsheet.htm

Some of the families that participated in the study had different views. Two families in particular brought law suits against the KKI alleging that their respective children were poisoned, or were at least exposed to the risk of being poisoned, by lead dust due to the negligence of the KKI researchers. They also alleged that they were not fully informed of the risks of the research and that the KM failed to warn them in a timely manner of the children's exposure to the known presence of lead. In August of 2001 the Maryland Court of Appeals unanimously overturned a lower court decision that would have barred the suits from going forward. Six of the seven judges signed on to an opinion that offered a sweeping indictment of the lead paint study.

Writing for these six judges, Judge Dale R. Cathell criticized the basic design of the study:

> Otherwise healthy children, in our view, should not be enticed into living in, or remaining in, potentially lead-tainted housing and intentionally subjected to a research program, which contemplates the probability, or even the possibility, of lead poisoning or even the accumulation of lower levels of lead in blood, in order for the extent of the contamination of the children's blood to be used by scientific researchers to assess the success of lead paint or lead dust abatement measures (p. 7).

To the court, the language of the consent form did not provide a clear and complete explanation that the purpose of the study was to measure the efficacy of the abatement procedures by measuring the extent to which the children's blood was being contaminated. As a result, it was not clear that the parents understood that the very design of the research presupposed the accumulation of lead in their children's blood.

The extent to which the families that participated in this study understood its design and purpose is a question that was disputed before the court. Judge Cathell was clear, however, that in the court's view "parents, whether improperly enticed by trinkets, food stamps, money or other items, have no more right to intentionally and unnecessarily place children in potentially hazardous nontherapeutic research surroundings, than do researchers. In such cases, parental consent, no matter how informed, is insufficient" (p. 7). In fact, the majority went even further, stating that, "We hold that in Maryland a parent, appropriate relative, or other applicable surrogate, cannot consent to the participation of a child or other person under legal disability in nontherapeutic research or studies in which there is any risk of injury or damage to the health of the subject" (pp. 89–90).

As a result of this decision, the substantive legal issues raised by these lawsuits will be argued before a trial court. But many observers were surprised by the scope and severity of the Appeals Court opinion. In the estimation of the court, the KKI lead paint study was similar to research abuses of the past in which vulnerable populations were knowingly subjected to harmful or poisonous substances, not for some direct benefit to themselves, but in order to generate generalizable scientific data. Those who agree with the court will argue that children from low-income inner city families are already disadvantaged in ways that their more affluent middle and upper class counterparts are not. The high prevalence of lead in their living quarters, and the significant threat it poses to their mental and physical health, is simply one particularly visible way in which the opportunity range of these children is unfairly limited by their poverty. Why should the fact that poverty consigns many of these children to toxic housing conditions justify providing them with less stringent research protections than would be extended to children from more affluent and socially mobile families? Does their poverty and lower-income social status make the lead to which they were exposed in this study less toxic, or the risks to their health less profound or important?

In defense of this study, the KKI has argued that the methods they employed "were then believed to be the best practices within high-risk housing" and that the interventions and follow up provided by the study "were greater than those children would have received without the Study and likely would not have occurred without the Study." They estimate that the lead reduction measures implemented in these properties improved them by approximately 80% over all other existing housing alternatives in these neighborhoods. They also note that "The Court was silent with respect to the obligations of various levels of government that tolerated the evidence of lead paint for decades, and a society that does not offer realistic options for low income families to move out of high risk neighborhoods."

Relative to the thousands of families living in non-abated houses, the subjects of this study could reasonably be said to have benefited by their participation. Furthermore, one reason for the inaction of the public and private sectors in the face of this pervasive public health hazard is a reluctance to pay the high cost of lead abatement procedures whose relative merits over less expensive alternatives have not been clearly quantified. From this point of view, the KKI can be seen as a well-intentioned agent of social reform seeking to provide clear data on effective means of curbing a public health problem that will otherwise persist and continue to damage the lives of innocent lower-income inner-city children.

In ruling that parents and guardians cannot consent to the participation of children in research that poses *any* degree of risk, the Maryland Court of Appeals enunciated an ideal for research protections that could threaten the permissibility of important pediatric research. Is this standard too high? The current federal regulations permit research on children that is a minor increment over minimal risk, where minimal risk is defined as "the probability and magnitude of harm or discomfort anticipated in the research are not greater in and of themselves than those ordinarily encountered in daily life or during the performance of routine physical or psychological examinations or tests." Would the KKI lead paint study be permissible in high-risk neighborhoods of Baltimore City, but not in newer, wealthier suburbs, because the inner city children are exposed to higher risks of lead poisoning in their daily lives whereas their suburban counterparts are not?

Even after the legal questions raised by this case are settled, other ethical issues will likely remain. In particular, this case raises troubling questions about the role of research into health problems that are due, in large part, to social and economic inequalities between populations. When the ultimate goal is to get local and federal agencies to spend the money it will take to alleviate the lead hazards in low-income neighborhoods, is it permissible to conduct research in which the protections afforded to subjects fall below standards that are enjoyed by wealthier members of society? Should the way a trial is designed be determined by whether or not the social will exists to spend significant amounts of money to improve the housing conditions of largely low-income inner city populations? Is there a guarantee that the social will exists to spend smaller, but still significant amounts of money to reduce, but not eliminate such hazards? Should it be required before such research can begin that there be an agreement in place guaranteeing that some money will be spent to implement an effective lead abatement strategy in the places where research is conducted? In criticizing the design of this study are critics washing their hands of the larger public health and social justice issues that the researchers were hoping this study would address?

While the Court of Appeals compared the KKI study to the infamous Tuskegee Syphilis Study, the above questions suggest that a more instructive comparison might be the internationally sponsored short course AZT trials that were conducted in developing countries in collaboration with entities from the developed world (See Part 5, Section 3). In both cases the proposed research was designed to be responsive to a health problem that disproportionately affects one population, but not some others. Furthermore, in both cases a major reason for this difference is economic. Many developing countries cannot afford the full course of AZT—known as the 076 protocol—that is the current standard of care in the developed world. In response, researchers designed a study to find a shorter and more economical regimen of AZT that would offer some significant, but not optimal, protection against mother-to-child transmission of HIV. Similarly, many low-income inner city families cannot afford to pay for complete lead abatement or to move to safer, but more expensive, housing. In response, researchers from the KKI designed a study to quantify the efficacy of several affordable methods of removing or controlling lead paint exposure in low-income housing units without removing the hazard completely. Is this a fair comparison? Does it make a difference to the moral evaluation of these studies that many of the countries that hosted the short-course AZT trials are themselves technologically and economically underdeveloped whereas the U.S. is one of, if not the, wealthiest and most technologically advanced nation in the world?

As medical research is deployed to alleviate health problems that are rooted in economic disparities between populations, the line between studying an illness or disease and exploiting economic deprivations is blurred. As more is learned about the social determinants of health and the impact of social inequalities on health status, the more pressing these issues will become. One of the challenges posed by the Kennedy Krieger lead paint study, and the short course AZT studies, is to find a framework for evaluating clinical research that is responsive to these realities, and to the important moral principles they bring into conflict.

RESEARCH ON CHILDREN AND THE SCOPE OF RESPONSIBLE PARENTHOOD

Thomas H. Murray

The voluntary consent of the human subject is absolutely essential.

—The Nuremberg Code

To attempt to consent for a child to be made an experimental subject is to treat a child as not a child. . . . If the grounds for this are alleged to be the presumptive or implied consent of the child, that must simply be characterized as a violent and false presumption.

—Paul Ramsey, *The Patient as Person*

Consent is the heart of the matter.

—Richard McCormick, "Proxy Consent in the Experimentation Situation"

What obligations do parents have to their children? On the whole, bioethics has not grappled with the nuances of parental obligations and duties. Sometimes its treatment of issues even seems to lack common sense. Part of the problem has been that bioethicists have considered mostly life-or-death decisions. But sometimes we create our own difficulty by the way we frame the problem. Nowhere has this been more true than in discussions of research on children, in which a history of morally abominable research, mostly on adults, led to the problem—and solution—being framed in terms that were simply irrelevant to children.

When the tools we have at hand are poorly suited for the job, the work is more difficult and the result inferior. We have some useful distinctions for understanding the ethics of research on children. But we have also been stuck with some downright clumsy contraptions. The problems become inescapable when we try to make sense of a morally complex proposal, like one to study the impact of human growth hormone on children with short stature.

A CONTROVERSIAL STUDY OF GROWTH HORMONE

Our bodies produce human growth hormone, or hGH, as part of the normal processes of growth. Children whose bodies cannot produce it do not grow as do other children. Unless they receive hGH somehow, they will become adults with extremely short stature. In a society that values height, those children can suffer severe disadvantages and discrimination.

But not all short children lack hGH. Height is like many other natural characteristics: people vary in how much of it they have. A few are very tall or very short; some are a bit taller or shorter than average; most are near the average. Some of the children who are much shorter than average have no

Reprinted with permission from Thomas H. Murray, *The Worth of a Child* (Berkeley, CA: University of California Press, 1996), pp. 70–95, 194–195.

Editor's note: Most footnotes have been deleted. Students who want to follow up on sources should consult the original article.

discernible lack of hGH. Nor do they have any of the other signs that often accompany dwarfism caused by the absence of hGH. They are short, in all likelihood, because their parents are short, just as other children are well muscled because their parents are well muscled.

The quandary is this: short stature is a problem for children and adults not merely when it is a disease. In a world constructed for adults of a particular height range, being short enough (or, for that matter, tall enough) to fill outside the range is like having a disability. The world is harder to navigate when you are the "wrong" size. There is nothing intrinsically wrong with being substantially shorter or taller than average; the world could be made to fit a broader range of sizes. But for now at least it is not. And so extreme short stature can be a disability.

For most short children, the problem takes another form. Parents understand that short stature can make life tougher for their child; children can be very cruel to those who look or act "different." Furthermore, the adult world is "heightist." Tall people get many advantages, just by virtue of their height. Most parents want to give their children whatever advantages they can. If they can make a short child taller, why not? Many parents seem to have reasoned this way, because many have sought growth hormone for their children who are not lacking it but who are nonetheless short.

The increasing use of hGH for children who are not hGH-deficient prompted the National Institutes of Health (NIH) to approve a research project to study the effects of hGH injections on such children. The study raised enough questions that NIH asked a special panel to consider its ethical acceptability.

The study was originally planned to include eighty children ages nine through fifteen with normal levels of hGH but well below average height for their age. Each child receives three injections a week for as long as seven years. The study has a control group. Children in that group are treated exactly like the children in the experimental group, except that the injections they receive—600 to 1,100 over the life of the study—contain no hGH. Let me put that another way: None of the children in this study were ill. Some of them will receive as many as one thousand or more injections of a potent hormone; the others will get the same number of shots of salt water.

The special panel concluded that this study was acceptable. The panel's reasoning clung closely to the language of the regulations governing research on children. There are problems with the panel's strategy. A good ethical result is unlikely if the regulations lack a sound moral foundation. When we lack vigorous moral concepts for analyzing problems, we are tempted to take refuge in legalisms. A look at the moral debate at the time the regulations were written reveals that they were built on a flawed effort to understand the ethics of research with children.

THE NATIONAL COMMISSION AND THE NUREMBERG CODE

Research on children covers a lot of moral ground. When a child has a grave disease and there is no good standard treatment, the child's only hope may be an experimental therapy. The novel therapy might carry its own substantial risks. But if previous research indicates that the experimental treatment is promising, and there is no solid alternative, then involvement of that child in research makes good moral sense. What makes the case persuasive is the hope that the particular child may benefit.

The ethics of research become more complex as the possibility of benefit to each of the children involved in the research becomes murkier. There are moral complexities, to be sure, when parents are asked to allow an experimental therapy to be used on their child who is suffering from disease. In most relevant respects, though, such a decision is not that different from other choices parents must make about treatment for their ill child. The uncertainty involved in experimental treatments is greater, of course, but we can never eliminate uncertainty. The crucial question in acceding to either standard or experimental treatment is the same: Will this benefit my child?

Another class of research studies has been more controversial: so-called nontherapeutic research, or in plainer language, research intended to gain knowledge but not to benefit its subjects directly. For example, the parents of a healthy, normal newborn might be asked to allow their child to serve as a control subject in a study of the physiology of some awful disease that strikes other babies. Perhaps the researchers want to monitor your baby's blood pressure more carefully than would otherwise be done for a healthy newborn; perhaps they want to draw an extra drop of blood from a heel prick, or a sample of blood from a vein; or perhaps in a study of infant heart disease, they want to insert a catheter through your baby's artery and into the heart, where they can measure changes in pressures and gas concentrations while they administer powerful drugs. It does not require much sophistication in ethics or science to notice great differences between the last experiment and the others. What would moral common sense say about these proposed studies?

If we were assured that there was no risk of harm or discomfort in the first proposed study—more frequent monitoring of blood pressure—indeed that the baby would not even notice it, then we might well agree to allow our newborn to participate in the study. Even if we refused, it is difficult to see what criticisms could be made of parents who did agree. Parents who allow their children to be observed in this manner do not seem to be failing in any important parental duty.

At the other extreme, we would be highly suspicious if parents consented to exposing their healthy babies to the pain and risk of having catheters threaded into their hearts and given powerful drugs, all with no conceivable benefit to their child. We might suspect that the parents did not understand what was to be done to their babies, or were so blinded by awe or gratitude that they were powerless to refuse; or, if they did understand the risks, that they were lousy parents who were not protecting their infant from a completely unnecessary risk of grave harm.

Such were the issues facing the members of the National Commission for the Protection of the Human Subjects of Biomedical and Behavioral Research when they developed their recommendations regarding the ethics of research on children. Should parents be prohibited from consenting to any research that held no hope of benefiting their children? Or should such research be permitted, with restrictions and safeguards?

As with any reasonably complex issue, many morally relevant questions arise. The ones of greatest interest to us are the nature and scope of parents' obligations to their children and in particular whether parents are ever justified in allowing their child to be used to benefit the community. Must we always refuse to expose our children to any risks or discomforts except when they might benefit our child? In the absence of any substantial risk or discomfort, do we wrong our children by allowing them to be used for others' benefit?

What makes this controversy particularly interesting for bioethics is that the most forceful, convincing argument was for banning all nontherapeutic research. Nonetheless, the commission adopted a more moderate stance allowing nontherapeutic research of children if the risks approximated those encountered in daily life and if parents consented. The commission accepted this policy even though the arguments supporting it were notably weaker than the arguments favoring a complete ban on such research. Paul Ramsey, a brilliant, acerbic, and relentless Protestant theologian championed a ban. Richard McCormick, equally brilliant, gave the most thorough defense of the moderate view Their exchange over this issue illuminates the moral obligations of parents toward their children, even as it exemplifies the dangers of moral reasoning that fails to give full weight to context—in this case, both the historical context that shaped discussions of the ethics of research with human beings and the social context of parent-child relationships.

Ramsey opened his discussion by citing in full a classic text in bioethics, the first article of what has come to be known as the Nuremberg Code. The first sentence of the article is the key: "The voluntary consent of the human subject is absolutely essential." The second sentence is also worth citing in full: "This means that the person involved should have legal capacity to give consent; should be so situated as to be able to exercise free power of choice, without the intervention of any element of force, fraud, deceit, duress, overreaching, or other ulterior form of constraint or coercion; and should have sufficient knowledge and comprehension of the elements of the subject matter as to enable him to make an understanding and enlightened decision."[1] The remainder of the article discusses the sort of information a subject should be given.

If we take the Nuremberg Code seriously—if we accept this first article as a firm moral rule governing research—the implications for research on children are straightforward: there will be none. If the consent of the subject is "absolutely essential" and if this requires that the person "have legal capacity to give consent" and be able to reach "an understanding rand enlightened decision," all infants and young children are disqualified along with all youth below the age of legal consent and all adults with significant mental impairments.

Note that this blanket prohibition makes no distinction between research intended to help the child—an innovative therapy, for example—and the nontherapeutic research that troubled the commission. If we followed strictly the Nuremberg Code, all medical experiments on children would be banned, including all studies of promising treatments for children dying from diseases like leukemia and brain cancer. This defies moral common sense. What prompted the drafters of the Nuremberg Code to make such a stark and unqualified declaration?

The Nuremberg Tribunal's task was to try people accused of war crimes. Confronted with overwhelming evidence of astoundingly cruel, almost unimaginable treatment of human beings in the name of science, the tribunal had to articulate a set of standards by which to judge the abominable conduct of the accused who came before it. Grave evil had been done. The catalog of horrors was long and gruesome: prisoners left naked in freezing weather, or immersed in near-freezing water until they lost consciousness or died; wounds inflicted, then exacerbated with glass fragments or dirt to simulate battle injuries; prisoners infected with typhus, some even used as human viral cultures; the list goes on.

Faced with such an unconscionable register of horrors inflicted on people who were captives in the first place and never given any choice whether to participate, there is little wonder why the Nuremberg judges adopted voluntary consent as a clear and ringing first principle. When dealing with unmitigated evil, subtlety and nuance are less important than firmness and clarity. They might have reasoned this way: the Nazi experiments were morally atrocious because they inflicted terrible harms on unconsenting victims; no reasonable person would ever consent to such treatment; insisting that no person be used without his or her voluntary consent prevents the evils of coercion and of excessively risky or harmful experiments; therefore, a policy of voluntary consent will prevent morally monstrous research, like the Nazi experiments, from occurring in the future.

The judges at Nuremberg were not formulating timeless and detailed rules to govern all scientific research. They needed a set of principles for a specific task—trying war criminals for their barbarous treatment of prisoners in what was called, often very loosely, "science." The principles they articulated, the Nuremberg Code, served their purposes very well. In putting it this way, I intend no criticism of the court. To the contrary, I believe they showed admirable wisdom in formulating moral standards for research that would become the starting point for all later efforts. We should not fault them for failing to answer questions they were not asked, questions such as, what to do about children or others incapable of giving consent, or whether it makes a morally important difference if the research may or may not be intended to benefit the subject. Later bodies could deal with such questions. The Nuremberg court's emphasis on consent, though, would color all subsequent efforts to understand the ethics of research with human subjects.

By the time the national commission deliberated on the ethics of research with children, a new distinction and a new concept had entered the discussion. The distinction was between research intended to benefit the subject and research with no such intention—what are commonly referred to as therapeutic research and nontherapeutic research. The concept was proxy consent, that is, consent by someone other than the subject who, presumably, knows what the subject would have wanted or has the subject's best interests at heart. Much ink and even a little (symbolic) blood has been spilled by bioethicists arguing over the meanings and significance of these two ideas. I have no desire to add to the deluge of words. What I want to do is to show how readily even the most perceptive thinker can become bewitched by ethical abstractions and how appreciating moral common sense and social context can, in the best sense, disenchant. To do that, though, we must revisit the debate in some detail.

PAUL RAMSEY AND THE RESPONSIBILITIES OF PARENTHOOD

In his influential book *The Patient as Person,* Paul Ramsey began with a chapter on the ethics of research with children. Contrasting research on humans with research on animals, Ramsey asserts,

"Any human being is more than a patient or experimental subject; he is a *personal* subject—every bit as much a man as the physician-investigator." He then links consent to the fidelity that should characterize relationships between persons: "The principle of an informed consent is the *canon of loyalty* joining men together in medical practice and investigation." Though his language and metaphors are drawn from theology rather than law, his debt to the Nuremberg judges seems clear. Ramsey, though, is fully aware of the quandary created by Nuremberg: how to justify therapeutic research with children. Should children's inability to give a mature and understanding consent deprive them of experimental treatments that might help them? Ramsey articulates a principle that he never abandons: "From consent as a canon of loyalty in medical practice it follows that children, who cannot give a mature and informed consent, . . . should not be made the subjects of medical experimentation unless . . . it is reasonable to believe that [the experimental therapy] may further *the patient's own recovery*."

Ramsey is suspicious of the idea of "proxy" consent. Certainly, it is necessary at times for someone to decide, on a child's behalf, whether to administer some treatment that might benefit the child. Ramsey is adamant about what such proxy consent could not be: "To attempt to consent for a child to be made an experimental subject is to treat a child as not a child. It is to treat him as if he were an adult person who has consented to become a joint adventurer in the common cause of medical research. If the grounds for this are alleged to be the presumptive or implied consent of the child, that must simply be characterized as a violent and false presumption." The parents' duty is to safeguard their child's welfare, to be their child's protector. But the parent's consent on behalf of the child is not morally equivalent to an adult's consent on his or her own behalf. An adult can consent to participate in a risky experiment, but, Ramsey claims, "no parent is morally competent to consent that his child shall be submitted to hazardous or other experiments having no diagnostic or therapeutic significance for the child himself."

Ramsey is correct that consent has a different moral significance when it comes from the person directly affected, rather than from another presuming to speak for that person. Consent is an extremely powerful moral warrant, particularly in a liberal secular society that gives enormous moral weight to individuals and their preferences. Why are you riding Emily's bike? She said it was OK. What right do you have to demand money from me? Because we have a contract. I paint your house; you pay me $2,000. It is not much of an exaggeration to say that for some persons, inducting a few moral theorists, consent functions as a universal moral solvent, dissolving all moral dilemmas; as long as there is consent, no further moral justification is needed. Not everyone believes this. Outside of a few doctrinaire libertarians, debates over the appropriate scope and limits of individual liberty are taken very seriously. Are contracts for surrogate motherhood legitimate expressions of individual liberty? Should we be permitted to sell our babies? Our kidneys?

Ramsey's argument is that however potent you think consent is in justifying particular actions, children are incapable of consent. Fictions such as "proxy" consent can only disguise that fact. When consent is a necessary condition for something being morally acceptable—as the Nuremberg Code suggests is true for medical research—it would always be morally wrong to perform that action without genuine consent. Children cannot consent to participate in research. Therefore, without some other compelling moral justification, children cannot be subjects in research. What other justification is possible? Pursuing the child's own welfare. Thus therapeutic research for children can be justified; nontherapeutic research on children cannot.

Ramsey's suspicion of proxy consent contrasts with his enthusiastic embrace of the distinction between research that does and does not benefit the child. He sees this as decisive: "What is at stake here is the covenantal obligations of parents to children—the protection with which a child should be surrounded, and the meaning and duties of parenthood. . . . The issue here is the wrong of making a human being subject." As always, Ramsey chooses his concepts with care: children made the subject of research with no benefit to themselves are wronged even if no harm comes to them. The analogous concept in a law is a battery, an unconsented touching, and Ramsey explicitly pursues the parallel.

Here is where Ramsey runs into difficulties. Because he makes consent a moral fulcrum, he is compelled to defend the proposition that all research on children, however innocuous, that is not done with the hope of benefiting its child-subjects, is immoral and violates "the meaning and duties of parenthood." Our task would be easier if we could consult an authoritative list of parental duties. Lacking such a list, Ramsey employs several strategies to persuade us that parental duties include the obligation to protect our children from nontherapeutic research, even riskless research. He appeals to our ideals of parenthood: "A parent's decisive concern," he writes, "is for the care and protection of the child, to whom he owes the highest fiduciary loyalty, even when he also appreciates the benefits to come to others from the investigation and might submit his own person to experiment in order to obtain them." He expresses skepticism that there could be a scientific experiment that did not exceed "the ordinary risks of daily living." He echoes Kant in stating that "fidelity to a human child also includes never treating him as a means only, but always also as an end." He launches the rhetorical equivalent of a nuclear weapon by suggesting, in a somewhat opaque passage, that research even with "no *discernible* risks . . . imposed on subjects for the sake of supposable or actual good to come" puts us "back with the Nazis." Finally, he acknowledges that the problem is "the *use* of children in research, in which the risks are minimal or 'negligible,' but still not in their behalf medically. It is hard to see how this can be an expression of parental care (or of the state's care *in loco parentis*), or anything other than a violation of the nature and meaning of the responsibilities of parenthood as a covenant among the generations of men."

Is permitting one's child to be a subject in a scientific study where the risks are minimal or negligible "a violation of the nature and meaning of the responsibilities of parenthood"? A frightfully strong and austere conclusion: Could there be some flaw in Ramsey's reasoning? The best contemporary effort to find such a flaw, Richard McCormick's defense of minimally risky research on children, was at best only a partial success.

RICHARD MCCORMICK AND "VICARIOUS CONSENT"

McCormick, a Roman Catholic theologian, agrees with Ramsey that "consent is the heart of the matter."[2] But he points out that we take parents' consent to their children's medical treatment to be morally justifiable: Why cannot parental consent work as well in justifying the involvement of children in research? Saying as Ramsey does that it would amount to treating the child as an object does not provide an answer.

McCormick employs the concept of "vicarious consent" which, he says, is a close relative of proxy consent. Vicarious consent, he argues, "is morally valid precisely insofar as it is a reasonable presumption of the child's wishes, a construction of what the child would wish could he consent for himself." Many children are too young to express their wishes; we are loath to accept a young child's wishes in any event, unless we believe that honoring a particular one would not be opposed to the child's best interest. McCormick asserts that a sound understanding of what a child would wish requires asking, "Why *would* the child so wish?" His answer: "[The child] would choose he were capable of choice because he *ought* to do so."

By now McCormick's difficulties are obvious. He has made consent the moral centerpiece of his case and is trying to rescue the moral authority of parental consent by equating what a child *would* want with what it *ought* to want. McCormick is not completely lost for intellectual resources to buttress his case. He calls on natural law theory, a position closely associated with Catholic theology. Focusing on the values and goods that constitute or promote our flourishing as humans, McCormick claims that two assertions account for our willingness to allow parents to consent to therapy for their children: "(a) that there are certain values . . . definitive of our good and flourishing, hence values that we *ought* to choose and support if we want to become and stay human, and that therefore these are good also for the child; and (b) that these 'ought' judgments, at least in their more general formulations, are a common patronage available to all men, and hence form the basis on which policies can be built."

Another big step remains. McCormick needs to make a plausible case that the child—say, an infant whom researchers want to enroll in a study of pulmonary physiology—*ought* to want to volunteer for it. He argues: "To pursue the good that is human life means not only to choose and support this value in one's own case, but also in the case of others when the opportunity arises. . . . [T]he individual *ought* also to take into account, realize, make efforts in behalf of the lives of others also, for we are social beings and, the goods that define our growth and invite to it are goods that reside also in others." So infants and children *ought* to want to help others by, for example, participating as research subjects. McCormick tries to clinch the argument thus: "To share in the general effort and burden of health maintenance and disease control is part of our flourishing and growth as humans. To the extent that it is good for all of us to share this burden, we all *ought* to do so. And to the extent that we *ought* to do so, it is a reasonable construction or presumption of our to say that we would do so." He then concludes: "The reasonableness of this presumption validates vicarious consent."

McCormick has traveled a long way from the sort of infants and children of my acquaintance, most of whom recognize a sharp distinction between what they *should* do (in the eyes of their parents at least) and what they would or want to do. I accept that a crucial part of a parent's job is to help their children understand what they ought to do, and to develop a conscience and motivation that helps them want to do what they should do. In other words, bringing *should* and *would* into closer conjunction is one of the principal tasks of parenthood. The move from "ought" to "would" is an interminable battle fought between parents and children as well as within every person's psyche. Far from the "reasonable construction or presumption of our wishes" that McCormick optimistically maintains, presuming that a child want what it *would* want what it *should* want imputes capacities and preferences that most young children flatly lack.

CONSENT, PARENTAL DUTIES, AND THE ETHICS OF RESEARCH

In contrast to this awkward theoretical effort to rescue the concept of consent as a moral justification for nontherapeutic research on children, McCormick's practical conclusions seem eminently reasonable and wise. If the scientific experiments are "well designed," "cannot succeed unless children are used," and "contain no discernible risk or undue discomfort for the child," then McCormick believes "parental consent to this type of invasion can be justified."

Here is our quandary. On the one hand, we have an incisive, comprehensive analysis—Ramsey's—that reaches what seems to be an unreasonable conclusion: that no research on children which does not have direct benefit of its subjects as an aim is ethically justified. Ramsey's analysis would rule out the most innocuous research on children that might be hugely beneficial to other children. On the other hand, we have a nuanced but strained and unconvincing analysis—McCormick's—that reaches what seem to be very sensible conclusions. McCormick would permit nontherapeutic research on children under very strict circumstances, including no discernible risks, with parental consent.

The problem, I believe, is the shared way in which they formulated the problem. For both Ramsey and McCormick, the issue was the ethics of consent. Recall McCormick agreeing with Ramsey that "consent is the heart of the matter." The social and historical context helps us understand why this particular formulation of the ethics of nontherapeutic research with children suggested itself to both scholars. The horrifying history of Nazi experimentation, the primacy and availability of consent as a moral warrant for participating in research, and the focus on medical experimentation with its propensity for dramatic risks and bodily invasions combined to make consent look like *the* moral solution to unethical human experimentation. The fact that consent could be applied to children at best metaphorically did not deter scholars and researchers from trying to beat it into a shape that might justify research with children, as did McCormick, or writing it off—at least for nontherapeutic research—as a "false and violent presumption" as did Ramsey.

Consent, of course, is not the entirety of the ethics of research even with fully competent adult volunteers. The research must be competent, have some reasonable goal, impose no greater risks than are necessary, and protect subjects' confidentiality, among other considerations. In one of the episodes in Woody Allen's movie *Everything You Always Wanted to Know about Sex but Were Afraid to Ask,* a mad scientist appears. He brings Woody and his companion into the laboratory where he shows them his great experiment: he explains that he is exchanging the brains of a lesbian and a telephone repairman. Even if his two subjects had consented to this experiment (a point not clarified in the movie) it would still be unethical because, well, it's nuts. Even a competent experiment that exposed its subjects to more risk than necessary, or to great risk when there was no corresponding benefit to them such as cure of their disease, would be unethical. Consent may be a crucial concept in the ethics of research, but it is not the whole story. It must be a much smaller part of the story when the subjects of the research cannot give consent—children, for example.

If consent is not the entire, perhaps not even the most important, consideration in the ethics of experimentation with children, then Ramsey's and McCormick's formulation of the problem is defective. Rather than try to hammer consent into a shape that accommodates all of our ethical concerns about the involvement of children in research, we can reformulate the question. Let us ask under what circumstances, if any, parents are morally permitted to enroll their children in nontherapeutic research.

We will not expect to find the answer in any reshaped metaphor of consent. And we should not be embarrassed by that. Yes, it would be wrong to impose research on unconsenting adults. It would be wrong even if it caused them no harm; much worse if, like the Nazi experiments, it heartlessly tortured and killed. It is equally wrong to harm children in the name of research. Relying on parental consent is an important, if imperfect, bulwark against abuse; but it does not have the same moral status as an adult volunteer's consent to participate.

Both Ramsey and McCormick saw that the content of parents' obligations to their children was crucial. Ramsey simply failed to go beyond dismissive pronouncements. Recall what he wrote about parents who would permit their children to participate in minimally risky research: "It is hard to see how this can be an expression of parental care or anything other than a violation of the nature and meaning of the responsibilities of parenthood." There have been countless occasions when I have rebuked myself for failing to fulfill my responsibilities as a parent. I cannot say that having any of my children participate in riskless research would rank high among them. McCormick tried to stuff the huge and ungainly octopus of parental obligations into a sack labeled "vicarious consent: it was an awkward fit at best. He became entangled in the metaphor; his effort to cut his way out with natural law theory strained common sense.

If Ramsey and McCormick became prisoners to their framing of the problem, leaving themselves with, respectively, an extreme solution and an ill-fitting one, can our refraining do any better? When a problem does not yield to a head-on confrontation, a useful strategy is to try to capture its crucial features but move them into a different context. If the context of research raises inescapable echoes of Nuremberg, but our problem is what parents may or may not do with their children that is not directly to their child's benefit, let us look for analogous choices that parents face.

Your next door neighbors have been out of work for a year since the factory closed. They are good hardworking people and fine neighbors, but they are in terrible financial trouble at the moment. Their new baby has been sleeping in a dresser drawer since she came home four weeks ago, but she must move to a crib as soon as possible. They do not have one and cannot afford to buy one. Your two-year-old son will be ready to give up his crib in another six months. It is a bit early to move him into a youth bed: there is always the chance that he might fall out of it in his sleep, or get out of bed at night, wander around the house, and hurt himself. You weigh your neighbors' need and the small risks to your son, and you offer to lend them the crib.

Have you done the right thing?

Your generosity and compassion for your neighbors exposes your child to some slight risks—at the most, probably a small bump on the head. Ramsey's understanding of parenthood, with his exclusive focus on protecting children from any threats to their physical safety, implies that lending the crib would be morally unacceptable, "a violation of the nature and meaning of the responsibilities of parenthood." Surely that is too harsh a judgment. The ethics of neighborliness and charity may not strictly oblige you to lend the crib, but generosity such as this should be valued and is certainly morally permitted. We could jiggle the circumstances of the case to steer judgments toward the obligatory or the prohibited: if the risk to your own child was trivial and the benefit to your neighbors was life-saving or otherwise monumental, we would be more likely to conclude that a genuine moral obligation existed; if the risk to your child became substantial without major benefit to your neighbors (if, for example, the object to be lent was a gate preventing a dangerous tumble down a steep staircase), we would judge it a morally prohibited action, a violation of parental duties to safeguard one's child. The particular factors of the case always do and properly should affect our moral judgments. In the original version it seems fair to say that "what those parents did was morally permitted, despite the fact that it added an iota to the risks facing their own child. Under some circumstances, parents are morally permitted to do things that do not take protection of their own child's safety as the preeminent concern. Some people might argue that this case is different from volunteering your child for research. Our relations with our near neighbors are more intimate, the moral obligations more stringent, than those characterizing the relationship between parents and children, on the one hand, and researchers and those who might someday benefit from the research, on the other. Fair enough. Consider another case.

It is 4 P.M. on a Christmas Eve. Your baby has been cranky today, but has finally fallen asleep. You look forward to her and her parents (that is, you and your spouse) having a couple of peaceful hours. The phone rings. It is the director of the Christmas pageant at the church you visited for the first time last Sunday to see if it was the sort of place you and your family would like to attend regularly. One visit was not sufficient for you to make up your mind, but you had left your name and phone number with the friendly usher who had approached you and admired your baby. Back to the phone call: the pageant director (who also happened to be the amiable usher) is desperate and flattering: the infant who was to have played the part of Baby Jesus has chicken pox. (This actually happened to my wife in a pageant she coordinated.) Your lovely baby would be the perfect replacement. All the adults and children attending the pageant would be *sooo* disappointed if they had to substitute a doll for a live infant. Would you be willing to bring your darling to church in half an hour?

Some parents would probably decline, preferring to let their baby sleep and to enjoy the quiet themselves. I cannot see how they can be said to have any moral obligation to do this favor for these strangers. Other parents would accede, some happily, some reluctantly but moved by the prospective disappointment of the pageant's audience. Do the parents who disturb their baby's slumber to benefit these strangers violate their parental duties? The facts, as always, are important. Their baby may be unhappy for awhile, but she may find the colors of the costumes interesting. In all likelihood, she will go back to sleep soon afterward, only a little the worse for wear. The pageant will be successful and the audience gratified.

What we must decide is whether the parents are morally permitted to donate their infant's services to the pageant or whether they are morally forbidden to do so. This does not strike me as a terrible moral quandary. Of course, the parents may bring their baby to church that afternoon if they wish. The child suffers no great hardship from it, and some people derive a little good—enjoyment at the spectacle, perhaps a little religious edification, and, most of all, delight in watching the unalloyed joy of the children present. Even though there may be no direct benefit for their child, bringing her to the pageant falls well within the compass of permissible moral discretion. It also reminds us that no impenetrable barricade separates moral relationships within families from the moral world outside. We have special and strong moral obligations to those closest to us; but attending to our familial obligations does not mean ignoring all moral interests and relationships outside the family that might in any way, however insignificantly, affect the interests of those within the family circle. This would not merely put the family first but would put the family above everything else—a dangerously shortsighted view of moral life.

In both of these hypothetical cases parents accept some risk, discomfort, or inconvenience for their child, with no direct benefit for that child. Yet in neither case does it seem that the parents have acted immorally or irresponsibly toward their children. The accusation that they have treated their child as a means rather than an end makes no sense. Neither does any claim that they have violated their sacred parental duty.

Two points about parents' moral obligations to children emerge from these analogies. First, protecting a child's physical safety may be very important but is not the entirety of our moral obligations to our children; risks, especially very small ones, may be accepted in the service of other goods and values. Second, the goods and values that may justify accepting risks to our children can include those of other persons and need not always be limited to our child's immediate well-being.

Turn our conclusions on their head for a moment. Imagine a parent who took Ramsey's comments about parental responsibilities with respect to research and generalized them to the whole of parenthood. This parent would refuse to do anything that did not directly benefit the child, citing all the while a parent's moral duty. We have probably all known overprotective parents, but this case might reach new heights—or, rather, depths. The best description of this parental style is "smothering." Those of us with a more cynical bent might suspect that the parent is using purported parental duties as an excuse for avoiding other moral obligations, perhaps out of miserliness or laziness. At best, we would say that they show a lack of proportion or perspective in their moral judgments, that they suffer from an affliction that might be called moral myopia.

At no point in this discussion of parental duties outside the realm of research have we needed to invoke some fictitious or metaphorical notion of the child's own consent to analyze what the parent is permitted morally to do. If the debate over using children in nontherapeutic research has been bewitched by consent, a little disenchantment can be liberating. Consent *is* crucially important when it is genuinely possible—with competent adults. But different problems call for different analyses more suited to their particular circumstances. Children cannot consent; why try to understand the ethics of research with children through the concept of consent? If parental obligations are central as both Ramsey and McCormick acknowledge, then look directly at those obligations.

The cursory look we have taken suggests that involving children in activities that impose no significant hazards on those children but that may contribute substantially to other goods and values even though the child may not benefit directly is well within the circle of morally permissible parental discretion. Nontherapeutic research, when the risks are truly minimal and the benefits to others potentially substantial, is just that kind of activity.

Whether any particular study satisfies the criterion of minimal risk depends on the particulars of the study. Monitoring a baby's blood pressure, if it involved no invasiveness or discomfort, seems to qualify, as would a quick heel prick for a drop of blood. There might be some disagreement about taking repeated vials of blood by venipuncture: the risks are tiny, but the needle will sting. Threading catheters into the heart and injecting powerful drugs, though, is clearly well beyond what any responsible parent should allow: the pain and discomfort are substantial, the risks real and potentially catastrophic.

Where the risks are minimal and the study is competent and potentially significant, parents are permitted morally, but not obliged, to allow their child to participate: not because the child would consent or should consent—consent being an ill-fitting metaphor in this case—but because such participation does not violate the parents' duties to their offspring and because it enhances other goods and values prized by the community.

GROWTH HORMONE FOR SHORT STATURE REVISITED

Should the National Institutes of Health sponsor a. study that gives as many as 1,100 injections to children whose only "deviation" from normal is that they are short? We must consider two separate questions here. First, do parents who enroll their children in this experiment exceed the limits of parental discretion? Second, is it good, morally sound, public policy to encourage such an experiment?

Why would parents permit their children to participate in the study? The only plausible answer is that parents want to protect their children from the cruelty and discrimination experienced by people of short stature. Parents do all sorts of things to try to spare their children from pain or to give them whatever advantages they can provide. A drug that might make their child a little taller could be seen as just another measure parents take to help their children.

When a child's body cannot make a substance necessary for normal growth, development, or function, we say that the child suffers from a disease. Administering a drug that compensates for the missing substance is a benefit for that child, if it does more good than harm. A child who suffers from diabetes cannot make insulin. Responsible parents of such children do their best to promote their children's health by watching their diet, monitoring their blood sugar, and ensuring that they receive appropriate doses of insulin. Children who are short but who have no deficiency of hGH do not have a disease—unless we declare that all those who differ substantially from average on any human characteristic are similarly "diseased." So they are not like children with diabetes, for whom treatment with a drug is justified. A reason that justifies giving a potent drug to your child is that the child has a serious disease for which the drug is an effective treatment. Because short children with normal hGH do not have a disease, we need another good reason for giving them a drug. Perhaps hGH benefits children with short stature.

Unfortunately, the evidence that hGH actually benefits such children is scanty. Growth hormone does appear to accelerate growth, but what matters most to these children and their parents is the child's final adult height. Here the evidence is equivocal: despite the acceleration in growth velocity, the children may stop growing sooner and end up no taller as adults. Let us say that several years worth of hGH injections did add two or three inches to adult height. What sort of benefit is that?

If growth hormone does in fact increase the adult height of children with short stature, then the benefit is far different from the benefit a child with diabetes derives from insulin. A diabetic child's health and life are threatened by the inability to make insulin. A short child who makes normal hGH is not ill and does not suffer from any dire physiological imbalance. Short children with normal hGH are not in any special danger from disease. Growth hormone for such children is not a treatment for any physiological disease, and there is no particular medical benefit from it. But, it is true, being a bit taller for such children could mean that they will suffer fewer cruelties at the hands of other children and less discrimination as adults.

The benefit is entirely social. If it works at all, growth hormone in such cases works by blunting the impact of social prejudice against short people, not by dealing with the roots of prejudice. Those roots are left untouched. Instead, the use of growth hormone for children of short stature tacitly accepts heightism. Parents who seek it for their children understandably want to spare them from discrimination. But as their children benefit, other children, whose parents perhaps cannot afford the tens of thousands of dollars a year needed to pay for hGH, continue to bear the burden of discrimination. Indeed, as those who are fortunate enough to be able to afford hGH climb closer to average height, those left behind will stand out as even more "different."

Imagine that we discovered a possible "treatment" for another form of social prejudice—a hormone that reduces the amount of melanin in the skin. If it worked, giving it to children would cause them to have a lighter hue. It might diminish the amount of racial discrimination they will face by making them appear less different from the light-skinned majority. Does it make sense to deal with racial prejudice by trying to obliterate physical differences? Should we encourage biomedical fixes for complex social problems? Or would be we wiser to deal with the roots of prejudice?

Even if we were able to lay aside our concerns about justice and the sources of discrimination, to defend this research we need to consider the risks to the children involved and weigh them against the potential benefits. We can divide both risks and benefits into two categories: physical and psychological. The most obvious physical harms are the 600 to 1,100 injections each child in the study will receive. Half of the children will get hGH in their shots, half will receive nothing more than sterile salt water.

Consider first the children receiving the salt-water placebo. Other than the pain of the shots and the very remote chance of infection or other complications, the study exposes them to no other significant physical risks. But a thousand-plus injections is not a trivial matter. Anyone who can recall how as a child you regarded the prospect of a *single* injection will not dismiss lightly an experiment designed to give as many as 1,100 to each participant.

The physical benefits to such children are much less clear. They will receive a three-day workup by the researchers and regular follow-up by experts. This intensive medical scrutiny might uncover subtleties that normal health care did not. If that happened—and no one can say how likely it is—then children in the placebo group might benefit. Another possible benefit for the children receiving growth hormone is a so-called placebo effect. Sometimes people who receive a presumed inactive treatment nonetheless do better than those who receive nothing at all. In this study, finding a placebo effect would mean that the children injected with saline solution grew taller than they otherwise would have. The possibility of such a placebo effect was the primary reason offered by the experimenters for injecting salt water into half of the children. I know that the mind and body interact in often mysterious ways. But I must say that the likelihood that saline injections will make kids grow taller seems about as likely as pixie dust allowing them to fly. In any event, it seems fair to say that the likelihood of children in the control group benefiting by an increase in their adult height is remote. On purely physical grounds, then, the study brings more harms than benefits to the children in the control group.

To be fair, we should also look at the balance of psychological benefits and risks. The committee convened by the NIH identified two kinds of potential psychological benefits: "the possible gratification of participating in an important study" and "information that may later be useful to one as a parent."[3] I don't mean to downplay the satisfaction gained by doing something important that can aid others in distress. But these hypothetical psychological benefits are awfully insubstantial compared to the psychological risks.

Children learn what is important about them according to how we treat them. They can learn that their short stature is just one, relatively insignificant, aspect of who they are that pales in importance compared to their wit or expressiveness, the warmth of their smile, or any of hundreds of other details of character and appearance. Or children can learn that their short stature is such a grievous deficiency that it justifies hundreds of injections, regular visits to the doctor, great worry, and, for many, tens of thousands of dollars. Children, that is, can learn that their short stature is a central defining characteristic of their identity—one in which they will assuredly, even with hGH, come up short. The children who receive placebo injections will get this message just as surely as the children getting the drug. Unless salt water *is* a kind of pixie dust, these children will be no taller for all of the hundreds of injections they endure. But they will have learned that their short stature is a severe and crucial deficiency.

The children who receive hGH face a slightly different array of risks and benefits. A leading authority on pediatric endocrinology lists several possible hazards, including diabetes, hypertension, and abnormal growth of both soft and bony tissues, and reports that some children developed leukemia after treatment with hGH. Nevertheless, most experts appear to believe that hGH is reasonably safe. The significant hazards are either rare or unproved. The physical benefit, of course, would be an increase in adult height. But in what sense is increased height a benefit? Being short is not a physical illness, and being taller is not its cure. The point of trying to make children taller is to diminish psychological distress and social discrimination. Increasing height is the means, not the end. The important balance will be between the psychological and social risks and benefits.

If children who receive hGH gain a few inches in adult height, and if that gain diminishes the discrimination they experience at the hands of others, and if the intense focus on their short stature is more than offset by their pride at being less short than anticipated, then they may benefit on the whole. Of course, some, perhaps most, of the children who receive hGH will be no taller for their trouble. Even when the treatment is effective, the increase in height in unlikely to be dramatic. For a boy of 5′3″ or a girl of 4′10½″ a gain of even three inches will not bring them up to average height for their sex. Previous studies found that children with demonstrable hGH deficiency expected greater height gains than hGH treatment could deliver. The children, as well as their parents, experienced disappointment and a sense of failure. Nor were they any happier about themselves.[4] At best, the evidence that a child would benefit significantly from hGH treatment is equivocal. We do not know whether there will be any increase in final height. Even children who gain a few inches may find little comfort. They will still be shorter than average. Their self-confidence may be blighted by their failure to grow as tall as they and their parents thought was so vitally important.

Under the circumstances, do parents who enroll their children in this experiment exceed the limits of parental discretion? The most likely motive for a parent is the hope that his or her child might indeed be one of the fortunate few who would benefit from participating. I say "fortunate few" because the children would have to be lucky in three ways. They would have to be among those participants randomly assigned to receive hGH rather than saline solution. They would have to be one of the as yet unknown proportion of those receiving hGH who become significantly taller. And they would have to experience less discrimination and develop a more robust sense of self by virtue of that gain in height. The odds are not favorable. But then neither are the odds that any particular child will benefit significantly from music lessons. I suspect that most parents who enroll their children in music lessons hope that the child's latent musical gifts will blossom, that he or she will learn habits of dedication and lessons about the relationship of hard work and success that will last a lifetime, and that their perfected talent will provoke respect, if not awe, among their peers. I have no idea what the actual numbers are of children who reap such marvelous fruits from their musical experience compared to those for whom it becomes mainly an exercise in parent-child conflict. But it would not surprise me if the ratio of success to failure was roughly comparable to the ratio for children enrolled in this experiment—substantially less than half.

If we take the optimistic view about physical risks—that the serious ones are fanciful and the pain of the injections tolerable—and an equally optimistic view about the likelihood of social and psychological benefit, then we can draw a rough analogy between enrolling one's child in this experiment or in music lessons. The psychological risks are probably much greater in the experiment, but then so is the concern to spare your child from discrimination and damage to self-esteem.

I do not believe we can say that parents who enroll their children in this experiment clearly violate their obligations to their children. They hope that their children will benefit from participating, even if the benefit does not so clearly fall into the realm of the "therapeutic." I would have to say the same about the parents of dark-skinned children who wanted to spare them from discrimination by placing them in a (nonexistent and hypothetical) study of a skin-lightening hormone that was no more physically risky than hGH. On the other side, parents who choose not to use hGH for their short-stature children also act as responsible parents. They may look at the pain and risks involved and decide that it is more important to stress their child's strengths. (I would say exactly the same about parents who chose to emphasize their children's abilities and accomplishments as well as pride in their ethnic history rather than attempting to change the color of their skin.)

Deciding that parents do not choose wrongly by choosing either way is not the end of the story. We need to address the second question: Is it good, morally sound, public policy to encourage such an experiment? There are many reasons to say no. First, at least half had probably more than half of the children in the study are likely to be harmed more than helped by it. Second, if the study showed that some non-hGH-deficient children grew a few more inches, parents of other short children would have an additional incentive to seek growth hormone for their kids. Since their children are not ill, insurers would resist paying for such an expensive treatment, just as they oppose paying for certain kinds of cosmetic surgery. If insurers resisted successfully but hGH was still available to those who could afford it, then savvy, wealthy parents could get it for their children as just another of the advantages that money can buy. Nor would there be any reason to limit it to short children. If you can buy a few inches, and height confers a competitive advantage, then parents of average and tall children might also want to give their kids a leg up, so to speak. To the advantages of wealth would be added one more—enhanced height.

We do have options. We could adopt the egalitarian approach and make hGH available to all children at public expense. Unfortunately, this would do nothing to defeat heightism. Although average height would rise, there would still be a wide range with plenty of children at the lower end of the curve. Indeed, with a premium placed on height, discrimination against the relatively shorter might intensify. A few groups would benefit. Pediatric endocrinologists would be kept very busy. Investors in the drug companies that manufacture hGH would become wealthy. And a few others would profit, for example, fabric makers, because everyone would need larger sizes. On the whole, though, we would be worse off. Many mere children would get hundreds of shots, more of our national resources would go into making hGH, and discrimination against the relatively shorter would be reinforced rather than diminished. Not a pretty picture.

Perhaps the best result would be proof that growth hormone does nothing for short children who are not hGH-deficient. Parents would then have no reason to give it to their children, and the ugly scenarios would not have to be played out.

There are, and have been, other possibilities for controlling the nontherapeutic use of human growth hormone. The companies that make hGH could require that it be given only to children with medically demonstrable hGH deficiency. That is unlikely to happen. Companies want to sell more, not less, of their products. Indeed, the NIH experiment has corporate sponsorship. More plausibly, pediatricians could take a professional stand that firmly opposes hGH treatment for children not clearly suffering from disease or at great risk of disability. To their credit, pediatric professional societies have urged caution in the use of hGH. Nonetheless, persistent parents can usually find a physician willing to prescribe hGH for their child (who will, incidentally, probably be male, as were approximately 90 percent of the children enrolled in the NIH study). Firmer stands with tighter professional self-regulation is probably our best strategy for now.

HONORING THE WORTH OF A CHILD IN RESEARCH

How should we honor the worth of children in research? We should, of course, protect them from needless harm. We do that in at least two ways: by requiring researchers to demonstrate that the research is important and the risks minimal and by respecting parents' authority to protect and guide their children. We also honor children's moral worth by acknowledging that young children are not just tiny adults when it comes to the moral weight we should give to their consent. Young children's consent does not protect them from harm as well as an adult's consent. To say that a young child consented to participate in an extremely risky nontherapeutic study would never excuse our subjecting them to such unjustified risks.

A better acknowledgment of children's moral worth would be to see participation in nontherapeutic research as one of a class of activities in which parents and children are asked to contribute to the community's well-being and that involve minimal risks to the children. We honor children's worth here by protecting them from overzealous researchers and awestruck or uncaring parents and by recognizing that good rearing of children does not mean a phobic shielding from all imaginable dangers, but rather a sense of proportion that includes acting responsibly toward one's community.

Perhaps because the moral foundation for research on children has been so vague, even well-intentioned people trying to make sense of a proposal like the NIH study of growth hormone for children of short stature may take refuge in tenuous readings of regulations rather than ask the two questions I believe we need to ask: Do parents who enroll their children in this experiment exceed the moral limits of parental discretion? Is it good, morally sound, public policy to encourage such an experiment?

A preliminary look at the limits of parental discretion suggests that parents act within the bounds of good parenting when they consent to a wide range of research protocols for their children, including research likely to benefit their child but also research that might benefit others without being unduly risky to their children. Parents who enroll their children in the NIH growth hormone study are probing the boundaries of parental discretion. Many people might feel that they have stepped over that boundary. Even with a tentative yes to the question whether parents are morally permitted to enroll their children in such a study, the second question remains.

What may be permissible for individual parents may not be wise for us as a community. Encouraging hormonal treatment for social discrimination muddies the line between disease and disadvantage and prompts us to look for medical solutions for social problems. If hGH works in children with normal growth hormone levels, then we must make hard choices. If we permit parents to obtain hGH for their nondeficient children, we would face two equally unpalatable scenarios. We could either heap another, physically distinctive, inequality on top of the other inequalities wealth can buy. Or we could engage in a futile and expensive orgy of competition after which there would be the same number of winners and losers as before.

The most sensible course is to restrict this powerful drug to occasions when it treats disease. Professionals could accomplish this by self-regulation, bolstered, if needed, by laws to discourage the proliferation of hGH treatment for nontherapeutic uses. We should not thwart parents who want to do what is right for their children. But as a community we must recognize that there are situations, like arms races, when the effect of each individual party pursuing self-advantage makes everyone, collectively, worse off. We do not need an experiment on growth hormone for healthy children to show us that.

NOTES

1. Cited in Paul Ramsey, *The Patient as Person* (New Haven: Yale University Press, 1970), 1.
2. Richard A. McCormick, "Proxy Consent in the Experimentation Situation," *Perspectives in Biology and Medicine* 18, no. 1 (Autumn 1974): 9.
3. National Institutes of Health, *Report of the NIH Human Growth Hormone Protocol Review Committee,* 2 October 1992, 13.
4. Diane Rotnem, Donald J. Cohen, Raymond Hintz, and Myron Genel, "Psychological Sequelae of Relative 'Treatment Failure' for Children Receiving Human Growth Hormone Replacement," *Journal of the American Academy of Child Psychiatry* 18 (1979): 505–520.

IN LOCO PARENTIS: MINIMAL RISK AS AN ETHICAL THRESHOLD FOR RESEARCH UPON CHILDREN

Benjamin Freedman, Abraham Fuks, and Charles Weijer

While respect for rights is the hallmark of a liberal society, responsibility toward vulnerable persons unable to care for themselves or even speak on their own behalf is the mark of a humane society. And within the broad field of social ethics, bioethics in particular must focus upon such responsibilities: to the very old and very young, those muted or rendered incoherent by illness. Yet delineating the nature of that responsibility has proven to be among the most vexing problems bioethics has faced.

Agreement in principle upon the touchstone of responsibility toward the incompetent is elusive. Should we act in their best interests, or as they would have directed us to act? More difficult still is the application of such a standard, as when we attempt to describe what is required by the best interests of a particular handicapped newborn. Most difficult, perhaps, is the application of a standard under conditions of risk and uncertainty, when our ethical calculus, ill-grounded as it is, is put to work on shifting and statistically ill-defined values.

The ethics of clinical research in children seems tailor-made for addressing these moral quandaries. Is it ever ethical to expose children to risks associated with research? If it is, what are the ethical limits to such risk? How can a specific threshold to research risk be formulated, justified, and applied? These questions have preoccupied pediatric researchers and others for many years. Recent revisions of United States regulations regarding research with human subjects and the formulation of a "common

Reprinted with permission from *Hastings Center Report* 23, no. 2 (1993): 13–19.

Editor's note: Most footnotes have been deleted. Students who want to follow up on sources should consult the original article.

rule" applying to all federal departments involved with human research make it necessary to examine these questions.

The new definition provided in the "common rule" states, "'Minimal risk' means that the probability and magnitude of harm or discomfort anticipated in the research are not greater in and of themselves than those ordinarily encountered in daily life, or during the performance of routine physical or psychological examinations or tests. Finding that a research study poses only 'minimal risk' has some important procedural consequences for review. In this paper, though, we will focus upon another role: 'minimal risk' has some important procedural consequences for review. In this paper though, we will focus upon another role: 'Minimal risk' is the concept used in American regulation to serve as an anchoring measure of allowable risk (or—the other side of the coin—relative safety) in clinical research. The critical threshold of risk that may not be surpassed (short of special federal approval) is in fact one level higher: 'minor increment over minimal risk.' However, since the rule offers no independent definition or specification of 'minor increment,' attention must first be focused upon its anchor, 'minimal risk.' . . .

THE UBIQUITY OF RESEARCH RISK

In any ethical consideration of research, the question of the allowable maximum of research risk must inevitably arise. Every activity poses some risks to its participants, and research is no exception to this rule. Risk, commonly expressed as the magnitude of some harm multiplied by the probability of its occurrence, can never be eliminated. . . . Absolute safety can therefore never be guaranteed to participants in clinical research.

Ethics requires that clinical trials comparing two forms of treatment begin with an honest null hypothesis, a state of clinical equipoise—uncertainty in the expert clinical community concerning the comparative merits and disadvantages of each trial arm. As current United States regulations put it, a trial comparing, for example. standard therapy with a nonvalidated intervention may only be approved if "the risk is justified by the anticipated benefit to the subjects" and "the relation of the anticipated benefit to the risk is at least as favorable to the subjects as that presented by available alternative approaches." When this condition is satisfied, some will feel that while one trial arm may involve more *uncertainty* than another, no arm is *riskier* than any other.

However, comparative trials raise their own problems of specific research risk. Once the trial's arms are established tube in clinical equipoise, a second stage of analyzing research risks proceeds. Now those interventions that have no therapeutic warrant, hut that are required to answer the trial's scientific question, are separated from the treatment interventions. The risks associated with those interventions required purely for research purposes are tabulated and added separately. Their sum represents the incremental research risk of the study. . . .

The doctrine of informed consent to research constitutes one major response to the ethical challenge of research risks. Competent subjects with the capacity of understanding research risks and benefits, by consenting to serve as research subjects, voluntarily assume these risks. As the legal maxim states, *Volenti non fit injuria* (One who has agreed to an activity is not wronged by it). Conceivably the same justification applies to research upon persons who have while competent executed a valid advance directive permitting specified forms of research to be performed upon them when their competency should lapse. This stratagem, the research analogue to treatment's 'living will,' may in the future serve an important role in research upon Alzheimer's dementia.

But no such solution is available on behalf of incompetent subjects who were never competent—most importantly, infants and small children but also those suffering from congenital intellectual handicaps. Unless safety is understood in a relative sense, permitting some small risk that falls below a specified threshold, these incompetent persons could never be permitted to participate in clinical research—a situation that would in the long run leave them 'therapeutic orphans' and for that reason at even greater risk.

THE MEANING AND USE OF 'MINIMAL RISK'

What does 'minimal risk' mean in the medical literature? How is it understood by clinical investigators? How is it defined within the regulations, and what role does it play in ethically evaluating research upon children? As we will see, a purely definitional approach without reference to the ethical purpose underlying the threshold, is incapable of capturing anything significant by the term.

Which procedures are said in the medical literature to impose no more than minimal risk? Such highly invasive maneuvers as splenectomy, transthoracic enucleation of esophageal leiomyomas and pancreatic biopsies are all described as "of minimal risk." This characterization, on the surface so surprising, is nonetheless justifiable given the necessity for the procedure in the patient populations in question and the risks associated with alternative intentions. Clearly, the term cannot be defined without specifying a context: minimal risk to what end, from whose point of view; and under which situations? On a semantic level, 'minimal risk' is relational, context-dependent. To understand its meaning in the research context, we must examine that specific usage.

Even if we restrict the context to research interventions upon children, though, and even if we restrict our inquiry to investigators, significant disagreement remains. Janofsky and Starfield surveyed chairpersons of pediatric departments and directors of pediatric clinical research units in the United States to elicit their understanding of 'minimal risk,' 'minor increment over minimal risk,' and 'more than minor increment over minimal risk.'[1] (Recall that 'minor increment over minimal risk' is the critical threshold, determining whether a study could be approved by a local committee or would require approval by a special federal panel.) Respondents were asked to classify common research procedures as administered to pediatric subjects of different ages.

The results demonstrated serious disagreements among respondents: 14 percent thought tympanocentesis (puncturing of the ear drum) posed minimal risk or less, 46 percent classified this as a minor increment over minimal risk, and 40 percent thought it more than a minor increase. Expressed in practical terms, 40 percent thought research requiring tympanocentesis was inpermissible, despite the importance of the research, without the approval of a federally authorized panel of ethics experts In addition to the approval of the parents. (With regard to a population of research subjects aged one to four years, respondents came close to the three-way mathematical maximum of dissension: 34% thought it minimally risky, 31% a minor increment, 35% more than a minor increment.) While these are extreme examples, substantial scatter across the categories was the rule rather than the exception throughout the study.

It does not seem, therefore, that 'minimal risk' or the other thresholds it anchors may be clarified by examination of sense or signification within the medical literature, nor by usage of the community of clinical investigators. There appears so be no natural or uniform understanding of 'minimal risk' upon which we can draw. If that is the case we are left with only the definition of 'minimal risk' provided in the regulations: the risk of daily life or that encountered in routine physical or psychological examinations, Although other interpretations are possible, this definition seems to set the risks of daily life as the baseline and the risks of routine examinations as an example of the risks of everyday life most similar to the kinds of interventions found in research studies—routine immunizations, developmental testing, and the obtaining of urine and blood specimens. An intervention's satisfaction of the minimal risk standard can therefore be demonstrated in one of two ways: directly, by showing that it falls within the definition; or indirectly, by showing that it is relevantly similar to other interventions known to fall within the definition.

But how is the definition itself to be interpreted? What is meant. by 'the risks of everyday life'? As Kopelman notes, the risks of everyday life may be understood in several different ways; for example, it may refer to all the risks any person might encounter or so those that all of us encounter. She rightly rejects the first possibility. The fact that some people commonly face very high risks (parachuting, firefighting) could not justify allowing a similar level of risk in research upon children. The second characterization is much more restrictive, constituting a lowest common denominator of risk. Kopelman criticizes this interpretation of the risks of everyday life as follows:

> This interpretation assumes that we know the kinds of risks we all encounter and their probability and magnitude. Neither is obvious. Most of us drive cars, walk across busy streets, and fly in airplanes. Are these the everyday risks the definition refers to? How do we determine what risks are encountered routinely by all of us and estimate the probability and magnitude of these risks?[2]

In the passage two distinct claims are made, one concerning the difficulty in *identifying* the risks of everyday life, the difficulty in *quantifying* them. The first difficulty, though, is clearly exaggerated. While there will always be exceptions, within any given society daily life will present the bulk of its citizens with ordinary hazards at home, at work, at play, and in transit, crossing the street or taking a bath. It is not hard to identify this set of common social risks. We are, by definition, each acquainted with them; and, almost by definition, if we are unsure whether they belong within the set of common risks then they don't.

On quantification Kopelman seems on firmer ground. While we all ride in cars, few of us know the likelihood of our being in a fatal accident. And it is certainly true that IRBs or other research ethics bodies typically consider whether a given proposal is acceptable without recourse to actuarial charts of the risks of daily living.

Indeed, Kopelman could have posed a far more fundamental challenge to the concept. As noted above, the critical threshold for allowable research risk in children is not 'minimal risk' itself; but rather, 'a minor increase over minimal risk.' What meaning attaches to the qualification minor increase that is not defined, specified, or characterized in any way within the regulations? If, as Kopelman believes, these thresholds are quantitative measures, verbal surrogates for numbers expressing the probability and magnitude of potential harms of everyday life, the question is unanswerable, This strongly suggests that an alternative, nonquantitative understanding of 'minimal risk' is intended. To understand that, we need to turn to the basic principles that underlie committee research review.

THE PURPOSE OF 'MINIMAL RISK'

A number of parties must concur in the judgment that a clinical study is ethically appropriate before that study will proceed. The first and probably most important decision-maker is the investigator, who must consider before developing a protocol whether the task may be ethically achieved, how risks may be minimized, how the study's goals and risks may be explained, and so forth. If the study is done upon competent persons, their consent represents another ethical decision node. If the subjects are young children the agreement of parents is required, as well as the assent of the child herself to the extent that she is capable of giving it.

What role does a research ethics committee play? The institution within which research proceeds, both in itself and as society's agent, has its own obligation to treat subjects in a trustworthy capacity. Research review by the ethics committee is a concrete expression of this institutional fiduciary responsibility. In addition, as investigators are sometimes overly enthusiastic or bold, committee review of the ethics of research serves in part as a fail-safe mechanism to curb inappropriate zeal. For example, in assessing any protocol, the IRB must determine that its risk-to-knowledge ratio is reasonable and that the scientific importance of the undertaking is proportional to the risks subjects will be undergoing. These issues should have been considered by the investigators; and usually they do that. Nonetheless, the research committee is charged not to take that for granted, to serve as a backup in case the investigator has not competently discharged his or her personal and professional obligation. Again, it is the inalienable obligation of the investigators properly to inform subjects prior to their participation in a trial. The IRB, in reviewing the study's consent form, serves as a failsafe mechanism to ensure that the investigator's plan for informing subjects will satisfy ethical norms and the institution's own moral obligation to protect subjects.

The IRB plays the same backup role vis-à-vis parental (or guardian) approval of participation of a child (or other incompetent person) in research. Parents may be ignorant, apathetic, or merely inattentive. Cognizant of these and other possibilities, and of its own moral obligation to protect incompetent research subjects, the institution charges a review committee to act as surrogate for the scrupulous parent by filtering out those studies that would impose an unacceptable level of risk upon child participants. It is in this light that the threshold concept, 'minor increase over minimal risk,' needs to be understood. In applying this standard, the IRB is attempting to track those decisions that would be made by in-formed and scrupulous parents whose children are being invited to participate in research. This fail-safe measure does not ensure that parents will scrupulously evaluate studies; rather, it ensures that they will only have the opportunity to enroll a child in a study that could have passed such an evaluation.

Asking a parent to agree to the child's participation in research is asking for a decision for participation in a new situation, with new attendant risks. These decisions are not arrived at quantitatively, by calculating risks, but rather on a *categorial* basis. Consider another such choice. A child has been asked out to an overnight camping trip for the first time. The risks of the trip are not the risks of everyday life—it is a new experience. If the threshold of allowable risk never permitted anything other than the risks of everyday life, no new experiences could ever be enjoyed (something which itself in the not-very-long run would not be in the child's best interests). Rather, a mother asks herself, "Is the child ready for this? Should the child approach this by stages? *Are the risks sufficiently similar to those in my child's everyday life that I should allow this experience at this time?*" In discussions about whether to permit this involvement—with the mother resisting, and the child pressing—a certain logic may be discerned. Appealing to consistency, the child will say that he has been permitted, and successfully undergone, situations relevantly and roughly similar though not identical—while the parent will focus upon difference.

In other words, the parental decision to permit exposure to new risks is not itself governed by, but rather anchored to, the risks of everyday life. And this point is of course exactly mirrored in our understanding of the regulations, in which the upper threshold of research risk is not governed by, but anchored to, the concept of minimal risk. Almost by definition, exciting and important research ventures into the unknown. A prohibition on such research involvement would be to the long-term detriment of this child and other children, just as a prohibition on new experiences is harmful to children over the long term. Therefore, the limit is set as a 'minor increase over minimal risk.' This limit is not quantitative, but represents a categorical judgment that focuses upon the comparison of new experiences to those of everyday life. It is this form of discussion that needs to take place in research ethics committees considering the approval of research involving children.

JUSTIFYING AND APPLYING THE THRESHOLD

Because children and their situations differ, a judgment anchored to the risks of everyday life, whether arrived at by parent or IRB, must be made relative to the child's actual situation. A diabetic child's everyday life includes pinprick blood tests, and additional such tests required by a study protocol represent much less of a variation in that child's daily life than in the life of a healthy child. This relativistic understanding of minimal risk, held by the National Commission for the Protection of Human Subjects (with the exception of Commissioner Turtle), is in fact the current interpretation of the regulations.

We should also point out that by choosing the risks of everyday life as an anchor to an acceptable level of research risk, less net added risk is imposed upon the child than might be thought. The risks of research are to a degree substitutive, rather than additive: research risks are undergone, but the risks of alternative activities are forgone. Normal, healthy subjects of research would otherwise he pursuing their normally risky daily lives; anti ill subjects who are not enrolled in research studies may nonetheless receive treatments and diagnostic tests under the rubric of therapy that are similar to those they would have experienced in research. Furthermore, although in principle any given level of risk associated with an activity can be reduced, there is substantial empirical evidence that past a certain point individuals cease efforts at risk reduction, and the efforts of third parties to reduce risk yield severely diminishing returns. When cars have more safety features built in, for example, people seem to feel free to drive in a riskier fashion. Insurance companies have long since identified the problem under the phrase "moral hazard": property owners who are insured against damage or theft take fewer contingencies. People do differ in their propensity to trade off safety for other goods, but by specifying a threshold at or near the risks of everyday life we approximate a lowest common denominator of risk, the level at which most reasonable people feel 'safe enough' so that their choices can be made without considering the small risk repercussions.

The concept, 'risks of everyday life,' has normative as well as descriptive force, reflecting a level of risk that is not simply accepted but is deemed socially acceptable. Without defining the scope of parental authority and discretion within the law, therefore, we may be reasonably certain that the risks of everyday life fall within those bounds. There is, however no precise legal analogue to this level. Questions of child abuse deal with risks and is arms far above this threshold; so does the question of parental refusal of medical treatment for a child on religious grounds. In some ways, the closest analogy arises in disputes over child custody, which consider and weigh the risks of a child's transferring to a new school, being exposed to (or shielded from) church teachings, and so on. But these cases, inevitably are resolved on the relative basis of which parent is the better custodian rather than on the basis of whether parentally imposed risks fall beneath a threshold of acceptability.

One last aspect of the 'risks of everyday life' should be discussed: its flexibility, in conformity to time and circumstance. Kopelman sees this as a serious drawback: "the risks to children living in Belfast and Edinburgh are different; but we would not want to have this automatically influence what sort of research we think we would be 'not too risky' for them."[3] In our understanding developed above, the example is inapt—parental concern in Belfast may not be less than in Edinburgh—but the point that standards diverge across cultures is true.

However, this flexibility of the threshold is to our minds an advantage. Any society's notion of what demands on children are allowable changes over time. The routine labor expectations of children fifty years ago are considered exploitative now, and those made one hundred years ago would not be actionable child abuse. The same is true of exposure to risk. Given the huge historical and geographical differences among cultures as to the degree to which children should be protected from risk or engaged in life's risky activities, only the most parochial would maintain that the currently prevailing view in Western Europe and North America is necessarily the one right approach. The ethical evaluation of research can and must insist upon the rigorous protection of subjects, but cannot in so doing lose all reference to common social norms. An ethics of research must be sufficiently flexible as to incorporate and accommodate cultural variance, as is done when the risks of everyday life' is used as a categorical anchor for research risk.

Intercultural variance does, however, raise a very distasteful possibility. A Western researcher. frustrated by restrictions upon his or her own research, might go shopping for a community whose children are sufficiently destitute and underprotected that even exposure to heinous risk falls within the expected daily routine. Exploiting their miserable conditions of life, this researcher would claim simply to be accommodating cultural differences.

This stratagem would be precluded by recognizing that research in these circumstances is governed not by cultural but by intercultural ethics. It follows from what we have said that because cultures differ in the degree of protection to which their children are entitled, a research project might be ethical in culture A and unethical in culture B. But when a researcher from culture B contemplates doing research upon children from culture A, the question is, Whose values should be controlling? Some students of intercultural research ethics have adopted a "both-and" approach: in cross-cultural research the norms of both groups A *and* B must be respected. Such a requirement would eliminate, on ethical grounds, the prospect of a researcher's shopping for a useful risk pool.

The final question remaining is that of applying the standard. When is the aggregated risk of research interventions an. increase above a minor increment over minimal risk? The status of many of the most common research interventions, for example, blood sampling, dietary restrictions and other measures listed by the National Commission is easily settled: they are associated with routine physical examinations and so are of minimal risk. Some other interventions not on that list because not associated with the risks of everyday life of healthy persons are minor interventions common to the lives of all ill children within the relevant class. In accepting the principle of commensurate risks, it follows that the form, and perhaps also the sum, of research risk for ill children may exceed that imposed upon their healthy counterparts. The question. Is this research risk sufficiently similar to their daily experience? could not receive the same answer in two groups whose daily experience of risk is so different as the healthy and the ill. On the other hand, some interventions—for example, liver biopsies—are so risky and unfamiliar that no colorable case could be made on their behalf.

What are the hard cases the threshold needs to address? One kind of problem is posed by the reiteration of minimally risky procedures for research purposes. One or two venipunctures are minimally risky; four, arguably so, but still not more than a minor increase over minimal risk. But what of five, ten, forty, or any number in between? Similarly, when testing a new treatment for meningitis it is acceptable to perform one lumbar puncture on a sick child to satisfy the protocol's scientific needs, but not five. Where is the break point? Another set of problems is posed by those procedures (arterial punctures performed upon healthy children, for example) that are qualitatively different from common procedures, although of low risk.

It is not to be expected that the threshold definition of minimal risk as the risk of everyday life will settle each of these questions in an unambiguous and nonarbitrary fashion. Neither this nor any other threshold definition is self-interpreting; each will require the exercise of judgment. But we can require that the threshold define the terms of the argument, the kinds of questions that will need to be posed in the committee's deliberations. This the threshold can do. The arguments will parallel those familiar to any parent considering allowing a child to undergo a new experience. The committee, acting *in loco parentis,* will need to debate whether the demarcated research intervention is similar to a common experience of this child, and whether the incremental research risks are similar to the risks this child or others like him runs on a routine basis. The debate takes place within a context recognizing that the committee owes a fiduciary duty to these subjects, and that this duty entails imposing upon a child no risks substantially above a socially defined minimum for any scientific end, however worthy.

If the above analysis is sound, it may shed light upon our broader responsibilities to children and other incompetent persons as well. All cases of medical intervention occur under conditions of relative uncertainty; because of patient variability treatment is always an experiment in nature. And so, in clinical treatment as well as research, those concerned with the care of the patient—doctors, nurses, members of the institution's ethics committee. among others—may acknowledge their fiduciary responsibility to act *in loco parentis.* In doing so, we suggest, the same kinds of considerations we have raised for clinical research reappear. Risk is always present and seems more appropriately dealt with in categorical rather than quantitative fashion; the allowable limits of risk will always, ineluctably, rely upon a social consensus that varies over time and geographical setting. This consensus itself fuzzy at the edges, is better at identifying those numerous and varied acts contrary to a person's best interests than at defining the one course of action dictated by them.

REFERENCES

1. Jeffrey Janosky and Barbara Starfield, "Assessment of Risk in Research on Children," *Journal of Pediatrics* 98, no. 5 (1981): 842–846.
2. Loretta Kopelman, "Estimating Risk in Human Research," *Clinical Research* 29 (1981): 1–8, 4.
3. Loretta Kopelman, "When Is the Risk Minimal Enough for Children to Be Research Subjects?" in *Children and Health Care: Moral and Social Issues,* ed. Loretta Kopelman and John Moskop (Dordrecht: Kluwer, 1989), p. 91.

DRUG-FREE RESEARCH IN SCHIZOPHRENIA: AN OVERVIEW OF THE CONTROVERSY

Paul S. Appelbaum

The ethics of psychiatric research—in particular drug-free research on schizophrenia—have been the focus of intense interest in the last two years. We have witnessed a proliferation of professional conferences on the topic, often with coverage in the lay press. The American Psychiatric Association has organized a work group to formulate ethical guidelines for psychiatric researchers. At the federal level, the National Institute of Mental Health has indicated its interest in funding research that explores the ethical issues involved in studies of persons with psychiatric disorders.

Why this sudden interest in the ethics of psychiatric research, an area that has been quiescent for nearly a decade and a half? This paper explores the context from which much of this interest has grown: drug-free research on schizophrenia. I consider the roots of the controversy, the nature both of the disorder and of the research that lies at the core of the debate, and the ethical issues that have been raised.

WHY THE CURRENT PROMINENCE OF ISSUES RELATED TO DRUG-FREE RESEARCH IN SCHIZOPHRENIA?

In May 1994, the federal Office of Protection from Research Risks (OPRR) issued a report on its investigation of complaints against a leading group of schizophrenia researchers at the University of California at Los Angeles (UCLA) Medical School. The subjects on whose behalf complaints were filed had participated in a series of studies using Prolixin decanoate, a long-acting, injectable form of a standard antipsychotic agent.

Subjects in the UCLA studies initially went through a one-year, fixed-dose study in which they received injections every two weeks. On the successful completion of the first study, subjects who were willing to continue in the research were enrolled in a second, more controversial protocol. Each subject was assigned, in a randomized, double-blind fashion, to continue the same dose of Prolixin or to receive a placebo injection. After twelve weeks, the groups crossed over, with those subjects who had received active medication now getting placebo, and vice versa. Subjects who were still stable after an additional twelve weeks were then assigned to a withdrawal protocol. The medications were stopped and subjects were followed for at least one year, or until a serious exacerbation or psychotic relapse occurred. The goal of the study was to identify predictors of successful functioning without antipsychotic medication.

Two subjects who had been enrolled in the withdrawal protocol ran into trouble. One subject committed suicide after completion of the formal one-year drug withdrawal study, while continuing to be followed by the research team in a drug-free state. A second person, a young college student, experienced a severe psychotic relapse that began not long after the medication was discontinued. During this period, he left school, began to hallucinate, and threatened to kill his parents when he became convinced that they were possessed by the devil. He and his parents alleged that, despite repeated appeals to the research team, it took nine months before he was put back on medication.

In the wake of these episodes, allegations were made to OPRR that the drug withdrawal protocols in which the subjects had been enrolled were unethical because they virtually guaranteed that subjects would relapse; that proper informed consent had not been obtained from the subjects; and that the investigators, who were also the subjects' clinicians, had not monitored their conditions closely enough

IRB, Vol. 18, No. 1, 1–5.

Editors' note: All notes have been deleted. Readers who wish to follow up on sources should consult the original article.

and had been too slow about pulling them off the protocol and restarting medications.

OPRR's investigation concluded that the design of the research was not unethical, since it comported with current clinical and scientific standards. However, the agency determined that the informed consent obtained from subjects was inadequate, because the consent documents failed to describe clearly the differences between being in the research project and receiving ordinary clinical care. Although UCLA's monitoring of subjects' clinical status was deemed to be acceptable, OPRR also found that subjects should have been informed that their clinicians simultaneously were acting as investigators in the study.

Far from settling the controversy regarding drug-free research in schizophrenia, the OPRR report stimulated renewed consideration of the issues. The controversy was widely covered in the popular media, congressional hearings were held, and a lawsuit was filed against UCLA by the family of one of the subjects. Before considering the ethical issues raised by participants in the debate over drug-free research, however, it may be helpful to know a bit more about schizophrenia and its treatment.

WHAT IS SCHIZOPHRENIA AND HOW IS IT TREATED?

Schizophrenia is a major mental disorder characterized by periods of psychosis or detachment from reality. Patients typically experience hallucinations, delusions, disorganized thinking and behavior, and social withdrawal. Psychiatrists only make a diagnosis of schizophrenia after symptoms have been present for at least six months, but most patients will suffer from the effects of the disorder for the rest of their lives. Periods of relative remission, in which withdrawal and restricted emotions are the most notable characteristics, are frequently punctuated by acute exacerbations, marked by the most florid psychotic symptoms. Persons with schizophrenia experience considerable agony as a result of their disorder; lifetime rates of suicide approximate 10 percent.

Treatment of schizophrenia, once limited to lifetime custodial care, was revolutionized in the mid-1950s by the introduction of the first effective medications for the disorder, the phenothiazine antipsychotics. These drugs—including Thorazine, Mellaril, and Prolixin—appear to have a specific effect on psychotic symptoms, rather than merely "tranquilizing" the patient. Their mechanism of action is believed to involve blockade of brain dopamine receptors, but this continues to be an area of active investigation. Administration of the medications can lead to resolution of acute psychotic episodes and a diminished likelihood of recurrence over time. Eighty percent or more of patients with schizophrenia get some benefit from the medications, and many of those who are resistant to phenothiazines have benefited from other classes of drugs more recently introduced.

On the other hand, it is clear that currently available antipsychotic medications are a mixed blessing. Though they usually are effective in diminishing symptoms, complete remission is uncommon. Even when maintained on medication, most patients will experience periodic breakthroughs of their psychosis. Moreover, the success achieved by the medications is purchased at the price of substantial side-effects. Acutely, many patients experience drug-induced parkinsonism, muscle spasms called dystonias, feelings of inner restlessness associated with a need to move ("akathisia"), and akinetic states in which the motivation to move and even to think is diminished. Less frequently, patients may experience a potentially fatal hypermetabolic state known as "neuroleptic malignant syndrome"; the most popular of the newer medications, clozapine, can cause dangerous (or life-threatening) suppression of white blood cells (agranulocytosis).

The most profound of the long-term side-effects of the phenothiazine-type medications (and those that act similarly, like Haldol) is tardive dyskinesia. This syndrome is characterized by involuntary muscular movements affecting the face, limbs, and trunk, and sometimes other muscle groups as well. Ranging in intensity from mild to occasionally disabling, tardive dyskinesia occurs in 4 to 5 percent of patients on neuroleptic medication each year. Though it sometimes remits when the medications are stopped, it is often irreversible; patients with tardive dyskinesia may be faced with the choice of continuing the medications, with a possible worsening of the syndrome, or discontinuing them, only to experience an exacerbation of their schizophrenic symptoms. Other delayed neuromuscular syndromes may occur as well.

On balance, though, most patients with schizophrenia tolerate the side-effects of the drugs, both acute and long-term, as a lesser evil compared with untreated schizophrenia.

WHY CONDUCT DRUG-FREE RESEARCH IN SCHIZOPHRENIA?

Given the availability of reasonably effective drugs for the treatment of schizophrenia, and the distress associated with acute episodes of the disorder, one might wonder on what basis researchers perform studies with patients who have been taken off their medication. Three justifications are commonly given.

First, it has been known for many years that some schizophrenic patients can have their medication discontinued without experiencing relapse for a substantial period of time. If such patients could be identified in advance, they would be spared the negative effects of the medication, without undue risk of relapse. At this time, though, there are no good predictors for identifying this patient group. Indeed, developing such markers was the major goal of the UCLA project that stimulated the controversy over drug-free research. To identify patients who do well without medications, the most obvious design is to study subjects in a drug-free state.

Second, the limitations of the current medications point to the desirability of developing new compounds that might be more effective or carry fewer risks. When these new drugs are tested, subjects' current medications are often stopped for a period of several weeks to allow them to wash out of the body, thus minimizing the risk of adverse drug-drug interactions. The medication-free period may also provide a baseline against which the new drug's therapeutic and side-effects can be assessed. Once the trial of the new medication begins, one group of subjects will usually be assigned randomly to receive an inactive placebo, so that their response can be compared with those subjects receiving the new medication.

Third, drug-free research may be helpful in elucidating the pathophysiology of schizophrenia. . . .

WHAT ARE THE RISKS OF DRUG-FREE RESEARCH?

The major risk of taking clinically stable research subjects off their antipsychotic medications is that they will suffer a relapse of their disorder. The most recent analysis of studies involving discontinuation of medication in schizophrenia indicates an overall relapse rate of 54.8 percent during an average follow-up period of 9.7 months. In comparison, 16.6 percent of patients maintained on medication are likely to relapse during the same period of time. Most episodes of relapse occur in the first year after discontinuation. Forty-four percent of subjects off medication will relapse in the first three months, with the total at two years approaching 80 percent.

Efforts to limit the risk of relapse, for example, by eliminating subjects who may be likely to suffer exacerbation of their conditions, are hampered by the absence of reliable predictors. The only significant correlate of likelihood of relapse is the amount of time subjects have been off their medications. Even prolonged stabilization on antipsychotic medications does not seem to reduce the risk of an acute episode once the medications are discontinued. One factor frequently associated with research protocols, however, appears to magnify the risk of relapse: abrupt discontinuation of medication induces a threefold greater risk of relapse than gradual discontinuation over a period of weeks to months.

The effects of a psychotic episode on patients with schizophrenia are not limited to the profound psychic suffering that often accompanies psychosis. Patients may engage in high-risk behaviors, such as assault and suicide attempts. A relapse may destabilize their psychosocial situations, costing them their jobs, housing, and the support of family and friends. Some evidence suggests intermittent use of medications increases the risk of tardive dyskinesia compared with uninterrupted treatment. Most controversially, it has been suggested that psychotic episodes themselves have a "toxic" effect on patients, increasing the likelihood of further episodes in the future and decreasing the long-term effectiveness of existing medications. These claims have been challenged by other researchers, and are by no means generally accepted.

SHOULD WE DO DRUG-FREE STUDIES IN SCHIZOPHRENIA?

Given the risks associated with withdrawal or withholding of medication from patients with schizophrenia, a lively debate is under way about the legitimacy of this form of research. Arguments against drug-free research take a variety of forms. Some advocates for mentally ill persons would ban all studies involving prolonged drug-free periods on the grounds that they threaten subjects with an unacceptable likelihood and level of harm. These critics invoke the provisions of the Nuremberg Code, which demand that researchers avoid unreasonable degrees of risk for research subjects.

Most commentators, however, including the National Alliance for the Mentally Ill, the country's largest advocacy group for persons with mental disorders, have not gone so far as to endorse an absolute ban on drug-free studies. Not only do they fear that progress on the treatment of schizophrenia will be stymied, but they shy away from the implied stigmatization of persons with mental illness. After all, competent persons, even those with major illnesses, generally are allowed to consent to research that induces risk, at times even serious risk. To suggest that persons with mental illness, alone among other competent adults, should not be permitted to participate in risky research labels them as unable to play an equal role in making decisions about their lives.

Thus, most of the criticisms of drug-free research have taken a somewhat narrower approach, looking either to negate some of the justifications for the research or to modify the conditions under which it takes place. Among the suggestions that have been made are that researchers abandon routine use of placebo control groups in clinical trials of new medications; that reasonable precautions be taken to prevent harm to subjects; and that more intensive informed consent procedures be employed.

Use of Placebo in Medication Trials

Drug-free research in schizophrenia has become a lightning rod for discussion of a broader issue in the ethics of experimental design: the legitimacy of using placebo in trials of new medications for serious disorders, when reasonably effective medications are already available. Opponents of placebo use argue that medical ethics, as embodied in the Declaration of Helsinki, require that "[i]n any medical study, every patient—including those of a control group, if any—should be assured of the best proven diagnostic and therapeutic method." This statement, it is claimed, "effectively proscribes the use of a placebo as control when a proven therapeutic method exists." Since the practical question inherent in the development of a new medication is whether it is superior to existing drugs anyway, design of clinical trials should be changed so that new medications are compared with the best current treatments. A more moderate group of critics is willing to permit subjects to consent to participation in placebo-controlled trials, as long as they are aware of the risks of forgoing standard treatment (or even promising experimental treatment). They argue, however, that once potential subjects are well informed about these matters, it is difficult to imagine that many of them would agree to participate in the placebo-controlled study.

Proponents of placebo use, including the U.S. Food and Drug Administration, note that placebos may not be dispensed with quite as easily as some critics suggest. The most problematic situations that arise without the use of placebo controls occur when no differences are detected in the efficacy of the new medication and standard treatment. Such findings might indicate that both medications are equally effective, prompting a search for other advantages of the new drug, perhaps a reduced rate of side effects. Alternatively, however, the results may simply mean that in the circumstances of this particular study, real differences between the medications were obscured, with each appearing to be equally ineffective with this sample.

A variety of methodologic difficulties could underlie the failure to detect real differences between the drugs. Actual differences may have existed, but poor measurement techniques might have precluded them from being detected. Alternatively, each medication may have truly failed to have much effect because of peculiarities of the sample. This is a particular problem in schizophrenia research, where study samples seem to be drawn increasingly from treatment-resistant populations. It is, after all, persons who have not benefited from existing treatments who are most likely to seek opportunities to try new medications. Whereas the failure to find a difference between new and current treatments in this population could be interpreted as their being equally effective, in fact the results may be due to the selection of an atypical study sample resistant to the effects of all medications. Whether the study's conclusions can be relied upon would only be evident with the inclusion of a placebo control group.

Mechanisms of Reducing Risks To Subjects

If drug-free studies are to continue, whether as part of clinical trials or other research, the ethics of research demand that attention be given to means of minimizing the risks faced by subjects. Carpenter and colleagues have suggested several approaches that may be helpful. First, high-risk subjects could be excluded from entry into the study. Although it is impossible at this point to identify those subjects at greatest risk of relapse, individual subjects' histories may help to identify those who are likely to face the greatest risk of harm from psychotic deterioration. This group might include patients with histories of disastrous consequences from deterioration, or those in marginal social situations. Patients who have done exceptionally well on existing treatment might also be excluded, unless the study rationale specifically required their participation, and other safeguards were included.

Who should make these decisions? The National Commission for the Protection of Human Research Subjects suggested that IRBs could require that a "person who is responsible for the health care of a subject" determine that participation will not interfere with that care—a recommendation that could be extended here to insuring that unreasonable risk does not arise. When the potential subject's clinician is also involved in the research, an independent clinical judgment attesting to the appropriateness of including the patient could be required.

In addition, Carpenter and colleagues note that research milieux can be designed with enhanced psychosocial treatments available, since these may mitigate the effects of taking patients off medication. They point to the importance of close monitoring for early signs of relapse, since restarting medication will usually, though not always, prevent the development of a full-fledged psychotic episode. Use of the shortest possible medication-free period, and a study design that offers some benefits to all participants, even those receiving placebo, are also suggested. The latter might be accomplished, for example, by offering subjects in the placebo group the opportunity for an open trial of the new medication at the conclusion of the double-blind study. A final suggestion comes from investigators who have reviewed the literature on relapse after drug withdrawal: slowly tapering medications, rather than stopping them abruptly, appears to reduce the risk of subsequent relapse.

Informed Consent Procedures in Drug-Free Research

Much of the criticism of the UCLA studies and similar projects has focused on the procedures they used to get consent from prospective subjects. OPRR's investigation highlighted several inadequacies in the UCLA disclosures. Jay Katz has extended this critique to point to several problems with consent that are particularly likely to arise in research of this sort. He notes that, consistent with physicians' general dislike for discussing adverse consequences with patients, investigators often will be reluctant to describe clearly the probability of relapse and the severity of the symptoms that might be expected. For the same reason, and because it may facilitate recruitment, investigators may blur the distinction between the treatment being provided by the research project and the care patients would otherwise receive.

Katz also points to investigators' reluctance to disabuse subjects of the idea that research procedures are designed primarily to benefit them, rather than for the purpose of generating generalizable research findings. This "therapeutic misconception" appears to be widespread among research subjects. The risk may be especially great when the subjects' treating clinicians are also the investigators in the project. Indeed, one of the subjects turned complainant in the UCLA study was quoted as saying that he was delighted to get into the research program "because I thought I was going to get the premier treatment, while they did a little research on the side." Extra attention from IRBs may be warranted to insure that investigators communicate information targeted specifically at these common problems in investigators' disclosure and subjects' understanding. Persons independent of the research project could be used, for example, to supplement the information potential subjects receive to insure that it is complete and unbiased.

The rationale for allowing patients with schizophrenia to participate in drug-free studies presumes their competence to consent to research. Reassuring data came from a study of a small group of psychiatric patients, most with schizophrenia, showing that their decisions about participation in hypothetical research projects that varied systematically in their risk-benefit ratios were no different from those of a medically ill group. More recent data suggest, however, that hospitalized schizophrenics as a group are at elevated risk of having their capacities to consent impaired, compared with persons with other psychiatric and medical disorders and with matched controls from the general population. Although comparable data from research settings are lacking, there is good reason to believe that similar problems are likely to appear there too. Indeed, some of the information that should be communicated to subjects in drug-free trials may be particularly difficult for persons with schizophrenia to understand. Denial of the presence or seriousness of their illness, for example, is extremely common in schizophrenics, rendering it more difficult for them to accept that drug withdrawal may result in psychotic relapse. The difficulty that many patients have with abstractions could impair their ability to grasp the negative consequences of decompensation (e.g., "If I become symptomatic again, my family and friends may reject me.")

Given the risks inherent in drug-free studies, and the complexities of the consent process, it may be worth verifying the assumption of subjects' competence by screening potential participants for decision-related capacities. Since capacities exist on a spectrum, higher-risk studies might be limited to patients with better decisionmaking performance. Inclusion of lower-functioning groups, which may be necessary for scientific reasons, may require additional safeguards.

Also of concern is the probability that as subjects in a drug-free condition begin to experience more symptoms, they may lose the decisionmaking capacities they had at the start of the study. One of the UCLA subjects again provides a good example. As he became increasingly delusional, he lied to his caregivers regarding his symptoms, believing "if I told the doctors I was having hallucinations, they would have me arrested or assassinated." Thus, although all subjects at the start of the study may understand the safeguards available, including their right to withdraw at any point, precisely at the time when those safeguards become relevant, subjects may lose the capacity to invoke them. This suggests the desirability of creating mechanisms (e.g., through a durable power of attorney) whereby substitute decisionmakers can act on patients' behalf, if necessary, when they are unable to do so.

CONCLUSION

There are sound reasons to perform drug-free research in schizophrenia. To justify the risk of relapse by subjects in recent studies, however, careful attention must be given to insuring appropriateness of the design, minimization of risks, and adequacy of informed consent.

THE UCLA SCHIZOPHRENIA RELAPSE STUDY

Jay Katz

A research study conducted at the Neuropsychiatric Institute of the University of California, Los Angeles (UCLA), which began in the early 1980s . . . [and was still in progress at the time this article was published in the Fall of 1993—eds.] illustrates the problems I have discussed.* To orient the reader, I briefly summarize three facts about the design of the experiment and two facts about its aftermath that are of concern to me: (1) The study required schizophrenic patients who had recovered from their psychotic disorders to be withdrawn from medication even though "[i]t is generally accepted that maintenance antipsychotic medication will benefit a substantial proportion of chronic schizophrenics."[1] (2) The study expected to produce a relapse (recurrence of symptomatology) in many patient-subjects in order to attain its objective to predict better relapse, particularly of those who would exhibit such severe symptoms as "bizarre behavior, self-neglect, hostility, depressive mood and suicideability."[2] (3) The informed consent form signed by the participants was inadequate in disclosing to the subjects the risks which their participation entailed. (4) The IRB approved the research protocol and informed consent form without asking the investigators for clarifications that might have led the IRB to better protect the subjects of research. (5) The subsequent response to the review of the study by the National Institutes of Health's Office for the Protection of Research Risks (OPRR) did not go far in remedying the problems which came to OPRR's attention.

I also want to emphasize at the outset that my analysis is limited to a review of one of the research protocols, including the informed consent form approved by UCLA's IRB, the action taken by the OPRR, once parents of one of the subjects had lodged a complaint about the study and a perusal of the psychiatric literature pertinent to the research project.[3] I cannot address what might have been disclosed to the subjects in conversations between them and the investigators; about that I have no knowledge. I can only note that the data available from the protocol and the OPRR review hardly suggests that scrupulous attention was paid at any point to full disclosure and consent.

The UCLA experiment was designed to make an important contribution to a better understanding of the need for continuous medication following patients' recovery from a recent onset of schizophrenic disorder. Thus, the research project sought to identify patients who can function without medication because antipsychotic medication can cause tardive dyskinesia, a syndrome consisting of involuntary and potentially irreversible movements for which no known treatment exists.[4]

All potential patient-subjects were being followed in UCLA's After Care Clinic.[5] The study, according to the protocol, consisted of two sequential phases.[6] In the first phase, lasting for twenty-four weeks, the patient-subjects were randomized, in a double-blind design, to one of two groups. The first group received a standardized dose of 12.5 mgm of prolyxin decanoate, an antipsychotic medication, every two weeks, while the second was injected with a placebo, an inert, therapeutically ineffective substance. After twelve weeks, the injections given to members of each group were reversed so that those who had been receiving medication now received a placebo, and vice versa. In the second phase, "all clinically appropriate patients" received no medication, i.e., those who were still on prolyxin were also deprived of the active drug.[7]

The patient-subjects were then followed for at least one year unless "1) the subject withdraws

---

Saint Louis University Law Journal, Vol. 38:1, pp. 41–51. Used with permission of the publisher.

Editors' note: In a previous section of this article, deleted here, Professor Katz had argued for greater public visibility of the decisions made in the conduct of human experimentation, and had warned against the tendency of local institutional review boards to place the needs of research above the rights and interests of patients.

Editors' note: The article has been edited and the notes renumbered.

permission for the study or 2) clinical relapse or psychotic exacerbation occurs."[8] Criteria for psychotic relapse included "[high scores on test measures] for hallucinations, unusual thought content, or conceptual disorganization; [for] psychotic exacerbation [fairly severe recurrence of symptomatology; and] for relapse-other type, [high scores] on scales of *bizarre behavior; self-neglect, hostility, depressive mood, and suicidability*."[9] Apparently the patient-subject's therapist was authorized in the first double-blind phase of the study to break the code for "clinical reasons" but the protocol contained no information, and therefore the IRB could not know, as to when the therapist might take such action. Clearly the intent was to tolerate severe recurrences in symptomatology. Once that had happened "the patient [would] be withdrawn from the study."[10]

The investigators noted in the protocol's section on "Potential Benefits" that since "no study shows 100% relapse in schizophrenics withdrawn from antipsychotics, unquestioned maintenance treatment may for any particular patient involve much risk and little benefit. At present, there is little consistent data regarding predictive factors for patients at low risk of relapse without pharmacotherapy."[11] In that section the investigators also stated

> that clinical relapse or psychotic exacerbation can be expected to occur in at least some of our patient subjects. *However, since most of our patients have been requesting drug withdrawal for months, and since our knowledge as to which acute schizophrenic patients will relapse following drug withdrawal is very meager, we feel this risk is justified, especially in view of the risk of tardive dyskinesia with long-term antipsychotic use.* Withdrawal from antipsychotic medication one year after the psychotic episode is not unusual in standard psychiatric practice for patients with acute, nonchronic schizophrenia, since little clear evidence exists regarding longer-term prophylactic effects for this nonchronic population.[12]

It is true that many schizophrenic patients complain about the side effects of antipsychotic medication. However, therapists who believe that such treatment is clinically indicated generally do their level best to impress on patients the need for remaining on medication or to encourage its resumption as soon as symptoms recur. In the UCLA study, on the other hand, all patients were withdrawn from medication, indeed required to do so, for research purposes until the needs of the study, and not those of the individual patient, had been satisfied.[13] The expectation of relapse was an integral aspect of the research design; it was not an unfortunate consequence of treatment but one which the investigators deliberately induced. This is particularly problematic because of the continuing controversy in psychiatric circles as to whether relapse leads to additional, at times irreversible, injury.[14]

The consent form submitted to the IRB for review and approval informed prospective patient-subjects that "the purpose of this study is to take people like me off medication in a way that will give the most information about the medication, its effects on me, on others and on the way the brain works."[15] It mentioned that an inactive substance (placebo) or an (active) medication would be randomly administered during the first phase and that then "all medication will be stopped and that I will continue to receive regular care at the UCLA After Care Clinic."[16] Stating it in that way could only confuse potential subjects. In the same sentence they were told that medication would be stopped and that they would continue to receive regular care, without alerting them in most explicit language that "regular care" was compromised by the withdrawal of medication.[17]

Moreover, the patient-subjects were not informed at the beginning of the study that already during the first phase they would not necessarily receive optimal individual treatment, but only a *standardized* dose of 12.5 mg of prolyxin. Such a standardized dose can itself lead either to a return of symptomatology or produce unnecessary side effects because it is known that the amount of prolyxin must be tailored to the individual needs of patients with some requiring larger or smaller amounts of medication.[18] The consent form then goes on to describe in considerable detail the psychological tests that would be administered to the patient-subject during the study period. That aspect of the research could have been presented in a more abbreviated fashion and surely, in light of other omissions, did not deserve the space it was given.

With respect to significant risks and benefits the following information was provided:

> I understand that during blood drawing, I may experience pain from the needle prick, a small amount of bleeding, infection or black and blue marks at the site

> of the needle mark which will disappear in about 10 days.
>
> I understand that because of the withdrawal of active medication, I may become worse during this study and that either a relapse of my initial symptoms or new symptoms may occur. I understand that I will not be charged for the active medication or the placebo that I am provided during this study. If I do show a significant return of symptoms, I understand the clinic staff will use active medication again to improve my condition. If I would require hospitalization during this study, although this is not likely, I understand that the clinic staff would help to arrange an appropriate hospitalization but the research project would not pay for the hospitalization.
>
> I understand that I may benefit from this study by being taken off medication in a careful way while under close medical supervision. The potential benefits to science in this study are that it will increase my doctor's knowledge of the relationship between the medication, its effect on people such as myself, and on the way the brain functions in certain forms of mental illness.
>
> I understand that my condition may improve, worsen or remain unchanged from participation in this study.[19]

No information was provided as to what constituted a "significant return of symptoms," that it could mean a return of hallucinations, conceptual disorganization, self-neglect, depressive mood, or suicidal ideation. Potential patient-subjects under the care of mental health professionals in an Aftercare Clinic might very well have believed that "significant" did not encompass such dire consequences. Moreover, while it was acknowledged that "I *may* become worse," the consent form of July 1988 did not state that at that time it was known that of those patient-subjects enrolled in the study so far, eighty-eight percent had suffered a relapse.[20]

In light of the high relapse rate it was misleading to aver "that my condition *may* improve, worsen or remain unchanged." The odds favoring relapse were far too great; few subjects would "improve" or "remain the same." Finally, it is not only ironic but also misleading that the risks of a needle prick were discussed in such exquisite detail. Such a forthcoming and honest acknowledgement could only leave patient-subjects with the impression that the investigators would disclose any other risks in similar detail and with similar candor.

The informed consent form should have highlighted in bold face that the primary objective of the study was to advance knowledge for the sake of future patients and, depending on outcome, only of value to some of the subjects' future well-being. The form, further, should have acknowledged that the study was not designed to attend to their *individual* therapeutic needs, and that the subjects exposed themselves to considerable risks. Moreover, the patient-subjects were not presented with any information about the merits of not joining the research project. They were deprived of considering that alternative. To be sure, the informed consent form must be supplemented by the oral informed consent process[21] and the latter may be more important than the former in providing patient-subjects with meaningful disclosures, particularly since the forms are generally written in such incomprehensible language. When, however, as in this instance, the written document provided incomplete information, and with insufficient candor, patient-subjects who are intent on reading it are deprived of crucial information. From a different perspective, the consent form, as written, cannot help but create concerns, though most difficult to substantiate, as to whether the oral informed consent was similarly flawed.[22]

After complaints about the study had come to OPRR's attention[23] and it had discussed the problem with UCLA, a letter from OPRR detailed "the agreed-upon actions" which UCLA would now take:

> [P]rovide (a) more detailed information regarding the risks associated with lengthy withdrawal of antipsychotic medication, including information regarding the likely rates of exacerbation or relapse and the consequences thereof; (b) an indication that, in the event of such exacerbation or relapse, it is likely that antipsychotic medication will need to be resumed; (c) a description of the risks associated with continued fixed dose medication treatment; and (d) a disclosure of alternative courses of treatment . . . .[24]
>
> . . . .
>
> The Continuing Care Brochure will be modified to ensure that it accurately reflects the parameters of the After Care Program's research protocols.[25]

In addition, OPRR required the following additional actions:

> (1) No new subjects should be enrolled in this research until the revised Informed Consent Documents have

been reviewed and approved by the UCLA Institutional Review Board (IRB).

(2) The revised IRB-approved Informed Consent Documents should be used to obtain renewed consent from all subjects currently participating in this research, including subjects for whom clinical monitoring constitutes the only research involvement.

(3) Copies of the revised IRB-approved Informed Consent Documents and of the revised Continuing Care Brochure should be forwarded to OPRR as soon as possible.

(4) UCLA should consider, and OPRR strongly recommends, contacting former research subjects in writing to provide them with the additional information included in the revised Informed Consent Documents. Copies of such communications with former subjects should be forwarded to OPRR as soon as they become available.[26]

OPRR did not insist that UCLA stop the research project immediately, or at least, that the patient-subjects be examined by independent psychiatrists in order to assess their individual treatment needs. In light of what already had transpired, such an opportunity would have made it easier for patient-subjects to decide whether they wished to continue in, or withdraw from, the study. Moreover, in light of the serious deficiencies in the informed consent form,[27] which is one of the prime responsibilities of IRBs to review,[28] OPRR did not institute a thorough investigation of the practices of UCLA's IRB. OPRR's evaluation was sufficiently critical of the IRB process to suggest that the IRB's review of other research proposals may be similarly flawed.[29] Undertaking such an investigation was even more pressing in this case since several subject-patients suffered severe schizophrenic relapses,[30] and one young man allegedly committed suicide.[31]

The revised informed consent form, while an improvement over the previous one, continues to leave patient-subjects uninformed, *inter alia,* about the *specific* severity of relapse which they might suffer, mentioning only "difficulties in relationship with others and problems with work or school"; or what specific "psychotic symptoms or severe symptoms" will lead to providing medication once again. It does not present in any meaningful detail the advantages and disadvantages of participating in the study or receiving customary treatment for their condition. The consent form did not state with sufficient clarity that the primary objective of the study was to conduct research for the sake of future patients, perhaps of benefit to those enrolled in this study *in the future,* and that it was not therapy for the subject's individual *present* needs. While the consent form now admits that "70-80% of patients who have entered this study in the past have experienced a psychotic exacerbation or relapse within one year" and that "I may become worse during the study," it says nothing about what subjects specifically should consider, and reflect on, before exposing themselves to these risks. On the other hand, with respect to benefits it is noted that withdrawal of medication will keep them from "developing tardive dyskinesia which involves abnormal movements of the face, hands, legs or trunk." And the form goes on to emphasize, "I may benefit from this study by being taken off medication in a careful way while under close medical supervision."[32] The risks deserved at least similar detailed explication and prominence.

What transpired in this study is not unique to UCLA; it is symptomatic of the flawed nature of current regulations and current practices protecting the human rights of research subjects. These flaws, as I have argued throughout this article, extend from the Federal Regulations themselves[33] to the supervision of projects by IRBs and OPRR. Thus, my analysis of UCLA's consent form should not be taken merely as a critique of the nature and depth of the information that was or was not included in the written document, but, more importantly, as a critique of the entire informed consent process. The problems with this study, as with many others, are: (1) subject-patients' consent was manipulated; (2) trivial and non-trivial risks were insufficiently distinguished; (3) the severity of predictable risks was not highlighted nor was the incidence of their likelihood disclosed; and (4) the risks and benefits of non-participation were neither sufficiently disclosed nor satisfactorily discussed. Under these circumstances, patient-subjects were not offered a meaningful choice whether or not to participate in the study.

NOTES

1. Keith H. Nuechterlein & Michael Gitlin, Research Protocol for Developmental Processes in Schizophrenic Disorders Project: Protocol; Double Blind Crossover

and Withdrawal of Neuroleptics in Remitted, Recent-Onset Schizophrenia, HSPC #86-07-336 1,6 [hereinafter Protocol] (on file with author). In a 1988 article the investigators gave a clear account of these research objectives:

> The present study is a prospective examination of prodromal signs and symptoms of schizophrenic relapse, using a systematic and carefully controlled research design. One important improvement over the previous studies is that relapse was defined as the elevation of psychiatric symptoms to the severe or extremely severe level. Thus, minor symptom fluctuations that might often be inconsequential were not considered relapses. In contrast to the studies that defined the period of observation by the necessity to increase medication to avoid a possible relapse, we can be certain that any prodromal changes that we isolated actually did precede a clear relapse.

Kenneth L Subotnik & Keith N. Nuechterlein, *Prodromal Signs and Symptoms in Schizophrenic Relapse,* 97 J. Abnormal Psychology 405, 406 (1988).

2. *Id.*
3. These and all other discussed unpublished documents are in the possession of the author and available upon request.
4. In some patients symptoms of tardive dyskinesia disappear within several months after antipsychotic drugs are withdrawn, but withdrawal of antipsychotic medication does not guarantee that symptoms will vanish. In some patients, symptoms may persist indefinitely. Dorland's Illustrated Medical Dictionary 517–18 (27th ed. 1988).
5. *See infra* note 32 and accompanying text.
6. Protocol, *supra* note.
7. Protocol, *supra* note, at 4.
8. *Id.* at 6.
9. *Id.* (emphasis supplied).
10. *Id.*
11. *Id.* at 7.
12. Protocol, *supra* note, at 8.
13. The protocol does not make clear whether all the patient-subjects had been on medication for at least one year when enrolled in the study, which, according to the investigators, is the time when "in standard psychiatric practice" patients are often taken off medication. *Id.*
14. Although the issue is far from settled, many psychiatrists believe that relapse can be permanently harmful to patients: "[S]ome patients are left with a damaging residual if a psychosis is allowed to proceed unmitigated." Richard J. Wyatt, *Neuroleptics and the Natural Course of Schizophrenia,* 17 Schizophrenia Bulletin 325, 347 (1991). "[N]euroleptic drugs . . . if they fully control all acute episodes, may protect against the otherwise inevitable decline of mental function." R. Miller, *Schizophrenia as a Progressive Disorder: Relations to EEG, CT, Neuropathological and Other Evidence,* 33 Progress Neurobiology 17, 35 (1989).
15. Keith Nuechterlein, Informed Consent Agreement for Patients (Version 1): Double-Blind Drug Crossover and Withdrawal Project 1 (July 1988) [hereinafter Consent Agreement I] (on file with author).
16. *Id.*
17. Being absolutely clear on this point was important since the subjects were recruited from the Continuing Care Program of The Neuropsychiatric Institute UCLA. The brochure, given to patients enrolled in this program, contained the following information:

> THE CONTINUING CARE PROGRAM . . .
> . . . is a specialty service combining treatment, research, and training in the care of the individual with psychotic symptoms. Jointly sponsored by NIMH, UCLA, Camarillo-NIP, and the Clinical Research Center, the Program offers continuing care to people who are experiencing their first psychotic episode.
>
> The Program includes inpatient and outpatient treatment as well as an active follow-up evaluation of each person. Fully integrated with these services is a research project aimed at increasing understanding and knowledge of the factors that are related to relapse and remission.
>
> PURPOSE
> The goal of the Program is to assist persons in making a successful adaptation to life in the community and to improve their daily living and social skills. An equally important goal is to facilitate the family's coping skills for dealing with mental illness. Where appropriate, consultation with other community agencies and social support networks is provided.
>
> . . . .
>
> AFTERCARE CLINIC
> A range of outpatient services are offered through the Aftercare Clinic at the UCLA Neuropsychiatric Institute. Following discharge, patients and their families are provided:
>
> *Group Therapy:* in small groups, patients learn problem-solving skills and interpersonal effectiveness.
>
> *Family Education:* counseling is aimed to upgrade the entire family's coping skills and understanding of the illness, and to facilitate use

of resources both within the family and the community.

Medication is administered at the lowest optimal dose to maximize coping with symptoms and stressors and to minimize side effects.

PARTICIPATION

. . . is voluntary by patients and families in both the research and the clinical services. It is expected that a voluntary agreement to participate for a minimum of two years be made at the point a patient joins the Program.

UCLA Neuropsychiatric Institute, Continuing Care Program of the Mental Health Clinical Center 1–3 (on file with author). Since the Aftercare program serves dual objectives, treatment and research, any experimental interventions needed to be specified and differentiated from therapy with the greatest of care, particularly whenever the research component compromised therapeutic intentions.

18. See *Physician's Desk Reference* 619 (47th ed. 1993) ("Appropriate dosage of Prolyxin Decanoate (Fluphenazine Decanoate Injection) should be individualized for each patient. . . . The optimal amount of the drug and the frequency of administration must be determined for each patient, since dosage requirements have been found to vary with clinical circumstances as well as with individual response to the drug."); *Textbook of Neuropsychiatry* 682 (Stuart C. Yudosky & Robert E. Hales eds., 2d ed. 1991) ("Blood levels vary widely in different patients given the same dose of a neuroleptic. . . . [T]here is no established correlation between serum concentration and clinical response."); Robert F. Asarnow & Stephen R. Marder, *Differential Effect of Low and Conventional Doses of Fluphenazine on Schizophrenic Outpatients with Good or Poor Information-Processing Abilities,* 45 Archive Gen. Psychiatry 822 (1988).
19. Consent Agreement I, *supra* note 15, at 2.
20. Of the 24 patients who entered the drug withdrawal period, 21 have ultimately had psychotic exacerbations or relapses. ranging from 17 to 123 weeks after the last fluphenazine administration. For these 21 exacerbation/relapses plus the 3 psychotic exacerbations during the placebo phase of the crossover, the mean time to exacerbation/relapse is 33 weeks. Of these 24 patients who have developed an exacerbation/relapse after medication discontinuation, 5 exacerbation/relapses occurred after 60 or more weeks (21%), 6 after 40-59 weeks (25%), 7 after 20–39 weeks (29%), 4 after 10-19 weeks (17%), and 2 after less than 10 weeks (8%). Three more remain well after 104, 30 and 23 weeks. Keith H. Nuechterlein, Grant Application: Developmental Processes in Schizophrenic Disorders, RD I MH 37705-07, 1, 84 (Nov. 15, 1988) (on file with author).
21. UCLA claims to have presented much of the information required for informed consent to patient-subject's orally. Department of Health and Human Services (DHHS) regulations at 45 C.F.R. ß 46.117 require, however, that the elements of legally effective Informed Consent (specified at 45 C.F.R. ß 46.116 (1992)) be embodied in the *written* Informed Consent Document.
22. The special care that, I believe, must be given to the informed consent process whenever the research-therapy distinction is in danger of being compromised, is illustrated by a comment made by my respected colleague and friend Robert J. Levine who read an earlier draft of this paper:

> My perception of the investigators' motivation continues to be very different from yours. I see this as an instance of opportunistic research. The physician-investigators did not expose subjects to the risks of withdrawal from medication in order to do research. Rather, in the light of their reading of the results of observations published by others, they decided that it would be in the medical interests of these patients to have their medications withdrawn. Although they knew that some of them would develop symptoms, they could not predict which. What they planned to do was to keep a careful record of their observations of those who developed symptoms. They further made plans to remove patients from the study and treat them if certain specific criteria were met.

Letter from Robert J. Levine to Jay Katz (Sept. 24, 1993) (quoted by permission). Viewing the "motivation" of the investigators as "opportunistic research" in the service of the "medical interests of these patients" cojoins therapy and research. In the UCLA study the patient-subjects' medical interests were subordinated to the inflexibility of the research design. It is this fact that needed to be highlighted in the consent form, notwithstanding any accompanying therapeutic motivations of the investigators. Viewing research also as treatment invites confusion in the minds of all participants as to who they are: physicians or investigators, patients or subjects. In turn, it makes it easier for investigators to take license because of their "benevolent therapeutic intentions." Furthermore, the "specific criteria [for removal from the study]" noted by Levine included relapse to the severest level of psychosis, an unacceptable criterion for clinical practice. Long before that point is reached psychiatrists would urge their patients to resume taking medication. Thus, I would argue that the physician-investigators' conduct was motivated by their research interest, even though they might eventually also bestow benefits on their subjects or future patients. If I am correct, then the patient-subjects' medical interests are in this instance different from, and should not be conflated with, the investigators' research interests.

23. The complaint was lodged by Bob and Gloria Aller, parents of one of the subjects. The story of Greg's participation in, and gradual deterioration during, the study is graphically described in a recent article: Eventually, he not only dropped out of college, but also

> took out a carving knife, walked to the door of his mother's kitchen, [and thinking that] "my mom was possessed by the devil," . . . "[m]y plan was to scare the devil out of her literally." The Allers began barricading their bedroom door at night [A few days later] he moved out, [and when he saw Nuechterlein's partner, Dr. Michael Gitlin, Greg kept this information from him, and thus Gitlin] noted "Moved out from parents. Says no symptoms present. Finishing the semester."

James Willwerth, *Tinkering with Madness,* 42 TIME 41–42 (Aug. 30, 1992). It took five more months, and the article describes what happened during that interval, before he was remedicated at UCLA. *Id.*

24. Letter from J. Thomas Puglisi, Acting Chief, Compliance Oversight Branch of the Office for Protection from Research Risks (OPRR) to Richard Sisson, Senior Vice Chancellor of Academic Affairs at the University of California Los Angeles 1 (Aug. 19, 1992) (on file with author).
25. *Id.* at 2.
26. *Id.*
27. Even after modifying the consent forms initially used, UCLA continues to deny any wrongdoing and contends that the forms and process used to obtain initial consent were appropriate. *See* Letter from Richard Sisson, Senior Vice Chancellor of Academic Affairs at the University of California Los Angeles to J. Thomas Puglisi, Acting Chief, Compliance Oversight Branch of the OPRR 4-5 (Sept. 17, 1992) (on file with author).
28. Federal Regulations instruct IRBs to "determine that all of the following requirements are satisfied: . . . (4) Informed consent will be sought from each prospective subject . . . in accordance with, and to the extent required by § 46.117." 45 C.F.R. § 46.111(4) (1992).
29. The copy of the letter from OPRR to UCLA, made available to me through the Freedom of Information Act, excluded three paragraphs. They may have contained additional criticisms of UCLA'S conduct in this case. See *supra* note 24.
30. Subotnik & Nuechterlein, *supra* note.
31. One participant in the UCLA project committed suicide on March 28, 1992, after being taken off psychotropic medication. Sandy Rovner, *Ethics Concerns Raised in Schizophrenia Study,* WASH. POST, Sept 29, 1992, at H7. The Federal Regulations require that "[w]here appropriate, the research plan makes adequate provision for monitoring the data collected to insure the safety of subjects." 45 C.F.R. § 46.111(6) (1992). The protocol, however, did not describe in sufficient detail the special monitoring that would be provided, even though some of the research subjects could suffer a severe relapse. The protocol only stated that "a member of the clinic staff will meet regularly as needed" with the patient. See *supra* note.
32. Keith Nuechterlein, Informed Consent Agreement for Patients: Double-Blind Drug Crossover and Withdrawal Project 3 (Sept 1992) (on file with author).
33. Shamoo and Irving recently noted that recommendations by various Federal Commissions to consider persons with mental illness as members of a vulnerable group who deserve special protection whenever they participate in research were not implemented. They learned that "[this] outcome was the result in large part of opposition from researchers on mental disorders who claimed that the population in question were no more vulnerable than most persons with severe medical disorders and that the suggested limitations would seriously restrict research on mental disorders." Shamoo and Irving concluded that "the issue of using persons with mental illness as human research subjects has been lost in the shuffle, due in part to the lobbying effort of some researchers on mental disorders." They also raise the important question, "what was the justification for delegating to local IRBs the essential responsibilities for affording protections for persons with mental illness . . . ?" Adil F. Shamoo & Dianne N. Irving, *Accountability in Research Using Persons With Mental Illness* 1, 2(1994) (forthcoming article, on file with author).

RECOMMENDED SUPPLEMENTARY READING

GENERAL WORKS

Brody, Baruch A. *Ethical Issues in Drug Testing. Approval, and Pricing: The Clot-Dissolving Drugs.* New York: Oxford University Press, 1995.

Dresser, Rebecca. *When Science Offers Salvation: Patient Advocacy and Research Ethics.* New York: Oxford University Press, 2001.

Foster, Claire. *The Ethics of Medical Research on Humans.* Cambridge: Cambridge University Press, 2001

IRB: A Review of Human Subjects Research. Hastings-on-Hudson, NY: Hastings Center.

Kahn, Jeffrey P.; Mastroianni, Anna C.; and Sugarman, Jeremy; eds. *Beyond Consent: Seeking Justice in Research.* New York: Oxford University Press, 1998.

Katz, Jay; Capron, Alexander M.; and Glass, Eleanor Swift; eds. *Experimentation with Human Beings.* New York: Russell Sage Foundation, 1972.

Levine, Robert J. *Ethics and Regulation of Clinical Research.* 2nd ed. New Haven, CT: Yale University Press, 1988.

The National Bioethics Advisory Commission. *Ethical and Policy Issues in Research Involving Human Participants.* Bethesda MD, 2001.

Rothman, David J. *Strangers at the Bedside: A History of How Law and Bioethics Transformed Medical Decision Making.* New York: Basic Books, 1991.

Shamoo, Adil E. and Resnik, David B. *Responsible Conduct of Research.* New York, Oxford University Press, 2002.

Thompson, Andrew, and Temple, Norman J. eds. *Ethics, Medical Research, and Medicine: Commercialism Versus Environmentalism and Social Justice.* Boston: Kluwer Academic Publishers, 2001.

Vanderpool, Harold Y., ed. The *Ethics of Research Involving Human Subjects: Facing the 21st Century.* Frederick, MD: University Publishing Group, 1996.

Veatch, Robert. *The Patient as Partner: A Theory of Human Experimentation Ethics.* Bloomington: Indiana University Press, 1987.

BORN IN SCANDAL: THE ORIGINS OF U.S. RESEARCH ETHICS

Annas, George J., and Grodin, Michael A., eds. *The Nazi Doctors and the Nuremberg Code: Human Rights in Human Experimentation.* New York: Oxford University Press, 1992.

Caplan, Arthur L., ed. *When Medicine Went Mad: Bioethics and the Holocaust.* Clifton, NJ: Humana Press, 1992.

Fairchild, Amy L. and Bayer, Ronald. "The Uses and Abuses of Tuskegee." *Science* 284 (May 7, 1999): 919–921.

Human Radiation Experiments: Final Report of the Advisory Committee on Human Radiation Experiments. New York: Oxford University Press, 1996.

Jonas, Hans. "Philosophical Reflections on *Experimentation with Human Subjects.*" In *Experimentation with Human Subjects,* edited by Paul Freund. New York: Braziller, 1970.

Jones, James. *Bad Blood: The Tuskegee Syphilis Experiment: A Tragedy of Race and Medicine.* Rev. ed. New York: Free Press, 1993.

Lasagna, Louis. "Some Ethical Problems in Clinical Investigation." In *Human Aspects of Biomedical Innovation,* edited by E. Mendelsohn, et al. Cambridge, MA: Harvard University Press, 1971.

Lederer, Susan E. *Subjected to Science: Human Experimentation in America before the Second World War.* Baltimore: The Johns Hopkins University Press, 1995.

Lifton, Robert Jay. *The Nazi Doctors: Medical Killing and the Psychology and Genocide.* New York: Basic Books, 1986.

Moreno, Jonathan D. *Undue Risk: Secret State Experiments on Humans.* New York: Routledge, 2001.

Reverby, Susan M. ed. *Tuskegee's Truths: Rethinking the Tuskegee Syphilis Study.* Chapel Hill: University of North Carolina Press, 2000.

Rothman, David J. "Were Tuskegee & Willowbrook "Studies in Nature'?" *Hastings Center Report* 12 no. 2 (1982): 5–7.

Shuster, Evelyne. "Fifty Years Later: The Significance of the Nuremberg Code." *The New England Journal of Medicine* 337, no. 20 (November 1997): 1436–1440.

Thomas, Stephen B., and Quinn, Sandra Crouse. "The Tuskegee Syphilis Study, 1932 to 1972: Implications for HIV Education and AIDS Risk Education Programs in the Black Community." *American Journal of Public Health* 81, no. 11 (November 1991): 1498–1504.

"Trusting Science: Nuremberg and the Human Radiation Experiments." *Hastings Center Reports* (symposium; September, October 1996).

"Twenty Years After: The Legacy of the Tuskegee Syphilis Study." *Hastings Center Report* (November–December 1992): 29ff.

THE ETHICS OF RANDOMIZED CLINICAL TRIALS

Appelbaum, Paul S., et al. "False Hopes and Best Data: Consent to Research and the Therapeutic Misconception." *Hastings Center Report* 17, no. 2 (April 1987): 20–24.

Brody, Baruch A. "Conflicts of Interest and the Validity of Clinical Trials." In *Conflicts of Interest*, edited by Roy G. Spece, Jr., David S. Shimm, and Allen E. Buchanan. New York: Oxford University Press, 1996.

Christakis, Nicholas. "Ethics Are Local: Engaging Cross-Cultural Variation in the Ethics for Clinical Research." *Social Sciences in Medicine* 35, no. 9 (1992): 1079–1091.

Freedman, Benjamin, Weijer, Charles, and Glass, Kathleen C. "Placebo Orthodoxy in Clinical Research I: Empirical and Methodological Myths." *Journal of Law, Medicine, and Ethics* 24 (1996): 243–251.

Freedman, Benjamin, Glass, Kathleen C., and Weijer, Charles. "Placebo Orthodoxy in Clinical Research II: Ethical, Legal, and Regulatory Myths." *Journal of Law, Medicine and Ethics* 24 (1996): 252–259.

Fried, Charles. *Medical Experimentation: Personal Integrity and Social Policy*. New York: American Elsevier, 1974.

Gifford, Fred. "Community-Equipoise and the Ethics of Randomized Clinical Trials." *Bioethics* 9, no. 2 (April 1995): 127–148.

———. "Freedman's 'Clinical Equipoise' and 'Sliding-Scale All Dimensions—Considered Equipoise.'" *The Journal of Medicine and Philosophy* 25, no. 4 (August 2000): 399–427.

Ijsselmuiden, Carel B., and Faden, Ruth. "Research and Informed Consent in Africa: Another Look." *New England Journal of Medicine* 326, no. 12 (March 19, 1992): 830–834.

Kadane, Joseph B., ed. *Bayesian Methods and Ethics in a Clinical Trial Design*. New York: John Wiley & Sons, Inc., 1996.

Kopelman, Loretta. "Randomized Clinical Trials, Consent and the Therapeutic Relationship." *Clinical Research* 31 (1983): 1–11.

Levine, Carol, Dubler, Nancy N., and Levine, Robert. "Building a New Consensus: Ethical Principles and Policies for Clinical Research on HIV/AIDS "*IRB A Review of Human Subjects Research* 13, nos. 1–2 (January–April 1991): 1–17.

Levine, Robert J. "Uncertainty in Clinical Research." *Law, Medicine and Health Care* 16, nos.3–4 (Winter 1988): 174–182.

Marquis, Don. "Leaving Therapy to Chance." *Hastings Center Report* 13, no. 4 (1983): 40–47.

Miller, Bruce. "Experimentation on Human Subjects: The Ethics of Random Clinical Trials." In *Health Care Ethics*, edited by Donald VanDeVeer and Tom Regan. Philadelphia, PA: Temple University Press, 1987.

Miller, Franklin G., and Brody, Howard. "What Makes Placebo-Controlled Trials Unethical?" *American Journal of Bioethics*, forthcoming.

Schaffner, Kenneth F.,, ed. "Ethical Issues in the Use of Clinical Controls." *Journal of Medicine and Philosophy* 1, no. 4 (November 1986).

Tannsjo, Torbjorn. "The Morality of Clinical Research—A Case Study." *Journal of Medicine and Philosophy* 19 (1994): 7–21.

Weijer, Charles. "The Ethical Analysis of Risk." *Journal of Law, Medicine & Ethics*, 28 (2000): 344–361.

ETHICAL ISSUES IN INTERNATIONAL RESEARCH

Angell, Marcia. "The Ethics of Clinical Research in the Third World." *New England Journal of Medicine* 337, no. 12 (September 18, 1997): 847–849.

Annas, George J., and Grodin, Michael A. "Human Rights and Maternal-Fetal HIV Transmission Prevention Trials in Africa." *American Journal of Public Health* 88 (1998): 560–563.

Benatar, Solomon R. "Justice and Medical Research: A Global Perspective." *Bioethics* 15, no. 4 (August 2001): 333–340.

Benatar, Solomon R., and Singer, Peter A. "A New Look at International Research Ethics." *British Medical Journal* 321 (2000):824–826.

Brody, Baruch A. *The Ethics of Biomedical Research: An International Perspective*. New York: Oxford University Press, 1998.

Del Río, Carlos. "Is Ethical Research Feasible in Developed and Developing Countries?" *Bioethics* 12 (1998):328–330.

De Zulueta, Paquita. "Randomized Placebo-Controlled Trials and HIV-Infected Pregnant Women in Developing Countries. Ethical Imperialism or Unethical Exploitation?" *Bioethics* 15, no. 4 (August 2001): 289–311.

Grady, Christine. "Science in the Service of Healing." *Hastings Center Report* 28, no. 6 (1998) 34–38.

King, Nancy M. P. "Experimental Treatment: Oxymoron or Aspiration?" *Hastings Center Report* (July–August 1995): 6–15.

Levi, Jeffrey. "Unproven AIDS Therapies: The Food and Drug Administration and ddI." In *Biomedical Politics*. Washington, DC: Institute of Medicine, (1991)" 9–42.

Levine, Robert J. 'The 'Best Proven Therapeutic Method' Standard in Clinical Trials in Technologically Developing Countries." *IRB: A Review of Human Subjects Research* 20, No. 1 (1998): 5–9.

London, Alex John. "Equipoise and International Human-Subjects Research." *Bioethics* 15, no. 4 (August 2001): 312–332.

Luna, Florencia. "Is 'Best Proven' a Useless Criterion?" *Bioethics* 15, no. 4 (August 2001): 273–289.

Macklin, Ruth. "After Helsinki: Unresolved Issues in International Research." *Kennedy Institute of Ethics Journal* 11, no. 1 (March 2001):17–36.

The National Bioethics Advisory Commission. *Ethical and Policy Issues in International Research: Clinical Trials in Developing Countries.* Bethesda MD, 2001.

Resnik, David B. "The Ethics of HIV Research in Developing Nations." *Bioethics* 12 (1998): 286–306.

Schuklenk, Udo, and Ashcroft, Richard. "International Research Ethics." *Bioethics* 14 (2000): 158–172.

Shamoo, Adil E., and Keay, Timothy J. "Ethical Concerns about Relapse Studies," *Cambridge Quarterly of Healthcare Ethics* 5 (1996): 373–386.

Varmus, Harold, and Satcher, David. "Ethical Complexities of Conducting Research in Developing Countries." *New England Journal of Medicine* 337 (1997): 1003–1005.

Wendler, Dave. "Informed Consent, Exploitation and Whether It Is Possible to Conduct Human Subjects Research Without Either One." *Bioethics* 14, no. 4 (2000): 310–393.

RESEARCH ON CHILDREN AND OTHER "VULNERABLE" POPULATIONS

Dresser, Rebecca A. "Wanted: Single, White Male for Medical Research." *Hastings Center Report* 22, no. 1 (January–February, 1992): 24–29.

Dubler, Nancy, and Sidel, Victor W. "On Research on HIV Infection and AIDS in Correctional Institutions." *Milbank Quarterly* 67, no. 2 (1989): 171–207.

Glantz, Leonard H. "Research with Children." *The American Journal of Law & Medicine* 24, nos. 2–3 (1998): 213–244.

Grodin, Michael, and Glantz, Leonard E., eds. *Children as Research Subjects: Science, Ethics and Law.* Oxford: Oxford University Press, 1994.

Kass, Nancy E, et al. "Harms of Excluding Pregnant Women from Clinical Research: The Case of HIV-Infected Pregnant Women." *The Journal of Law, Medicine and Ethics* 24, no. 1 (Spring 1996): 36–46.

Kopelman, Loretta M. "Children as Research Subjects: A Dilemma," *Journal of Medicine and Philosophy* 25, no.6 (2000): 745–764.

Kopelman, Loretta M., and Moskop, John C., eds. *Children and Health Care: Moral and Social Issues.* Boston: Kluwer Academic Publishers, 1989.

Mastroianni, Anna C.; Faden, Ruth; and Federman, Daniel; eds. *Women and Health Research: Ethical and Legal Issues of Including Women in Clinical Studies.* Vols. I and 2. Washington, DC: National Academy Press, 1994.

Merton, Vanessa. "The Exclusion of Pregnant, Pregnable, and Once-Pregnable People (a.k.a.

Women) from Biomedical Research." *American Journal of Law and Medicine* 19, no.4 (1993): 369–451.

Miller, Franklin G., and Rosenstein, Donald L. "Psychiatric Symptom-Provoking Studies: An Ethical Appraisal." *Biological Psychiatry* 40 (1997): 403–409.

National Bioethics Advisory Commission. *Research Involving Persons with Mental Disorders That May Affect Decisionmaking Capacity*. Rockville, MD: 1999.

Tauer, Carol A. "The NIH Trials of Growth Hormone for Short Stature." *IRB* 16, no. 3 (1994): 1–9.

Williams, Peter C. "Ethical Principles in Federal Regulations: The Case of Children and Research Risks." *Journal of Medicine and Philosophy* 21, no. 2 (1996): 1771–183.

RESOURCES IN BIOETHICS

DATABASES AND WEB RESOURCES

Bioethics.net
Center for Bioethics at the University of Pennsylvania
http://ajobonline.com/
Keep up-to-date on breaking bioethics issues, explore resources in Bioethics for Beginners, explore links to bioethics journals and their tables of contents, look for a job in bioethics, and view the current offerings of the *American Journal of Bioethics, AJOB.*

Bioethics Resources on the Web
The National Institutes of Health
http://www.nih.gov/sigs/bioethics/
Compendious list of links to resources including: Academic centers and programs, governmental agencies, educational sites and resources, bioethics documents including federal regulations, journals in bioethics and health law, bibliographical and database resources, and specific sections on research ethics, ethics and human genetics, and more.

ELSI: Ethical, Legal, and Social Issues in the Human Genome Project
http://www.ornl.gov/hgmis/elsi/elsi.html
Explore educational materials on the human genome project including publications, teaching aids, posters, online animation, links to videos, webcasts, presentations, career enhancement resources for teachers, and an array of valuable links.

Ethics Updates
Edited by Lawrence M. Hinman
http://ethics.acusd.edu/
This cite is organized by topics in ethics and contains expansive bibliographies, access to important publications, video and multimedia resources, case studies, and course materials including syllabi.

The National Library of Medicine
http://www.nlm.nih.gov/
Search a wide array of databases including MEDLINE/PubMed.

The National Reference Center for Bioethics Literature
Kennedy Institute of Ethics, Georgetown University
http://www.georgetown.edu/research/nrcbl/
Request a free bibliographical computer search online, or by calling the National Reference Center for Bioethics Literature at 1-800-633-3849.

Access an annotated bibliography of bioethics resources on the web and explore links to education and teaching resources.

Access bibliographical resources on a variety of bioethics topics including Basic Resources in Bioethics, Assisted Suicide and the Right to Die, Human Cloning, Ethics and Human Genetics.

Scope Notes Series: View the wide array of topics covered in this series of review essays and annotated bibliographies, and access selected Scope Notes online.

ENCYCLOPEDIAS AND REFERENCE WORKS

Becker, Lawrence C., and Charlotte B., eds. *Encyclopedia of Ethics.* New York: Routledge, 2001. 3 vols.

Burley, Justine, and Harris, John, eds. *A Companion to Genetics.* Oxford: Blackwell Publishers, 2002.

Chadwick, Ruth, ed. *Encyclopedia of Applied Ethics.* San Diego, CA: Academic Press, 1998. 4 vols.

Craig, Edward, ed. *The Routledge Encyclopedia of Philosophy.* New York: Routledge, 1998. 10 vols. Available online at: http://www.rep.routledge.com/index.html.

Edwards, Paul, ed. *Encyclopedia of Philosophy.* New York: Macmillan, 1967.

Goodin, Robert E., and Pettit, Philip, eds. *A Companion to Contemporary Political Philosophy.* Oxford: Blackwell Publishers, 1995.

Kuhse, Helga, and Singer, Peter. *A Companion to Bioethics.* Oxford: Blackwell Publishers, 1998.

Murray, Thomas H., and Mehlman, Max, eds. *Encyclopedia of Ethical, Legal, and Policy Issues in Biotechology.* New York: Wiley-Interscience, 2000. 2 vols.

Reich, Warren R., ed. *Encyclopedia of Bioethics.* 3rd ed. New York: MacMillan, forthcoming 2003. 5 vols.

Singer, Peter, ed. *A Companion to Ethics.* Oxford: Blackwell Publishers, 1993.

Zalta, Edward N. ed. *Stanford Encyclopedia of Philosophy* at http://plato.stanford.edu/.

INSTRUCTIONAL AIDS

A Right to Die? The Dax Cowart Case. Interactive CD-ROM by David Andersen, Robert Cavalier, and Preston K. Covey. New York: Routledge, 1996.

Dax's Case: Who Should Decide? An hour-long film about the burn patient discussed in the case study in Part 3, Section 2 of this text. Produced by Concern for Dying and available from Filmakers Library, 124 E. 40th St., New York, NY 10016, 212-808-4980, or from Choice in Dying, 200 Varick St., New York, NY 10014.

The Issue of Abortion in America. Interactive CD-ROM By Robert Cavalier, Preston Covey, Elizabeth A. Style, & Andrew Thompson. New York: Routledge, 1998.